Second Edition

NEUROLOGICAL
SURGERY *Volume 6*

A Comprehensive Reference
Guide to the
Diagnosis and Management of
Neurosurgical Problems

Edited by

JULIAN R. YOUMANS, M.D., Ph.D.

Professor, Department of Neurological Surgery,
School of Medicine, University of California
Davis, California

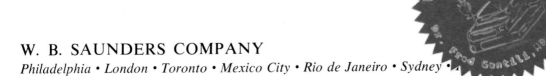

W. B. SAUNDERS COMPANY
Philadelphia • London • Toronto • Mexico City • Rio de Janeiro • Sydney •

W. B. Saunders Company: West Washington Square
Philadelphia, PA 19105

1 St. Anne's Road
Eastbourne, East Sussex BN21 3UN, England

1 Goldthorne Avenue
Toronto, Ontario M8Z 5T9, Canada

Apartado 26370—Cedro 512
Mexico 4, D.F., Mexico

Rua Coronel Cabrita, 8
Sao Cristovao Caixa Postal 21176
Rio de Janeiro, Brazil

9 Waltham Street
Artarmon, N.S.W. 2064, Australia

Ichibancho, Central Bldg., 22-1 Ichibancho
Chiyoda-Ku, Tokyo 102, Japan

Library of Congress Cataloging in Publication Data

Youmans, Julian Ray, 1928–
  Neurological surgery.

  1. Nervous system—Surgery.   I. Title.
[DNLM: 1. Neurosurgery.   WL368 N4945]
RD593.Y68   1980   617′.48
ISBN 0-7216-9662-7 (v. 1)   80-21368

Volume 1	ISBN	0-7216-9662-7
Volume 2	ISBN	0-7216-9663-5
Volume 3	ISBN	0-7216-9664-3
Volume 4	ISBN	0-7216-9665-1
Volume 5	ISBN	0-7216-9666-X
Volume 6	ISBN	0-7216-9667-8
Six Volume Set	ISBN	0-7216-9658-9

Neurological Surgery—Volume Six

Last digit is the print number: 9   8   7   6   5   4   3   2

Contributors

MARSHALL B. ALLEN, JR., M.D., F.A.C.S.

Intracerebral and Intracerebellar Hemorrhage, Sympathectomy

Chairman of Department of Neurological Surgery, Medical College of Georgia. Chief of Neurological Surgery, Eugene Talmadge Memorial Hospital; Consultant, University Hospital and Veterans Administration Hospital, Augusta, Georgia; Dwight D. Eisenhower Army Medical Center, Fort Gordon, Georgia; and Central State Hospital, Milledgeville, Georgia.

CHARLES E. BRACKETT, M.D., F.A.C.S.

Pulmonary Care and Complications, Arachnoid Cysts, Subarachnoid Hemorrhage, Post-Traumatic Arachnoid Cysts, Cordotomy

Professor of Neurological Surgery, Chairman of Department of Neurological Surgery, University of Kansas Medical Center, College of Health Sciences and Hospital. Chief of Neurological Surgery Service, University of Kansas Medical Center; Attending Staff, Kansas City Veterans Administration Hospital, Kansas City, Missouri.

VERNE L. BRECHNER, M.D., F.A.C.A.

Conduction Anesthesia Techniques

Clinical Professor of Anesthesiology, School of Medicine, University of California at Los Angeles. Attending Staff in Anesthesiology, Center for Health Sciences, University of California at Los Angeles, Los Angeles, California; Medical Director, Centinela Pain Management Center, Inglewood, California.

FERNANDO CABIESES, M.D., Ph.D., F.A.C.S.

Parasitic and Fungal Infections

Professor of Neurological Surgery (Ret.), School of Medicine, Universidad de San Marcos. Chief, Neurological Surgery Unit, Peruvian Armed Forces, Anglo-American Hospital, and Hospital 2 de Mayo, Lima, Peru.

WILLIAM F. COLLINS, M.D., F.A.C.S.

Physiology of Pain

Harvey and Kate Cushing Professor of Surgery, Chief of Section of Neurological Surgery, Yale University School of Medicine. Neurological Surgeon-in-Chief, Yale–New Haven Medical Center, New Haven, Connecticut.

WILLIAM S. COXE, M.D., F.A.C.S.

Viral Encephalitis

Professor of Neurological Surgery, Washington University School of Medicine. Assistant Neurological Surgeon, Barnes and Allied Hospitals; Attending Neurological Surgeon, St. Louis City Hospital; Consultant, Veterans Administration Hospital, St. Louis, Missouri.

BENJAMIN L. CRUE, JR., M.D.

Stereotaxic Mesencephalotomy, Trigeminal Tractotomy

Clinical Professor of Surgery (Neurological Surgery), University of California, School of Medicine at Los Angeles, Los Angeles, California. Director, New Hope Pain Center, Alhambra Community Hospital, Alhambra, California.

RICHARD A. DE VAUL, M.D.

Pain Refractory to Therapy

Associate Professor of Psychiatry, The University of Texas Medical School at Houston. Attending Staff, Hermann Hospital and Memorial Southwest Hospital, Houston, Texas.

ELDON L. FOLTZ, M.D., F.A.C.S.

Affective Disorders Involving Pain

Professor of Neurological Surgery, School of Medicine, University of California at Irvine. Chief of Section of Neurological Surgery, University of California Medical Center, Irvine, California.

PHILIP L. GILDENBERG, M.D., Ph.D., F.A.C.S.

Pain Refractory to Therapy

Professor of Neurological Surgery and Chief of Division of Neurological Surgery, University of Texas Medical School at Houston. Chief of Neurological Surgery, Hermann Hospital, Houston, Texas.

SIDNEY GOLDRING, M.D., F.A.C.S.

Epilepsy in Adults

Professor of Neurological Surgery and Co-Head of Department of Neurology and Neurological Surgery, Washington University School of Medicine. Neurosurgeon-in-Chief, Barnes Hospital and St. Louis Children's Hospital, St. Louis, Missouri.

STANLEY J. GOODMAN, M.D., F.A.C.S.

Bacterial Infections

Associate Clinical Professor of Neurological Surgery, University of California, School of Medicine at Los Angeles, Los Angeles, California. Attending Staff, South Bay Hospital; San Pedro Peninsula Community Hospital, San Pedro, California; Community Hospital of Gardena, Gardena, California; Kaiser Hospital, Harbor City, California; Wadsworth Veterans Administration Hospital, Los Angeles, California; Little Company of Mary Hospital and Harbor General Hospital, Torrance, California.

JOHN R. GREEN, M.D., F.A.C.S.

Epilepsy in Children

Adjunct Professor of Surgery (Neurological Surgery), University of Arizona College of Medicine, Tucson, Arizona. Director, Barrow Neurological Institute of St. Joseph's Hospital and Medical Center, Phoenix, Arizona.

JULES HARDY, M.D., F.R.C.S.(C.), F.A.C.S.

Indications for and Results of Hypophysectomy, Transsphenoidal Hypophysectomy

Professor of Neurological Surgery, Chairman of Division of Neurological Surgery, University of Montreal Faculty of Medicine. Neurosurgeon, Notre Dame Hospital and University of Montreal Hospital, Montreal, Quebec.

NELSON HENDLER, M.D.

Psychiatric Aspects of Pain

Assistant Professor of Psychiatry, The Johns Hopkins University School of Medicine. Psychiatric Consultant, Chronic Pain Treatment Center, Johns Hopkins Hospital, Baltimore, Maryland; Clinical Director, Mensana Clinic, Stevenson, Maryland.

PETER J. JANNETTA, M.D.

Micro-Operative Decompression for Trigeminal Neuralgia, Cranial Rhizopathies

Professor of Neurological Surgery, Chairman of Department of Neurological Surgery, University of Pittsburgh. Active Staff, Presbyterian–University Hospital and Children's Hospital of Pittsburgh; Senior Attending Neurological Surgeon, Montefiore Hospital; Senior Consultant, Veterans Administration Hospital, Pittsburgh, Pennsylvania.

ROBERT B. KING, M.D., F.A.C.S.

Cephalic Pain

Professor of Neurological Surgery, Chairman of Department of Neurological Surgery, State University of New York, Upstate Medical Center College of Medicine, Syracuse, New York. Chief of Neurological Surgery, State University Hospital of Upstate Medical Center; Attending Neurological Surgeon, Crouse-Irving Memorial Hospital; Consultant, Neurological Surgery, Veterans Administration Hospital. Syracuse, New York.

CAROLE C. LA MOTTE, Ph.D.

Physiology of Pain

Assistant Professor of Neuroanatomy and Neurological Surgery, Sections of Neuroanatomy and Neurological Surgery, Yale University School of Medicine, New Haven, Connecticut.

HUN JAE LEE, M.D.

Parasitic and Fungal Infections

Late Professor of Neurological Surgery, Chairman of Department of Neurological Surgery, Yonsei University College of Medicine. Late Chief of Neurological Surgery, Yonsei Medical Center, Seoul, Korea.

JOHN D. LOESER, M.D.

Dorsal Rhizotomy

Professor of Neurological Surgery, University of Washington School of Medicine. Attending Physician, University Hospital, Veterans Administration Hospital, Harborview Medical Center, and Children's Orthopedic Hospital, Seattle, Washington.

DONLIN M. LONG, M.D., Ph.D., F.A.C.S.

Tumors of Skull, Chronic Pain, Pain of Spinal Origin, Pain of Visceral Origin, Peripheral Nerve Pain

Professor of Neurological Surgery, Chairman of Department of Neurological Surgery, The Johns Hopkins School of Medicine. Neurological Surgeon-in-Chief, Johns Hopkins Hospital, Baltimore, Maryland.

JOSE GERARDO MARTIN-RODRIGUES, M.D.

Tuberculoma and Syphilitic Gumma

Head of Neurosurgical Service, Department "Sixto Obrador," Centro Especial "RAMON Y CAJAL," Ministry of Health and Social Security, Madrid, Spain.

WILLIAM H. MORETZ, M.D., F.A.C.S.

Sympathectomy

President, Medical College of Georgia; Professor of Surgery, Medical College of Georgia. Attending Surgeon, Eugene Talmadge Memorial Hospital and University Hospital, Augusta, Georgia.

BLAINE SANDERS NASHOLD, JR., M.D., F.A.C.S.

Stereotaxic Mesencephalotomy, Trigeminal Tractotomy

Professor of Neurological Surgery, Duke University School of Medicine. Attending Neurological Surgeon, Duke University Hospital, Durham, North Carolina.

SIXTO OBRADOR, M.D.

Tuberculoma and Syphilitic Gumma

Late Professor of Neurological Surgery, Facultad de Medicina, Universidad Autonoma. Late Director and Chief of Department of Neurological Surgery, Centro Especial "RAMON Y CAJAL" of the Spanish Social Security, Madrid, Spain.

GEORGE A. OJEMANN, M.D.

Abnormal Movement Disorders

Professor of Neurological Surgery, University of Washington School of Medicine. Attending Physician, University Hospital and Harborview Medical Center; Consultant, Veterans Administration Hospital, Seattle, Washington.

RUSSELL H. PATTERSON, JR., M.D., F.A.C.S.

Extradural Dorsal Spinal Lesions, Metastatic Brain Tumors, Hypophysectomy by Craniotomy

Professor of Neurological Surgery, Cornell University Medical College. Attending Surgeon-in-Charge, Department of Neurological Surgery, The New York Hospital, New York, New York.

ROBERT A. RATCHESON, M.D., F.A.C.S.

Stereotaxic Surgery

Harvey Huntington Brown, Jr., Professor of Neurological Surgery; Director of Division of Neurological Surgery, Case Western Reserve University School of Medicine. Director of Division of Neurological Surgery, University Hospitals of Cleveland, Cleveland, Ohio.

HUBERT L. ROSOMOFF, M.D., D. Med. Sc., F.A.C.S.

Stereotaxic Cordotomy

Professor of Neurological Surgery, Chairman of Department of Neurological Surgery, University of Miami School of Medicine. Chief of Neurosurgical Service, Jackson Memorial Hospital; Attending Neurological Surgeon, Veterans Administration Hospital; Medical Director, Pain and Back Rehabilitation Program, University of Miami Hospital and Diagnostic Clinic, Miami, Florida.

FRANK A. ROWE, M.D.

Parasitic and Fungal Infections

Resident, Neurological Surgery, University of California at Davis Medical Center at Sacramento, Sacramento, California.

HOWARD A. RUSK, M.D., F.A.C.P.

Rehabilitation

Distinguished University Professor, New York University. Founder, Institute of Rehabilitation Medicine, New York, New York.

GEORGE HEINRICH SELL, M.D.

Rehabilitation

Late Associate Professor of Clinical Rehabilitation Medicine, New York University School of Medicine. Late Acting Clinical Director, Institute of Rehabilitation Medicine, New York University Medical Center; Late Associate Attending Physician, Bellevue Medical Center, New York, New York.

ALVIN D. SIDELL, M.D.

Epilepsy in Children

Senior Pediatric Neurologist, Director of Electroencephalography Laboratory, Barrow Neurological Institute, St. Joseph's Hospital and Medical Center, Phoenix, Arizona.

W. EUGENE STERN, M.D., F.A.C.S.

Preoperative Evaluation, Prevention and Treatment of Complications; Bacterial Infections

Professor of Surgery/Neurological Surgery, University of California, School of Medicine at Los Angeles, Los Angeles, California. Chief of Neurological Surgery, University of California Los Angeles Center for Health Sciences; Neurological Surgeon Consultant, Wadsworth Veterans Administration Hospital, Harbor General Hospital, St. John's Hospital, Los Angeles, California, and Santa Monica Hospital, Santa Monica, California.

WILLIAM H. SWEET, M.D., D.Sc., D.H.C., F.A.C.S.

Intracerebral Stimulation for Pain, Primary Affective Disorders

Emeritus Professor of Surgery, Harvard Medical School. Senior Neurosurgeon, Massachusetts General Hospital; Consulting Neurosurgeon, New England Deaconess Hospital, Massachusetts Eye and Ear Infirmary, Waltham Hospital, and Milton Hospital, Boston, Massachusetts.

JOHN M. TEW, JR., M.D., F.A.C.S.

Percutaneous Rhizotomy for Trigeminal, Glossopharyngeal and Vagal Pain

Adjunct Professor of Anatomy, University of Cincinnati College of Medicine. Chairman of Department of Neurological Surgery, Good Samaritan Hospital; Attending Neurological Surgeon, Christ Hospital, Cincinnati, Ohio.

JOHN S. TYTUS, M.D., F.A.C.S.

Medical Therapy, Minor Procedures, and Craniotomy for Trigeminal Neuralgia; Glossopharyngeal and Geniculate Neuralgias

Clinical Associate Professor of Neurological Surgery, University of Washington School of Medicine. Attending Neurological Surgeon, Virginia Mason Hospital, King County Hospital, and Children's Orthopedic Hospital, Seattle, Washington.

JOHN M. VAN BUREN, M.D., Ph.D.

Stereotaxic Surgery

Professor of Neurological Surgery, University of Miami School of Medicine. Chief of Neurological Surgery, Veterans Administration Hospital; Attending Neurological Surgeon, Jackson Memorial Hospital, Miami, Florida.

ARTHUR A. WARD, JR., M.D.

Abnormal Movement Disorders

Professor of Neurological Surgery, Chairman of Department of Neurological Surgery, University of Washington School of Medicine. Attending Neurological Surgeon, University Hospital, Harborview Medical Center; Consultant, Veterans Administration Hospital, Children's Orthopedic Hospital, Seattle, Washington.

PHILIP RALPH WEINSTEIN, M.D., F.A.C.S.

Indications for and Results of Hypophysectomy, Stereotaxic Hypophysectomy

Professor of Neurological Surgery, University of Arizona School of Medicine. Chief of Neurological Surgery, University of Arizona Hospital; Attending Neurological Surgeon, Tucson Medical Center; Consultant, Barrow Neurological Institute, St. Joseph's Hospital, Tucson, Arizona.

KEASLEY WELCH, M.D., M.S., F.A.C.S.

Sensory Root Section for Trigeminal Neuralgia

Franc D. Ingraham Professor of Neurosurgery, Harvard Medical School, Neurosurgeon-in-Chief, Children's Hospital Medical Center; Division Chief (Neurosurgery), Department of Surgery, Peter Bent Brigham Hospital and Women's Hospital, Boston, Massachusetts.

LOWELL E. WHITE, JR., M.D.

Affective Disorders Involving Pain

Professor of Neuroscience, University of South Alabama. Attending Neurological Surgeon, University of South Alabama Medical Center, Providence Hospital, Mobile, Alabama.

CHARLES B. WILSON, M.D., F.A.C.S.

Dural Fistulae, Chemotherapy, Sellar and Parasellar Tumors, Indications for and Results of Hypophysectomy, Stereotaxic Hypophysectomy

Professor of Neurological Surgery, Chairman of Department of Neurological Surgery, University of California. School of Medicine at San Francisco. Chief of Neurological Surgery, University Hospital, San Francisco, California.

R. LEWIS WRIGHT, M.D., F.A.C.S.

Infections of Spine

Attending Neurological Surgeon, St. Mary's Hospital and Stuart Circle Hospital, Richmond, Virginia.

JULIAN R. YOUMANS, M.D., Ph.D., F.A.C.S.

Diagnostic Biopsy, Cerebral Death, Cerebral Blood Flow, Trauma to Carotid Arteries, Glial and Neuronal Tumors, Lymphomas, Sarcomas and Vascular Tumors, Tumors of Disordered Embryogenesis, Peripheral and Sympathetic Nerve Tumors, Parasitic and Fungal Infections.

Professor of Neurological Surgery, University of California, School of Medicine at Davis, Davis, California. Attending Neurological Surgeon, University of California Davis Medical Center at Sacramento, Sacramento, California; Consultant in Neurological Surgery, United States Air Force Medical Center, Travis Air Force Base, California; Veterans Administration Hospital, Martinez, California.

RONALD F. YOUNG, M.D.

Cephalic Pain

Associate Professor of Neurological Surgery, University of California, School of Medicine at Los Angeles. Chief of Division of Neurological Surgery, Harbor General Hospital, Torrance, California; Attending Neurological Surgeon, University of California Hospital, Los Angeles, California.

Contents

———————— VOLUME SIX ————————

XI. **Infections**... **3321**

Chapter 110
CRANIAL AND INTRACRANIAL BACTERIAL INFECTIONS................ 3323
S. J. Goodman and W. E. Stern

Chapter 111
VIRAL ENCEPHALITIS.. 3358
W. S. Coxe

Chapter 112
PARASITIC AND FUNGAL DISEASES OF THE CENTRAL NERVOUS
SYSTEM.. 3366
F. A. Rowe, J. R. Youmans, H. J. Lee, and F. Cabieses

Chapter 113
TUBERCULOMA AND SYPHILITIC GUMMA.................................. 3441
S. Obrador and J. G. Martin-Rodriguez

Chapter 114
INFECTIONS OF THE SPINE AND SPINAL CORD 3449
R. L. Wright

XII. **Pain**... **3459**

Chapter 115
PHYSIOLOGICAL ANATOMY OF PAIN...................................... 3461
C. C. LaMotte and W. F. Collins

Chapter 116
PSYCHIATRIC CONSIDERATIONS OF PAIN.................................. 3480
N. Hendler

Chapter 117
GENERAL CONSIDERATIONS IN THE MANAGEMENT OF CHRONIC
PAIN.. 3523
D. M. Long

Chapter 118
CEPHALIC PAIN.. 3531
R. B. King and R. F. Young

Chapter 119
GENERAL CONSIDERATIONS, MEDICAL THERAPY, AND MINOR
OPERATIVE PROCEDURES FOR TRIGEMINAL NEURALGIA.............. 3554
J. S. Tytus

Chapter 120
TREATMENT OF TRIGEMINAL NEURALGIA BY PERCUTANEOUS
RHIZOTOMY.. 3564
J. M. Tew, Jr.

Chapter 121
TREATMENT OF TRIGEMINAL NEURALGIA THROUGH TEMPORAL
CRANIOTOMY.. 3580
J. S. Tytus

Chapter 122
TREATMENT OF TRIGEMINAL NEURALGIA BY SECTION OF THE
SENSORY ROOT IN THE POSTERIOR FOSSA................................. 3586
K. Welch

Chapter 123
TREATMENT OF TRIGEMINAL NEURALGIA BY MICRO-OPERATIVE
DECOMPRESSION.. 3589
P. J. Jannetta

Chapter 124
GLOSSOPHARYNGEAL AND GENICULATE NEURALGIAS.................. 3604
J. S. Tytus

Chapter 125
TREATMENT OF PAIN OF GLOSSOPHARYNGEAL AND VAGUS
NERVES BY PERCUTANEOUS RHIZOTOMY.................................... 3609
J. M. Tew, Jr.

Chapter 126
PAIN OF SPINAL ORIGIN... 3613
D. M. Long

Chapter 127
PAIN OF VISCERAL ORIGIN.. 3627
D. M. Long

Chapter 128
PAIN OF PERIPHERAL NERVE INJURY.. 3634
D. M. Long

Chapter 129
MANAGEMENT OF PAIN BY CONDUCTION ANESTHESIA
TECHNIQUES... 3644
V. L. Brechner

Chapter 130
DORSAL RHIZOTOMY.. 3664
J. D. Loeser

Chapter 131
STEREOTAXIC CORDOTOMY.. 3672
H. L. Rosomoff

Chapter 132
CORDOTOMY BY OPEN OPERATIVE TECHNIQUES.......................... 3686
C. E. Brackett

Chapter 133
STEREOTAXIC MESENCEPHALOTOMY AND TRIGEMINAL
TRACTOTOMY.. 3702
B. S. Nashold, Jr., and B. L. Crue, Jr.

Chapter 134
SYMPATHECTOMY... 3717
M. B. Allen, Jr., and W. H. Moretz

Chapter 135
AFFECTIVE DISORDERS INVOLVING PAIN................................. 3727
E. L. Foltz and L. E. White, Jr.

Chapter 136
INTRACEREBRAL ELECTRICAL STIMULATION FOR THE RELIEF OF
CHRONIC PAIN... 3739
W. H. Sweet

Chapter 137
MANAGEMENT OF CHRONIC PAIN REFRACTORY TO SPECIFIC
THERAPY.. 3749
P. L. Gildenberg and R. A. DeVaul

XIII. Neurophysiological and Ablative Procedures................. 3769

Chapter 138
CRANIAL RHIZOPATHIES... 3771
P. J. Jannetta

Chapter 139
PRINCIPLES OF STEREOTAXIC SURGERY................................. 3785
J. M. Van Buren and R. A. Ratcheson

Chapter 140
ABNORMAL MOVEMENT DISORDERS..................................... 3821
G. A. Ojemann and A. A. Ward, Jr.

Chapter 141
NEUROSURGICAL ASPECTS OF EPILEPSY IN CHILDREN AND
ADOLESCENTS 3858
J. R. Green and A. D. Sidell

Chapter 142
NEUROSURGICAL ASPECTS OF EPILEPSY IN ADULTS..................... 3910
S. Goldring

Chapter 143
NEUROSURGICAL ASPECTS OF PRIMARY AFFECTIVE DISORDERS.... 3927
W. H. Sweet

Chapter 144
INDICATIONS FOR AND RESULTS OF HYPOPHYSECTOMY.............. 3947
J. Hardy, P. R. Weinstein, and C. B. Wilson

Chapter 145
TRANSSPHENOIDAL HYPOPHYSECTOMY....................................... 3959
J. Hardy

Chapter 146
STEREOTAXIC HYPOPHYSECTOMY... 3973
P. R. Weinstein and C. B. Wilson

Chapter 147
HYPOPHYSECTOMY BY CRANIOTOMY... 3981
R. H. Patterson, Jr.

XIV.   Rehabilitation... 3987

Chapter 148
REHABILITATION FOLLOWING CENTRAL NERVOUS SYSTEM
LESIONS... 3989
G. H. Sell and H. A. Rusk

INDEX i

XI

INFECTIONS

CRANIAL AND INTRACRANIAL BACTERIAL INFECTIONS

BASIC CONSIDERATIONS

Despite the near elimination of several infectious diseases and the lowered morbidity and mortality rates for many others, infections continue to be an inherent part of human life. While certain specific microbial infections have been controlled, different ones are emerging as troublesome therapeutic and epidemiological problems. With the use of cytotoxic drugs, massive x-ray irradiation to treat malignant diseases, and immunosuppressive agents, infections caused by organisms previously considered saprophytic or commensal have increased. Moreover, although antimicrobial agents are successfully reducing the number of deaths associated with some common infections, other microbes are evolving into major causes of human disease.

To achieve an understanding of diagnostic procedures and therapeutic principles, general aspects of the host-organism relation must be studied, even though some of this information may not be specifically applicable to the individual patient who has an infection. *Bacteria, infection,* and *clinical disease* are not synonymous. Bacteria have been cultured from "clean" wounds at the time of operation. Growth of bacteria from clean wounds has no positive correlation with postoperative wound infection or the type of pathogens isolated from a subsequent infection.[1] Indeed, the multiplication of microorganisms within the host at normally sterile sites does not necessarily produce symptoms. In this case the host-organism relation is characterized as a "subclinical infection" or a "carrier state." The ratio of subclinical infection to overt clinical disease varies widely among microbial species.[6]

Host Factors: Resistance and Susceptibility

A group of host factors, collectively referred to as "resistance," or conversely, "susceptibility," influence the likelihood of disease and the outcome of infection once it is established. Hypothetically, the following metabolic and cellular factors are important in determining resistance: phagocytic function; the antibacterial activity of such substances as lysozymes, phagocytin, and other lysozomal enzymes; qualitative and quantitative alterations in serum proteins; disordered metabolism at the cellular level; the presence or absence of tissue-injury products influencing vascular permeability; the effects of tissue pressure; and similar processes. In experimental animals many factors can be shown to influence infection, e.g., sex, age, microbial strain, route of infection, the presence of specific antibodies or other diseases, the state of nutrition, exposure to ionizing radiation, high environmental temperature, the administration of certain compounds (such as mucin, nitrogen mustard, adrenal steroids, epinephrine and other vasopressors, and metabolic analogues), and xerosis. Many of these experimental variables are critically

S. J. GOODMAN AND W. E. STERN

important to man.[6,14,22] Clinically, several additional factors are known to lower resistance to infection, including alcoholism, diabetes mellitus, uremia and cirrhosis, deficiency or absence of immunoglobulins, defects in cellular immunity, and malnutrition.[14,22,23] Shock, long-term administration of adrenal cortical hormones, chronic lymphedema, ischemia, the presence of foreign bodies, obstruction of a hollow tube or viscus, agranulocytosis, various blood dyscrasias, and prolonged hospitalization are still other factors that cause greater susceptibility to infection.[6,14,22]

In addition to the general host factors contributing to resistance and susceptibility, recurring patterns of clinical phenomena predispose to cranial and intracranial infection, the latter occurring in relation to one or more of the following: (1) penetrating craniocerebral trauma; (2) compound depressed skull fracture; (3) basal skull fracture "internally compounded" (especially with cerebrospinal fluid rhinorrhea); (4) craniotomy; (5) "neighborhood" or contiguous infections of the paranasal sinuses, mastoids, scalp, or face; (6) intrathoracic infection (especially pulmonary empyema, abscess, and bronchiectasis); (7) right-to-left circulation shunts that bypass the pulmonary filter (congenital heart disease, especially cyanotic forms); (8) a distant, chronic septic focus (e.g., osteomyelitis, diverticulitis); (9) prior parenchymatous brain injury; (10) intracranial tumor; and (11) the presence of an intracranial "foreign" body, especially retained bone fragments, wood, prosthetic materials (shunt apparatus, other synthetic compounds), and occasionally, in-driven metallic fragments.

General Clinical Features

The symptoms and signs of infection are derived from the primary lesion and the systemic host response, and the neurological manifestations are prominently affected by the location of the process and its degree of circumscription or confinement. Questions to determine other influencing factors should be asked: Is the infection irritative (meningitis) or destructive to neural tissue (parenchymatous abscess)? Is cerebral edema or hydrocephalus present? Is the integument (scalp, bone) involved? Signs and symptoms of central nervous system involvement can be observed because toxins are liberated by bacteria at remote sites (e.g., botulism, tetanus), but unfortunately, the mechanisms that produce most "constitutional" signs and symptoms of human infection are unknown.

A secure diagnosis of infection requires direct demonstration of the causative organism or proof of its presence by indirect means. The organism may be seen microscopically in appropriate fluid, within leukocytes, in bone marrow, or within tissue. The microscopic analysis can be extended by fluorescence and dark-field techniques. Organisms can be isolated by inoculating appropriate material onto suitable media with proper regard to the environment (temperature, oxygen, and carbon dioxide levels). They can be isolated by inoculation of appropriate material into mice or guinea pigs. Blood cultures should be obtained if bacteremia is suspected or if there is a possibility of intravascular infection (bacterial endocarditis, mycotic aneurysm, suppurative thrombophlebitis). Bacteria entering the bloodstream are promptly removed from circulation by phagocytosis. Because of this phenomenon, a shaking chill and fever may occur 30 to 90 minutes after the vascular influx of microorganisms, but a blood culture may still be negative. Blood cultures should therefore be taken at intervals when bacteremia is suspected; two to four cultures daily for two or three days are usually sufficient to establish such a diagnosis. Immunological tests are available for detecting microorganisms: for example, serological measurements of antibody titer (a rapid rise or fall of the titer indicates a recent contact with the antigen) and skin tests (bacterial or tuberculin) for delayed hypersensitivity.

With intracranial infections that contaminate the free cerebrospinal fluid pathways, such as leptomeningitis or unobstructed ventriculitis, the causative organism can be demonstrated by sampling cerebrospinal fluid obtained by lumbar puncture. In other intracranial infections an examination of this type will not reveal the organism and may, as in the case of parenchymatous abscess, precipitate a lethal brain herniation syndrome (e.g., herniation of the posterior temporal gyrus or uncus, of the cingulate gyrus, or of the cerebellar tonsil).

The diagnostic evaluation of a patient

with suspected intracranial infection must include several considerations: Is there evidence of increased intracranial pressure? Is there evidence of obstructive hydrocephalus or the potential thereof? Is there evidence of a posterior fossa mass? Is there evidence of a lateralized cerebral hemispheric mass? A goal of the initial diagnostic studies should be to establish whether the process is focal and localizable by techniques that will avoid precipitating an internal herniation syndrome. The value of computed tomography as a screening device deserves emphasis; alternative or supplemental testing can then be used as required (electroencephalography, radioactive nuclide scanning, cerebral angiography).

Antimicrobial Agents

Several major factors must be considered in the selection and administration of antimicrobial agents. Although a microorganism may be "sensitive" to a particular antibiotic on a culture medium, therapy is guided better by the semiquantitative concept of microorganism susceptibility in which the concentration of the drug required for antibacterial effectiveness is determined. The clinical decision can then be made whether or not that required concentration can be attained. Dilution methods of susceptibility testing are the most accurate and are expressed in terms of the minimum inhibitory concentration (MIC) required to inhibit growth after overnight incubation. Since the size and turnover rate of the "reservoir" (i.e., the cerebrospinal fluid compartment) will vary from patient to patient and will greatly influence the final antibiotic concentration in the fluid, the determination of minimum inhibitory concentration and attainable antibiotic levels is of considerable help when intrathecal or intraventricular routes are used to administer an aminoglycoside such as gentamicin in the treatment of a gram-negative meningitis or ventriculitis. Whenever possible, cranial and intracranial infections should be treated with *bactericidal* rather than *bacteriostatic* drugs.[88] Bactericidal agents include the penicillins, cephalosporins, polymyxins, and vancomycin. Bacteriostatic agents are the tetracyclines, sulfonamides, chloramphenicol, erythromycin, and lincomycin.[50]

The *route of administration* of an antibiotic is related, in general, to the severity of infection. Oral administration is restricted to treatment of mild infections, whereas parenteral therapy is used when the infection is severe. The choice of intravenous or intramuscular therapy will depend on the specific antibiotic and considerations of pain, phlebitis, and other local tissue reactions at the site of administration. Selection of the antibiotic must take into account *blood-brain and blood–cerebrospinal fluid penetration*. Entrance of substances from blood into cerebrospinal fluid is determined by physical and chemical properties, which include lipid solubility, ionization, molecular size, and protein binding. The blood–cerebrospinal fluid barrier is partially incompetent during meningeal inflammation. As a result, there is an unpredictable, variable increase in penetration of substances from the blood to the fluid. The physical and chemical properties determining the rate of entry of substances from blood to brain are less well known. In general, the blood–cerebrospinal fluid barrier is more readily traversed by antibiotics than is the blood-brain barrier. In fact, chloramphenicol is the only commonly employed antibiotic that penetrates the blood-brain barrier in microbiologically significant amounts. Gentamicin does not readily cross from blood to cerebrospinal fluid despite meningeal inflammation. Intrathecal or intraventricular administration of gentamicin should be combined with intramuscular use if a gram-negative meningitis or ventriculitis leads to the selection of that antibiotic.

The patient should be questioned about antibiotic allergy, and the toxicity of the drug must be considered. The aminoglycosides may be nephrotoxic. If renal function is impaired from either pre-existing disease or prior antibiotic use, the dose must be decreased because the reduced renal clearance prolongs the half-life of the drug. Guidelines based on serial determinations of the serum creatinine are available that indicate specific antibiotic reduction schedules. Antibiotic neurotoxicity originally referred to a drug's capacity to cause central nervous system irritability (convulsions, myoclonic jerks, hyperreflexia) subsequent to its cortical application or to parenteral administration sufficiently vigorous for high cerebrospinal fluid levels to accumulate.[48,55,84] "Penicillin convulsions" were described and systematically studied at the end of World War II.[84] Antibiotic neurotoxicity has also been defined in terms of pleocytosis, periventricular inflammation, and behavioral changes in animals studied by ventriculocisternal perfusion of different antibiotics.[87] When several antibiotics are used simultaneously, antibiotic synergism or antagonism may occur, but usually two antibiotics have an indifferent combined effect.

Specific antimicrobial agents are numerous; some of the most important and commonly used drugs are reviewed here, mainly to indicate the categories from which selections are made.[43] The treatment of specific infections is discussed later.

Penicillins

Penicillinase-susceptible penicillins include penicillin G and certain broad-spectrum penicillins. Penicillin G is still widely used and has the favorable property that, in large intravenous doses (20 million units per day), it produces high blood levels and effective penetration of cerebrospinal fluid. A number of broad-spectrum penicillins are available, such as ampicillin and carbenicillin. Ampicillin is an efficient and effective antibiotic that maintains a higher blood level than penicillin G because of a lower renal clearance rate; moreover, its concentration of available free antibiotic at the site of infection is higher because serum protein binding of ampicillin is less than the binding of penicillin G. The incidence of hypersensitivity reactions with ampicillin is comparable to that with penicillin G. Blood levels considerably higher than those of ampicillin can be attained with carbenicillin (which has a still lower renal clearance rate), and these high blood levels (in the range of 100 μg per milliliter) are bactericidal against *Pseudomonas, Proteus, Enterobacter,* and several other gram-negative organisms.

Penicillinase-resistant penicillins have greatly enhanced the effectiveness of antistaphylococcal chemotherapy inasmuch as over three fourths of nosocomial infections are due to *Staphylococcus aureus,* which is penicillinase-producing.[80] There has been a progressive rise in nonnosocomial staphylococcal infections caused by penicillinase-producing organisms, and the current estimates are that 85 per cent of community-acquired infections stem from such

bacteria.[39,42] Three parenteral preparations of comparable therapeutic efficacy are available: methicillin, oxacillin, and nafcillin. Although oral agents are available (nafcillin, oxacillin, cloxacillin, dicloxacillin) and may be used for mild soft-tissue infections, they are most commonly used with central nervous system infections to complete therapy that was begun parenterally. Sufficiently high blood levels can be achieved with these penicillinase-resistant penicillins to be effective against pneumococci and most streptococci, so both types of penicillins need not be used against these organisms. Ampicillin should be used, however, if enterococci or *Neisseria* is suspected.

Cephalosporins

Like the penicillins, the cephalosporins are bactericidal and are effective against a wide spectrum of organisms: group A and viridans streptococci, pneumococci, penicillin G–sensitive and resistant *Staphylococcus aureus, Neisseria,* and most strains of the following gram-negative organisms: *Escherichia coli, Proteus mirabilis, Klebsiella,* and *Hemophilus influenzae.* Penetration of the blood–cerebrospinal fluid and blood-brain barriers by the cephalosporins is poor, but effective antibiotic concentrations in spinal fluid can be maintained by intrathecal administration. There is approximately a 10 per cent risk of allergic reaction to cephalosporins in patients who are allergic to penicillin. This figure excludes patients with a prior history of anaphylaxis to any of the penicillins, who probably should not be given cephalosporin therapy. Cephalosporins can be administered intravenously, intramuscularly, and orally. In patients with nonanaphylactic penicillin allergy who have staphylococcal meningitis, successful treatment response can often be achieved with combined intravenous cephalothin (12 gm per day) and intrathecal cephaloridine (12.5 to 50 mg per day).

Aminoglycosides

The aminoglycosides include streptomycin, neomycin, kanamycin, and gentamicin.[41] Streptomycin and neomycin are used by neurosurgeons for open and closed, clean or infected wound irrigation, but their systemic use is rare because of a variety of potential toxic effects. Kanamycin is effective against staphylococci and most gram-negative bacilli except *Pseudomonas*. The nephrotoxic blood level is sufficiently close to the therapeutic blood level that antibiotic blood levels should be followed closely and dosage adjusted carefully to the serum creatinine value. Kanamycin is most often used as part of a multiple antibiotic approach to serious infection while awaiting culture results. Gentamicin is similar to kanamycin in its antibacterial spectrum, and it is also effective against *Pseudomonas*. Its toxicity and the need for careful dosage adjustment resemble those for kanamycin. Since gentamicin is so effective in gram-negative infections yet crosses the blood–cerebrospinal fluid barrier so poorly, intrathecal or intraventricular administration may be required in treating gram-negative meningitis or ventriculitis.

Chloramphenicol

Chloramphenicol is bacteriostatic. It crosses the blood–cerebrospinal fluid and blood-brain barriers exceedingly well and has a broad spectrum of activity. With the increasing identification of anaerobic organisms involved in brain abscess and subdural empyema, it is now realized that *Bacteroides fragilis* is a common anaerobic pathogen. Over half the strains of this organism are resistant to the penicillins. On the other hand, almost all *Bacteroides* strains are susceptible to chloramphenicol. As a result, there is renewed interest in the use of this antibiotic with cranial and intracranial infections, despite the occurrence of

aplastic anemia in approximately 1 of 25,000 persons receiving it.[8,85,93] A less serious problem is the chloramphenicol protein synthesis inhibition with doses larger than 2 gm per day, an effect that is reversible and clinically manifested by leukopenia, anemia, and thrombocytopenia. This reversible hematological toxic effect can be monitored simply by twice weekly blood counts.

Other Antibiotics

Other agents may be considered and used in special circumstances. Parenteral clindamycin is active against *B. fragilis* and is not toxic to bone marrow. It lacks the broad gram-negative spectrum of chloramphenicol, however, and most importantly, it does not cross the blood-brain barrier. Its use in intracranial pyogenic infections is therefore limited.[20] The *polymyxins, tetracyclines,* and *sulfonamides* are used infrequently in treating cranial and intracranial infections.

SPECIFIC CLINICAL ENTITIES

For consideration of specific pyogenic entities, the schema of Turner and Reynolds provides an excellent recapitulation of the potential routes that infection may take once the process is established in or adjacent to the cranium (Fig. 110–1).[82] (Further illustration of these features can be found in Figure 110–12.) The hematogenous mode as a pathway should also be kept promi-

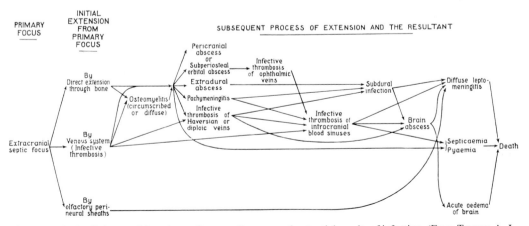

Figure 110–1 Schema of the primary focus, pathways, and potential results of infection. (From Turner, A. L., and Reynolds, F. E.: Intracranial Pyogenic Diseases. Edinburgh, Oliver & Boyd, 1931. Reprinted by permission.)

nently in mind in the establishment of the initial focus.

Subgaleal Abscess

Subgaleal abscess is a purulent infection of the subgaleal space, and while strictly it is neither cranial nor intracranial, its importance demands its inclusion. Infection beneath the galea aponeurotica may spread rapidly, with the potential of occupying an area limited only by the boundaries of the galea along the frontalis, temporalis, and occipitalis muscles. Pathogenetic mechanisms include hematogenous spread from distant septic foci, contaminated inoculations associated with drug abuse, and spread from a focus of calvarial osteomyelitis. The most common mechanism is the colonization of organisms in the subgaleal space following scalp trauma. Examples of note are accidental lacerations and puncture wounds, and puncture wounds from skeletal traction or other immobilization devices, needle electrode insertion for fetal monitoring, and use of pediatric scalp vein needles. Unless secondary to spread from subpericranial infection contiguous to osteomyelitis of the skull, the process usually remains confined to the subgaleal space. The potential exists, however, for spread to adjacent tissue (bone) and deeper layers (epidural, subdural, and subarachnoid spaces) via a propagating thrombophlebitis or by direct access as afforded by an underlying skull fracture.

Subgaleal abscess most often causes local tenderness and warmth as well as systemic symptoms and signs of sepsis. There may be localized or generalized scalp edema, puffy eyelids, and prominent cervical adenopathy. Although the diagnosis of subgaleal abscess is usually self-evident, it is at times subtle. The significance of purulent drainage from a repaired laceration must be stressed so that extensive subgaleal spread of infection can be prevented by early treatment. In a newborn infant, subgaleal abscess appearing as a complication of fetal electrocardiographic monitoring may be misinterpreted as cephalohematoma or as caput succedaneum.

Preventive management deserves comment in view of the observation that the most frequent cause of subgaleal abscess is inadequate initial debridement and closure of a scalp laceration. If the wound is properly converted from a contaminated (not infected) wound to a clean wound by debridement, buried suture material is permissible. Alternatively, the use of a full-thickness single suture closure with or without an end-on-end mattress design may be employed. A sterile dressing should be applied to prevent secondary contamination.

Operative drainage with debridement and cleansing of the purulence in the subgaleal space constitute the basic treatment of subgaleal abscess. Multiple incisions may be necessary to permit through-and-through drainage and irrigation, and to insure access to all reaches of the purulent process. In planning incision placement, the clinical signs of the scalp will guide the surgeon, who must also take into consideration scalp blood supply and cosmetic consequences. Subgaleal drains are recommended and may be combined with soft rubber catheters for daily irrigation over several days. The drainage wounds are loosely closed. (The authors usually employ a mixture of bacitracin 500 units per milliliter, neomycin 1.0 per cent, and polymyxin 0.1 per cent.) Appropriate antibiotic therapy should be administered systemically for one week and orally for an additional week.

The bacteriological character of subgaleal abscess involves polymicrobial pathogens, chiefly *Staphylococcus epidermidis, Streptococcus,* and anaerobic cocci.[33] Therefore, in conjunction with drainage, combined therapy with methicillin and penicillin is the initial treatment of choice. When patients are allergic to penicillin, clindamycin and cephalothin are excellent alternatives. The polymicrobial etiology of subgaleal abscess supports the idea that bacterial synergism may be an important factor in the pathogenesis of serious soft-tissue infections.

Subgaleal abscess can be necrotizing to underlying pericranium as well as to the overlying scalp. If a scalp defect leaves bone exposed, denuded, and shiny when the infection has been controlled, granulation tissue coverage over the bone can be encouraged by placing an array of twist drill holes into the diploic space through the necrotic outer table. After the bone is covered with granulation tissue, the area may be covered with a split-thickness graft or a rotation flap. Secondary calvarial osteomyelitis remains a prominent danger until the bone is safely covered.

Osteomyelitis

Osteomyelitis of the skull may result from hematogenous spread of bacteria from a distant septic focus, from thrombophlebitic spread in relation to a contiguous infection (especially frontal sinusitis), from fetal monitoring, from direct bacterial inoculation into bone (trauma, skeletal traction), and from contamination during craniotomy.[3,68,79,90] Scalp defects from any cause, including ionizing irradiation, failure of skin grafts, and the like, set the stage for inoculation. Calvarial osteomyelitis causes local pain, tenderness of the overlying scalp, scalp edema (as well as eyelid edema in frontal bone involvement), occasionally scalp erosion with bone exposure, and sometimes redness and warmth. The occurrence of any delayed wound drainage must raise the concern of bone involvement. Figure 110–1 demonstrates that infection established in bone (osteomyelitis) may spread in several directions, one of which is through the outer table to produce a subperiosteal tumefaction of purulence that is readily detected clinically (Pott's "puffy tumor"). The process may be fulminating and spreading, as seen in association with acute frontal sinusitis, or it may be more localized and sclerosing (Figs. 110–2 and 110–3). It may be multifocal and in the chronic state may produce skull sclerosis and thickening, forming sequestra of dead bone.[79] The systemic signs and symptoms will be proportional to the intensity and extent of the bone infection as well as to the presence of any contiguous process, but are often surprisingly meager. Basal skull osteomyelitis may cause the now rarely encountered Gradenigo's syndrome of petrous pyramiditis (ipsilateral abducens paresis and unilateral head pain from trigeminal nerve involvement). Infection may involve the clivus, and thus possible access through transoral procedures should be remembered.[2]

Acute calvarial osteomyelitis may involve several bones, does not respect bony sutures, and may spread subpericranially and epidurally or by the mechanism of retrograde thrombophlebitis to deeper intracranial tissues. Several organisms can be responsible. *Staphylococcus aureus* and anaerobic streptococci lead the list, but Staphylococcus epidermidis and *Serratia marcescens* are found; and the report of *Arachnia propionica* with its gram-positive branching filaments and sulfur granules reminds us of the occurrence of osteomyelitis owing to *Actinomyces*.[2,60]

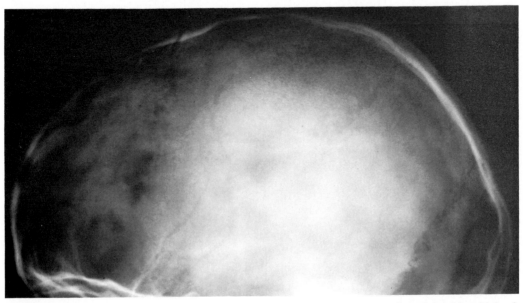

Figure 110–2 Frontal osteomyelitis (*Staphylococcus aureus*) secondary to acute frontal sinusitis, with headache, scalp swelling, and somnolence.

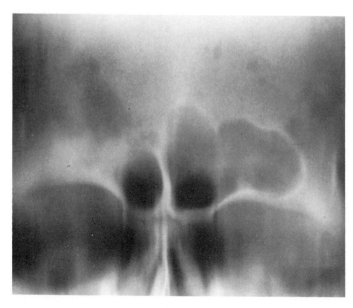

Figure 110–3 Frontal osteomyelitis (*Micrococcus*) secondary to sinusitis with soft-tissue swelling. Note loss of mucoperiosteal delineation of right frontal sinus and sclerosis of supraorbital bone.

Osteomyelitis following craniotomy involves the bone flap and, in contradistinction, usually spares the surrounding cranium (Fig. 110–4). Such an infection is often indolent and may become manifest only as poor healing of the scalp or as a secondary breakdown of previously healed scalp after the sutures are removed. There may be no pus. The scalp defect may be only millimeters in length, and usually there will have been an attempt at secondary closure. Delayed wound dehiscence may occur after hair has regrown, and the patient may complain only of continued formation at one site of a scab that flakes off with shampooing or hair brushing. There may be local scalp erythema and edema, and local tenderness. If purulence can be demonstrated, the seriousness of this lesion is immediately appreciated. The same serious implications are present when a craniotomy scalp wound does not heal per priman or when the healed scalp breaks down secondarily.

Tuberculous osteitis (osteomyelitis) usually causes a painless lump if the flat

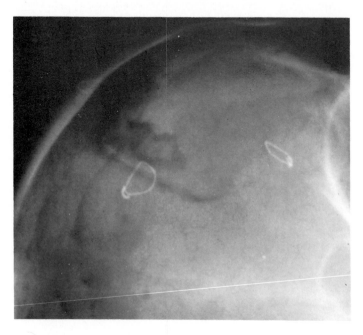

Figure 110–4 Osteomyelitis of bone flap (*Staphylococcus aureus*) eight months following craniotomy for aneurysm. Note limitation of infection to the flap.

bones are involved, but the basal bones may be the site of infection. Discrete punched-out areas without sclerosis are seen radiologically. Typically a disease of the young, it is rarely primary. The differential diagnostic considerations must include syphilis and neoplasm (usually metastatic), and the same may be said for osteomyelitis of other bacterial origin.[61]

Almost all cases of calvarial osteomyelitis should be treated with antibacterial medication and excision of the infected bone. Radiological guides to the amount of bone removal needed are less useful than the pathological condition revealed at the time of operation. Bone that is dead (sequestrum) must be removed, and preferably, all bone in which infection is visible or apparent to the feel of the rongeur. Such abnormal tissue should be excised back to healthy, bleeding margins. As one encounters hard, sclerotic bone, the decision to perform further excision becomes more difficult; however, if the bone exudes purulence or is soft and does not bleed, it should be sacrificed.

Clinical evaluation should include an immediate Gram stain and culture of drainage from any local wound or material from accessible neighboring or distant possible sources of infection. Both aerobic and anaerobic organisms should be searched for; moreover, tuberculosis and fungi as possible etiological agents should not be overlooked. Radiological changes identifiable in plain studies may lag weeks to months behind the clinical manifestations of bacterial infection of bone (Fig. 110–5). Polytomography will often be helpful at an earlier date (cf. Figs. 110–3 and 110–5C). Radioactive isotope bone scanning may also be useful to demonstrate abnormal sites of reactive bone. Computed tomography is an excellent screening tool to detect unsuspected extensions of the infection and, with cerebral angiography, must be considered if there are clinical indications of intracranial involvement. The duration of the infection and the organism involved will influence radiological findings that may reveal varying mixtures of osteolytic and osteoblastic changes and possibly bone sequestra. The early changes of blurring of the mucoperiosteal margins of accessory sinuses and the small areas of lucency (motheaten appearance) should be searched for in acute cases. Calvarial osteomyelitis secondary to hematogenous spread may mimic, radiologically, a neoplastic metastasis.

Osteomyelitis involving the bone flap of a craniotomy should be suspected if bone is exposed in the management of soft-tissue infection. Bone that loses its vascularity, its sheen, and its ivory color is suspect. In the authors' experience, once evidence exists of infection involving any portion of the bone flap, it requires removal of the entire plate. Nibbling procedures are usually doomed to fail (Fig. 110–6).

Inasmuch as bone flap osteomyelitis reveals itself slowly, large-dose antistaphylococcal therapy should be started whenever a tender small scalp dehiscence occurs and cannot be explained by a local stitch abscess or minor trauma. Most bone flap osteomyelitis is due to coagulase-positive *Staphylococcus*. Antibiotic therapy may sterilize a soft-tissue scalp infection and, possibly, early osteomyelitis in a still-vascularized osteoplastic flap. If scalp breakdown continues, however, or if radiological changes appear, the bone flap should be removed.

After bone excision, the site of infection should be widely drained, and the drains usually accompanied by soft irrigation catheters so that for the initial days the wound can be irrigated with local antibiotic compounds, as described in the section on subgaleal abscess. In such wound management suction-irrigation techniques have been effective.[26] The scalp may be loosely approximated with wire about the drains and catheters to prevent severe retraction. If drainage and irrigation devices are used they should be brought out of well-placed stab wounds and drainage must be adequate. Catheters are removed gradually, as are the drains, and the local management can be judged adequate if repeated cultures are sterile. Biopsy, Gram stain, and culture data will assist in selecting the appropriate antibiotic regimen to be used (this may be necessary for many weeks following operative treatment). Osteomyelitis occurring as a sequel to a contiguous infection of the paranasal sinuses or mastoid region necessitates operative eradication of the primary focus of disease. Bony defects that result from operative treatment of osteomyelitis should not be repaired by cranioplasty until

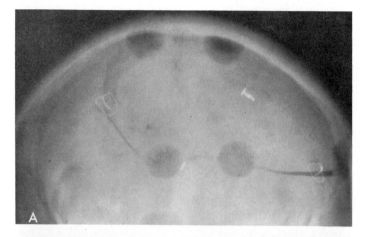

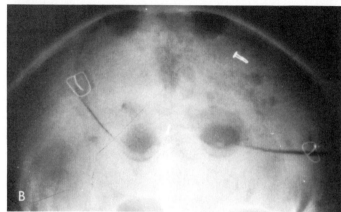

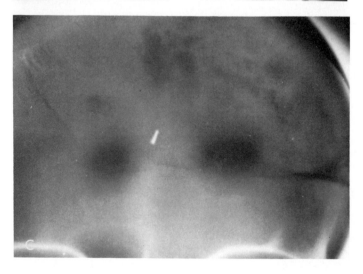

Figure 110–5 *A.* Suspected bone flap infection three months postcraniotomy. Note minimal changes. *B.* Comparison films nine months postcraniotomy. *C.* Tomography at nine months postcraniotomy.

6 to 12 months have elapsed from the time of wound closure. (Management of craniotomy infections is discussed in Chapter 29.)

Because of the considerable morbidity involved in postcraniotomy bacterial osteomyelitis of the bone flap, it must be distinguished from aseptic necrosis. Osteomye-litis of the bone flap requires removal of the flap, several weeks of treatment, and cranioplasty one year after good-quality scalp healing. Aseptic necrosis is more likely to occur with a free bone flap. It usually is not associated with scalp wound problems, nor is it accompanied by local or systemic signs

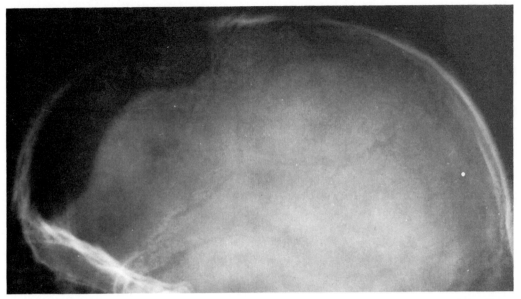

Figure 110-6   Postexcision cranial defect from removal of infected bone visualized in Figure 110-2.

of infection. Radiological changes may be similar in aseptic necrosis and in bone flap osteomyelitis; in both, the earliest changes appear at the margins of the bone flap. Osteomyelitis, however, tends to cause progressive lysis and mottling along peripheral zones of the flap as shown in Figure 110-4, whereas aseptic necrosis typically appears as diffuse mottling and rarefaction of the entire flap. If radiological changes occur in association with a nonhealing tender scalp or with a breakdown of a once-healed scalp, a presumptive diagnosis of osteomyelitis should be made. Repeated attempts should be made to isolate an organism, although the only positive culture may be from the bone flap itself (see Chapter 29).

Epidural Abscess

Epidural abscess usually forms, intracranially, as a sequel to osteomyelitis of the calvarium, and its management is accomplished by observing the principles set forth for that condition. It is also encountered in about 20 per cent of patients with subdural empyema as an associated finding.[9] It forms adjacent to mastoiditis and accessory nasal sinusitis, and may follow direct implantation as a sequel to a penetrating wound of scalp and skull. It is a recognized complication of an operative site infection after craniotomy. Its occurrence in association with a congenital dermal sinus (lesions that are rarer in the cranium than in the spine) should be remembered.[25] Liquid pus may be encountered, or a combination of purulence and a carpet or tumefaction of infected granulation tissue. The dura mater is usually an excellent barrier to the spread of infection to deeper layers except through thrombophlebitis involving emissary dural and intradural venous channels. Infection in the epidural space may, however, cause sites of dural thinning and necrosis. Operative treatment must acknowledge this potential with gentle technique, but in general, the infected, soft granulation tissue can be lightly scraped from the outer dural layer. As with most infections and purulence resulting from a contiguous site of infection (e.g., osteitis-osteomyelitis, mastoiditis), the primary site of trouble should be eradicated. Evacuation of the epidural pus is usually accomplished as an integral part of such eradication.

Subdural Empyema

Subdural empyema is a purulent infection of the subdural space that usually progresses rapidly and fatally if untreated. Less acute forms of subdural purulence do occur, as can be expected from a more favorable balance between the virulence of the infective organism and the host's resistance.

In both children and adults, the most frequent cause of infection in the subdural space is extension of paranasal sinusitis through emissary veins and retrograde thrombophlebitis, or of mastoiditis through mucosa, bone, and dura mater.[53,77] In infants, subdural empyema most often occurs as an infection of the subdural space secondary to bacterial meningitis.[27] Sterile neighborhood subdural effusions with membrane formation are also well recognized in these circumstances, and whether sterile or infected, such effusions are bilateral in a large proportion of patients.[25] In all age groups, subdural empyema can stem from direct contamination in penetrating wounds and operative procedures. It may also follow intrathoracic purulence and stem from neighborhood processes outside the skull (subgaleal abscess or facial infection) or inside the skull (spontaneous or operative rupture of a brain abscess).[47,53,77] Pus in the subdural space has the potential for rapid extension over the brain convexity and into the interhemispheric cleft.[53,89] It may spread bilaterally, it may occur in multiple sites, and in a small proportion of cases, it may extend over the cerebellum.[9,25] Although the carpet of pus may be only 5 to 8 mm in thickness, and the total volume of pus seemingly small, nevertheless, intracranial hypertension occurs owing to the interrelated factors of cerebral edema, septic and aseptic cortical vein thrombosis, and thrombosis (septic and aseptic) of major venous sinuses.

The patient is usually quite sick, his condition septic and toxic. A history of acute frontal sinusitis (often following swimming), severe headache, and rapid neurological deterioration with seizures and coma constitute a common constellation and should remind the physician of the fulminating capabilities of this process. A depressed sensorium, hemiparesis, dysphasia, oculomotor deficit, papilledema, and signs of meningeal irritation are typical findings. A clue to the nature of the process may be found on physical examination if evidence for frontal sinusitis, mastoiditis, or scalp infection is present. The particular syndrome in each patient will be determined by the intracranial mass effect from subdural pus and cerebral edema, the location of the mass effect, the degree of subarachnoid inflammation (either as a sterile parameningeal response or as an associated bacterial meningitis), and the extent of subjacent cortical involvement.

Other associated purulent processes may share in the picture: brain abscess, leptomeningitis, and osteomyelitis. Some fever and peripheral blood leukocytosis are encountered in the majority of cases.

The differential diagnosis in such an acute problem would include viral encephalitis, bacterial meningitis, ventriculitis, brain abscess (with or without rupture into the cerebrospinal fluid pathways), septic cavernous sinus thrombosis, and possibly a rupture of a neoplasm containing materials such as cholesterol.

Radiological studies include views of the skull, accessory sinuses, mastoid region, and chest to identify foci of disease (Fig. 110–7). Electroencephalographic slowing

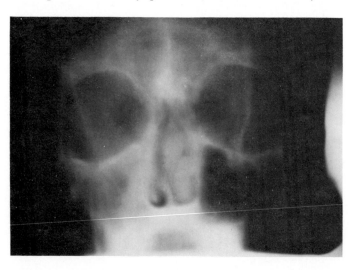

Figure 110–7 Pansinusitis associated with acute subdural empyema.

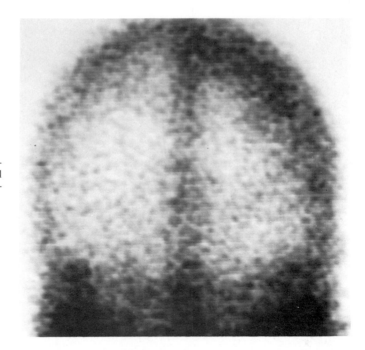

Figure 110–8   Technetium radio-isotope scan in acute frontoparietal subdural empyema following pansinusitis.

may be expected but is not diagnostic, and a radionuclide brain scan can be helpful in a minority of cases (Fig. 110–8).[47] Computed tomography may provide sufficient detail upon which to base an operation, although cerebral angiography continues to be a highly useful study for such lesions, including parafalcine collections (Fig. 110–9). Small-volume collections of pus requiring urgent operative drainage may be located in a frontal or occipital site in such a way that angiographic oblique views are required for adequate visualization. Subdural empyema appears as an avascular extracerebral mantle angiographically, and the presence or absence of an interhemispheric component should be specifically noted (Fig. 110–10). Computed tomography may reveal the degree and extent of cerebral edema in addition to the presence and location of an extracerebral collection. It demonstrates a crescent-shaped area of decreased density and mass effects, and with contrast enhancement (an essential step), a rimlike crescent of increased density may be seen adjacent to the parenchyma.[44] Calcification in the cavity wall in a chronic case has been reported.[21]

Lumbar puncture for cerebrospinal fluid examination is expendable, hazardous, and nondiagnostic and should not be performed until the emergency CT scan or cerebral angiogram has excluded an operatively treatable mass lesion. It should be reserved for patients for whom it is the critical test required to establish a diagnosis (meningitis). In the absence of prior meningitis or operation, the fluid may reveal from 0 to more than 1300 white cells, chiefly mononuclear, and a normal or moderately elevated protein content (300 mg per 100 ml).[9] If the abscess occurs as a postoperative complication, a greater percentage of polymorphonuclear cells may be evident, as well as a higher protein value. If the empyema is associated with partially treated leptomeningitis, many more white cells are to be expected.[47] The revelation of an extracerebral, avascular mass leads to the presumptive diagnosis of subdural empyema. Antibiotic therapy should be started immediately when the patient arrives in the operating room.

Acute subdural empyema is a surgical emergency. As a closed-space infection it requires prompt evacuation of as much pus and necrotic debris as possible. Since the exudate is often applied as an adherent layer to arachnoid, and since septa traversing the subdural space frequently occur as a response to the subdural infection, thereby producing loculations, any evacuation by burr hole technique alone must accommodate such exigencies. Under these circumstances the pus may be neither easily debrided nor indirectly irrigated out through burr openings that are widely separated. In

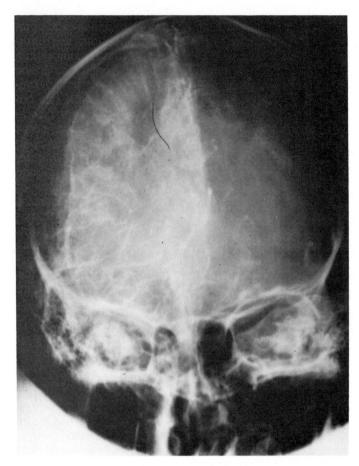

Figure 110–9 Cerebral angiogram of acute subdural empyema (alpha-hemolytic streptococcus) following pansinusitis.

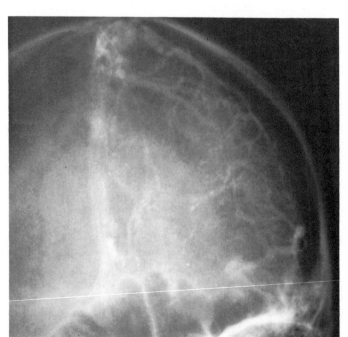

Figure 110–10 Cerebral venogram in acute subdural empyema (beta-hemolytic streptococcus) following suspected acute sinusitis.

such cases an osteoplastic bone flap, centered upon the thickest portion of pus, as indicated by the preoperative studies, permits more complete, prompt initial therapy of the empyema. Whether evacuation is by bone flap or multiple burr holes or craniectomy, several catheters and drains should be distributed over the exposed empyema cavity, the dura mater closed around them, the bone flap secured, and the scalp closed.[47,53,67] The authors prefer a generous bone flap for initial mechanical debridement. The basic principles for the control of raised intracranial pressure as outlined in the discussion of acute brain swelling in chapters 24 and 29 pertain in the operative management. The catheter and drain system, brought out through scalp incisions, is utilized for twice-daily irrigation with a debriding solution. The authors prefer a triple antibiotic solution of bacitracin 500 units per milliliter, neomycin 1.0 per cent, and polymyxin 0.1 per cent. The irrigation is then slowly withdrawn over several days and finally discontinued approximately one week after operation. As the dura mater and scalp are being closed, the surgeon must verify that, in fact, the irrigation and drainage system successfully distributes the solution over the entire subdural cavity (with special attention to parafalcine collections) and that drainage occurs without risking raised intracranial pressure.

If there is a high index of suspicion regarding the lesion, the initial antibiotic therapy in subdural empyema is begun empirically without Gram stain or culture data.

The bacteriological findings most commonly encountered will assist in preliminary therapy pending precise data. The aerobic organisms tyically found in empyema associated with sinusitis and mastoiditis are the streptococci. For empyema following craniotomy or head injury, the *Staphylococcus, Streptococcus,* and *Enterobacter* species are common. Anaerobic organisms have been found as causative in approximately 12 per cent of cases. (The anaerobic and microaerophilic streptococci and *Bacteroides* lead the list.) For cases of subdural empyema following or associated with leptomeningitis, the leaders are *H. influenzae, N. meningitides,* and the pneumococcus. The frequency of "sterile" cultures (27 per cent) suggests that with more sophisticated anaerobic studies the yield of

anaerobes may be increased.[47,53,93] Preoperative antibiotic therapy should include penicillin for pneumococcus and aerobic streptococci, methicillin for penicillinase-producing staphylococci, and chloramphenicol for *Bacteroides fragilis.* The surgeon must also be alert to the conduct of the bacteriological evauation. An experienced individual must be assigned the task of interpreting the initial Gram stain material because this will be a critical guide for antibiotic therapy. Fastidious anaerobic culture inoculation must be started promptly. Antibiotic therapy is modified as the results from the bacteriological laboratory become available.

The diffusely spreading "empyematous" lesion already described is an acute and highly dangerous process. There appear also to be more localized subdural purulent collections (more appropriately called abscesses than empyemas) for which the pathogenesis and the management are similar to that just outlined. Whether the bacterial etiology differs is not certain, but the process has a more sanguine outlook if properly treated.

Subdural empyema has a mortality rate of 25 to 40 per cent.[9,25] It is to be hoped that results can be improved if clinical recognition is prompt and wide evacuation is afforded.

A final comment would be to emphasize the importance of eradicating any treatable primary focus from which the empyema was derived.[67]

Meningitis

Bacterial meningitis is a purulent infection of the subarachnoid space. In adults the infection is usually contained entirely within the subarachnoid space, but in the newborn it frequently extends into the subdural space as subdural effusion or subdural empyema, i.e., leptomeningitis, or into the brain, i.e., meningoencephalitis. Untreated bacterial meningitis is nearly always fatal. Antimicrobial therapy has dramatically improved the outlook for patients with meningeal infections, but still an appreciable number of patients die, even though treated adequately and promptly. The reasons for these therapeutic failures remain enigmatic. The fallibility of culturing techniques notwithstanding, many patients are found to have sterile cerebrospinal fluid prior to death, indicating that multiplying bacteria per se may not be the cause of death. While some organisms invading the meninges produce an endotoxin that may be deleterious to the host, *Diplococcus pneumoniae* is a notable exception. The mortality rate associated with pneumococcal meningitis is at least as high as with other pathogens, making it unlikely that endotoxin plays an important role in most of the deaths. It seems probable that death in meningitis is often related to severe intracranial hypertension stemming from acute hydrocephalus and from severe cerebral edema.[18,28,38,54]

With the exceptions of postcraniotomy and post-traumatic meningitis, the antecedent of bacterial meningitis is an infection elsewhere, especially the bloodstream, respiratory tract, paranasal sinuses, mastoids and ears, and even the pituitary fossa.[24] Thus, except for those previously ill, the premature or sick infant, and the debilitated or aged, the typical patient with meningitis (regardless of the causative organism) has suffered some form of recent acute febrile illness, the vast majority being infections about the head or septicemia. These patients generally report fever and lethargy, confusion, headache, vomiting, or stiff neck to suggest the diagnosis of meningitis. A single such symptom is often the only warning of meningitis in a patient with an otherwise ordinary infection of the respiratory tract. In children under 1 year of age, the symptoms are largely behavioral and require individual interpretation. Listlessness and vomiting are the major symptoms. Neck stiffness and fever may not be prominent or may be absent. Some patients develop confusion, lethargy, and steady deterioration of consciousness within the first day of headache. Other patients have slowly progressive symptoms of meningitis over a period of several days after an upper respiratory tract infection. In still other patients, there may be a one- to three-week separation between respiratory tract symptoms and the first meningeal symptoms.

Patients with meningococcal meningitis may evidence clear signs of meningeal irritation, fever, depressed consciousness, and widespread petechial eruptions. In addition, seizures, hemiparesis, and signs of extensive central nervous involvement such as absence of oculovestibular reflexes, fixed midstage pupils, and abnormalities in respiration may occur. Hyponatremia due to inappropriate secretion of antidiuretic hormone occurs frequently.

Once the possibility of meningitis is suspected, examination of the cerebrospinal fluid is required. Since lumbar puncture is potentially hazardous with localized intracranial suppurative mass lesions (brain abscess or subdural empyema), cerebral angiographic or computed tomographic studies should be obtained if the clinical situation warrants them. In cases in which meningitis is associated with intracranial hypertension, or in which there are both meningitis and localized pus, the lumbar puncture should be performed only as the intracranial hypertension is being treated with steroids, osmotic diuretics, antipyretics, anticonvulsants, and respiratory support.

Protein and glucose determinations, differential cell count, appropriate cultures, and Gram stain should be performed. A cerebrospinal fluid pleocytosis preponderantly composed of polymorphonuclear cells (over 90 per cent) is frequently associated with untreated bacterial meningitis. The same response can, however, occur early in viral, tuberculous, or fungal meningitis.[66] A predominant cerebrospinal fluid lymphocytosis can occur with viral or fungal or parasitic infections, with central nervous system syphilis, with central nervous system collagen vascular disease, with meningeal carcinomatosis, and with partially treated bacterial meningitis.[81] Cerebrospinal fluid lymphocytosis may occur with an occult (or obvious) neighborhood *extradural* infection, i.e., as a parameningeal response to calvarial osteomyelitis, interspace infection in the spine, and similar entities.

The importance of a Gram stain in every case of suspected meningitis cannot be overemphasized. It will give positive results 75 per cent of the time in patients with culture-proved bacterial meningitis.[78] The test is inexpensive, simple, rapid, and often diagnostic. The absence of visible bacteria on smear does not exclude the possibility of bacterial meningitis, however, and therefore, results of the cerebrospinal fluid culture are important. Although the yield may be low, acid-fast smear and India ink preparation should be done routinely on cerebrospinal fluid; and cultures for bacteria, fungi, mycobacteria, and viruses should be obtained. Meningococci are fastidious organisms, and for successful culture results the cerebrospinal fluid must be inoculated at the bedside onto chocolate agar plates previously warmed to 25°C. If the patient has already received antibiotic therapy, the culture may grow no organisms despite clinical features and other findings indicative of bacterial meningitis. It is common for the cerebrospinal fluid pressure to be elevated (over 300 mm of water) in patients with untreated bacterial meningitis. Also, there is a polymorphonuclear pleocytosis (usually hundreds of cells), increased protein, and hypoglycorrhachia (less than 30 mg per 100 ml glucose). If anaerobic organisms are cultured from cerebropinal fluid, the presumptive diagnosis would be a leaking abscess, inasmuch as such organisms are rare in uncomplicated meningitis.

Therapy for bacterial meningitis is based on knowledge of the predominant pathogens isolated in this disease. In the adult population, *Diplococcus pneumoniae* and *Neisseria meningitidis* are the most common bacteria isolated from the cerebrospinal fluid, and for these two organisms intravenous penicillin G in doses up to 20 million units per day is the drug of choice. Ampicillin also may be used with almost equal efficacy. If patients are allergic to penicillin, 4 gm per day of chloramphenicol given intravenously is the alternative agent. The cephalosporins may also have a role in the treatment of staphylococcal meningitis in patients allergic to penicillin, and is administered intravenously and intrathecally.[30] In a patient whose immune responses are suppressed or who has neoplastic disease, unusual pathogens such as *Listeria* or gram-negative bacilli are usually isolated. When the patient is presumed to have bacterial meningitis, and a definitive identification of the organism is not available, the initial antimicrobial therapy will have to be effective against these pathogens. In cases of gram-negative bacillary meningitis, parenteral gentamicin alone may not suffice, and intrathecal or intraventricular supplementation may be required.[45,70] An acceptable regimen would be gentamicin given intravenously at a dosage of 5 mg per kilogram of body weight per day with intrathecal gentamicin administered every 18 to 24 hours in a dosage of 4 to 8 mg.

In the pediatric patient, *H. influenzae, Neisseria meningitidis,* and *Diplococcus pneumoniae* are the major bacteria recovered from the cerebrospinal fluid. Therefore, ampicillin is the drug of choice until specific identification of the organism can be made. The recommended dosage for ampicillin is 200 to 300 mg per kilogram of body weight per day. Chloramphenicol can be substituted in penicillin-allergic patients. Also, in areas where there is a high incidence of ampicillin-resistant *H. influenzae,* both ampicillin and chloramphenicol can be given until sensitivity studies are completed. Meningitis in the neonate and premature infant is chiefly due to *E. coli* and other enterobacteria. Additional bacteria infecting this age group are *Pseudomonas, D. pneumoniae, Staphylococcus, Streptococcus,* and opportunistic pathogens. Before an etiological diagnosis is established, the drugs of choice are ampicillin and gentamicin, or, alternatively, chloramphenicol and kanamycin.

Bacterial meningitis continues to cause a high mortality rate in the very young and very old, in patients with cancer or immunological deficiencies or debilitating disease, and in those in whom the course is fulminant. For example, the overall mortality rate in neonates and premature infants is 60 per cent, and at least half of the survivors are left with residual neurological damage. Moreover, there is increasing psychometric evidence that intellectual and behavioral defects may be a major concomitant of bacterial meningitis in childhood. Permanent cranial nerve palsies are also frequently encountered as postmeningitic sequelae.

The neurosurgeon often manages patients in whom bacterial meningitis may be suspected following cranial trauma or cranial operations. In both cases *all* the classic signs and symptoms of bacterial meningitis can be duplicated by noninfectious disorders. Depressed consciousness can be due to the cranial trauma, a pre-existing neurological disorder, or the recent operation. The clinical and cerebrospinal fluid findings indicative of arachnoid inflammation can be quite similar whether the inflammation stems from bacteria or from chemical agents such as blood, air, irrigating, fluids, or tissue coagulum.

Post-Traumatic Meningitis

Post-traumatic *chemical* meningitis is seen frequently in any busy emergency room. Blunt head trauma causes varying degrees of bleeding into the subarachnoid space, which in turn may cause headache, stiff neck, and vomiting. Low-grade fever may be present. An altered state of consciousness in the patient with chemical meningitis can be caused by the head trauma or some pre-existing condition such as drug abuse. There are, however, many diagnostic considerations: for example, the alcoholic with minor head trauma is peculiarly prone to develop pneumococcal meningitis, or the headache and altered state of consciousness could be due to subdural hematoma or aneurysmal rupture. Since patients with post-traumatic chemical meningitis (or subarachnoid hemorrhage meningitis) demonstrate clinical syndromes dominated by neurological abnormalities rather than by septic signs and symptoms, the diagnosis will generally be correctly achieved after appropriate neuroradiological studies are done. Physicians should be alert to the possible misinterpretations of cerebrospinal fluid findings whenever a lumbar puncture is performed to confirm suspected bacterial meningitis and instead find indications of subarachnoid hemorrhage.

Post-traumatic *bacterial* meningitis occurs as a complication of compound skull fractures associated with dural and arachnoid lacerations. The risk of contaminating the subarachnoid space is obvious when blunt or penetrating injury to the convexity of the skull causes a compound fracture directly exposing the brain. Less obvious but equally important is the risk of bacterial meningitis with basal skull fracture. Small hairline fractures across the cribriform plate, frontal sinus, or lateral petrous pyramid can connect the body surface with the subarachnoid space. Patients with any signs of basal skull fracture should be carefully inspected for air-fluid levels in paranasal sinuses (brow-up and brow-down lateral skull x-rays), for intracranial air (often only a small bubble of air in the chiasmatic or pontine cistern, as shown in Figure 110–11), and for cerebrospinal fluid otorrhea or rhinorrhea (careful checking of external auditory canals, nares, and oropharynx).

The organisms encountered in *penetrating* wounds are nonpneumococcal and in-

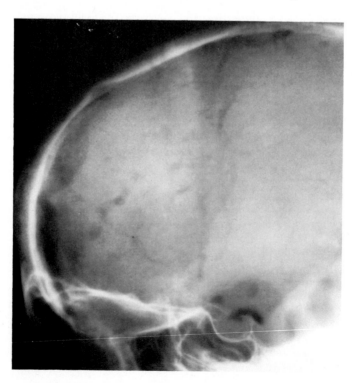

Figure 110–11 Pneumocranium in association with postcraniotomy paradoxical eustachian tube–cerebrospinal fluid rhinorrhea. Note air frontally and above dorsum sellae.

clude *Staphylococcus, Streptococcus,* and the gram-negative bacillary group. In *nonpenetrating* injuries, *D. pneumoniae* is the typical organism responsible, but *N. meningitidis* and the *Hemophilus* species are also encountered. Such information assists in the planning of antibacterial protocols.[34,43]

Bacterial meningitis can complicate basal skull fracture even when no frank cerebrospinal fluid leak has been observed; moreover, it can complicate basal skull fracture weeks, months, or years following a posttraumatic episode of cerebrospinal fluid rhinorrhea.

The use of lumbar puncture to assist healing at the site of cerebrospinal fluid rhinorrhea is controversial, as is the use of prophylactic antibiotics to avoid bacterial meningitis.[37,40,56] When careful, consistent, frequent punctures are done with vigorous drainage of fluid, the magnitude of the rhinorrhea appears to diminish correspondingly. Clinical information has neither clearly refuted nor supported the use of antibiotics. The administration of antimeningitic levels of antibiotics effective against common nasal pathogens seems reasonable, since cerebrospinal fluid rhinorrhea is a "contaminated wound" with respect to the central nervous system. Antibiotic therapy should continue until there is no further detectable rhinorrhea.

Postcraniotomy Meningitis

Bacterial meningitis can occur subsequent to craniotomy, a number of factors such as length of operation, reoperation, drains left in situ for more than 48 hours, and the presence of a cerebrospinal fluid fistula being responsible for this increased risk.[3,90] Postoperative meningitis adds significantly to the morbidity and mortality rates; these nosocomial infections frequently involve unusual and resistant microorganisms, and the patients may have preinfectious debilitating conditions.

Postcraniotomy aseptic meningitis may closely resemble bacterial meningitis. Fever, meningismus, and polymorphonuclear pleocytosis and persistent low glucose levels in the cerebrospinal fluid may occur. Although often associated with operations in the posterior fossa, this syndrome has been observed after various neurosurgical procedures. The cause of postcraniotomy aseptic meningitis is not known, and although blood and the breakdown products thereof have been suspect, the syndrome is not uniquely related to underlying brain disease, operative technique, length of operation, fourth ventricular entrance, whether the dura mater is left open or is closed, subarachnoid blood, or radiotherapy (see Chapter 29).[17]

Ventriculitis

Bacterial ventriculitis is characterized by ventricular pleocytosis (usually in the hundreds), low glucose level in ventricular fluid, and recovery of bacteria from the ventricles. Ventriculitis may occur in association with bacterial meningitis, the presence of ventricular shunting devices, external ventriculostomies, penetrating wounds, and myelomeningoceles.[57,73,76] Along with meningitis it is the most common associated finding in patients dying from brain abscess.[5] The explanation of ventriculitis in association with brain abscess is often found in the leaking or more dramatic rupture of the abscess into the adjacent ventricle. The rupture occurs in that portion of an abscess wall proximal to the ventricle, which appears to be the thinnest, thus favoring spillage of purulent matter. The ependymal inflammation accompanying ventriculitis may cause partial or complete aqueductal obstruction and may elicit the formation of single or multiple purulent webs that span the ventricles, thereby creating loculations. At times the ependymal inflammatory obstructions can be reversed with antibiotic therapy, but occasionally permanent obstructive ventricular coaptations remain as sequelae to the inflammatory process.

There is no specific ventriculitis syndrome, but the diagnosis should be suspected in patients with known meningitis who have had a poor clinical or laboratory response to the usual therapy, who are severely ill, who are infected with an unusual organism, or who suffer persistently high intracranial pressure. It should also be considered in any patient treated for hydrocephalus with an indwelling ventricular shunt in whom a febrile, toxic central nervous system infection occurs. In patients with external ventriculostomies or in those sustaining penetrating injuries to the ventricular space, bacterial ventriculitis should be considered when there is an unaccountable fever. Ventriculitis may be unexpectedly diagnosed at the time of ventriculography in patients with myelomeningocele. The risk of bacterial contamination and low-grade ventricular infection is sufficiently great in patients with weeping or open myelomeningocele lesions that ventricular fluid should be analyzed before the shunt is placed internally.

Thus the nonspecific clinical syndrome of bacterial ventriculitis is that of fever, considerable toxicosis accompanied by altered consciousness, and a deteriorating clinical course. At times fluid and electrolyte abnormalities occur, as well as changes in vital signs. The particular clinical course will be determined by the underlying disorder (e.g., meningitis, blunt head trauma leading to ventriculostomy for intracranial pressure monitoring), the magnitude of ependymal inflammation (third ventriculitis with hypothalamic derangements, fourth ventriculitis with brain stem derangements), and the magnitude of accompanying hydrocephalus. If available, computed tomography may assist diagnosis of the entity by demonstrating a contrast enhancement of the ependyma of the ventricle.[65]

Aseptic ventriculitis may follow operative entrance into the ventricular system, and the surgeon should be alert to such a possibility after procedures on intraventricular meningiomas, arteriovenous malformations, third ventricular colloid cysts, and the like. The syndrome may resemble bacterial ventriculitis, but the clinical intoxication is less, there is less peripheral leukocytosis, and, empirically, the risk of bacterial infection in elective intraventricular procedures is reassuringly low. Aseptic ventriculitis can be reduced by avoiding spilling blood into the ventricles or retracting an intraventricular surface, and possibly by irrigating with an artificial cerebrospinal fluid instead of the more commonly employed saline solutions. Postoperative steroids will be helpful in reducing the impact of aseptic ventriculitis.

When ventriculitis is suspected, ventricular fluid must be obtained for complete analysis. If there is an existing internal or external ventricular drain, it can be used for obtaining the fluid sample. In urgent situations, the ventricle should be directly tapped; this can relieve pressure, provide material for analysis, and prevent the false-negative results that can occur when lumbar fluid is sampled. Since ventriculitis can cause intraventricular blocks, the specific anatomy of the ventricles should be followed by computed tomography.

The microbial flora in ventriculitis is related to the clinical circumstances. Ventriculitis complicating external ventriculostomy is due to organisms frequently encountered in nosocomial infections. Ventriculitis complicating myelomeningocele stems from the organisms frequently infecting neonates. Ventriculitis accompanying internal ventricular shunting is caused by the organisms that usually infect shunt tubing.

When the diagnosis of ventriculitis is confirmed, previously placed ventricular catheters should be removed promptly, since microorganism colonization on foreign bodies is particularly resistant to sterilization. If the ventricular pathways are unobstructed and if the organism is sensitive to an antibiotic with good blood-brain and blood–cerebrospinal fluid distribution, then therapy may be restricted to the administration of systemic antibiotics. Conversely, if there is an obstructive hydrocephalic component or the organism is sensitive only to poorly penetrating antibiotics, or both, daily ventricular taps are needed for drainage and for combined systemic and intraventricular administration of drugs. The authors have had some success with through-and-through perfusion of antibiotic solutions delivered into one lateral ventricle and removed via the other. The outflow channel must be an unimpeded pathway to a sterile but vented reservoir to avoid iatrogenically produced elevations in ventricular pressure. As obstructive hydrocephalus develops, ventriculitis becomes a "pyocephalus" requiring both drainage and antibiotic therapy. The therapy of ventriculitis in neonates and infants will generally require systemic and intraventricular therapy because of both the frequency of gram-negative infections and the frequency of obstructive hydrocephalus. Successful therapy requires adjustment of the intraventricular dosage until the ventricular antibiotic level exceeds the minimum inhibitory concentration by severalfold. Ventriculitis that complicates external ventriculostomy in an adult without obstructive hydrocephalus may be managed by systemic antibiotic therapy alone, depending on the organism involved. Occasionally the ventricular puncture site may have to be varied if multiple loculations develop. The particular risk of bacterial ventriculitis complicating external ventriculostomy in adult patients can be reduced by meticulous wound and dressing care, by limiting use of the drainage system to a period of 72 hours, and by maintaining a strictly "closed system" technique. Additional protection may be provided by the prophylactic use of parenteral antistaphylococcal medication while the external catheter remains indwelling.[76,91]

Brain Abscess

Brain abscess is a purulent infection of brain parenchyma and is, invariably, tissue-destructive, existing as a mass lesion. The host-organism relationship varies in such a manner that a spectrum of pathological findings is seen in large series. It may be so balanced that only a small nidus of infection occurs, with surrounding dystrophic calcification visible on plain skull x-rays. It may provoke development of a thick-walled collagenous capsule containing an inner granulation tissue zone with central necrosis and pus. Liquid pus may be only partially surrounded by a thin boundary or wall, or a small amount of pus may merge with an area of severe edema having no macroscopic boundary, an area of "cerebritis."[53]

The thick-walled abscesses are usually secondary to penetrating trauma and retained foreign bodies such as bone, or to contiguous middle ear or mastoid disease; less often are the thick-walled lesions due to frontal sinusitis. Abscesses secondary to cyanotic congenital heart disease and those hematogenously spread from a purulent thoracic process or more remote focus are frequently quite thin-walled. Surrounding edema is a common characteristic of all forms of abscess except, perhaps, for the most chronic, very thick-walled forms. Solitary lesions are not infrequently multiloculated, and multiple lesions may occur, especially when hematogenous spread from a distant site occurs.

In the hierarchy of pathogenetic mechanisms responsible for brain abscess, some variations are to be found among series, but most surveys reveal common features.[53,58,74,83] *Frontal accessory nasal sinusitis and middle ear disease or mastoiditis* head most lists (Fig. 110–12). Beller and co-workers, for example, found that 51 of 89 cases were due to contiguous sites of infection.[5] The abscess is adjacent to the contiguous bony focus and often is "attached" to the dura mater at the site of the infection's spread from bone through meninges and into parenchyma. Such a "stalk" may be noted at the time of excision. With otogenic sources, the temporal lobe and the cerebellum are the sites of abscess in a ratio of approximately 3:2. Indeed, the vast majority of cerebellar abscesses stem from infective otogenic disease.[75] *Metastatic spread* may occur with *general sepsis* from a *purulent intrathoracic source* (of which empyema, pneumonia, bronchiectasis, and lung abscess are notable examples), from pyogenic dental processes, furuncles, distant osteomyelitis, endocarditis, or infected

Figure 110–12   Routes for spread of infection from mastoid and middle ear focus to parameningeal tissues and brain. (From Nager, G. T.: Mastoid and paranasal sinus infections and their relations to the central nervous system. Clin. Neurosurg., *14*:293, 1967. Reprinted by permission.)

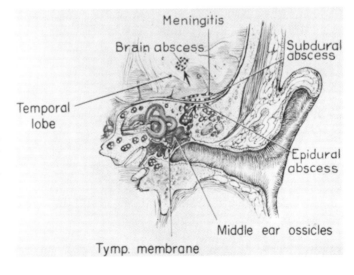

prosthetic devices (heart valves). Erasmus, in his series, found 37 single nonencapsulated lesions, 61 single encapsulated abscesses, 21 multiloculated collections, 12 unilateral but multiple (discrete) abscesses, and 10 bilateral multiple processes. Of the multiple discrete abscesses, the vast majority were due to systemic causes rather than to contiguous foci.[25] *Cyanotic congenital heart disease* (usually in the absence of bacterial endocarditis) or other processes associated with a lesser or greater circulation shunt is a third mechanism. *Penetrating trauma,* including *craniotomy,* may give rise to abscess formation, especially in the presence of retained intradural foreign material. An abscess may develop as a sequel to or in association with *leptomeningitis,* cranial osteomyelitis, or similar inflammatory processes. Finally, the *origin* may be *unknown;* an unexplained group of abscesses remains in almost all series. In the survey of Beller and co-workers, the figure was 19 per cent. In these cases no primary origin could be established.

Clinical Presentation

The clinical syndrome in a particular patient is the product of the forces involved in the host-organism interaction, the size and number of the lesions (if multiple), the specific brain sites involved, and the neighborhood anatomical disturbances involving ventricles, venous sinuses, and cisterns.

Some symptoms and signs are directly related to the particular location of the abscess or abscesses. For example, a pontine abscess causes specific brain stem manifestations distinguishable from an abscess in another locale. Abscesses in certain locations (brain stem, cerebellum, cerebral hemisphere) can distort the aqueduct of Sylvius and cause obstructive hydrocephalus. Abscesses adjacent to ventricular walls may leak or rupture and produce ventriculitis. There can be septic spread from the abscess to other tissue layers and, through rupture or thrombophlebitis, the production of leptomeningitis, major venous sinus thrombophlebitis, or subdural empyema. The observation that the portion of a cerebral hemispheric abscess closest to the ventricle tends to have the thinnest (and presumably the weakest) wall may explain the occurrences of ventricular rupture in such lesions. The clinical syndromes are thus

quite diverse: there is no single "typical" brain abscess syndrome, and there is no constellation of symptoms pathognomonic of brain abscess. The nonspecificity of symptoms and signs can be appreciated from the review of Morgan and associates, who found, among 88 consecutive patients, headache in 70 per cent, altered consciousness in 66 per cent, hemiparesis in 38 per cent, and seizures in 32 per cent.[62] Nevertheless, in reviewing their personal experience, the authors have noted that patients with brain abscess usually present with one of four recognizable syndromes, and although these syndromes are not specific for abscess, they are useful guides, emphasizing the often ominous and precarious balance in the intracranial mass dynamics.[92]

Type I—Rapid Focal Mass Expansion

Patients in this group present with the symptoms and signs of a rapidly progressive localized intracranial mass lesion advancing, usually over days but occasionally during a few hours or, by contrast, over several weeks. The precise pattern of focal disease to be encountered will depend upon the location of the abscess: a temporal lobe abscess will cause an early superior homonymous quadrantanopia; a cerebellar abscess will cause ipsilateral signs of cerebellar hemisphere deficit. Both may evidence low-grade fever, mild signs of meningeal irritation, and sufficient clouding of consciousness that subtle changes such as early visual field deficit may be missed. In respect to systemic signs of infection, the data of Morgan and co-workers are valuable: Among 88 consecutive patients with brain abscess, the temperature was above approximately 38°C in 44 per cent, and there was a peripheral white blood count higher than 15,000 in 38 per cent.[62] It is important to appreciate that there may be no signs of sepsis in the presence of a potentially lethal abscess. In one series of 89 patients, 40 had no symptoms or signs of an infective process, but only those associated with a space-occupying mass.[5] Because of the temporal profile, these lesions can be misinterpreted (in half of the authors' patients) as malignant neoplasms or spontaneous intracerebral hematomas. An initially correct clinical diagnosis will usually be made in the remaining patients because of singularly important clues: cyanotic congenital heart disease or other causes of right-to-left circulation shunts, intrathoracic purulent processes, skull osteomyelitis, and other contiguous sites of infection such as otitis media or accessory nasal sinusitis.

Type II—Intracranial Hypertension

These patients present with symptoms and signs of neurological deterioration associated with intracranial hypertension. Prominent symptoms include headache, nausea, vomiting, obtundation, memory loss, and personality change. Papilledema is a commonly encountered sign. Some patients have varying degrees of localizing or lateralizing neurological deficits, but the major clinical syndrome is that of increased intracranial pressure. The correct diagnosis will be made in approximately half of these cases; malignant glioma and meningitis will often be diagnosed in the remainder.

Type III—Diffuse Destruction

Patients in this category present with a rapidly destructive component; i.e., there is major neurological deterioration out of proportion to the clinical estimate of intracranial pressure. They continue to deteriorate in the absence of a brain herniation. The correct diagnosis will depend upon neuroradiological studies.

Type IV—Focal Neurological Deficit

The temporal profile progresses so slowly that the lesion is often interpreted as a slowly growing neoplasm in half the patients.

Diagnosis

Although the mortality rate may have declined following the introduction of antibiotics, it has remained unchanged and high (about 40 per cent) since that time.[4,74,83] Abscesses from purulent intrathoracic disease and those hematogenously spread are frequently more acute in their course, causing more deaths than those associated with direct implantation from trauma or derived from a contiguous bony focus.[53,83] The patient's preoperative state of consciousness remains the best guide to the prediction of short-term outcome. Factors contributing to death declare the importance of massive cerebral edema, brain stem compression, rupture into a ventricle with ventriculitis, meningitis, missed loculations and multiple lesions, delay in diagnosis and moribund states on admission, diagnostic failures, and technical failures such as the inability to localize the lesion at the time of operation.[5,25,74,83]

In the pursuit of timely diagnosis, knowledge of the various predisposing factors for the development of brain abscess often assists in heightening the suspicion for this infection.[51] *Pericranial* infection, as the most common identifiable source of infection preceding the development of brain abscess, should be looked for (cf. Fig. 110–2). *Hematogenous or metastatic spread* of infection from a distant focus as the second most commonly encountered cause demands examination for intrathoracic purulent infections and infections at other peripheral sites (skin, abdomen, heart). *Congenital heart disease* with a right-to-left shunt is usually associated with cyanosis.[10,71] The accompanying cerebral intravascular stasis, combined with bacteremia that bypasses lung filtration, is probably the important pathogenic mechanism. Clinical awareness should be acute in dealing with such patients, as it should be in dealing with those with similar shunting mechanisms such as pulmonary arteriovenous malformations. Neurological abnormalities in infants and children under the ages of 3 or 4 years who have cyanotic congenital heart disease generally stem from other mechanisms (polycythemia, hypoxia, thrombosis). After this age, brain abscess is a likelier explanation. Known *cranial trauma* or *craniotomy* is usually self-evident.

The initial diagnostic evaluation must include plain x-rays of the skull and chest, standard blood counts, determination of erythrocyte sedimentation rate, blood cultures, and additional pertinent screening studies to elucidate a suspected septic source suggested by a comprehensive bedside history and physical examination. Plain roentgenograms of the skull are recommended irrespective of the precision of subsequently utilized tests. They can reveal sinus and mastoid disease, a pineal shift, signs of chronic pressure, and gas in an abscess cavity.[64] Isotope brain scanning may reveal a focal area or areas of parenchymatous blood-brain barrier incompetency.[74] New and co-workers found nine out of nine

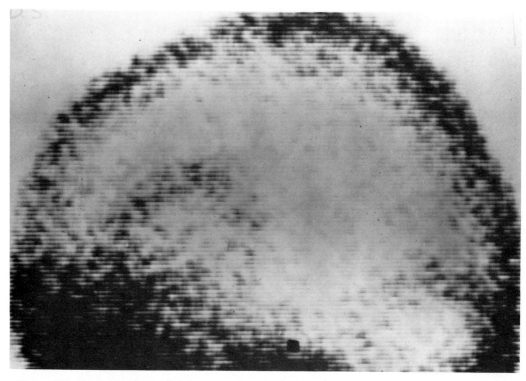

Figure 110–13 Technetium radioisotope scan in acute frontal abscess (*Hemophilus* sp.) six years following penetrating gunshot wound.

radionuclide scans positive, usually in a nonspecific pattern (only one of the nine showed a "ring" of uptake surrounding a "cooler" center of lesser uptake) (Fig. 110–13).[64] Electroencephalography may localize high-amplitude slow waves, which frequently occur over abscess.[58] Among 45 electroencephalographic studies on patients harboring brain abscesses, Beller and associates found only 14 in which the focal abnormalities were in agreement with more definitive studies, notably angiography.[5] Cerebral angiography usually localizes an avascular mass (composed of abscess and surrounding edema in indeterminate proportions), and in a later arterial phase occasionally reveals a neovascular or granulation tissue rim (blush) around a central necrotic zone (Fig. 110–14).[64,65] Computed tomography is accorded the premier position as a screening and localizing procedure (Fig. 110–15).[49] It may reveal either a low-density core or a higher-density vascular "capsule," a low-density periabscess "cerebritis," an infusion-enhanced abscess wall, or perhaps some mixture of all these components. Both an unenhanced and an enhanced scan should be obtained; only oc-

casionally will an unenhanced scan show a rim of higher density surrounding an area of low density. A low-density area of 0 to 15 Hounsfield units surrounded by a capsule that can be enhanced with contrast, 32 to 74 units, is the characteristic finding.[64]

If gas is present, it will be evidenced by very low attenuation figures (−200 to −340). The diagnostic yield exceeds 90 per cent in recent reports.[21,64] Nielsen and Gyldensted found decreased attenuation in all their 22 abscess cases. Contrast enhancement occurred in 18 of the 22, with a ring formation.[65] The differential diagnostic considerations based upon the CT findings include malignant glioma, metastatic neoplasm, infarction, postoperative changes, focal encephalitis (viral), fungal abscesses, and tuberculomas.[21,64] Both angiography and computed tomography will disclose the mass displacements of midline structures and ventricles.

Clinical surveys repeatedly review the catastrophe of major herniation syndromes following lumbar punctures in brain abscess patients.[15,32,74] When the diagnostic tests are scheduled, lumbar puncture is best deferred until neuroradiological studies are

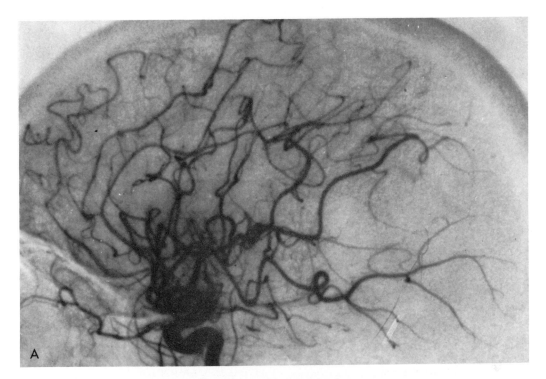

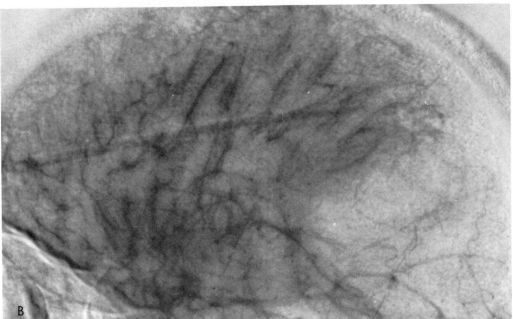

Figure 110–14 *A.* Mid–arterial phase cerebral angiogram of posterior parietal abscess (anaerobic and microaerophilic streptococcus) from unidentified source. *B.* Later arterial phase demonstrating a vascular mass.

complete and the diagnosis of abscess is excluded. In the report by Morgan and associates, there was information concerning lumbar cerebrospinal fluid findings in 44 patients. Two thirds of these patients had protein values greater than 50 mg per 100 ml (half were between 50 and 100 and half were greater than 100 mg per 100 ml). The white blood cell counts were: 0 to 5 in 41 per cent, 6 to 100 in 20 per cent, and more than 100 cells in 39 per cent. The findings are not diagnostic.[62]

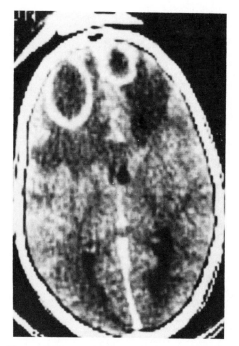

Figure 110-15 Bilateral frontal lobe abscesses (*Eikenella corrodens* and *Bacteroides fragilis*) secondary to acute frontal sinusitis and osteomyelitis. Note extensive edema and posterior displacement of both lateral ventricles.

The selection and timing of the diagnostic studies will be determined by the urgency of the clinical status of the patient, but an economy of effort is urged. The differential diagnostic considerations will probably include primary glioma, metastatic neoplasm, hemorrhagic infarction, necrotizing vasculitis, hemorrhage from focal vascular disease, and focal viral encephalitis.

Causative Organisms

Cure for brain abscess (like any other abscess) can only be achieved dependably by operative excision or drainage, concomitant antibiotic therapy, and eradication of any existing septic focus. Antibiotic therapy, alone, will often fail to sterilize the abscess: organisms can be recovered within the abscess despite therapeutic concentrations of antibiotics *within the abscess*.[11] Whenever possible, systemic antimicrobial therapy is begun preoperatively to reduce the associated surrounding cerebritis and minimize local tissue contamination during operative manipulation.

Four factors appear to be pre-eminent determinants of the ultimate microbial flora of brain abscess: the primary source of infection or conditions predisposing to brain abscess; the age of the patient; the patient's underlying disease or immune status; and previous use of antibiotics.

Primary Source of Infection and Predisposing Factors

Chronic otitis media, mastoiditis, and paranasal sinustis are all associated with mixed anaerobic and aerobic organisms. The predominant anaerobes are streptococci (anaerobic and microaerophilic), and *Bacteroides* species (including *B. fragilis*) are also found. *Staphylococcus aureus* and *Streptococcus viridans* are the aerobes that are commonly isolated. Organisms frequently associated with metastatic spread from distant foci have been anaerobic and microaerophilic streptococci, *Fusobacterium*, staphylococci, *Klebsiella*, *Diplococcus*, and occasionally *Actinomyces* and *Nocardia*. The distant focus may remain occult; it is only after the diagnosis of abscess has been made that some cases of endocarditis are suspected.

The presence of a coagulase-positive staphylococcal brain abscess or meningitis in the absence of cranial injury or infected peripheral foci should strongly suggest infective endocarditis, especially if the patient is young and has a history of drug abuse. Brain abscess associated with cranial trauma or operation tends to stem from *Staphylococcus aureus;* occasionally aerobic gram-negative bacilli, especially *Pseudomonas aeruginosa*, can be found in these infections. In cyanotic congenital heart disease the "normal" bacteremia is not efficiently filtered out of the circulation by the lungs, and thus bacteria reach peripheral sites, including the brain. Therefore, microbial flora in brain abscess associated with congenital heart disease or other lesions with right-to-left circulation shunting will depend on the type of peripheral infection and bacteremia involved (Fig. 110-16).[54,58,74,83]

Age of Patient

Neonatal infections are generally due to gram-negative bacilli and *Staphylococcus aureus*. Children up to the age of 10 years often become infected with *Hemophilus influenzae*, commonly in the upper respira-

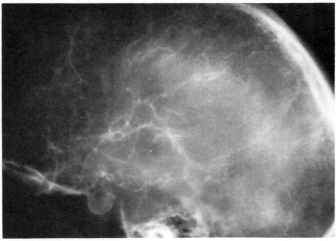

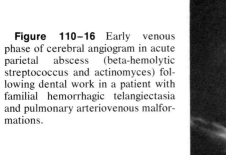

Figure 110-16 Early venous phase of cerebral angiogram in acute parietal abscess (beta-hemolytic streptococcus and actinomyces) following dental work in a patient with familial hemorrhagic telangiectasia and pulmonary arteriovenous malformations.

tory tract, ears, and sinuses. At the other end of the age spectrum, older patients may be more prone to gram-negative and staphylococcal infections, perhaps because of frequent hospital admissions with greater risk of hospital-acquired infections, or owing to associated diseases.

Underlying Disease or Immune Status

Certain disease states are associated with particular types of infecting organisms, for example, sickle cell disease with *Salmonella* or pneumococci; alcoholic liver disease with pneumococci, *Klebsiella*, or *E. coli;* prostheses (heart valves, ventriculojugular shunts, and the like) with coagulase-negative or -positive staphylococci; heroin addiction with *Staphylococcus aureus, Candida,* or gram-negative bacilli, especially *Pseudomonas;* and burns, with infections caused by *Pseudomonas aeruginosa.* Additionally, patients with lymphoma or leukemia or cancer, or with abnormal immune defense mechanisms secondary to drug therapy (steroids, antineoplastic agents), can develop brain abscess owing to unusual microorganisms. The patient whose immune surveillance is suppressed is more susceptible to "opportunistic" pathogens than is one in whom it is intact. The fungi are especially troublesome in such a setting, as they are in patients with diabetes mellitus. The actinomycotic organisms, *Nocardia asteroides,* and *Aspergillis* are particularly worrisome etiological agents associated with a very high mortality rate.[63,86] *Mucor* only very rarely forms sup-

purative lesions, but numerous other fungi do.[29]

Previous Use of Antibiotics

Often, patients are given antibiotics for various types of infections before the clinical onset of brain abscess. Under these conditions, it is predictably difficult to anticipate the type of microbial flora that might be found at the time brain abscess is diagnosed. The usual aerobic and anaerobic flora of the primary disease or factors predisposing to brain abscess may be replaced by other less common microorganisms. This frequently occurs in the hospital patient who is receiving antibiotics and in whom the usual mouth and respiratory tract microbial flora have been replaced by gram-negative bacilli or staphylococci.

In clinical experience the typical organisms isolated from brain abscess in the past have been streptococci and staphylococci.[5,74,83] Many brain abscesses, however, have failed to yield bacteria when material was cultured. Improvement in culture techniques has led to the awareness that although aerobic cultures may demonstrate bacteria in half the patients with brain abscess, a higher overall yield of a confirmed organism results if careful anaerobic techniques are also applied. Thus, the "sterile" cultures reported in brain abscess may be, in part, due to the failure to recover anaerobes.[35] Anaerobes are fastidious microorganisms that survive only under conditions of low oxidation-reduction potential (oxygen-free environment). The collection of the brain abscess material in oxygen-free transport containers is therefore important. Failure to adhere to this practice will result in poor yield of anaerobes regardless of whatever sophisticated anaerobic culture method is subsequently used. Cultures for fungi should also be obtained.

Antibiotic Therapy

The initial antibiotic therapy is empirically selected preoperatively or intraoperatively before specific culture and sensitivity information can be available. Most brain abscesses will harbor organisms that are sensitive to penicillin. In the absence of clinical clues to the contrary, penicillin G is the drug of choice and should be administered intravenously in four to six divided doses totalling 20 million units a day. If a staphylococcus is suspected, a penicillinase-resistant penicillin (such as methicillin) should be added. If the patient has a definite penicillin allergy, chloramphenicol should be substituted for penicillin in a dose of 4 gm a day administered intravenously. The cephalosporins, especially cephalothin (Keflin) and clindamycin (Cleocin) do not cross the blood-brain barrier very well and therefore are not recommended.

The single most important diagnostic tool available when a decision concerning antibiotic therapy is being made is the Gram stain. At the time of drainage of the brain abscess, the abscess fluid must be studied via this procedure. The presence of thin nonpleomorphic gram-negative bacilli suggests *Bacteroides;* moreover, the possibility of *B. fragilis* cannot be excluded. The latter organism is resistant to penicillin, and over half the strains are not susceptible to tetracycline. Chloramphenicol is the drug of choice for the initial therapy, before sensitivity data are available in this situation. Organisms that are gram-positive branching rods might suggest *Actinomyces* or *Nocardia*, the latter often being weakly acid-fast and requiring sulfonamide therapy, while the former is best treated with penicillin. Large gram-positive cocci are usually staphylococci, and methicillin or nafcillin is indicated. Once the culture data are available, necessary adjustments in chemotherapy can be made.

Operative Management

There are two basic operative techniques available for treating brain abscess,

namely, drainage (aspiration) and excision. Each approach has certain advantages and disadvantages; excision can follow aspiration; each may have its appropriate timing and suitability. It is suggested that outcome is not closely correlated with the method used.[83] The report of Choudbury and associates, however, warrants recognition of their excellent results from excision.[19]

Aspiration

A burr hole is strategically placed that provides: (1) the shortest distance between dural opening and abscess, (2) a safe trajectory between dura mater and abscess that does not traverse crucial structures (neural, vascular, or ventricular), and (3) a route that avoids infected bone, paranasal sinuses, and scalp wounds. If the first burr hole does not satisfy all these requirements, a second is placed. The burr hole is then used as a route for intermittent retapping of the abscess or for placement of a soft catheter to permit intermittent "fractional" drainage (aspiration). A meticulous sterile technique is mandatory. A large, blunt 16- or 14-gauge cannula is advanced by experienced "dead reckoning" or with fluoroscopic aid or with stereotaxic techniques until the abscess is entered. Often the surgeon can "palpate" the tough collagen abscess wall before the cannula "pops" into the central cavity; occasionally, a more difficult situation exists wherein the cannula advances through surrounding abnormally soft brain, and the only tactile clue for abscess is the softer, liquid necrotic abscess core. Whether pus spontaneously drains through the cannula as the stylet is withdrawn depends on the size of the cannula, the accuracy of placement, the amount and consistency of pus, and the intracranial pressure. If no pus drains out and the surgeon is reasonably confident that the cannula is properly placed, irrigating fluid can be added gravitationally to determine whether, in fact, the cannula tip is in a cavity. Gentle, small-volume syringe-pressured instillations and aspirations can provide mechanical irrigation. A triple-antibiotic solution of bacitracin 500 units per milliliter, polymyxin 0.1 per cent, and neomycin 1.0 per cent is used for abscess irrigation, although controlled data are unavailable to support its efficacy. If an indwelling catheter is to be utilized, the medication can be started in the operating room after the initial cannula entrance; as the cannula is withdrawn, the exact same trajectory is matched by the entering catheter (e.g., No. 10 Red Robinson or equivalent diameter soft pliable silicone tube) in an effort to follow the cannula track through the abscess wall. Occasionally the catheter must be passed through a cannula. After the catheter is attached to a suitable connector extracranially, it may be used for intermittent irrigation and drainage as needed. The frequency of intermittent cannulation or fractional catheter drainage is determined by the size of the abscess and the neurological signs and symptoms.

The aspiration technique requires precise knowledge of the abscess location and size and shape as well as of the presence of loculations of "daughter" abscess formation for recannulation to be safe and accurate. Imaging of the abscess can be most satisfactorily performed by computed tomography. This is the procedure of choice when the instrumentation is available; a complete scan is not necessary, but contrast enhancement is. In circumstances in which computer scanning is not possible, the otherwise obsolete procedure of marking is strongly recommended whereby the abscess can be visualized on plain skull x-rays (Fig. 110–17). Such marking may be done with air, but for longer-term progress audit, microbarium sulfate with or without povidone-iodine (1 part Micropaque, 4 parts povidone-iodine) can be instilled into the abscess at the time of initial operative localization.[12,59] Thorium dioxide has been an excellent marker with distinct advantages, but its radioactivity and its rare leakage into the subarachnoid pathways have removed it from the armamentarium.[12,72] Since abscess formation involves widespread tissue changes (necrosis, gliosis, collagen formation, granulation tissue production, edema formation) and since the shape is seldom uniformly spherical, abscess imaging has been a difficult task, requiring the simultaneous use of several anatomical diagnostic techniques combined with daily measurements and comparisons during the early therapeutic phase. The computer scan has made this job easier.

Aspiration techniques are simple. The burr hole can be placed with local anesthesia, and thereafter repetitive manipulation of the abscess cavity can be a bedside procedure. Successful aspiration therapy achieves prompt three-dimensional diminution of the abscess that will be unequivocal within days. The goal is for the only remnant of the abscess to be a sterile collagen-glial core. In some instances, aspiration two or three times one or two days apart may achieve the goal. In other cases the authors have aspirated intermittently six or more times to control the lesion. Rapid improvement should be documented clinically as well as radiologically, and the clinical and radiological evaluation will determine whether aspiration is to be followed by excision. The presence of a catheter or the reintroduced cannula may cause a periventricular abscess to discharge into the ventricle with grave consequences. The danger of ventricular spill is partly related to the peculiarity that the thinnest part of the abscess wall is next to the ventricle, i.e., is subependymal. As the abscess wall changes its configuration, an indwelling catheter, fixed to the integument, may lose its ideal central location, penetrate the abscess boundary, and inoculate additional brain tissue. More superficial abscesses may rupture into a cistern, or the convexity subarachnoid space may become contaminated during manipulation. Daughter abscesses may be undetected. Radiological internal marking, if used as the only means of following improvement of an abscess, may obscure an enlarging, contiguous, but unmarked daughter abscess. Skill and clinical acumen are required to correlate the clinical course with the neuroanatomical and pathophysiological problem. Again, the CT scan is of inestimable value.

Excision

Excision or "radical extirpation" refers to complete operative removal of the abscess. To the extent that there is an organized wall there will be a readily identifiable interface between brain and abscess, permitting abscess removal with minimal damage to surrounding brain. Radical extirpation should remove all infected material and thus assume the lowest abscess recurrence rate. Abscesses may be encountered as tumor masses, and their true nature be discovered only at the time of or after resection. Such may be the case with thick-walled lesions adjacent to a contiguous focus or with those secondary to a retained foreign body, examples of which may be found decades after the penetrating injury. For resection of the preoperatively diag-

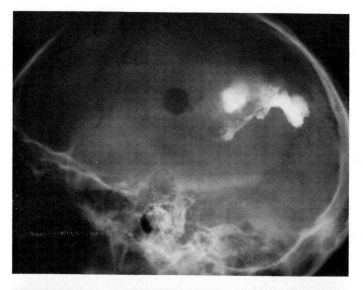

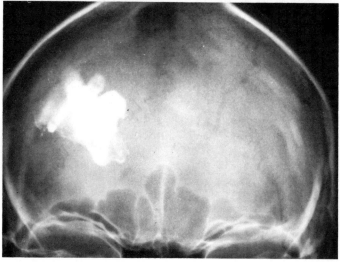

Figure 110–17 Microbarium sulfate "pyogram" of multiloculated abscess (same patient as Figure 110–16). Foul-smelling pus was aspirated, and the lesion was subsequently totally excised.

nosed abscess, a generous osteoplastic or "free" bone flap is turned as for the management of a benign neoplasm (Fig. 110–18). Measures to control intracranial mass dynamics are adopted as needed for each case. Antibiotic coverage is presupposed and, in any case, should be initiated before operation. The abscess is approached with its configuration in mind, and the wall is defined by blunt and gentle dissection. Sharp penetrating instruments should be avoided, although a fibrous "stalk" between the abscess and an adjacent dural or bony focus may require cutting after coagulation or clipping. One avoids entering the necrotic center, but if spillage occurs, the dissection should continue and the purulent material be thoroughly irrigated out. Alert observa-

tion for small nubbins and loculations will avoid leaving such troublesome tissue behind. The mass is removed intact, and closure techniques standard for neoplasms are employed. No compromise of closure of each layer in proper Cushing fashion is accorded in the abscess. The antibiotic therapy appropriate to the organism, when known, is continued. Although highly effective and favored by many when applicable, this method of treatment, cannot be used for all lesions.[53,74] The abscess may be too hazardously deep (in thalamus or brain stem, for example), or the lesion may be so large and thin-boundaried as to invite certain rupture.[52] There may be intense surrounding cerebral edema that precludes safe brain retraction. If aspiration is elected

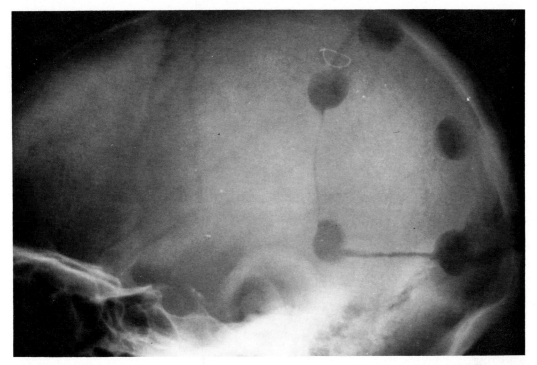

Figure 110–18 ''Free'' parieto-occipital bone flap designed for total excision of multiloculated abscess (alpha-hemolytic streptococcus) secondary to hematogenous spread from diverticulitis.

as the initial step, radical extirpation remains available as a secondary procedure. Under such circumstances, the initial procedure reduces the dangerous mass, yields the benefits of organism identification, permits optimal chemotherapy, achieves a virtually sterilized operative field, contributes to the resolution of cerebral edema, and makes neurological improvement possible. Antibiotic therapy is maintained for four weeks after the total excision.

Recent reports by the group from Derby are offered as a strong rebuttal to these arguments.[19] They document 24 consecutive abscesses treated by excision with one death and minimal morbidity, a notable record. On careful perusal, it is to be observed that in their early cases aspiration preceded resection, a sequence that was abandoned with the advent of computed tomography. More important to note, however, is that in this presentation, to the extent that data are available, there were few if any abscesses from thoracogenic spread owing to congenital heart disease or other hematogenous origin. It is in these latter cases, in particular, that the large, thin-walled lesions occur for which aspiration may be safer in the initial stages. Nevertheless, the series referred to is an excellent one and, if replicated with a broader population of patients, could be a compelling defense of primary excision.

The clinical circumstances should influence the operative technique selected. Brain abscess is usually a surgical emergency and the more profound the neurological illness, the more expeditious and less manipulative should be the therapy. For example, children with cyanotic congenital heart disease and brain abscess tolerate craniotomy poorly and, in general, are best treated, as least initially, by repeated abscess aspiration (Fig. 110–19).[31]

For large and thin-walled abscesses that have been diagnosed as such preoperatively, the authors prefer to aspirate initially, using the technique of intermittent tapping with a cannula. For less acute and thick-walled lesions, direct excision is undertaken.

In the management of the altered intracranial mass dynamics, the therapeutic armamentarium as reviewed in Chapter 29 is mobilized. It is the authors' usual practice to utilize high-dosage glucocorticoids (dex-

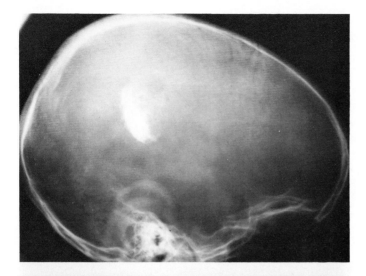

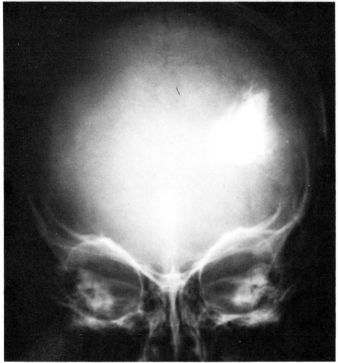

Figure 110–19 Pyogram (microbarium sulfate) of brain abscess (alpha-hemolytic streptococcus) in a 6-year-old child with cyanotic congenital heart disease. Repeated tapping of thin-walled sac was followed by recovery.

amethasone), acknowledging that such compounds may alter the host antibiotic-organism interrelations.[69]

A controversial issue exists regarding whether a preabscess phase of "cerebritis" can be successfully treated by chemotherapy alone. First, there is meager evidence that a clinical phase of bacterial cerebritis is usually antecedent to abscess. On the contrary, the particular host-organism interaction from the beginning can be remarkably indolent in one patient and very

inflammatory in the next. Second, since there is neither single nor combined study pathognomonic for abscess, the same diagnostic limitation pertains to the recognition of an "early abscess." Apparent chemotherapy cures of abscess may, in fact, have been superfluous antibiotic therapy during viral encephalitis or during septicemia and cerebral vasculitis. A recent report by Berg and co-workers suggests that the nonoperative cure of brain abscesses can be based upon computer scan information and clinical presentations.[7] The CT findings characteristic of brain abscess have been reviewed in this chapter, and it should be noted that they are based upon operatively or pathologically confirmed cases. That similar findings may occur in patients who do not harbor suppurative sacs of pus is also clear. It may be difficult to refute the claim of cure if the illness has been interpreted as "abscess" when in fact it is not, and the patient recovers. Experience with high mortality rates associated with nonoperatively treated abscesses leads one to recommend operative therapy for abscess. In a particular patient there may well be controversy regarding antibiotic selection and the timing (and type) of operation, but the guiding principle should be that chemotherapy and operation, *combined*, are needed.[13] Computer scan data that are suggestive of abscess have been found reversible without purulent breakdown. It is the authors' practice, however, to operate on all patients in whom, by utilizing all data, a diagnosis of abscess is made. Such a course seems safer than to entertain the nebulous diagnosis of cerebritis or to wait for an abscess to "wall off" or "ripen."

Regardless of the modes of operative treatment or types of antibiotic used, the mortality rate of patients with brain abscess is directly related to the neurological status of the patient when therapy is begun,[15,46] although several other factors such as the patient's age, the multiplicity of lesions, and the cause of the infection also influence survival.[16,46,83]

Patient evaluation must be expedited safely, and antibiotic and operative therapy must be started relatively early in the unfolding sequence of pathophysiological events. Epilepsy is a common late complication of brain abscess, with a frequency of 30 per cent or higher, and is not significantly altered by the particular operative or antibiotic therapy employed.[15,25,62,83] Other patterns of long-term neurological deficit can be correlated with the particular locations of the brain abscess.[15,74]

REFERENCES

1. Ad Hoc Committee on Trauma, National Academy of Sciences, National Research Council: Postoperative wound infections—the influence of ultraviolet irradiation of the operating room and of various other factors. Ann. Surg., *160*:suppl.:1–192, 1964.
2. Albright, L., Toczek, S., Brenner, V. J., and Ommaya, A. K.: Osteomyelitis and epidural abscess caused by arachnia propionica. Case report. J. Neurosurg., *40*:115–119, 1974.
3. Balch, R. E.: Wound infections complicating neurosurgical procedures. J. Neurosurg., *26*:41–45, 1967.
4. Ballantine, H. T., Jr., and White, J. C.: Brain abscess. New Eng. J. Med., *248*:14–19, 1953.
5. Beller, A. J., Sahar, A., and Praiss, I.: Brain abscess. Review of 89 cases over a period of 30 years. J. Neurol. Neurosurg., Psychiat., *36*:757–768, 1973.
6. Bennett, I. L., and Petersdorf, R. G.: An approach to infectious diseases. *In* Wintrobe, M. M., et al., eds.: Principles of Internal Medicine. 6th Ed. New York, McGraw-Hill Book Co., 1970, pp. 724–732.
7. Berg, B., Franklin, G., Cuneo, R., Boldrey, E., and Strimling, B.: Nonsurgical cure of brain ulcers: Early diagnosis and follow-up with computerized tomography. Ann. Neurol., *3*:474–478, 1978.
8. Best, W.: Chloramphenicol-associated blood dyscrasias. A review of cases submitted to the American Medical Association Registry. J.A.M.A., *201*:181–188, 1967.
9. Bhandari, Y., and Sarkari, N. B. S.: Subdural empyema: A review of 37 cases. J. Neurosurg., *32*:35–39, 1970.
10. Bhatra, R., Tandon, P. N., Baneyi, A. K., and Prakash, B.: Brain abscess and congenital heart disease. Acta Neurochir., *33*:233–239, 1976.
11. Black, P., Graybill, J. R., and Charache, P.: Penetration of brain abscess by systemically administered antibiotics. J. Neurosurg., *38*:705–709, 1973.
12. Blinderman, E. E.: An evaluation of micropaque barium sulphate as a radiographic marker for cerebral abscess. J. Neurosurg., *21*:867–873, 1964.
13. Brewer, N. S., MacCarty, C. S., and William, E. W.: Brain abscess: A review of recent experience. Ann. Intern. Med., *82*:571–576, 1975.
14. Burke, J. F.: Clinical determinants of host susceptibility to infection in surgical patients. *In* Brachman, P. S., and Eickhoff, T. C., eds.: Proceedings of the International Conference on Nosocomial Infections. Chicago, American Hospital Association, 1971, pp. 169–172.
15. Carey, M. E., Chou, S. N., and French, L. A.: Long-term neurological residue in patients surviving brain abscess with surgery. J. Neurosurg., *34*:652–656, 1971.
16. Carey, M. E., Chou, S. N., and French, L. A.: Experience with brain abscesses. J. Neurosurg., *36*:1–9, 1972.
17. Carmen, P. W., Fraser, R. A. R., and Stein, B. M.: Aseptic meningitis following posterior fossa surgery in children. J. Neurosurg., *41*:44–48, 1974.
18. Carpenter, R. R., and Petersdorf, R. G.: The clinical spectrum of bacterial meningitis. Amer. J. Med., *33*:262–275, 1962.
19. Choudbury, A. R., Taylor, J. C., and Whitaker, R.: Primary excision of brain abscess. Brit. Med. J., *2*:1119–1121, 1538–1539, 1977.

20. Chow, A. W., Ota, J. K., and Guze, L. B.: Clindamycin plus gentamycin as expectant therapy for presumed mixed infections. Canad. Med. Ass. J., *1105*:1225–1229, 1976.

21. Claveria, L. E., duBoulay, G. H., and Moseley, I. F.: Intracranial infections: Investigation by computerized axial tomography. Neuroradiology, *12*:59–71, 1976.

22. Cluff, L. E.: Medical determinants of nosocomial infections. *In* Brachman, P. S., and Eickhoff, T. C., eds.: Proceedings of the International Conference on Nosocomial Infections. Chicago, American Hospital Association, 1971, pp. 164–168.

23. Cruise, P.: Infection surveillance—identifying the problems and the high-risk patient. Southern Med. J., *70*:suppl.:1:4–8, 1977.

24. Domingue, J. N., and Wilson, C. B.: Pituitary abscesses. Report of seven cases and review of literature. J. Neurosurg., *46*:601–608, 1977.

25. Erasmus, J. F. P.: Cranial and spinal pyogenic disease—with notes in 415 personal cases (Part I—General observations; Part II—Aspects of diagnosis and treatment). S. Afr. Med. J., *40*:416–419, 433–437, 1966.

26. Erickson, D. L., Seljeskog, E. L., and Chou, S. N.: Suction-irrigation treatment of craniotomy infections. J. Neurosurg., *41*:265–267, 1974.

27. Farmer, T. W., and Wise, G. R.: Subdural empyema in infants, children and adults. Neurology (Minneap.), *23*:254–261, 1973.

28. Fergin, R. D., and Dodge, P. R.: Bacterial meningitis—newer concepts of pathophysiology and neurologic sequelae. Pediat. Clin. N. Amer., *23*:541–556, 1976.

29. Fetter, B. K., Klintworth, G. K., and Hendry, W. S., eds.: Mycoses of the Central Nervous System. Baltimore, Williams & Wilkins Co., 1967.

30. Fisher, L. S., Chou, A. W., Yoshikawa, T. T., and Guze, L. B.: Cephalothin and cephaloridine therapy for bacterial meningitis. Ann. Intern. Med., *82*:689–693, 1975.

31. French, L. A., and Chou, S. N.: Treatment of brain abscesses. Advances Neurol., *6*:269–275, 1974.

32. Garfield, J.: Management of supratentorial intracranial abscess. A review of 200 cases. Brit. Med. J., *2*:7–11, 1969.

33. Goodman, S. J., Cahan, L., and Chou, A. W.: Subgaleal abscess. A preventable complication of scalp trauma. Western J. Med., *127*:169–172, 1977.

34. Hand, W. L., and Sanford, J. P.: Post-traumatic bacterial meningitis. Ann. Intern. Med., *72*:869–874, 1970.

35. Heineman, H. S., and Braude, A. I.: Anaerobic infection of the brain. Observation on eighteen consecutive cases of brain abscess. Amer. J. Med., *35*:682–697, 1963.

36. Heineman, H. S., Braude, A. I., and Osterholm, J. L.: Intracranial suppurative disease. Early presumptive diagnosis and successful treatment without surgery. J.A.M.A., *218*:1542–1547, 1971.

37. Hoff, J. T., Brewin, A., and Sang, H.: Antibiotics for basilar skull fracture. Letter to Editor. J. Neurosurg., *44*:649, 1976.

38. Horenstein, S., and Schreiber, D. J.: Clinical features of bacterial meningitis. Advances Neurol., *6*:141–159, 1974.

39. Hughes, G., Chidi, C., and Macon, W., IV: Staphylococci in community-acquired infections. Ann. Surg., *183*:355–357, 1976.

40. Ignelzi, R. J., and Vander Ark, G. D.: Analysis of the treatment of basilar skull fractures with and without antibiotics. J. Neurosurg., *43*:721–726, 1975.

41. Jackson, G. G.: Present status of aminoglycoside antibiotics and their safe effective use. Clin. Ther., *1*:200–215, 1977.

42. Jessen, O., Rosendal, K., Bulow, P., Faber, V., and Eriksen, K. R.: Changing staphylococci and staphyloccal infections. A ten-year study of bacteria and causes of bacteremia. New Eng. J. Med., *281*:627–635, 1969.

43. Jones, S. R., Luby, J. P., and Sanford, J. P.: Bacterial meningitis complicating cranial-spinal trauma. J. Trauma, *13*:895–900, 1973.

44. Joubert, M., and Stephanov, S.: Computerized tomography and surgical treatment in intracranial suppuration. Report of 30 consecutive unselected cases of brain abscess and subdural empyema. J. Neurosurg., *47*:73–78, 1977.

45. Kaiser, A. B., and Zell, A. M.: Aminoglycoside therapy of Gram-negative bacillary meningitis. New Eng. J. Med., *293*:1215–1220, 1975.

46. Karandanis, D., and Shulman, J. A.: Factors associated with mortality in brain abscess. Arch. Intern. Med. (Chicago), *135*:1145–1150, 1975.

47. Kaufman, D. M., Miller, M. H., and Steigbigel, N. H.: Subdural empyema: Analysis of 17 recent cases and review of the literature. Medicine (Balt.), *54*:485–498, 1975.

48. Keener, E. B., and Perot, P. H.: Antibacterial drugs topically applied to the central nervous system. Arch. Neurol. (Chicago), *3*:665–676, 1960.

49. Keogh, A. J.: Computerized transverse axial tomography for the early diagnosis and follow-up of intracranial abscess. J. Neurol. Neurosurg. Psychiat., *39*:920–921, 1976.

50. Kirby, W. M. M., and Petersdorf, R. G.: Chemotherapy of infection. *In* Thorn, G. W., Adams, R. D., Braunwald, E., Isselbacher, K., and Petersdorf, R. G., eds.: Harrison's Principles of Internal Medicine. 8th Ed. New York, McGraw-Hill Book Co., 1977, pp. 775–789.

51. Krayenbuhl, H. A.: Abscess of the brain. Clin. Neurosurg., *14*:25–44, 1967.

52. Law, J. D., Lehman, R. A. W., Kirsch, W. M., and Ohni, G.: Diagnosis and treatment of abscess of the central ganglia. J. Neurosurg., *44*:226–232, 1976.

53. Le Bean, J., Creissard, P., Harispe, L., and Redondo, A.: Surgical treatment of brain abscess and subdural empyema. J. Neurosurg., *38*:198–203, 1973.

54. Lerner, P. I.: Selection of antimicrobial agents in bacterial infections of the nervous system. Advances Neurol., *6*:169–202, 1974.

55. Lerner, P. I., Smith, H., and Weinstein, L.: Penicillin neurotoxicity. Ann. N.Y. Acad. Med., *145*:310–318, 1967.

56. Lewin, W.: Cerebrospinal fluid rhinorrhea in nonmissile head injuries. Clin. Neurosurg., *12*:237–252, 1964.

57. Lorber, J., Kalhan, S. C., and Mahgrefle, B.: Treatment of ventriculitis with gentamycin and cloxacillin in infants born with spina bifida. Arch. Dis. Child., 34:178–185, 1970.

58. Martin, G.: Non-otogenic cerebral abscess. J. Neurol. Neurosurg. Psychiat.36:607–610, 1973.

59. Maxwell, J. A., and DeLong, W. B.: Use of micropaque barium in the radiographic visualization of brain abscess. Case report. J. Neurosurg., 28:280–282, 1968.

60. McCallum, J. E., Brand, E., and Selker, R. G.: Osteomyelitis of the skull in chronic granulomatous disease of childhood. Case report. J. Neurosurg., 40:764–766, 1974.

61. Miles, J., and Hughes, B.: Tuberculous osteitis of the skull. Brit. J. Surg., 57:673–679, 1970.

62. Morgan, H., Wood, M. W., and Murphey, F.: Experience with 88 consecutive cases of brain abscess. J. Neurosurg., 38:698–704, 1973.

63. Mukoyama, M., Gimple, K., and Poser, C. M.: Aspergillosis of the central nervous system. Report of a brain abscess due to A. fumigatus and review of the literature. Neurology (Minneap.), 19:967–974, 1969.

64. New, P. F. J., Davis, K. R., and Ballantine, H. T., Jr.: Computer tomography in central abscess. Radiology, 121:641–646, 1976.

65. Nielsen, H., and Gyldensted, C.: Computer tomography in the diagnosis of central abscess. Neuroradiology, 12:207–217, 1977.

66. Oill, P. A., Yoshikawa, T. T., and Yamauchi, T.: Infectious disease emergencies—Part I: Patients presenting with an altered state of consciousness. Western J. Med., 125:36–46, 1976.

67. Osgood, C. P., Dujouny, M., Hohn, E., and Postic, B.: Delayed post-traumatic subdural empyema. J. Trauma, 15:916–921, 1975.

68. Overturf, G. D., and Balfour, G.: Osteomyelitis and sepsis: Severe complications of fetal monitoring. Pediatrics, 55:244–247, 1975.

69. Quartey, G. R. E., Johnston, J. A., and Rozdisky, B.: Decadron in the treatment of cerebral abscess. An experimental study. J. Neurosurg., 45:301–310, 1976.

70. Rahal, J. J., Jr., Hyams, P. J., Simberkoff, M. S., et al.: Combined intrathecal and intramuscular gentamycin for Gram-negative meningitis. Pharmacologic study of 21 patients. New Eng. J. Med., 290:1394–1398, 1974.

71. Raimondi, A. J., Matsumoto, S., and Miller, R. A.: Brain abscess in children with congenital heart disease. J. Neurosurg., 23:588–595, 1965.

72. Robert, C. M., Jr., Stern, W. E., Brown, W. J., Greenfield, M. A., and Bartson, J. R.: Brain stem abscess treated surgically with special note upon the employment of thorium dioxide. Surg. Neurol., 3:153–160, 1975.

73. Salmon, J. H.: Ventriculitis complicating meningitis. Amer. J. Dis. Child., 124:35–40, 1972.

74. Samson, D. S., and Clark, K.: A current review of brain abscess. Amer. J. Med., 54:201–210, 1973.

75. Shaw, M. D. M., and Russell, J. A.: Cerebellar abscess. A review of 47 cases. J. Neurol. Neurosurg. Psychiat., 38:429–435, 1975.

76. Smith, R. W., and Alksne, J. F.: Infections com-plicating the use of external ventriculostomy. J. Neurosurg., 44:567–570, 1976.

77. Stern, W. E., and Boldrey, E. B.: Subdural purulent collections. Surg. Gynec. Obstet., 95:623–630, 1952.

78. Swartz, M. N., and Dodge, P. R.: Bacterial meningitis—A review of selective aspects. I. General clinical features, special problems and unusual meningeal reaction mimicking bacterial meningitis. New Eng. J. Med., 272:725–730, 1965.

79. Thomas, J. N., and Nel, J. R.: Acute spreading osteomyelitis of the skull complicating frontal sinusitis. J. Laryng., 91:55–62, 1977.

80. Thompson, R. E. M., Harding, J. W., and Simon, R. D.: Sensitivity of Staphylococcus pyogenes to benzyl penicillin and BRL 1241. Brit. Med. J., 5200:708–709, 1960.

81. Tourtellotte, W. W.: Cerebrospinal fluid examination in meningoencephalitis. Mod. Treatm., 4:879–897, 1967.

82. Turner, A. L., and Reynolds, F. E.: Intracranial Pyogenic Diseases. A Pathological and Clinical Study of the Pathways of Infection from the Face, the Nasal and Paranasal Air Cavities. Edinburgh, Oliver & Boyd, 1931, p. 271.

83. Van Alphen, H. A. M., and Dreissen, J. J. R.: Brain abscess and subdural empyema. Factors influencing mortality and results of various surgical techniques. J. Neurol. Neurosurg. Psychiat., 39:481–490, 1976.

84. Walker, A. E., Johnson, H. C., and Kollros, J. J.: Penicillin convulsions: The convulsive effects of penicillin applied to the cerebral cortex of monkey and man. Surg. Gynec. Obstet., 81:692–701, 1945.

85. Wallerstein, R., Condit, P. K., Kasper, C. K., Brown, J. W., and Mornson, F. R.: Statewide study of chloramphenicol therapy and fatal aplastic anemia. J.A.M.A., 208:2045–2050, 1969.

86. Weiss, M. H., and Jane, J. A.: Nocardia asteroides brain abscess successfully treated by enucleation. Case report. J. Neurosurg., 30:83–86, 1969.

87. Weiss, M. H., Kurze, T., and Nulsen, F. E.: Antibiotic neurotoxicity. Laboratory and clinical study. J. Neurosurg., 41:486–489, 1974.

88. Wherle, P. F.: Pitfalls in the management of central nervous system infections. J. Florida Med. Ass., 57:16–18, 1970.

89. Wilkins, R. H., and Goree, J. A.: Interhemispheric subdural empyema. Angiographic appearance. J. Neurosurg., 32:459–462, 1970.

90. Wright, R. L.: A survey of possible etiologic agents in postoperative craniotomy infections. J. Neurosurg., 25:125–132, 1966.

91. Wyler, A. R., and Kelly, W.: Use of antibiotics with external ventriculostomies. J. Neurosurg., 37:185–187, 1972.

92. Yoshikawa, T. T., and Goodman, S. J.: Brain abscess. Western J. Med., 121:307–319, 1974.

93. Yoshikawa, T. T., Chou, A. W., and Guze, L. B.: Role of anaerobic bacteria in subdural empyema. Amer. J. Med., 58:99–104, 1975.

111

VIRAL ENCEPHALITIS

Diseases of viral origin occasionally mimic expanding central nervous system lesions. The ones that most often prompt neurosurgical consideration are acute necrotizing encephalitis and acute hemorrhagic leukoencephalitis. These entities as well as certain aspects of other viral diseases having special neurosurgical significance are discussed in this chapter.

ETIOLOGY AND PATHOLOGY

Acute encephalitis (encephalomyelitis) results from direct invasion of the central nervous system and its membranes by a host of well-known viruses. Except for the rabies virus, probably none is neurotropic in the sense of having special affinity for neurons. Others such as herpes and mumps viruses cause relatively benign illnesses that may become severe when the central nervous system is involved. Encephalitis can also develop as an aftermath of exanthematous viral diseases, prophylactic inoculations, or obscure illnesses of probable viral origin, and has been variously called postinfectious, parainfectious, or allergic. Although the latter term implies a known cause, the pathogenesis of this condition remains in question.

The histopathological changes of these two categories of encephalitis oftentimes overlap because of the similarities of neural tissue response to a variety of insults. There are, however, certain features of possible differential value. Viral encephalitis may produce diffuse edema (acute toxic encephalopathy), mild to severe meningeal inflammation, swelling or disintegration of cortical neurons, glial nodule formation, perivascular inflammation in cortex and white matter, perivascular demyelination, fibrin-oid changes in the walls of capillaries and blood vessels, and focal cortical or white matter hemorrhages.* Acute necrotizing encephalitis is usually caused by herpes simplex virus, type 1. Electron microscopic studies of tissues from such cases may show herpes simplex virus particles. If the disease progresses, focal coalesence of areas of edema, necrosis and hemorrhage may produce mass effects sufficient to require neurosurgical attention.[6,8,11,30-32]

The pathological changes of postinfectious encephalitis, of which hemorrhagic leukoencephalitis is an example, usually affect white matter more than gray. Generalized edema, widespread focal inflammatory changes, perivascular inflammation, demyelination, and hemorrhages, occurring alone or in combination, may be found in any portion of the central nervous system, though the cerebral hemispheres are usually most severely involved. Sometimes these lesions are centered predominantly in centrum ovale and subcortical white matter of one hemisphere, causing massive shifts of intracranial structures. Secondary pathological changes incident to hemisphere and axial displacements may ensue as with other large intracranial masses.

SYMPTOMS AND SIGNS

A differentiation of viral encephalitides on clinical grounds alone is almost impossible without laboratory assistance. Most begin with malaise, mild fever, myalgia, and respiratory or gastrointestinal symptoms. Neurological symptoms appear either immediately, or after a brief period of improvement. In some, rapid neurological

---

* See references 4, 7, 10, 17, 43, 48.

W. S. COXE

deterioration accompanied by high fever evolves within 24 to 48 hours, leading to death. More commonly, a slower progression is the case, with such symptoms as headache, stiff neck, photophobia, chills, fever, nausea, and vomiting ushering in more serious symptoms of restlessness, confusion, hallucinations, lethargy, and coma. However, contrasting states of marked confusion and memory loss in otherwise alert patients may also be characteristic of viral encephalitis. Focal or generalized seizures are a frequent accompaniment, and only rarely does papilledema develop. Signs of diffuse or multifocal cerebral hemisphere dysfunction usually predominate, but facial masking, cranial nerve paresis, dysarthria, dysphagia, and ataxia may signify simultaneous involvement of brain stem and cerebellum. In this connection it is important to remember that symptoms of midbrain decompensation do not necessarily indicate viral involvement of the brain stem, but may be secondary to compression from transtentorial herniation. Occasionally encephalitis causes primary cerebellar or brain stem syndromes.* In the former, children and young adults are more frequently affected, the symptoms varying from mild to severe ataxia and dysmetria without clinical or x-ray evidence of increased intracranial pressure. Brain stem encephalitis, also rare, produces a spectrum of symptoms ranging from mild vertigo and cranial nerve palsy to states of coma associated with long-tract signs.

Some nervous system diseases with a subacute or chronic course have come to be recognized as viral infections.[42,48] As an example, there is little doubt that measles virus or a "measles-like" virus is the cause of subacute sclerosing panencephalitis.[1,25,35,41,47] This disease occurs most frequently in young people and follows an insidious course of intellectual and personality deterioration eventually ending with hypertonus and coma. Convulsions, hemiparesis, and visual disturbances may occur during the course of the disease, requiring consideration of brain tumor as a possible cause.

Primary viral myelitis is less common with the diminished incidence of poliomye-

litis, but other viruses can produce a similar neurological picture, one not usually confused with surgical disorders.[7,40] On the other hand, the syndromes of acute transverse myelitis following exanthematous infections, vaccinations, or mild respiratory infections are more troublesome diagnostic problems. The thoracic cord is affected most frequently, symptoms appearing rapidly, with mild muscular aching, fever, malaise, paresthesias in the lower extremities, and girdle sensations, progressing rapidly to paraparesis. Cord lesions may become complete, but islands of sensation usually persist below a sharp dermatomal level. When the syndrome is one of ascending myelitis it may be difficult to distinguish from ascending polyneuritis (polyradiculopathy, Guillain-Barré syndrome). In the latter conditions, progression of symptoms is slower, bladder and bowel functions are often spared, and sensory disturbances are much less severe.

DIFFERENTIAL DIAGNOSIS

The clinical manifestations of viral and postinfectious encephalitis can simulate a number of illnesses including meningitis (bacterial, tuberculous, or fungal), parasitic diseases, meningeal carcinomatosis, occlusive vascular disease (either arterial or venous), poisoning, metabolic disorders, seizure disorders, benign intracranial hypertension, Behçet's syndrome, and psychiatric illness. For our purpose it is of importance to recognize that on rare occasions certain encephalitides can also mimic brain abscess, tumor, and hemorrhage, and that even with the help of a variety of diagnostic aids, a clear differentiation may not be possible without resorting to operative exploration and biopsy. With brain abscess, progression of symptoms is usually not so rapid unless rupture into the subarachnoid space or ventricle occurs. Fever, often present at the inception of abscess formation, is frequently absent as signs of increased intracranial pressure and focal neurological symptoms develop. With viral infections, fever is common, often persistent and may be associated with more diffuse neurological disturbance. Subdural empyema can be easily confused with viral illnesses, since the course may be characterized by headache, seizures, high

---

* See references 4, 9, 14, 23, 33, 34, 45.

fever, and delirium. The spinal fluid findings with brain abscess and viral encephalitis are often identical, showing slight monocytic response and increased protein and normal sugar content. Rupture of an abscess into spinal fluid pathways, however, usually provokes a much higher cell count of polymorphonuclear type and chemical changes of bacterial meningitis.

Brain tumors rarely account for diagnostic confusion. Necrosis, swelling, or hemorrhage within gliomas of the corpus callosum or hypothalamus may engender the rapid appearance of confusion, memory impairment, lethargy, delirium, tremulousness, autonomic instability, and other signs suggesting a diffuse process. Similar changes within temporal lobe tumors may mimic features observed in herpes simplex encephalitis, which commonly involves temporal and rhinencephalic structures. Some cystic or metastatic tumors produce meningeal reactions identical with encephalitis and present a special problem when the clinical picture is not typical of tumor. Cerebellar tumors in children might also be confused with acute cerebellar ataxia of childhood, a syndrome caused by a number of viral infections (polio, varicella, ECHO type 9, infectious mononucleosis).[12,23,33,34] The rapidity of onset, absence of signs of increased intracranial pressure, normal skull films, the presence of opsoclonic eye movements, and characteristic spinal fluid changes of viral encephalitis would, however, be unusual for most tumors presenting in this region.[12,45] With increasing access to computed tomographic scanning, the question of tumor versus encephalitis may be answered quickly and without risk to the patient. If the technique is available, more hazardous diagnostic procedures may be avoided.

Intracranial hemorrhages, either subarachnoid or intracerebral, are usually signaled by sudden headache and meningismus or catastrophic neurological deficit in previously normal individuals, and are rarely mistaken for encephalitis. Some types of encephalitis produce bloody spinal fluid and rapidly progressive symptoms of diffuse or focal cerebral dysfunction, but the number of red cells is usually much lower and the onset less dramatic. Posttraumatic hemorrhages are ordinarily recognized from historical data or clinical features uncommon to infections. Again a CT scan may prove quite helpful, but if there is any doubt about the diagnosis, cerebral angiography should be performed.

Spinal cord syndromes of viral or parainfectious origin offer equally pressing diagnostic problems, the differential categories being the same: infectious, neoplastic, and vascular. Spinal epidural abscess requires early diagnosis since surgical decompression is necessary to prevent irreparable cord damage.[3] Spinal rigidity and tenderness to pressure or percussion, discovery of possible sources of infection, increased white blood count, and fever suggest spinal suppuration rather than myelitis from other causes. Patients with spinal canal tumors usually have prolonged histories and insidiously progressive neurological symptoms, oftentimes resulting in delayed discovery. Viral diseases would, therefore, hardly be considered among possible diagnoses when the patient reaches the stage of neurosurgical consultation, but review of the history may indicate that some early symptoms were regarded as sequelae of viral illnesses. This is particularly true of intramedullary tumors of childhood in which a paretic or poorly developed extremity was ascribed to "old poliomyelitis." Cord compression from metastatic tumors or lymphomas may appear rapidly, though at a rate of development hardly comparable to that of inflammatory myelitis. The absence of prodromal symptoms or fever, and the presence of pain on movement or percussion of the back would also suggest tumor rather than myelitis.

Certain vascular diseases of the spinal cord are also sources of diagnostic confusion.[40] Occlusion of the anterior spinal artery causes a variety of neurological deficits depending upon the level of occlusion and variations in the collateral circulation. The illness may appear abruptly or progress over a period of several days. Pain, often the presenting symptom, may be intense, with a radicular quality at or near the area of maximal cord involvement, or diffusely distributed, particularly over the lower body areas. The pattern of sensory loss is variable, but unlike myelitis, dissociated sensory changes usually occur with loss of pain and temperature sense and preservation of posterior column function. Motor paresis may be complete or partial. These features, plus the absence of fever, signs of brain stem or cerebral involvement, and lack of pleocytosis in spinal fluid, are useful differential points.

Syndromes incident to rupture of vascular anomalies of the cord are too varied to warrant detailed consideration here and are discussed in the section on vascular anomalies of the cord. Again, the outstanding features are abrupt onset, back pain with either radicular or diffuse distribution, and changing neurological function without evidence of diffuse disease or infection. If rupture occurs in the subarachnoid space, spinal fluid findings will clearly suggest the cause.

DIAGNOSTIC STUDIES

Routine laboratory tests are of little aid in arriving at specific diagnoses either for diseases of viral origin or the surgical conditions considered as diagnostic possibilities. The white blood count may be normal or elevated to 25,000 or 30,000 in the acute phase of both viral and allergic encephalitis, but similar levels may be attained with acute bacterial infections, brain abscess, subdural empyema, and occasionally subarachnoid hemorrhage. The sedimentation rate is usually elevated in all. Urinalysis is usually normal though proteinuria and microscopic hematuria are sometimes found with acute hemorrhagic leukoencephalitis. Spinal fluid examination usually shows pleocytosis of from 20 to several hundred lymphocytes, normal to increased protein, and normal sugar content. Significant variation from these characteristic values can occur, leading to doubts of viral etiology. Cell count may rise well above 1000 per cubic millimeter, and glucose fall as low as 20 mg per 100 ml.[44] Protein levels above 200 mg per 100 ml are suggestive of polyneuritis or a compressive cord lesion. Xanthochromia and a significant number of red cells may be found with herpes simplex or acute hemorrhagic leukoencephalitis, bringing into consideration more common causes of subarachnoid hemorrhage. Spinal fluid pressure is usually normal, but may be high, particularly in those with evidence of expanding lesions. In addition to these studies, attempts should be made to isolate virus from blood and spinal fluid. If facilities are not immediately available for handling specimens, they should be frozen, preferably at $-20°$ C, for shipment to the proper laboratory. Acute phase and convalescent sera should be obtained, frozen, and subjected to appropriate procedures for antibody detection (e.g., neutralization tests, complement fixation, fluorescent antibody staining). Serological tests are of limited value in the acutely ill patient, since the tests rely on the demonstration of a rise in antibody titers from the acute to the convalescent stage. Moreover, it should be noted that false negative results may prove misleading. Of additional interest in laboratory differentiation of bacterial from viral infections is the determination of circadian periodicity of blood amino acids. It has been shown that the well-defined periodicity normally present in man is reversed with viral infections. In the presence of bacterial infections, the absolute concentrations of amino acids may be altered, but circadian periodicity generally remains undisturbed.[16]

Electroencephalography can be of value when slow high-voltage activity is present in noncomatose patients, and particularly if extreme slowing is present in the alert patient with acute encephalitis.[7,10,18] Focal slowing may occur with viral infections, but also should heighten suspicion of other focal processes. Isotopic brain scans can show focal uptake in encephalitis and therefore have little value in differential diagnosis. If uptake is extraordinarily heavy, brain abscess or tumor is a more likely possibility.

Encephalitic processes may cause evidence of diffuse unilateral swelling or specific lobar involvement, findings identical to those in a number of conditions that require operative intervention. Echoencephalography is helpful in detecting midline brain shifts, but nothing else. Before the advent of computed tomography (CT), cerebral angiography used to be the most accurate method of defining the locus of mass effect, the extent of cerebral shift, and in some instances the nature of the lesion itself. Tumor was suspected when the angiogram demonstrated a diffuse area of hyperemia with increased brain stain or "blush" together with an early vein. Where computed tomography is available it is usually performed prior to angiography. Besides demonstrating a mass effect, when this is present, the tomogram shows a decrease in density of the brain parenchyma, which is presumed to represent edema, and in some cases may show contrast enhancement. Because of the noninvasiveness of the technique it can be repeated at short intervals when required. This is most helpful in, for example, the diagnosis of herpes encephalitis when a significant change in the appearance of the lesion over a short period of time can be demonstrated. When the lesions are multifocal, computed tomography may show multiple or bilateral areas of decreased density (Fig. 111–1). It has been reported, however, that diffuse brain swelling may be misleading because of the absence of ventricular displacement, and also because of the occasional absence of any alteration in brain density on the tomogram. In these cases, one may be alerted when the lateral ventricles are small or barely visualized. Pneumoventriculography provides a valuable but less desirable method of study for several reasons. The maneuvers required are awkward to perform upon the acutely ill and uncooperative patient, and might cause additional aggravation of his condition. Since the ventricles may be displaced and smaller than normal, direct ventricular puncture may prove difficult and hazardous if multiple needle passes are required. Since the same information is obtained by the noninvasive technique of computed tomography, pneumoventriculography should not be considered in the diagnosis of herpes encephalitis where CT is available.

Positive contrast myelography offers the

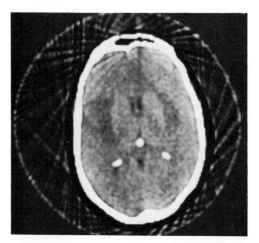

Figure 111–1 Computed tomographic scan in a patient with herpes encephalitis. There are bilateral areas of decreased density in the deep part of both temporal lobes extending into the external capsules. The left is larger than the right, causing a slight shift of the third ventricle.

best method for differentiation of compressive cord lesions from transverse myelitis of viral, postinfectious, or vascular occlusive cause, though it should be kept in mind that manometric and contrast media blocks are sometimes found in myelopathy of viral origin.[36] Myelography will often disclose vessel patterns of arteriovenous anomalies, particularly if the supine position is always included during the study. Selective aortography with subtraction techniques should also be used when this diagnosis is suspected to delineate feeding vessels as well as the disposition of the anomaly itself.

CONDITIONS SOMETIMES REQUIRING OPERATIVE MANAGEMENT

At present there are no specific antiviral medications of proved therapeutic value for encephalitis. For patients developing signs of increased intracranial pressure, steroid hormones and dehydrating agents may be useful adjuncts to combat edema and inflammation. On the other hand, steroids possibly can hasten the spread of viral infection and must be used with caution when the cause of the encephalitis is not clear.

Operations are rarely performed upon patients in whom encephalitis is considered as a primary diagnosis, but rather are done when more common surgical problems are suspected. As a result, their main value resides in diagnostic biopsy and occasionally therapeutic decompression for certain patients with acute hemorrhagic leukoencephalitis and acute necrotizing (herpes simplex) encephalitis. The latter disease affects any age group, but when older children and adults are stricken, one side of the brain is frequently more involved, producing symptoms and x-ray findings characteristic of an expanding hemispheric mass process most often centered within temporal lobe and other rhinencephalic areas.* In newborns and infants, diffuse destruction is common and may be but one part of widespread systemic infection. The course is acute and rapid, often suggesting hemorrhage or fulminant infection. Most patients either die within a few days or weeks, or are left with serious residual neurological

---

* See references 6, 8, 11, 15, 30, 31.

deficit regardless of any therapeutic measures. Pathological study may show type A Cowdy intranuclear inclusions in areas of edema, but these may be found with other viral infections. The best laboratory means of diagnosis are isolation of virus from brain or spinal fluid and demonstration of specific antigen in central nervous system cells by immunofluorescence.[28] Since viruses are seldom isolated from the spinal fluid, brain biopsy specimens may prove of great value. Elevation of antibody titer is also helpful diagnostically, a fourfold or greater rise being sufficient to establish diagnosis for most viral infections. With herpes simplex encephalitis, however, such an elevation is not necessarily diagnostic since it may only represent reactivation of a latent herpes infection unrelated to coexistent nervous system disease.[47] Moreover, cases of herpes simplex encephalitis have been described with less than a fourfold rise of antibody titer. Also, several cases of recurrent herpes encephalitis have been reported that suggest reactivation of a latent herpes infection, though serological tests on these patients have been inconclusive.[37]

Even when acute necrotizing encephalitis is suspected, removal of areas of hemorrhage and necrosis may be lifesaving if irreversible brain stem compression seems imminent. Prompt histological study of the tissues removed should be done and other specimens rapidly frozen and prepared for fluorescent antibody staining for virus antigen and bound human antibody. Unfrozen tissue or spinal fluid should be inoculated into established cell cultures. If the diagnosis of herpes can be made early, consideration should be given to the use of antiviral agents. Several years ago iododeoxyuridine was tried, but with little success on herpes encephalitis. This agent received most attention for creating involvement corneal epithelial rather than deeper tissues. Cytosine arabinoside has been found effective in tissue culture and experimental keratitis. Results in human encephalitis remain inconclusive, and its immunosuppressive complications may outweigh any virocidal effect.[19,31] The most promising antiviral drug being tried for herpes encephalitis at present is adenosine arabinoside. It must be emphasized that before the drug can be administered, tissue confirmation of herpes infection must be obtained. This requires biopsy early in the course rather than after severe neurological deterioration has occurred. A recent placebo-controlled study in 28 biopsy-proved cases supports the efficacy of the drug in patients suspected of having type 1 herpes simplex encephalitis. It is suggested that this treatment be started after biopsy but before virological confirmation is obtained, since therapy may then be terminated in those who do not prove to have herpes encephalitis.[43a]

Hemorrhagic leukoencephalitis, usually considered of postinfectious etiology, is an equally acute disease characterized by edema, small hemorrhages, necrosis, and perivascular demyelination within white matter. Since these changes are usually widespread, involving both cerebral hemispheres and other portions of the central nervous system, the symptom complex does not usually suggest a surgical disorder. However, for the few patients who develop severe unilateral hemispheric signs leading to operative intervention, the management is similar to that described for acute necrotizing encephalitis. Contrast studies may show more generalized hemispheric swelling, similar in many respects to diffusely infiltrating gliomas, or multiple metastatic lesions, findings which make a decision for operative intervention less sure. Nevertheless, a generous internal decompression centered in the anterior frontal white matter or in combination with partial temporal lobe resection and bony decompression, may help tide some patients through the acute phase of the disease. The texture of brain tissue encountered can either be soft, edematous, and easily suctioned, or somewhat firm and tough, reminiscent of an infiltrating glioma. Concomitant administration of dehydrating agents and large doses of steroids has been used during and after operative intervention. A few patients have recovered, but others have succumbed within a few days or months despite all medical and surgical measures.[13,29,32] It is also likely that there are many patients with this condition who have a less malignant course and recover spontaneously without benefit of tissue diagnosis.

A few additional sequelae of viral infections may have surgical implications. Chronic forms of encephalitis may be responsible for epileptogenic foci found in specimens removed surgically in treatment of focal seizures.[2,20] Though proof of active viral infection in these cases is lacking, histological changes are typical of chronic encephalitis of known viral etiology. Patients having these findings are likely to show clinical evidence of more widespread and progressive neurological deterioration than patients with epilepsy from other causes.

Enlargement of ventricles resulting from widespread cerebral damage follows some episodes of encephalitis, particularly type 2 herpes simplex infections in the newborn. Poor circulation of cerebrospinal fluid over the cerebral convexity may be demonstrable by pneumoencephalography and radioiodinated serum albumin cisternography, findings similar to other forms of cummunicating hydrocephalus, though the reasons for this are not clear. Thus far, shunt operations have had no beneficial effect upon a few cases so treated.

Aqueductal stenosis in childhood and adolescence may also result from mumps encephalitis with associated ependymitis. The lesion has been produced experimentally and presumably may be the cause in some patients presenting with this diagnosis in later life. These patients, of course, may derive great benefit from cerebrospinal fluid diversion.

For patients with acute transverse myelitis, laminectomy is probably justifiable in the rare event that myelographic obstruction is demonstrated. Decompression carried out to exclude the possibility of a mass lesion could have a beneficial effect.

REFERENCES

1. Adams, J. M., Baird, C., and Filloy, L.: Inclusion bodies in measles encephalitis. J.A.M.A., 195:290–298, 1966.
2. Aguilar, M. J., and Rasmussen, T.: Role of encephalitis in pathogenesis of epilepsy. Arch. Neurol., 2:663–676, 1960.
3. Altrocchi, P. H.: Acute spinal epidural abscess vs. acute transverse myelopathy. Arch. Neurol., 9:17–25, 1963.
4. Baker, A. B.:Viral encephalitis. In Baker, A. B., ed.: Clinical Neurology. 2nd Ed. New York, Hoeber Medical Division, Harper & Row, 1962, vol. 2, pp. 811–858.
5. Baker, A. B.: Secondary forms of encephalitis. In Baker, A. B., ed.: Clinical Neurology. 2nd Ed. New York, Hoeber Medical Division, Harper & Row, 1962, vol. 2, pp. 859–927.
6. Bennett, D. R., ZuRhein, G. M., and Roberts, T. S.: Acute necrotizing encephalitis. Arch. Neurol., 6:96–113, 1962.
7. Berg, L. F.: Viral and post viral encephalomyelitis: A survey with neurosurgical orientation. Clin. Neurosurg., 14:101–122, 1967.
8. Bergouignan, B., Julien, J., Vital, C., and Duvert, M.: Acute necrotizing encephalitis: Electron microscopic visualization of herpes virus. Presse Méd., 76:709–714, 1968.
9. Bickerstaff, E. R.: Brain-stem encephalitis. Brit. Med. J., 1:1384–1387, 1957.
10. van Bogaert, L., Radermecker, J., Hozay, J., and Lowenthal, A., eds.: Encephalitides: Proceedings of a Symposium on the Neuropathology, Electroencephalography and Biochemistry of Encephalitides. Amsterdam, Elsevier Pub. Co., 1961.
11. Carmon, A., Behar, A., and Beller, A. J.: Acute necrotizing hemorrhagic encephalitis presenting clinically as a space-occupying lesion. J. Neurol. Sci., 2:328–343, 1965.
12. Cogan, D. G.: Ocular dysmetria; flutter-like oscillations of the eyes and opsoclonus. A.M.A. Arch. Ophthal., 51:318–335, 1954.
13. Coxe, W. S., and Luse, S. A.: Acute hemorrhagic leukoencephalitis. J. Neurosurg., 20:584–596, 1963.
14. Curnen, E. C., and Chamberlin, H. R.: Acute cerebellar ataxia associated with poliovirus infection. Yale J. Biol. Med., 34:219–233, 1961–1962.
15. Dodge, P. R., and Cure, C. W.: Acute necrotizing encephalitis with intranuclear cellular inclusions. A non-fatal case of probable herpetic etiology diagnosed by biopsy. New. Eng. J. Med., 255:849–853, 1956.
16. Feigin, R. D.: Blood and urine amino acid aberrations. Physiologic and pathological changes in patients without inborn errors of amino acid metabolism. Amer. J. Dis. Child., 117:24–47, 1969.
17. Fields, W. S., and Blattner, R. J.: Viral Encephalitis. Springfield, Ill., Charles C Thomas, 1958.
18. Gibbs, F. A., Gibbs, E. L., Spies, H. W., and Carpenter, P. R.: Common types of childhood encephalitis: Electroencephalographic and clinical relationships. Arch. Neurol., 10:1–11, 1964.
19. Gilout, D. M., Johnson, M. T., Luby, J. P., and Sanford, J. P.: Herpes virus hominis type 1 encephalitis treated with cytarabine, an unresolved problem in encephalitis. Medicine, 32:331–338, 1973.
20. Gupta, P. C., Roy, S., and Tandon, P. N.: Progressive epilepsy due to chronic persistent encephalitis. Report of four cases. J. Neurol. Sci., 22:105–120, 1974.
21. Harland, W. A., Adams, J. H., and McSeveney, D.: Herpes simplex particles in acute necrotizing encephalitis. Lancet, 2:581–582, 1967.
22. Herndon, R. M., Johnson, R. T., Davis, L. E., and Descalzi, L. R.: Ependymitis in mumps virus meningitis. Electron microscopic studies of cerebrospinal fluid. Arch. Neurol., 30:475–479, 1974.
23. Hoyne, R. M.: Involvement of the CNS in infectious mononucleosis. Report of a case with ataxia and nystagmus. Arch. Neurol. Psychiat., 63:606–610, 1950.
24. Itabashi, H. H., Bass, D. M., and McCulloch, J. R.: Inclusion body of acute inclusion encephalitis. Arch. Neurol., 14:493–505, 1966.
25. Jabbour, J. T., Garcia, J. H., Lemmi, H., Gag-

land, J., Duenas, D. A., and Sever, J. L.: Subacute sclerosing panencephalitis. A multidisciplinary study of eight cases. J.A.M.A., 207:2248–2254, 1969.

26. Johnson, R. T.: The pathogenesis of herpes viral encephalitis. J. Exp. Med., 119:343–356, 1964.

27. Johnson, R. T.: Virus invasion of the central nervous system. Amer. J. Path., 46:929–943, 1965.

28. Johnson, R. T., Olson, L. C., and Buescher, E. L.: Herpes simplex virus infections of nervous system. Problems in laboratory diagnosis. Arch. Neurol., 18:260–264, 1968.

29. Litel, G., and Ehni, G.: Acute hemorrhagic encephalitis—treatment with corticosteroids and dehydrating agents. J. Neurosurg., 33:445–452, 1970.

30. MacCallum, F. O., Potter, J. M., and Edwards, D. H.: Early diagnosis of herpes simplex encephalitis by brain biopsy. Lancet, 2:322–334, 1964.

31. Marshall, W. J. S.: Herpes simplex encephalitis treated with idoxuridine and external decompression. Lancet, 2:579–580, 1967.

32. Martins, A. N., Kempe, L. G., and Hayes, G. J.: Acute hemorrhagic leucoencephalitis (Hurst) with a concurrent primary herpes simplex infection. J. Neurol. Neurosurg. Psychiat., 27:493–501, 1964.

33. Marzetti, G., and Midulla, M.: Acute cerebellar ataxia associated with ECHO type 6 infection in two children. Acta Paediat. Scand., 56:547–551, 1967.

34. McAllister, R. M., Hummeler, K., and Coriele, L. L.: Acute cerebellar ataxia. Report of a case with isolation of type 9 ECHO virus from cerebrospinal fluid. New Eng. J. Med., 261:1159–1162, 1959.

35. Meulen, V. ter, Katz, M., and Müller, D.: Subacute sclerosing panencephalitis. A review. Curr. Top. Microbiol. Immun., 57:1–38, 1972.

36. Miller, J. D., and Ross, C. A. C.: Encephalitis: Four year survey. Lancet, 1:1121–1126, 1968.

37. Milstein, J. M., and Biggs, H. E.: Recurrent encephalitis with elevated titers for herpes simplex. Arch. Neurol., 34:434–436, 1977.

38. Olson, L. C., Buescher, E. L., Artenstein, M. S.,
and Parkman, P. D.: Herpes virus infections of the human central nervous system. New Eng. J. Med., 227:1271–1277, 1967.

39. Parker, J. D., and Anderson, W. B.: Myelitis simulating spinal cord tumor Amer. J. Roentgen., 95:942–946, 1965.

40. Plum, F.: Myelitis and myelopathy. In Baker, A. B., ed.: Clinical Neurology. 2nd Ed. New York, Hoeber Medical Division, Harper & Row, 1962, pp. 1679–1742.

41. Resnick, J. S., Engel, W. K., and Sever, J. L.: Subacute sclerosing panencephalitis: Spontaneous improvement in patient with elevated measles antibody in blood and cerebrospinal fluid. New Eng. J. Med., 279:126–129, 1968.

42. Schwerdt, P. R., Schwerdt, C. E., Silverman, L., and Rubinstein, L. J.: Virions associated with progressive multifocal leukoencephalopathy. Virology, 29:511–514, 1966.

43. Waksman, B. H., and Adams, R. D.: Infectious leukoencephalitis. J. Neuropath. Exp. Neurol., 21:491–518, 1962.

43a. Whitley, R. J., Soong, S. J., Dolin, R., Galasso, G. J., Ch'ien, L. T., Alford, C. A., and the Collaborative Study Group: Adenine arabinoside therapy of biopsy-proved herpes simplex encephalitis: National Institute of Allergy and Infectious Disease collaborative antiviral study. New Eng. J. Med., 297:289–294, 1977.

44. Wilfert, C. M.: Mumps meningoencephalitis with low cerebrospinal-fluid glucose, prolonged pleocytosis and elevation of protein. New Eng. J. Med., 280:855–859, 1969.

45. Winkler, G. F., Sweeney, V. R., Baringer, J. R., and Cogan, D. G.: An acute syndrome of ocular oscillations and truncal ataxia. Trans. Amer. Neurol. Ass., 91:96–99, 1966.

46. Wooley, C. F.: Intracranial hypertension associated with recovery of a Coxsackie virus from CSF. Neurology, 10:572–574, 1960.

47. Zeman, W., and Kolar, O.: Reflections on the etiology and pathogenesis of subacute sclerosing panencephalitis. Neurology, 18:1–7, 1968.

48. Zimmerman, H. M.: Infections of the nervous system. Res. Publ. Ass. Nerv. Ment. Dis., XLIV. Baltimore, Md., Williams & Wilkins Co., 1968.

112

PARASITIC AND FUNGAL DISEASES OF THE CENTRAL NERVOUS SYSTEM

The parasitic and fungal diseases of the central nervous system are of increasing importance in the field of neurological surgery. They are being diagnosed with increasing frequency and represent what many consider to be the most common disease entities in the world, presenting a health problem of enormous international medical, social, and economic significance. It is estimated that they, in conjunction with the protozoan diseases, may infect as many as four to six hundred million people at any given time.[341] Of those infected, an estimated three million die annually. International travel has changed the traditional epidemiological patterns of diseases once thought to be exclusively restricted to endemic areas. Additionally, advances in cancer chemotherapy and organ transplantation have added new diagnostic challenges in patients whose immune responses are compromised. Fortunately, increased awareness and better diagnostic methods have improved the once bleak prognosis of many of these diseases.

Parasitic and fungal diseases manifest themselves primarily in the pulmonary and gastrointestinal systems. Some of them—leishmaniasis, malaria, pneumocystosis, diphyllobothrium infections, streptomycosis—so rarely come to the attention of the neurosurgeon that they do not warrant discussion in this chapter. Involvement of the central nervous system by any of them without systemic involvement elsewhere is uncommon. Conversely, the onset of neu-rological dysfunction in patients with known parasitic or fungal diseases should suggest the possibility of dissemination to the central nervous system. Infection by protozoan, parasitic, and fungal organisms should be a routine consideration in the differential diagnosis of meningitis and brain abscess as well as in infections of the spinal axis.

Parasitic disease implies a host-organism relationship, the criteria of which are fulfilled by many organisms, including the bacteria, viruses, and rickettsiae. Historically, however, "parasitic disease" usually has been taken to mean those infections due to protozoa and helminths. The same confusion applies to the classification of the fungal diseases. Such entities as actinomycosis and nocardiosis, although traditionally grouped with the fungal diseases, actually have bacteria as their causative agents.

Fungi are common in the environment, but relatively few are pathogenic. An important characteristic of those that are pathogenic is their dimorphism, or ability to assume two different forms in vivo under different environmental conditions, thus enhancing the pathogenicity of the organism. Mycotic diseases generally are not transmitted from one person to another, nor are they contagious from animal to man. Epidemics commonly arise from an environmental source, and the mechanism of inoculation is often inhalation—an important public health consideration. A few

F. A. ROWE, J. R. YOUMANS, H. J. LEE, AND F. CABIESES

of the entities—such as *Candida albicans* and *Actinomyces israeli,* which are normal flora of the mouth or gastrointestinal tract —are endogenous and capable of producing autoinfection under appropriate circumstances.

AMEBIASIS

Amebiasis is a parasitic disease caused by infection with *Entamoeba histolytica.* It primarily involves the gastrointestinal tract, and the clinical symptoms are usually limited to this area. The intestinal form of the disease may produce serious extraintestinal complications, however, one of which is infection of the central nervous system. Cerebral amebiasis due to *E. histolytica* should not be confused with primary amebic meningoencephalitis, a disease caused by any of several species of free-living amebae.

While these two entities appear to be relatively similar in etiology, they differ in almost all other fundamental aspects, including treatment and prognosis. Differential diagnosis is critical.

Epidemiology

It is estimated that roughly 10 per cent of the world's population may harbor *E. histolytica.*[317] Estimates of infection rates vary considerably from country to country and within certain subpopulations. The rate in the United States has been estimated at between 1 and 5 per cent.[263] Owing to improvement of public health measures and more reliable laboratory identification methods, however, these estimates have been steadily revised downward over the past 20 years, reflecting the steadily decreasing percentage of the general population that is now infected with *E. histolytica.*[213] Endemic foci still exist in certain sections of the country, however, particularly among such subpopulations as institutionalized patients, and within these particular groups infection rates may be considerably higher.

Despite the relatively common occurrence of hepatopulmonary and intestinal forms of the disease, cases of cerebral amebiasis are rather rare. Orbison has esti-

mated that approximately 1 per cent of all symptomatic cases of amebiasis eventually develop brain abscess.[263] The highest reported incidence to date is in Mexico, where cerebral involvement was found in 17 of 210 documented cases of amebiasis (an incidence of 8.1 per cent).[228] Some investigators have computed incidence rates for cerebral involvement in terms of those cases also manifesting hepatic or pulmonary involvement or both.[77,147,263] This extrapolation, although biased, is quite reasonable, since it is from this group that most if not all cases of cerebral amebiasis originate. There have been reports of amebic brain abscess for which no apparent focus of antecedent disease could be found, but this obviously does not preclude the possibility that such a focus would either be small enough to be missed at autopsy or would heal sufficiently to prevent unequivocal histopathological confirmation.[112,263]

Several species of amebae are capable of infecting man, but of these parasitic species only *E. histolytica* is considered pathogenic.[317] The organism exists in two primary forms: the cystic form and the trophozoite.[11,321] The cystic form is responsible for maintaining the organism outside the gastrointestinal tract. It resists most environmental changes and is the form most frequently responsible for transmission of the disease.[11,317,321] The trophozoite is motile and invasive, but only rarely serves as the infecting vector.

Two important points concerning the epidemiological features of the disease should be noted. First, transmission nearly always requires ingestion of the cystic form of the organism.[321] Second, hygienic conditions, which usually reflect the level of economic development within an endemic area, dictate prevalence of the disease.[54,321]

Direct human to human spread is possible but, as noted previously, represents an infrequent mode of transmission.

The cerebral form of the disease, like most other forms, is seen in nearly every age group. There appears to be no racial predominance not explained by environmental or geographic factors. Adult males are more likely to develop the more severe hepatic and intestinal forms of the disease as well as amebic brain abscess.[359] No reason other than possible greater occupational exposure has been postulated.

Pathogenesis

The life cycle of *Entamoeba histolytica* is extremely complex and only rarely involves the central nervous system. Further, cerebral amebiasis almost never exists in the absence of antecedent disease.[112,228,263]

From its primary focus in the gastrointestinal tract the organism is hematogenously disseminated to other sites including the liver and lung. Cerebral amebiasis is usually secondary to spread from these "primary" sites.[112,228] The organisms are seeded to the central nervous system and in all likelihood establish abscesses by means of pathophysiological mechanisms that are similar to those seen in hepatopulmonary forms of the disease. The underlying mechanism involves an embolic and thrombotic process causing occlusion, infarction, and eventual neurolysis. The neurolytic process is due not only to the lytic enzymes released by the amebae themselves but also to those released by the host in response to the destructive process.[11,116] It is somewhat unusual in that, at least initially, it appears to occur in the absence of any inflammatory reaction.

The organism gains access to the central nervous system by one of two possible routes. The first is through the arteries, a route that is suggested because the lesions are multiple, are frequently in the distribution of the middle cerebral artery, and often follow open drainage procedures utilized in treating hepatopulmonary forms of the disease.[112,228,263] A second route of access is Batson's plexus, which would explain the apparent absence of extraintestinal primary lesions in cases of apparently primary cerebral disease. Both mechanisms are reasonable, and in all probability both are utilized, although the latter to a significantly lesser degree.

The pathological process that will ultimately result in the formation of cerebral abscesses is initiated by thrombosis of the vessels to and subsequent infarction of the affected area. Initially, there is little evidence of an inflammatory reaction; reactive gliosis is virtually absent, and the borders of the lesion are poorly defined. The lesions may appear as confluent hemorrhagic areas. The term "acute abscess," then, characterizes the histopathological status of the brain tissue prior to necrosis and cavitation following infarction of the cortex.

Eventually, however, necrosis and cavitation do take place. The necrosis resembles the necrotic liquefaction of hepatic lesions. Progression to chronic stages of abscess formation takes place over a variable period of time during which the abscess may form a thin fibrous wall. The capsule structure seldom becomes as extensive as that of a bacterial abscess but nevertheless is of a consistency that is amenable to operative removal. Grossly, the structure closely resembles other types of abscess. The tissue adjacent to the lesion may manifest moderate to severe cerebral edema. The abscesses are usually multiple and may be multilocular. They are most frequently located in the frontal lobes and basal ganglia.[226] Brain stem and cerebellar lesions are rare.[112] In many cases, particularly those in which the abscess is located over the convexity, the accompanying meningitis may be quite significant from both the clinical and the pathological standpoint. The meningitis, however, is not characterized by any unique pathological features that would aid in the diagnosis. The cellular response initially consists predominantly of polymorphonuclear cells, but with time lymphocytes and mononuclear cells predominate.

The amebae themselves, if present, are most often located at the periphery of the lesions. They are seldom observed in the cerebrospinal fluid unless rupture into the ventricular system has occurred.[112]

Clinical Manifestations

Cerebral amebiasis almost invariably presents as a late complication of the disease. The time lapse between the appearance of gastrointestinal or pulmonary symptoms and neurological symptoms may be quite long—so long, in fact, that rarely the patients may be otherwise clinically asymptomatic when the neurological symptoms become evident. In the more common clinical presentation, however, the patient develops dysentery and subsequently hepatic abscess. Following a variable incubation period, he experiences the onset of neurological symptoms ranging from severe headache to sudden hemiplegia. As with all forms of brain abscess, the range and extent of the deficits depend upon location of the lesion. Severe headache refractory to most analgesics is common. The pain, as with many kinds of brain abscess, may be localized over the area of the abscess.[261] Focal seizures are not uncommon and may be followed by persistent focal deficits ranging from paresis to complete hemiplegia. Various cranial nerve malfunctions, most commonly of the second, third, and seventh cranial nerves, are frequent.[112] In comparison with the hepatopulmonary forms of the disease, neurological symptoms usually progress more swiftly. In approximately 50 per cent of cases the onset of neurological symptoms is quite rapid.[263] When this occurs the progression of symptoms also tends to be rapid. Acute decompensation may take place over as little as 12 hours.

Diagnosis and Laboratory Findings

The diagnosis of cerebral amebiasis is established by identifying the trophozoites of E. histolytica in biopsy specimens from the lesions themselves or much less frequently in the cerebrospinal fluid. Care should be taken when collecting the samples. The use of cotton swabs is not recommended as this tends to desiccate the organisms and decrease the probability of transfer and hence detection in standard wet preparations. Syringes or glass pipets are usually more effective. Samples should be viewed for several minutes. The organism is extremely sensitive to both physical and chemical stimuli and generally reacts by an abrupt cessation of activity. Several minutes may pass before activity is resumed.

Morphologically, the trophozoite is relatively distinctive. The organism usually measures 10 to 20 μ in diameter in culture but may appear larger when actively feeding in tissues. The nucleus is round with a small central karyosome. Cellular debris consisting of red or white blood cells may be observed throughout the otherwise homogeneous cytoplasm. In fresh unstained preparations the fingerlike pseudopodia can usually be seen and thus will demonstrate the motility.

The cystic form of the organism is not generally found in extraintestinal tissues. It should be searched for in stool specimens from patients with any form of amebiasis and their contacts, as it represents the most important potential source for transmission of the disease. The cyst usually measures 5 to 20 μ in diameter.

Laboratory culture of E. histolytica is extremely difficult.[247] Singh has provided an excellent review of the subject.[321] In brief, the organisms grow best under anaerobic conditions in an acidic environment in which the redox potential is kept between -300 and -500 mv.

Several serological tests are available to help to confirm a diagnosis of cerebral amebiasis. Included are: indirect hemagglutinating antibody, complement fixation, agar gel differentiation, and indirect immunoflourescent antibody. Since such a high percentage of patients will have had either active or occult hepatic, intestinal, or pulmonary involvement, the tests will be positive in the overwhelming majority of patients and thus will not specifically indicate cerebral amebiasis. Initial cerebrospinal fluid analysis usually reveals a moderate neurophilic pleocytosis whose cell count may approach several thousand. Eosinophils are not usually present to any significant degree. Glucose and protein levels show no consistent pattern. The motile trophozoite of the organism has not yet been reported isolated from cerebrospinal fluid obtained via lumbar puncture. It should be noted that concurrent bacterial infections are not unusual occurrences, and the type and extent of the laboratory investigations should reflect this.

The radiographic investigation of amebic brain abscess is subject to the same constraints that limit investigation of other types of brain abscesses. Plain skull films seldom reveal any unusual findings. Computed tomography appears to be the most useful radiographic technique, but very little has been reported on the specific findings in cerebral amebiasis. In its absence the more traditional techniques of brain scanning, ventriculography, and angiography may be used with the appropriate precautions.

Ancillary diagnostic methods such as electroencephalography frequently reveal nonspecific abnormalities that help little in narrowing the differential diagnosis.

Treatment

As with most forms of brain abscess, the optimal management of cerebral amebiasis requires careful integration of operative and medical therapy. Although cures have been reported with either medical or operative therapy alone, most authors recommend a combined approach.[112,228]

Several drug regimens are available for use in non–central nervous system forms of the disease, but none has consistently proved successful in treating amebic brain abscess adequately. It is quite difficult to estimate which pharmacological agents, if any, will reliably attain acceptable therapeutic levels within the nervous system. For this reason the effectiveness of chemotherapeutic treatment alone is limited, and operative drainage in combination with medical therapy offers the most consistently reliable means of effective treatment. Among the drugs used to treat amebiasis are emetine hydrochloride, metronidazole, chloroquine, tetracycline, diiodohydroxyquin (Iodoquinol), diloxanide furoate, and dihydroemetine.

Generally, treatment of amebic abscess should include a luminal drug as well as adequate medication for the almost invariably present hepatic abscess. An acceptable regimen might include an initial course of metronidazole followed by a course of emetine or dehydroemetine and chloroquine if indicated. Emetine should be avoided if extensive myocardial damage is known to be present. Steroids and immunosuppressive drugs are usually contraindicated. Their risk-to-benefit ratio must be carefully weighed before use of these agents is even considered. Multi-drug regimens offer the opportunity to lower dosages in order to take advantage of the synergism ordinarily observed or in some cases to circumvent toxic side effects associated with higher dosages.

Clinical status permitting, most authors agree that in the ideal situation medical therapy may precede operative therapy.[112,228] The operative treatment requires special consideration of the rather common tendency for these cases to be complicated by secondary bacterial infection. For this reason, some authors have recommended a closed aspiration technique to minimize this possibility.[112]

Prognosis

In the past, amebic brain abscess was almost invariably fatal. More recently, cures have been reported.[112,228] Still, the mortality rate for cerebral amebiasis is so high and the morbidity is so great that there is little to be lost by pursuing the most aggressive combination of medical and operative therapy available. The prognosis can be improved by minimizing the effect of exogenous factors. To this end treatment of primary forms of the disease (hepatopulmonary and intestinal) must be intensive.

TOXOPLASMOSIS

Toxoplasmosis is one of the most widely distributed protozoan infections found in man. The etiological agent is *Toxoplasma gondii,* an obligate intracellular parasite that produces a wide spectrum of disease in both mammalian and avian hosts. The vast majority of toxoplasmic infections in humans are asymptomatic, and evidence of clinical disease is unusual.

Epidemiology

The organism has a worldwide distribution and exists as a coccidian of cats, which are considered the definitive hosts. Cats appear to acquire the disease by ingesting infected meat, and the oocysts are passed in cat feces. Other animals may also acquire the infection by the same route, but only in felines are the gametogenic and schizogenic reproductive cycles completed, thereby creating the infectious form of the organism. The pathways by which humans acquire the infection are generally unknown, although the vehicles of infection appear to be cystic and oocystic forms of the organism. Such potential sources of infection as undercooked meat have been identified, although epidemiological studies would suggest that other sources are possible.[30,128]

Pathology

Toxoplasma exists in three forms: the trophozoite, the cyst, and the oocyst. The oocyst is responsible for transmission of the disease but otherwise does not participate in the disease process in humans. It is formed in the cat, excreted in the feces, undergoes a period of maturation, and thereafter becomes infective. The oocyst may survive in moist soil for up to one year.

Both the cyst and the oocyst are infective, and their consumption is responsible for completion of the life cycle of the organism.

The propensity for most cases of toxoplasmosis to present subclinically initially correlates well with several histopathological features of the disease, most notably, the virtual absence of tissue response to intact cyst structures. In addition, the extraneural cysts rarely cause mechanical problems unless they are located within or near vital structures.

Central nervous system involvement, however, almost invariably produces symptoms that parallel the severity of the infection. While the incidence of central nervous system disease in the general population is ordinarily quite low, it may approach 50 per cent in certain subpopulations such as those patients with malignant disease or other conditions that compromise the immune system. In almost all cases of fatal toxoplasmosis the presence of neurological lesions can be demonstrated, although they may not be the immediate cause of death.[82] The selective vulnerability of the brain may be associated with the relatively less effective immune response in the central nervous system in comparison with other organ systems. The brain is also considerably more sensitive to the edema produced by inflammatory processes.

Clinical Manifestations

As with many of the fungal entities, a distinction must be drawn between infection and clinical disease. Serological surveys have demonstrated that the overwhelming majority of infections are asymptomatic. The factors that determine which cases of infection will result in clinical disease are poorly understood, although it is clear that a distinct minority of patients are subject to these various factors.

The most severe cases of disease appear in hosts with compromised immune responses, and in contrast to the rather benign forms of the disease that appear in normal hosts, disease in debilitated hosts is often fatal. Encephalitis and its attendant complications are the most frequent causes of death. The clinical course does not conform to a consistent profile. Some cases of central nervous system disease pursue a rapid fulminating course, whereas others pursue a protracted chronic course.

Variable clinical patterns are the rule rather than the exception, and their classifications frequently overlap. The lack of a distinctive clinical syndrome makes clinical diagnosis difficult. Neurological manifestations are often attributed to the underlying primary disease. The syndrome associated with congenital toxoplasmosis is often so severe that the fetus will be spontaneously aborted.

The clinical presentation of acquired disease is usually complex. Varying degrees of altered sensorium ranging from confusion to coma are almost invariably present. Encephalitic and meningoencephalitic forms often demonstrate meningeal signs such as headache and stiff neck in combination with seizure activity.

Focal deficits are present to some degree in a large percentage of patients (more than 50 per cent) with all forms of the disease but tend to dominate the clinical picture in patients with mass lesions.[340]

The association of acquired central nervous system toxoplasmosis with malignant disease has been well documented, although it is seen most frequently in association with Hodgkin's disease.[73,350] In this context a variety of constitutional symptoms, unrelated to toxoplasmosis as such, are part of the clinical picture.

Diagnosis

Antemortem diagnosis of toxoplasmosis requires careful interpretation of all available laboratory data. Isolation of the parasite from noncerebral human tissue or blood does not in itself unequivocally substantiate acute infection, since organisms may remain viable in latent foci for long periods. Organisms have also been recovered from asymptomatic subjects for more than one year following the initial infection. The documentation of trophozoites in cerebral tissue, however, may be considered a confirmation of acute disease.

Although the organism stains with both Wright and Giemsa stains, light microscopy may not provide adequate visualization. In cases in which serological examination is equivocal, electron microscopy may prove invaluable in detecting the parasites within cerebral lesions.[283]

Supportive confirmation of central nervous system toxoplasmosis relies heavily on immunological testing and, in particular, the demonstration of rising antibody titers by complement fixation, the Sabin dye test, or indirect fluorescent antibody techniques. Careful attention must be paid not only to the presence or absence of antibodies but to the various patterns that are observed.

In those cases in which the immunological profile must be relied upon heavily to confirm or support the diagnosis, serial titers assessing the status of IgA, IgG, and IgM components should be drawn. Although some information can be obtained from a single examination, the most useful information is generally obtained from serial measurements. Plasma specimens should be obtained at two-week intervals.

In cases of active disease, the diagnostic yield of brain biopsy is reasonably good, but the risk entailed in performing the procedure, even though small, should limit its use to those clinical situations in which other diagnostic modalities have failed to provide a diagnosis or the clinical status of the patient necessitates immediate diagnosis.

In acquired disease cerebrospinal fluid findings are usually mildly abnormal and nonspecific. Protein levels may be elevated but rarely exceed 200 mg per 100 ml and may be accompanied by a moderate mononuclear pleocytosis. Glucose values are usually normal. Cerebrospinal fluid analysis in infants with the congenital form of the disease will show a considerably different profile. Protein levels are not infrequently measured in the grams per 100 ml range.[140] Few entities, most notably *E. coli* meningitis, achieve levels of this magnitude. Cellular measurements may also be more dramatic.

In comparison to the neuroradiological findings of acquired disease, the radiographic findings of congenital toxoplasmosis are quite distinctive. Intracranial calcifications are seen in 30 to 60 per cent of cases.[81] The calcifications are of four types: nodular, linear, curvilinear, and irregular. Nodular calcifications vary in size from minute to several millimeters in diameter and have no particular parenchymal predisposition. Linear calcifications, on the other hand, tend to outline the shape of the lateral ventricles, and the curvilinear ones are primarily distributed throughout the basal ganglia and thalamic areas. Irregular calcifications of various sizes whose primary distinction is their large size constitute the fourth category; these may be located in any of several parenchymal locations. Although one particular type of calcification may predominate, the more usual case will reveal varying combinations of the different types. In general, the calcifications will most likely be located in the parietal and frontal areas, though no anatomical region is exempt. Cerebellar and cord calcifications are particularly unusual.[82]

Neuroradiological examinations other than skull films should primarily be directed at assessing ventricular size and cerebrospinal fluid flow. Computed tomography is probably the procedure of choice for investigation of almost all the abnormalities associated with central nervous system toxoplasmosis. Angiography confirms the avascularity of mass lesions and will occasionally demonstrate concurrent vasculitis, but in general, findings are rarely of etiological significance.

Electroencephalography usually reveals nonspecific abnormalities. Diffuse slow-wave delta activity is a common finding.[215]

Isolation trials may be helpful but often take longer than is feasible for results to be confirmed. The sediment obtained from cerebrospinal fluid samples is injected intraperitoneally into laboratory mice, which are subsequently bled. The blood is then analyzed for the appearance of antitoxoplasma antibodies.

Treatment

The primary mode of treatment of toxoplasmosis is chemotherapeutic, and to date the most effective regimen appears to be the combination of sulfadiazine and pyrimethamine. Both agents are particularly helpful in central nervous system forms of the disease because they penetrate the blood-brain barrier and because all central nervous system forms of disease require intensive treatment. Therapy should be particularly aggressive in the patient whose immune response is compromised.

The risk-to-benefit ratio of using corticosteroids in toxoplasmosis must be carefully weighed. Because of the intense inflammatory response often seen in acute stages, relatively large doses of steroidal medications may be necessary. Experimental evidence seems to indicate, however, that steroids may be involved in the reactivation of latent cystic foci. If steroids are required they should be tapered as quickly as possible. With appropriate treatment 80 per cent of patients may be expected to improve or undergo complete remission.

Prognosis

The prognosis of central nervous system toxoplasmosis must first and foremost be considered within the context of the major disease entities (congenital versus acquired) caused by the organism. Congenital toxoplasmosis produces a spectrum of disease ranging from relatively benign to lethal.

The key component affecting the prognosis of patients with acquired toxoplasmosis appears to be the immunological status of the patient. In debilitated patients whose immune responses are depressed, the clinical course is much more likely to be acute and fulminating, whereas in those patients capable of mounting an appropriate immune response the disease is more likely to be subacute. The second major factor affecting prognosis is the prompt institution of appropriate chemotherapy. Although cases of survival have been reported in untreated patients, this very much represents the exception rather than the rule. This is particularly true in patients with underlying neoplastic disease, a large percentage of whom may be treated and cured when specific treatment is given.

TRYPANOSOMIASIS

There are two major diseases of trypanosomal origin. The first, African trypanosomiasis, is more commonly referred to as sleeping sickness. The second is American trypanosomiasis, known by the eponym Chagas' disease.[327] Both are parasitic diseases whose etiological agents are *Trypanosoma gambiense* and *Trypanosoma cruzi* respectively. The organisms have a wide distribution and may produce profound and debilitating effects on the central nervous system. Their pathophysiological effects are primarily of neurological rather than neurosurgical importance. The ultimate pathological response of nervous tissue to invasion by trypanosomal organisms is multifocal neuronal damage and eventual

depopulation. There appears to be some modification of intracellular metabolic mechanisms, which either liberates toxic substances or impairs cellular metabolism, in addition to the actual structural damage that is produced by the invading organism. Regardless of the mechanism utilized, the pathological end point is the same, and the result is extensive neuronal damage. The broad clinical spectrum and the profound neurological consequences of these diseases virtually assure that cases of trypanosomiasis will come to the attention of the neurosurgeon. In general, however, neither disease produces pathological effects that lend themselves to primary neurosurgical therapy, and hence, they merit only brief consideration. Several excellent monographs and review articles detail their pathophysiological and clinical aspects.[10,328]

CYSTICERCOSIS

Cysticercosis is a parasitic disease that is usually produced by infestation with the larval stage of *Taenia solium*, the pork tapeworm. The larva bears the specific name *Cysticercus cellulosae* from which the disease entity takes its name. The infection is of particular interest to the neuroscientist because the organism shows a remarkable predilection for nervous tissue and may produce some of the most dramatic clinical manifestations associated with parasitic disease of the central nervous system.

Epidemiology

The epidemiological parameters that characterize cysticercosis are generally nonspecific. The age range is quite broad, although the peak incidence occurs between the second and fourth decades.[65] The entity is observed equally among the sexes.[19] *T. solium* has a worldwide distribution, but prevalence rates for the different forms of the disease vary considerably. Cysticercosis is most common in Eastern Europe, Asia, Africa, U.S.S.R., Mexico, and South America but practically nonexistent in the United States and Canada.[3,19,330] Although the actual number of reported cases is relatively small, the incidence of disease in the United States appears to be highest among Mexican-Americans.[115] Infection rates are highest among populations whose dietary habits include the ingestion of raw or inadequately cooked pork containing the larvae of the organism. Ova may also contaminate vegetables and fruits, which serve as ideal sources of infection because they are often consumed uncooked. Man serves as both the definitive and intermediate hosts for the adult tapeworm and for its larvae.

The life cycle of the organism is relatively simple. Human taeniasis occurs when the larvae are ingested in inadequately cooked infected pork. During the process of digestion, the larvae are released from the infected meat and become attached to the mucosa of the intestine. Over a period of weeks, the larva will develop into an adult tapeworm. The adult worm produces eggs containing an embryonal form of the organism termed the oncosphere. The eggs are excreted in feces, where the embryos may remain viable for several weeks. The oncospheres are consumed by swine and released during the process of digestion. They then penetrate the mucosa of the bowel and are carried via the mesenteric circulation to various tissue sites, where they develop into the larval form of the organism, completing the cycle.

The infestation of human tissues with the larvae (i.e., the development of cysticercosis) follows a similar pattern. The key pathophysiological requirement that must be fulfilled to produce cysticercosis is for the eggs to reach the stomach. This occurs via several routes including contaminated food or reverse peristalsis or, as a result of poor personal hygiene, via the fecal-oral route. This latter form of infection is most commonly seen among the pediatric age group and may produce fulminating disease.[115] Between 10 and 25 per cent of patients with cysticercosis concurrently harbor the adult tapeworm.[53,109]

Five types of cerebral cysticercosis have been described on the basis of their anatomical area of involvement as well as histopathological features. They are the racemose meningobasal), the cystic (parenchymal), the mixed (cerebromeningeal), the intraventricular, and the spinal.[65] This classification is particularly useful because it emphasizes the relationship between the anatomical location and the development of particular histopathological forms.

Racemose cysticercosis is characterized by the presence of vesicles. The vesicles, however, are irregular in shape and send out fingerlike projections that insinuate themselves throughout the subarachnoid space.[135] The structures may outgrow the cisterns, extending into the ventricles or invading the parenchyma itself. On rare occasions, they extend into the spinal subarachnoid space. The internal structure resembles the cystic form with two exceptions: the vesicular membrane is often quite irregular in thickness, and the racemose form generally does not contain the scolex.[135] In the racemose form the parasite is located in the leptomeninges, where its growth is not limited by parenchymal constraints. The racemose form produces its pathophysiological effects primarily by disrupting cerebrospinal fluid flow, causing hydrocephalus and increased intracranial pressure.[115] Cranial nerve deficits may also be seen.[135]

The cystic form generally occurs in parenchymal locations.[342] The lesion itself consists of a vesicle, usually measuring less than 1.5 cm in diameter. Within this fluid-filled vesicle, the scolex may be found. The cyst is structured so that the embryo does not come into direct contact with the host. Metabolic byproducts of the embryonal organism are excreted via a pore. These toxins are responsible for producing an intense inflammatory response that results in the formation of a zone of granulation tissue around lesions of some duration. The tissue response is relatively mild while the larva remains viable, but becomes considerably more intense when the organism dies.[6]

The structures of the mixed form possess characteristics of both the foregoing. Although intraventricular cysticerci may be seen in any of the types of disease, exclusive involvement of the ventricular system is rare.[110,135]

Spinal involvement may be intramedullary or extramedullary. Intramedullary forms present with symptoms suggestive of a spinal cord tumor. Extramedullary involvement resembles any of several compressive lesions. In either case, the signs and symptoms are not specific for cysticercosis in particular. Leptomeningeal forms of the disease are more common than either intramedullary or epidural forms.[131] The pathogenetic mechanisms involved in the production of spinal disease are similar to those in the production of intracranial disease.

Clinical Manifestations

The clinical presentation of central nervous system cysticercosis encompasses a wide spectrum of neurological dysfunction ranging from mild headache to profound motor and sensory deficits. Disturbances in the sensorium are also seen and range from mild to severe. The extent and severity of the disease is roughly proportional to the number of larvae present and their location.[6,217,351] The clinical presentation often closely resembles that of neoplastic or vascular occlusive disease.

The onset of clinical manifestations does not occur within any certain prescribed time period. Symptoms may begin within months of infection or may not occur for several years, the average period being five years. Approximately 80 per cent of patients will demonstrate symptoms within seven years.[196] The meningobasal form of the disease is slightly more common than the other forms and may produce a wide range of clinical manifestations.[217] Since the process is usually basilar in location, communicating hydrocephalus is not uncommonly part of the sequelae.[135]

The cystic form of the disease produces a clinical syndrome congruous with the presence of mass lesions. Seizure activity and focal deficits may dominate the clinical picture.[217] As the disease progresses, the vesicles may disintegrate, producing an intense inflammatory response.

Diagnosis

The diagnosis of cerebral cysticercosis depends heavily on radiographic and immunological evidence, which supports rather than confirms it. Definitive diagnosis is generally accomplished by identifying the parasite in nervous tissue, but if this cannot be done, ancillary tests may provide a high degree of certainty.

A provisional diagnosis may be made by utilizing complement fixation tests on cerebrospinal fluid. These will be positive in 64 to 88 per cent of patients.[124,157,281] Carbajal and associates report that the examination approaches 97 per cent accuracy.[65] Additional analysis of the cerebrospinal fluid usually reveals a lymphocytic pleocytosis. Cerebrospinal fluid eosinophilia is observed in about 50 per cent of patients, although the degree varies considerably. The degree of eosinophilia correlates relatively closely with the activity of the disease.[6,157,253]

Plain skull radiographs often reveal the presence of calcified cysticerci. In up to 40 per cent of those patients in whom the disease has been present for some time, calcifications may be observed, although most studies note these findings in a much smaller percentage.[110,196,330] The calcifications usually consist of punctate masses measuring 2 to 4 mm in diameter. Calcification is more likely to be seen with the cystic form.

The most useful neuroradiological examination is computed tomography. The cystic structures usually contain fluid of approximately the same density as cerebrospinal fluid. When the cysts are located within the parenchyma proper they are usually visualized. Intraventricular cysts, however, may be difficult to visualize even in advanced disease. As would be expected, cysts that have undergone calcification are readily visualized. The degree of edema present is dependent upon whether the integrity of the vesicle has been disrupted.

Angiography will confirm the presence of an avascular mass. Ventriculography or pneumoencephalography may be necessary in order to assess the extent of intraventricular disease.

The preferred sites for deposition of the larval organisms are skeletal muscle and nervous tissue. In disease of some duration, x-ray studies of the soft-tissue detail of skeletal muscle tissue, particularly thigh muscles, may reveal multiple calcifications, a finding that is considered characteristic of cysticercosis.[115,196] The soft-tissue calcifications are usually irregular in shape, varying from ovoid to linear.

Treatment

No specific chemotherapeutic agent is available to eradicate the cysticerci, although promising results have been noted in experimental studies utilizing mebendazole.[49] Treatment, therefore, is directed at amelioration of the various symptoms produced by the disease. Steroids are particularly useful in controlling the inflammatory response, and anticonvulsant medications are usually effective as far as seizure activity is concerned.[115,135,157,217]

Operative intervention may be helpful in those patients who present with localized disease.[135] The cystic lesions are amenable to removal from both parenchymal and intraventricular sites.[63,235] Multiple cysts and racemose lesions do not lend themselves to effective operative therapy unless it is to treat the various complications of the disease such as hydrocephalus. Procedures to ameliorate cranial nerve involvement may also be required.[135]

Prognosis

The prognosis of neurocysticercosis is poor. The majority of lesions are multiple and not amenable to operative removal. The usual clinical course is characterized by progressive deterioration and eventual death. Intensive supportive care will occasionally allow cystic lesions to calcify and thereby effect a cure, but these cases are unusual. Racemose forms of the disease have a particularly poor prognosis. Spinal cases, on the other hand, have a better prognosis because of the location of the lesion and because they are diagnosed earlier.

HYDATID DISEASE (ECHINOCOCCOSIS)

Echinococcosis, caused by the larval or hydatid stage of the dog tapeworm *Taenia echinococcus,* has been recognized as a disease entity since antiquity. Hippocrates and Galen made reference in their writings to hepatic forms of it.[102] By the seventeenth century the belief that it was caused by an animal was firmly established. The first report of a case of cerebral hydatid disease is attributed to Guesnard, while vertebral echinococcosis was first described by Chaussier in 1807.[71] Although many of the fundamental aspects of the disease were reasonably well characterized in these early writings, the terms used to describe various pathological aspects of the cerebral and vertebral forms often were used interchangeably when, in fact, the manifestations differ substantially. These inconsistencies still persist to some degree. For example, the term "hydatid cyst" should be reserved to describe cerebral lesions. The same term applied to vertebral lesions implies pathogenetic and histopathological similarities that are inappropriate. Most authors prefer the term "hydatidosis" when referring to bony involvement.[13,138,287]

Hepatic and pulmonary forms of the disease are the most common and account for almost 85 per cent of the cases.[27] Involvement of the central nervous system proper is seen in only 2 to 3 per cent of patients. Arana-Iñiguez presented a series of 102 cases of central nervous system forms of the disease, of which 76 were cerebral, 8 were cranial, and 18 were vertebral.[15]

Hydatid disease is caused either by ingestion of the hexacanth embryo (also termed scolex) or ingestion of eggs that may be present on infected foodstuffs. Infection in children commonly takes place via accidental contamination with feces of dogs harboring the adult worm *Echinococcus granulosus.* In adults, the disease is most commonly contracted by ingesting eggs on contaminated foodstuffs. The usual hosts for the adult worms are dogs, wolves, and foxes. Cattle, sheep, and hogs serve as intermediate hosts. Man also may serve as an intermediate host. The life cycle of the worm is modified in response to the host that ingests it. If the scolex is ingested by the definitive host it will attach itself to the intestinal mucosa, and the adult worm will form. If the scolex is ingested by an intermediate transport host, however, a larval stage of the organism called the hydatid will form. In definitive hosts, the adult worm achieves a maximum length of 10 mm. Eggs are released from the adult worms into the feces of canines. Following ingestion by man, the egg capsule is digested, releasing the hexacanth oncosphere in the jejunum, where it penetrates the intestinal mucosa and passes into the portal circulation. Most (65 per cent) become entrapped in the small intrahepatic venules, but others pass to the lungs (20 per cent), central nervous system (2 to 3 per cent), bone (4 to 5 per cent), and other sites.[22] Following distribution to these various structures the embryo begins the transformation into the vesicular structure that will eventually become the cyst. In healthy individuals large numbers of these oncospheres are destroyed by normal host defense mechanisms. In debilitated individuals, however, the embryos may disseminate widely, increasing rapidly in size. Over a period of weeks they form unilocular cystic structures that may achieve several millimeters in diameter. Cysts tend to grow larger in organs such as the liver and spleen, attaining sizes up to 15 cm in diameter. The cysts are somewhat smaller in the brain, but cysts measuring up to 12 cm in diameter have been reported.[104]

After several months the cyst wall differentiates into an internal granular layer (endocyst) and an outer cuticular laminated nonnuclear layer termed the ectocyst. The host reacts by forming an adventitial fibrous capsule, and the entire lesion usually becomes well encapsulated. The cavity of the cyst contains hydatid fluid with daughter cysts, brood capsules, and scolices. The endocyst has a germinal layer from which brood capsules arise. These may become separated from the cyst wall and remain free within the cystic cavity. Some develop internal buds that form scolices with suckers and hooks. The brood capsule and scolices that lie within the fluid of the cyst are referred to as hydatid sand, an important feature both radiographically and pathologically.

Epidemiology

Involvement of the central nervous system in echinococcal infections is rare. The association of cerebral lesions with systemic involvement elsewhere (primarily hepatic or pulmonary) is not invariable (early observations place it at 80 per cent).[102] On the basis of more recent studies, however, this percentage has been revised downward.[198] Nevertheless, a diligent effort should be made to rule out foci elsewhere if the nervous or osseus systems are found to be involved. The distinct types of echinococcosis affecting the central nervous system include cerebral, vertebral, and cranial forms.

Echinococcosis has a worldwide distribution, being most common in the sheep and cattle raising countries of South America (Uruguay and Argentina), Australia, and South Africa. The disease is also relatively common in Europe and Central Asia. It is unusual in North America, and in the United States the majority of reported cases have occurred in immigrant populations.[198] A greater incidence has been noted in Alaskan villages where contact with dogs is perhaps more frequent than elsewhere — in some it has been estimated at 25 per cent of the population.[22] Endemic foci also exist in the lower Mississippi valley and some of the sheep raising areas of the western United States.

Most authors believe that the single most important epidemiological factor in spreading the disease is direct contact with dogs that shed ova in their feces.[22] It may also be transmitted via contaminated food and water.

Cerebral Echinococcosis

Cerebral echinococcosis is considered a childhood disease, and indeed, an estimated 50 to 75 per cent of cases involving the central nervous system occur in the pediatric age group.[102] Sixty-five per cent of cysts occur in children between the ages of 5 and 10 years.[13] Up to 5 per cent of children contracting other forms of the disease will eventually demonstrate cerebral lesions.[103] Those cases appearing in adults were once thought to represent childhood infections with long latent periods. For many years it was thought that these lesions were possibly "as old as the patient." Recently, however, Beard has suggested that this assertion may be an exaggeration.[37] By reviewing epidemiological data he has shown that adults may be relatively susceptible and should, therefore, be considered in public health measures directed at eradication of the disease. Characteristically, the lesions are long-standing and chronic, antedating the onset of clinical symptoms by a considerable period of time in many cases but not to the extent previously thought. There appears to be no sex bias in cerebral forms of the disease.[26]

Pathogenesis and Pathology

In humans the majority of cysts occur in the liver (65 per cent) and lungs (20 per cent). Cerebral cysts usually are single and supratentorial, and tend to occur in the distribution of the middle cerebral arteries.[201] As the cyst grows, a subtle asymmetry of the cranium may be noted and may be demonstrated in a number of ways clinically, e.g., by transillumination or with a tuning fork. Those cysts that develop within the cerebral tissue can attain large sizes because they encounter relatively little resistance. Multiple cysts occur either by embolization of multiple larvae or by spontaneous cyst rupture.[266] Iatrogenic spread can occur during investigative procedures such as ventriculography or at operation.[14]

As with any expanding mass lesion, compressive forces of the mass itself produce a number of effects including dissection, stasis, and in the case of larger masses, necrosis. In the early stages of development the cysts are usually well tolerated by the nervous system because they neither infiltrate the parenchyma nor disrupt the vasculature through compression. Mild inflammation is seen in both cerebral and vertebral lesions. In cerebral forms this is reflected in the formation of an adventitial layer surrounding the lesion. In vertebral forms of the disease the increased blood flow as a result of the inflammation leads to decalcification.

The predilection for white matter is undisputed, but the exact reason for this is not known.[187] Intraventricular cysts have also been described but are considered unusual.[201] The localization of cysts is relatively evenly divided between frontal, temporal, and parietal lobes. Less than 3 per cent are seen in the cerebellum. Approximately 5 per cent will attain sizes great enough to affect an entire hemisphere.[13]

Clinical Manifestations

Clinical manifestations of cerebral hydatid cysts are primarily those related to increased intracranial pressure. Headache accompanied by vomiting is a prominent symptom in both adults and children. As the disease process advances, ill-defined focal deficits and varying degrees of sensory loss may be noted. In children the progression of symptoms usually takes place over several months, at which time a remission of symptoms often appears to take place. The remission is more apparent than actual, however, as pathological processes continue. It is merely a reflection of the ability of children to accommodate increased intracranial pressure more readily. Papilledema and visual field defects are not uncommon, and often the progression is to

blindness. Visual field changes are usually hemianopic and are seen in 35 per cent of the cases. Papilledema has been reported in up to 84 per cent of patients in some series, and optic atrophy in 14 per cent.[100] Evidence of pyramidal tract dysfunction was noted in almost 90 per cent of patients. In early series over half the patients presented with hemiparesis, but this is now seen less frequently, as the disease is usually diagnosed earlier. Mental changes were noted in 25 per cent of children, and seizure activity in approximately one patient in five, although estimates from some studies have ranged as high as 50 per cent.[308,338] Hydrocephalus, initially mild, may become severe, and ophthalmoscopy frequently reveals secondary optic atrophy. Some authors consider childhood and adult forms of the disease separately because of the different progression of symptoms.[13,201] The adult clinical history is certainly less well defined. Evidence of increased intracranial pressure dominates the symptom complex in both groups, however, and as would be expected, is tolerated less well in adults. This inability of the typical adult patient to tolerate the increased intracranial pressure is evidenced by the faster progression of symptoms. Visual disturbances are seen less frequently than in children, but their progression is more rapid. Motor dysfunction ranging from mild cerebellar signs to hemiparesis is seen in 75 per cent of patients. In the adult, mental changes are more frequent than in children, but this may be due to the adult's greater ability to appreciate and describe them. These changes are quite diverse and usually improve with removal of the cyst.[13] Seizures are less frequent than in children but still have an incidence of approximately 10 per cent.

Diagnosis

A detailed clinical examination should be the first diagnostic step. Increased head circumference is frequent in children, as is the "cracked pot" sign. Transillumination may be helpful, as may tuning fork localization.

A successful laboratory diagnosis of echinococcosis is dependent on a relatively high index of suspicion for the disease, as laboratory tests are quite specific. Nonspecific findings such as an elevated sedimentation rate and eosinophilic pleocytosis are supportive evidence but add little to a definitive diagnosis.

If Casoni's intradermal skin test and Weinberg's complement-fixation test as well as the eosinophil count are supportive, the diagnosis can be made in 85 per cent of cases. If the full immunological panel is added to the investigation the false positive rate is usually less than 5 per cent. If all of the serological tests are negative, a diagnosis of echinococcosis is extremely unlikely.[12]

Definitive diagnosis is dependent upon identification of the parasite or its body parts in the lesion. A preoperative diagnosis is not necessary, however, to begin implementation of appropriate treatment. Biopsy procedures are contraindicated because they serve only to jeopardize a potentially acceptable operative result through possible contamination. Cerebrospinal fluid obtained via lumbar puncture usually is normal unless the cyst has ruptured, producing an elevation in protein and moderate pleocytosis. Eosinophilic pleocytosis is rarely observed. Since the symptom complex is dominated by evidence of increased intracranial pressure and since the findings are nonspecific, lumbar puncture is not advised.

Arana-Iñiguez has proposed that a reasonable epidemiological investigation should proceed as follows: The initial investigations might include radial double diffusion or latex agglutination tests. Positive results in either of these could be confirmed by immunoelectrophoresis and immunofluorescence, while negative ones may be confirmed by electrosyneresis.[13]

Preoperative localization of the lesion is particularly important in this disease because if the cyst is ruptured at operation, scolices capable of disseminating the infection may be released. The operative approach must be meticulously planned in order to avoid this contamination, and thus a thorough radiographic investigation is not only advisable but mandatory.

Plain skull radiographs frequently show evidence of increased intracranial pressure and mass effect. In children, particularly, diastasis of the sutures, erosion of the sella, and thinning of the bone overlying the lesion may be observed. Oblique films of the area of suspected disease may demonstrate this thinning. Calcification of the cyst wall has been observed but is unusual.

Radionuclide scanning frequently shows evidence of a lesion with decreased isotope uptake, but none of the findings are pathognomonic. Gallium scanning may reveal increased uptake if the cyst is infected. Prior to the introduction of computed tomography, angiography was the procedure of choice. The typical findings include an avascular mass with moderate to marked stretching (depending on the size of the cyst) of otherwise normal appearing vessels. Rarely, if surrounding tissue is inflamed, a blush may be noted, but this is seldom of the degree seen with tumors. Angiographic findings in the adult differ from those in pediatric patients. In general, the cysts are somewhat smaller in adults, and therefore the findings are less dramatic than those seen in children. Vessel displacement is invariably less owing to the smaller size, and this should be taken into consideration lest minor but significant changes be overlooked. Angiography has provided a correct preoperative diagnosis in 35 to 60 per cent of reported cases.[14]

The most preferable mode of investigation at this time is computed tomography. The examination usually reveals an intraparenchymal lesion with a clearly defined margin. The margin can rarely be enhanced. There is usually significant ventricular shift, and hydrocephalus may be pronounced.[1] Cerebral edema is conspicuous in its absence, and this fact is helpful in differentiating the lesion from brain abscess and cystic tumors.[230,249] The cyst fluid has roughly the same density as cerebrospinal fluid, but hydatid sand, if present, may decrease the attenuation.

Postoperative CT scans reveal that re-expansion of the brain substance is limited. Extra-axial collections of fluid may persist for a long time, but seldom behave as mass lesions.[1] Within several weeks a compensatory shift of midline structures to a more normal position takes place. The site of the cyst defect itself usually will remain for a long time, although it is often smaller than the cyst itself.[265]

Various patterns of dysfunctional electrical activity have been detected. A common one is that of an electrically silent focus surrounded by a zone of delta activity.[133] This nonspecific delta rhythm is observed in 70 per cent of patients. Epileptogenic foci are also found in approximately 70 per cent of preoperative recordings and nearly 90 per cent of postoperative recordings. Despite these statistics, seizures occur in fewer than 20 per cent of the patients. An interesting finding of some note is that, following evacuation of the cyst, the delta wave activity tapers off significantly. Its reappearance may indicate recurrence of the cyst.[13]

Therapy

Medical treatment has virtually no place in the treatment of central nervous system forms of the disease. Primary efforts must be directed toward alleviating the effects of the mass lesion.

Successful operative treatment of cerebral echinococcosis depends upon complete removal of the unruptured cyst. Advances and refinements in the various radiographic methods of investigation have allowed meticulous planning of the operative approach. Analysis of the physical properties of the cyst itself has also contributed significantly. The wall of the cyst is relatively pliable. Arana-Iñiguez has suggested that this is an important physical property that may be utilized at operation because the structure can be forced through an opening smaller than its actual resting dimensions.[13] Hydrostatic expulsion, that is, the forcing of saline beneath the cyst in order to displace it outward, is a technique that has been used with some success. If the contents are not under pressure, some surgeons recommend puncture of the cyst with a small-gauge needle and drainage followed by careful dissection of the cyst wall from the surrounding parenchyma.[201] While it is possible to remove the cyst under these circumstances without gross contamination of the operative field, the chances are obviously, nevertheless, increased. The importance of removal of the cyst in toto is demonstrated by the fact that a cubic centimeter of fluid from a hydatid cyst may contain as many as 400,000 scolices, thus virtually assuring contamination if the cyst wall is ruptured.[100] If removal of the cyst can be accomplished without rupture a cure can be anticipated. If accidental rupture of the cyst should occur, irrigation with hypertonic saline (3 per cent) is recommended in the hope of destroying those organisms present in the operative field through osmotic desiccation.[265]

While the only satisfactory treatment is operative, none of the procedures employed is completely benign. Serious sequelae have been noted as a result of or following the operation. Visual disturbances occur and vary from hemianopia to complete blindness. The cysts are often quite large, and the rapid decompression caused by their evacuation may cause significant autoregulatory problems in an already compromised vascular state. This potential complication should be anticipated in the postoperative period.

Prognosis

The prognosis of the cerebral form of the disease depends upon several factors. These include: the location and size of the lesion; the presence of single or multiple lesions; and the presence of contamination, either spontaneous or iatrogenic.

In the traditional sense, the lesions themselves are benign and noninvasive. They exert their pathological effects through physical compression of and mechanical disruption of blood flow to neuronal elements. As would be expected, early operative treatment of lesions before permanent neurological damage has taken place improves the prognosis considerably. As with all mass lesions, location in a nonvital area also improves prognosis. The effect of multiple lesions on the prognosis is obvious.

Of those factors that are under the direct control of the neurosurgeon, the single most important is the avoidance of contamination. Typically, the lesions of cerebral echinococcosis are single and accessible, thus setting the stage for curative operative therapy if the technique is meticulous and the cyst is removed completely.

Cranial Hydatid Disease

Localization of hydatid disease exclusively within the bones of the cranium is exceptionally rare. Osseous lesions account for only 4 to 5 per cent of all hydatid disease, and cranial bone lesions for only 2 to 3 per cent of those.[99,154,155] In contrast, nearly 50 per cent of osseous lesions are vertebral.[9] The remainder are located in the long bones of the body. Although considered by some to be a separate disease entity, the pathological processes in the creation of lesions of the cranial vault are essentially identical to those seen in vertebral hydatidosis.

Cranial hydatid disease produces infiltrative lesions quite similar to the vertebral lesions. The bony deformities range from those almost exclusively confined to the outer table of the skull to those with such extensive intracranial progression that they behave like cerebral mass lesions.[302] The osteolytic lesions usually begin with involvement of the diploë, and growth is bidirectional, causing a widening of the diploic space.[302] The internal layer of the skull is preferentially violated. Once this bony barrier is violated there is little resistance to further development. As with vertebral forms of the disease, multiple vesicular structures form, often achieving considerable size. The dura rarely is violated. If the outer layer of the skull is pierced, large subgaleal effusions appear that are capable of forming fistulae.[302] Frontal bone lesions have been reported to erode into the sinuses.[13] The bony lesions are by no means restricted to the peripheral calvarium. Basilar portions of the skull may also be affected, and cranial nerve involvement is frequent with basilar lesions.[12] Multiple nerves are usually affected but in no consistent pattern.

Diagnosis

The initial investigation should include plain skull films. If a lesion is located peripherally, tangential views of the skull may be helpful. This should be followed by computed tomography, which should effectively define the intracranial extent of the disease. Angiography may be required if the intracranial extent of the lesion justifies it. Other diagnostic studies such as electroencephalography and radionuclide scanning rarely add significantly to the diagnostic evaluation. The battery of biological tests should also be included in the initial investigation.

Prognosis

The prognosis is directly dependent upon the location of the lesion. Since treatment is directed at complete extirpation of the affected bone, patients with lesions of the peripheral vault fare quite well. If contamination of the operative field can be avoided, operative complications and the mortality rate should be minimal.

Obviously, the treatment options available for patients with basilar disease are more limited. Although the efficacy of medical treatment with fluoromebendazole has not yet been definitively established, it may represent the only mode of therapy available. If medical therapy is decided upon, it should be aggressive, and possible side effects should be carefully monitored. Steroidal medications have been found helpful in treating cranial nerve palsies associated with basilar involvement.

Vertebral Hydatidosis

Vertebral hydatidosis is considered a different pathological entity by many authors because the pathophysiology of the disease differs significantly from that of its cerebral counterpart.[293,348] Although intradural hydatid cysts have been documented, they appear to be the exception rather than the rule.[67] Spinal cord involvement is almost always the result of vertebral disease of primary osseous origin. Vertebral hydatidosis, like most forms of bony disease, is more common in older adults. An estimated 40 per cent of cases occur in the 30- to 50-year-old age group.

The lesions seen in vertebral hydatidosis show several remarkable characteristics:

1. The vertebral lesions differ from the cerebral lesions in that they are microvesicular and invasive. The single unilocular cyst such as is seen in the brain or liver has not been described in bone. The original nidus of infection produces necrosis. The destructive process that follows produces diverticula by exogenous vesiculation in an irregular fashion at the margin of the lesion, forming contiguous cystic lesions. Cerebral lesions develop in tissue that offers little resistance to the expansion of the hydatid cyst. Bone, however, offers considerable resistance to their expansion, and thus the gross appearance of the lesions is substantially different.[99]

2. The destructive process is nearly always aseptic, forming cells containing cellular debris and fat. Secondary bacterial infection may occur, but is considered rare.

3. The invasive process is relentlessly

progressive. The normal barriers that prevent progression in many other diseases do not appear as effective in hydatidosis. The initial stages of the invasive process are slow and may, in fact, take place over months or years.[99] Patients are usually clinically asymptomatic during this stage, remaining so until the bony erosion is complete enough to provide access to the vertebral canal. Access is obtained when the periosteum undergoes destruction, releasing the microvesicular elements into the spinal canal. Generally, it is mechanical factors that determine whether the vesicles remain in clumps or form multiple individual lesions.

4. The actual pathological mechanism producing symptoms is one of compression rather than invasion. The vesicles themselves show virtually no tendency toward spontaneous fistula formation or dural disruption. Additionally, the compression takes place not only by the increasing size of individual vesicles but also by the continuing release of vesicles that by sheer numbers cause compression. Generally, the vesicles increase in size rather slowly. This accounts for the insidious onset of clinical symptoms and also correlates well with the remarkable functional recovery that can follow early decompression.

5. Although all parts of the vertebra may be affected, there appears to be a special predilection for the pedicle and centrum. Bony hydatid disease exhibits some of the same characteristics as other osseous abnormalities in that lesions preferentially affect the more highly vascularized bones or portions thereof. Thus, in vertebral hydatidosis the centrum and pedicle are the most commonly affected portions of the vertebra.[287]

6. Both intraspinal invasion and extraspinal invasion take place. The intraspinal process, of primary interest to the neurological surgeon, usually takes place posteriorly. Violation of the dura is unusual but has been reported. Invasion of the cord parenchyma is not uncommon, however, if the dura has been opened at a previous operation. The abscesses that develop actually provoke little inflammatory reaction.

7. Approximately 50 per cent of vertebral lesions develop in the thoracic area, 20 per cent in the sacral area, and 29 per cent in the lumbar area.[287] Cervical involvement occurs but is much less common. In the thoracic area it is generally the lower third of the region that is affected.[13] Secondary invasion of the canal may take place from various paravertebral locations (costal or mediastinal or paraspinal muscle and the like). As would be expected, these lesions have a slightly better prognosis than those that originate within the vertebrae themselves.

Clinical Manifestations

The initial symptoms of vertebral hydatid disease consist of radicular pain, motor deficits, or both in 95 per cent of the patients. Rarely, paravertebral swelling is present. It is often painless, however, and often remains undetected until other symptoms intervene. As with most cases of cord compression, sensory and sphincter disturbances follow if decompressive treatment is not initiated. In some cases the onset of symptoms will be abrupt. The rapid onset of neurological dysfunction usually implies vascular compromise, and as would be expected, functional recovery in these cases is usually less than complete. Acute decompensation should also suggest possible pathological fracture. The sequence in which symptoms usually progress is not characteristic of disease of bone.[13]

Diagnosis

Completely normal spine films virtually exclude the diagnosis of vertebral hydatidosis. Advances in computed tomography of the spine should add significantly to the diagnostic regimen available to the clinician. The diagnosis is made primarily on the basis of radiographic data, but other parameters also should be examined. Cerebral spinal fluid examination usually reveals several abnormal findings, but none that might be considered pathognomonic. Serological tests on the cerebrospinal fluid are positive in 95 per cent of the cases.[366]

Therapy

The immediate objective of operative therapy is decompression. The invasive nature of the disease makes complete extirpation of the affected bone an unlikely possibility in most cases. Nevertheless, at operation a meticulous effort should be made to evacuate all of the hydatid material from the operative site, since fistulae may form. (It should be noted that while there is no tendency toward formation of spontaneous fistulae, the operative site represents a considerably different situation.) Irrigation of the wound with hypertonic saline (3 per cent) for five minutes at the end of the operative procedure has been recommended.[278]

The operative approach and extent are most often dictated by the radiological extent of bony involvement, which unfortunately provides only an inexact estimate of the true extent of involvement. Microscopic evidence of disease extends beyond the radiographic lesion in almost all cases. Because of this finding, most authors recommend as radical a procedure as possible.[278] The technical aspects of vertebrectomy, prosthesis insertion, and other radical procedures usually do not require modification because of any special disease characteristics except that they should be aggressive. Recently, more radical excisions of bone and restorations with methylmethacrylate and other synthetic prostheses as well as autogenous bone grafts have been attempted. Although a few case reports cite promising results, adequate definitive data are not yet available.[138,139]

Prognosis

There are three major factors that determine the prognosis of vertebral hydatid disease. The first is the rapidity of onset. As has been stated before, rapid neurological decompensation suggests vascular compromise. Recovery is rarely as complete or as quick as that seen in the more slowly progressive forms. Second is prompt operative treatment. If those patients with more slowly progressive forms are taken as a group, their prognosis improves in direct relationship to the promptness with which decompressive operative intervention is instituted. Thus, patients who have progressed to complete paraplegia prior to the institution of therapy fare less well than those whose deficits are less profound at the time treatment starts. The third factor is recurrence of the disease. It is imperative that the physician and his patient understand two fundamental aspects of the therapy: (1) decompression is the only acceptable mode of therapy, but while it does eliminate the mechanical compressive forces, it almost never eradicates the bony

disease, and therefore, (2) recurrence is not only a possibility but a likely probability. About three fourths of the patients will have recurring symptoms of varying degrees within two years of their initial operation.[13] A few patients have remained asymptomatic for years, but in general, the course is one involving multiple operations over a period of years. This inability to completely eradicate the bony form of the disease is probably the single most important factor adversely affecting the prognosis.

SCHISTOSOMIASIS

Schistosomiasis was described in 1850 by the German pathologist Bilharz—hence its informal designation bilharziasis.[40] It is one of the most widely distributed of the parasitic infestations, affecting an estimated 200 to 300 million people.[26,54,193]

The term "schistosomiasis" designates those diseases caused by digenetic trematodes belonging to the family Schistosomatidae. Three species—*Schistosoma mansoni, S. haematobium,* and *S. japonicum* are the primary pathogens in man. These flukes, also informally known as blood flukes because they inhabit the circulatory systems of many mammals, are capable of producing lesions throughout the human body, including the central nervous system.

Etiology and Life Cycle

As with many parasitic infections, the liver plays a central role in the life cycle of the worm. The portal, mesenteric, or vesicular venous systems serve as the primary repository for the adult worm, which measures 1 to 2 cm in length. The adult worms may remain viable for as long as 30 years (average 5 to 10 years) producing up to 3000 eggs per day (the number depending on the species) for the duration of their life span. The eggs remain viable for approximately three weeks, during which time they secrete an enzymatic substance that destroys surrounding tissue. A few find their way into the bladder or bowel and are excreted. Once in fresh water, the eggs hatch, producing miracidia, which invade the specific snail host appropriate to the species.[325] The miracidia remain in the snail host for six to eight weeks, during which time they are transformed into their infective larval form called cercariae. The cercarious form of the organism is capable of penetrating human skin. Direct contact with the organism at this stage while bathing, swimming, or working in infected water provides the opportunity for infection.

Epidemiology

The disease is primarily endemic to three continents—Africa, South America, and Asia—and is restricted by the habitat of its snail hosts. Major endemic foci also exist in Puerto Rico, the Antilles, Japan, and the Philippines. Wright estimates that the disease may be endemic in as many as 72 countries.[362] The absence of the appropriate snail hosts in Europe and North America accounts for the relative rarity of the condition in these areas. Industrial development, particularly with regard to the harnessing of water resources in endemic areas, has led to a dramatic increase in the incidence of the disease as breeding places for its snail hosts have increased.[91,150] Indeed it has been estimated that in endemic areas infection rates among indigenous populations may approach 90 per cent.[280] Although involvement of the central nervous system is rare in comparison with the other protean clinical manifestations of the disease, recent case reports citing an increase in central nervous system involvement tend to support these statistics. The disease is seen most often among young people and children, the average age being less than 30 years.[144,237] Certain forms of the disease (spinal) have a peculiar unexplained sex distribution (male-to-female ratio of 6:1).[296,298]

Pathogenesis and Clinical Manifestations

The initial symptom of infection may be pruritus, or "swimmers itch," occurring within several hours of exposure. This usually abates quickly. A quiescent asymptomatic period usually follows during which time the adult worms mate. The onset of ovulation in the female is usually accompanied by an illness resembling a severe viral infection. The symptoms, which may be quite severe but nonspecific, may include fever, malaise, diarrhea, and hematuria.

The first report of a case of cerebral schistosomiasis is attributed to Yamagiwa.[365] He originally considered the cause of the lesion to be *Paragonimus westermani*. It was not until some years later that the eggs found in brain necropsy material were identified as those of *S. japonicum*. Brain involvement is due predominantly to *S. japonicum*. In contrast, egg deposits within the spinal cord are primarily those of *S. haematobium* and *S. mansoni*. These tropisms have led to the establishment of two clinical forms of central nervous system involvement: the cerebral form and the spinal form.

Cerebral Schistosomiasis

The cerebral form may have an acute or chronic presentation. Of the three species of *Schistosoma*, *S. japonicum* produces the largest number of eggs, and the eggs are smaller than those of *S. mansoni* or *S. haematobium*. These two factors may facilitate their wider dissemination and the more frequent brain involvement.

Once the eggs are deposited in the brain they produce an inflammatory reaction characterized by intense lymphocytic and microglial infiltration. Adjacent astrocytes hypertrophy, and there is marked formation of glial fibers. Eventually a fibrocaseous mass, often simulating a tumor or diffuse inflammatory process, is formed. Eggs have been recovered from all parts of the brain, and lesions range from minute miliary foci to large granulomas. Large granulomas often resemble neoplastic tissue. The granulomatous formation may be due to metabolites of the living ova rather than to the worm itself, which produces a much less intense reaction. Large granulomas often appear to form around large numbers of ova. This relatively localized deposition of eggs would suggest deposition in situ. The miliary lesions are probably produced by egg embolization. Gelfand examined the brains of 50 patients with visceral or urinary forms of the disease and found eggs present in the brains of 28 of them. Most of these patients were asymptomatic, which suggests that central nervous system involvement may be present but clinically inapparent.[148] Blankfein estimated that 2 to 4 per cent of patients with schistosomiasis will demonstrate cerebral complications.[43]

An immunological basis relating the severity of the disease to acute rather than chronic exposure to the organism has been postulated but not yet proved. The theory, advanced by Levy and co-workers, suggests that nonimmune subjects may present with fulminating forms of the disease while residents of endemic areas may remain neurologically asymptomatic despite the presence of widely disseminated ova in the brain.[224]

The acute cerebral form of the disease usually presents clinically as an encephalopathy, and symptoms are frequently fulminating. Meningitic signs including fever, meningismus, and headache are common, as are pyramidal tract signs.[285] Personality changes as well as generalized disturbances of sensorium are also common.[186,373]

Chronic forms of the disease are usually due to the presence of granulomatous mass lesions. Accordingly, a symptom complex including evidence of increased intracranial pressure and neurological symptoms may appear at long intervals (two to four years) following the initial infestation when the disease process is otherwise subclinical. Disturbances of the sensorium ranging from disorientation to coma are common.[224,237] Seizures, both focal and generalized, are also relatively common.[146] Marcial-Rojas and Fiol reviewed the literature in 1963 and found 99 cases. Of these, 72 had cerebral lesions and 17 presented initially with seizure activity.[237] Several cases of acute hemiplegia have been reported in association with the disease.[222,223,373] Various reported focal deficits correspond to lesion location.

Spinal Schistosomiasis

Although both arterial and venous routes have been implicated in the entrance of the organism into the central nervous system, most authors favor venous routes.[126,142,237] In spinal forms of the disease the anastomotic channels of Batson's plexus, as well as the anterior radicular artery, have been suggested.[143]

The pathological changes observed within the spinal cord involve not only the gray and white matter but the vasculature as well.[160] No specific histopathological feature is invariably found. In some cases of infarction the eggs appear to cause no tissue reaction at all. In others the reaction may be of the diffuse inflammatory type.

Spinal schistosomiasis usually presents in one of three ways: as an intramedullary tumor, as acute cord compression with acute transverse myelitis, or as a radiculopathy. Of the three types, the myelitic presentation is more common. Most frequently, the presenting symptom is pain—either local or radicular. This is usually followed by weakness of the lower extremities and sphincter disturbances. The sequence and progression of symptoms, however, is not invariable. The prognosis worsens if the disease is acute and the symptom complex is rapidly progressive. Those cases due to granuloma formation presenting as extrinsic masses usually respond well to operative decompression.[178] In schistosomal radiculopathy, pain, low in the back or sciatic in distribution, is usually more prominent than in the myelitis, in which motor disturbances predominate.

Diagnosis and Laboratory Findings

Diagnosis is established by isolation of ova in the stool, urine, or biopsy material. Stool concentration and other special concentration techniques may be required. In approximately 80 per cent of acutely ill patients, ova will be present in stool specimens.[43] Rectal biopsy is probably the single most reliable isolation technique when repeated stool specimens are negative. Viability of the eggs should be demonstrated to substantiate active infection unequivocally.

Ancillary tests include complement fixation, circumoval precipitin and indirect fluorescent antibody tests. Intradermal skin tests are also available.[305] Eosinophilia is common, being found in up to 60 per cent of patients.[72]

Involvement of the central nervous system without active involvement of other body systems is distinctly unusual. Confirmation of central nervous system disease is dependent upon isolation of eggs and more rarely the worm itself in brain tissue or along the spinal axis.[171] Isolation of the ova from cerebrospinal fluid obtained via lumbar puncture is extremely unusual; cerebrospinal fluid obtained from a patient with schistosomiasis will usually show an increase in protein and a slight increase in the lymphocyte count, but up to two thirds of patients have completely normal cerebrospinal fluid. The electroencephalogram may be helpful. Patients presenting with focal deficits often reveal a pattern of discrete cortical abnormalities that corresponds with histopathological lesions that have been found at autopsy. This pattern may be helpful in localizing lesions in which operative removal is considered.

Angiography and radionuclide brain scans have not been extensively used in evaluation of cerebral forms of the disease. As would be expected, however, these studies are most helpful when large granulomas are present. It is anticipated that computed tomographic examination will provide much useful information and perhaps become the definitive study in investigating cerebral forms of the disease.

Myelography in patients with symptoms of transverse myelitis is almost invariably normal. In those presenting with chronic granulomatous myelitis, the myelogram most often demonstrates an intramedullary mass with or without a complete block.

A presumptive diagnosis is often based on positive immunological studies. The intradermal skin test gives positive results in 90 per cent of infected patients.[16] Complement fixation tests are positive in approximately 75 per cent of patients with acute or chronic infections.[113,178] Unfortunately these examinations can continue to show positive values long after active infection has passed and treatment has been instituted. Numerous new bioassay and immunoassay techniques have been developed but are not yet in general use.[170]

Treatment

Several groups of drugs are available to treat schistosomal infection. The drugs, although not entirely species specific, do differ in their effectiveness against the different species.[337]

Niridazole is the agent of choice against *S. haematobium*.[32] Stibophen may also be used.

The trivalent antimonials are preferred in *S. mansoni* infections.

Hycanthone has been used effectively in both *S. mansoni* and *S. haematobium* infections.[199,326] Its primary advantage is that only a single intramuscular injection is required.

Schistosoma japonicum infection is the most difficult of the types to treat. It does not respond to hycanthone or metrifonate. It also responds poorly to most of the trivalent antimonials. At the present time the antimonial tartrates are recommended, although they do produce more severe side effects.[169,199]

Treatment of spinal forms of the disease is dictated by the mode of presentation. Patients with clinical evidence of acute cord compression with rapid progression of symptoms require decompression. Concurrent chemotherapy is mandatory.[219]

Operative resection of large granulomas may become necessary and should also be accompanied by concurrent chemotherapy.[87]

Steroid therapy has been recommended as a useful adjunct to chemotherapy.[219]

Prognosis

In endemic areas it is common for up to 90 per cent of the indigenous population to be infected and yet remain relatively asymptomatic. Quite probably the central nervous system forms of the disease are more frequent than the symptomatic cases would indicate.

The mechanisms contributing to the pathogenesis of the lesions are primarily immunological in nature. Most likely the immunological status of the patient is intimately related to the severity of the complications associated with the disease. There are some species differences in the response to the various pharmacological agents used in treatment. Also, their marked toxicity limits the most effective use of many of these agents in seriously ill patients. Untreated symptomatic cerebral schistosomiasis is often fatal, yet autopsy studies suggest that a substantial number of patients with this disease can remain asymptomatic.

The prognosis of spinal schistosomiasis depends primarily on how rapidly treatment is instituted after the onset of neurological symptoms. As with most mass lesions, delay in treatment frequently leads to progressive loss of function. If all function has been lost at the time of operative decompression, it is unlikely to return.

PARAGONIMIASIS

Paragonimiasis was originally described as a disease entity in 1880 by Manson, who suggested that the lung fluke might be the cause of benign hemoptysis seen commonly among natives of the Far East.[236] It was not until 1887, however, that Otani described the first case of cerebral paragonimiasis.[264]

Etiology

The causative agent of paragonimiasis is one of several species of trematode worms belonging to the genus *Paragonimus*. The importance of any single species as a causative agent varies from one endemic area to another, but *Paragonimus westermani* has the widest distribution and is generally considered to be the most important pathological agent infecting man.[57,244,282]

Paragonimus westermani (0.8 to 1.4 cm in length, 4 to 6 mm in width, and 3.5 to 5 mm in thickness) is oval in shape, reddish-brown in color, and has been likened in appearance to a coffee bean. Its life cycle requires a final host (man and other mammals) as well as two intermediate hosts. The adult worm lays eggs in cysts located in the peripheral lung tissue. The operculated eggs reach the bronchioles, where they are expectorated in the sputum or swallowed and passed via the feces. Under favorable conditions the eggs develop into ciliated free-swimming miracidia. The mature miracidia then hatch and burrow into snails (the first intermediate host), where they develop into free-living microcercariae. These larvae in turn invade crustacea, usually crabs and crayfish, which serve as the second intermediate host. Man is infected by ingestion of the parasitized host. In the Orient, consumption of uncooked crustaceans is not uncommon.[179] In Korea, fresh crab juice is used as a home remedy for measles; and in the Cameroons, for infertility.[90] Delicacies such as pickled crab and "drunken crab" (raw crabs soaked in wine prior to consumption) are popular among many of the natives.

Once ingested, the mature metacercariae lose their covering in the duodenum and penetrate the intestinal wall, reaching the abdominal cavity in three to six hours. They remain in the abdominal cavity for several days before migrating through the portal vein, liver, and diaphragm to reach the pleural cavity and lungs, where they become encysted in peripheral alveolar tissue. The adult worm provokes an exudative granulomatous reaction with gradual development of a fibrotic encapsulated cyst. The cysts may eventually abscess and over several years gradually calcify. Ectopic sites of encystation include the liver, kidneys, eyes, subcutaneous tissues, genitalia, and central nervous system. Of these ectopic sites, the brain is by far the most common, accounting for an estimated 50 per cent of reported cases.[70,179,183]

Epidemiology

Paragonimus westermani is widely distributed throughout southeast Asia and the Far East, the principal endemic areas being Japan, Korea, China, Formosa, the Philippines, and Thailand. Isolated foci of other species exist in Africa and South America. Additional species known to cause disease include *P. africanus* (Cameroons, Nigeria, Congo), *P. mexicanus*, *P. peruvianus*, *P. caliensis* (Central and South America), *P. skrjabini* and *P. heterotremus* (China). The number of species that are documented causes of human paragonimiasis is steadily increasing. Most of these species are probably capable of invading the central nervous system, although virtually all cases of cerebral paragonimiasis reported thus far appear to be due to *P. westermani*. In addition to human hosts several other mammals, predominantly feline, serve as reservoirs. More than 80 per cent of reported cases implicate insufficiently cooked crustaceans as vectors. Only one autochthonous case has been reported in North America, but numerous heterochthonous cases have been reported, particularly among military personnel and tourists returning from endemic areas.[204]

Age and sex incidence data derived from numerous studies show that cerebral paragonimiasis is more common among young adult men (average age less than 30 years).[179] Epidemiological factors contributing to this are thought to be primarily related to socioeconomic aspects of diet, with men being more likely to ingest infected crustaceans. Weakened host resistance, especially among children who may be exposed not only through diet but also during play, may also be a contributing factor. Although few studies provide sufficiently detailed epidemiological data, Sadun suggests that the probability of infection is greater in the families of infected individuals than in the general population in endemic areas because of common dietary habits and food sources.[300]

The age range for onset of symptoms varies from 1 to 45 years. Average duration of symptoms is 5.5 years, although in some cases symptoms have persisted for as long as 26 years.[257]

Cerebral Paragonimiasis

Pathogenesis and Clinical Manifestations

Paragonimiasis has been called endemic hemoptysis—a term once thought to denote its primary clinical manifestation.

Many ectopic forms of the disease exist, however, and the symptom complex is usually dominated by the most extensively involved system. Clinical manifestations of the disease in its most common form are primarily pulmonary. They usually have an insidious onset and are nonspecific, preceding the onset of cerebral symptoms (the most common ectopic form) in 69 per cent of cases.[204,257] In some patients, in fact, pulmonary symptoms may be so minimal or nonspecific so as to be overlooked, making cerebral signs and symptoms appear primary. Recognition of this fact is especially important in facilitating diagnosis of the disease.

The reported incidence of cerebral infection from pulmonary paragonimiasis varies. Estimates range from 0.8 to 26.6 per cent.[70,163,259] This apparent discrepancy is due to two major factors: (1) Incidence rates and prevalence of the entity vary from one endemic area to another, the highest estimates coming from the most heavily infected areas; and (2) while pulmonary symptoms of paragonimiasis may be overlooked, cerebral symptoms rarely are. In general, cerebral symptoms tend to be more severe and incapacitating, necessitating treatment. Specialty centers, therefore, are likely to see skewed populations with a disproportionate number of patients with cerebral involvement. In recent years the incidence in most endemic areas has decreased because of intensive public health measures.

The mode of entrance of the organism into the cranial cavity has not been established. Several theories have been postulated, and theoretically two general routes are available: (1) arterial-venous egg embolization and (2) invasion of the perivascular or perineural structures by the worm itself.[319,367]

Egg embolism from the lungs or other ectopic sites to the central nervous system has also been considered a possible mode of pathogenesis and was proposed by Yumoto and Nagayoshi.[368] Clinical findings such as the sudden onset of hemiplegia would seem to support the theory.

Regardless of the mode of intracranial entrance, once the worm is within the cranial cavity it begins its migration, leaving in its tracks spawned eggs and metabolic waste products that produce an inflammatory reaction. The most frequent localization of these lesions is in the posterior parietal, temporal, and occipital lobes. These locations suggest that the worm may migrate through the lateral sinus. Involvement of the brain stem, frontal lobe, and intraventricular spaces as well as the spinal axis has also been reported. Posterior fossa involvement is distinctly unusual.[179]

In the acute phase (stage I) of cerebral paragonimiasis the symptoms are those of meningitis and include vomiting, meningismus, fever, and headache. The condition of the patient may vary from nearly asymptomatic to acutely ill. In many of the cases these acute inflammatory symptoms will regress over a period of six to eight weeks even without treatment, only to recur paroxysmally. The recurrence of symptoms is probably due to reinfection rather than to some cyclic symptom complex.

In other cases, however, the disease course is rapid and fulminating, resulting in death. The largest proportion of deaths due to cerebral paragonimiasis occur during this stage.

As the disease progresses to stages II and III a deterioration of the sensorium is generally noted. Visual aberrations are commonly noted, a high incidence (80 per cent) of homonymous hemianopia in some series and optic atrophy with impaired visual acuity (32 per cent).[179,257] The incidence of papilledema is approximately 16 per cent. Sensory and motor disturbances varying from subjective dysesthesias to the sudden onset of hemiplegia have been reported.

Kim and Walker proposed a clinical classification based on four modes of presentation.[204] Oh has proposed a similar clinical classification of the disease that has six forms: (1) the meningitic form in which patients present with meningitic signs, (2) the subacute and encephalitic form characterized by the slow progression of neurological deficits without evidence of increased intracranial pressure, (3) the tumorous form characterized by the progression of focal neurological deficits with evidence of increased intracranial pressure, (4) the dementing form characterized by a nonprogressive dementia, (5) the epileptic form characterized by the presence of seizures with nonprogressive neurological deficits, and (6) the hemiplegic form characterized by the acute onset of hemiplegia.[257]

This clinical classification effectively summarizes the myriad presentations of the disease but does not imply either a temporal or invariable progression of symptoms. No clear progression of symptoms characteristic of cerebral paragonimiasis alone has been described.

The most common form, on the basis of the most frequently noted symptom in almost all series, is the epileptic form. Seizure activity, which may be focal (75 per cent) or generalized (25 per cent), is seen in 95 per cent of patients either at the onset or during progression of the disease.[259]

Diagnosis

Definitive diagnosis of cerebral paragonimiasis is difficult. The demonstration of either eggs or the adult worm in cerebral tissue represents unequivocal proof but requires biopsy, which is rarely indicated. Demonstration of the ova in cerebrospinal fluid is difficult and exceedingly unusual.

Because of the difficulty in establishing a definitive diagnosis, Oh formulated diagnostic criteria based on a composite of the various investigative procedures employed by many centers (Table 112–1).[255]

A history of travel in an endemic area or ingestion of raw crustaceans is a simple but important diagnostic consideration. The simplest and most direct means of establishing the diagnosis is egg isolation. Spu-

TABLE 112–1   DIAGNOSIS OF PARAGONIMIASIS

Paragonimiasis
  Suggestive findings
    Positive intradermal paragonimiasis test
  Highly suggestive findings
    Positive complement-fixation test in serum
    Cystonodular type lesions in chest x-ray films
  Confirmatory findings
    Demonstration of the paragonimus ova in sputum, stool, gastric juice, and any other body fluid or tissue specimen
    Demonstration of paragonimiasis worm in any tissue specimen
Cerebral paragonimiasis
  Suggestive findings
    Abnormal spinal fluid findings
    Intracranial radiological calcifications other than type 4
    Focal electroencephalographic abnormality
  Highly suggestive findings
    Abnormal colloidal gold reaction in spinal field
    Increase of gamma globulin in spinal fluid
    Eosinophilia in spinal fluid
    Type 4 "soap bubble" calcification on skull x-ray films
  Confirmatory findings
    Demonstration of ova in spinal fluid, either lumbar or ventricular
    Positive complement-fixation test in spinal fluid
    Histological evidence of *Paragonimus* ova or worm in brain tissue

tum and stool specimens are usually the most productive. Isolation of the eggs may be difficult to demonstrate early in the course of the disease but they are usually found in the sputum or feces of infected patients. Twenty-four-hour specimens are preferable. When difficulty is encountered in demonstrating the eggs, gastric juice and pleural fluid specimens should be examined. The diagnostic yield may be improved by subjecting the patient to bronchoscopy, thoracentesis and, in unusual cases, open biopsy procedures.

Several ancillary diagnostic procedures are available for screening, follow-up, or tentative confirmation in the absence of egg isolation in the body tissues or fluids. Complement-fixation tests are available, and the results correlate roughly with the degree of active infection. They are positive in the majority of patients with cerebral paragonimiasis. If therapy is successful they are usually negative within six months. Intradermal skin tests are also available, but reactions remain markedly positive after the active phase of the infection has passed, and therefore they are primarily used for epidemiological screening only. Eosinophilia is a frequent but not invariable finding.[204,243] Leukocytosis, elevated sedimentation rate, and microcytic anemia have also been reported, but in no consistent or pathognomonic pattern.[204,259] Cerebrospinal fluid findings may vary from completely normal to markedly abnormal and may correlate with the degree of cerebral involvement. Demonstration of the ova in the cerebrospinal fluid is extremely unusual. The probability of isolating ova is highest in ventricular fluid specimens. Complement-fixation tests of spinal fluid will be positive in approximately 40 per cent of patients.[257] Immunoelectrophoresis and bioassay techniques have been reported but are not yet available for widespread clinical use.

Radiology

Approximately 50 per cent of patients with cerebral paragonimiasis have calcifications demonstrable with plain skull films. The incidence varies between 39 and 70 per cent in several reported studies.[141,204,256]

Plain films also frequently show evidence of increased intracranial pressure, demonstrating mild diastasis of the sutures, erosion of the posterior clinoid processes, and rarely, increased convolutional markings.

Angiography is seldom helpful in differentiating paragonimiasis from other space-occupying lesions. The absence of tumor blush or abnormal feeder vessels should aid in the differentiation from brain tumors. It is noteworthy that if a mass is present the shift is frequently toward the side of the lesion, owing to the cortical atrophy usually present at this stage.

Usually it is difficult to introduce air into the subarachnoid space because of the chronic arachnoiditis that follows the meningitic phase of the disease. If the study is successful, two major abnormalities may be observed: (1) ventricular deformity and enlargement with or without evidence of porencephaly and (2) subcortical atrophy, usually more pronounced on the side of the lesion. The studies are almost never normal.

Computed tomography is becoming a method of choice, and characteristic cyst-like structures are usually easily appreciated.

Electroencephalography

The electroencephalogram is almost invariably abnormal.[271] Epileptogenic patterns are the most common finding, and nearly all these patients will exhibit clinical seizures sometime during the course of the disease if not treated. Asymmetry of background activity and focal slowing, often corresponding to lesion location, are also observed. No specific findings are considered diagnostic.

Pathology

The pathological anatomy of cerebral paragonimiasis correlates well with its clinical presentation. Three distinct histopathological stages of the disease exist: stage I, the meningoencephalitic form; stage II, the granulomatous form; and stage III, the organization-calcification form.[258]

Stage I, the meningoencephalitic stage, is one of early reactive inflammation. An exudative reaction takes place around the migrated fluke, eggs, and toxic metabolic waste products. This produces an inflammatory response, which may result in a necrotizing granulomatous reaction.

Stage II, the granulomatous stage, is characterized by the formation of multiloculated granulomas filled with necrotic debris and ova. There is proliferation of dense collagen fibers, which line the granulomas. The cystoid lesions become progressively more necrotic. The lesion eventually becomes well-encapsulated by the proliferation of dense hyaline collagen fibers, which line the granulomas. It is during this stage that the parenchymal gliotic changes become more apparent.

Stage III is one of organization and calcification. As the disease progresses the central portion of the granuloma may undergo necrosis, forming a localized encapsulated abscess. The lesions tend to coalesce and often form lesions several centimeters in diameter that may eventually calcify.

Treatment

Operative treatment of cerebral paragonimiasis was first reported by Kawai in 1939.[200] Since that time numerous reports have appeared.[179,204] Since the lesions are frequently multiple and not grossly apparent, complete excision may not be either possible or practical, and therefore concomitant chemotherapy is recommended in all cases.[179,244] Treatment with bithionol (2,2'-thiobis (4,6-dichlorophenol)) is recommended.[207,244] The dosage of 30 to 50 mg per kilogram given on alternate days for one month is generally considered adequate. Hepatotoxicity is considered the major side effect of the drug, and initiation of therapy should be preceded by a complete battery of liver function tests. Pulmonary symptoms usually respond quickly, with resolution of infiltrates within three to five months. The cure rate for pulmonary paragonimiasis following adequate treatment has been reported as between 84 and 100 per cent.[257] The effect of bithional on cerebral paragonimiasis is less clear, although Oh has reported that the drug is effective in the acute stages of the disease but not in the chronic phases.[254] More than one course of treatment is sometimes necessary. Complement-fixation tests may be used to follow the patient in the post-treatment period to assess efficacy of treatment. A decompressive operation is rarely required because the cerebral atrophy that is present in the late stages of the disease usually compensates adequately. Lesions in the frontal lobe and anterior parts of the parietal and temporal lobes are more likely to develop fulminating symptoms with marked mass effect, especially during the granulomatous encapsulation stage. If operative therapy is to be successful it must be undertaken before irreversible neurological damage has taken place. Several authors have reported lessened seizure activity postoperatively.[179,257] Those patients in whom seizure activity was lessened or absent postoperatively tended to be those treated early in the disease process. Those in the advanced stages of the disease rarely become seizure-free, and most require lifelong anticonvulsant therapy. The operative mortality rate has improved considerably in recent years and is estimated at 5.5 per cent.[257]

Prognosis

The prognosis of the disease is dependent on the stage in which it is treated. Patients with pulmonary involvement alone usually fare well. Pulmonary lesions resolve spontaneously in 5 to 10 years, and often a single bithionol treatment is sufficient. Cerebral paragonimiasis has a less favorable prognosis, and data regarding it must take into account the natural history of the disease. The average duration of symptoms is approximately five years. Seventy-five per cent of fatalities, however, occur within two years of the onset of symptoms.[259] This figure demonstrates, as would be expected, that most of the patients who die from the disease do so during the initial phases. Well-localized unilateral lesions can often be operatively excised, but recurrence is not uncommon despite gross total excision of abnormal-appearing tissue as well as preoperative and postoperative chemotherapeutic supplementation. Lesions that are widespread and bilateral are considered inoperable, as is brain stem involvement, which is inevitably fatal.

Spinal Paragonimiasis

The classification of spinal paragonimiasis as a separate disease entity is based on a practical consideration of the anatomy of the spine and spinal cord.

Spinal paragonimiasis is rare in comparison to cerebral paragonimiasis. Most reports show it to account for 3 to 5 per cent of central nervous system involvement with paragonimiasis.[76,257] The highest reported estimate is 13 per cent. Concurrent cerebral and spinal involvement is even more unusual.[255]

The epidemiological features of spinal paragonimiasis are similar to those of cerebral paragonimiasis. The disease is most commonly seen in young adult men, although the age range is quite broad (ages 5 to 65 years).[255] The average duration of symptoms is approximately one year, but there is considerable variation.

Clinical Manifestations

The symptoms observed in cases of spinal paragonimiasis are remarkably similar to those of many other granulomatous diseases. Their onset usually is insidious and they tend to occur over relatively long periods of time. While their order of progression is quite well defined and consistent, their temporal sequence is not. Symptoms have been reported to last for up to six years in some cases. The typical patient presents with weakness of and radicular pain in the lower extremities progressing to spastic paraplegia, which develops over a variable period of time. Sensory changes usually occur late in the disease. Back pain is relatively common, but point tenderness over the area of the lesion is not. There are reports of remissions in the degree of deficit, ranging from slight to nearly complete, but in the main, the situation is one of progressive deterioration if treatment is not instituted.

Pathogenesis

Spinal lesions of paragonimiasis exhibit several characteristics that help to delineate the pathogenesis of the disease more clearly. Most frequently the lesions are located in the lower thoracic (54 per cent) and lumbar areas.[259] Cervical location is unusual. The typical extradural location of most lesions supports the theory of direct migration of the parasite via intercostal nerves or vessels. Single or multiple cysts may form. They are usually surrounded by granulomatous tissue and may extend over several vertebral segments. In fact, according to Oh, in approximately 50 per cent of cases the lesion will extend over 4 segments and has been reported to extend over as many as 16 segments.[244a] Those cases with intradural involvement are usually extramedullary and likely to show cerebral involvement also.

Pathology

The histopathological processes of spinal paragonimiasis are quite similar to those instrumental in producing cerebral lesions. There is a tendency for the cystic structures that are formed to be multiple and to remain in relative contiguity with one another. These cystic structures often contain dark yellow to chocolate colored material, the only recognizable elements in the lesion being eosinophils and ova in various stages of decomposition. These cystic structures are usually surrounded by granulomatous tissue. At the interface of the two layers, giant cells of various types are usually seen. Varying degrees of inflammatory cell infiltration have been observed during the different phases of development but are generally less prominent than that seen in cerebral infections.

Diagnosis

A preoperative diagnosis of spinal paragonimiasis is unusual. Serious consideration of the entity in the differential diagnosis of extradural mass lesions is neither practical nor appropriate under most circumstances. Of paramount importance are the patient's residence in or travel to an endemic area and his dietary habits. If after consideration of these factors, parasitic disease is still a possibility, the choices are limited. In fact, spinal schistosomiasis is probably the only other reasonable possibility, and one should be able to distinguish that entity on the basis of the clinical presentation, which is almost invariably more acute than spinal paragonimiasis. Extradural tumors usually mimic the symptoms of paragonimiasis most closely, and it is for these that the entity is most frequently mistaken.

Laboratory Findings

The majority of the laboratory findings do not differ significantly from those of cerebral paragonimiasis. Examination of cerebrospinal fluid is likely to show an elevated protein content (average 100 mg per 100 ml). The glucose level as well as the other commonly measured metabolic parameters is usually within normal limits. Eosinophilia is rare, but represents an important aid if present, as it strongly suggests parasitic rather than tumoral involvement. In those cases in which the cell count is elevated (10 lymphocytes per cubic millimeter) lymphocytes usually predominate. Neither *Paragonimus* ova nor the adult specimen have been recovered in the spinal fluid.

Radiology

Characteristically, plain x-rays of the spine are normal. Abnormalities reported by various authors are nonspecific.[76,319] In contradistinction to cerebral lesions, calcification rarely is encountered. This is not likely the result of an altered mechanism of histopathogenesis, since the finding is so common in cerebral forms of the disease, but rather of the fact that patients with symptoms of progressive cord compression invariably seek treatment before the disease process is allowed to reach the stage in which calcium is deposited.

The typical extradural block consisting of a serrated feathered effect above or below the level of obstruction is seen on the myelogram but is not pathognomonic of the disease. It is almost invariably complete. Although numerous cystic structures are often present, these are rarely seen on mye-lography, most likely because of the arachnoiditis that usually is present.

Treatment

Although few fatalities have been reported that can be attributed solely to spinal paragonimiasis, their rarity should not imply that the disease process is benign. If it is allowed to progress, neurological deficits are profound and debilitating. Depending on the time course and the promptness with which operative treatment is initiated, however, a nearly complete remission of symptoms may be achieved. Although it should accompany operative treatment in all cases, treatment with bithionol alone is not adequate.[259]

TRICHINOSIS

Trichinosis is a widely distributed parasitic disease caused by invasion of the larval form of *Trichinella spiralis*. The organism is one of several nematodes capable of infecting the human central nervous system.

Epidemiology

The geographic distribution of trichinosis probably is broader than that of any of the other parasitic diseases, although prevalence rates are quite variable.

The majority of human infections can be traced to consumption of inadequately cooked pork and pork products, although other hosts such as rabbits, walruses, foxes, and bears have also been implicated.[86,354] There are no intermediate hosts. Both the larval and adult stages of the organism complete their developmental cycles within the same animal.

Clinical Manifestations

Trichinosis causes a myriad of symptoms and mimics a number of different entities as the disease progresses through its various clinical stages. The typical symptom complex is usually initiated by the onset of gastrointestinal symptoms. These symptoms include nausea, diarrhea, and abdominal cramping; appear within 48 hours of ingesting the infected meat; and usually abate upon completion of the enteric phase. Early signs of muscle invasion appear within seven days and include periorbital and facial edema, chemosis, subconjunctival and retinal hemorrhages, and the development of subungual splinter hemorrhages. The muscle involvement may cause severe myalgia. Involvement of the diaphragm is occasionally so severe as to produce dyspnea. Myocarditis may be reflected in significant electrocardiographic abnormalities including ST-T wave anomalies.[282] The myositis associated with trichinosis may be so severe that it simulates flaccid paresis.[210]

Central nervous system involvement is probably the most serious complication of the disease and occurs only in the most severe infections. Between 6 and 17 per cent of patients with clinically symptomatic gastrointestinal disease develop evidence of neurological dysfunction.[363]

The neurological signs and symptoms are so nonspecific as to be of little etiological significance, although the deficits themselves may be quite profound. Patients with central nervous system symptoms are, however, likely to show clinical evidence of disease elsewhere, which may help considerably to narrow the differential diagnosis.

In contradistinction to many of the other parasitic organisms, *Trichinella spiralis* shows no predilection for any particular site within the nervous system. The most frequent clinical presentation is that of a localized encephalitis associated with varying degrees of meningitis. The clinical picture reflects the histopathological progression of the disease from a diffuse meningitis to a relatively localized encephalitis. In the early stages, headache, neck pain, and impairment of cognitive function will dominate the symptom complex. Fully 75 per cent of patients will demonstrate an altered sensorium.[86] As the disease progresses, cranial nerve findings may be noted. Dysfunction is most likely to involve the sixth and seventh cranial nerves and may be aggravated by involvement of the extraocular muscles themselves. In those cases in which the disease is allowed to progress, potentially irreversible focal motor deficits ranging from as minimal as transient hemifacial weakness to as profound and debilitating as dense quadriplegia will dominate the clinical picture.

Pathological reflexes associated with lower motor neuron dysfunction may be seen in 20 to 25 per cent of patients.[86]

Pathology

The clinical course of the disease may be divided into three phases: the invasive (enteric), migratory (hemolymphatic), and encystment (parenteral) phases.

The invasive phase is initiated by ingestion of the organism in insufficiently cooked meat products. The meat contains the encysted larvae. Following ingestion the cystic structure undergoes destruction in the stomach, liberating the free larvae, which migrate to the small intestine, where they penetrate the mucosa and undergo a period of maturation. The enteric phase is usually completed within seven days. Within a short time the male and female organisms copulate. The male dies, but the viviparous female begins producing larvae within 7 to 10 days, a process that may continue for up to four months. Each female may produce 3000 offspring. These larvae are deposited in the mucosa of the gastrointestinal tract and subsequently migrate via hemolymphatic routes—the migratory phase of the disease. The encystment phase usually follows within two to three weeks. During this period the larvae mature. During the maturation process the larvae become resistant to peptic digestion. They eventually encyst within skeletal muscle. The predilection for this particular anatomical site is thought to be related to the large proportion of end-arteries in skeletal muscle. Other organs with similar vascular architecture (brain, myocardium) also show large numbers of organisms. The only permanent repository for the encysted form, however, is skeletal muscle. The severity of the disease appears to be roughly proportional to the number of larvae ingested.

The wide range of clinical neurological dysfunction associated with central nervous system trichinosis confirms the diverse pathophysiological capabilities of the organism. The larvae themselves can invade tissues and may produce vasculitis and hemorrhage or thrombotic or embolic phenomena or a combination of these.

The pathological findings are not distinctive and usually confirm the presence of a diffuse meningoencephalitis. The larvae may be located in the meninges, in the perivascular space, or within granulomatous lesions located in the parenchyma. They have also been located within the vasculature as emboli and have been demonstrated within the layers of the retina.

Within the brain, the typical encystment of the larvae does not take place, but significant glial and fibroblast proliferation may be produced. The microglial nodules that develop rarely attain significant size. The granulomatous nodules are usually found in the subcortical white matter and may contain young larvae. Occasionally, free *Trichinella* larvae unassociated with any cellular response are found.

Diagnosis

Definitive diagnosis of trichinosis requires demonstration of the larva in the blood, cerebrospinal fluid, or muscle. Muscle biopsy is the most useful procedure to accomplish this. The deltoid and gastrocnemius are the sites most frequently used. A positive examination will demonstrate the presence of cysts, or larvae or both.

The most consistent supportive laboratory finding is the eosinophilic pleocytosis that usually appears within 7 to 10 days. The proportion of cells may approach 50 per cent in cases of moderate severity.[282] The eosinophilia is so consistent that it is often utilized as a prognostic factor. Its absence or sudden decrease has traditionally been regarded as a poor prognostic sign and is often seen in patients whose condition is preterminal.

Serological studies that may support the diagnosis include the precipitin reaction and the indirect fluorescent antibody, complement-fixation, bentonite-flocculation, and latex-agglutination tests. It is important to obtain baseline examinations, since changes in titers may be observed as the disease progresses. In the presence of active infection, most of the tests will become positive within three weeks and may remain positive for years. The bentonite-flocculation, immunofluorescent antibody, and latex-agglutination tests are the examinations of choice, since they are both sensitive and specific.

Investigation of the cerebrospinal fluid is most helpful if the larvae are observed. This occurs in approximately 25 per cent of cases.[210] Approximately half of all specimens will have normal glucose, protein, and cell count. The remainder will be nonspecifically abnormal. The larvae are more likely to be observed in centrifuged specimens. Electromyographic studies may confirm the presence of lower motor neuron disease or anterior horn cell degeneration. The muscular weakness is more often due to acute myositis, however, and electromyography will usually reflect this.

Treatment

Treatment with corticosteroids may produce dramatic results in patients with trichinosis, and the beneficial effects are not restricted to an amelioration of central nervous system symptoms. In addition to improvement of the neurological status there is also marked improvement of constitutional symptoms. When the dosage is adequate, the fever usually abates quite rapidly, and the patient obtains relief from myalgias. The recommended dosage of methylprednisolone is 40 to 60 mg per day.[92]

Corticosteroids are usually given in combination with thiabendazole, an antihelminthic agent of the benzimidazole group. In addition to its larvicidal capabilities the drug also appears to have analgesic as well as anti-inflammatory capabilities. This agent is especially important, since it appears to be effective during not only the enteric phase of the disease but the parenteral phase as well. This factor alone portends a disproportionate significance, since the vast majority of cases are diagnosed after encystation has taken place. The thiabendazole appears to facilitate destruction of the cystic structure and to disrupt larval metabolism. The recommended dosage is 50 mg per kilogram per day in divided doses. Both agents are given until symptoms subside or significant toxic side effects appear. This usually requires a period of 7 to 10 days. The patient should be observed during this period because the release of protein breakdown products may produce a Herxheimer-like reaction.[64] Steroid dosage should be tapered when the drug is discontinued. The side effects associated with the use of thiabendazole may be bothersome but rarely necessitate termination of the treatment. They are primarily gastrointestinal in nature and include nausea, vomiting, and abdominal cramping. Occasionally, dermatitis will be produced.

Prognosis

The prognosis of the disease improved dramatically with the introduction of effective chemotherapy. The organism is capable of producing a wide range of pathological effects; and the longer the central nervous system phase of the disease persists without treatment, the more significant the morbidity and the higher the mortality rate to be expected. The overall death rate for untreated central nervous system involvement may approach 50 per cent. As would be expected, the longer the deficits are allowed to persist, the greater is the likelihood that they will become irreversible despite appropriate treatment at later stages in the disease. The mortality rate in patients who receive early and appropriate therapy is negligible.

ANGIOSTRONGYLIASIS

"Angiostrongyliasis" is the term given to the disease entity caused by *Angiostrongylus cantonensis*, the rat lungworm. It is more commonly known as eosinophilic meningitis—a term that stems from its most remarkable biological characteristic, the eosinophilic pleocytosis that is invariably observed in the spinal fluid. Although the existence of an eosinophilic meningitic syndrome had been noted prior to the identification of angiostrongyliasis, its etiology had not been definitively established.[339] Nomura and Lin were the first to report the presence of parasites in a patient with eosinophilic meningitis.[252] The disease was further characterized in 1948 by Bailey, who emphasized its eosinophilic character.[24] Epidemics in New Caledonia in 1950–1951 further demonstrated the clinical manifestations of the disease, and the life cycle of the worm was investigated.[234] In 1961 Alicata proposed that the entry of *Angiostrongylus cantonensis* into the central nervous system caused the entity, and hence it has often been termed Alicata's disease.[8]

Epidemiology

The disease is primarily restricted to the Far East and many of the Pacific Islands, including Hawaii. It is more common in men (male-to-female ratio is 2.6 to 1).[195] Racial differences have also been noted and are most likely due to dietary habits.[286] Although the organism and its hosts are widespread in many populous areas, the specific dietary habits as well as the relatively complicated life cycle of the parasite requiring obligate passage through certain hosts restricts spread of the disease. It occurs in all age groups.

Etiology

Angiostrongyliasis is caused by *Angiostrongylus cantonensis*, the rat lungworm, which is only one of the many nematode parasites producing disease in man. The life cycle of the organism is complicated, utilizing both obligate and paratenic hosts. Where there is little consumption of the paratenic hosts (raw crabs, shrimp, and the like), and where sanitation measures effectively isolate water and foodstuffs from contamination with rat feces, the incidence of the disease is very low.

In the natural cycle of the organism the adult worm resides in the pulmonary arteries of the rat. Undeveloped eggs are expelled from the adult female and embolized to the pulmonary arterioles, where they develop for approximately six days and subsequently hatch into first-stage larvae. These larvae migrate through respiratory passages to the pharynx, where they are expectorated or swallowed and eliminated in the feces. The larvae then infect snails or slugs in which they undergo further changes. The cycle ordinarily completes itself when the rat ingests the snail host. It is, however, expanded when intermediate transport hosts (primarily crustaceans and fish) become infected. Although larvae development is not thought to progress to the adult form in these hosts, the number and range of dietary vectors through which man may be infected is increased considerably. Infection in man takes place by ingesting either the snail hosts, paratenic hosts such as crabs or freshwater prawns, or less frequently, contaminated water or vegetables that harbor the metastrongyloid form of the organism.

Following ingestion the worm invades the gastric mucosa, thus gaining access to the vascular and lymphatic systems and eventually entering the pulmonary vasculature. The larvae are thought to gain access to the central nervous system in two ways: directly via the circulation or indirectly by initially invading skeletal muscle and subsequently migrating along peripheral nerves. In animals such as the rat, after a variable period of time some of the worms enter the subarachnoid space, where they enter the intracranial venous system and migrate once again to the pulmonary musculature. In man, however, it appears that the worm does not complete the cycle of migration back to the pulmonary arterioles, but rather dies within the central nervous system. The failure of the worm to migrate back to its natural habitat (the lung) is the single most important histopathogenic factor in the production of eosinophilic meningitis.

The microscopic findings in the brain are the results of both the worm's presence and of its migration. Parenchyma surrounding the migratory path of the worm shows degenerating tissue as well as cellular infiltrates of eosinophils and neutrophils. Neuronal degeneration frequently is seen. Generally the lesions are considerably less hemorrhagic than in other forms of parasitic infection. The leptomeninges show extensive cellular infiltrates consisting of eosinophils, mononuclear cells, lymphocytes, plasma cells, and some neutrophils. The infiltration is most marked over the basilar portions of the brain. Charcot-Leyden crystals, which are thought to arise from the cytoplasm of macrophages that have phagocytized eosinophilic leukocytes, are also seen. Vascular lesions have also been described and consist of perivascular infiltration as well as intraluminal changes suggestive of prethrombotic lesions. Despite their appearance these lesions seldom lead to vessel necrosis.

Clinical Manifestations

Central nervous system dysfunction is usually the first evidence of infection. Prodromal symptoms are uncommon. The more characteristic clinical picture is initial presentation as a full blown meningoencephalitis.[311] Fever is observed in approximately two thirds of the cases, but it is usually a consistently low-grade temperature elevation as opposed to the more marked elevations seen in viral or bacterial meningoencephalitides.[191] Headache, which is almost invariably present, is severe. It is often accompanied by evidence of mild to moderate meningeal irritation. Kernig's and Brudzinski's signs, however, are usually absent. Visual aberrations may be seen in up to 50 per cent of the patients.[195] A typical presentation of the disease includes various cranial nerve palsies, especially peripheral facial palsies, which are seen in an estimated 3 to 7 per cent of cases.[294] Dysfunction of cranial nerves VI, VII, IX, and XII has also been noted.

Patients often describe paresthesias and dysesthesias, most often in a radicular distribution, but nondermatomal distributions may be seen as well. Schollhammer and coworkers described "pins and needles" paresthesia when the skin was touched lightly or rubbed with a volatile liquid.[311] These dysesthesias may be the result of posterior meningoradiculitis. Some authors consider these algoparesthesias so characteristic as to permit clinical diagnosis.[191]

Animal experiments have clearly implied that the size of the inoculum (the number of infecting larvae) correlates reasonably well with the severity of the disease. It is apparent from the case histories, however, that clinically symptomatic infections may be produced by ingestion of only a relatively few larvae. The incubation period varies, depending on a number of factors that include the size of the inoculum and the immunological status of the host. In the majority of cases, the incubation period is approximately two weeks although it may be as long as 30 days in some cases and as short as 2 to 3 days in others.[9,286]

Diagnosis

Definitive diagnosis is made by identifying the organism in the cerebrospinal fluid.[184,286] This is rarely accomplished, however, and most often the diagnosis is inferred from a positive dietary history, the characteristic clinical syndrome, and the eosinophilic pleocytosis in the cerebro-

spinal fluid. So essential is the demonstration of this eosinophilic pleocytosis that the diagnosis cannot be made without it.

The eosinophilic reaction is not an immediate response. The latency of the response depends primarily on the immune status of the infected individual. In some cases, when the incubation period is prolonged, the diagnosis may be missed because of this latency. If the index of suspicion for the disease is high, the cerebrospinal fluid should be examined on several occasions. The cell count is variable. It may approach several thousand cells in severe cases but ranges between 100 and 1000 cells in two thirds of the cases.[195] The proportion of eosinophils may approach 75 per cent of the total cell count but is usually much lower.[195] Punyagupta and associates have suggested that the pleocytosis should at least exceed 20 cells per cubic millimeter and account for at least 10 per cent of the cells.[286] Of paramount importance is the fact that cerebrospinal fluid examination must include at least one staining technique that is capable of visualizing eosinophils. Giemsa's or Wright's stains are satisfactory. Cerebrospinal fluid will also frequently show a moderate increase in protein (averaging less than 100 per cent). It ranges from being colorless to quite turbid. The opening pressure is elevated in approximately half the cases. The blood usually demonstrates an analogous elevation of the eosinophil count averaging about 10 per cent.

The persistence of eosinophilia in the cerebrospinal fluid is common and may continue for weeks after the active phase of the infection has passed. There does not appear to be any direct attenuation of the cell count correlating with the disappearance of clinical symptoms.

Several immunological tests including fluorescent antibody and indirect hemagglutination tests have been designed and developed to detect A. *cantonensis* infection.[74] The high degree of cross-reactivity between similar antigenic components present in other parasitic organisms has made it difficult to isolate sufficiently specific antigens.

The differential diagnosis of the disease is important in that some entities that mimic eosinophilic meningoencephalitis have significantly higher mortality rates and require different treatment regimens. The eosinophilic pleocytosis noted in the cerebrospinal fluid is also seen in other diseases—parasitic and otherwise. Several helminthic diseases in which the eosinophilia is also seen include paragonimiasis, schistosomiasis, gnathostomiasis, cystercercosis, and echinococcosis. For the most part, however, these diseases exhibit characteristic features that are readily discerned through laboratory or radiographic investigation. Noninfectious diseases affecting the central nervous system, including Hodgkin's disease and polyarteritis nodosa, should also be included.[125,306]

Radiographic studies are almost invariably normal. Electroencephalography usually shows generalized nonspecific abnormalities.

Treatment

The general course of the disease is protracted over several weeks or months in most patients but usually results in spontaneous recovery. Numerous antiparasitic compounds have been tried without success.[322,355] Thiabendazole has been found to control larval invasion of the brain, but has little effect against adult worms.[84,250] Symptomatic treatment is recommended for the various neurological symptoms of the disease. Repeated lumbar puncture can be used to control intracranial pressure in those patients with hydrocephalus. Shunting procedures are rarely required because the course of the disease is relatively short. Many cases of increased intracranial pressure are due to cerebral edema and respond reasonably well to steroids. Steroids also are effective in cases of isolated cranial nerve involvement.

Prognosis

The prognosis of the disease is good. The mortality rate due to the disease itself is low. Punyagupta and associates estimated a rate of approximately 1.2 per cent, which may even be somewhat high.[334] Even in the most severe of cases intercurrent peripherally related complications are more likely to be the direct cause of death than the disease itself.[295]

ACTINOMYCOSIS

Actinomycosis is one of several granulomatous diseases capable of infecting the central nervous system. The most frequent causative agent, *Actinomyces israelii*, is considered part of the normal flora and becomes pathogenic only when it invades sites other than its usual habitat in the tonsillar crypts and gingival margins.

Because of its unusual form and structure, classification of the organism presented a dilemma for taxonomists, and the organism was initially grouped with the fungi. It has subsequently been reclassified as a funguslike bacterium.[209]

Epidemiology

Cases of human actinomycosis have been reported from all over the world.[276] Infection usually arises from an endogenous source—carious teeth, the gingival margins, and the tonsillar crypts being the most frequent sites of isolation.

The disease has been reported in nearly all age groups, though it is most common between the first and third decades.[168] Male agricultural workers have a higher than usual incidence, and the male-to-female ratio is approximately 2 to 1. Numerous occupational variables have been studied, but none has yet been conclusively proved to be a definite predisposing factor.

Pathogenesis and Clinical Manifestations

Human actinomycosis usually produces an abscess in the region of the jaw or pharynx, arising from its endogenous site in the buccal cavity. The organism has a remarkable proclivity to form abscesses and subsequently sinus tracts. The tracts extend by contiguity, rarely respecting tissue planes, and form multiple cutaneous fistulae. The process of forming fistulae is usually accompanied by an intense fibrotic reaction. While this fibrosis prevents spread of infection, it also forms a considerable barrier to pharmacological treatment. Additionally, since the organism forms clusters, it is necessary to achieve drug levels high enough to suppress even those organisms confined within the granules.

Most cases involve the cervicofacial, the thoracic, or the abdominal area. Infection in other sites does occur, however. Central nervous system involvement is a rare complication of primary disease. Numerous articles describe lesions of the brain and spinal cord thought to be due to actinomycosis, but in fewer than 30 has the diagnosis been established by culture.[47,175] Sanford and Voelker reviewed 587 cases of actinomycosis reported in the United States, citing an incidence of brain and spinal cord involvement in 1.3 per cent.[304] More recent surveys place the incidence of all forms of central nervous system involvement at approximately 3 per cent.[58,356]

Central nervous system actinomycosis rarely appears as an isolated entity. The mechanism of infection is relatively straightforward. Access to the central nervous system is obtained either by direct extension from contiguous foci or via hematogenous dissemination. Involvement by direct extension favors basilar locations, with progression via the orbit, auditory canal, or sinuses. Hematogenous dissemination is usually the result of spread from a primary focus in the lung. Hematogenous dissemination is by far the most frequently implicated mechanism of involvement.

Actinomyces is capable of causing a wide range of pathophysiological effects. The most common form of central nervous system disease produced is the brain abscess, which may be single, multiloculated, or multiple.

Intracranial abscesses are usually caused by direct extension of the infection from adjacent bone. The mandible and middle ear are common primary sites. The abscesses are usually well encapsulated and can be easily identified by computed tomography, which is the diagnostic procedure of choice.

Meningitis may, but does not usually, accompany brain abscess formation. It will more likely be seen in those cases in which access to the central nervous system is obtained by direct extension. It may, of course, also be seen following abscess rupture.

The clinical symptoms associated with central nervous system actinomycosis reflect the pre-eminence of brain abscess as its most common neurological form. The symptom complex is usually dominated by focal deficits and evidence of increased in-tracranial pressure. It is not sufficiently distinctive, however, to allow differentiation from other forms of brain abscess on the basis of the clinical findings with the exception, perhaps, that it appears to develop more slowly than pyogenic forms of the disease.

The gross appearance of actinomycotic brain abscesses is much like that of other forms of brain abscess. The capsule is usually well defined, and the contents grossly consist of white or yellow pus. The granules may be present throughout the abscess. The microscopic findings are not particularly distinctive. There is usually an outer zone that consists of granulation tissue and a lymphocytic cellular infiltrate. The organisms, which tend to be basophilic when stained, may be scattered throughout. The granules of actinomycosis tend to be broader (over 3 μm in diameter) than those found in other similar diseases, particularly nocardiosis. Nocardial granules tend to lack the radiating fringe of eosinophilic clubs that characterize those seen in actinomycosis. Accurate morphological identification requires experience.

Spinal abscesses may be caused by direct extension or by hematogenous spread. In both instances the most common primary site is the lung. Involvement of the spinal axis usually takes the form of epidural abscess and is frequently associated with concurrent osteomyelitic involvement of the vertebral column. Ernst and Ratjen estimated that bony structures are involved in 15 per cent of cases, and vertebral involvement is specifically estimated at 5.5 per cent.[123] The vertebrae themselves usually show irregular surface erosion with scattered areas of new bone formation. They may be involved in the absence of any cerebral disease. In those cases in which cerebral disease is present concurrently, evidence of mastoiditis, sinusitis, or osteomyelitis of the skull should be searched for.

Patients with vertebral actinomycosis usually present with a chronic debilitating illness. Back pain is often present, and cutaneous fistulae are almost invariably present. Paravertebral subcutaneous abscesses are quite common. Any portion of the vertebrae may be involved. In contradistinction to tuberculosis, however, the intervertebral disc space is usually spared.[216] The differential diagnosis should include blastomycosis, tuberculosis, nocardiosis, and metastatic carcinoma. The onset of neurological symptoms is usually gradual, occurring over a period of weeks. Spinal cord compression occurs in less than 10 per cent of cases and, when present, is usually due to epidural abscess formation.[216] Vertebral collapse is unusual.[79]

Diagnosis and Laboratory Findings

Actinomyces israelii belongs to the order Actinomycetales. It is a microaerophilic organism consisting of thin branching filaments. Gram stain preparations reveal a gram-positive central filamentous mass. Often a surrounding area of gram-negative material is seen, but this is thought to represent reactive lipoid material laid down by the host. The organism tends to grow in colonies in the tissues, eventually forming what are commonly referred to as sulfur granules, although they do not contain sulfur. These distinctive granules are often helpful as diagnostic aids.

Diagnosis of non–central nervous system forms of the disease is usually relatively easy once the characteristic cutaneous fistulae develop. Collections of pus near fistulous openings often reveal the characteristic "sulfur granules." The granules may be found by diluting the pus in sterile saline and filtering the sediment. Although usually described as yellow, the granules may be white, black, cream colored, or brown. Samples should be stained both by Gram's method and the modified Ziehl-Neelsen technique. A confirmatory identification depends upon noting the distinctive branching filaments.

The status of *Actinomyces israelii* as normal flora compromises the use of laboratory culture as a definitive means of diagnosis. This is particularly true of sputum specimens. Isolation of the organism from cerebrospinal fluid is unusual. For all practical purposes a positive cerebrospinal fluid culture result may be considered diagnostic.

Analysis of cerebrospinal fluid almost invariably yields results that are abnormal but nonspecific. Protein is frequently increased to a moderate degree, and polymorphonuclear pleocytosis may be seen. The cell count rarely exceeds 1000 per cubic millimeter. Glucose levels are rarely significantly depressed.

Chest radiographs, particularly those showing periosteal proliferation of the ribs and pulmonary consolidation in association with one another, may be quite helpful, as this combination is rarely seen in other disease entities. Involvement of the vertebral column also presents a characteristic picture that has been described as a coarse sieve and is due to absorption and then reformation of new bone. Intervertebral discs are usually spared. Myelographic investigation of those cases of spinal involvement that present as epidural abscess often reveals a complete block, but the radiographic picture is not pathognomonic.

Treatment

The presence of neurological manifestations in central nervous system actinomycosis implies a grave prognosis. Recently, however, advances in the early radiographic diagnosis of the disease have improved the outlook for patients. Intracranial actinomycotic brain abscess is treated by operative excision or decompression accompanied by intense antibiotic therapy. Lane and co-workers reported good results with antibiotic and steroid therapy without operative decompression in two cases of vertebral actinomycosis.[216] The combination of decompression with adjunctive antibiotic therapy is recommended, however. Penicillin remains the antibiotic of choice, although it is inconvenient in that treatment must be parenteral and prolonged. The nature of the pathological process with its extension fibrosis makes it difficult to achieve adequate in vivo drug levels. Doses of 10 to 20 million units per day in divided doses for a minimum of six weeks are recommended. Treatment may be required for as much as one year or longer. Tetracycline antibiotics are also very effective and may be helpful, especially in patients allergic to penicillin. Recommended dosage is 500 mg orally every six hours. Their use in cerebrospinal forms of the disease is somewhat limited because of poor penetration of the blood-brain barrier.

Prognosis

The prognosis is relatively good in the two major primary forms of the disease (cervicofacial and abdominal), with recovery rates estimated at 90 per cent and 80 per cent respectively.[156] Involvement elsewhere usually implies widespread dissemination, and the prognosis is guarded.

PETRIELLIDIOSIS

This rare fungal entity is caused by *Petriellidium* (*Allescheria*) *boydii,* an organism first described by Saccardo in 1911.[299] In 1921, Boyd and Crutchfield were the first to isolate the organism from a mycetoma in man.[52] Although it is a common cause of mycotic mycetoma in temperate areas, reported cases of central nervous system involvement are rare.

Epidemiology

The fungus has been isolated from soil and sewage, and most of the cases of the usual pedal form of the disease are seen among agricultural workers. The majority of cases have been reported from tropical and subtropical locations.[315] There appears to be no age, sex, or racial predilection.

Pathogenesis and Clinical Manifestations

P. boydii usually gains access to the subcutaneous tissues via cutaneous inoculation. Subcutaneous abscesses and sinus tracts are formed through which mycotic granules grossly visible to the naked eye are extruded. The area of involvement usually shows suppuration with extensive fibrosis. While the organism is most commonly isolated from pedal mycetomas, it has also been isolated from pulmonary lesions, sputum specimens, thyroid gland, and brain. Whether this reflects a preference for vascular tissue on the part of the organism, is a result of generalized hematogenous dissemination, or reflects some as yet unknown pathophysiological mechanism is unclear.

Although nervous system lesions occur without an identifiable primary focus, isolated involvement of the central nervous system is distinctly unusual.[130] Unlike the forms found elsewhere in the body, which tend to be intermittently progressive, those in the central nervous system, although slow, usually are relentless in their progression.

The specific pathophysiological mechanisms involved in production of central nervous system forms of the disease have yet to be completely characterized. Three pathological types—brain abscess, meningitis, and granulation tissue interspersed throughout the subarachnoid space—have been described.

Diagnosis and Laboratory Findings

As with most of the fungal diseases, definitive diagnosis is based on morphological identification of the organism in tissue. The mycelial form of the organism has been cultured from or identified in specimens obtained from all types of lesions. The organism grows well on Sabouraud's agar. It is initially white but later turns light gray. It produces granules that vary in color. Microscopic examination reveals intertwined septate hyphae or round encysted forms termed chlamydospores. The structure differs, depending on the source from which the specimen is isolated. Serological studies using immunodiffusion techniques are available to confirm the presence of the disease. This is especially important, since mixed infections are not uncommon. Cerebrospinal fluid findings have been reported in only a few cases and, while definitely abnormal, they lack specific etiological significance.[132] They generally include a neutrophilic pleocytosis and increased protein. The sugar content may be low but is more likely to be in the normal range.

Treatment

Amphotericin B has been used in the treatment of auricular forms of the disease, but has not been found to be particularly effective in central nervous system disease. It does, however, represent one of the few treatment options available. Localized lesions should undergo operative debridement. Recently, estrogens have been used, but their role is experimental and their efficacy has not been established.

Prognosis

Although the disease is characterized by periods of spontaneous remission, the usual clinical course is one of progressive deterioration. Most reported cases of central nervous system involvement have proved fatal.[132] Secondary infections are an important cause of complications and death.

ASPERGILLOSIS

Aspergillosis is one of the more commonly encountered mycotic infections of the central nervous system, which as a group are rather rare entities. The disease is produced by relatively few of the more than 350 species of the *Aspergillus* group.[231] Approximately eight species are pathogenic in man, the most important being *Aspergillus fumigatus,* which accounts for almost 90 per cent of human infections.[370]

Epidemiology

The pathogenic *Aspergillus* species have a worldwide distribution. Because the organism thrives at the higher temperatures produced by bacterial fermentation, its habitat usually consists of moist decomposing plant matter. Early in this century, aspergillosis was considered an occupational disease of wig makers, furriers, pigeon handlers, and stockyard workers. It was later discovered that the organism is ubiquitous and that, while persons in certain occupations are more likely to receive a heavier inoculum at any one time, the disease is by no means restricted to these groups. The organism is not infrequently encountered as a laboratory contaminant. The disease is, however, infrequent in comparison with the number of persons who are exposed, supporting the contention that the organism's pathogenicity is relatively low unless host resistance has been significantly altered. The organism is opportunistic, and as would be expected, it is seen much more frequently in association with disease entities or conditions that alter host resistance (e.g., leukemia, neoplastic disease, steroid or immunosuppressive therapy.).[241]

There is no age or race predilection.[241] Several studies have, however, confirmed a preponderance of the disease in men.[246]

Factors other than occupational have not been implicated.

The true incidence of central nervous system involvement is unknown. Although localization exclusively within the central nervous system has been observed, this represents the exception rather than the rule.[277] In disseminated disease more than one site is usually involved (brain and kidney in two thirds of cases). Fetter and associates estimated that neurological lesions may be present in 60 to 70 per cent of these patients.[130] A recent review cites a much lower estimate (approximately 13 per cent), but this report summarizes a group of patients who were carefully and continuously observed for fungal diseases because of their debilitated or compromised immune state, and thus it does not represent the general population.[271]

Although the entity is still considered rare, its incidence appears to be increasing. Responsible factors may be a greater awareness of the disease itself, the availability of laboratory techniques to diagnose it, the use of immunosuppressive agents and antibiotics that may predispose to opportunistic infection, and the increased longevity of patients with depressed immune responses.

Pathogenesis and Clinical Manifestations

The portal of entry for the fungus in most forms of the disease is almost invariably the respiratory tree, where the disease may remain localized or become disseminated to various ectopic sites, which include the skin, kidney, brain, gastrointestinal tract, and eye.[51] In the central nervous system, however, three major routes are implicated: hematogenous dissemination from a primary source (e.g., lung) or by direct vascular access (blood transfusions or self-administration of narcotics), contiguous spread from an adjacent focus (orbit, paranasal sinuses, mastoid cells) or iatrogenic spread (during neurosurgical procedures, instillation of intrathecal antibiotics, lumbar puncture).[127,271,364,375]

Hematogenous dissemination is by far the most frequent means of access.[176,231] Although it was once believed to be usually via the posterior circulation, more recent studies suggest that both anterior and posterior circulations are essentially equally involved.[271] Lesions associated with hematogenous dissemination tend to be more acute and necrotizing, and this is undoubtedly related to the organism's ability to invade blood vessels and produce thrombosis and infarction.[290] Those infections caused by local extension from contiguous sites tend to be more chronic.

Five major forms of the disease occur in the central nervous system: (1) meningitis; (2) meningoencephalitis; (3) abscesses, cranial and extracranial and single or multiple; (4) single solid granuloma without abscess formation; and (5) primary vascular disease, which includes such varied presentations as occlusion of the internal carotid artery and subarachnoid hemorrhage secondary to rupture of mycotic aneurysms.

Of the five major groups, abscesses and meningitis account for nearly 80 per cent of the cases.[246]

Because of the wide spectrum of pathogenic mechanisms displayed by the organism, the clinical manifestations are also quite varied. It is unusual for neurological symptoms alone to predominate.

Meningitis usually is less fulminating than bacterial types, although the patient may be quite ill not only because of nervous system involvement but because the disease often is disseminated throughout the body. Symptoms are nonspecific, usually consisting of headache, nuchal rigidity, and altered sensorium. The course is more likely to be fulminating if the meningitis accompanies brain abscess. If the course is fulminant from the onset, the prognosis is grave. The meningoencephalitic form of the disease presents in a similar manner, mimicking a hemorrhagic leukoencephalitis. Disturbances in the level of consciousness in both forms of the disease may be aggravated by the azotemia caused by renal involvement. In other respects the patient's condition often resembles septic shock. *Aspergillus fumigatus* is one of the few fungi producing an endotoxin that is both histotoxic and hemotoxic.[176]

Brain abscesses and granulomas tend to act as space-occupying lesions. The most common symptoms include headache, seizures, and focal deficits associated with the particular anatomical area that is involved. Evidence of increased intracranial pressure is quite common. The abscesses vary in size and frequently are multiple.[185,374]

Infections of the spinal axis involving *Aspergillus* are rare.[185,316] So few cases have been reported, in fact, that generalizations are difficult. Nevertheless, it is obvious that this form of the disease is considerably less common than cerebral involvement. It usually occurs in the presence of disseminated disease.[174,185] The presenting feature is likely to be extradural compression in the thoracic region.[185] Whether entrance to the spinal axis is obtained by direct extension or by hematogenous dissemination has not been clearly delineated. Both routes are possible. Most of the reported cases have occurred in patients with disseminated disease who are debilitated and whose immune response is suppressed, or in those patients receiving corticosteroids or broad-spectrum antibiotics.[371]

Granulomas tend to form in patients who have been infected with the fungus for some time and are more likely to form in those with concurrent infections of the orbit, mastoid cells, or paranasal sinuses. The formation of granulomas in patients with acute disseminated disease or end-stage neoplastic disease is extremely rare. Granulomatous lesions tend to be chronic and sclerosing, and like those of other granulomatous diseases, show a predominance of mononuclear cell infiltrations. Granulomatous lesions of the cranial nerves have also been reported.[173] A remarkably constant feature, regardless of the histological variations, is the degree of vascular invasion and secondary thrombosis and infarction. Unusual clinical presentations of this form of the disease include trigeminal nerve neuroma, trigeminal neuralgia, and nonpulsating exophthalmos mimicking retro-orbital neoplasia.[189,310,376]

Numerous reports have described subarachnoid hemorrhage secondary to mycotic aneurysm, but relatively few cases are well documented.[5] Many fungi are difficult to culture, and specimens may be mishandled if this potential cause is not considered in the differential diagnosis from the outset. Without confirmation by culture, definitive diagnosis usually is not possible. Presumptive diagnosis, however, based on the morphological characteristics of the aneurysm may be made. Fungal mycotic aneurysms tend to be relatively large and generally arise from major arterial trunks. In contradistinction, bacterial mycotic aneurysms usually are smaller and most frequently are situated at peripheral branches of the middle cerebral artery.[182,292]

Although the entity of fungal mycotic aneurysm still is considered to be rare, the incidence appears to be increasing. Probably this is due not only to improved culture techniques and diagnostic methods, but also to the increased use of various chemotherapeutic agents that alter or suppress the immune response. Considering the pathophysiological mechanisms of the organism, it is not surprising that most of these cases are due to *Aspergillus*. The organism is capable of blood vessel invasion that results in thrombosis—ideal conditions for aneurysm formation. Despite these favorable circumstances, formation of aneurysms secondary to fungal infection remains an unusual complication of the disease. Three deaths due to rupture of mycotic aneurysms of the internal carotid artery have been reported.[246]

Diagnosis

Ideally, diagnosis consists of microscopic identification of *Aspergillus* from the involved site corroborated by culture verifications from the same site. Diagnosis by this means is rarely possible for two reasons. The first is that aspergillosis frequently involves vital centers and biopsy for examination and culture is not possible. Second, the *Aspergillus* group is ubiquitous and is not infrequently encountered as a laboratory contaminant. A single positive culture obtained from a source other than a "deep tissue" site is usually not considered to be diagnostic proof. Cultures of blood, sputum, and other body fluids, including the cerebrospinal fluid, are rarely positive even when meningitis is present.[371] Several specimens of each fluid should be examined. The structure of the organism depends upon the oxygen tension. The rather characteristic conidiophore is seen only during periods of growth as a saprophyte where the organism is exposed to air (predominantly in pulmonary lesions).[371] The more usual form consists of uniform-appearing septate hyphae. Biopsy of suspected tissue often confirms the presence of these characteristic hyphae and frequently aids in the diagnosis. Biopsy, however,

often is not a practical alternative in central nervous system lesions, and therefore culture of suspected tissue is mandatory.[371]

Cerebrospinal fluid examination usually is nonspecifically abnormal. Most often the fluid is clear with a moderate neutrophilic pleocytosis. Cell counts usually average about 500 cells per cubic millimeter, but counts as high as 8000 cells per cubic millimeter have been reported.[246] The protein usually is increased into the 100 to 300 mg per 100 ml range.[189,240,260,376] The opening pressure is elevated in those forms that present as mass lesions. Other parameters usually are normal. Several ancillary immunological tests including immunodiffusion, complement fixation, immunoelectrophoresis, and immunofluorescence are also available. Although if positive they do tend to lend considerable support to the diagnosis, they are of little use if they are not. Several authors have found them unreliable in cases of invasive aspergillosis.[241,371] As with many of the fungal diseases, the diagnosis is most often inferred from a combination of supportive laboratory evidence and clinical findings.

Plain radiographs of the skull seldom are helpful in providing specific clues. Signs of increased intracranial pressure may be present, and bony destruction has been reported, but this is not the usual case. Intracranial calcification has also been reported but is unusual.[188]

Radionuclide brain scans are frequently positive, showing uptake if areas of abscess or granuloma formation are present, but this is not invariable.[241,318,352]

Angiography reveals findings consistent with the primary disease. In abscess and granuloma formations an avascular mass is usually seen. Aneurysmal dilatations or thrombosis or both may be seen in cases of mycotic arteritis.

Most reported cases of spinal cord involvement have implicated epidural abscess as the predominant pathological feature. Myelographic findings are not specific for this particular entity.

Computed tomography is useful in locating mass lesions, but the findings, usually solid lesions without a significant amount of edema, are not pathognomonic.[344] The lesions show moderate contrast enhancement. Calcification may or may not be present and does not appear to differ from that found in other granulomatous diseases.

Treatment

Treatment is directed at the fundamental underlying disease. Localized lesions have been successfully excised from the lung, brain, and spinal axis. Concurrent treatment with amphotericin B is recommended, although its value has not been unequivocally established in systemic infections. Obtaining drug levels that are capable of inhibiting the organism within the central nervous system is difficult. Another complication of treatment is that frequently the patients are receiving multiple pharmacological agents that may potentiate the various side effects of amphotericin B. Experimental data have suggested that drug regimens such as amphotericin B and 5-fluorocytosine or rifampin or both would be helpful, but they have not been confirmed clinically.[18,206] Combination therapy appears to exhibit synergistic activity in vivo, making it preferable to the use of the individual agents. Intrathecal instillation of amphotericin B has also been tried, but its use is experimental, and some authors consider it to be too toxic.[346] None of the currently available pharmacological regimens is completely satisfactory. A specific effort should be made to restore the host's defense mechanisms, since this is one of the major predisposing factors.

Operative treatment of brain and epidural abscesses due to *Aspergillus* does not differ significantly from procedures for those due to other causes with the exception of the chemotherapy. The use of corticosteroids is discouraged except when absolutely necessary, since they appear to enhance tissue invasion and dissemination of the fungus.

Prognosis

The prognosis of the disease is intimately related to the general health of the patient, which is the single most important prognostic factor. The almost invariable association of disseminated aspergillosis with a compromised immune state or debilitating illness makes selection and analysis of other specific prognostic factors difficult. Nevertheless, some generalizations may be made: (1) Disseminated disease is almost invariably fatal. (2) The presence of renal involvement alone, because it is exceptionally difficult to eradicate, implies an unfavorable prognosis. (3) Meningitic forms of the disease, if fulminant from the outset, have a poor prognosis. (4) Meningitic forms of the disease in combination with brain abscess also have a poor prognosis. (5) Multiple brain abscesses have a less favorable prognosis than single lesions. (6) The prognosis of all central nervous system forms of the disease, chemotherapeutic advances notwithstanding, is extremely poor.

BLASTOMYCOSIS

North American blastomycosis, also known as Gilchrist's disease, is a fungal disease caused by *Blastomyces dermatitidis*. It was first described in 1896 and was originally thought to be tuberculous in origin.[151] The entity should be differentiated from European and South American blastomycosis, whose etiological agents are not members of the *Blastomyces* genus. The preferred designation of these entities is cryptococcosis and paracoccidioidomycosis respectively.

Epidemiology

While the disease may occur in widely separated geographic locations, the most heavily endemic areas are located in the south central part of the United States.[262]

Central nervous system blastomycosis is secondary to systemic dissemination. The majority of cases of systemic disease occur in middle-aged adult men, but the age range extends from infancy through the ninth decade.[262] The male-to-female ratio ranges from as low as 6:1 to as great as 15:1.[130] There does not appear to be any definite racial predilection, although the disease is somewhat more common in blacks.[220]

The organism is thought to be a soil saprophyte. Accordingly, the disease appears to be more common among those whose occupations require prolonged or frequent exposure to the soil. Transmission of the disease by contagion appears possible but probably is not a significant risk factor. The majority of infections are contracted by inhalation of the infectious agent from environmental sources.[262]

Pathogenesis and
Clinical Manifestations

Three clinical forms of blastomycosis are generally recognized.[220] The first is a primary localized cutaneous form that results in skin lesions, is extremely rare, and may exist in the absence of pulmonary involvement. Its potential as a source for central nervous system infection is limited. The lesions themselves are produced by direct inoculation of the organism into the skin. The majority of tegumentary lesions are due to systemic dissemination, however, rather than direct inoculation. The presence of a dermatological lesion should prompt a thorough investigation to determine the primary source and the extent of the spread. The absence of the characteristic skin lesions does not exclude systemic dissemination, however, since only 25 per cent of patients with disseminated disease develop the obvious skin lesions.[202] The skin lesions resemble those caused by other fungal diseases (paracoccidioidomycosis, actinomycosis, coccidioidomycosis) at various stages of development. Mature lesions, however, have a distinctive appearance that allows reasonably facile identification.

Pulmonary forms of the disease constitute the second disease category and vary from a relatively benign self-limited infection to a severe and progressively debilitating illness. The primary portal of entry is the respiratory tract itself. Although the lung is the most common primary site of infection, this may be difficult to demonstrate radiographically and may not be evident clinically. In those patients in whom pulmonary infection does become symptomatic, the onset of symptoms is frequently insidious, with cough and chest pain. The associated constitutional symptoms resemble tuberculosis, but actual cavitary disease occurs in relatively few patients. Pulmonary lesions of some type are found in up to 95 per cent of autopsies on patients with blastomycosis.[158] Acute lesions may consist of infiltrates and consolidation, whereas chronic lesions tend to be fibronodular.[220]

In a minority of cases, the pulmonary infection progresses to systemic generalized disease capable of infecting several organ systems including the central nervous system. Systemic disease represents the third major disease classification. The mechanism of dissemination is primarily hematogenous.

Direct extension from sources such as the paranasal sinuses and other contiguous osseous locations may also occur.[165] Primary central nervous system disease, however, does not occur, and for all practical purposes involvement of the central nervous system is considered a complication of systemic disease.

Estimates of involvement of the central nervous system vary from 3 to 10 per cent of all cases.[130,158] If the patient population is restricted to those with disseminated disease, the incidence may approach 33 per cent.

The clinical presentation of blastomycosis of the central nervous system usually falls into one of three major categories: meningitis, mass lesions (cerebral and spinal), and meningoencephalitis.

The first two categories encompass 90 per cent of the cases.[59,158,245] A substantial number of patients present with a combination of histopathological findings suggesting that more than a single pathophysiological mechanism is operative. In those cases in which one clinical form predominates, however, meningitis is more common.

Blastomycosis may spread by direct extension, but the organism does not generally invade the dura. Several cases confirming the presence of epidural mass lesions as a result of skull involvement have been reported.[130,158]

The most common signs and symptoms of central nervous system involvement are headache, convulsions, memory deficits, various focal deficits, and altered sensorium.[59,220,221]

Spinal cord compression by an epidural mass is the most readily recognized clinical presentation. It closely resembles similar syndromes produced by tuberculosis and metastatic carcinoma of the lung, although this particular manifestation is seen relatively more frequently in blastomycosis.[158]

The propensity of the organism to extend to the posterior elements of the vertebral body accounts for the relatively greater frequency of blastomycosis presenting in this manner. Multiple segments may be involved, since the organism appears capable of dissecting under the spinal ligaments. This produces pathological changes similar to those seen in tuberculous spondylitis. Pathological changes in the disc space are also seen, most commonly a marked narrowing. Since multiple levels are usually involved, vertebral collapse is not uncommon. The radiographic findings are so similar to those of the tuberculosis that no distinction between the two entities can be made radiologically. Most cases require histological diagnosis. The thoracic portion of the cord is most often affected, and disease in this location is almost invariably accompanied by paravertebral or pulmonary involvement.[158] Occasionally, pleural fistulae are demonstrated. The tendency to metastasize to multiple intracerebral and spinal sites resembles the clinical patterns seen in tuberculosis and carcinoma of the lung.

Diagnosis

The diagnosis of blastomycosis of the central nervous system may be difficult to establish. Brain biopsy may be required because identification and culture confirmation are more likely if a tissue source is used. Lacking this, ventricular or cisternal fluid will often yield good results. Smears of cerebrospinal fluid may yield positive results in up to 50 per cent of cases.[158] The presence of the organism has only rarely been confirmed by cerebrospinal fluid culture.[59,158] Cultures may take four to eight weeks to become positive.[245] Cerebrospinal fluid is quite often abnormal, but in a nonspecific manner. Leukocytic pleocytosis is common, and protein levels are usually moderately elevated. Glucose levels tend to be normal.

Immunological tests are of little use in specific confirmation of the disease. Cross-reactivity with histoplasmosis and coccidioidomycosis antigens is common.[220]

The neuroradiological procedures that are used to evaluate central nervous system blastomycosis may reveal definite evidence of neuropathological changes, but they are seldom of any etiological changes, but they are seldom of any etiological significance. Morgan and associates noted contrast enhancement of a blastomycotic granuloma on CT scan, but the lesion otherwise resembled any of several other types of lesions of varying causes.[245]

Cerebral blastomycosis invariably presents either subsequently to or concurrently with obvious involvement elsewhere. Up to 90 per cent of patients with the various forms of central nervous system disease also have disseminated disease, and it may be possible to isolate the organism from several sources.[221]

Treatment

Untreated systemic disease is almost invariably fatal. Although a few other chemotherapeutic agents are available, the drug of choice for the treatment of blastomycosis is amphotericin B. The cumulative dosage required for cure is variable. Leers has recommended that the total not exceed 5 gm.[220] The majority of cases will require less. Insufficient total dosage, however, frequently results in relapse. Patients who receive a cumulative dosage of less than 1.5 gm appear to be especially vulnerable.[220,272] The renal status of the patient requires constant monitoring. Those with a normal baseline renal status should tolerate dosages in the range of 2 to 4 gm without difficulty. Most strains of *B. dermatitidis* are sensitive to amphotericin B, and dosages in the range of 2 to 3 gm are sufficient. Whenever possible, analysis of cerebrospinal fluid flow dynamics allows the clinician to assess the efficacy of intrathecal treatment.

Prognosis

The recent literature attests to the fact that, like the prognoses for many of the other systemic mycoses, that for all forms of blastomycosis improved following the introduction of amphotericin B. In earlier reports of involvement of the central nervous system, mortality rates regularly exceeded 90 per cent.[59,165] With appropriate treatment, this rate has been reduced to 15 per cent and can be expected to improve as neuroradiological techniques, particularly computed tomography, make earlier diagnosis possible.[60]

CANDIDIASIS

Candidiasis (candidiosis, moniliasis, candidosis) is a fungal disease caused by any of several species belonging to the genus *Candida*. The disease encompasses a broad clinical spectrum varying from self-limited dermatological infections to fatal endocarditis or meningitis. Once it was believed to be rare, but in recent years a dramatic increase in incidence has been noted.[181] Candidiasis is now considered by some authors to be the most common mycotic disease affecting the central nervous system.[273] The increase is related to concurrent increase in several factors that predispose to its development—among them the increased use of indwelling catheters, broad-spectrum antibiotics, corticosteroid medications, and cytotoxic immunosuppressive agents.[20,136,314] Although *Candida* fulfills many of the criteria for opportunistic organisms, it is by no means restricted to a debilitated patient population. Approximately 25 per cent of patients present with no apparent predisposing factor.

Epidemiology

Candida species have a worldwide distribution and colonize several avian and mammalian hosts, including man. Although some 80 species are included in the genus *Candida* only eight are considered pathogenic, and of these, two—*Candida albicans* and *Candida tropicalis*—cause the majority of human disease.[4] *Candida albicans* can be consistently isolated from numerous body sites in as many as 50 per cent of otherwise healthy individuals. Central nervous system forms of the disease are seen twice as frequently in males as in females. For reasons that are not entirely clear, the disease affects younger age groups. A substantial percentage of the cases have been reported among the neonatal population, a phenomenon that is probably due to immaturity of immunological defense mechanisms.

An unusual feature of candidiasis, unlike the other fungal entities, is its potential for transmission as contagion. Animal-to-man transmission may also be possible because numerous animals also harbor the organism as part of their normal flora.

Although several authors have noted the possibility of primary central nervous system candidiasis, the issue is of little practical importance because it is rare and its documentation does not require modification of the treatment plan.[211,336]

Pathogenesis

The anatomical findings associated with *Candida* infection of the central nervous system are diverse, reflecting a wide range of pathological changes.[42] The majority of cases present as leptomeningitis. The duration of the infection will, to some extent, determine the range of pathological findings. The cellular reaction varies from a scant perivascular collection of cells to a picture that closely mimics pyogenic meningitis. In these cases there may be extensive deposition of exudate and heavy infiltration of polymorphonuclear cells. It may be possible to identify the organism among the leukocytic collection of cells.

The organism is also capable of producing a granulomatous meningitis that, at least grossly, closely resembles tuberculous meningitis. The granulomatous changes may be observed in the leptomeninges as well as in the ependymal surfaces of the ventricles and the choroid plexus. The friable lesions resemble tubercles and may be distributed extensively over the surface of the meninges and throughout the subarachnoid space. Cases of pachymeningitis have also been reported.[23]

Within the brain parenchyma itself the organism produces a variety of lesions ranging in size from minute to several centimeters in diameter. The mass lesions are most often granulomatous in nature, but occasionally abscesses are formed. Minute glial nodules have also been observed, as have various degrees of encephalitis as well as areas of hemorrhagic infarct.

Brain abscesses due to *Candida* infection are more frequently seen in the white than in the gray matter. The initial lesion may appear as acute encephalitis that later progresses to the traditional abscess structure and is accompanied by formation of frank pus and dense infiltration by inflammatory cells. The formation of the capsular structure takes place over a relatively long period of time. Consequently, definite capsules are only seen in lesions that are relatively long-standing. The more pathogenic of the *Candida* species appear to have a definite vascular tropism. Lacking the invasive capabilities of such organisms as *Mucor*, they nevertheless are capable of causing thrombosis by provoking inflammatory changes in the walls of the artery. Infarction secondary to an embolic phenomenon is not uncommon, especially in those cases in which concurrent endocarditis exists. The sequence of infarction followed by necrosis predisposes to the development of abscesses as well as the postinfarction gliotic changes that usually take place. The pathological changes of spinal lesions closely parallel those seen in the parenchyma, and lesions in the meninges demonstrate similar histological features.

Clinical Manifestations

Although the majority of patients with *Candida* infection of the central nervous system present with meningitis, they also may have meningoencephalitis, brain abscess, and granulomatous mass lesions.

The clinical presentation is quite similar to that observed in the other fungal meningitides. The syndrome is usually initiated by the onset of progressive severe headache followed by nuchal rigidity, fever, nausea, and vomiting. The clinical picture ranges from virtually asymptomatic to deathly ill. The symptoms may progress more rapidly in those cases in which obstructive hydrocephalus makes a significant contribution, and in them nausea and vomiting are usually more prominent and papilledema is frequently observed. As in many of the mycotic diseases, extension of the meningitic process into the perivascular space produces a meningoencephalitis that can be exceptionally debilitating. The majority of parenchymal lesions, however, are the result of hematogenous dissemination.

Diagnosis

Definitive diagnosis depends heavily on identification of the fungus in tissue. Positive identification of the organism in cerebrospinal fluid is possible in only about half the cases. Laboratory culture provides positive identification in an additional 25 per cent of patients. Culture of all specimens is mandatory because species identification cannot be made from direct smears in many cases and also because of the close resemblance to other fungal organisms. *Candida* species display several important morphological features that make relatively rapid identification possible. In general the organisms appear round to oval, measuring 5 to 10 μ in diameter. Budding may be observed as well as the true mycelium or the pseudomycelium. Grossly, the organisms appear as white colonies. *Candida albicans* produces chlamydospores that enable it to resist a wide range of environmental changes.

Invasion of the central nervous system by *Candida* is almost invariably secondary to spread from a primary source. It is imperative to identify the primary focus in order to formulate a rational treatment plan. This requires blood and urine cultures, at least, and careful consideration of other potential sites. The results of cultures often require careful interpretation, since transient fungemia is not a rare finding, particularly in patients who are debilitated or whose immune responses are compromised, or following open heart procedures.

Except for culture, investigation of the cerebrospinal fluid is not consistently informative. Although the results may be quite striking, they are seldom consistent. Nevertheless, the following generalizations may be noted. The fluid is usually clear and colorless. There is usually a neutrophilic pleocytosis that may approach several thousand cells in the early stages of the disease but often shifts to a monocytic pleocytosis if the disease has been present for a long time. Protein is usually increased and, although it may approach several hundred milligrams per 100 ml, it usually averages slightly over 100 mg per 100 ml. Glucose may be utilized by the yeast, and this is reflected in the lower than expected values that are frequently seen.

Treatment

Amphotericin B is the drug of choice for the treatment of candidiasis. 5-Fluorocytosine may also be utilized alone but is more frequently used in combination with amphotericin B.[180] If an abscess or granulomatous mass requires drainage or removal, concurrent drug therapy should be given.

Prognosis

Mass lesions of the brain and brain abscesses, in particular, have a very poor prognosis.[42,101,322] The mortality rate among this group may approach 95 per cent. The increasing use of computed tomography is expected to improve the prognosis by making earlier diagnosis and more effective follow-up possible. The various forms of meningeal involvement, for the most part, also share a rather bleak prognosis. Although it appears that many cases of *Candida* meningitis are relatively benign and self-limited, a substantial percentage of the patients, estimated at between 15 and 25 per cent, succumb to the disease despite treatment.

CLADOSPORIOSIS

Cladosporiosis is a fungal infection by any of the species belonging to the genus *Cladosporium*. The disease is commonly grouped under the more inclusive name "chromomycosis" ("Chromoblastomycosis"), which is a general term denoting a variety of infections produced by any of several species of pigmented soil fungi belonging to the family Dematiaceae. As a group these fungi represent a collection of rather common saprophytes with only latent pathogenic potential insofar as their effect on the nervous system is concerned. The majority of species in the family produce the pigmented verrucous skin lesions that are the most common pathological manifestations observed in humans. *Cladosporium trichoides* is the exception to this generalization and has, in fact, only rarely been implicated as a cause of dermal chromomycosis. Its peculiarly neurotropic character appears unique among the members of this family.[130] The term "cladosporiosis" is also used synonymously with the more general term "cerebral chromoblastomycosis." Although not precise in its implications, this term is acceptable from a practical standpoint for two reasons. The first is that the overwhelming majority of the cases are caused by *Cladosporium trichoides*. The second equally important reason is that the central nervous system form of the disease usually exists in the absence of other definable lesions.

Epidemiology

Although the dermatological forms of the chromomycoses occur predominantly in tropical regions, cerebral chromoblastomycosis appears to have a wider distribution, occurring in temperate areas as well.[130] The majority of cases have been reported from outside the United States but from no particular geographic location. Epidemiological data regarding the disease are somewhat sparse, but there appears to be no age or race predilection.[335] Regarding sexual distribution, males appear to predominate, but this may be related to occupation.[335]

Pathogenesis and Clinical Manifestations

The causitive agent, *Cladosporium trichoides* (bantianum) is ubiquitous, being found in soil and on vegetation. Most cases involving the nervous system appear to be limited to the brain and have no readily discernible primary focus.[130] This is in contradistinction to the other fungi with which the organism is grouped, which often cause obvious skin lesions. The fungus can produce a wide spectrum of pathological changes varying from cerebral abscess to osseous cranial involvement.[114] The most frequently seen lesion is the cerebral abscess, which is usually multilocular and well encapsulated. In cases with exclusive central nervous system involvement, frontal lobe lesions are most frequent. The remainder appear to be equally distributed among the occipital, temporal, and parietal lobes. Posterior fossa and brain stem involvement is extremely rare. The multiplicity and random distribution of the lesions strongly suggest that entrance into the central nervous system takes place by hematogenous dissemination.

Clinical manifestations are nonspecific and consistent with those of a mass lesion. Headache, nausea, and vomiting are invariably present. Visual disturbances including papilledema, diplopia, decreased visual acuity, and visual field defects are common. Focal deficits are variable and reflect the diverse location of the lesions throughout the central nervous system. The cerebral lesions may be well encapsulated, and if so, may be quite amenable to operation.

Meningitis has also been reported and tends to be of the basilar type. It is often accompanied by the development of hydrocephalus.[130]

Diagnosis

Definitive diagnosis depends upon identification of the organism in tissue, which is usually readily accomplished without special staining techniques. The cerebral lesions frequently are darkly pigmented and should be examined in both stained and unstained preparations. The organism appears in routine hematoxylin and eosin stains as brown septate hyphae measuring 1 to 3 μ in width. Species identification is not possible on the basis of histological sections alone and requires that the organism be grown on Sabouraud's agar.

The opening cerebrospinal fluid pressure usually is elevated, glucose is usually normal, and protein is moderately increased.[129] The cell count usually is elevated and neutrophils predominate. The organism has not yet been isolated by spinal fluid culture.

Radiographic and angiographic investigation has yet to reveal any invariably consistent or pathognomic features.

Treatment

Operative drainage and excision is the accepted treatment. No universally effective chemotherapeutic regimen is known. Binford and associates reported the survival of one patient following treatment with penicillin and sulfadiazine.[44] Both amphotericin B and 5-fluorouracil have been used with some success in skin lesions but have not yet been reported successful in treatment of cerebral forms of the disease. The use of 5-fluorocytosine has been proposed because of its excellent penetration of the blood-brain barrier, but its efficacy has yet to be established.[239a]

Prognosis

Cladosporiosis is almost invariably fatal. The time course is usually over a matter of months. No practical preventative measures have been described. The only long-term survivors have received prompt operative therapy.

COCCIDIOIDOMYCOSIS

Coccidioidomycosis is a fungal infection produced by the dimorphic fungus *Coccid-*

ioides immitis. This fungus is considered a natural inhabitant of soils in the lower Sonoran life zone.[269] In the United States, this corresponds to the central valley of California, Arizona, New Mexico, West Texas, and Utah. The organism has also been found in several comparable geographic areas of Central and South America but not nearly to the extent to which it has been found in the American Southwest.[118] In general, the distribution of the disease correlates closely with the ecological niche of the organism. Up to 80 per cent of the inhabitants of endemic areas are infected, but the majority of cases remain asymptomatic.[227,269]

Coccidioides immitis is dimorphic. Its two forms consist of spherules, which produce endospores, and hyphae, which produce infectious arthrospores. Infection may occur when the arthrospore becomes airborne and is inhaled. In most cases the infection is benign, but under some circumstances the organism is capable of producing exceptionally debilitating and even fatal disease.

Since the natural repository of the arthrospore is the soil, the infection rate is higher among those who by virtue of their work (agricultural workers, archeologists) are more frequently exposed to the infectious arthrospores. Coccidioidal infections have been reported in virtually all age groups ranging from neonates to the elderly.[269] The more severe forms tend to occur in adults.

The arthospores produced in culture are highly infectious, and cultures should be handled with extreme care. Other potential sources of infection such as sputum, exudates, dressings, and the like should also be subject to careful handling. Person-to-person transmission of the disease probably does not occur, however, and it is unnecessary to isolate patients with the disease.[269]

Pathogenesis and Clinical Manifestations

Coccidioidomycosis is generally a respiratory infection caused by inhalation of the arthrospore. Once inhaled, the arthrospore undergoes morphological changes in the lung, forming the thin-walled spherule. Within this spherule, endospores develop that are eventually liberated when the spherule ruptures. In the vast majority of patients this process produces a relatively localized inflammatory response with a correspondingly benign and self-limited clinical course. In approximately 35 per cent of patients, however, significant pulmonary lesions develop.[269] These foci provide a source from which the disease may become hematogenously disseminated.

Extrathoracic dissemination occurs in fewer than 1 per cent of all patients who develop the disease.[118,130] Of these, approximately one third to three quarters develop coccidioidal meningitis—the predominant form of the disease in the central nervous system. Other types of lesions (granulomas and abscesses) have been reported but are considered unusual.[111] These lesions generally do not manifest any anatomical preference. The meningitic process, however, is predominantly basilar in location and often produces a noncommunicating hydrocephalus, which is probably the most serious pathological consequence of the disease. The meningitis may be accompanied by prominent cerebrovascular changes severe enough in some cases to produce clinically evident thrombosis and infarction.[208] The spectrum of the central nervous system disease is further broadened by the occasional appearance of osteolytic lesions that may involve neural structures. This particular phenomenon is more frequently observed in lesions of the spinal axis.[360]

Coccidioidal meningitis is almost invariably preceded by involvement of the respiratory system, but this may be appreciated only in retrospect, since neurological symptoms appear so late in the course of the disease. Clinically, the pulmonary disease mimics tuberculosis. Following an incubation period, the patient notes the onset of fever, malaise, and anorexia. Later a dry cough develops, and this is accompanied by chest pain.

Infection of the central nervous system with *C. immitis* usually produces a subacute meningitis lacking many of the usual clinical characteristics associated with a meningitic process.[69,118] Headache is the predominant symptom and is accompanied by varying degrees of altered sensorium. Focal deficits have been reported but are considered unusual.

Diagnosis

The diagnosis of central nervous system coccidioidomycosis requires demonstration of the endosporulating spherule in cerebral tissue or fluid, or culture from the same sources. While cerebrospinal fluid culture results are confirmatory, they are positive in only 20 to 40 per cent of cases.[69,118] The yield may be improved if repeated large-volume specimens are obtained.

The cerebrospinal fluid profile of patients with coccidioidal meningitis is almost invariably abnormal. Glucose levels are frequently depressed, and protein levels are often elevated. The cellular response initially consists of polymorphonuclear leukocytes but eventually manifests a lymphocytic predominance. Occasionally a moderate eosinophilia (5 to 10 per cent) is noted.[69,118] Several serological examinations may provide valuable supportive information. IgM precipitins are a particularly useful indicator in acute illness, since they appear in approximately 90 per cent of patients within four weeks of infection.[269] Levels may be expected to diminish thereafter if the disease does not become chronic or disseminate from pulmonary sites. Complement-fixing antibodies (IgG) appear somewhat later in the course of the disease but persist for much longer periods.[269]

Skin tests are of little use in diagnosing the central nervous system forms of the disease for two reasons. The first is that in endemic areas almost all residents eventually show positive skin test reactivity.[269] The second is that patients with disseminated forms of the disease may be anergic. A positive test is useful in indicating prior exposure but does not constitute evidence of active infection. Neuroradiographic investigation may produce results that are quite striking but not pathognomonic.

Treatment

Amphotericin B is the most effective treatment for all forms of coccidioidomycosis. Systemic as well as intrathecal administration is required in disease of the central nervous system. The duration of therapy is dictated by the clinical response and may be followed by serial measurements of complement-fixing antibodies in serum and cerebrospinal fluid. Effective treatment may require a commitment to months or even years of therapy.[269] The most frequent complication of central nervous system coccidioidomycosis for which neurosurgical consultations are sought is the development of hydrocephalus. Most cases require the placement of shunting devices. The nature of the pathophysiological process is such that periodic obstruction of the device is to be expected. Additional complications associated with the mechanical dissemination of the disease are not uncommon.

Steroids may reduce amphotericin-induced arachnoiditis, thereby promoting better tolerance of intrathecal administration of the drug. Although limited low-dosage regimens do not appear to produce the same range of undesirable effects, it is probably best to avoid them whenever possible.[96,111]

Prognosis

Prior to the introduction of amphotericin B, coccidioidomycosis of the central nervous system was almost invariably fatal.[270,333] This agent has improved the outlook, but the overall mortality rate among patients with disseminated disease still approaches 40 per cent.[118] The death rate may be further augmented by inclusion of those patients who die as a result of complications associated with the various forms of treatment. The best therapeutic results can be expected when the diagnosis is made relatively early and treatment is aggressive. Under these conditions up to 30 per cent of infected patients may be cured.[270]

CRYPTOCOCCOSIS

Cryptococcosis is the most common mycotic infection affecting the central nervous system.[130] In many respects—its clinical spectrum and the pattern and extent of pathological involvement—it typifies mycotic involvement of nervous tissue, but it also displays some unique pathophysiological features that enable it to exert a profound and debilitating effect on the nervous system.

Cryptococcosis has been recognized as a disease entity since late in the last century.[61] As with many of the fungal organisms, early reports attempting to clarify morphological and physiological details often failed to use consistent terminology, spawning a myriad of misnomer eponyms, many of which continue to be perpetuated in the literature today.

Epidemiology

Cryptococcus neoformans, the etiological agent of cryptococcosis, has a worldwide distribution. There appear to be few restrictions on its ecological habitat. It has been isolated from numerous natural reservoirs, including man, though more consistently from the excreta of pigeons.[226] Although the genus consists of many species, C. neoformans is the only one that is considered pathogenic. Most strains of the organism do not exhibit significant pathogenicity unless the immune status of the host has been significantly compromised. The organism is exceptionally resistant to desiccation and apparently may remain viable for years under the most adverse conditions.[75] The disease does not appear to be contagious. Cryptococcosis is more frequently seen in males, but otherwise its epidemiological profile is unremarkable.[117]

Pathology

Cryptococcosis bears many of the hallmarks of fungal disease in general. Although other sites including the skin and mucous membranes may be utilized, the respiratory tract is considered the primary portal of entry.[374] From these primary sites the organism may undergo hematogenous dissemination to any of a number of secondary locations including the brain, spinal cord, and meninges. Primary disease involving the central nervous system in the absence of disease elsewhere is a relative rarity, although the primary focus may be difficult to isolate.[203]

Cellular rather than humoral mechanisms are the primary line of defense, although there is evidence to suggest that in infected patients these mechanisms may be modified.[68] The exact pathophysiological mechanism is not entirely understood but is thought to involve an antigenic polysaccharide contained in the capsule of the organism itself. This polysaccharide is antiphagocytic and may be capable of blunting the immune response.

Clinicopathologically, cryptococcosis generally falls into one of three general categories: meningitis, meningoencephalitis, or intracranial mass lesions.[197]

The location of the meningitic process is frequently basilar. Characteristically, the cellular response is minimal in comparison with the number of organisms, but there may be extensive deposition of a gelatinous exudate that may originate from the polysaccharide components of the capsule.

Meningeal involvement ranges from relatively localized to diffuse and extensive. Owing to the blunted inflammatory response, edema is not a prominent feature. The cellular response consists of histiocytic macrophages, lymphocytes, and giant cells. The neutrophilic response is not extensive unless pyogenic infection is also present.

The meningoencephalitis associated with cryptococcosis is the result of extension of the meningitic process into the perivascular space. The cellular reaction here may also vary from minimal to extensive. A relatively distinct pathological finding associated with this phase of the disease is the formation of cystlike cavities. Although most frequently located in the superficial cortical layers, the lesions may be found in deeper cerebral locations also. In the majority of cases these cystic structures do not produce extensive cellular damage but rather displace nervous tissue. The structures contain large numbers of organisms in a gelatinous matrix. The displacement of the neural elements may produce the appearance of an increase in microglia and astrocytes that is more apparent than real. The overall effect is to produce a honeycombed appearance. The cystic structures are usually small and uniformly sized, although cysts large enough to produce mass effects have been described. Similar lesions created in the basal ganglia are probably embolic in origin but produce morphologically identical lesions.

The granulomatous lesions of cryptococcosis do not exhibit the extensive caseous necrosis found in other fungal diseases. The lesions are frequently multiple and usually accompanied by cellular infiltration with lymphocytes, plasma cells, and macrophages. They often contain contiguous cystic spaces with large numbers of organisms and are usually surrounded by a capsule infiltrated by microglia and lymphocytes.

Clinical Manifestations

In contradistinction to many of the mycotic diseases, none of the usual clinical syndromes of cryptococcosis are characterized by long prodromal periods. Following the onset of symptoms, however, the clinical course may be protracted. One of the most consistent findings is that evidence of the primary disease is often lacking even after the appearance of neurological symptoms. The rather benign clinical course associated with extraneural forms of the disease may be the result of the organism's failure to incite the strong immunological response seen with many of the other mycotic diseases. It is likely that the majority of primary infections of the lung are benign and clinically asymptomatic.

Although *C. neoformans* is capable of producing a variety of tissue reactions, the majority of cases are characterized by the development of meningitis. The onset of clinical symptoms may be acute but more frequently is insidious. The syndrome almost invariably begins with a progressively severe headache followed by a typical meningeal complex of symptoms including nausea, vomiting, nuchal rigidity, fever, and later, evidence of increased intracranial pressure.[106] The symptom complex may wax and wane somewhat, often causing delays in diagnosis and treatment because of apparent spontaneous clinical improvement. Untreated infections may persist in this subacute state for weeks or months. The majority of these infections will cause death within six months if appropriate treatment is not instituted, however.

The meningoencephalitic process pursues a similar clinical course and, in fact, is often seen in conjunction with meningitis. The symptoms closely resemble those of tuberculous meningitis. Neuro-ophthalmic complications are frequent and include papilledema, optic atrophy, and extraocular muscle paresis. An unusually large number of patients will display markedly altered sensorium and significant personality disturbances.

As intracranial mass lesions, cryptococcal granulomas may present in a variety of ways and frequently mimic abscesses or tumors. These lesions are not restricted to the brain parenchyma, although their appearance along the spinal axis is considered unusual. They can occur in the absence of any meningeal involvement.

Localizing deficits are observed with these space-occupying lesions; their extent, of course, depends on the anatomical location. In the majority of cases the signs and symptoms of increased intracranial pressure tend to dominate the clinical picture. Hydrocephalus is an important complication of all three forms of the disease but is more likely to be seen in chronic cases of meningitis.

Diagnosis

There are several species of *Cryptococcus*, but only *C. neoformans* is considered pathogenic. Cultures are positive in up to 95 per cent of cases if performed with 5 to 7 ml of cerebrospinal fluid on the appropriate media.[62,214]

The capsule of the *C. neoformans* can be readily recognized in India ink preparations because it appears as a halo around the organism, and up to 70 per cent of cases can be diagnosed by utilizing this method alone.[117] Since it is the only encapsulated yeast affecting the nervous system, its definitive identification by this method is considered justification to begin treatment. Generally, however, the capsular structure itself does not stain well. Occasionally, it is demonstrated with hematoxylin and eosin, but alcian blue and mucicarmine stains usually afford better resolution. Rarely, the capsule structure is so minimal that no staining technique will demonstrate it. In these cases the organism closely resembles a lymphocyte, and diagnosis from such specimens is unlikely unless all specimens are cultured.

Cerebrospinal fluid analysis reveals lymphocytic pleocytosis in 97 per cent of patients, hypoglycorrachia in 45 per cent, increased protein in 90 per cent, and an elevated opening pressure in 64 per cent.[62]

Both sera and cerebrospinal fluid should be analyzed for cryptococcal antigen and antibody. In minimally symptomatic or asymptomatic cases the cryptococcal antigen may not be detected, perhaps suggesting that only the more malignant cases produce significant results. The titer corresponds roughly with the disease activity, often falling with treatment and corresponding clinical improvement. Anticryptococcal antibody and cryptococcal antigens share an inverse relationship. The antibody is found early in central nervous system disease and also during treatment. If the treatment is successful, the antibody should be in excess of the declining antigen. More than 90 per cent of patients with positive cultures will show demonstrable antigen.[161]

Utilizing a combination of direct microscopy, culture, and immunodiagnostic methods improves the diagnostic accuracy considerably, providing antemortem diagnosis in up to 95 per cent of patients.[62,161,214]

Standard neuroradiological procedures may be used to investigate the lesions of cerebral cryptococcosis. Computed tomography is most helpful in diagnosing cryptococcal granulomas, which appear as discrete lesions of relatively uniform density.[343] Some enhancement of the capsular structure may be expected in contrast studies, but not to the degree that is observed in pyogenic abscesses. Ventriculography, pneumoencephalography, and angiography do not reveal any distinctive features of etiological significance. If computed tomography is not available brain scans may be utilized to try to localize space-occupying lesions and in fact may be more helpful in cases in which the meningoencephalitic component is more prominent. The lesions rarely calcify, and therefore skull radiographs are rarely useful.

Treatment

The treatment of central nervous system cryptococcosis is primarily chemotherapeutic and consists of three pharmacological agents: amphotericin B, 5-fluorocytosine, and miconazole.[97,347]

Amphotericin B is considered the first-line drug of choice even though it must be administered intravenously, is expensive, and usually produces serious side effects. Its administration requires careful supervision and constant monitoring of the renal status, preferably by serial measurement of creatinine clearance. Nephrointoxication is produced in more than 80 per cent of the patients in whom it is used.[242] Intrathecal administration of the drug may be required. Cerebrospinal fluid flow studies may help to assess the efficacy of this form of treatment. Patients with shunts require particularly careful assessment, since cerebrospinal fluid outflow may be too rapid to allow therapeutic levels of the agent to accumulate.

Although clinical experience with 5-fluorocytosine is less extensive than with amphotericin B, some outstanding clinical results have been produced by utilizing the drug alone or in combination with amphotericin B.[347] It has the distinct advantages of oral administration and a significantly lower incidence of side effects. The most serious side effect is bone marrow supression.

The third pharmacological agent that may be used in the treatment of cryptococcal meningitis is miconazole. Its use has been rather limited, and there are reports of both failure and success following its use.[97] It does appear that intraventricular administration of the agent offers a higher probability of success, since cerebrospinal fluid penetration is poor with intravenous administration. At the present time its use is indicated primarily in those cases in which other forms of therapy including amphotericin B and 5-fluorocytosine have failed.

Localized granulomatous lesions may be amenable to operative resection. There is little question that symptomatic mass lesions require treatment, the extent of which is governed by traditional neurosurgical considerations: the anatomical location of the lesion, the potential for successful removal, and the extent of the neurological deficit that may be anticipated. The removal of asymptomatic lesions, however, is controversial. It appears that organisms may remain viable in granulomatous lesions despite the presence of apparently effective chemotherapeutic levels. This may provide a continuing source for reinfection, thus precipitating recurrent episodes of meningitis that produce significant morbidity and cause deaths themselves. Communicating hydrocephalus, a relatively frequent complication of chronic meningitis, may also require therapy. The judicious assessment of these various factors and the utilization of selected neurosurgical techniques offer the potential to further improve the prognosis of all forms of the disease.

Prognosis

As many as 50 per cent of cases occur in individuals whose immune responses are compromised, and as would be expected, this population does not generally respond exceptionally well to treatment.[130] Prior to the introduction of amphotericin B, neurological forms of cryptococcal disease were almost invariably fatal. The introduction of this as well as other antifungal agents has dramatically reduced the number of deaths and the morbidity attendant on the disease. Despite these advances, the mortality rate approaches 40 per cent in some patient populations, and as many as 25 per cent of patients suffer relapses following completion of chemotherapeutic therapy.[62] Diamond and Bennett noted that the prognosis is adversely affected by (1) the presence of lymphoreticular malignant disease; (2) continuing corticosteroid therapy; (3) cerebrospinal fluid findings showing a high opening pressure, a low glucose level, less than 20 leukocytes per cubic millimeter, and the presence of the organism detected on smear; (4) isolation of the organism from extraneural sites; and (5) high titers of cryptococcal antigen in cerebrospinal fluid and serum.[107]

Cryptococcemia, multiple site isolations, or both indicate an especially poor prognosis. Blood, sputum, and urine cultures should routinely be included in the initial evaluation as well as in subsequent follow-up examinations, since this may be the first indication of relapse. Culture of specimens from other sites should be performed as indicated.

Patients who were more likely to relapse are usually those in whom the organism is isolated extraneurally and who have high cryptococcal antigen titers that persist at elevated levels even in the post-treatment period. Since untreated cases of cryptococcosis are invariably fatal, the most important prognostic factor is the early and aggressive diagnosis of the disease.

HISTOPLASMOSIS

Histoplasmosis is a widely distributed mycotic infection caused by the dimorphic fungus *Histoplasma capsulatum*. The organism was first described in 1906 by Darling, a U.S. Army pathologist working in Panama.[88,89] It was not until many years later that De Monbreun demonstrated that the organism originally described by Darling was actually the yeast phase of a fungus.[95]

Epidemiology

Although histoplasmosis has been reported from many parts of the world and indeed appears to have a nearly worldwide distribution, it is most heavily endemic in the midwestern United States. Its prevalence among some patient populations located in the Ohio and Mississippi river valleys may approach 90 per cent.[218] The more benign forms of the disease may occur in any age group, but the more severe forms appear to follow a bimodal age distribution with the peaks occurring at the extremes of the age range.[218,324] According to several studies, the first peak occurs in children less than one year of age and the second in adults between the fifth and sixth decades.[324] Among the infant population the sex distribution is equal, but among adults, men are more frequently affected in a ratio of 3 to 1.[291] The predominance of males may be due to greater occupational exposure.

Estimates of the incidence of histoplasmosis are based primarily on retrospective sources of information such as chest x-rays or histoplasmin skin tests. On this basis, it has been estimated that as many as 40 to 60 million people in the continental United States have had the infection.[7] The estimated number of new cases exceeds 500,-000 per year in the United States alone.[309]

Central nervous system histoplasmosis is rare in comparison with other forms of the disease. Cases have been reported in which the presence of antecedent disease could not be unequivocally established, but in the overwhelming majority, central nervous system involvement is a complication of disseminated histoplasmosis.[80] Between 10 and 25 per cent of all patients with the disseminated disease develop clinically apparent neurological complications, as compared with 7.5 per cent of those with other forms of histoplasmosis.[78,218,312,324] Although the majority of cases are subclinical, the presence of neurological symptoms in the absence of other symptoms is extremely rare.

Pathogenesis

H. capsulatum is a pathogenic fungus. Granted, its pathogenicity is enhanced in the immunologically compromised host, but to infer that this is the only circumstance in which this organism has a significant pathogenic effect is not justified. In the majority of reported cases the fungus appears to have utilized one of four portals of entry: nasopharyngeal, pulmonary, gastrointestinal, or tegumentary.

In the overwhelming majority of cases the primary focus is pulmonary.[162] The existence of primary cerebral histoplasmosis is controversial; if it does exist, it is extremely rare. Tynes and associates reported 25 cases of *Histoplasma* meningitis; in only two was there no definite evidence of *Histoplasma* involvement outside the central nervous system.[345] In all there are perhaps only two other well-documented reports of primary disease.[152,194]

Three types of histopathological cerebral lesions have been described: miliary granulomas, meningitis, and histoplasmomas.

The miliary granulomas of histoplasmosis closely resemble those seen in tuberculosis. Well-established granulomatous lesions may be accompanied by a moderate amount of inflammation and caseation necrosis. Epithelioid cells and occasional giant cells may be observed in the surrounding tissue. Extensive phagocytosis usually prevents a significant inflammatory response until the lesion is reasonably well established.

The meningitic process runs the gamut from insignificance (occasional organisms in leptomeningeal macrophages that produce no symptoms) to extensive and lethal involvement.

The third lesion produced in cerebral histoplasmosis is the pathological counterpart of the tuberculoma. It is focal and destructive, producing the relatively discrete lesions that have been termed histoplasmomas.

More extensive pathological classifications have been proposed but their usefulness is debatable, since in essence, they reflect the various degrees of the pathological process rather than isolated disease processes.[78]

Clinical Manifestations

Most cases of histoplasmosis present in one of three general categories: as acute primary disease, as chronic cavitary disease, or as progressive disseminated disease.[162,291,324] Perhaps as many as 95 per cent of all cases fall into the first category, and the majority of these are inapparent, subclinical, or completely benign.[218,291,324] Symptoms, which are usually nonspecific, resemble those seen in viral syndromes and include fever, cough, and occasionally chest pain. The infection is almost invariably self-limited, usually resolving within 10 to 14 days even without treatment.

The chronic cavitary form of the disease is usually limited to the lungs, and its clinical and pathological manifestations closely resemble tuberculosis. Hematogenous dissemination may be either localized or general. It is unclear whether these two distinctions are part of the same process or represent slightly different pathophysiological mechanisms. Generalized dissemination is certainly more frequent and produces a fulminating clinical course. Clinically, cerebral histoplasmosis mimics any of several mycotic infections. The disease most commonly presents as meningitis with headache, nuchal rigidity, and seizures. Less frequently, it presents as an intracranial mass lesion. In these cases sensory and motor deficits are likely to dominate the clinical picture.

Diagnosis

The diagnosis of histoplasmosis may be confirmed by any of several methods. Serological and skin testing procedures have limited potential for individual diagnosis, especially in endemic areas.[275] Serological tests may be more helpful, particularly in the otherwise normal host. More frequently, confirmation is by identification of the fungus in tissue or cultural isolation from the body tissues or fluids.

Biopsy of any of several tissues may provide supportive evidence in the absence of cultural confirmation. Likely tissue sources include lung, liver, skin, buccal mucosa, and bone marrow. Of these, bone marrow aspirates are most likely to yield positive results.

Treatment

The mainstay of treatment of central nervous system histoplasmosis is amphotericin B. Despite potentially hazardous side effects a single course of therapy is more effective than successive short courses, as relapses are more likely to occur with the latter. Since the pathological process has a predilection for the basilar aspect of the

brain, obstructive hydrocephalus may limit the effectiveness of chemotherapeutic treatment.

The duration of the therapy depends upon the severity of the disease. Usually it is at least 10 weeks, but it may be three or four months in cases in which side effects warrant a reduction in dosage and extend the time needed to administer the cumulative dosage. Recurrent infections usually require another full course of treatment. The question of concurrent use of glucocorticoids is unresolved. Their primary purpose is to ameliorate troublesome but nonlethal side effects of amphotericin B such as nausea and vomiting. They may, however, also inactivate or decrease the effectiveness of amphotericin B. The mechanism by which amphotericin B and the other polyene antibiotics in general exert antifungal activity is by binding the sterol moiety in the cell membranes of sensitive fungi.

Neurosurgical therapy is usually limited to the resection of granulomatous mass lesions or the placement of shunting devices in those patients who develop obstructive hydrocephalus. Concurrent chemotherapy must accompany both procedures.

Prognosis

Since infection of the central nervous system with *H. capsulatum* almost invariably occurs along with disseminated disease, the prognosis must be considered within this context. In the absence of chemotherapy with amphotericin B, nearly 90 per cent of patients with progressive disseminated histoplasmosis may be expected to succumb, as may 50 per cent of those with chronic pulmonary forms of the disease.[130,346a] Early aggressive systemic chemotherapy substantially reduces this rate. Despite aggressive therapy, a mortality rate approaching 25 per cent can be anticipated.[346a] The death rate peaks occur in infancy and among adults in the fifth and sixth decades.

Although *H. capsulatum* is not generally considered an opportunistic organism, factors that depress the immune response do appear to predispose to the development of disseminated disease in a select group of patients.[309,346a] Disease due to reactivation of endogenous foci appears to be particularly debilitating.[360a] The concurrent existence of other mycotic or granulomatous diseases, particularly tuberculosis, further worsens the prognosis. As with most mycotic diseases, delay in diagnosis also clearly affects the prognosis adversely. Since the most common manifestation of central nervous system histoplasmosis is basilar meningitis, the complications of obstructive hydrocephalus may persist long after apparent eradication of the actual infection.

NOCARDIOSIS

Nocardiosis is a chronic to subacute suppurative infection caused by members of the genus *Nocardia*. The etiological organism of the disease was first described by Nocard in 1888, and hence the entity bears his name.[251] Eppinger is credited with isolating the organism in man in 1890.[120] He described a case of disseminated disease in which the central nervous system lesion consisted of purulent meningitis in combination with brain abscess—the most common pathological form of the disease seen when the nervous system is involved.

From the time of its discovery the genus presented problems for taxonomists attempting to classify the organism. In fact, the *Nocardia* species as well as the closely related *Actinomyces* were originally classified and later consistently misrepresented as fungi, although they were in fact bacteria. Together with the genus *Actinomyces,* they are even now referred to as the fungus-like bacteria.[209]

Epidemiology

The infection is uncommon in comparison with other types of infection. It is estimated that approximately 500 to 1000 cases occur in the United States in any one year.[36] As with many of the fungal diseases, a high percentage of the cases have been reported in debilitated or immunologically compromised individuals, prompting designation of the organism as "opportunistic."[149] There is no question that the immunologically compromised state facilitates both the occurrence and the progression of the disease, but it should be noted that a high percentage of cases, variously esti-

mated at 15 to 50 per cent, occur in the absence of any apparent predisposing factors.[36,181,267] In between one third and one half of patients with systemic disease, the central nervous system is involved.

There are numerous nonhuman hosts for the organism, including cattle, goats, cats, dogs, and marsupials, but there is no evidence for human-to-human or animal-to-human transmission.

Pathology

The basic features that characterize and establish the actinomycetes as bacteria are morphological, structural, and physiological. The last is important, since growth is inhibited by any of several antibacterial agents including the penicillins, tetracyclines, and sulfonamides, which are ineffective against fungi.

Primarily, central nervous system involvement takes the form of cerebral abscess, occasionally single but more frequently multiple, often accompanied by purulent meningitis.[153,288] Meningitis in the absence of brain abscess is unusual.* The meningitic process is most evident at the basal aspect of the brain and does not as a rule exhibit any unusual pathological features not seen in other similar diseases. Nocardial abscesses are usually small but frequently coalesce to form large multilocular lesions.

Grossly the abscesses resemble other types of brain abscess. The intense fibroblastic reaction seen with other organisms, however, is not usually seen with *Nocardia,* and hence most nocardial abscesses lack well-defined capsules.[130]

Microscopically, the abscesses are not particularly remarkable in appearance. They lack the strong tendency toward the formation of giant cells seen in most other abscess conditions, and there is virtually no granuloma formation. Secondary scarring is minimal. The abscesses usually are purulent and contain necrotic brain, polymorphonuclear leukocytes, glial cells, and rare multinucleated giant cells.[251] In the early stages they may contain branching hyphae. Older lesions are more likely to contain the segmented forms of the organism.[320]

---

* See references 46, 66, 85, 122, 153, 205.

Clinical Manifestations

In general, nocardial infections tend to be chronic, and this is reflected in the clinical presentation. Acute disease is seen, however, particularly in debilitated or immunologically incompetent patients.[130,320] Prodromal pulmonary symptoms almost invariably precede the onset of neurological symptoms. Like many of the fungal diseases whose portal of entry is the lung, however, initial symptoms are often insidious and nonspecific, and may be overlooked. They may include intermittent production of thick purulent sputum and fever. Rarely, when the abscess extends into the pleural space, pleuritic-type chest pain may be quite prominent. Constitutional symptoms vary from minimal to extensive and may in some cases dominate the clinical picture. These include night sweats, anorexia, generalized malaise, weight loss, and fever.

Central nervous system symptoms are also quite nonspecific and have little etiological significance. The neurological picture is usually dominated by signs and symptoms associated with meningitis. When the abscesses become larger the symptoms are typically those associated with expanding mass lesions—such as headaches, visual aberrations, and decreased sensorium. A few authors have reported concurrent spinal axis involvement.[121,357] Clinical symptoms in these cases included pain, often unusual in character and nondermatomal in distribution, followed by motor deficits of varying degrees. Bony involvement (osteolytic lesions) is usually also present in these cases, and a certain amount of local pain in the area of the osseous lesion may be noted. The intervertebral disc space is usually preserved.[130] Osteolytic lesions of the cranial bones have been reported.[137]

Diagnosis

The diagnosis of nocardiosis is not difficult. An increasing awareness of fungal disease in general has increased the index of suspicion for the entity among clinicians. The culture requirements and staining procedures are reasonably simple. The single most important factor in making the diagnosis of nocardiosis is not a laboratory method or examination but merely the inclusion of the disease in the differential diagnostic considerations.

Nocardia is neither a member of the normal flora in the human nor a frequent laboratory contaminant.[320] In obtaining specimens it is important to remember that, in contrast to the closely related microaerophilic or anaerobic *Actinomyces,* most of the pathogenic *Nocardia* species are aerobic; culture under strictly anaerobic conditions is unacceptable. The organism may not grow for three or four days following inoculation. Cultures should be maintained past the 72-hour limit usually imposed. Maintaining the cultures for as long as two weeks may be necessary.

The morphological characteristics in conjunction with identification by culture usually form the basis of diagnosis. Occasionally it becomes necessary to resort to biochemical or serological methods. Biochemical methods, while quite accurate, are expensive and not generally available. Serological methods are readily available, but almost invariably numerous cross-reactions with mycobacterial antigens make their interpretation difficult. For this reason serodiagnostic efforts have been limited and should be attempted only by qualified laboratories. Its form and structure are so important in identification of the organism that it may be well to consider transporting specimens to a laboratory experienced in fungal identification rather than risk misdiagnosis.

Pulmonary infection is frequently associated with other forms of the disease. Therefore, sputum cultures must be included in the diagnostic evaluation even if pulmonary symptoms are minimal or lacking. Coexisting disease, particularly tuberculosis, may cloud the diagnosis. Inappropriate or less than desired responses to traditionally effective forms of therapy, especially in cases of suspected tuberculosis, should prompt vigorous diagnostic efforts to discover coexistent disease. It should be noted that despite the close morphological relationship between *Nocardia* species and the Mycobacteriae, antituberculous therapy is not effective in treatment of nocardiosis.

Other diagnostic studies are of limited value. Cerebrospinal fluid is usually nonspecifically abnormal. Opening pressure is elevated in those cases of symptomatic mass lesions. The fluid is usually clear, showing only a moderate neutrophilic pleocytosis (average 1000 cells). Protein is only slightly increased in most cases, while sugar levels are frequently decreased.

Radiographic investigation often reveals a plethora of findings, but the majority are nondiagnostic and etiologically nonspecific. This includes computed tomography, which reveals the presence of the typical rim enhancement of the lesions characteristically seen with most brain abscesses.[297] Angiography has on occasion revealed abscesses so vascular that they resembled a typical tumor blush.[55] Myelography usually reveals findings characteristic of epidural abscess.

The combination of pulmonary and neurological symptoms should help to narrow the differential diagnosis considerably. Diagnostic consideration should include tuberculosis, bronchogenic carcinoma, bacterial pulmonary abscess, and a few of the fungal entities such as actinomycosis and aspergillosis.

Treatment and Prognosis

The best results with treatment of central nervous system nocardiosis have been obtained by combining appropriate chemotherapy with evacuation of the abscesses if they are present.[212,276] The central nervous system is rarely involved in the absence of disseminated disease, and therefore large series of patients with nocardiosis of that system exclusively do not exist. The prognosis for forms of the disease affecting the central nervous system must therefore be considered in the context of systemic dissemination, which may be seen in as many as half the patients. The overall mortality rate for all forms of the disease ranges between 50 and 60 per cent.[320] If dissemination, particularly to the brain, has taken place, the rate may be as high as 80 per cent. In Ballenger and Goldring's series of 29 patients with nervous system involvement, 5 patients survived—4 of them following operative intervention.[29] Factors affecting the prognosis adversely include multiplicity of abscesses, debilitating disease, or immunological compromise.

Sulfonamides are universally recommended for treatment of all forms of the disease including those in the central nervous system. The sulfa drugs, in general, are estimated to attain cerebrospinal fluid concentrations between one third and one half peak plasma concentrations. The recommended serum concentration is 15 to 20 mg per 100 ml.[297] The exact dosage required to produce this level will vary from patient to patient and with the particular agent that is selected. Relapses are not uncommon, and a prolonged course of treatment is invariably required. For patients with brain abscess, therapy for a minimum of a year is advisable. Palmer and associates have recommended lifelong therapy for patients with brain involvement.[267] Careful monitoring of the patient's renal status should be included as part of the routine follow-up.

PARACOCCIDIOIDOMYCOSIS

Paracoccidioidomycosis is one of several systemic fungal diseases caused by dimorphic fungi. The etiological agent of the disease is *Paracoccidioides brasilienses*—a thermally dimorphic organism originally described by Lutz in 1908.[233]

Epidemiology

P. brasiliensis is thought to be a soil saprophyte endemic to portions of South America and Mexico.[225] The majority of cases have been reported from Brazil, where paracoccidioidomycosis is considered to be a major systemic mycosis.[229] Several thousand cases encompassing the entire clinical spectrum have been reported from this region, the majority of them in young adult men.

Pathogenesis and Clinical Manifestations

The primary focus of the disease is usually pulmonary, though dissemination to other organ systems can and usually does occur. As opposed to other mycotic diseases, however, in which the initial infection is benign, heals spontaneously, and subsequently confers some degree of immunity, paracoccidioidomycosis appears to be capable of maintaining latent foci that provide endogenous sources of reinfection. The development of the self-limited benign illness may confer some degree of immunity, which possibly limits progression of the disease until the host's immunological defense mechanisms are compromised. In these cases the disease may make its appearance long after initial exposure to the organism has taken place, and the incubation period may be impossible to determine.[279]

Despite the high incidence of pulmonary involvement, pulmonary symptoms rarely dominate the clinical picture. The disease usually manifests itself in one of three characteristic clinical forms: mucocutaneous, lymphangitic, or systemic.[303] A fourth "mixed" category has been proposed, but this reflects the extent of the disease process rather than any distinct pathophysiology.

The prodromal symptoms of primary pulmonary disease are nonspecific and resemble those of a benign viral disease.

The tegumentary lesions are quite distinctive in appearance and are most frequently found in the nasal and oral region and the buccal mucosa. Since dissemination takes place via hemolymphatic routes, regional lymphatic tissue is usually involved to a significant degree.

Central nervous system forms of the disease vary in their presentation. Four distinct clinical syndromes have been described: mass lesions, meningitis, meningoencephalitis, and meningoradiculitis.

The space-occupying lesions may consist of solitary or multiple granulomas. If multiple, they are occasionally confluent. The lesions usually have necrotic centers surrounded by epithelioid giant and plasma cells as well as lymphocytes. The granulomatous reaction is frequently accompanied by pyogenic abscess formation or inflammation or both. Granulomatous lesions have also been observed in the meninges and choroid plexus. The meningitic process usually is basilar in location.[130]

The symptoms that accompany any of these syndromes usually are nonspecific. Evidence of increased intracranial pressure is usually prominent, and papilledema may be extensive. Other symptoms include headache, vomiting, seizures, and altered sensorium.

Laboratory Diagnosis

An extensive battery of tests is available to diagnose paracoccidioidomycosis, but the cornerstone of the diagnostic regimen continues to be identification of the organism in tissues. Its distinctive structure, generally as a refractile body measuring 10 to 60 μ in diameter, makes microscopic diagnosis relatively easy.[291] The organism reproduces by budding, and these buds are located in a circumferential fashion around its periphery. In the classic orientation, the organism resembles a pilot's wheel. Multiple buds must be seen, however—a single bud is not acceptable for diagnosis because organisms of this conformation resemble *Blastomyces dermatitidis* too closely to permit unequivocal differentiation.

In the absence of morphological identification of the organism, serological tests may be used. In general, they are of limited value for diagnosis but may be used to follow the clinical course and the response to chemotherapy.

Cerebrospinal fluid findings are almost always nonspecifically abnormal. Meningitic forms of the disease tend to produce a lymphocytic pleocytosis, whereas parenchymatous forms produce a mononuclear response. Immunodiagnostic procedures performed on the cerebrospinal fluid produce a profile quite similar to serological surveys.

Treatment

The appropriate treatment of central nervous system paracoccidioidomycosis may be surgical or medical.

The medical options available to treat paracoccidioidomycosis are rather limited. Sulfa drugs have been recommended for several forms of the disease, but their use has been limited in the central nervous system forms.[225] The preferred pharmacological agent is amphotericin B. There is no question that amphotericin B produces rapid regression of symptoms, but its potential for providing a definitive cure needs to be evaluated further.

Every lesion must be assessed to determine its suitability for operative removal. The characteristics of the disease itself constitute no special mitigating circumstances that require consideration beyond the currently accepted criteria for operative treatment of mass lesions. Concurrent chemotherapy is recommended with all operative procedures.

Prognosis

The prognosis for central nervous system paracoccidioidomycosis has improved considerably since the introduction of amphotericin B.[248,291] The major obstacle to effective treatment is still the fact that the majority of cases are diagnosed late in their course, thereby reducing the potential effectiveness of any chemotherapeutic regimen.

PHYCOMYCOSIS

Phycomycosis is any one of several diseases caused by members of the Phycomycetae class. Although the term is often used synonymously with the more widely accepted designation "cerebral mucormycosis," this usage is not an entirely accurate application of precise taxonomic terminology. The class Phycomyceta includes the Mucoraceae family to which the genera *Mucor*, *Rhizopus*, and *Absidia* belong. The overwhelming majority of cases of phycomycosis are caused by members of this family. Rare cases are due to the Mortierellaceae family, which also belongs to the Phycomyceta class, however, and the term "mucormycosis" as applied to these cases is inappropriate.[35,145] From the clinical standpoint the term "cerebral mucormycosis" is more widely recognized and more germane to a discussion of the disease as it affects the nervous system. For all practical purposes this term accurately describes the majority of cases and is used hereafter.

Paltauf was the first to describe mucormycosis as a disease entity in humans.[268] The case was somewhat atypical in that it involved the gastrointestinal tract and lungs as well as the brain, which is not the usual pattern. It was not until 1943 that Gregory and co-workers described the syndrome that is recognized today as cerebral mucormycosis.[167]

Epidemiology

Members of the Mucoraceae family have a wide geographic distribution. The organism is ubiquitous, is commonly isolated from spoiled bread and fruit, and is also a frequent laboratory contaminant.[105] The disease has been reported in all age groups and appears to have no racial, sexual, or occupational predilection.[130] Certain subpopulations, however, particularly persons with diabetes, are more likely to develop the disease.[25] Other predisposing factors include leukemia, cyanotic heart disease, primary immunodeficiency diseases, multiple myeloma, renal disease, cirrhosis, and prolonged administration of antibiotics, antimetabolites, or corticosteroids.[50] In primary disease, access to the tissues is usually gained by inhalation.

Pathology

Members of the Mucoraceae family are the organisms most frequently isolated in cerebral mucormycosis. Specifically, it is the genus *Rhizopus* that is responsible for the majority of cases. The actual species implicated in decreasing order of frequency are *R. oryzae*, *R. arrhizus*, and *R. nigricans*.[25]

In cerebral tissue the form and structure of the organism are quite constant; it is invariably seen in its mycelial form. Meticulous examination of the microscopic sections is mandatory because the organism has a tendency to twist and coil on itself, causing considerable distortion. The distorted shapes may be mistaken for spores and thus alter diagnostic considerations. Of the fungi, the *Rhizopus* most closely resembles *Penicillium* and *Aspergillus* morphologically, but in general, the branching is more irregular and the hyphae are of larger diameter.[130]

A prominent feature almost invariably observed in cerebral lesions is invasion of the vasculature.[130] This is usually accompanied by significant destruction of blood vessels, extensive enough in some cases to produce large aneurysms.[329] The vascular pathological changes are not unlike those produced in aspergillosis. The angiotropic character of the organism provides reasonably direct hematogenous access to the central nervous system. Vessels of nearly any caliber, including the carotid artery, may be affected. In the majority of cases, however, the organism gains the central nervous system by direct extension from a contiguous focus—specifically the paranasal sinuses. Other routes are also possible[130]

The organism is truly opportunistic. Quite limited under normal circumstances, its pathogenicity is significantly enhanced by factors that compromise the host's resistance, the two major ones being the presence of acidosis and the presence of granulocytopenia.[25,34,167]

The association of cerebral mucormycosis with diabetic ketoacidosis is well established and quite frequent but not invariable. Any condition that favors the development of acidosis, such as dehydration in infants, predisposes to development of the disease.

Several pathological processes are caused by mucormycosis. In general, the overall picture is one of acute meningoencephalitis.[105] In the terminal stages, infarction accompanied by the formation of multiple abscesses takes place.

The histopathological progression of the disease is intimately related to the sequential appearance of clinical symptoms. The three primary patterns of involvement—rhinological, orbital, and cerebral—reflect not only the clinical sequence in most cases but also the anatomical progression of the disease.

Clinical Manifestations

Rhinological Involvement

Rhinological involvement almost always occurs in the presence of concurrent sinusitis. Any or all of the sinuses (frontal, maxillary, ethmoid, sphenoid) may be involved, and of these the sphenoid and ethmoid sinuses are the most frequent locations of primary disease.[284]

In the early stages symptoms are nonspecific. Purulent drainage is usually seen and may be accompanied by epistaxis. The symptoms closely resemble those caused by acute bacterial sinusitis. As the disease progresses, however, the more characteristic pathological features become more apparent. Ischemia produced by direct vascular involvement may produce necrosis and eventual gangrene. Perforation of the turbinates and septum may take place, and epistaxis may be so severe as to require operative treatment.

Orbital Involvement

It is during the stage of orbital involvement that the disease is most often diagnosed. The symptoms are quite characteristic and therefore generally more easily recognized. The clinical presentation is that of an orbital cellulitis, and the symptoms almost invariably progress rapidly. The patient initially notes severe pain in the orbital or nasal region. Eventually proptosis, chemosis, visual aberrations ranging from blurring of vision to blindness, sensory abnormalities (particularly in the distribution of the trigeminal nerve), and pupillary abnormalities develop. Funduscopic changes are usually quite prominent and often include central retinal artery occlusion with its characteristic attendant sequelae.[274,331]

The orbital adipose tissue provides an ideal medium for the development of abscesses. Pathological examination usually reveals thrombosis of the ophthalmic, ciliary, and central retinal arteries. Other orbital contents including the extraocular muscles and their sheaths may also be invaded. The globe itself, however, is not usually violated, and panophthalmitis is rare. Vascular compromise of periorbital vessels may also take place, producing disfiguring soft-tissue necrosis.

Cerebral Involvement

If the disease has progressed to the point at which orbital involvement is obvious, cerebral involvement will have taken place in 65 to 80 per cent of the cases.[130,134,284]

The frontal and temporal lobes by virtue of their proximity to the sinuses are the cerebral locations most commonly affected. The mental changes that are almost invariably present at this stage reflect this anatomical relationship. Hypophyseal and cerebellar involvement occurs also.

In the cerebral stage, eye findings may continue to dominate the clinical picture.

Eventually, however, the signs and symptoms of acute meningoencephalitis become more obvious.

Cranial nerve findings, usually multiple and homolateral, are frequent. Acute meningeal signs are not particularly prominent. Motor and sensory deficits vary from minimal to profound, depending on the extent of involvement.

In the typical clinical picture, progression of the disease takes place along the nasal-orbital-cerebral axis; however, other forms do exist. Primary involvement may occur in the pulmonary, gastrointestinal, and renal systems. Hematogenous dissemination may take place from any of these sources, causing cerebral lesions in the absence of any prodromal orbitonasal pathological changes. These cases may be difficult to diagnose since the cerebral lesions often are located deep in intraparenchymal tissues that are difficult to obtain biopsies from or to treat by operation.

Diagnosis

Members of the genus *Rhizopus* are frequent laboratory contaminants and their isolation does not necessarily reflect infection. On the other hand, neither is the organism considered part of the normal flora, and its development in a culture cannot be ignored. Should the organism be isolated, an extensive effort should be made to document its presence in tissue.

On appropriate culture media (e.g., Sabouraud's dextrose agar) the organism grows well and is usually easily identified. Material for culture should be taken from biopsy specimens to rule out unequivocally the possibility of laboratory contamination. The organism has not been cultured from spinal fluid.[130]

Microscopic identification of the *Rhizopus* may be more difficult. Several sections of each specimen should be examined to ascertain morphological details accurately. Several stains may be used to visualize the organism. The standard fungi stains (e.g., Gridley, methenamine silver) are acceptable, and others of some use are hematoxylin and eosin, periodic acid–Schiff, and acridine orange.

Examination of the cerebrospinal fluid usually reveals a neutrophilic pleocytosis and elevated glucose and protein levels.[105,130]

Radiographic examination should begin with a skull and sinus series. Sinus films in infected patients usually show thickened paranasal linings, absence of fluid levels in the erect position, and irregular focal destruction of the bony walls of one or more paranasal sinuses.[164]

Cerebral angiography has not been used extensively to evaluate cerebral mucormycosis. The relatively few complete studies have almost invariably revealed diffuse vasculitis.[31,39,284] In a high percentage of patients there is evidence of thrombosis. Parmentier and associates state that 50 per cent of patients with cerebral involvement will have thrombosis of the internal carotid artery on the side of the involved paranasal sinus. The thrombosis tends to occur at the level of the cavernous sinus.[274] Orbital venography is not particularly helpful because the organism appears to have a definite predilection for the arteries.

Computed tomography may be extremely helpful in delineating the extent of involvement, especially when operative procedures, which invariably need to be extensive, are being planned. In addition to the standard views obtained routinely, orbital cuts should be specified to delineate the full extent of orbital disease.

Additional diagnostic studies such as electroencephalography and radionuclide scanning rarely contribute significantly to the diagnosis.

Treatment

Early diagnosis of cerebral mucormycosis provides the only hope for effective treatment. Any of the following symptoms or signs in a diabetic patient should prompt investigation to rule out mucormycosis: orbital cellulitis, ophthalmoplegia, ecchymotic nasal lesions, epistaxis, and unilateral headache or eye pain.

Once the diagnosis is made, the institution of treatment is urgent because the disease usually pursues a rapidly progressive course.[44]

Several different therapeutic regimens have been recommended but all include at least these four components:

1. Predisposing factors such as diabetic ketoacidosis and neutropenia must be corrected.

2. The extent of the disease should be determined and the appropriate operative treatment instituted as soon as the metabolic status of the patient is stable. The thrombotic process that initiates infarction of naso-orbital tissues is usually quite extensive. The necrosis and gangrene that invariably follow make the affected tissue unsalvageable. If this tissue is not removed promptly it continues to provide a nidus for continuing infection not only with the etiological organism but with other opportunistic and secondary pathogens as well. The demarcation between viable and nonviable tissue is usually quite obvious, and nothing is to be gained by delaying appropriate therapy. The operative procedure may range from simple excision of localized tissue to exenteration of the orbit accompanied by excision of diseased cerebral tissue. Regardless of the procedure, an approach combining the expertise of the otorhinolaryngological, the ophthalmological, and the neurological surgeons yields the most acceptable therapeutic and cosmetic results.

3. The third key element in the therapeutic regimen is the administration of amphotericin B, which should be instituted immediately. Local irrigation of the affected area is not sufficient. Systemic administration of the drug, despite its numerous side effects, is mandatory. Maximum cumulative dosages of 2 to 3 gm have been recommended, but "cures" have been reported with much less.[2,33] The minimal amount required to provide effective treatment is not known. The large doses usually produce significant renal intoxication, and therefore renal status must be carefully monitored before, during, and after treatment, preferably with serial measurements of creatinine clearance.

Several other chemotherapeutic agents including 2-hydroxystilbamidine and clotrimazole have been used but are still considered less satisfactory than amphotericin B.[44]

4. Corticosteroids, which favor fungal dissemination, should be avoided. Other medications, including antimetabolites, cytotoxic drugs, and even antibiotics, should be discontinued if possible.

Prognosis

The prognosis of cerebral mucormycosis is intimately related to the accompanying medical problems that predispose the patient to develop the disease. If the diabetes or acidosis (or both) cannot be adequately controlled, the clinical course is usually rapidly fulminating, and the prognosis is poor. With aggressive diagnostic and therapeutic efforts, however, cures may be anticipated.[31,215a] In those patients who do survive, morbidity is primarily related to the degree of vascular involvement and the extent of associated thrombosis and infarction, which may be extensive.[130,185a,286b] When involvement of the vasculature is extensive, mycotic aneurysms may develop.[185a] These aneurysms frequently involve major arterial structures and their rupture usually produces serious sequelae. Cavernous sinus infection and thrombosis may also occur, producing additional morbidity in the form of ocular palsies and blindness.[109a]

SARCOIDOSIS

Sarcoidosis is a multisystem granulomatous disease of unknown etiology. It is characterized by the formation of noncaseating granulomas, proliferation of lymphoid tissue, and depression of cell-mediated immunity. Although the disease most commonly manifests itself with perihilar lymphadenopathy, pulmonary infiltration, and skin and eye lesions, numerous other systems including the central nervous system may be affected. Immunological defects, whether primary or secondary, are cardinal features of the disease and play a key role in diagnosis. Various infective and environmental sources have been implicated as causative agents but none has yet been established as the definitive cause. Histological changes similar to those seen in several fungal diseases, beryllium disease, tertiary syphilis, and several other entities are also observed in sarcoidosis. It is possible that several agents are capable of inciting the common pathological process.

Epidemiology

Although sarcoidosis is considered a disease of young adults, it occurs in all age groups. The patients usually are between 20 and 40 years of age.[192,358] The average duration of symptoms is 2.6 years. The distribution of the disease is worldwide. Its true incidence is difficult to estimate for several reasons, among them the dependence on sophisticated immunological testing for diagnosis, which makes the disease more easily diagnosed where these tests are more readily available. Statistics also vary considerably with the population under study. In the United States, for example, sarcoidosis is 10 times as prevalent among blacks as among whites.[192] In Great Britain a prevalence of 20 cases per 100,000 population has been reported.[38] Certain subgroups, however, contribute disproportionately. For example, the prevalence among Irish women in London is estimated at 200 cases per 100,000—a figure 10 times that for the population as a whole. Various other racial predilections have also been reported.[190] The disease is more common in women. Incidence rates are roughly double those found in men, and hormonal factors have been implicated.[192] Familial associations have also been reported, and a recessive mode of inheritance has been postulated but not yet confirmed.

Central nervous system lesions account for approximately 5 per cent of disseminated disease.[323] Isolated central nervous system lesions are extremely rare, although neurological dysfunction is often the presenting symptom. It has been estimated that only 1 per cent of patients with central nervous system sarcoidosis show clinical neurological complications.[289,307] Central nervous system forms of the disease may regress spontaneously, as do other forms, prior to being diagnosed. Therefore, the incidence of subclinical disease may actually be considerably higher.

Pathogenesis and Clinical Manifestations

Sites of involvement by sarcoidosis are protean. Neurological manifestations are variable, and lesions have been identified throughout the central and peripheral nervous systems. In general, peripheral nerve and cranial nerve lesions suggest disease of more recent onset, whereas central nervous system lesions usually represent a longer-standing process.

Symptoms related to the central nervous system usually fall into five broad overlapping categories: (1) signs and symptoms associated with meningitis, (2) seizure activity, (3) signs and symptoms of hydrocephalus, (4) mental changes, and (5) hypothalamic–pituitary axis dysfunction.

Basal meningitis is the most common intracranial form. Involvement of the basilar meninges is usually quite extensive and results in a relatively high rate of involvement of the cranial nerves, pituitary gland, and hypothalamus. Cranial nerve involvement, in fact, accounts for approximately 50 per cent of neurological manifestations.[92,358] The second, seventh, and eighth cranial nerves are most commonly affected, and bilaterality is not an infrequent feature. The frequency with which the seventh cranial nerve alone is affected is increased by the relatively common syndrome of concurrent parotid gland involvement.[232,238]

Seizures are observed in 5 to 18 per cent of patients.[358] The grand mal type is most frequent and may be quite resistant to even the most vigorous anticonvulsant therapy. Concurrent steroid therapy may help to provide effective seizure control.[166] Seizures have been observed in nearly all pathological forms of the disease, but as would be expected, more frequently in those patients with mass lesions.

Hydrocephalus frequently occurs in patients with neurosarcoidosis. Many mechanisms to explain the development of hydrocephalus have been postulated. Granulomatous infiltration of the choroid plexus has been observed and may alter cerebrospinal fluid production and dynamics.[192] Outflow obstruction in the form of stenosis of the aqueduct or at various points along the outflow tract has also been noted.[232] The clinical symptoms produced by any of these mechanisms, however, are not unique, appearing quite similar to those observed in the other disease entities that also produce hydrocephalus.

Mental changes almost invariably accompany all intracranial sarcoidosis and may be produced by non–central nervous system forms as well. The pathophysiological mechanisms responsible for these changes are myriad and may require the coordinated effort of many medical specialties to assess properly the degree to which each is implicated. For example, sarcoid of the lungs frequently causes pulmonary insufficiency and may contribute to carbon dioxide narcosis. Liver involvement, depending on the degree of infiltration, may produce hepatic encephalopathy; and renal involvement, uremia. In addition, treatment may require prolonged high-dosage steroid administration, and steroid-induced psychosis has been reported on numerous occasions.[172,193]

Involvement of the hypothalamic-pituitary axis is also quite common, and symptoms associated with dysfunction of this axis may occur in 35 to 50 per cent of patients with neurosarcoidosis.[177] Both neurohypophyseal and adenohypophyseal involvement may be observed. The former is usually more evident. Visual disturbances, including bitemporal hemianopia, optic atrophy, and papilledema may occur.

Unfortunately, owing to the relative rarity of neurosarcoidsis, comprehensive and definitive reports regarding its histopathology are few. Basically, the disease may be categorized into three, often coexistent, pathological forms: basilar meningitis, granulomatous mass lesions, and granulomatous angiitis.

Sarcoid meningitis does not usually produce any unique histopathological findings, although involvement may be quite extensive.

Sarcoid granulomas within the brain usually are multiple.[177] Solitary lesions mimicking neoplasms are rare.[21] Histologically the lesions resemble tuberculomas, but central caseation necrosis is absent, and the granulomas rarely coalesce. These lesions appear to have no particular predilection regarding intracranial location.

Peripheral neuropathies are common and are probably the result of an extension of the granuloma formation process. Neuropathies may be observed in up to 15 per cent of patients with the disseminated disease.[358] No specific distribution or pattern of involvement predominates. In general, peripheral neuropathies only superficially resemble multiple symmetrical polyneuritis. Sensory symptoms are usually more prominent than motor symptoms and may be accompanied by large areas of hypalgesia—often in a bizarre distribution.[238] Generally, nerve conduction studies reveal prolonged conduction velocity.

Granulomatous angiitis presents with necrotizing lesions of blood vessels accompanied by ischemic or hemorrhagic infarction of the parenchyma. The differential diagnosis from other forms of granulomatous angiitis may be quite difficult. The vascular changes are observed most frequently in conjunction with the basilar meningitis.

Diagnosis

Initial laboratory evaluation of the patient suspected of having sarcoidosis should include, at a minimum, chest x-ray; electrocardiogram; hematology panel, urinalysis, blood urea nitrogen and serum calcium determinations, and liver enzyme profile. Because of the relatively high frequency of asymptomatic fundus granulomas, an ophthalmological examination should also be included. Additional diagnostic evaluations such as pulmonary function tests, nerve conduction studies, and electromyography may be performed as indicated.

A cardinal feature of the disease is the altered immunological status of the patient. General findings may include leukopenia, eosinophilia, and elevated sedimentation rate. Abnormal immunoglobulin patterns are observed frequently.[192]

Since pulmonary involvement is so common, chest x-ray and pulmonary function studies should be included in the evaluation. Serious parenchymal changes are observed in more than 50 per cent of patients. Bilateral hilar adenopathy with right paratracheal node involvement is a common pattern. Pulmonary function tests usually demonstrate restrictive disease with decreased compliance and loss of effective diffusing surface.

Biochemical abnormalities include abnormal calcium metabolism, usually manifested by hypercalcemia and hypercalciuria. This is most often transient and may be related to altered vitamin D metabolism. Alkaline phosphatase is increased when there is extensive hepatic involvement.[192]

Investigation of mass lesions should include skull films and computed tomography. Angiography, ventriculography, and pneumoencephalography may be necessary to complete the evaluation, particularly if the pituitary–hypothalamic axis is affected. Radiographically, pathological granulomatous involvement of the pituitary gland may be difficult to establish. Calcification is almost never seen, and the sella is usually not enlarged.[93,166] Calcification is also unusual in other forms of the disease in which there are mass lesions. The granulomatous masses are usually enhanced by contrast injection on CT examination.[93]

Lumbar puncture usually produces nonspecifically abnormal findings. Opening pressure frequently is elevated. Protein generally is increased (average approximately 250 mg per 100 ml), and almost invariably there is an accompanying moderate pleocytosis (average 80 to 100 cells).

Treatment

Spontaneous remission of the disease has been observed; central nervous system involvement, however, usually requires treatment.[166,353] Long-term therapy with small doses of steroids may be useful.

Operative resection of certain granulomatous mass lesions is dictated by the clinical status of the patient and the anatomical area of involvement.

Severe cases of basilar meningitis often are complicated by the development of hydrocephalus, and patients should receive long-term follow-up to detect this complication. Shunting procedures may be required.

Prognosis

In the majority of patients, the prognosis is good, and there is a tendency for symptoms to undergo amelioration over time. Cranial nerve lesions, which constitute a majority of the symptomatic lesions, often respond well to steroid treatment; therefore, the prognosis for these individual lesions is good. Intracranial mass lesions, both supratentorial and infratentorial, also respond well to steroid therapy, and these patients may be maintained for long periods on small doses of steroids. Operative decompression of symptomatic mass lesions is not contraindicated if medical therapy fails and usually it is tolerated reasonably well. As with other forms of granulomatous disease, the presence of multiple lesions implies a less favorable prognosis.

Involvement of the hypothalamic-pituitary axis has a somewhat less favorable prognosis if only from the standpoint that these patients are subject to a series of complications if not carefully and continuously monitored. If the basilar meningitic process persists for a long time, infiltration of the brain stem may take place, altering the prognosis dramatically for the worse. The outcome in these cases is invariably fatal. Generally, as would be expected, the prognosis is better for peripheral than for central nervous system lesions.

Vertebral Sarcoidosis

The incidence of osseous involvement in disseminated sarcoidosis varies considerably from approximately 5 per cent to more than 30 per cent, depending on the population under study.[159,239,261,372] It usually affects the phalangeal bones of the hands and feet but may also involve the long bones; ribs, nasal bones, pelvis, cranial vault, and vertebrae.[45,48,108,159,349] Cases involving the vertebrae or spinal cord are rare. The same epidemiological features that characterize other forms of the disease also apply to the vertebral form. There is a definite racial predilection, the disease being far more common in blacks. The age range is also similar, with the majority of patients falling into the 15- to 35-year-old category.[28] In contrast to other forms of the disease, however, males and females appear to be equally affected.

The clinical presentation of vertebral sarcoidosis is quite variable. Many patients are neurologically asymptomatic at the time the lesion is discovered, but symptoms as severe as tetraplegia secondary to cervical collapse have been reported.[119] In those who are symptomatic, back pain is a rather common feature and may be accompanied by pronounced constitutional symptoms that make the patient appear acutely ill. Presentation with spinal cord symptoms and documented histological cord involvement is rare indeed. Several cases have been reported in which clinical symptoms suggested the diagnosis, but only rarely has histological confirmation been obtained. Severe arachnoiditis causing a cauda equina syndrome has also been reported.[361] Symptoms vary according to which portion of the cord is affected, and no definite anatomical predilection has been observed.

Antemortem diagnosis is uncommon;

however, some cases have been confirmed by vertebral biopsy. Since treatment regimens differ considerably for the granulomatous diseases, an effort should be made to obtain histological confirmation whenever possible.

The pathogenic mechanisms of sarcoidosis generally do not produce lesions that require special investigative techniques different from those used to evaluate other granulomatous diseases. Radiographic investigation is extremely important, and plain spine films usually provide the most significant information. Two types of lesions, osteosclerotic and osteolytic, may be observed.[28,48,56,313,369]

The two types of lesions may be seen alone but more commonly occur in conjunction with one another.[28,56] Lesions frequently involve more than one vertebral body and are typically located in the thoracic region.[28,313] Lumbar and cervical lesions have been reported but are distinctly unusual. Diseased vertebrae are not necessarily adjacent.[56] The disc space is usually preserved, but severe pathological narrowing has been observed.[28,56,313] Associated radiographic findings may include lytic lesions of the phalangeal bones of the hands and feet, and hilar adenopathy. Myelography, at least, should be performed before any operative procedure is undertaken. Computed tomography of the spine may also be quite helpful.

Because of the wide variability of presenting symptoms and the frequent paucity of supporting data the differential diagnosis is broad and should include tuberculosis and other fungal infections, the pyogenic forms of vertebral osteomyelitis, and metastatic disease as well as lymphoma, Hodgkin's disease, and leukemia.[28,56]

No uniform regimen specifically directed at treatment of vertebral sarcoidosis is universally recommended. Spontaneous resolution of the bony lesion may take place, and clinical symptoms may improve, but the more usual situation is that bony lesions stabilize rather than resolve, while clinically, the patients tend to improve over the course of time. Complications secondary to the primary disease are the usual cause of deterioration. Rarely, if bony destruction is extensive, stabilization procedures may be required. The decision to use steroids should be carefully tailored to the clinical situation. Their use, while producing dramatic results in other forms of the disease, has not been unequivocally established in vertebral forms. If steroids are used, careful monitoring for the development or reactivation of tuberculosis is mandatory.[28]

REFERENCES

1. Abbassiour, K., Sahmat, H., Ameli, N. O., and Tafazob, M.: Computerized tomography in hydatid cysts of the brain. J. Neurosurg., 49:408–411, 1978.
2. Abramson, E., Wilson, D., and Arky, R. A.: Rhinocerebral phycomycosis in association with diabetic ketoacidosis. Ann. Intern. Med., 66:735, 1967.
3. Acha, P. N., and Aguilar, F. J.: Studies on cysticercosis in Central America and Panama. Amer. J. Trop. Med. Hyg., 13:48–53, 1964.
4. Ackerman, N. B. and Kronmueller, J.: The importance of Candida as an infectious agent. Surg. Gynec. Obstet., 140:65–68, 1975.
5. Ahuja, G. K., Jain, N., Vijayaraghavan, M., and Roy, S.: Cerebral mycotic aneurysm of fungal origin. J. Neurosurg., 49:107–110, 1978.
6. Ahuja, G. K., Roy, S., Kamla, G., and Virmani, V.: Cerebral cysticercosis. J. Neurol. Sci., 35:365–374, 1978.
7. Ajello, I.: Coccidioidomycosis and histoplasmosis—A review of their epidemiology and geographic distribution. Mycopathologia, 45:221–230, 1971.
8. Alicata, J. E.: Angiostrongylus cantonensis (Nematoda: Metastrogylidal) as a causative agent of eosinophilic meningitis of man in Hawaii and Tahiti: Canad. J. Zool., 40:5–8, 1962.
9. Alicata, J. E., and Brown, R. W.: Preliminary observations on the use of an intradermal test for the diagnosis of eosinophilic meningoencephalitis in man caused by Angiostrongylus. Canad. J. Zool., 40:119–124, 1962.
10. Allencar, A.: Chagas' disease. In Minckler, J., ed.: Pathology of the Nervous System. New York, McGraw-Hill Book Co., 1972, pp. 2559–2565.
11. Al-Nakeeb, S. M.: Description and biology of enteric amebae. In Padilla y Padilla, C. A., and Padilla, G. M., eds.: Amebiasis in Man. Springfield, Ill., Charles C Thomas, 1974, pp. 10–36.
12. Arana-Iñiguez, R.: Hydatid echinococcosis of the nervous system. In Spillane, J. D., ed.: Tropical Neurology. London, Oxford University Press, 1973, pp. 408–417.
13. Arana-Iñiguez, R.: Echinococcosis. In Vinken, P. J., and Bruyn, G. W., eds.: Handbook of Clinical Neurology. Vol. 35. Amsterdam, Elsevier-North Holland, Inc., 1978, pp. 175–208.
14. Arana-Iñiguez, R., and San Julian, J.: Hydatid cysts of the brain. J. Neurosurg., 12:323–335, 1955.
15. Arana-Iñiguez, R., and Surri, J.: Echinococcosis of the nervous system. In Van Bogaert, L., Pereyra Kafer, J., and Poch, G. F., eds.: Tropical Neurology. Buenos Aires, Lopez, 1963, pp. 91–111; Rev. Neurol. B. Aires, 20:155–175, 1962.

16. Arean, V. M.: Schistosomiasis—a clinicopathologic evaluation. *In* Sommers, S. C., ed.: Pathology Annual, Vol. 1. New York, Appleton-Century-Crofts, 1966, pp. 68–126.

17. Armitage, F. L.: Amoebic abscess of the brain, with notes on a case following amoebic abscess of the liver. J. Trop. Med. Hyg., *22*:69–76, 1919.

18. Arroyo, J., Medoff, G., and Kobayashi, G. S.: Therapy of murine aspergillosis with amphotericin B in combination with rifampin or 5-fluorocytosine. Antimicrob. Agents Chemother., *11*:21–25, 1977.

19. Arseni, C., and Samitca, D. C.: Cysticercosis of the brain. Brit. Med. J., *2*:494–497, 1957.

20. Ashcraft, K. W., and Leape, L. L.: Candida sepsis complicating parenteral feeding. J.A.M.A., *212*:454–456, 1970.

21. Aszkanazy, C. L.: Sarcoidosis of the central nervous system. J. Neuropath. Exp. Neurol., *11*:392–400, 1952.

22. Ayres, C., Davey, L. M., and German, W. J.: Cerebral hydatidosis: Clinical case report with a review of pathogenesis. J. Neurosurg., *20*:371–377, 1963.

23. Bader, G.: Candidose. *In* Die Viszeralen Mykosen. Jena, Fischer, 1965, pp. 95–156.

24. Bailey, C. A.: An epidemic of eosinophilic meningitis, a previously undescribed disease, occurring in Ponape, Eastern Carolines. U.S. Naval, Med. Res. Instit., Project NM 005007, Rep. nr. 7, 1948.

25. Baker, R. D.: The pathologic anatomy of mycosis. *In* Handbuch der speziellen pathologischen Anatomie und histologie. Vol. 3, Part 5. Berlin-Heidelberg-New York, Springer Verlag, 1971.

26. Balasubramanium, V., Ramanujan, P. B., and Ramamurthi, B.: Hydatid disease of the nervous system. Neurology India, *18*:suppl. 1:92–95, 1970.

27. Balding, D. L.: Textbook of Parasitology. 3rd ed., New York, Appleton-Century-Crofts, 1965, pp. 626–640.

28. Baldwin, D. M., Roberts, J. G., and Croft, H. E.: Vertebral sarcoidosis. A case report. J. Bone Joint Surg., *56-A*:629–632, 1974.

29. Ballenger, C. N., Jr., and Goldring, D.: Nocardiosis in childhood. J. Pediat., *50*:145–159, 1957.

30. Bamford, C. R.: Toxoplasmosis mimicking a brain abscess in an adult with treated scleroderma. Neurology (Minneap.), *25*:343–345, 1975.

31. Bank, H., Shibolet, S., Gilat, T., Altmann, G., and Heller, H.: Mucormycosis of the head and neck structures: A case with survival. Brit. Med. J., *1*:766–768, 1962.

32. Barry, M.: Clinical trials of hycanthone in the treatment of bilharziasis. Cent. Afr. J. Med., suppl.:33–35, 1970.

33. Battock, J. D., Grausz, H., Bobrowsky, M., and Littman, M. L.: Alternate-day amphotericin B therapy in the treatment of rhinocerebral phycomycosis (mucormycosis)., Ann. Intern. Med., *68*:122–137, 1968.

34. Bauer, H., and Sheldon, W. H.: Leukopenia and experimental mucormycosis. Amer. J. Path., *33*:617–618, 1957.

35. Baum, J. L.: Rhino-orbital mucormycosis occur-

ring in an otherwise apparently healthy individual. Amer. J. Ophthal., *63*:335–339, 1967.

36. Beaman, B. L., Burnside, J., Edwards, B., and Causey, W. A.: Occurrence of nocardial infections in the United States during a 24 month period (1972–1974). J. Infect. Dis., *134*:286–289, 1976.

37. Beard, T. C.: Evidence that a hydatid cyst is seldom "as old as the patient." Lancet, *2*:30–32, 1978.

38. Beeson, P. B.: Sarcoidosis. *In* Beeson, P. B., McDermott, W., and Wyngaarden, J. B., eds.: Cecil Textbook of Medicine. 15th Ed. Philadelphia, W. B. Saunders Co., 1979, pp. 209–216.

39. Bentwich, Z., Rosen, F., Ganor, S., and Herman, G.: Chronic rhinocerebral mucormycosis (phycomycosis) with occlusion of the left internal carotid artery. Israel J. Med. Sci., *4*:977–981, 1968.

40. Bilharz, T., Wein. Med. Wochenschr. *6*:49–52, 65–68, 1856.

41. Binford, C. H., Thompson, R. K., Gorham, M. E., and Emmons, C. W.: Mycotic brain abscess due to Cladosporium trichoides, a new species: Report of a case. Amer. J. Clin. Path., *22*:535–542, 1952.

42. Black, J. T.: Cerebral candidiasis: Case report of brain abscess secondary to Candida albicans and review of literature. J. Neurol. Neurosurg. Psychiat., *33*:864–870, 1970.

43. Blankfein, R. J., and Chirico, R. M.: Cerebral schistosomiasis. Neurology (Minneap.), *15*:957–967, 1965.

44. Blatrix, C., Vergez, A., Geslin, P., et al.: Mucormycose naso-orbito-cérébrale. Presse Méd., *78*:2113–2117, 1970.

45. Bloch, S., Movson, I. J., and Seedat, Y. K.: Unusual skeletal manifestations in a case of sarcoidosis. Clin. Radiol., *19*:226–228, 1968.

46. Bojalil, L. F., Garcia-Ramos, E., and Gonzalez-Mendoza, A.: Infeccion humana por Nocardia asteroides in Mexico. Mycopathologia, *16*:97–103, 1962.

47. Bolton, C. F., and Ashenhurst, E. M.: Actinomycosis of the brain: Case report and review of the literature, Canad. Med. Ass. J., *90*:922–928, 1964.

48. Bonakdarpour, A., Levy, W., and Aegerter, E. E.: Osteosclerotic changes in sarcoidosis. Amer. J. Roentgen., *113*:646–649, 1971.

49. Borgers, M.: Morphological changes in cysticerci of *Taenia taeniaeformis* after mebendazole treatment. J. Parasitol., *61*:830–843, 1975.

50. Borlund, D. S.: Mucormycosis of the central nervous system. Amer. J. Dis. Child., *97*:852–856, 1959.

51. Boshes, L. D., Sherman, L. C., Hesser, G. J., Milzer, A., and MacLean, H.: Fungus infection of the central nervous system. Arch. Neurol. Psychiat. (Chicago), *75*:175–197, 1956.

52. Boyd, M. F., and Crutchfield, E. D.: A contribution to the study of mycetoma in North America. Amer. J. Trop. Med., *1*:215–289, 1921.

53. Brailsford, J. F.: Cysticercus cellulosae: Its radiographic detection in the musculature and the central nervous system. Brit. Med. J., *14*:79–93, 1941.

54. Bran, J. L.: Epidemiology. *In* Padilla y Padilla,

C. A., and Padilla, G. M., eds.: Amebiasis in Man. Springfield, Ill., Charles C Thomas, 1974, pp. 37–43.

55. Brine, J. A.: Human nocardiosis: A developing clinical picture. Med. J. Aust., *1*:339–342, 1965.

56. Brodey, P. A., Pripstein, S., Strange, G., and Kohout, N. D.: Vertebral sarcoidosis. A case report and review of the literatures. Amer. J. Roentgen., *126*:900–902, 1976.

57. Brown, H. W.: Basic Clinical Parasitology. 4th Ed. New York, Appleton-Century-Crofts, 1975.

58. Brown, J. R.: Human actinomycosis. A study of 181 subjects. Hum. Path., *4*:319–330, 1973.

59. Buechner, H. A., and Clawson, C. M.: Blastomycosis of the CNS. II. A report of nine cases from the Veterans Administration Cooperative study. Amer. Rev. Resp. Dis., *95*:820–826, 1967.

60. Busey, J. F. et al.: Blastomycosis. I. A review of 198 collected cases from Veterans Administrations Hospitals. Amer. Rev. Resp. Dis., *89*:659 –672, 1964.

61. Busse, O.: Ueber parasitare Zelleinschlisse und ihre Zuchtung. Zbl. Bakt. (Orig), *16*:175–180, 1894.

62. Butler, W. T., Alling, D. W., Spickard, A., and Utz, J. P.: Diagnostic and prognostic value of clinical and laboratory findings in cryptococcal meningitis. New Eng. J. Med., *270*:59–67, 1964.

63. Cabieses, F.: Parasitic and fungal disease of the brain. *In* Youmans, J. R., ed.: Neurological Surgery. Vol. 3. Philadelphia, W. B. Saunders Co., 1973, pp. 1563–1565.

64. Campbell, W., and Blair, L.: Chemotherapy of *Frichinella spiralis* infections (a review). Exp. Parasitol., *35*:304–334, 1974.

65. Carbajal, J. R., Palacios, E., Azar-Kia, B., and Churchill, R.: Radiology of cysticercosis of the central nervous system including computed tomography. Radiology, *125*:127–131, 1977.

66. Carlile, W. K., Holley, K. E., and Logan, G. B.: Fatal acute disseminated nocardiosis in a child. J.A.M.A., *184*:477–480, 1963.

67. Carrea, R., and Murphy, G.: Primary hydatid cyst of the spinal cord. Acta Neurol. Latino-amer.. *10*:308–312, 1964.

68. Case Records of the Massachusetts General Hospital, Case 27-1976. New Eng. J. Med., *295*:34 –42, 1976.

69. Caudill, R. G., Smith, C. E., and Reinarz, J. A.: Coccidioidal meningitis: A diagnostic challenge. Amer. J. Med., *49*:360–364, 1970.

70. Chang, H. T., Wang, C. W., Yu, C. F., Hsu, C. F., and Fang, J. C. U.: Paragonimiasis: A clinical study of 200 adult cases. Chinese Med. J., *77*:3–9, 1958.

71. Chaussier. Un cas de paralysie des membres inferieurs. J. Med. Chir. Pharmacol., *14*:231–237, 1807.

72. Cheever, A. W.: Schistosomiasis and neoplasia. J. Nat. Cancer Inst., *67*:13–28, 1978.

73. Cheever, A. W., Valsamis, M. P., and Rabson, A. S.: Necrotizing toxoplasmic encephalitis and herpetic pneumonia complicating treated Hodgkin's disease. New Eng. J. Med., *272*:26–29, 1965.

74. Chen, S. N., and Suzuki, T.: Fuorescent anti-

body and indirect haemagglutination tests for Angiostrongylus cantonensis infection in rats and rabbits. J. Form. Med. Ass., *73*:393–400, 1974.

75. Cheng, W. F.: Cryptococcosis: Report of a case. Chinese Med. J. (Peking), *74*:374–386, 1956.

76. Chung, H. L., et al.: Recent advances in diagnosis of paragonimiasis. Chinese Med. J., *74*:1 –16, 1956.

77. Clark, H. C.: The distribution and complications of amebic lesions found in 186 post mortem examinations. Amer. J. Trop. Med., *5*:157–171, 1925.

78. Cooper, R. A., and Goldstein, E.: Histoplasmosis of the central nervous system. Amer. J. Med., *35*:45–57, 1963.

79. Cope, V. Z.: Actinomycosis of the bone with special reference to infection of the vertebral column. J. Bone Joint Surg., *33-B*:205, 1951.

80. Couch, J. R., Abdou, N. I., and Sagawa, A.: Histoplasma meningitis with hyperactive suppressor T cells in cerebrospinal fluid. Neurology (Minneap.), *28*:119–123, 1978.

81. Couvreur, J., and Desmonts, G.: Congenital and maternal toxoplasmosis. A review of 300 congenital cases. Develop. Med. Child. Neurol., *4*:519–530, 1962.

82. Couvreur, J., and Desmonts, G.: Toxoplasmosis. *In* Vinken, P. J., and Bruyn, G. W., eds.: Handbook of Clinical Neurology. Infections of the Nervous System. Part III. Amsterdam, North Holland Publishing Co., 1978.

83. Crossland, N. O.: Integrated control of trematode diseases. Advances Drug Res., *12*:53–88, 1977.

84. Cuckler, A. C., Egerton, J. R., and Aluata, J. E.: Therapeutic effect of thiabendazole on Angiostrongylus cantonensis infection in rats. J. Parasitol., *51*:392–396, 1965.

85. Cupp, C. M., Edwards, W. M., and Cleve, E. A.: Nocardiosis of the central nervous system: Report of two fatal cases. Ann. Intern. Med., *52*:223–229, 1960.

86. Dalessio, D. J., and Wolfe, H. G.: Trichinella spiralis infection of the central nervous system. Arch. Neurol. (Chicago), *4*:407–417, 1961.

87. Dar, J., and Zimmerman, R. R.: Schistosomiasis of the spinal cord. Surg. Neurol., *8*:416–418, 1977.

88. Darling, S. T.: A protozoon general infection producing pseudotubercles in the lungs and focal necrosis in the liver, spleen and lymph nodes. J.A.M.A., *46*:1283–1285, 1906.

89. Darling, S. T.: Histoplasmosis, a fatal infectious disease resembling kala azar found among natives of tropical America. Arch. Intern. Med. (Chicago), *2*:107–123, 1908.

90. Dastur, D. K., and Lalitha, V. S.: Pathological analysis of intracranial space-occupying lesions in 1000 cases, including children. J. Neurol. Sci., *15*:397–427, 1972.

91. Davis, A.: Clinically available antischistosomal drugs. J. Toxicol. Environ. Health, *1*:191–201, 1975.

92. Davis, M. J., Cilo, M., Plaitakis, A., and Yahr, M. D.: Trichinosis: Severe myopathic involvement with recovery. Neurology (Minneap.), *26*:37–40, 1976.

93. Decker, R. E., Mardayat, M., Marc, J., and Ra-

sool, A.: Neurosarcoidosis with computerized tomographic visualization and transsphenoidal excision of a supra- and intrasellar granuloma. J. Neurosurg., 50:814–816, 1979.

94. Delaney, P.: Neurologic manifestations in sarcoidosis. Review of the literature with a report of 23 cases. Ann. Intern. Med., 87:336–345, 1977.

95. De Monbreun, W. A.: The cultivation and cultural characteristics of Darling's Histoplasma capsulatum. Amer. J. Trop. Med., 14:93–125, 1934.

96. Deresinski, S. C., and Stevens, D. A.: Coccidioidomycosis in compromised hosts. Medicine (Balt.), 54:377–395, 1975.

97. Deresinski, S. C., Lilly, R. B., Levine, H. B., Galgiani, J. N., and Stevens, D. A.: Treatment of fungal meningitis with miconazole. (Abstract) Amer. Rev. Resp. Dis. (suppl.), 113:71, 1976.

98. De Tribolet, N., and Zander, E.: Intrancranial sarcoidosis presenting angiographically as a sub-dural hematoma. Surg. Neurol., 9:169–171, 1978.

99. Deve, F.: L'Echinococcose Osseuse. Montevideo, Montevedere & Co., 1948.

100. Deve, F.: L'Echinococcose Primitive. Maladie Hydatique. Paris, Masson & Cie., 1949.

101. DeVita, V. C., Utz, J. P., Williams, T., and Carbone, P. P.: Candida meningitis. Arch. Intern. Med. (Chicago), 117:527–535, 1966.

102. Dew, H. R.: Hydatid Disease. Its Pathology, Diagnosis and Treatment. Sydney, The Australasian Medical Publishing Co., Ltd., 1928.

103. Dew, H. R.: Hydatid disease of the brain. Surg. Gynec. Obstet., 59:312–329, 1934.

104. Dharker, S. R., Dharker, R. S., Vaishya, N. D., Sharma, M. L., and Chaurasia, B. D.: Cerebral hydatid cysts in central India. Surg. Neurol., 8:31–34, 1977.

105. Dhermy, P.: Phycomycosis. In Vinken, P. J., and Bruyn, G. W., eds.: Handbook of Clinical Neurology. Vol. 35. Infections of the Nervous System. Part III. Amsterdam, North Holland Publishing Co., 1978, pp. 541–555.

106. Diamond, R. D., and Bennett, J. E.: Disseminated cryptococcosis in man: Delayed lymphocyte transformations in response to cryptococcus neoformans. J. Infect. Dis., 127:694–697, 1973.

107. Diamond, R. D., and Bennett, J. E.: Prognostic factors in cryptococcal meningitis. Ann. Intern. Med., 80:176–181, 1974.

108. Dinn, J. J.: Neurosarcoidosis. Irish J. Med. Sci., 140:266–273, 1971.

109. Dixon, H. B. F., and Hargreaves, W. H.: Cysticercosis (Taenia Solium): further 10 years' clinical study covering 284 cases. Quart. J. Med., 13:107–121, 1944.

109a. Dollman, C. L., and Herd, I. A.: Acute pancreatitis in pregnancy complicated by renal cortical necrosis and cerebral mucormycosis. Canad. Med. Ass. J., 81:562–564, 1969.

110. Dorfsman, J.: The radiologic aspects of cerebral cysticercosis. Acta Radiol. [Diagn.] (Stockholm), 1:836–842, 1963.

111. Drutz, D. J., and Catanzaro, A.: State of the art: Coccidioidomycosis. Part I. Amer. Rev. Resp. Dis. 117:559–585, 1978.

112. Duma, R. J.: Amoebic Infections. In Vinken, P.

113. Dunston, T. H. J., and Pepler, W. J.: A new complement fixation test for schistosomiasis. S. Afr. Med. J., 39:162, 1965.

114. Duque, O.: Cladosporiosis cerebral experimental. Rev. Lat. Amer. Anat. Path., 7:101–110, 1963.

115. Dyck, P., Ramseyer, J. C., and Doyle, J. B., et al.: Cysticercus cyst of temporal lobe presenting as a tentorial pressure cone. West. J. Med., 125:317–320, 1976.

116. Eaton, R. D. P., Meerovitch, E., and Costerton, J. W.: The functional morphology of pathogenicity in Entamoeba histolytica. Ann. Trop. Med. Parasit., 64:299–304, 1970.

117. Edwards, V. E., Sutherland, J. M., and Tyrer, J. H.: Cryptococcus of the central nervous system. Epidemiological, clinical and therapeutic features. J. Neurol. Neurosurg. Psychiat., 33:415–425, 1970.

118. Einstein, H. E.: Coccidioidomycosis of the central nervous system. Advances Neurol., 6:101–105, 1974.

119. Engle, E. A., and Cooney, F. D.: Tetraplegia secondary to cervical sarcoidosis. Case report. J. Neurosurg., 50:665–667, 1979.

120. Eppinger, H.: Uber eine neve pathogene Cladothrix und eine durch sie hervorgerufene Pseudotuberculosis (cladothricia). Beitr. Path. Anat., 9:287–328, 1891.

121. Epstein, S., Holden, M., Feldshuh, J., and Singer, J. M.: Unusual cause of spinal cord compression: Nocardiosis. N.Y. J. Med., 63:3422–3427, 1963.

122. Erchul, J. W., and Koch, M. L.: Cerebral nocardiosis with co-existent pulmonary tuberculosis. Amer. J. Clin. Path., 25:775–781, 1955.

123. Ernst, J., and Ratjen, E.: Actinomycosis of the spine: Report of two cases. Acta Orthop. Scand., 42:35, 1971.

124. Escobar, A.: Cerebral cysticercosis. New Engl. J. Med., 298:403–404, 1978.

125. Evans, R. J. C., and McElwain, T. J.: Eosinophilic meningitis in Hodgkin's disease. Brit. J. Clin. Pract., 23:382–384, 1969.

126. Faust, E. C.: An inquiry into the lesions in schistosomiasis. Amer. J. Trop. Med., 28:175–199, 1948.

127. Feely, M., and Steinberg, M.: Aspergillus infection complicating transsphenoidal yttrium-90 pituitary implant. Report of two cases. J. Neurosurg., 46:530–532, 1977.

128. Feldman, H. A.: Toxoplasmosis. New Eng. J. Med., 279:1370–1375, 1431–1437, 1968.

129. Fetter, B. F., and Klintworth, G. K.: Uncommon fungal diseases. In Vinken, P. J., and Bruyn, G. W., eds.: Handbook of Clinical Neurology. Vol. 35. Infections of the Nervous System Part III. Amsterdam, North Holland Publishing Co., 1978, pp. 563–564.

130. Fetter, B. F., Klintworth, G. K., and Hendry, W. S.: Mycoses of the Central Nervous System. Baltimore, Williams & Wilkins Co., 1967, pp. 63–74.

131. Firemark, H. M.: Spinal cysticercosis. Arch. Neurol. (Chicago), 35:250–251, 1978.

132. Forno, L. S., and Billingham, M. E.: Allescheria

J., and Bruyn, G. W., eds.: Handbook of Clinical Neurology. Infections of the Nervous System. Part III, Vol. 35. Amsterdam, North Holland Publishing Co., 1978, pp. 25–65.

boydii infection of the brain. J. Path., *106*:195–198, 1972.

133. Fuster, B.: The EEG in hydatid cysts of the brain. *In* Van Bogaert, L., Pereyra Kafer, J., and Poch, G. F., eds.: Tropical Neurology. Buenos Aires, 1963, pp. 128–139.

134. François, J., and Ruyssellaere, E.: Les mycoses oculaires. Bull. Soc. Belge Ophthal., *148*:363–380, 1968.

135. Franco-Ponce, J.: Neurocysticercosis. *In* Subirana, A., and Espadaler, J. M., eds.: Neurology: Proceedings of the Tenth International Congress on Neurology. Barcelona, Spain, September 8–15, 1973. New York, American Elsevier, 1974, pp. 234–250.

136. Freeman, J. P., David, P. L., and MacLean, L. D.: Candida endophthalmitis associated with intravenous hyperalimentation. Arch. Surg. (Chicago), *108*:237–240, 1974.

137. Freese, J. W., Young, W. G., Sealy, W. C., and Conant, N. F.: Pulmonary infection with N. asteroides: Findings in eleven clinical cases. J. Thorac. Cardiovasc. Surg., *46*:537–547, 1963.

138. Fregeiro, O., and Pol Deus, J.: Vertebral hydatidosis: Vertebrectomy and methylmethacrylate substitution. Acta. Neurol. Latinoamer., *24*:169–182, 1978.

139. Fregeiro, J. O., Navarro, E., Pol, J., and Arana-Iñiquez, R.: Vertebral hydatidosis: Treatment by vertebrectomy with substitution by methylmethacrylate. *In* Fifth International Congress of Neurosurgery (Tokyo). Excerpta Medica, 1973.

140. Frenkel, J. K.: Toxoplasmosis. *In* Minkler, J. K., ed.: Pathology of the Nervous System. Vol. 3. New York, McGraw-Hill Book Co., 1972, pp. 2521–2538.

141. Galatius-Jensen, F., and Uhm, I. K.: Radiological aspects of cerebral paragonimiasis. Brit. J. Radiol., *38*:494–502, 1965.

142. Gama, C.: Compression granuloma of spinal cord caused by Schistosoma mansoni ova; epiconus, conus medullaris; cauda equina; Report of a case. J. Int. Coll. Surg., *19*:665–671, 1953.

143. Garcia, E. G.: Advances in pathophysiology of schistosomiasis japonica: A review. Southeast Asian J. Trop. Med. Public Health, *7*:306–309, 1976.

144. Garcia-Palmieri, M. R., and Marcial-Rojas, R. A.: The protean manifestations of schistosomiasis manosi. Ann. Intern. Med., *57*:763–775, 1962.

145. Gass, J. D. M.: Acute orbital mucormycosis. Arch. Ophthal. (Chicago), *65*:214, 220, 1961.

146. Gawish, N.: Bilharziasis of the central nervous system in human beings and experimental animals. Egypt J. Bilharz, *3*:115–119, 1976.

147. Gehlen, J. N.: Amebiasis complicated by liver, lung and brain abscesses. Minn. Med., *17*:18–22, 1934.

148. Gelfand, M.: Schistosomiasis in South Central Africa. Juta & Co., Ltd. Cape Town, South Africa, 1950, p. 194.

149. Georg, L. K.: Nocardia species as opportunists and current methods for their identification. *In* Prier, J. E., and Friedman, H., eds.: Opportunistic Pathogens. Baltimore, University Park Press, 1974, pp. 177–201.

150. Ghaly, A. F., and El-Banhawy, A.: Schistosomiasis of the spinal cord. J. Path., *111*:57–60, 1973.

151. Gilchrist, T. C., and Stokes, W. R.: The presence of an oidium in the tissues of a case of pseudolupus vulgaris. Bull. Johns Hopkins Hosp., *7*:129–133, 1896.

152. Gilden, D. H., Miller, E. M., and Johnson, W. G.: Central nervous system histoplasmosis after rhinoplasty. Neurology (Minneap.), *24*:874–877, 1974.

153. Gilligan, B. S., Williams, I., and Perceval, A. K.: Nocardial meningitis: A report of a case with bacteriological studies. Med. J. Aust., *2*:747–752, 1962.

154. Goinard, P., and Descuns, P.: Les kystes hydatiques du névraxe. Rev. Neurol. (Pairs), *86*:369–415, 1952.

155. Goinard, P., Descuns, P., and Cerace, G.: Le kystes hydatiques du cerveau. Sem. Hôp. Paris, *26*:658–661, 1950.

156. Goldsand, G., and Braude, A. I.: Anaerobic infections. Disease-a-Month (Chicago), pp. 1–62, November, 1966.

157. Goni, P.: Cysticercosis of the nervous system: III. Clinical findings and treatment. J. Neurosurg., *19*:641–643, 1962.

158. Gonyea, E. F.: The spectrum of primary blastomycotic meningitis: A review of central nervous system blastomycosis. Ann. Neurol. *3*:26–39, 1978.

159. Goobar, J. E., Gilmer, W. S., Caroll, D. S., and Clark, G. M.: Vertebral sarcoidosis. J.A.M.A., *178*:1162–1163, 1961.

160. Goodman, H. C.: Immunology and tropical diseases: Challenges and opportunities. Ann. Immun. (Paris), *129*:267–274, 1978.

161. Goodman, J. S., Kaufman, L., and Koenig, M. G.: Diagnosis of cryptococcal meningitis. Value of immunologic detection of cryptococcal antigen. New Eng. J. Med., *285*:434–436, 1971.

162. Goodwin, R. A., and Des Prez, R. M.: Pathogenesis and clinical spectrum of Histoplasmosis. Southern Med. J., *66*:13–25, 1973.

163. Grauman, H., Grauman, T., and Shin, S. W.: Pulmonary and extrapulmonary paragonimiasis. Korean Med. J., *8*:85–98, 1957.

164. Green, W. H., Goldberg, H. I., and Wohl, G. T.: Mucormycosis infection of the craniofacial structures. Amer. J. Roentgen. *101*:802–806, 1967.

165. Greer, A. E.: North American blastomycosis of a nasal sinus. Dis. Chest, *38*:454, 1960.

166. Greggs, R. C., Markesbery, W. R., and Condemi, J. J.: Cerebral mass due to sarcoidosis. Regression during corticosteroid therapy. Neurology (Minneap.), *23*:981–989, 1973.

167. Gregory, J. E., Golden, A., and Haymaker, W.: Mucormycosis of the central nervous system. Bull. Johns Hopkins Hosp., *73*:405–419, 1943.

168. Harvey, J. C., Cantrell, J. R., and Fisher, A. M.: Actinomycosis: Its recognition and treatment. Ann. Intern. Med., *46*:868–885, 1957.

169. Hawking, F.: Helminthiasis. Trematode infections. Trop. Dis. Bull., *66*:965–982, 1969.

170. Hayashi, M., Kumakura, T., and Minai, M.: Epidemiological studies of brain dysfunction in the schistosomiasis-endemic area, with special ref-

erence to EEG findings. Brain Nerve, *28*:493–499, 1976.

171. Hayashi, M., Kumakura, T., Nosenas, J., and Blas, B.: Clinical studies of cerebral schistosomiasis Japonica in the Leyte Island, (The Philippines)—in comparison with same disease in the Kofu City area. Brain Nerve, *29*:425–432, 1977.

172. Haynes, R. C., and Larner, J.: Adrenocorticotrophic hormone; adrenocortical steroids and their synthetic analogs: Inhibitors of adrenocortical steroid biosynthesis. *In* Goodman, L. S., and Gilman, A., eds.: The Pharmacological Basis of Therapeutics. New York, Macmillan Publishing Co., 1975.

173. Hedges, T., and Leung, L. S.: Parasellar and orbital apex syndrome caused by aspergillosis. Neurology (Minneap.), *26*:117–120, 1976.

174. Hefferman, A. G., and Asper, S. P., Jr.: Insidious fungal disease: A clinicopathological study of secondary aspergillosis. Bull. Johns Hopkins Hosp., *118*:10–26, 1966.

175. Heineman, H. S., and Brande, A. I.: Anaerobic infection of the brain. Amer. J. Med., *35*:682–697, 1963.

176. Henrici, A. T.: Endotoxin from Aspergillus fumigatus. J. Immun., *36*:319–338, 1939.

177. Herring, A. B., and Urich, H.: Sarcoidosis of the central nervous system. J. Neurol. Sci., *9*:405–422, 1969.

178. Herskowitz, A.: Spinal cord involvement with Schistosoma mansoni. J. Neurosurg., *36*:494–498, 1972.

179. Higashi, K., Aoki, H., Takebayashi, K., Morioka, H., and Sakata, Y.: Cerebral paragonimiasis. J. Neurosurg., *34*:515–27, 1971.

180. Hill, H. R., Mitchell, T. G., Matsen, J. M., and Quie, P. G.: Recovery from disseminated candidiasis in a premature neonate. Pediatrics, *53*:748–752, 1974.

181. Hoeprich, P. D., ed.: Infectious Diseases: A Modern Treatise of Infectious Processes. 2nd Ed. Hagerstown, Md., Harper & Row, 1977.

182. Horten, B. C., Abbot, G. F., and Parro, R. S.: Fungal aneurysms of intracranial vessels. Arch. Neurol. (Chicago), *33*:577–579, 1976.

183. Hosokawa, S., Morita, K., Fugii, M., Mori, W., and Geshi, T.: One clinic and histopathology of cerebral parasitism of the human lung fluke, Paragonimus westermani. Amer. J. Hyg., *1*:63–78, 1921.

184. Hsiek, H. C.: Angiostrongylus cantonensis and eosinophilic meningitis or meningoencephalitis due to its infection. Taiwan Clin. Med., *3*:1–5, 1967.

185. Hughes, W. T.: Generalized aspergillosis. Amer. J. Dis. Child., *112*:262–265, 1966.

185a. Hutter, R. V.: Phycomycetous infection (mucormycosis) in cancer patients: A complication of therapy. Cancer, *12*:330–350, 1959.

186. Iuchi, M.: Clinical observation of 25 cases of chronic schistosomiasis japonica with abnormal behavior type of hepatocerebral syndrome. Naika, *26*:727–733, 1970.

187. Ivanisevich, O., and Rivas, C. I.: Equinococosis hidatica. Bueno Aires, Minist. Educ. Justicia, 1961–1962.

188. Iyer, S., Dodge, P. R., and Adams, R. D.: Two cases of aspergillus infection of the central nervous system. J. Neurol. Neurosurg. Psychiat., *15*:152–163, 1952.

189. Jackson, J. J., Earle, K. M., and Kuri, J.: Solitary Aspergillus granuloma of the brain: Report of two cases. J. Neurosurg., *12*:53–61, 1955.

190. James, D. G., Neville, E., Siltzbach, L. E., Turiaf, J., et al.: A worldwide review of sarcoidosis. Ann. N.Y. Acad. Sci., *278*:321–334, 1976.

191. Jenny, B., Biot, J., Fouquet, T. J., and Mafart, Y.: La meningite à eosinophiles. Etude de 62 cas, dont 51 chez des sujets transplantés a Tahiti. Med. Trop. (Marseille), *29*:330–340, 1969.

192. Johns, C. J.: Disease of uncertain etiology, sarcoidosis. *In* Thorn, G. W., Adams, R. D., Braunwald, E., Isselbacher, K. J., and Petersdorf, R. G., eds.: Principles of Internal Medicine. New York, McGraw-Hill Book Co., 1977, pp. 1119–1123.

193. Jones, J. E., and Thomas, J. A.: Pharmacology of the adrenocorticoids. *In* Bevan, J. A., ed.: Essentials of Pharmacology. Hagerstown, Md, Harper & Row, 1976.

194. Juba, A.: Uber eine seltene Mykose (durch Histoplasma capsulatum verursachte Meningoencephalitis) des Zentralnervensystems. Psychiat. Neurol., *135*:260–266, 1958.

195. Jundrak, K., and Alicata, J. E.: A case of eosinophilic meningoencephaltis in Vietnam, probably caused by Angiostrongylus cantonenis. Ann. Trop. Med. Parasit., *59*:294–300, 1965.

196. Kahn, P.: Cysticercosis of the central nervous system with amyotrophic lateral sclerosis: Case report and review of the literature. J. Neurol. Neurosurg. Psychiat., *35*:81–87, 1972.

197. Kaplan, M. H., Kosen, P. P., and Armstrong, D.: Cryptococcosis in a cancer hospital. Clinical and pathological correlates in forty-six patients. Cancer, *39*:2265–2274, 1977.

198. Katz, A. M., and San, C. T.: Echinococcus disease in the United States. Amer. J. Med., *25*:759–770, 1958.

199. Katz, N.: Clinical evaluation of niridazole and hycanthone in schistosomiasis mansoni endemic areas. J. Toxicol. Environ. Health, *1*:203–209, 1975.

200. Kawai, N.: Ein erfolgreich operierter Fall von Lungenegelerkrankung des Gehirns (Paragonimiasis s. Distomiasis cerebri). Deutsch. Z. Chir., *252*:705–710, 1939.

201. Kaya, U., Ozden, B., Tucker, L., and Tarcan, B.: Intracranial hydatid cysts: Study of 17 cases. J. Neurosurg., *42*:580–584, 1975.

202. Kepron, M. W., Schoemperlen, Hershfield, E. S., Zylak, C. J., and Cherniack, R. M.: North American blastomycosis in Central Canada. A review of 36 cases. Canad. Med. Ass. J., *106*:243–246, 1972.

203. Khan, M. A., and Sbar, S.: Cryptococcal meningitis in steroid treated systemic lupus erythematosus. Postgrad. Med. J., *51*:660–662, 1975.

204. Kim, S. K., and Walker, A. E.: Cerebral paragonimiasis. Acta Psychiat. Neurol. Scand., *36*:suppl. 153:1–85, 1961.

205. King, R. B., Stoops, W. L., Fitzgibbons, J., and Bunn, P.: Nocardia asteroides meningitis. A case successfully treated with large doses of

sulfadiazine and urea. J. Neurosurg., *24*:749–751, 1966.

206. Kitahara, M., Kobayashi, G. S., and Medoff, G.: Enhanced efficacy of amphotericin B and rifampicin combined treatment of murine histoplasmosis and blastomycosis. J. Infect. Dis., *133*:663–668, 1976.

207. Kitamura, K., and Nishimura, K.: Diagnosis and treatment of cerebral paragonimiasis. Clin. Neurol., *3*:376–381, 1963.

208. Kobayashi, R. M., Coel, M., Niwayama, G., and Trauner, D.: Cerebral vasculitis in coccidioidal meningitis. Ann. Neurol., *1*:281–284, 1977.

209. Kobayashi, G. B.: Actinomycetes: The fungus-like bacteria. *In* Davis, B. D., et al., eds.: Microbiology. Harper & Row, Hagerstown, Md., 1973, pp. 872–879.

210. Kramer, M. D., and Aita, J. F.: Trichinosis with central nervous system involvement. A case report and review of the literature. Neurology (Minneap.), *22*:485–491, 1972.

211. Krayenbühl, H., and Uhlinger, A.: Isolierte Moniliasis des Zentralnervensystems. Schweiz. Arch. Neurol. Psychiat., *80*:316–322, 1957.

212. Kreuger, E. G., Norsa, L., Kennedy, M., and Price, P. A.: Nocardiosis of the central nervous system. J. Neurosurg., *11*:226–233, 1954.

213. Krogstad, D. J., Spencer, H. C., Jr., Healy, G. R., Gleason, N. N., Sexton, D. J., and Herron, C. A.: Amebiasis: Epidemiologic studies in the United States. Ann. Intern. Med., *88*:89–97, 1978.

214. Kunz, L. J.: Diagnosis of cryptococcal meningitis. New Eng. J. Med., *285*:1488, 1971.

215. Lalisse, A., Mises, J., and Durand, C. H.: Les altérations électro-encéphalographiques dans la toxoplasmose congénitale et acquise. Ann. Pediat. (Paris), *11*:41–46, 1964.

215a. Landau, J. W., and Newcomer, V. D.: Acute cerebral phycomycosis (mucormycosis): Report of a pediatric patient successfully treated with amphotericin B and cycloheximide and a review of pertinent literature. J. Pediat., *61*:363–385, 1962.

216. Lane, T., Goings, S., Fraser, D. W., Ries, K., Pettrozzi, J., and Abrutyn, E.: Disseminated actinomycosis with spinal cord compression: Report of two cases. Neurology (Minneap.), *29*:890–893, 1979.

217. Latovitzki, N., Abrams, G., Clark, C., Mayeux, R., Ascherl, G., and Sciarra, D.: Cerebral cysticercosis. Neurology (Minneap.), *28*:838–842, 1978.

218. Lawrence, R. M., and Goldstein, E.: Histoplasmosis. *In* Vinken, P. J., and Bruyn, G. W., eds.: Handbook of Clinical Neurology. Infections of the Nervous System Part III, Vol. 35. Amsterdam, North Holland Publishing Co., 1978, pp. 503–515.

219. Lechtenberg, R., and Vaida, G. A.: Schistosomiasis of the spinal cord. Neurology (Minneap.), *27*:55–59, 1977.

220. Leers, W. D.: North American blastomycosis. *In* Vinken, P. J., and Bruyn, G. W., eds.: Handbook of Clinical Neurology. Infections of the Nervous System. Part III, Vol. 35. Amsterdam, North Holland Publishing Co., 1978.

221. Leers, W. D., Russell, N. A., and Laroye, G.: Cerebellar abscess due to Blastomyces derma-

titidis. Canad. Med. Ass. J., *107*:657–660, 1972.

222. Levy, L. F.: Bilharziasis of the spinal cord. Cent. Afr. J. Med., *15*:223, 1969.

223. Levy, L. F., and Taube, E.: Two further cases of spinal bilharziasis. Cent. Afr. J. Med., *15*:52, 1969.

224. Levy, L. F., Baldachin, B. J., and Clain, D.: Intracranial Bilharzia. Cent. Afr. J. Med., *21*:76–84, 1975.

225. Linares, G., Baker, R. D., and Linares, L.: Paracoccidioidomycosis in the United States (South American blastomycosis). Arch. Otol. (Chicago), *93*:514–518, 1971.

226. Littman, M. L., and Schneierson, S. S.: Cryptococcus neoformans in pigeon excreta, in New York City. Amer. J. Hyg., *69*:49–59, 1959.

227. Littman, M. L., Horowitz, P. L., and Sweden, J. G.: Coccidioidomycosis and its treatment with amphotericin B. Amer. J. Med., *24*:568, 1958.

228. Lombardo, L., Alonso, P., Arroyo, L. S., Brandt, H., and Mateos, J. H.: Cerebral amebiasis: Report of 17 cases. J. Neurosurg., *21*:704–709, 1964.

229. Londero, A. T., and Ramos, C. D.: Paracoccidioidomycosis. A clinical and mycologic study of forty-one cases observed in Santa Maria, RS, Brazil. Amer. J. Med., *52*:771–775, 1972.

230. Lott, T., El Gammal, T., Dasilva, R., Hank, D., and Renolds, J.: Evaluation of brain and epidural abscesses by computed tomography. Radiology, *122*:371–376, 1977.

231. Luke, J. L., Bolande, R. P., and Gross, S.: Generalized aspergillosis and aspergillus endocarditis in infancy. Report of a case. Pediatrics., *31*:115–122, 1963.

232. Lukin, R., Chambers, A., and Soleimanpour, M.: Outlet obstruction of the fourth ventricle in sarcoidosis. Neuroradiology, *10*:65–68, 1975.

233. Lutz, A.: Uma mycose pseudococcidica localizada no boca e observada no Brazil. Contribuicao ao conhecimenta das hyfoblastomycoses americans. Brasil Med., *22*:121, 1908.

234. Mackerras, M. J., and Sandars, D. F.: The life history of the rat lungworm angiostrongylus cantonensis (Chen) (Nematoda: Metastrongylidae). Aust. J. Zool., *3*:1–21, 1955.

235. Madrazo, I., Sanchez, J. M., Leon, J. A. M.: Pipette suction for atraumatic extraction of intraventricular cysticercosis cysts. J. Neurosurg., *50*:531–532, 1979.

236. Manson, P.: On endemic hemoptysis. Lancet, *1*:532–534, 1883.

237. Marcial-Rojas, R. A., and Fiol., R. E.: Neurologic complications of schistosomiasis. Ann. Intern. Med., *59*:215–230, 1963.

238. Matthews, W. B.: Sarcoidosis of the nervous system. J. Neurol. Neurosurg. Psychiat., *28*:23–29, 1965.

239. Maycock, R. L., Bertrand, P., Morrison, C. E., and Scott, J. H.: Manifestations of sarcoidosis. Amer. J. Med., *35*:67–89, 1963.

239a. McGill, H. C. Jr., Brueck, J. W.: Brain abscess due to Hormodendrum species: Report of a third case. Arch. Path. (Chicago), *62*:303–311, 1956.

240. McKee, E. E.: Mycotic infection of brain with arteritis and subarachnoid hemorrhage: Report

of a case. Amer. J. Clin. Path., *20*:381–384, 1950.

241. Meyer, R. D., Young, L. S., Armstrong, D., and Yu, B.: Aspergillosis complicating neoplastic disease. Amer. J. Med., *54*:6–15, 1973.

242. Miller, R. P., and Bates, J. H.: Amphotericin B toxicity, a follow-up report of 53 patients. Ann. Intern. Med., *71*:1089–1095, 1969.

243. Mitsuno, T., Siko, T. S., Inanaga, K., and Zimmerman, L. E.: Cerebral paragonimiasis: A neurosurgical problem in the Far East. J. Neuro. Ment. Dis., *116*:685–714, 1952.

244. Miyazaki, J., and Nishimura, K.: Cerebral paragonimiasis. *In* Hornabrook, R. W., ed.: Topics in Tropical Neurology. Philadelphia, F. A. Davis, 1975, pp. 109–132.

244a. Moon, T. J., Yoon, B. Y., and Hahn, Y. S.: Spinal paragonimiasis. Yonsei Med. J. *5*:55–61, 1964.

245. Morgan, D., Young, R. F., Chow, A. W., Mehringer, C. M., and Itabashi, H.: Recurrent intracerebral blastomycotic granuloma: Diagnosis and treatment. Neurosurgery, *4*:319–324, 1979.

246. Mukoyama, M., Gumple, K., and Poser, C. M.: Aspergillosis of the central nervous system. Report of a brain abscess due to A. fumigatus and review of the literature. Neurology (Minneap.), *19*:967–974, 1969.

247. Neal, R. A.: The in vitro cultivation of Entamoeba problems of in vitro culture. *In* Fifth Symposium of the British Society of Parasitiology. Oxford-Edinburgh, Blackwell Scientific Publications, 1967.

248. Negroni, P.: Prolonged therapy for paracoccidioidomycosis: Approaches, complications and risks. Paracoccidioidomycosis. Proc. First Pan Amer. Symp. PAHO-WHO Scientific Publ., *254*:147–155, 1972.

249. New, P. F. J., Davis, K. R., and Ballantine, H. T., Jr.: Computed tomography in cerebral abscess. Radiology, *121*:641–646, 1976.

250. Nishimura, K.: Experimental studies on the chemotherapy of rat lungworm Angiostrongylus cantonensis in rats. Chemoterapia, *10*:164–175, 1965.

251. Nocard, M. E.: Note sur la maladie des oeufs de la Guadeloupe. Connue sous le nom de farcin. Ann. Inst. Pasteur (Paris), *2*:293–302, 1888.

252. Nomura, S., and Lin, S. H.: *In* Beaver, P. C., and Rosen, L., eds.: Memorandum on the first report of Angiostrongylus in man by Nomura and Lin, 1945. Amer. J. Trop. Med., *13*:589–590, 1964.

253. Obrador, S.: Clinical aspects of cerebral cysticercosis. Arch. Neurol. Psychiat. (Chicago), *59*:457–468, 1948.

254. Oh, S. J.: Bithionol treatment in cerebral paragonimiasis. Amer. J. Trop. Med., *16*:585–590, 1967.

255. Oh, S. J.: Spinal paragonimiasis. J. Neurol. Sci., *6*:125–140, 1968.

256. Oh, S. J.: Roentgen findings in cerebral paragonimiasis. Radiology, *90*:292–299, 1968.

257. Oh, S. J.: Cerebral paragonimiasis. J. Neurol. Sci., *8*:27–48, 1969.

258. Oh, S. J.: Cerebral and spinal paragonimiasis. J. Neurol. Sci., *9*:205–236, 1969.

259. Oh, S. J.: Paragonimiasis in the central nervous system. *In* Vinken, P. J., and Bruyn, G. W., eds.: Handbook of Clinical Neurology. Vol. 35. Amsterdam, North Holland Publishing Co., 1978.

260. Olsen, S., Eriksen, K. R., Stenderup, H., and Balslov, J. T.: A case of aspergillosis cerebri. Ugeskr. Laeg., *124*:1881–1884, 1962.

261. Olsen, T. G.: Sarcoidosis of the skull. Radiology, *80*:232–236, 1963.

262. O'Neill, R. P., and Penman, R. W.: Clinical aspects of blastomycosis. Thorax, *25*:708–715, 1970.

263. Orbison, J. A., Reeves, N., Leedham, C. L., and Blumberg, J. M.: Amebic brain abscess. Review of the literature and report of five additional cases. Medicine (Baltimore), *30*:247–282, 1951.

264. Otani, S.: An autopsy case of paragonimiasis. Tokyo Igakkhai Zasshi, *1*:458–463, 507–511, 1887.

265. Ozgen, T., Erbengi, A., Berton, V., Saglam, S., Ozdemer, G., and Punor, T.: The use of computerized tomography in the diagnosis of cerebral hydatid cysts. J. Neurosurg., *50*:339–342, 1979.

266. Paillas, J. E., Bonnal, J., and Acquaviva, R.: Formes neurochirurgicales des parasitoses intracraniennes. Encycl. Med.-chir. neurol. *53*:1–6, 1970.

267. Palmer, D. L., Harvey, R. L., and Wheeler, J. K.: Diagnostic and therapeutic considerations in Nocardia asteroides infection. Medicine (Balt.), *53*:391–401, 1974.

268. Paltauf, A.: Mycosis mucorina. Virchow. Arch. Path. Anat., *102*:543–564, 1885.

269. Pappagianis, D.: Coccidioidomycosis. *In* Hoeprich, P. D., ed.: Infectious Diseases: A Modern Treatise of Infectious Processes. Hagerstown, Md., Harper & Row, 1977.

270. Pappagianis, D., and Crane, R.: Survival in coccidioidal meningitis since introduction of amphotericin B. *In* Ajello, L., ed.: Third International Symposium on Coccidioidomycosis. Miami, Symposia Specialists, 1977.

271. Park, C. S.: Electroencephalography of cerebral paragonimiasis. J. Kor. Med. Ass., *10*:684–689, 1967.

272. Parker, J. D., Doto, I. L., and Tosh, F. E.: A decade of experience with blastomycosis and its treatment with amphotericin B. A National Communicable Disease Center Cooperative Mycoses Study. Amer. Rev. Resp. Dis., *99*:895–902, 1969.

273. Parker, J. C., McCloskey, J. J., Solanki, K. V., and Goodman, N. L.: Candidosis: The most common postmortem cerebral mycosis in an endemic fungal area. Surg. Neurol., *6*:123–128, 1976.

274. Parmentier, N., Balasse, E., Pirart, J., and Vanderhaeghen, J. J.: Mucormycose orbitaire. Arch. Ophtal. (Paris), *25*:689–704, 1965.

275. Parsons, R. J., and Zarafonetis, C. J. D.: Histoplasmosis in man. Reports of seven cases and a review of 71 cases. Arch. Intern. Med. (Chicago), *75*:1, 1945.

276. Peabody, J. W., and Seabury, J. H.: Actinomycosis and nocardiosis. A review of basic differences in therapy. Amer. J. Med., *28*:99–115, 1960.

277. Pena, C. E.: Aspergillosis. *In* Baker, R. D., ed.: The Pathologic Anatomy of Mycoses. Human

Infection with Fungi. Berlin, Springer Verlag, 1970, pp. 762–831.

278. Perez Fontana, V.: El cloruro de sodio en la profilaxsis de la hidatidosis. Arch. Int. Hidatid. *13*:355, 1953.

279. Perry, H. O., Kierland, R. R., and Weed, L. A.: South American blastomycosis: Further observations on a case previously reported. Derm. Trop., *3*:79–84, 1964.

280. Pitchford, R. J.: Influence of living conditions on bilharziasis infection rates in Africans in the Transvaal. Bull. WHO, *18*:1088–1091, 1958.

281. Pinto Pupo, P.: Cysticercosis of the nervous system: Clinical manifestations. Rev. Neuropsiquiat. (S. Paulo), *28*:70–82, 1964.

282. Plorde, J. J.: *In* Thorne, G. W., et al., eds.: Harrison's Principles of Internal Medicine 8th ed. New York, A Blakiston Publication. McGraw Hill Book Co., 1977.

283. Powell, H. C., Gibbs, C. J., Jr., Lorenzo, A. M., Lampert, P. W., and Gadjusek, D. C.: Toxoplasmosis of the central nervous system in the adult. Electron microscopic observations. Acta Neuropath (Berlin), *41*:211–216, 1978.

284. Price, D. L., Wolpow, E. R., and Richardson, E. P., Jr.: Intracranial phycomycosis: A clinicopathological and radiological study. J. Neurol. Sci., *14*:359–375, 1971.

285. Prokovskii, V. I.: Acute phase of intestinal schistosomiasis with involvement of the central nervous system. Med. Parazit. (Mosk.), *44*:157–159, 1975.

286. Punyagupta, S., Bunnag, T., Juttijudata, P., and Rosen, L.: Eosinophilic meningitis in Thailand. Epidemiologic studies on 434 typical cases and the etiologic role of Angiostrongylus cantonensis. Amer. J. Trop. Med. Hyg., *19*:950–958, 1970.

286a. Punyagupta, S., Juttijudata, P., Bunnag, T., and Comer, D.: Two fatal cases of eosinophilic myeloencephalitis, a newly recognized disease caused by Gnathostoma spinigerum. Trans. Roy. Soc. Trop. Med. Hyg., *62*:801–809, 1968.

286b. Rao, V. R. K., Pillai, S. M., Mathews, G., and Radhakrishnan, V. V.: Cerebral mucormycosis—a case report. Neuroradiology, *15*:291–293, 1978.

287. Rayport, M., Wisoff, H. S., and Zaiman, H.: Vertebral echinococcosis. J. Neurosurg., *21*:647–659, 1964.

288. Rezek, P. R., and Millard, M.: Autopsy Pathology. Springfield, Ill., Charles C Thomas, 1963.

289. Ricker, W., and Clark, M.: Sarcoidosis, a clinical pathologic review of 300 cases, including 22 autopsies. Amer. J. Clin. Path., *19*:725, 1949.

290. Rifkind, D., Marchioro, T. L., Schneck, A. A., and Hill, R. B., Jr.: Systemic fungal infections complicating renal transplantation and immunosuppressive therapy. Amer. J. Med., *43*:28–38, 1967.

291. Rippon, J. W.: Medical Mycology—The Pathogenic Fungi and the Pathogenic Actinomycetes. Philadelphia, W. B. Saunders Co., 1974.

292. Roach, M. R., and Drake, C. G.: Ruptured cerebral aneurysms caused by microorganisms. New Eng. J. Med., *273*:240–244, 1965.

293. Robinson, R. G.: Hydatid disease of the spine and its neurological complications. Brit. J. Surg., *47*:301–306, 1960.

294. Rosen, L., Loison, G., Larget, J., and Wallace, G.: Studies on eosinophilic meningitis. 3. Epidemiologic and clinical observations on Pacific Islands and the possible etiologic role of Angiostrongylus cantonenis. Amer. J. Epidem., *85*:17–44, 1967.

295. Rosen, L., Chopell, R., Laquear, G., Wallace, G. D., and Weinstein, P. P.: Eosinophilic meningolungworm of rats. J.A.M.A., *179*:620–624, 1962.

296. Rosenbaum, R. M., Ishii, N., Tanowitz, H., and Wittner, M.: Schistosomiasis mansoni of the spinal cord. Report of a case. Amer. J. Trop. Med. Hyg., *21*:182–184, 1972.

297. Rosenblum, M. L., and Rosegay, H.: Resection of multiple nocardial brain abscesses: Diagnostic role of computerized tomography. Neurosurgery, *4*:315–318, 1979.

298. Ross, G. L., Norcross, J. W., and Harrax, G.: Spinal cord involvement by Schistosomiasis mansoni. New Eng. J. Med., *246*:823–826, 1952.

299. Saccardo, P. A.: Torula fungine bantiana. Ann. Mycol., *10*:320–321, 1912.

300. Sadun, E., and Buck, A.: Paragonimiasis in South Korea—immunodiagnostic, epidemiologic, clinical, roentgenologic and therapeutic studies. Amer. J. Trop. Med. Hyg., *9*:562–599, 1960.

301. Saeki, S.: An autopsy case of ectopic infestation of lung fluke. Trans. Soc. Path. Jap., *43G*:678–679, 1954.

302. Samiy, E., and Zadeh, F. A.: Cranial and intracranial hydatidosis with special reference to roentgen-ray diagnosis. J. Neurosurg., *22*:425–433, 1965.

303. Sampaio, S. A. P.: Clinical manifestations of paracoccidioidomycosis. Proceedings of the First Pan American Symposium, Medellin (Colombia). Pan American Health Organization. Scientific Publication No. 254, 1972, pp. 101–108.

304. Sanford, A. H., and Voelker, M.: Actinomycosis in the United States. Arch. Surg. (Chicago), *11*:809–841, 1925.

305. Saxe, N., and Gordon, W.: Schistosomiasis of spinal cord and skin. S. Afr. Med. J., *49*:57–58, 1975.

306. Sayk, J.: Klinischer Beitrag zur Liquoreosinophilie und Frage der allergischen Reaktion im Liquorraum. Deutsch. Z. Nervenheilk., *177*:62–72, 1957.

307. Scadding, J. G.: The nervous system in sarcoidosis. *In* Sarcoidosis. London, Eyre, Spottiswoode, 1967.

308. Schantz, P. M., Von Reyn, C. F., Weltz, T., Anderson, F. L., Schultz, M. G., and Kagan, I. G.: Epidemiologic investigation of echinococcus in American Indians living in Arizona and New Mexico. Amer. J. Trop. Med. Hyg., *26*:121, 1977.

309. Schlaegel, T. F.: Ocular Histoplasmosis. Current Ophthalmology Monographs. New York, Grune & Stratton Inc., 1977.

310. Schnyder, H. K.: Aspergillose der Schadelbasis. Pract. Otorhinolaryng. (Basel), *10*:402–421, 1948.

311. Schollhammer, G., Aubry, P., and Rigaud, J. L.: Quelques reflexions sur la meningite a eosino-

philes a Tahiti. Etude clinique et luologique de 165 observations, propos d'un cas atypique. Bull. Soc. Path. Exot., 59:341–349, 1966.

312. Schulz, D. M.: Histoplasmosis of the central nervous system. J.A.M.A., 151:549–551, 1953.

313. Schumacker, H. R.: Sarcoidosis. In Hollander, J. L., ed.: Arthritis and Allied Conditions: A Textbook of Rheumatology. 8th Edition. Philadelphia, Lea and Febiger, 1972, pp. 1295–1302.

314. Seelig, M. S.: The role of antibiotics in the pathogenesis of Candida infections. Amer. J. Med., 40:887–917, 1966.

315. Selby, R.: Pachymeningitis secondary to Allescheria boydii. J. Neurosurg., 36:225–227, 1972.

316. Seres, S. L., Ono, H., Benner, E. J.: Aspergillosis presenting as spinal cord compression. J. Neurosurg., 36:221–224, 1972.

317. Shaffer, J. G., Shlaes, W. H., Radke, R. A., and Palmer, W. L.: Amebiasis: A Biomedical Problem. Springfield, Ill., Charles C Thomas, 1962.

318. Shapiro, K., and Tabaddor, K.: Cerebral aspergillosis. Surg. Neurol., 4:465–471, 1975.

319. Shimizu, F.: A case of cerebral paragonimiasis which was diagnosed as brain tumor. Tokyo Iji Shinski, 72:474–475, 1955.

320. Shuster, M., Klien, Pribor, H. C., and Kozub, W.: Brain abcess due to Nocardia. Arch. Intern. Med. 120:610–614, 1967.

321. Singh, B. N.: Pathogenic and Non-Pathogenic Amoeba. New York, John Wiley & Sons, 1975.

322. Smit, A. M.: La meningite à eosinophiles à Kisaran (Indonesie) et le probleme de son etiologie. Bull. Soc. Path. Exot., 55:722–730, 1962.

323. Smith, L. H., Jr., Farnham, G. F., and Baringer, J. R.: Sarcoidosis of the nervous system. Calif. J. Med., 113:61, 1970.

324. Smith, J. W., and Utz, J. L.: Progressive disseminated histoplasmosis. Ann. Intern. Med., 76:557–565, 1972.

325. Smithers, S. R., and Terry, R. J.: The immunology of schistosomiasis. Advances Parasitol., 7:41–93, 1969.

326. Soulsby, E. J.: Cell mediated immunity in parasitic infections. J. Parasitol., 56:534–547, 1970.

327. Spina-Franca, A., and Mattosinho-Franca, I. C.: Chagas' disease and the nervous system. In Spillane, J. D., ed.: Tropical Neurology. London, Oxford University Press, 1973, pp. 397–407.

328. Spina-Franca, A., and Mattosinho-Franca, I. C.: Chagas' disease. In Subirana, A., Espadaler, J. M., and Burrows, E. H., eds.: Neurology. Proceedings of the Tenth International Congress of Neurology, Barcelona, Spain, September 8–15, 1973. Amsterdam, Excerpta Medica, 1974, pp. 227–233.

329. Stehbens, W. E.: Atypical cerebral aneurysms. Med. J. Aust., 1:765–766, 1965.

330. Stepien, L.: Cerebral cysticercosis in Poland. Clinical symptoms and operative results in 132 cases. J. Neurosurg., 19:505–513, 1962.

331. Straatsma, B. R., Zimmerman, L. E., and Gass, J. D. M.: Phycomycosis. Lab. Invest., 11:963–985, 1962.

332. Stroder, J., Kuhner, U., and Farber, D.: Candida albicans Meningitis im Sauglingsalter. Deutsch. Med. Wschr. 100:1196–1199, 1975.

333. Sung, J. P.: Treatment of disseminated coccidioidomycosis with miconazole. Western J. Med., 124:61–64, 1976.

334. Deleted in proof.

335. Symmers, W. S.: A case of cerebral chromoblastomycosis (cladosporiosis) occurring in Britain as a complication of polyarteritis treated with cortisone. Brain, 83:37–51, 1960.

336. Symmers, N. S.: Septicaemic candidosis. In Winner, H. I., and Hurley, R., eds.: Symposium on Candida Infections. Edinburgh-London, E. & S. Livingstone, 1966, pp. 196–213.

337. Tan, J. S.: Common and uncommon parasitic infections in the United States. Med. Clin. N. Amer., 62:1059–1081, 1978.

338. Tarcan, B.: Hydatid cysts of the brain. J. Int. Coll. Surg., 36:334, 1961.

339. Toledo, P., and Unceta, F.: Sindrome me ingea con pleocitosis eosinophilica. Rev. Clin. Bilbao, 4:134–135, 1929.

340. Townsend, J. J., Wolinsky, J. S., Baringer, J. R., and Johnson, P. C.: Acquired toxoplasmosis. A neglected cause of treatable nervous system disease. Arch. Neurol. (Chicago), 32:335–343, 1975.

341. Trelles, J. O.: Parasitic diseases in tropical neurology. In Vinken, P. J., and Bruyn, G. W., eds.: Handbook of Clinical Neurology. Part III, Vol. 35. Amsterdam, Elsevier—North Holland Publishing Co., 1978.

342. Trelles, J. O., and Trelles, L.: Cysticercosis of the nervous system. In Vinken, P. J., and Bruyn, G. W., eds.: Handbook of Clinical Neurology. Infections of the Nervous System Part III, Vol. 35. Amsterdam, North Holland Publishing Co., 1978.

343. Tress, B., and Davis, S.: Computed tomography of intracerebral toruloma. Neuroradiology, 17:223–226, 1979.

344. Tully, R. J., and Watts, C.: Computed tomography and intracranial aspergillosis. Neuroradiology, 17:111–113, 1979.

345. Tynes, B. S., Crutcher, J. C., and Utz, J. P.: Histoplasma meningitis. Ann. Intern. Med., 59:615–621, 1963.

346. Utz, J.: Current and future chemotherapy of the central nervous system—fungal infections. Advances Neurol., 6:127–132, 1974.

346a. Utz, J. P.: Histoplasmosis. In Hoeprich, P. D., ed.: Infectious Diseases. Hagerstown, Md., Harper & Row, 1977, pp. 383–388.

347. Utz, J. P., Garriques, I. L., Sande, M. A., Warner, J. F., Mandell, G. L., McGehee, R. F., Duma, R. J., and Shadomy, S.: Therapy of cryptococcosis with a combination of flucytosine and amphotericin B. J. Infect. Dis., 132:368–373, 1975.

348. Vengsarkar, U. S., and Abraham, J.: Hydatid disease of the spine. J. Postgrad. Med., 11:133–136, 1965.

349. Vesely, D. L., Maldonodo, A., and Levey, G. S.: Partial hypopituitarism and possible hypothalamic involvement in sarcoidosis. Report of a case and review of the literature. Amer. J., 62:425–431, 1977.

350. Vietzke, W. M., Gelderman, A. H., Grimley, P. M., and Valsamis, M. P.: Toxoplasmosis com-

plicating malignancy. Cancer, *21*:816–827, 1968.

351. Virmani, V., Ray, S., and Kamla, G.: Pseudolateralized epileptiform discharges in a case of diffuse cerebral cysticercosis. Neuropadiatrie, *8*:196–203, 1977.

352. Visudhipan, P., Bunyaratavej, S., and Khantanaphar, S.: Cerebral aspergillosis. J. Neurosurg., *38*:472–476, 1973.

353. Walker, A. G.: Sarcoidosis of the brain and spinal cord. Postgrad. Med. J., *37*:431, 1961.

354. Walker, A. T.: Trichiniasis: Report of an outbreak caused by eating trichinous bear meat in the form of "jerkey." J.A.M.A., *98*:2051, 1932.

355. Watts, M. B.: Five cases of eosinophilic meningitis in Sarawak. Med. J. Malaya, *24*:89–93, 1969.

356. Weese, W. C., and Smith, I. M.: A study of 57 cases of actinomycosis over a 36-year period. Arch. Intern. Med. (Chicago), *135*:1562–1568, 1975.

357. Welsh, J. D., Rhoades, E. R., and Jaques, W.: Disseminated nocardiosis involving the spinal cord. Case report. Arch. Intern. Med. (Chicago), *108*:73–79, 1961.

358. Wiederholt, W. C., and Siekert, R. G.: Neurological manifestations of sarcoidosis. Neurology (Minneap.), *15*:1147–1154, 1965.

359. Wilcocks, C., and Manson-Bahr, P. E.: Manson's Tropical Diseases. 17th ed. Baltimore, Williams & Wilkins Co., 1972.

360. Winter, W. G., Larson, R. K., Zettas, J. P., and Libke, R.: Coccidioidal spondylitis. J. Bone Joint Surg., *60*:240–244, 1978.

360a. Wiseley, R. J., and Davey, W. N.: Endogenous exacerbation of histoplasmosis after apparent recovery from an acute pulmonary infection. Ann. Rev. Resp. Dis., *103*:546–551, 1971.

361. Wood, E. H., and Bream, C. A.: Spinal sarcoidosis. Radiology, *73*:226–233, 1959.

362. Wright, W. H.: Schistosomiasis as a world problem. Bull. N.Y. Acad. Med., *44*:301–312, 1968.

363. Wright, W. H., Jacobs, L., and Walton, A. C.: Studies on trichinosis. XVI. Epidemiological considerations based on the examination for trichinae of 5313 diaphragms from 189 hospitals in 37 states and the District of Columbia. Public Health Rep., *59*:669–681, 1944.

364. Wybel, R. E.: Mycosis of cervical spinal cord following intrathecal penicillin therapy: Report of a case simulating cord tumor. Arch. Path. (Chicago), *53*:167–173, 1952.

365. Yamugiwa, K.: Beitrag zur Aetiologie der Jacksonschen Epilepsie. Virchow. Arch. Path. Anat., *119*:447–460, 1890.

366. Yarzabal, L. A., and Capron, A.: Aportes de la inmunologico de la hidatidosis. Torax, *20*:160, 1971.

367. Yokogawa, S., and Suemori, S.: An experimental study of the intracranial parasitism of the human lung fluke, Paragonimus westermani. Amer. J. Hyg., *1*:63–78, 1921.

368. Yumoto, Y., and Nagayoshi, Y.: A contribution to the pathology of paragonimiasis, especially on the embolism of various organs by worm eggs entering into the great circulation. Nehai Igaku, *1*:585–603, 1943.

369. Young, D. A., and Laman, M. L.: Radiodense skeletal lesions in Boeck's sarcoid. Amer. J. Roentgen., *114*:553–558, 1972.

370. Young, R. C., Jennings, A., and Bennett, J. E.: Species identification of invasive aspergillosis in man. Amer. J. Clin. Path., *58*:554–557, 1972.

371. Young, R. C., Bennett, J. E., Vogel, C. L., Carbone, P. P., and DeVita, V. T.: Aspergillosis: The spectrum of the disease in 98 patients. Medicine (Balt.), *49*:147–173, 1970.

372. Zener, J. C., Alpert, M., and Klainer, L. M.: Vertebral sarcoidosis. Arch. Intern. Med. (Chicago), *111*:696–702, 1963.

373. Zilberg, B.: Unusual manifestations occurring in the early stages of bilharziasis in children. Cent. Afr. J. Med., *16*:524, 1970.

374. Zimmerman, L. E.: Fatal fungus infections complicating other diseases. Amer. J. Clin. Path., *25*:46–65, 1955.

375. Zinneman, H. H.: Sino-orbital aspergillosis—report of a case and review of the literature. Minn. Med., *55*:661–664, 1972.

376. Ziskind, J., Pizzolato, P., and Buff, E. E.: Aspergillosis of the brain: Report of a case. Amer. J. Clin. Path., *29*:554–559, 1958.

TUBERCULOMA AND SYPHILITIC GUMMA

This chapter shows how social and economic conditions influence medical disease. Even in the relatively short history of modern operations on the brain, the inflammatory lesions of tuberculous and syphilitic origin have been greatly reduced.

TUBERCULOMAS

Macewen did the first operation for tuberculoma in 1883.[72] A few years later Horsley and others reported further examples of such conditions. In 1893 Starr reviewed 300 brain tumors from the literature and his own material, and remarked on the frequency of tuberculomas (52 per cent).[70] Cushing stated that at the turn of the century tuberculomas represented about 30 to 40 per cent of all intracranial space-occupying lesions.[24]

Incidence

In the large neurosurgical series assembled during the first half of this century, tuberculomas represent about 1.7 per cent of the lesions.[24,25] In 1967, Olivecrona, in reviewing his large number of 5250 space-occupying lesions, found that only 0.9 per cent were tuberculomas.[62] There is no doubt that intracranial tuberculomas are decreasing in most countries. During the first years of the senior author's neurosurgical practice in Mexico, he saw several tuberculomas. Later, in the first thousand cases of space-occupying lesions operated on in Madrid (between 1946 and 1956), tuberculomas represented about 7 per cent, while in the following thousand cases of space-occupying lesions that were operated on, the proportion of tuberculomas dropped to 0.6 per cent. In his series of 5400 space-occupying lesions treated in Madrid in the past 30 years, there were 82 cases of tuberculoma (1 per cent) verified either at operation (79) or at postmortem examination (3).

Although the decreasing incidence of cerebral tuberculosis represents the general trend throughout the world, during the 1950's and 1960's some countries in eastern Europe, the Middle East, and South America reported an incidence of 8 per cent or more.[2-5,32,41,66] Even in 1968, about 20 per cent of the intracranial space-occupying lesions in India were tuberculomas. There has, however been a drop to 12 per cent in the past five years.[38,64,69]

Etiology and Pathology

Hematogenous spread from tuberculous lesions of other parts of the body accounts for the origin of most cerebral tuberculomas. At the Institute of Neurosurgery in Chile, 72 per cent of autopsies performed on patients with tuberculomas revealed tuberculosis elsewhere in the body. Wilson stated that if there was no evidence of tuberculosis in other parts of the body the search could be taken as incomplete because tuberculomas are never the primary lesion of a tuberculous infection.[82]

At operation, the tuberculomas usually appear as nodular or irregular avascular masses localized beneath the cerebral or cerebellar cortex, although some are more superficial and adherent to the dura. They vary greatly in size. Some are very small,

---

S. OBRADOR AND J. G. MARTIN-RODRIGUEZ

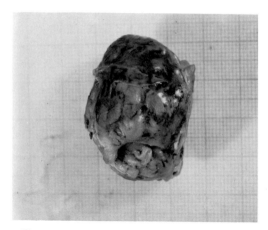

Figure 113–1 Operative specimen of a cerebral tuberculoma.

the size of a pea, while others are much larger (Fig. 113–1). Cerebral edema is nearly always present around the lesion and is quite severe in some cases.

Histologically, the tuberculomas give a typical picture of granulomatous lesions with necrotic areas and Langhans cells (Fig. 113–2). The tubercles have caseous centers and more rarely form real tuberculous abscesses. Sinh and co-workers remarked on some more unusual forms, such as meningocortical tuberculomatosis and the conglomeration of small tubercles.[69]

Because of the hematogenous spread, multiple tuberculomas are frequent. In cases that have been operated on, additional tuberculomas may remain undetected without producing symptoms, and eventually they may be cured, especially with modern antibiotics and chemotherapy. Statistics give the presence of known multiple intracranial tuberculomas as varying from 10 per cent to 33 per cent of the cases. In the senior author's series, multiple tuberculomas were found in 14 cases (18 per cent). Tuberculous meningitis, together with or related to intracranial tuberculomas, occurs in about 3 per cent of patients.[2]

Diagnosis

The clinical recognition of tuberculosis rests mainly on the evidence of the general disease. In many patients, it is very difficult to establish the nature of the lesion. In most series, the presence of tuberculous lesions in other organs or a definite history of tuberculous disease appears in only about

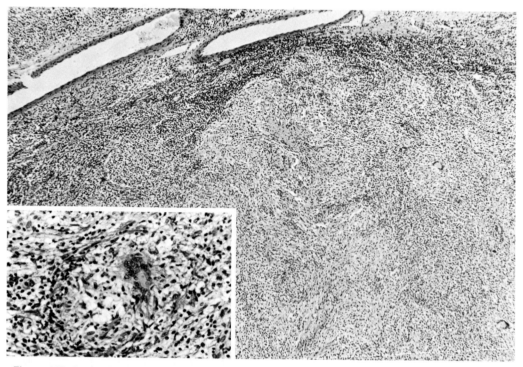

Figure 113–2 Cerebral tuberculoma. Hematoxylin-eosin, 32 ×. Nodule formed by numerous follicles separated from the brain tissue by a layer of connective tissue and abundant blood vessels. (*Inset*) At higher magnification (320 ×), a follicle with numerous epithelioid cells and a typical Langhans cell.

half the patients operated on for intracranial tuberculomas.

Intracranial tuberculomas often affect children or young people, and 60 per cent of the authors' cases, as reported by Villarejo and co-workers, were under 20 years of age.[77] Sixty per cent are in the posterior fossa. In most series, about two thirds of the tuberculomas are in the cerebellum and about one third are in the cerebral hemispheres. Since the infection is disseminated through the blood stream, the reason for the greater incidence in the posterior fossa is not understood. The cerebellum either is specially susceptible to the formation of tubercles or has different vascular and circulatory conditions that are responsible for the development of the lesions.

As in any other type of intracranial tumor, the usual symptoms and signs due to the increase of intracranial pressure and to the localization of the lesion are observable. Practically all the patients with infratentorial tuberculomas and most with supratentorial ones (around 80 per cent) have a definite increase of intracranial pressure. Different forms of epilepsy appear in 70 to 85 per cent of the cases with supratentorial localization. Other hemispherical disturbances, such as motor, sensory, or speech disorders, may be observed in about 50 to 70 per cent of these cases. Cerebellar signs are recorded in about 70 to 80 per cent of the infratentorial lesions. Interesting types of infratentorial tuberculomas are those in the brain stem or the pons and those expanding to the cerebellopontine angle that produce a clinical picture related to these two localizations. According to Chediack and Carrizo, general symptoms such as asthenia, weakness, and perspiration occur in 56 per cent of the cases, fever in 40 per cent, and abnormal white count in 60 per cent.[17] Findings related to the tuberculous bacteremia were present in 50 per cent of the authors' cases.[77] Calcification of the tuberculomas, which is visible in plain x-rays, is observed in up to 6 per cent of cases.[64] X-ray studies of the chest yielded positive findings of tuberculosis in 50 per cent of the patients.

The cerebrospinal fluid examination is normal in about half the patients. The other half have an increase of cells and protein content with positive globulin reactions. Electroencephalographic studies are useful mainly for the localization of the supratentorial masses.

In recent years carotid angiography has been used as a routine method and usually demonstrates the avascular supratentorial lesion (Fig. 113–3). Ramamurthi and Varadarajan reported its use in identifying the lesion in a group of patients with evidence of tuberculous lesions and progressive neurological disability but without increase of

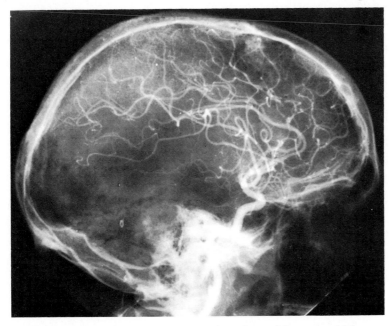

Figure 113–3 Carotid angiogram in tuberculoma of the temporal lobe.

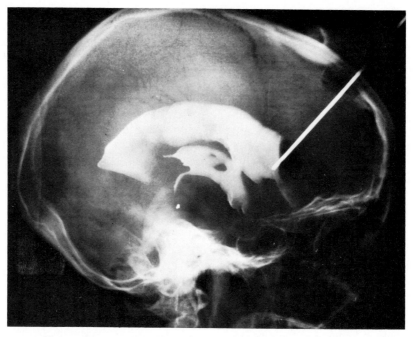

Figure 113–4 Iodoventriculogram in tuberculoma of the cerebellum.

intracranial pressure.[64] A positive contrast ventriculogram is useful in studying infratentorial lesions that have caused hydrocephalus (Fig. 113–4).

Computed tomography (CT) is a valuable tool in the diagnosis of tuberculomas. It can easily demonstrate one or more lesions and localize them accurately. The most common features are those of a cystic mass that is indistinguishable from any other abscess. The unenhanced image usually shows an area of low attenuation, but after the intravenous administration of a contrast medium the enhancement is demonstrated in the capsule of the lesion (Fig. 113–5A and B). Small lesions (less than 1 cm) can sometimes appear as a homogeneous and dense mass (Fig. 113–5C). Occasionally calcification can be seen within the lesion.[18]

Treatment and Results

In 1932 Cushing stated, "When a tuberculoma is surgically removed from the cerebellum, no matter with what care, a tuber-

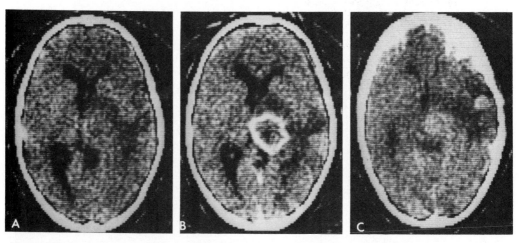

Figure 113–5 *A.* Unenhanced scan, CT level 2A, showing an area of low attenuation deep in the right thalamus with distortion of the midline structures. *B.* After intravenous administration of a contrast medium, CT level 22A, a capsular ring is demonstrated in the right thalamus. *C.* Enhancement in CT level 11B shows a small lesion in the right temporal lobe. (Courtesy of Dr. L. E. Claveria.)

culous meningitis is likely to ensue within three months.[24] This statement was valid until streptomycin was available for the treatment of tuberculosis. Streptomycin avoids the development of tuberculous meningitis after the removal of intracranial tuberculomas, as was demonstrated nearly 30 years ago.[60] With the addition of isoniazid to the antituberculous regimen, the medical treatment has assumed even greater importance during the postoperative period.

The operative removal of an intracranial tuberculoma should be followed by postoperative administration of streptomycin, 0.5 to 1 gm daily, by intramuscular injection for two or more months and isoniazid, 5 to 10 mg per kilogram, by oral or intramuscular daily administration for three to five or more months according to the condition of the patient. Para-aminosalicylic acid may be added to this regimen as well as the new antituberculous agents such as ethambutol, rifamycin, and capreomycin; and when there are signs of meningeal infection, corticosteroids are very useful. Currently, intrathecal steroids are not used as frequently as in earlier years.

Postoperative mortality following the removal of tuberculomas, mainly due to late meningeal spread of the infection, reached between 50 and 70 per cent of cases.* The prognosis for tuberculomas located in the cerebellum was especially poor. With the use of the specific drug treatment, the postoperative mortality rate has decreased to 10

---

* See references 2, 5, 32, 62, 66, 76.

or 15 per cent. As shown in the long follow-up of several years, if the tuberculoma can be removed, about 80 per cent of the patients will have a long-term recovery.

There are some tuberculomas in which only palliative operations and medical treatment can be given. Lesions in the pons and brain stem, as shown in Figure 113–6, and some multiple forms that cannot be removed are the most obvious examples. Some authorities believe that patients with focal neurological disturbances of probable tuberculous origin (with some angiographic changes but without a great increase of intracranial pressure) should first be treated with specific drug treatment.

Finally, in deciding whether to operate, many factors have to be considered. These factors include the general condition of the patient, the evolution of the disease, and the existence and importance of symptoms of other tuberculous lesions in the body, such as the presence of multiple cerebral tubercles and the like. The operative treatment and medical therapy of the tuberculomas represent only a part of the care of these patients with widespread tuberculous lesions in other parts of the body,

SYPHILITIC GUMMAS

As with tuberculomas, Macewen also did the first operation for cerebral gummas.[72] Later, Starr, Horsley, and others reported further examples of such conditions.[70] At the turn of the century gummas were so frequent that before the development of the

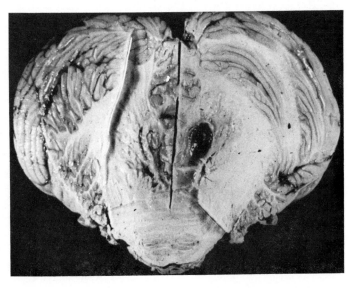

Figure 113–6 Autopsy specimen showing a tuberculoma in the pons.

Wassermann test, most patients with signs of a brain tumor were submitted to preliminary medical antisyphilitic treatment before the diagnosis of a neoplasm was made.

Incidence

In the large neurosurgical series assembled during this century, gummas represent about 0.6 per cent.[24] In 1945 Dandy remarked that gummas were very rare.[25] In reviewing his large number of brain tumors, Olivecrona found only one case of gumma.[62] At present gummas of the brain are so unusual that many neurosurgeons have never had occasion to treat one.

Etiology and Pathology

Gummas grow from miliary formations in the subcortical areas and may invade the dura through the vascular system and an extensive development of connective tissue. Sometimes they start in the meninges (luetic meningeal encephalitis) and spread into the brain.[7] According to Zülch and Christensen, the gummas may have a central necrotic area and a peripheral layer of connective tissue and giant cells.[83]

Diagnosis

Cerebral gummas are so rare that no clinic has a broad clinical experience with them. In the authors' series of space-occupying lesions there was not a single example of syphilitic gumma. Bailey mentioned that gummatous intracranial lesions may exist with a negative Wassermann reaction in the blood and cerebrospinal fluid.[7] As with tuberculomas, carotid angiography has been used as the routine method of diagnosis. It usually demonstrates the avascular supratentorial lesion similar to the types shown in Figure 113–3.

Treatment and Results

Classic opinions about the treatment of cerebral gummas are conflicting. Horsley and Cushing insisted upon their resistance to antisyphilitic treatment and the necessity of early operation. On the other hand, Dandy believed that these lesions usually melted after antisyphilitic treatment; therefore, operative removal was advised only when no improvement occurred. Because of the extreme rarity of these lesions now, there are no definite data regarding their treatment.

REFERENCES

1. Anderson, J. M., and MacMillan, J. J.: Intracranial tuberculoma, an increasing problem in Britain. J. Neurol. Neurosurg. Psychiat., 38:194–201, 1975.
2. Arseni, C.: Two hundred and one cases of intracranial tuberculoma treated surgically. J. Neurol. Neurosurg. Psychiat., 21:308–311, 1958.
3. Asenjo, A., Fierro, J., and Carrizo, F.: Tratamiento de los tuberculomas cerebrales. Neurocirugía (Santiago), 19:394–407, 1961.
4. Asenjo, A., Valladares, H., and Fierro, J.: Tuberculomas cerebrales (Revisión de 152 casos). Rev. Ap. Respir. Tuberc. (Santiago), 4:3–32, 1949.
5. Asenjo, A., Valladares, H., and Fierro, J.: Tuberculomas of the brain: Report of hundred and fifty-nine cases. Arch. Neurol. Psychiat. (Chicago), 65:146–160, 1951.
6. Bagchi, A.: Intracranial Tumours of Infancy and Childhood. Springfield, Ill., Charles C Thomas, 1952.
7. Bailey, P.: Intracranial Tumors. Springfield, Ill., Charles C Thomas, 1933.
8. Bailey, R. H.: Cerebral tuberculoma. Proc. Roy. Soc. Med., 31:1164–1167, 1938.
9. Balaparameswararao, S., and Dinakar, I.: Tuberculomas of the brain. Int. Surg., 57:216–220, 1972.
10. Bannister, C. M.: A tuberculous abscess of the brain. Case report. J. Neurosurg., 33:203–206, 1970.
11. Bedi, H. K., Devpura, J. C., and Bomb, B. S.: Clinical tuberculoma of pons representing as Foville's syndrome. J. Indian Med. Ass., 61:184–185, 1973.
12. Berlin, L.: Tuberculoma of the brain. Amer. J. Roentgen., 90:1185–1192, 1963.
13. Bernstein, T. C., Krueger, E. G., and Nayer, H. R.: Tuberculoma of the brain. Surgical removal in the presence of widespread tuberculosis. Amer. Rev. Tuberc., 62:654–666, 1950.
14. Borne, G.: Trigeminal neuralgia as the presenting symptom of a tuberculoma of the cerebellopontine angle. Case report. J. Neurosurg., 28:480–482, 1968.
15. Capon, A., Noterman, J., Hubert, J. P., Klatersky, J., and Flament-Durand, J.: Multiple tuberculomas of the brain. Acta Neurochir. (Wien), 32:303–312, 1975.
16. Castro, M., and Lepe, A.: Cerebral tuberculoma. Acta Radiol. [Diagn.] (Stockholm), 1:821–827, 1963.
17. Chediack, C., and Carrizo, F. E.: Clínica de los

tuberculomas encefálicos. Neurocirugía (Santiago), *19*:365–372, 1961.

18. Clavería, L. E., Boulay, G. H. du, and Moseley, I. F.: Intracranial infections: Investigation by computerized axial tomography. Neuroradiology, *12*:59–71, 1976.

19. Collomb, H., Courson, B., and Dumas, M.: Stenosis of the aqueduct of Sylvius of tubercular origin. Etiopathogenic discussion apropos of a case. Bull. Soc. Med. Afr. Noire Lang. Franc., *13*:204–207, 1968.

20. Constantinidis, J.: Calcified and ossified bilateral tuberculoma in the centrum ovale of the brain. Ann. Anat. Path. (Paris), *15*:197–205, 1970.

21. Courville, B. C.: Pathology of the Central Nervous System. 2nd Ed. Palo Alto, Calif., Pacific Press, 1945.

22. Cuneo, M. H., and Rand, C. W.: Brain Tumors of Childhood. Springfield, Ill., Charles C Thomas, 1952.

23. Cushing, H. W.: The intracranial tumours of preadolescence. Amer. J. Dis. Child., *33*:551–584, 1927.

24. Cushing, H. W.: Intracranial Tumors. Springfield, Ill., Charles C Thomas, 1932.

25. Dandy, W. E.: Surgery of the Brain. Hagerstown, Md., W. F. Prior Co. 1945.

26. Dastur, D. K.: Neurotuberculosis. *In* Minckler, J., ed.: Pathology of the Nervous System. New York, McGraw Hill Book Co., 1969.

27. Dastur, D. K., and Iyer, C. G. S.: Pathological analysis of 450 intracranial space occupying lesions. Indian J. Cancer, *3*:105–115, 1966.

28. Dastur, D. K., and Udani, P. M.: The pathology and pathogeneis of tuberculous encephalopathy. Acta Neuropath., *6*:311–326, 1966.

29. Dastur, H. M.: A tuberculoma review with some personal experiences. I. Brain. Neurol. India, *20*:111–126, 1972.

30. Dastur, H. M., and Desai, A. D.: A comparative study of brain tuberculomas and gliomas based upon 107 case records of each. Brain, *88*:375–396, 1965.

31. Dastur, H. M., Desai, A. D., and Dastur, D. K.: A cystic cerebral tuberculoma treated surgically. J. Neurol. Neurosurg. Psychiat., *25*:370–373, 1962.

32. Descuns, P., Garre, H., and Pheline, C.: Tuberculomas of the brain and cerebellum. J. Neurosurg., *11*:243–250, 1954.

33. Doege, T. C.: Tuberculosis mortality in the United States, 1900–1960. J.A.M.A., *192*:1045–1048, 1965.

34. Donoso, P., and Von Benewitz, A.: Historia natural y patología de los tuberculomas encefálicos. Neurocirugía (Santiago), *19*:359–364, 1961.

35. Evans, G. F., and Smith, C. F.: Tuberculous abscess of the brain. Amer. Rev. Tuberc., *24*:292–299, 1931.

36. Evans, H. S., and Courville, C. B.: Calcification and ossification in tuberculoma of the brain. Arch. Surg., *366*:637–659, 1938.

37. Garland, H. G., and Armitage, J.: Intracranial tuberculoma. J. Path. Bact., *37*:461–471, 1933.

38. Glasauer, F. E.: Intracranial tumors in Southeast Asia. Surg. Neurol., *6*:257–260, 1976.

39. Gonzalez Revilla, A.: Intracranial tuberculomas: Experience with ten consecutive cases. J. Neurosurg., *9*:555–563, 1952.

40. Herishanu, Y.: Convergence nystagmus in brain stem tuberculoma. Ophthalmologica, *163*:98–101, 1971.

41. Higazi, I.: Tuberculoma of the brain: A clinical and angiographic study. J. Neurosurg., *20*:378–386, 1963.

42. Hossmann, K. A., and Schutz, H.: Tuberculoma in the region of an old cerebral gunshot wound. Acta Neurochir. (Wien), *14*:254–263, 1966.

43. Jacques, S., Freshwater, D., and Randle, R. E.: Supratentorial tuberculoma: A case report and review. Bull. Los Angeles Neurol. Soc., *39*:56–59, 1974.

44. Kocen, R. S., and Parsons, M.: Neurological complications of tuberculosis. Quart. J. Med., *39*: 17–30, 1970.

45. Lehrer, H., Bhatrahally, V., and Gerolamo, R.: Tuberculoma of the brain. Amer. J. Roentgen., *118*:594–600, 1973.

46. Leibrock, L., Epstein, M. H., and Rybock, J. D.: Cerebral tuberculoma localized by EMI scan. Surg. Neurol., *5*:305–306, 1976.

47. Lepe, A., and Castro, M.: Radiología del tuberculoma cerebral. Neurocirugía (Santiago), *19*:377–389, 1961.

48. Luse, S. A.: Pathology of chronic inflammation in the nervous system. Clin. Neurosurg., *14*:227–238, 1966.

49. Martin, P. H.: Abcès tuberculeux de l'encéphale. Acta Neurol. Belg., *64*:1036–1039, 1964.

50. Mathai, K. V., and Chandy, J.: Tuberculous infections of the nervous system. Clin. Neurosurg., *14*:145–177, 1966.

51. Matson, D. D.: Neurosurgery of Infancy and Childhood. Springfield, Ill., Charles C Thomas, 1967.

52. Matus, A., and Chediack, C.: Complicaciones y secuelas de los tuberculomas encefálicos. Neurocirugía (Santiago), *19*:373–376, 1961.

53. Maurice-Williams, R. S.: Tuberculomas of the brain in Britain. Postgrad. Med. J., *48*:678–681, 1972.

54. Michel Zamora, M., and Sigüenza, P.: Tuberculomas del encéfalo. Neurocirugia (Santiago), *18*:104–110, 1960.

55. Mobius, W.: Differential diagnostische Probleme bei Tuberculomen des Gehirns. Deutsch. Med. Wschr., *94*:2281–2284, 1969.

56. Moore, G. A., and Thomas, L. M.: Infections including abscesses of the brain, spinal cord, intraspinal and intracranial regions. Surg. Annu., *6*:413–437, 1974.

57. Nath, K., and Prakash, C.: Tuberculoma of the brain. J. Indian Med. Ass., *27*:435–437, 1958.

58. Northfield, D. W. C.: The Surgery of the Central Nervous System. Oxford, Blackwell Scientific Publications, 1973.

59. Obrador, S.: Intracranial tuberculomas. A review of 47 cases. Neurochirurgia, *1*:150–157, 1959.

60. Obrador, S., and Urquiza, P.: The value of streptomycin in the surgical treatment of intracranial tuberculoma. J. Neurol. Neurosurg. Psychiat., *13*:66–70, 1950.

61. Odeku, E. L., and Adeloye, A.: Cerebral tuberculoma in Nigerian patients. Trop. Geogr. Med., *21*:293–304, 1969.

62. Olivecrona, H.: The surgical treatment of intracranial tumors. *In* Handbuch der Neurochirur-

gie. Vol. 4, Part 4, Berlin, Springer-Verlag, 1967.

63. Rab, S. M., Bhatti, I. H., and Ghani, A.: Tuberculous brain abscess. Case report. J. Neurosurg., *43*:490–494, 1975.

64. Ramamurthi, B., and Varadarajan, M. G.: Diagnosis of tuberculomas of the brain. Clinical and radiological correlation. J. Neurosurg., *18*:1–7, 1961.

65. Rao, B. D., Subrahamanayam, M. V., and Sathe, N. M.: Cerebral tuberculoma simulating a cystic glioma. A case report. J. Neurosurg., *20*:172–173, 1963.

66. Revilla, A. G.: Intracranial tuberculomas. J. Neurosurg., *9*:555–563, 1952.

67. Rouzaud, M., Gouaze, A., Degiovanni, E., Santini, J. J., and Medelsi, M.: Les formes chirurgicales de la tuberculose cérébrale. A propos de trois observations dont un abcès tuberculeux. Sem. Hôp. Paris, *47*:3063–3066, 1971.

68. Sibley, W. A., and O'Brien, J. L.: Intracranial tuberculomas. A review of clinical features and treatment. Neurology (Minneap.), *6*:157–165, 1956.

69. Sinh, G., Pandya, S. K., and Dastur, D. K.: Pathogenesis of unusual intracranial tuberculomas and tuberculous space-occupying lesions. J. Neurosurg., *29*:149–159, 1968.

70. Starr, M. A.: Brain Surgery. New York, William Wood & Co., 1893.

71. Steimle, R., Jacquet, G., Bonneville, J. F., and Cedillo-Arce, L.: Tuberculomes cérébraux d'allure primitive. Neurochirurgie (Paris), *19*:555–560, 1973.

72. Stern, W. E.: Surgery of the craniocerebral infections. *In* Walker, A. E., ed.: A History of Neurological Surgery. Baltimore, Williams & Wilkins Co., 1951.

73. Sumra, R. S., Mongia, S. K., Roy, S., and Pathak, S. N.: Tuberculoma of the brain stem: Control of relapses by steroid therapy. Case report. J. Neurosurg., *39*:402–404, 1973.

74. Thiebaut, F., and Philippides, D.: Tubercules de l'encephale en forme d'abcès. Neurochirurgie (Paris), *6*:377–378, 1960.

75. Thrush, D. G., and Barwick, D. D.: Three patients with intracranial tuberculomas with unusual features. J. Neurol. Neurosurg. Psychiat., *37*:566–569, 1974.

76. Valladares, H., and Poblete, R.: Tuberculomas del encéfalo. Neurocirugía (Santiago), *22*:69–74, 1964.

77. Villarejo, F., Soto, M., and Dabdoub, C.: Posterior fossa tuberculomas. Presented at the Fifth Congress of the European Society for Paediatric Neurosurgery. Stessa, Italy, 1976.

78. Villavicencio, C., Peña, A., and Chediack, C.: El E.E.G. en los tuberculomas encefálicos. Neurocirugía (Santiago), *19*:390–393, 1961.

79. Weigel, B.: Tuberculoma as rare cause of apoplexy-like hemiparesis. J. Ges. Inn. Med., *28*:535–537, 1973.

80. Wendt, F., Siedschalg, W. D., and Unger, R. R.: Intracerebral tuberculomas. Zbl. Neurochir., *30*:51–60, 1969.

81. Wilkerson, H. A., Ferris, E. J., and Mugia, A. L.: Central nervous system tuberculosis a persistent disease. J. Neurosurg., *34*:15–22, 1971.

82. Wilson, K.: Neurology. Baltimore, William Wood Co., 1940.

83. Zülch, K. J., and Christensen, E.: Pathologische Anatomia der raumbeengenden intrakraniellen Prozess. *In* Handbuch der Neurochirurgie. Vol. 3. Berlin, Springer-Verlag, 1956.

114

INFECTIONS OF THE SPINE AND SPINAL CORD

Infections involving the spinal cord and cauda equina are much less frequent than intracranial infections. Often they are misdiagnosed until severe neurological damage has occurred. Generally the chance of recovery is directly related to the degree of neurological impairment existing prior to operation: A patient whose infection is detected and operated upon in a stage of minimal dysfunction of the nervous system has the best chance of useful recovery. Hence a heavy burden of responsibility rests with the attending surgeon or physician in the diagnosis and treatment of patients with these lesions.

EXTRADURAL ABSCESS

Bacterial infections in the spinal extradural space are relatively uncommon.[7,13,20,21,22,24,28] Perhaps for this reason there are delay in diagnosis and irreversible neurological sequelae in a high percentage of cases.

The earliest pathological description of spinal extradural abscess was by Morgagni in 1583. Nineteenth century physicians and surgeons created many synonyms for this condition, such as perimeningitis spinalis, peripachymeningitis, epimeningitis spinalis, meningitis spinalis externa, and purulent perimeningitis. Macewen, in 1885, was probably the first to diagnose such a lesion during life and operate on the patient. By 1926 only 25 cases had been recorded in medical literature.[13] Since that time this condition has been diagnosed with increased frequency.

Infection in the spinal extradural space is blood-borne in most instances from sepsis at various distant sites. Furuncles and urinary tract infections have been especially common sites of primary infection. *Staphylococcus aureus* has been the causative organism in most cases. Other organisms including streptococci, pneumococci, *Pseudomonas,* and the typhoid bacillus are less frequently the cause. Rarely fungi may cause extradural granulomas that compress the cord. It seems likely that septic thrombophlebitis of the vertebral venous plexus (often called Batson's plexus) is a factor in many cases.[4,23] Less commonly it may spread directly from adjacent osteomyelitis of the spine or mediastinal or retroperitoneal abscesses. Occasionally it results from bacterial contamination at the time of spinal puncture or in association with a congenital midline dermal sinus.[40] In approximately one third of these cases, there is no history of antecedent infection or contamination.

The initial symptom in patients with spinal extradural abscess is back pain. This is often severe and is located at the area of infection. There may be pain radiating along the distribution of adjacent nerve roots, producing girdle pains around the torso when the lesion is thoracic in location or in the extremities when cervical or lumbosacral areas are involved. This is followed by signs and symptoms of spinal cord or cauda equina compression, such as paresthesias, increasing weakness with eventual paraplegia, and loss of sphincter control. The rapidity of progression may vary considerably in this disorder, and the two varieties of extradural abscesses, acute and chronic, are classified on this basis. Around two thirds are of the acute variety.

In acute extradural abscesses the entire clinical picture evolves over several hours

---

R. L. WRIGHT

or within a few days. There are often fever, tachycardia, peripheral leukocytosis, and local tenderness on firm palpation over the involved area of the spine. Progression from the stage of pain to complete paraplegia is rapid, and few cases are suspected until significant weakness of limbs, sensory loss, and sphincter disturbances have occurred. In chronic cases the same sequence of pain followed by signs of increasing spinal cord compression occurs, but the progression is slower so that weeks or months may elapse before paraplegia occurs. In this latter form fever and leukocytosis are often absent. The reason why some cases progress faster than others is not known. Since the extent of recovery is usually directly related to the patient's neurological status at the time of operation, every effort should be made to diagnose the lesion as early as possible in its clinical evolution. The cauda equina seems to withstand compression better than the spinal cord, and even with severe paresis the outlook for recovery following treatment of lumbar or sacral extradural infections is particularly favorable.

Patients suspected of having spinal extradural abscesses should have a careful neurological examination and history, x-rays of the spine, and a myelogram. X-rays will show, in a minority of cases, associated vertebral osteomyelitis. Lumbar puncture for myelography should be carefully performed, and aspiration of the extradural space should be done before the subarachnoid space is entered. In some instances purulence will extend to the lumbar region; if pus is obtained from the needle, it should not be advanced further lest meningitis result. If no purulent material is obtained, however, the needle is advanced to the subarachnoid space, where pressure and careful manometric determinations are done. It is important to remember that with a properly placed 18-gauge spinal needle, bilateral jugular compression will result in a prompt rise in pressure to more than 400 mm of water and a prompt fall to the original level on release if no block is present. In the presence of a block, no more than 2 to 3 ml of cerebrospinal fluid should be removed below the lesion. Virtually always there will be increased protein and white blood cells. In acute lesions these may be polymorphonuclear leukocytes, but lymphocytes often predominate in chronic abscesses. Almost all patients with extradural spinal abscesses will demonstrate a complete block on Queckenstedt's maneuver, and myelography can then be done with only 2 to 3 ml of iophendylate (Pantopaque) (Fig. 114–1).

Preoperative marking of the spine at the level of the block is best done at this time by inserting a needle into the appropriate spinous process or interspinous ligament under sterile precautions, and then cutting the hub off the needle at a level at which the retained fragment will be covered with skin. Prior to laminectomy many surgeons prefer to outline the entire length of spinal compression by concomitantly performing a cisternal myelogram to delineate the superior extent of the lesion. Operation should follow promptly.

Standard bilateral laminectomy is the procedure of choice in the absence of extensive osteomyelitis. Dandy has emphasized that most spinal extradural abscesses occur posterior to the dura because a true

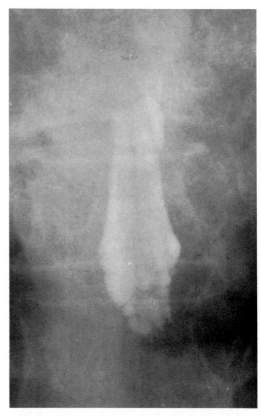

Figure 114–1 Myelogram showing block at T11 caused by extradural abscess. Meninges and spinal cord are compressed in diameter. There was no evidence of involvement of adjacent vertebral bodies in this case.

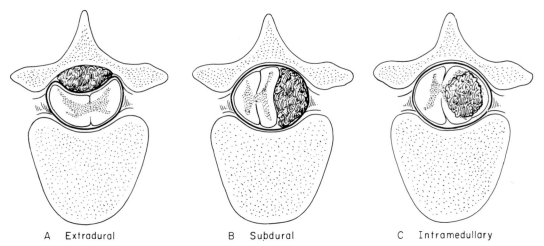

A   Extradural   B   Subdural   C   Intramedullary

Figure 114–2   Varieties of pyogenic intraspinal abscesses.

extradural space is usually not present anteriorly (Fig. 114–2A). It is vital that laminectomy be carried out over the entire extent of infection, and this can vary from one to many spinal segments. The purulent material and extradural fat should be radically stripped from the dura. Usually this is an easy maneuver. It is best accomplished by using a blunt dissector such as a dental spatula and by gently teasing away infectious material. Gram-stained smears should be examined and bacterial cultures planted.

The appearance of extradural abscesses varies with their age. In the acute state there is loculated pus with extensive hyperemia and polymorphonuclear infiltration in extradural fat. Later this process becomes altered so that friable infectious granulation tissue may be all that is found. The surgeon occasionally mistakes this shaggy gray tissue for metastatic extradural tumor. Extreme care should be taken not to injure the dura. Hemostasis should be achieved with electrocoagulation and repeated packing of the extradural space with thrombin-soaked cottonoid patties. Foreign material such as gelatin foam or oxidized cellulose gauze should not be left in septic wounds. The wound should then be copiously irrigated with saline and topical antibiotic solutions (such as bacitracin at a concentration of 1000 units per milliliter).

Whether the operative wound should be closed remains a point of debate. Some neurosurgeons prefer to leave it open, changing gauze packs at frequent intervals, and allowing healing to occur by secondary intention. Others recommend delayed clo-

sure after several days of open drainage. Most surgeons, however, have preferred to close the wound, leaving two rubber catheters extending to the extradural space. One each is brought through cephalad and caudal ends of the incision. Paravertebral muscles and subcutaneous tissues are closed with catgut, and the skin with sutures of stainless steel wire. The deeply placed catheters are left for five to seven days. In addition to providing drainage, they are used for the daily instillation of antibiotic solutions.

Systemic antibiotic therapy should begin preoperatively or intraoperatively as soon as the diagnosis of spinal abscess seems likely. The majority of these are caused by *Staphylococcus aureus*. Antibiotics may be modified on the basis of bacterial smears, cultures, and sensitivity tests, but their vigorous administration should continue at least four weeks in all cases of spinal abscess. In the absence of extensive osteomyelitis causing instability of the spine, rehabilitation training and ambulation should begin in the early postoperative period.

SUBDURAL ABSCESS

Localized abscesses in the spinal subdural space are rare (Fig. 114–2B)[8,17] Many of these are associated with congenital dermal sinuses, but some arise by hematogenous spread from sepsis at distant sites.[40] The manifestations may be similar to those of spinal extradural abscess. Pain may be entirely absent in some cases if adjacent nerve roots are not involved. Meningitis may occur as the result of leakage.

Diagnosis is confirmed by myelography, and operation should follow promptly. After the dura is opened the abscess should be evacuated completely by aspiration to prevent massive contamination of subarachnoid space. If a thin capsule is present an effort should be made to excise it; the operative site is then irrigated with saline and very dilute antibiotic solutions such as bacitracin in a concentration of 500 units per milliliter. A rubber drain is left at the site and the dura is reconstructed around this. The remainder of the wound is closed carefully with buried catgut sutures and wire for the skin. The drain should be removed within three or four days lest a cerebrospinal fluid fistula result. Vigorous systemic antibiotic therapy should continue at least four weeks, and rehabilitation training should commence early in the postoperative period.

INTRAMEDULLARY ABSCESS

Abscesses within the spinal cord are also of infrequent occurrence and may develop by hematogenous spread from distant septic sites, from penetrating injuries, or in association with congenital dermal sinuses (Fig. 114–2C).[15,38,40] ''Pyogenic myelitis'' is a synonym. In some cases there has been no history of antecedent sepsis. Among the blood-borne infections of this type, urinary tract infections and pneumonitis have been frequent antecedent factors. A wide variety of organisms has been recovered including *Staphylococcus, Streptococcus,* pneumococcus, *Klebsiella,* and coliform bacilli.

Symptoms have usually been progressive weakness, sensory loss, and disturbances of sphincter control. Pain has varied considerably in degree and is sometimes absent. At times, however, there is severe back pain with associated limitation of motion at the involved area of the spine. Fever and peripheral leukocytosis may or may not be present. Lumbar puncture has characteristically shown a complete or partial block and elevated protein content; cerebrospinal fluid cells and sugar may be normal or abnormal, depending on whether leakage into the subarachnoid space has occurred. Diagnosis of the exact level is by myelography, which shows enlargement of

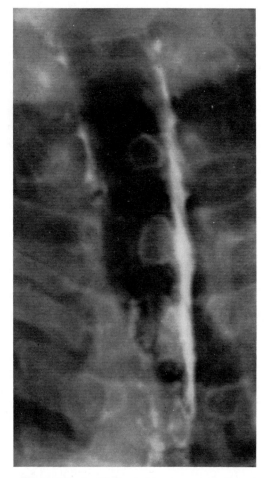

Figure 114–3 Myelographic appearance of cervical intramedullary abscess. The cord shadow is widened and no contrast material passed cephalad to C5-C6.

the cord shadow (Fig. 114–3). Combined lumbar and cisternal myelography will be desirable in most instances in which there is a total block to ascertain the entire extent of the enlargement of spinal cord.

If the diagnosis of infection seems probable preoperatively, antibiotic agents with broad-spectrum coverage should begin preoperatively or intraoperatively. A wide variety of organisms can be responsible for this lesion. Laminectomy, performed in the usual manner, should extend over the entire length of the abscess. The dura is opened in the midline and the posterior and lateral borders are carefully inspected to search for any subdural collection or other mass lesion. Aspiration of the cord is then done at an avascular site at the area of maximal enlargement. If purulent material is obtained it is immediately examined by gram-staining, and bacterial cultures are planted. From the meager pathological descriptions of fatal cases of intramedullary abscess, there seems to be little tendency for it to form a capsule as does its intracranial counterpart. Moreover, radical removal of these abscesses cannot be safely done in the spinal cord. Aspiration at several sites or small dorsal myelotomy incisions should be made until no more purulent material can be obtained. In most instances it will not be possible to close the dura because of spinal cord enlargement; foreign bodies such as dural substitutes should not be used in this instance. Instead the muscles and subcutaneous tissues should be tightly closed with multiple catgut sutures and the skin with fine stainless steel wire. Antibiotics as judged appropriate on the basis of sensitivity tests should continue for four to six weeks because of the high incidence of recurrent intramedullary abscesses. In the presence of severe swelling of the spinal cord the administration of glucocorticosteroid compounds (such as methylprednisolone or dexamethasone) is of value to lessen inflammatory edema. These drugs combined with antibiotics have proved of marked benefit in treatment of cerebral edema associated with brain abscesses, and there has been no indication of enhanced infection.

Patients with severe neurological deficits have often made good recoveries after drainage of intramedullary spinal abscesses, as compared with those in whom cord compression had been caused by extradural abscesses. Hence no effort should be spared in the aggressive treatment of these individuals.

OSTEOMYELITIS

The majority of cases of spinal osteomyelitis do not concern the neurosurgeon because in less than one fourth of them is function of the nervous system impaired. Infection usually reaches vertebrae by a hematogenous route and involves vertebral bodies to a greater extent than laminae or spinous processes.[36] Many cases are secondary to urinary tract infections or operative procedures on the urinary tract, but sepsis can spread from various other sites as well.[2,10,16,19,25] In some instances infection reaches the spine by direct extension from cervical, thoracic, or abdominal abscesses. *Staphylococcus aureus* is most often the causative organism, but others including *Escherichia coli, Pseudomonas,* and fungi may be the offenders. Uncommonly it results from external contamination from lumbar punctures or paravertebral nerve blocks, or follows spinal operations.[39]

Deep, boring back pain, local tenderness, and muscle spasm are the initial signs, and symptoms and are localized to the region of bony involvement. Osteomyelitis of the spine occurs less often in the cervical region than in thoracic or lumbar areas. Low-grade fever and peripheral leukocytosis may or may not be present, but erythrocyte sedimentation rate is usually elevated. Early in the clinical course of the disease x-rays may show no change, but eventually erosion of vertebral bodies with collapse will be seen (Fig. 114–4). Laminagrams of the spine will show the earliest changes. An important point in differentiation of vertebral erosion and collapse in osteomyelitis and metastatic tumor is that the former disorder characteristically involves the intervertebral disc, whereas metastatic tumors for some reason do not act in this manner (Fig. 114–5).

Vertebral osteomyelitis can compromise spinal cord function either by an associated extradural abscess or by severe bony deformity caused by collapse of multiple vertebrae. With progressive loss of strength, sensation, and sphincter control in a patient

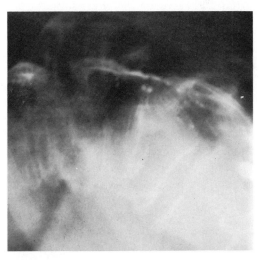

Figure 114–4 Roentgenographic appearance of osteomyelitis of the lower thoracic spine. In this lateral view are evidences of erosion and collapse of vertebral bodies with involvement of intervertebral discs.

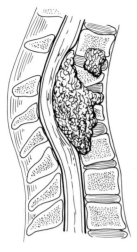 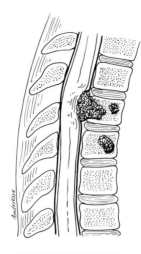

OSTEOMYELITIS   METASTATIC TUMOR

Figure 114–5 Vertebral erosion and collapse in infectious lesions of the spine is characterized by involvement of intervertebral discs. The discs are spared in cases of metastatic tumor.

suspected of having osteomyelitis, every effort should be made to establish and correct the cause. If bony erosion and deformity are modest in degree, it is likely that neurological impairment is being caused by an associated extradural abscess or granulation tissue. This should be dealt with promptly in the manner already discussed. If, however, there is severe kyphoscoliosis of the spine as a result of infection, then progressive paraparesis may be due primarily to bony impingement on the spinal canal. The conventional laminectomy approach in this instance may not adequately relieve pressure on the spinal cord and may further weaken stability of the spine. Such problems should be handled jointly with an orthopedic surgeon.[23,33] For surgical approaches to such deformities in the cervical region, an anterior approach for removal of the bony deformity is preferable. In the thoracic area an oblique posterior approach via costotransversectomy is useful (Fig. 114–6), and in the lumbar area a retroperitoneal approach as is done for lumbar sympathectomy is best. Necrotic bone and sequestra are removed and any associated abscesses drained. Infectious granulation tissue, if present, is removed from the extradural space. Bone grafts for fusion may be required when significant segments of the spinal column must be removed. Massive doses of appropriate systemic antibiotics should be begun prior to operation and subsequently altered if necessary on the basis of culture and sensitivity studies. After diseased bone impinging on the spinal canal has been carefully removed with fine cu-

rets and rongeurs, the wound is thoroughly irrigated with topical antibiotic solution; rubber catheter drains are left adjacent to the bone for several days to allow drainage and for instillation of antibiotics. The wound is closed with buried catgut sutures and stainless steel wire for the skin.

Postoperative immobilization is mandatory. In cervical cases in which extensive bony removal has been necessary, skeletal traction may be required. For patients with thoracic or lumbar involvement, absolute bed rest is mandatory; many orthopedists recommend a plaster jacket in such cases. Systemic antibiotic administration should continue for a minimum of four to six weeks. Ambulation and weight-bearing are not begun for a period of several weeks or months—until x-rays show evidence of stability and bony union of the involved section of the spine. In such chronic diseases, careful attention must be given to maintaining adequate nutrition and blood volume.

The result obtained in these patients depends in large part on the severity of neurological impairment prior to operative decompression of the spinal cord. When paraparesis has been mild to moderate in degree, functional recovery is often good. With total paraplegia and sensory loss, however, the chance for useful recovery is poor unless it comes soon.

TUBERCULOSIS

In the majority of cases, treatment of tuberculosis of the spine falls within the realm

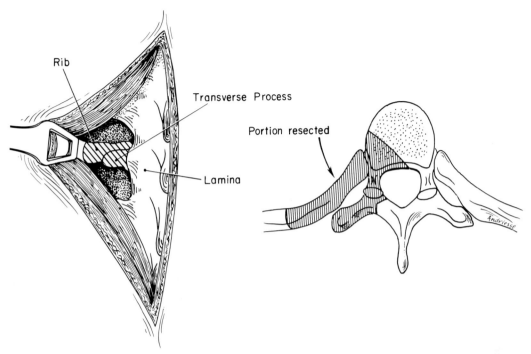

Figure 114-6   The technique of costotransversectomy as used in some cases of cord compression caused by infectious disease of the vertebral column. This procedure is indicated when the lesion lies anterior to the spinal cord and reduces the diameter of the spinal canal by vertebral compression and angulation or gibbus formation.

of orthopedic surgeons or physicians concerned primarily with infectious diseases. When paraparesis or paraplegia occurs in conjunction with vertebral collapse (a syndrome commonly called Pott's disease after Percival Pott, who described it in the eighteenth century), neurosurgical judgment is required.[1,14,23,25,29] Such neurological impairment occurs in approximately one fifth of patients with vertebral tuberculosis. The usual causes of spinal cord compression are tuberculous extradural abscesses (acute or chronic) or bony deformities caused by vertebral collapse and gibbus formation. The former is more common, but in a significant number of cases both are involved.

The thoracic spine is more frequently involved than cervical or lumbar areas. Symptoms occur and progress insidiously, and in most cases there is past history of pulmonary involvement. Increasing weakness and sensory loss are followed by difficulties with sphincter control. Spinal x-rays are similar to those in cases of bacterial osteomyelitis of other origin, with erosion and varying degrees of collapse of vertebral bodies, and with characteristic involvement of intervening intervertebral discs (see

Figs. 114-4 and 114-5). Associated paravertebral abscesses are common.

Operation for decompression of the spinal cord or cauda equina is indicated when there are progressive signs of spinal cord dysfunction not relieved by vigorous medical management or external devices to correct deformity (such as spica casts and traction). In cases of rapid onset and progression of neurological signs, decompression must be achieved promptly.

It is important to determine preoperatively whether constriction of the cord by caseous abscess or granulation tissue in the extradural space, or whether deformity of vertebral bodies anterior to the cord is chiefly to blame. Laminagrams and myelography may help in reaching this decision. Myelography will show a constriction of meninges in a total block, the picture characteristic of extradural obstruction; on lateral films it is often possible to determine whether the major obstruction in such cases is anterior or posterior to the spinal cord.

If cord compression seems due to tuberculous disease in the extradural space, then it is best treated by standard laminectomy and handling of the abscess as described in a preceding section on extradural abscesses. If it is due to angulation and compression of the spinal cord because of severely diseased vertebral bodies, then the anterolateral approach (costotransversectomy) and resection of the transverse process, pedicle, and the portion of vertebral body encroaching on the spinal canal is the best procedure (see Fig. 114–6). Such an operation leaves laminae and spinous processes intact. This type of procedure was introduced by Dott and was also advocated by Alexander over two decades ago.[1,14] Such procedures are best performed conjointly with an orthopedic surgeon so that he can judge the degree of instability of the spine and when necessary proceed with a lateral fusion once the sequestered and overgrown bone and granulation tissue have been resected to restore patency of the spinal canal. An alternative approach for correction of such bony deformity in the thoracic region is via left thoracotomy and excision of rib, pedicle, and portions of the vertebral body at the site of infection.[29]

Uncommon sites of severe tuberculosis deformity in cervical and lumbar regions of the spine may be approached by the anterior and retroperitoneal routes respectively.[33]

Postoperatively, antituberculous drugs are continued for a prolonged period (usually a minimum of 12 to 18 months). Immobilization after operation is also necessary for proper healing. If bone removal has been minimal and no fusion required, ambulation can usually be safely begun at an earlier date. Conversely, in the presence of instability or extensive bony removal and fusion, many months must elapse before mobilization. This decision is based on the time when bony regeneration appears solid on follow-up roentgenograms of the spine.

In North America, intradural spinal tuberculomas are so rare that most modern-day neurosurgeons will not encounter one. In other areas of the world they are more common. They may be either intramedullary or extramedullary.[3,6,8] In many instances a history of tuberculosis is remote or absent. Clinical symptoms are indistinguishable from those of other mass lesions compressing the spinal cord. Accurate localization by myelography and removal via the standard laminectomy approach are indicated. In most instances a precise diagnosis will not be made until after microscopic examination of the tumor mass. Antituberculous drugs should be administered to lessen the risk of postoperative tuberculous meningitis. Operative wounds can be safely closed with absorbable catgut sutures for the deeper layers in most instances. In situations in which large caseous abscesses are evacuated, external drainage should be employed in the immediate postoperative period and delayed closure should be considered.

Rarely, paraplegia caused by tuberculosis is seen in the absence of any of the aforementioned pathological causes. In these situations it is caused either by vasculitis or meningitis. In cases of vasculitis, decompressive laminectomy has little to offer. With meningitis, laminectomy and division of arachnoidal adhesions might be expected to give relief only in the rare cases in which there is a discrete block on the myelogram.

FUNGUS INFECTIONS

Fungus infections often involve the vertebral column, although compromised function of the nervous system is indeed rare.[5,11,35,37] Among the varieties of mycotic disease that have done this are actinomycosis, blastomycosis, coccidioidomycosis, and cryptococcosis.* In most instances bony involvement of the spine is secondary to direct spread from cervical, intrathoracic, or intra-abdominal infections, and when spinal cord dysfunction occurs it is caused by compression by extradural granulomas. A few instances of hematogenous spread with subdural and intramedullary spinal abscesses have been documented.

The pattern of bony erosion of vertebrae in these conditions varies somewhat from cases of tuberculosis or pyogenic osteomyelitis of the spine. In addition to involvement of vertebral bodies and adjacent intervertebral discs, there is frequently erosion of pedicles, transverse processes, and adjacent ribs. Radiographically, cortical surfaces of vertebrae often appear severely eroded, and cavity formation surrounded by a zone of increased density is commonly seen. With spinal cord or cauda equina compression that is progressive, decom-

---

* See references 9, 12, 18, 26, 27, 30, 31, 34.

pression by previously mentioned operative techniques is indicated. Definitive diagnosis is established by demonstration of the respective organisms on smears or histological sections from the affected parts and by culture. Serological tests are of little value. Specific antimicrobial treatment should be administered postoperatively.

SYPHILIS

Most physicians in North America will seldom encounter syphilitic involvement of the spinal cord. Osteomyelitis of the spine does rarely occur in syphilis, but the spinal cord is usually spared in such instances.[16] Gummas within the spinal canal are extraordinarily rare.[32] When they occur they should be dealt with like any other space-occupying intraspinal lesion with as complete a removal as it is technically possible to carry out. The exact diagnosis can be made only on microscopic examination of the tissue. Postoperative antiluetic therapy, usually penicillin, should be administered.

DISC SPACE INFECTIONS

In rare cases infection or inflammation of the intervertebral disc occurs after direct contamination of the involved disc by operation, lumbar puncture, or discography.[39-41] Occasionally, and especially in children, infection occurs in the absence of these procedures and is presumed to be of hematogenous origin. The lumbar spine is involved more frequently than other sites.

Severe low back pain is the initial complaint. Leucocyte count and temperature are normal or slightly elevated. Sedimentation rate, however, is elevated in nearly all cases. Physical examination characteristically shows limited back motion, and local tenderness and muscle spasm may be present.

X-rays may show no changes in the early stages. From two to six weeks after the onset of symptoms there will be lytic changes of varying degree in adjacent vertebral bodies and narrowing of the intervertebral disc space (Fig. 114–7). In many instances, follow-up x-ray studies will show bony fusion of the adjacent vertebrae.

Treatment consists of bed rest, immobilization, and analgesic medications. Serial x-ray studies are indicated to determine

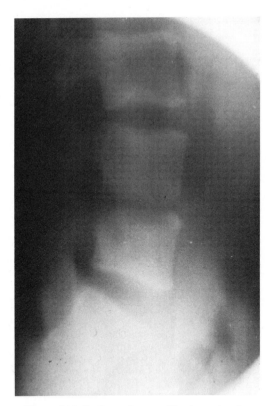

Figure 114–7 Lateral x-ray of lumbar spine showing disc space infection at L4–L5. There is erosion of the adjacent vertebral bodies and narrowing of the space. In this case, a 42-year-old man, there was no history of infection, operation, or lumbar puncture.

whether significant osteomyelitis is developing and to check on healing of the disease.

In most cases the clinical picture is one of gradual but progressive improvement over a period of weeks to several months. In the few cases that do not improve on conservative management, needle biopsy or aspiration of the involved intervertebral space is indicated for culture and sensitivity tests. Often there will be no bacterial growth. In about half the cases, however, cultures will show organisms of low virulence (especially *Staphylococcus epidermidis*). In these cases appropriate antibiotic therapy should be instituted and continued for several weeks. Although these patients may have a prolonged period of pain, the ultimate prognosis is good.

REFERENCES

1. Alexander, G. L.: Neurological complications of spinal tuberculosis. Proc. Roy. Soc. Med., *39*:730–734, 1946.

2. Ambrose, G. B., Alpert, M., and Neer, C. S.: Vertebral osteomyelitis. A diagnostic problem. J.A.M.A., 197:101–104, 1966.

3. Arseni, C., and Samitca, D. C.: Intraspinal tuberculous granuloma. Brain, 83:285–292, 1960.

4. Batson, O. V.: The function of the vertebral veins and their role in the spread of metastasis. Ann. Surg., 112:138–149, 1940.

5. Baylin, G. J., and Wear, J. M.: Blastomycosis and actinomycosis of the spine. Amer. J. Roentgen. 69:395–398, 1953.

6. Bertrand, I., Guillaume, J. M., Samson, M., and Gueguen, Y.: Tuberculome intramédullaire dorsal. Rev. Neurol., 98:51–54, 1958.

7. Bischof, W., and Nittner, K.: Pathogenesis, clinical findings and treatment of spinal epidural abscess. Zbl. Neurochir., 26:193–210, 1965.

8. Bucy, P. C., and Oberhill, H. R.: Intradural spinal granulomas. J. Neurosurg., 7:1–12, 1950.

9. Carton, C. A., and Mount, L. A.: Neurosurgical aspects of cryptococcosis. J. Neurosurg., 8:143–156, 1951.

10. Clawson, D. K., and Dunn, A. W.: Management of common bacterial infections of bones and joints. J. Bone Joint Surg., 49-A:164–182, 1967.

11. Cope, V. Z.: Actinomycosis of bone with special reference to infection of the vertebral column. J. Bone Joint Surg., 33-B:205–214, 1951.

12. Craig, W. McK., Dockerty, M. B., and Harrington, S. W.: Intravertebral and intrathoracic blastomycoma simulating dumb-bell tumor. Southern Surg., 9:759–766, 1940.

13. Dandy, W. E.: Abscesses and inflammatory tumors in the spinal epidural space (so-called pachymeningitis externa). Arch. Surg., 13:477–494, 1926.

14. Dott, N. M.: Skeletal traction and anterior decompression in the management of Pott's paraplegia. Edinburgh Med. J., 54:620–627, 1947.

15. Dutton, J. E. M., and Alexander, G. L.: Intramedullary spinal abscess. J. Neurol. Neurosurg. Psychiat., 17:303–307, 1954.

16. Epstein, B. S.: The Spine. A Radiological Text and Atlas. Philadelphia, Lea & Febiger, 1969.

17. Freedman, H., and Alpers, B. J.: Spinal subdural abscess. Arch. Neurol. Psychiat., 60:49–60, 1948.

18. Greenwood, R. C., and Voris, H. C.: Systemic blastomycosis with spinal cord involvement. J. Neurosurg., 7:450–454, 1950.

19. Henriques, C. Q.: Osteomyelitis as a complication in urology. Brit. J. Surg., 46:19–28, 1958.

20. Heusner, A. P.: Nontuberculous spinal epidural infections. New Eng. J. Med., 239:845–854, 1948.

21. Horwitz, N. A., and Rizzola, H. V.: Postoperative Complications in Neurosurgical Practice. Recognition, Prevention and Management. Baltimore, Md., Williams & Wilkins Co., 1967.

22. Hulme, A., and Dott, N. M.: Spinal epidural abscess. Brit. Med. J., 1:64–68, 1954.

23. Kirkaldy-Willia, W. H., and Thomas, T. G.: Anterior approaches in the diagnosis and treatment of infections of the vertebral bodies. J. Bone Joint Surg., 47-A:87–110, 1965.

24. Korbin, W. M.: Spinal epidural abscess: review of literature and report of case. Bull. Los Angeles Neurol. Soc., 23:21–26, 1958.

25. Langenskiöld. A., and Riska, E. B.: Pott's paraplegia treated by anterolateral decompression in thoracic and lumbar spine; report of twenty-seven cases. Acta Orthop. Scand., 38:181–192, 1967.

26. Lesne and Belloir: A propos d'un cas d'actinomycose médullaire. Ann. Méd., 12:329–336, 1922.

27. Ley, A., Jacas, R., and Oliveras, C.: Torula granuloma of the cervical spinal cord. J. Neurosurg., 8:326–335, 1951.

28. McLaurin, R. L.: Spinal suppuration. Clin. Neurosurg., 14:314–336, 1967.

29. Mathai, K. V., and Chandy, J.: Tuberculous infections of the nervous system. Clin. Neurosurg., 14:145–177, 1967.

30. Meyer, M., and Gill, M. B.: Mycosis of the vertebral column. A review of the literature. J. Bone Joint Surg., 17:857–866, 1935.

31. Rand, C. W.: Coccidioidal granuloma. Report of two cases simulating tumor of the spinal cord. Arch. Neurol. Psychiat., 23:502–511, 1930.

32. Ray, B. S.: Gumma simulating tumor of the cauda equina. J.A.M.A., 114:401–404, 1940.

33. Shaw, N. E., and Thomas, T. G.: Surgical treatment of chronic infective lesions of spine. Brit. Med. J., 1:162–164, 1963.

34. Smith, F. B., and Crawford, J. S.: Fatal granulomatosis of the central nervous system due to a yeast (Torula). J. Path. Bact., 33:291–296, 1930.

35. Utz, P.: Fungal infections of the central nervous system. Clin. Neurosurg., 14:86–100, 1967.

36. Wiley, A. M., and Trueta, J.: The vascular anatomy of the spine and its relationship to pyogenic vertebral osteomyelitis. J. Bone Joint Surg., 41-B:796–809, 1959.

37. Wilson, J. W., and Plunkett, O. A.: The Fungus Diseases of Man. Berkeley and Los Angeles, University of California Press, 1965.

38. Wright, R. L.: Intramedullary spinal cord abscess. J. Neurosurg., 23:208–210, 1965.

39. Wright, R. L.: Septic Complications of Neurosurgical Spinal Procedures. Springfield, Ill., Charles C Thomas, 1970.

40. Wright, R. L.: Congenital dermal sinuses. Progress in Neurological Surgery, vol. 4. Basel, S. Karger, 1971, pp. 175–191.

41. Wright, R. L.: Infections and infestations of the spine. In Practice of Surgery. Chapter 20, Neurosurgery, pp. 1–10. Hagerstown, Md., Harper & Row, 1972.

XII

PAIN

115

PHYSIOLOGICAL ANATOMY OF PAIN

The control of pain by operative procedures has been limited by a paucity of information concerning its anatomical and physiological correlates. Despite this, the observations and skill of many have combined to give the neurosurgeon an armamentarium of procedures to aid the patient in whom the experience of pain has lost any "protective" usefulness and has left only its debilitating effects.

In discussion of the physiological anatomy of pain, it is important to be continually aware of the multiple aspects of a painful experience. A given set of neurons may have a relevant function in pain by processing discrete pain information for purposes of identification, location, and quantification of the stimulus; or by relaying a diffuse, qualitative pain sensation; or by integrating sensory and motor events in response to the painful stimulus; or by contributing to arousal and escape behavior. The "pathways" for each of these aspects of the pain experience are no doubt partially overlapping; none have been defined completely.

This chapter is not designed to be a comprehensive summary of or review of the literature on all aspects of pain, but rather to assemble anatomical and physiological data that may relate to its control. The emphasis is toward more recent studies, and the intention is to provide an overview of current anatomical and physiological thought.

ASCENDING PATHWAYS

Peripheral Receptors and Nerves

Receptors are generally divided into free nerve endings and endings that are encapsulated by nonneural tissue.[7,12,35,161] Although classes of mechanoreceptive fibers have been positively associated with certain sensory organs (e.g., Pacinian corpuscle, Meissner's corpuscle, Merkel's disc, hair receptors), the receptors for most classes remain unidentified, particularly the receptors for warmth, cold, and pain. There is firm evidence that Krause's corpuscles and Ruffini's endings are both mechanoreceptors, and not thermoreceptors as formerly thought. The fine structure of many cutaneous nerve endings has been studied, but their function has not been identified. Hensel has shown that cold receptors in the cat's nose are served by thinly myelinated A fibers that divide into several nonmyelinated terminals within the stratum papillae. The fine bare receptive endings penetrate into the basal epidermal cells and contain many mitochondria, fine filaments, and microvesicles.[94] It is generally considered that pain receptors are also free nerve endings.

In the last 20 years recordings of single sensory peripheral nerve fibers (primary afferents) have revealed several classes that respond to noxious stimulation of their receptive fields. Within the class of "nociceptive" afferents are subclasses of nonmyelinated (C) and thinly myelinated (A-delta) afferents that are responsive to certain kinds of noxious stimulation. Some respond only to intense mechanical stimuli produced by pinching the skin or poking it with a sharp object. Others are entirely thermosensitive and respond only to noxious heating or to noxious stimulation that is either cold or hot. Another class of nociceptors is "mechanothermal" and responds to mechanical and cold or hot stimulation. One of the most common of these is the C-polymodal nociceptor; this class of

C. C. LaMOTTE and W. F. COLLINS

C fibers is responsive to mechanical, thermal, and chemical stimulations that are noxious.*

In addition to the nociceptive afferents, there are low-threshold primary afferents that are not only sensitive to innocuous stimulation but also respond to noxious stimulation of the skin. There are mechanosensitive fibers of large and small diameter that function primarily as position or velocity detectors at low intensities of mechanical stimulation but respond well to noxious intensities.[35] Since they are not selectively responsive to noxious stimulation, it is not likely that they transmit specific information about painful stimulation to the skin. Other classes of low-threshold primary afferents that may respond to noxious stimulation are the "warm" and "cold" fiber afferents. The warm afferents are C fibers and are selectively responsive to gentle warming of their cutaneous receptive fields and are suppressed by cooling. Warm fibers also respond to noxious heating, but their discharge is irregular and may cease altogether at higher temperatures.† Cold fibers conduct in the A-delta range, are selectively responsive to gentle cooling of their cutaneous receptive fields, and are suppressed by warming. They also have a response to noxious heat that may account for the "paradoxical cold" sensation that can be evoked by painful heating of the skin.[62,65,67,95,148]

Correlations of Peripheral Events and Sensation

Studies have only begun to relate peripheral neural events to the quality and intensity of painful sensation. A noxious stimulus often evokes a rapid pricking sensation followed by a burning or aching sensation. The results of nerve stimulation studies and nerve blocking experiments suggest that the first sensation is served by fibers conducting in the A-delta range, while the second sensation is mediated by C fibers. Collins, Nulsen, and Shealy showed that when only A-delta fibers were stimulated electrically in humans, sharp pain is felt. Repetitive stimulation of C fibers alone caused poorly localized and unbearable pain.[53] Recordings of single fibers in humans by Torebjörk and Hallin and by Van Hees and Gybels have demonstrated C fibers that were excited by pricking, itching, intense mechanical stimuli, noxious cold, heat, and histamine; activity in these fibers was correlated with simultaneous reports of pain.[221,225] Confirming evidence for the role of C fibers was found in a close correlation between the threshold for responses to noxious heating in C fibers in monkeys and the threshold for pain evoked by the same stimuli in humans.[135]

Primary afferents sensitive to noxious stimuli have graded responses to the increasing intensity of the stimulus; the increasing fiber response correlates with the increasing subjective magnitude of the sensation evoked in humans. The magnitude of pain evoked in humans and the frequency of discharge in nociceptive afferents in monkeys change as a function of time, however, even when the physical intensity of stimulation is held constant. The term "adaptation" is commonly used to describe a decrease in the magnitude of sensation or in neural response during sustained stimulation of constant intensity. When stimulus temperature is carefully controlled, a complete adaptation of pain in humans can be demonstrated for temperatures as high as 46°C.[88] The terms "suppression" and "fatigue" have been used to characterize the decrease in the magnitude of human pain and the neural reponse in nociceptive afferents, respectively, with repeated deliveries of a noxious stimulus. The time course of fatigue of the responses of C-polymodal nociceptors to repeated stimulation with noxious heat corresponds to the time course of suppression in the magnitude of pain evoked in humans by the same stimuli.[135,183]

Cutaneous hyperalgesia occurs in injured skin in the area reddened by vasodilation. There is a lower pain threshold for thermal and mechanical stimulation and also an increased pain sensitivity to suprathreshold stimuli. This state is termed "primary hyperalgesia" or "erythralgia" and is believed to be due to the release of a kininlike substance from injured cells.[47,89,142] This substance presumably acts on the endings of nociceptive afferents to lower their response thresholds. Two classes of fibers may contribute to the development of hy-

---

* See references 17, 23, 34, 78, 135, 170, 181, 220, 225.

† See references 63, 85, 95, 122, 130, 135, 211.

peralgesia. Both the C-polymodal nociceptors and the A-delta nociceptors develop an enhanced responsiveness to heat and a lower heat threshold after repeated heatings at high intensities.[18,23,38a,57,73]

Recently, the results of a study of causalgia patients have implicated the involvement of A-delta nociceptive afferents.[228] In patients who had experienced relief following a sympathectomy, the causalgic pain returned to the previously affected areas following an intradermal injection of norepinephrine. The pain that occurred following the injection was eliminated by application to the peripheral nerves of a pressure block sufficient to block A fibers. Thus causalgic pain may be due in part to an increase in the concentration of norepinephrine near the endings of A-delta nociceptors that sensitizes these fibers to mechanical stimuli. According to this hypothesis, a sympathectomy would result in a reduction in norepinephrine and thus a reduction of pain.

Chapman and co-workers showed that dorsal root stimulation leads to the release of a kininlike substance into the skin.[47] There is evidence that vasodilation resulting from electrical stimulation of the dorsal root is due to antidromic activity in C fiber afferents.[44,100] This antidromic activity can increase vascular permeability, presumably by the release of a chemical mediator, even in skin areas pretreated with cholinergic and adrenergic blocking agents.[109] This substance, if collected and injected intradermally, produces a sensation of burning pain. Polypeptides (bradykinin), amines (5-hydroxytryptamine), and prostaglandins evoke pain reactions themselves when introduced intradermally, intra-arterially, or intraperitoneally in man and animals. They can also excite mechanical and thermal nociceptors in skin and muscle.[84,86] These chemicals may alter the sensitivity of the nociceptors so that natural stimuli are more effective and therefore more painful. Prostaglandins potentiate the action of bradykinin and 5-hydroxytryptamine on sensory nerves, and one possible explanation of the analgesic effect of aspirin is that it interferes with the synthesis of prostaglandins. It is not known whether the sensitizing effect of prostaglandins is exerted directly by acting on the nerve membranes or indirectly by influencing the surrounding tissue. All substances known to excite nociceptive nerve endings or to enhance their responsiveness to natural noxious stimulation also affect vascular smooth muscle.[86]

Sensory Ganglia and Roots

The cell bodies of all somatic and visceral peripheral afferents are located in the dorsal roots and cranial nerve ganglia (except the cells of the mescencephalic trigeminal nucleus).[144] Within the dorsal root and trigeminal ganglion, the cells are arranged somatotopically. Recent studies using autoradiography, horseradish peroxidase, and physiological recording have mapped the relationship of groups of cells within a ganglion with their central processes within a root and with their spinal cord projections. In general, laterally located cells send their central processes into the rostral rootlets of their dorsal roots, and medially located cells send their processes into the caudal rootlets. Ganglion cells also have a distribution related to their modality, and can be grouped into classes based on their morphology and their suspected neurotransmitters. Large and small cells are found; the large cells are pale and probably give rise to myelinated axons. The small cells are dark and are probably the origin of nonmyelinated axons; they differ histochemically and ultrastructurally from the large cells. There is evidence that the small dark cells are nociceptive afferents. Recently, Hökfelt and associates have demonstrated that there are at least two subgroups of the small cells, one that contains a suspected transmitter, the peptide substance P, and another that contains the peptide somatostatin.[101] As is discussed later, these labeled cells have been demonstrated to enter the cord via Lissauer's tract and to be distributed to different regions of the spinal cord dorsal horn.

Since 1973, evidence has accumulated that from 25 to 35 per cent of the fibers of the spinal ventral roots of several species (man, cat, rat) are unmyelinated axons arising from sensory dorsal root ganglion cells.[51,150] Electrophysiological studies have located receptive fields of these fibers in both cutaneous regions and visceral structures; most fibers have high thresholds and may be nociceptive.[50,74] These primary afferents have been traced into the spinal gray matter and may terminate in both the dorsal and ventral horns.[132,146] The sensory fibers of the ventral root may provide an explanation for the fact that dorsal rhizotomy is not always successful in relieving pain.[52] The use of ganglionectomy as an alternative procedure has been suggested recently.[166]

Both myelinated and nonmyelinated dorsal root afferents are distributed somatotopically in the dorsal horn.[131] Physiological recordings of roots in cats and monkeys have shown a progressive representation of the limb. Proceeding rostrocaudally from C5 to T3, the roots supply the proximal preaxial, the distal preaxial, the distal postaxial, and finally the proximal postaxial limb dermatomes.[93,126,184]

Entry of Dorsal Roots into Spinal Cord

In cross sections of peripheral nerves and of dorsal rootlets, small bundles of nonmyelinated and thinly myelinated fibers appear to be randomly distributed among the larger-diameter myelinated fibers. At the entry of the dorsal rootlets into the spinal cord, however, the larger fibers converge into a medial bundle and enter the dorsal columns. The small myelinated and nonmyelinated fibers converge into two bundles, a larger bundle on the ventrolateral side of the rootlet and a second smaller bundle on the dorsomedial surface. The ventrolateral bundle directly joins the tract of Lissauer, while the dorsomedial bundle of small fibers turns sharply ventral and then also enters Lissauer's tract.[191,205,213] The large myelinated fibers that enter the dorsal columns send collateral branches into the dorsomedial region of the dorsal horn gray matter. These collaterals arise both at the level of the rootlet entry and along several segments rostral and caudal to this point. Similarly the small primary afferent fibers that enter Lissauer's tract may run rostrocaudally for one or two segments before entering the dorsal gray. The afferents are joined in Lissauer's tract by propriospinal axons that arise from nearby substantia gelatinosa neurons and re-enter the gray within one or two segments. Some of the collateral branches from the large-diameter afferents of the dorsal columns terminate in the substantia gelatinosa, but most terminate in Rexed laminae IV to VI and the intermediate and ventral gray matter.[194] The small myelinated (A-delta) and nonmyelinated (C) afferents, arising from the tract of Lissauer, are distributed mainly to laminae I, II, and III; fewer are found in IV and V.[131]

Substance P has been identified by immunohistochemical analysis in a subpopulation of small ganglion cells. It also has been found in axons of the dorsal roots, in Lissauer's tract, and in axon terminals of laminae I and II. A second group of small ganglion cells contains somatostatin; somatostatin-positive axons also have been demonstrated in Lissauer's tract and in axon terminals of lamina I. Thus, these peptides are associated with two populations of small ganglion cells, axons of Lissauer's tract, and the marginal and gelatinosal regions of the dorsal horn. Dorsal rhizotomy lowers the levels of substance P and somatostatin in the dorsal horn.[101,214] Electron microscopic histochemical analysis has shown substance P in axon terminals to be associated with large vesicles that may be peptide storage sites. The presence of many unlabeled small vesicles in the same terminals suggests these terminals may also contain another neurotransmitter and that substance P might be released with nerve impulses to act as a modulator rather than an initiator of synaptic events.[12a,172a]

Using multibarreled microelectrodes, Randic and Miletic have recorded the effects of substance P and somatostatin on the responses of single neurons in laminae I, II, and III. Cells that were activated by noxious mechanical or thermal stimulation or by a volley from A-delta or C fibers were excited by substance P, and their responses to peripheral stimuli were enhanced. In contrast, somatostatin depressed the activity of the cells. These authors suggest that substance P may have a role as an excitatory transmitter or modulator at the first synapse, while somatostatin may have an inhibitory modulating effect.[189,190]

Dorsal Horn and Nucleus Caudalis

The spinal dorsal horn and the nucleus caudalis of the trigeminal complex are similar morphologically and physiologically. Both consist of laminae that differ in the type of afferents and descending projections received, in their populations of projection neurons and interneurons, and in the ultrastructure of the neuropil. Aspects of the structural and synaptic morphology of the dorsal horn, especially the substantia gelatinosa, have been described in numerous studies using light and electron microscopic analysis and techniques of degeneration, Golgi staining, and autoradiography.* Several detailed studies also have been made of the substantia gelatinosa of the nucleus caudalis.[79-82,117,229] Cells of origin of the spinothalamic tract have been identified by several methods including (1) antidromic stimulation of the tract or the thalamus while recording caudally in the gray, (2) retrograde chromatolysis following severing of the tract, and (3) labeling of the cells following retrograde transport of horseradish peroxidase from the nerve terminals.† Single-unit recording of neurons throughout the dorsal horn has resulted in the classification of several types of cells by their responses to peripheral stimuli and electrical stimulation of primary afferents of peripheral nerves.‡

Lamina I

The marginal layer (lamina I) of the dorsal horn and of the nucleus caudalis contains large neurons that project to the ventral posterior and intralaminar nuclei of the thalamus and to the reticular formation. Recent physiological and anatomical evidence suggests that most afferents to the marginal layer are thinly myelinated (A-delta) fibers, although the area also receives some nonmyelinated (C) afferents.[127,131] Several types of cells have been found in lamina I, including neurons responding to (1) noxious mechanical stimuli, (2) noxious mechanical and thermal stimuli, (3) innocuous warming or cooling as well as noxious mechanical and thermal stimuli, and (4) both innocuous and noxious mechanical and thermal stimuli. Response latencies indicate a direct monosynaptic input from primary afferents.

Laminae II and III

The substantia gelatinosa (laminae II and III) is populated by many small interneurons; few projection (spinothalamic)

neurons have been found either anatomically or physiologically. The small-diameter primary afferents terminate heavily in this region, particularly the C afferents, and some collateral branches of large-diameter (A-beta) dorsal column afferents may also end in the deeper regions of the substantia gelatinosa.[127,131] Within the substantia gelatinosa are found large numbers of characteristic arrangements of the neuropil, called glomeruli, which are very likely of great importance in the integration and modulation of afferent input to the dorsal horn.[79,117,186,193,229] The typical substantia gelatinosa glomerulus consists of an outer ring of small-diameter dendrites and a few axonal endings that nearly surround a large central axon. The glomerulus is partially encapsulated by thin overlapping glial processes. Within the glomerulus is a central dark axonal ending of a C primary afferent that synapses on several different dendrites. There are also axoaxonic and dendrodendritic synaptic arrangements within the glomerulus. The relationships of the primary afferent terminals and of the dendrites and axons of the substantia gelatinosa interneurons to the glomerular components have been partially determined in the nucleus caudalis. One class of substantia gelatinosa interneuron in the nucleus caudalis, the "stalked" cell, has its dendrites within the substantia gelatinosa but projects its axon into lamina I. Its dendrites probably contribute to the glomerulus and receive excitatory synapses from the central C terminal. It may function as an excitatory interneuron that transmits information from the primary afferents ending in laminae II and III to the projection neurons in lamina I. The other classes of nucleus caudalis substantia gelatinosa neurons have their axons and dendrites confined within laminae II and III. Their axons probably form axoaxonic inhibitory synapses on the primary afferent endings of the glomeruli and form axodendritic synapses onto stalked cell dendrites in the glomeruli. These inhibitory local neurons could reduce transfer of primary afferent information to lamina I cells either by axoaxonic synapses on the primary afferent endings or by direct inhibitory contact on stalked cell dendrites.[80-82]

The functional role of the substantia gelatinosa has long been difficult to assess because of its complex synaptic relationships

---

* See references 92, 118, 131, 138, 186, 187, 193, 200, 209, 210, 213.

† See references: (1) 3, 175, 179, 223; (2) 75, 129, 157, 206; (3) 3, 222.

‡ See references 48, 87, 106, 127, 180, 182, 223, 234.

and because the small size of the neurons has made it very difficult to record unit activity. The once popular "gate control theory" proposed by Melzack and Wall has now been challenged by several subsequent studies.[153,163] Electrophysiological experiments have recently succeeded in recording from small numbers of substantia gelatinosa neurons and promise to clarify many speculations about the functions of this area.[43,96,127,232,236] The dominant primary afferent projection to the substantia gelatinosa appears to be from nonmyelinated (C) fibers, including polymodal nociceptive and low-threshold afferents.[127,146a,146b] Recent anatomical studies confirm the heavy distribution of nonmyelinated afferents to the substantia gelatinosa.[131,192] Cervero and colleagues found a common feature of the substantia gelatinosa neurons was a background discharge that could be altered by mechanical or noxious stimulation of the receptive field. Some cells had an excitatory field superimposed over an inhibitory field.[43] These cells project axons into Lissauer's tract for up to three segments. One theory to be tested is whether these neurons have a tonic inhibitory or excitatory influence, possibly via the glomeruli, on the projection neurons of laminae I, IV, and V, which often contribute dendrites to the substantia gelatinosa glomeruli. Thus the role of the substantia gelatinosa is complex; while receiving the majority of nonmyelinated primary afferents for distribution of sensory information, it also contributes to propriospinal connections for sensory integration.

Laminae IV, V, and VI

These laminae comprise the nucleus proprius of the spinal dorsal horn and the magnocellular layer of the nucleus caudalis. Many neurons of these areas project cephalad to the ventroposterior nucleus of the thalamus and to the reticular formation of the brain stem. Recording from this region has resulted in the identification of cells receiving input from slowly- or quickly-adapting, low-threshold mechanoreceptive afferents, from one or more classes of nociceptive afferents, and from both low-threshold and nociceptive afferents. Receptive fields are often larger than those of primary afferents, thus showing convergence. Noxious stimulation of their receptive fields evokes a prolonged discharge, and the response to noxious stimulation is usually graded with stimulus intensity.

Most of the axons of the projection neurons of the dorsal horn cross the midline of the cord and ascend to terminate in regions of the brain stem reticular formation and central gray matter or terminate in certain thalamic nuclei.

Brain Stem Reticular Formation

Areas of the reticular formation associated with ascending pathways of nociception have been identified either by single-unit recording from regions activated by A-delta or C peripheral fiber stimulation or anatomically by degeneration following anterolateral cordotomy or spinal commissural myelotomy. Degeneration from anterolateral cordotomy differs from that from the myelotomy, since the former interrupts not only spinothalamic axons but also the ventral spinocerebellar, spinotectal, spino-olivary, and spinolateral reticular tracts; and the latter interrupts the crossed spinothalamic fibers, the ventral spinocerebellar and the spino-olivary tracts; neither lesion is exclusive for nociceptive pathways.[119,152]

In the medulla and pons, the region of the nucleus reticularis gigantocellularis and the lateral reticular region receive anterolateral projections; those to the nucleus reticularis gigantocellularis appear to be mainly ipsilateral and derived from the deeper laminae of the spinal gray matter. Within the nucleus reticularis gigantocellularis, neurons of large receptive fields are found that can be activated only by noxious stimulation; other neurons are excited by either mechanical or noxious stimulation.[41,42,139,169]

In the mesencephalon, the anterolateral fibers project to the periaqueductal (central) gray matter and to the tegmental reticular formation lateral to the central gray.[119,152,162] Degeneration after myelotomy is heaviest in the ventrolateral part of the central gray and is continuous rostrally into the posterior hypothalamus, forming a long column extending through the mesencephalon into the diencephalon.[119] Stimulation electrically in humans of the periaqueductal gray elicits noxious somatic and visceral painful sensations accompanied by strong emotional reactions; stimulation more laterally in the tegmentum elicits similar but generally less intense reactions.[162]

Thalamus

The ventrobasal complex, the posterior complex, and the intralaminar thalamic nuclei receive both direct spinothalamic and indirect spinoreticulothalamic projections.[152] The ventrobasal complex is composed of the ventroposterolateral nucleus, which receives somatosensory projections representing the body, and the ventroposteromedial nucleus, which receives trigeminal somatosensory projections. The major input to the ventrobasal complex is from the somatotopically organized lemniscal projections of the dorsal column nuclei and of the main nucleus of the trigeminal complex. But additionally, cells of the spinal marginal layer and nucleus proprius project directly upon the more caudal parts of the ventrobasal complex in a detailed somatotopic pattern.[4,46,152,208] Golgi studies by Scheibel and Scheibel and degeneration studies by Bowsher have also demonstrated projections from the midbrain reticular formation.[29,199] Golgi studies have shown that reticular axons end on the soma and proximal dendrites of the ventrobasal complex neurons, whereas lemniscal axons end on distal portions of the dendrites.[28,199] The lemniscal properties of the ventrobasal complex neurons are reflected by their specific responses. Many respond to only one modality, including hair movement, touch, pressure, joint movement, warming, or cooling; a few have been found to respond to noxious stimulation of the tooth pulp.* There is a somatotopic organization and some general grouping of the cells by modality. A few nonspecific, "extralemniscal" units have also been identified. They often have bilateral fields and are polymodal, responding to various tactile, thermal, auditory, or nociceptive stimuli.[8,19,171,177]

The role of the ventrobasal complex in pain is unclear. Stimulation of the dorsal portion of it in awake humans results in localized, nonpainful tactile sensations.[195,215] Stimulation in the ventral and caudal regions can produce contralateral local-ized pain sensations in humans and monkeys.[21,91] Lesions of the ventrobasal complex, particularly the ventrocaudal region, produces changes in pain sensitivity, which may later be followed by hyperpathia.[71,195,201] These data and many studies of the lemniscal properties of the ventrobasal complex suggest that it is involved in localizing and identifying innocuous and noxious stimuli.

The posterior complex of the thalamus is an area caudal to the geniculate bodies and ventral to the pulvinar. It includes the magnocellular region of the medial geniculate, the suprageniculate-limitans nucleus, and an ill-defined region (the posterior nucleus) extending anteriorly from the medial geniculate body to the posterior region of the nuclear complex.[36,112,173] These regions differ both anatomically and physiologically.[19,59,60,110,156] Of particular interest to analysis of the somatosensory pathways is the medial region of the posterior nucleus.[36] This area receives projections from both the dorsal column nuclei and spinothalamic cells and also descending corticothalamic projections from the somatic sensory cortex. Cells of this area respond to somesthetic stimuli and project to the retroinsular area of the cortex, an area lying just posterior to the secondary somatosensory region of the cortex. The suprageniculate-limitans nucleus receives projections from the superior colliculus and projects to the granular insular cortex, which receives visual, auditory, and somesthetic stimulation. The lateral region of the posterior nucleus receives ascending auditory fibers and projects to the postauditory complex. The magnocellular region of the medial geniculate body projects widely to all areas of the auditory cortex.[36] Unlike the ventrobasal complex, most of the neurons are not somatotopically organized, have very large contralateral or ipsilateral receptive fields, and lack specific response characteristics. Many cells are polymodal, responding to some of several types of stimuli, including tactile, nociceptive, vestibular, or auditory. Most cells do respond to nociceptive stimuli.† Stimulation of the posterior complex in humans produces unpleasant sensations; in the monkey it can elicit pain responses, or contrary to this, increase pain thresh-

---

*See references 8, 22, 40, 173, 174, 177, 185, 204, 235, 237.

†See references 19, 59, 60, 66, 171, 173.

olds.[21,90] The role of the posterior complex in pain may be complex and also multifold, owing to its several components. Some cells can be inhibited by systemic injection of morphine.[203]

The intralaminar nuclei include the n. centrum median, the n. parafascicularis, the n. paracentralis, and the n. centralis lateralis. Anatomical and physiological evidence indicates that the nucleus centrum medianum does not receive spinothalamic fibers and may be more closely related to motor than to somatosensory functions. The other nuclei receive afferents from the reticular formation and from the marginal layer of the dorsal horn and nucleus caudalis. There is little or no lemniscal projection to the intralaminar nuclei. Like the cells of the posterior complex area, many of the intralaminar neurons are polymodal (usually including noxious stimuli) and have large contralateral or ipsilateral receptive fields.[2] Stimulation of these areas often evokes diffuse unpleasant sensations, anxiety, or sometimes diffuse pain.[90,195] Lesions in this region in humans can relieve intractable pain, and in animals, raise the pain threshold.[5,149,195] The cells can also be inhibited by morphine.[45]

Cortex

The primary and secondary somatosensory areas of the neocortex participate in nociception, but their roles are unclear. The primary somatosensory area consists of the postcentral gyrus, including its medial extension in the paracentral lobule. The secondary somatosensory area extends along the superior lip of the lateral sulcus, ventral to the primary somatosensory area and to the motor cortex. In many studies, the retroinsular region of the superior lip has been included as the most posterior region of the secondary somatosensory area, although Burton and Jones consider it to be a separate but related region.[36] The primary and secondary areas are somatotopically interconnected ipsilaterally and contralaterally; that is, parts of the primary and secondary somatosensory areas with similar peripheral receptive fields are interconnected, and there are also commissural connections to these somatosensory areas on the other side.[113-115] The ventrobasal complex of the thalamus projects somato-

topically to both the primary and secondary somatosensory areas.[49,115] The retroinsular cortical area receives a major projection from the medial region of the thalamic posterior nucleus.[36]

Most cells of the primary somatosensory area have small receptive fields and are modality specific, responding either to light touch, deep pressure, joint movement, hair movement, muscle stretch, warming, cooling, or tooth pulp stimulation. A few cells of this area have much larger, or often bilateral, receptive fields and can be excited by one or more stimuli, including pricking pain or pinch, deep pressure, hair movement, or light touch.* Electrical stimulation of the primary somatosensory area in humans produces well-localized sensations of pressure, temperature, tingling, or occasionally pain.[70,141,143] Removal of the postcentral gyrus results in some loss of somatic discriminative ability and can sometimes relieve pain or raise the pain threshold; however, hyperpathia may eventually follow.[70,136,141,196,230]

Both specific and nonspecific polymodal cells are found in the secondary somatosensory area, but the nonspecific cells are more common. The polymodal cells are mostly located posteriorly and medially, presumably in the retroinsular region. Many of the cells respond to noxious stimulation of their receptive fields, and stimulation of the secondary somatosensory area elicits localized painful sensations.[39,141,231] Lesions sometimes alter pain sensibility or relieve intractable pain while not affecting somatosensory discriminative capacity.[24,140] Pain and temperature sensitivity may, however, remain after removal of the entire primary somatosensory area and all but the posterior part or retroinsular cortex of the secondary somatosensory area.[20,176]

MODIFICATION OF PAIN

Modulating Pathways

Like other sensory systems, the relay nuclei of the "pain pathways" are sites of considerable modification of the sensory input originating in the periphery. The existence of these modulating systems has only

---

* See references 124, 158–160, 165, 178, 224, 226.

recently become known, and their analysis begun.

Control of the transmission of nociceptive information occurs first at the segmental level.* Electrical stimulation of the large-diameter cutaneous mechanoreceptors of the peripheral nerve can inhibit the excitation of spinothalamic neurons by both innocuous and injurious stimuli. This inhibition lasts only for the duration of the mechanoreceptor stimulation, and is probably mediated by dorsal column collaterals that enter the dorsal horn and act either directly or via interneurons on the spinothalamic cells. Central inhibition may not, however, be the only mechanism of reduction of pain of peripheral origin by transcutaneous electrical stimulation of peripheral nerves; local axonal blockade of A fiber afferents also occurs at stimulation levels required for pain relief.[38,216]

Within the brain stem, several areas, including the dorsal column nuclei, the nucleus magnocellularis, and the raphe nuclei, project to the spinal dorsal horn. Certain cells of the dorsal column nuclei project ipsilaterally to lamina I and to laminae IV and V of the dorsal horn.[37,58] Stimulation of these cells inhibits activity in nociceptive spinothalamic cells; this pathway may account in part for the putatively prolonged effects of dorsal column stimulation in relief of chronic pain.†

Two areas of the brain stem reticular formation may be important for inhibiting responses of spinothalamic neurons.[14] Recently the nucleus reticularis magnocellularis, located ventral to the nucleus reticularis gigantocellularis and lateral to the nucleus raphe magnus, has been found to project ipsilaterally to the dorsal horn and intermediate gray matter via the dorsolateral fasciculus, and to the ventral horn via the ventrolateral fasciculus. Little is known yet about this path, although it is thought to be inhibitory and to not be monaminergic. A second source of descending fibers is the nucleus raphe magnus, and studies indicate it may be very important for mechanisms of analgesia. The nucleus raphe magnus projects to structures that are nociceptive or receive visceral afferent input. These include the solitary nucleus, the dorsal motor nucleus of the tenth nerve, the marginal and gelatinosal laminae of the trigeminal nucleus caudalis and of the spinal cord, and also laminae V, VI, and VII of the spinal gray matter. The spinal pathway is bilateral, via the dorsolateral fasciculus, and immunohistochemical and physiological studies have shown these fibers to be serotoninergic.[61,69] Electrical stimulation of the raphe produces analgic behavior and inhibits nociceptive responses of spinothalamic cells in laminae I and V in the cat and monkey.[13,16,72,233] This inhibitory effect is reduced if the dorsolateral fasciculus is transected.

The raphe magnus appears to be closely linked to the periaqueductal gray matter; stimulation of the periaqueductal gray produces marked analgesia to almost all types of noxious stimuli in animals and in humans, apparently without affecting other sensory modalities.[101a,145,195a,195b] Electrical stimulation of the periaqueductal gray inhibits cells of the raphe magnus, lamina V cells of the dorsal horn, cells of the nucleus gigantocellularis, and areas of the medial and ventrobasal thalamus. Lesions of the raphe or of the dorsolateral fasciculus, however, abolish the analgesic effect of the stimulation. Thus the periaqueductal gray appears to exert part of its effect by way of the raphe pathway.

Cortical projections from the primary somatosensory and motor areas also descend to spinal laminae IV and V, as demonstrated with horseradish peroxidase labeling and with electrical stimulation.[55] The descending fibers appear to arise from the cortical layer V. The main effect of stimulation is to depress the discharge of spinothalamic cells in laminae IV and V during response to tactile input, but there is also some inhibition of the response to nociceptive input.

Opiates

There is considerable evidence that drugs, hormones, and neurotransmitters act at specific receptor sites consisting of large molecules located on the external surface of target cells. Recent studies have demonstrated that opiate effects result from binding to receptor sites in the brain and spinal cord.[83,207,208] Both biochemical and autoradiographic studies reveal marked re-

---

* See references 33, 76, 87, 107, 108, 227.
† See references 32, 76, 87, 99, 202, 212.

gional variations in the density of opiate receptors in the brains of several species. Highest levels of binding are observed in regions that subserve pain and regions of the limbic system not specifically related to pain.* Opiate receptors in the monkey brain are most dense in the major components of a widespread limbic circuit, including areas of the reticular formation, the hypothalamus, the mediodorsal thalamic nucleus, the septal nuclei, and the amygdala. The opiate receptors, however, are not distributed equally throughout the limbic pathways, but appear to be concentrated in certain groups of closely interrelated nuclei and not in others. Large numbers of opiate receptors also occur in those sensory and motor areas that are most directly linked to the limbic system. Components of the spinothalamic and spinoreticular systems provide a major sensory input to the system, and the substantia gelatinosa, the periaqueductal gray matter, and the intralaminar thalamic nuclei have high densities of opiate receptors. The opiate receptors in the substantia gelatinosa have been directly associated with the dorsal root afferents that terminate in that region.[133] Additionally, the motor areas of the forebrain (ventroanterior thalamic nucleus, rostral corpus striatum) that are less closely coupled with basic motor functions but associated with the limbic system are rich in opiate receptors. Inhibition of neural activity or behavioral analgesia following local microinjection of opiates has been observed in several areas with high levels of opiate receptor binding including the spinal cord dorsal horn, the nucleus reticularis gigantocellularis, the periaqueductal gray matter, the hypothalamus, the medial thalamus, and the cortex.[68,120,172,198]

Discovery of the existence of specific opiate receptor sites has led to a search for a natural opiatelike substance in the brain that acts at these sites. Investigators have isolated opiatelike factors from the brains of several species.[103,167,217,218] Two of these factors are closely related pentapeptides, methionine-enkephalin and leucine-enkephalin. The ratio of these two enkephalins differs from one brain region to the next, but the significance of this phenomenon is not known. Enkephalins are found in local interneurons and in nerve terminals in many of the same regions as opiate receptors in the brain and spinal cord, especially the substantia gelatinosa, the periaqueductal gray matter, the locus ceruleus, areas of the thalamus, and the amygdala.[68a, 197a,204a] Certain cells of the pituitary and hypothalamus also contain a high concentration of factors with opiatelike effects, called endorphins.[56,219] Endorphin cells in the hypothalamus project axons to many regions, including the nucleus accumbens, the septal region, the periaqueductal gray, and the locus ceruleus; there is little projection of endorphin axons to the lower brain stem or the spinal cord.[1a,25]

Understanding the role of these substances in pain modulation is one of the major challenges for the coming years. The enkephalins and the endorphins have many potential sites at which to modulate pain systems as well as to mediate many of the other pharmacological actions of opiates. It appears that some of the opiate analgesic effects may be both locally mediated and produced by activation of descending systems. In the spinal cord, enkephalinergic terminals presumed to arise from local neurons are heavily distributed in the substantia gelatinosa and marginal zones, often in close opposition to the soma and dendrites of the cells of these regions.[68a,197a,204a] Many of these same neurons appear to receive numerous projections of substance P terminals from primary nociceptive afferents.[132a] Local ionotophoresis of morphine and enkephalin inhibits the release of substance P from primary afferents and reduces the responses of dorsal horn neurons to painful stimulation of their receptive fields.[68,109a,155]

In addition to their local actions in the spinal cord, enkephalins and opiates may also act via the descending bulbospinal serotoninergic system arising from the raphe magnus. As described earlier, the raphe projects via the dorsolateral fasciculus to the spinal gray matter, and receives input from the periaqueductal gray matter; stimulation of either the periaqueductal gray or the raphe produces analgesia. There is also a high concentration of enkephalinergic terminals and cells and opiate receptors in the periaqueductal gray. Intracerebral injection of opiates or enkephalin into the periaqueductal gray produces analgesia similar to that produced by electrical stimu-

---

* See references 9, 10, 11, 98, 125, 134.

lation, and both are blocked by naloxone, or by lesion of the raphe magnus or the dorsolateral fasciculus.[1,12b]

CONCLUSION

A rapid proliferation of information on the functional anatomy and physiology of pain has occurred over the last decade. Several characteristics of the mechanisms of pain transmission and perception are becoming understood and serve as a foundation for future basic and clinical research.

Although the knowledge of structures and mechanisms of pain receptors remains minimal, both the classic studies of Lewis and more recent studies indicate that at least some nociceptors respond both to direct stimulation and to subsequent tissue changes resulting from inflammation and injury. These tissue changes may also activate receptors not usually responsive to noxious stimuli. Analysis of these mechanisms will be important for the understanding and treatment of inflammation and causalgia.

There is now considerable evidence that from the peripheral receptor level to the cortex many nuclei of the ascending pain pathways are organized both to preserve the specificity and the somatotopy of the pain sensations and also to integrate information from several types of sensory afferents. That is, within the nuclei are cells of small receptive fields specifically responsive to certain types of noxious stimuli and also polymodal cells, usually with larger receptive fields. Most research so far has concentrated on primary afferents and the cells of the spinal cord; similar studies are needed for analyzing the neural preservation of pain information at higher levels.

Of equal importance to the control of pain is consideration of the role of both local interneuron circuits and descending systems. For example, in the dorsal horn substantia gelatinosa, elaborate interrelationships of small interneurons with primary afferents and spinothalamic cells are critical for both the relay and the modification of sensory information. Further, projections from the periaqueductal gray matter via the raphe nucleus appear to exert profound effects on the activity of the spinothalamic cells.

Finally, the recent advances in techniques of immunohistochemistry and microelectrophoresis are revealing the variety of neurochemical interactions involved in several nuclei. The identification and localization of putative neurotransmitters and "modulators," such as substance P, somatostatin, and the newly found enkephalins and endorphins, is an important step toward more specific neuropharmacological approaches to pain treatment.

REFERENCES

1. Akil, H., Richardson, D. E., and Barchas, J. D.: Pain control by focal brain stimulation in man: Relationship to enkephalins and endorphins. In Beers, R. F., Jr., and Bassett, E. G., eds.: Mechanisms of Pain and Analgesic Compounds. New York, Raven Press, 1979, pp. 239–247.

1a. Akil, H., Watson, S. J., Berger, P. A., and Barchas, J. D.: Endorphins, β-LPH, and ACTH: Biochemical pharmacological, and anatomical studies. Advances Biochem. Psychopharmacol., 18:125–139, 1978.

2. Albe-Fessard, D., and Besson, J. M.: Convergent thalamic and cortical projections—The non-specific system. In Iggo, A., ed.: Handbook of Sensory Physiology. Vol. II. The Somatosensory System. New York, Springer-Verlag, 1973, pp. 489–560.

3. Albe-Fessard, D., Levante, A., and Lamour, Y.: Origin of spinothalamic tract in monkeys. Brain Res., 64:503–509, 1974.

4. Albe-Fessard, D., Boivie, D., Grant, G., and Levante, A.: Labelling of cells in the medulla oblongata and the spinal cord of the monkey after injections of horseradish peroxidase in the thalamus. Neurosci. Let., 1:75–80, 1975.

5. Albe-Fessard, D., Dondey, M., Nicolaidis, S., and LeBean, J.: Remarks concerning the effect of diencephalic lesions on pain and sensitivity with special reference to lemniscally mediated control of noxious differences. Confin. Neurol., 32:174–184, 1970.

6. Anderson, D. J., and Matthews, B., eds.: Pain in the Trigeminal Region. Amsterdam, Elsevier–North Holland Publishing Co., 1977.

7. Andres, K., and von During, M.: Morphology of cutaneous receptors. In Iggo, A., ed.: Handbook of Sensory Physiology. Vol. II. The Somatosensory System. New York, Springer-Verlag, 1973, pp. 3–28.

8. Angel, A., and Clarke, K. A.: An analysis of the representation of the forelimb in the ventrobasal thalamic complex of the albino rat. J. Physiol. (London), 249:399–423, 1975.

9. Atweh, S. F., and Kuhar, M. J.: Autoradiographic localization of opiate receptors in rat brain. I. Spinal cord and medulla. Brain Res., 124:53–67, 1977.

10. Atweh, S. F., and Kuhar, M. J.: Autoradiographic localization of opiate receptors in rat brain, II. The brain stem. Brain Res., 129:1–12, 1977.

11. Atweh, S. F., and Kuhar, M. J.: Autoradiographic localization of opiate receptors in rat brain. III. The telencephalon. Brain Res., *134*:393–405, 1977.

12. Bannister, L. H.: Sensory terminals of peripheral nerves. *In* Landon, D. N., ed.: The Peripheral Nerve. London, Chapman & Hall, 1976, pp. 396–463.

12a. Barber, R. P., Vaughn, J. E., Slemmon, J. R., Salvatrra, P. M., Roberts, E., and Leeman, S. E.: The origin, distribution and synaptic relationships of substance P axons in rat spinal cord. J. Comp. Neurol., *184*:331–352, 1979.

12b. Basbaum, A. I., and Fields, H. L.: Pain control; A new role for the medullary reticular formation. *In* Hobson, J. A., and Brazier, M. A. B., eds.: The Reticular Formation Revisited. New York, Raven Press, 1980, pp. 329–348.

13. Basbaum, A. I., Clanton, C. H., and Fields, H. L.: Opiate and stimulus-produced analgesia: Functional anatomy of a medullospinal pathway. Proc. Nat. Acad. Sci. U.S.A., *73*:4685–4688, 1976.

14. Basbaum, A., Clanton, C. H., and Fields, H. L.: Three bulbospinal pathways from the rostral medulla of the cat: An autoradiographic study of pain modulating systems. J. Comp. Neurol., *178*:209–224, 1978.

15. Basbaum, A. I., Marley, J. E., O'Keefe, J., and Clanton, C. H.: Reversal of morphine and stimulus produced analgesia by subtotal spinal cord lesions. Pain, *3*:43–56, 1977.

16. Beall, J. E., Martin, R. F., Applebaum, A. E., and Willis, W. D.: Inhibition of primate spinothalamic tract neurons by stimulation in the region of the nucleus raphe magnus. Brain Res., *114*:328–333, 1976.

17. Beck, P. W., Handwerker, H. O., and Zimmerman, M.: Nervous outflow from the cat's foot during noxious radiant heat stimulation. Brain Res., *67*:373–386, 1974.

18. Beitel, R. E., and Dubner, R.: The response of unmyelinated (C) polymodal nociceptors to thermal stimuli applied to the monkey's face. J. Neurophysiol., *39*:1160–1175, 1976.

19. Berkley, K. J.: Response properties of cells in ventrobasal and posterior group nuclei of cat. J. Neurophysiol., *36*:940–952, 1973.

20. Berkley, K. J., and Parmer, R.: Somatosensory cortical involvement in responses to noxious stimulation in the cat. Exp. Brain Res., *20*:363–374, 1974.

21. Berkley, K. J., and Smith, O. A., Jr.: Behavioral indices for neural systems involved in pain and fear responses in monkeys. Exp. Neurol., *26*:527–542, 1970.

22. Bertrand, G., Jasper, H., and Wong, A.: Microelectrode study of the human thalamus: Functional organization in the ventro-basal complex. Confin. Neurol., *29*:81–86, 1967.

23. Bessou, P., and Perl, E. R.: Response of cutaneous sensory units with unmyelinated fibers to noxious stimuli. J. Neurophysiol., *32*:1025–1043, 1969.

24. Biemond, A.: The conduction of pain above the level of the thalamus opticus. Arch. Neurol. Psychiat., *75*:231–244, 1956.

25. Bloom, F. E., Rossier, J., Battenberg, E. L. F.,

Bayon, A., French, E., Henrickson, S. J., Siggins, G. R., Segal, D., Browne, R., Ling, N., and Guillemin, R.: β-Endorphin: Cellular localization, electrophysiological and behavioral effects. Advances Biochem. Psychopharmacol., *18*:89–109, 1978.

26. Bonica, J. J., ed.: Advances in Neurology. Vol. 4. Pain. New York, Raven Press, 1974.

27. Bonica, J. J., and Albe-Fessard, D., eds.: Advances in Pain Research and Therapy. Vol. 1. New York, Raven Press, 1976.

28. Bowsher, D.: The termination of secondary somatosensory neurons within the thalamus of Macaca mulatta: An experimental degeneration study. J. Comp. Neurol., *117*:213–227, 1961.

29. Bowsher, D.: Etude comparée des projections thalamiques de deux zones localisées des formations réticulées bulbaires et mésencéphaliques. C. R. Acad. Sci. D (Paris), *265*:340–342, 1967.

30. Bradley, P. B., Briggs, P. B., Gayton, R. J., and Lambert, L. A.: Effects of micro-iontophoretically applied methionine-enkephalin on single neurones in rat brainstem. Nature, *261*:425–426, 1976.

31. Bresler, D. F., and Katz, R. L., eds.: The Management of Pain: Alternatives to Phamacological and Surgical Therapy. New York, Grune & Stratton, Inc., 1978.

32. Brown, A. G., and Martin, H. F.: Activation of descending control of the spinocervical tract by impulses ascending the dorsal columns and relaying through the dorsal column nuclei. J. Physiol. (London), *235*:535–550, 1973.

33. Brown, A. G., and Short, A. D.: Effects from the somatic sensory cortex on transmission through the spinocervical tract. Brain Res., *74*:338–341, 1974.

34. Burgess, P. R., and Perl, E. R.: Myelinated afferent fibers responding specifically to noxious stimulation of the skin. J. Physiol. (London), *190*:540–542, 1967.

35. Burgess, P. R., and Perl, E. R.: Cutaneous mechanoreceptors and nociceptors. *In* Iggo, A., ed.: Handbook of Sensory Physiology. Vol. II. The Somatosensory System. New York, Springer-Verlag, 1973, pp. 29–78.

36. Burton, H., and Jones, E. G.: The posterior thalamic region and its cortical projection in New World and Old World monkeys. J. Comp. Neurol., *168*:249–302, 1976.

37. Burton, H., and Loewy, A. D.: Projections to the spinal cord from medullary somatosensory relay nuclei. J. Comp. Neurol., *173*:773–792, 1977.

38. Campbell, J. N., and Long, D. L.: Transcutaneous electrical stimulation for pain: Efficacy and mechanism of action. *In* Bresler, D. F., and Katz, R. L., eds.: The Management of Pain: Alternatives to Pharmacological and Surgical Therapy. New York, Grune & Stratton, Inc., 1978.

38a. Campbell, J. N., Meyer, R. A., and LaMotte, R. H.: Sensitization of myelinated nociceptive afferents that innervate the monkey hand. J. Neurophysiol., *42*:1669–1679, 1979.

39. Carreras, M., and Andersson, S. A.: Functional

properties of neurons of the anterior ectosylvian gyrus of the cat. J. Neurophysiol., *26*:100–126, 1963.

40. Carreras, M., Mancia, D., and Pagni, C. A.: Unit discharges recorded from the human thalamus with microelectrodes. Confin. Neurol., *29*:87–89, 1967.

41. Casey, K. L.: Somatic stimuli, spinal pathways, and size of cutaneous fibers influencing unit activity in the medial medullary reticular formation. Exp. Neurol., *25*:25–26, 1969.

42. Casey, K. L.: Responses of bulboreticular units to somatic stimuli eliciting escape behavior in the cat. Int. J. Neurosci., *2*:15–28, 1971.

43. Cervero, F., Molony, V., and Iggo, A.: Extracellular and intracellular recordings from neurones in the substantia gelatinosa Rolandi. Brain Res., *136*:565–569, 1977.

44. Chahl, L. A., and Ladd, R. J.: Local oedema and general excitation of cutaneous sensory receptors produced by electrical stimulation of the saphenous nerve in the rat. Pain, *2*:25–34, 1976.

45. Chang, H. T.: Integrative action of thalamus in the process of acupuncture for analgesia. Sci. Sin., *16*:25–60, 1973.

46. Chang, H. T., and Ruch, T. C.: Topographical distribution of spinothalamic fibers in the thalamus of the spider monkey. J. Anat., *81*:150, 1947.

47. Chapman, L. F., Ramos, A. O., Goodell, H., and Wolff, H. G.: Neurohumoral features of afferent fibers in man: Their role in vasodilation, inflammation, and pain. Arch. Neurol. (Chicago), *4*:617–650, 1961.

48. Christensen, B. N., and Perl, E. R.: Spinal neurons specifically excited by noxious thermal stimuli: Marginal zone of the dorsal horn. J. Neurophysiol., *29*:293–307, 1969.

49. Clark, W. E. L., and Powell, T. P. S.: On the thalamocortical connexions of the general sensory cortex of Macaca. Proc. Roy. Soc., London, ser. B., *141*:467–487, 1953.

50. Clifton, G. L., Coggeshall, R. E., Vance, W. H., and Willis, W. D.: Receptive fields of unmyelinated ventral root afferent fibers in the cat. J. Physiol. (London), *256*:573–600, 1976.

51. Coggeshall, R. E., Coulter, J. D., and Willis, W. D.: Unmyelinated fibers in the ventral root. Brain Res., *57*:229–233, 1973.

52. Coggeshall, R. E., Applebaum, M. L., Facem, M., Stubbs, T. B. III, and Sykes, M. T.: Unmyelinated axons in human ventral roots, a possible explanation for the failure of dorsal rhizotomy to relieve pain. Brain, *98*:157–166, 1975.

53. Collins, W. F., Nulsen, F. E., and Shealy, C. N.: Electrophysiological studies of peripheral and central pathways. *In* Henry Ford Hospital Symposium: Pain. Boston, Little, Brown, & Co. 1966., pp. 33–45.

54. Costa, E., and Trabucchi, M., eds.: Advances in Biochemical Psychopharmacology. Vol. 18. The Endorphins. New York, Raven Press, 1978.

55. Coulter, J. D., Foreman, R. D., Beall, J. E., and Willis, W. D.: Cerebral cortical modulation of primate spinothalamic neurons. *In* Bonica, J.

J., and Albe-Fessard, D., eds.: Advances in Pain Research and Therapy. Vol. I. New York, Raven Press, 1976, pp. 271–277.

56. Cox, B. M., Opheim, K. E., Teschemacher, H., and Goldstein, A.: A peptide-like substance from pituitary that acts like morphine 2. Purification and properties. *In* Goldstein, A., ed.: The Opiate Narcotics. New York, Pergamon Press, 1975, pp. 25–30.

57. Croze, S., Duclaux, R., and Kenshalo, D.: The thermal sensitivity of the polymodal nociceptors of the monkey. J. Physiol. (London), *263*:539–562, 1976.

58. Crutcher, K. A., Humbertson, A. O., Jr., and Martin, G. F.: The origin of brainstem-spinal pathways in the North American opossum (Didelphis Virginiana). Studies using the horseradish peroxidase method. J. Comp. Neurol., *179*:169–194, 1978.

59. Curry, M. J.: The exteroceptive properties of neurones in the somatic part of the posterior group (PO). Brain Res., *44*:429–462, 1972.

60. Curry, M. J.: The effects of stimulating the somatic sensory cortex on single neurones in the posterior group of the cat. Brain Res., *44*:463–481, 1972.

61. Dahlstrom, A., and Fuxe, K.: Evidence for the existence of monoamine containing neurons in the central nervous system: I. Demonstration of monoamines in the cell bodies of brain stem neurons. Acta Physiol. Scand., *62*:suppl. 232:1–55, 1964.

62. Darian-Smith, I., Johnson, K. O., and Dykes, R.: "Cold" fiber population innervating palmar and digital skin of the monkey: Responses to cooling pulses. J. Neurophysiol., *36*:325–346, 1973.

63. Darian-Smith, I., Johnson, K. O., and LaMotte, C.: Peripheral neural determinants in the sensing of changes in skin temperature. *In* Kornhuber, H. H., ed.: The Somatosensory System. Stuttgart, G. Thieme, 1975, pp. 23–37.

64. DeReuck, A. V. S., and Knight, J., eds.: Touch, Heat and Pain. CIBA Foundation Symposium. Boston, Little, Brown & Co., 1966.

65. Dodt, E., and Zotterman, Y.: Mode of action of warm receptors. Acta Physiol. Scand., *26*:345–357, 1952.

66. Dong, W. K., and Wagman, I. H.: Modulation of nociceptive responses in the thalamic posterior group of nuclei. *In* Bonica, J. J., and Albe-Fessard, D., eds.: Advances in Pain Research and Therapy. Vol. 1. New York, Raven Press, 1976, pp. 455–460.

67. Dubner, R., Sumino, R., and Wood, W. I.: A peripheral "cold" fiber population responsive to innocuous and noxious thermal stimuli applied to the monkey's face. J. Neurophysiol., *38*:1373–1389, 1975.

68. Duggan, A. W., Hall, J. G., and Headley, P. N.: Morphine, enkephalin and the substantia gelatinosa. Nature, *264*:456–458, 1976.

68a. Elde, R., Hokfelt, T., Johansson, O., and Terenius, L.: Immunohistochemical studies using antibodies to leucine-enkephalin: Initial observations on the nervous system of the rat. Neurosciences, *1*:349–355, 1976.

69. Engberg, I., Lundberg, A., and Ryall, R. W.: Is

the tonic decerebrate inhibition of reflex paths mediated by monoaminergic pathways? Acta Physiol. Scand., *72*:123–133, 1968.

70. Erickson, T. C., Bleckwenn, W. J., and Woolsey, C. N.: Observations on the postcentral gyrus in relation to pain. Trans. Amer. Neurol. Ass., *77*:57–59, 1952.

71. Ervin, R. R., and Mark, V. H.: Stereotactic thalamotomy in the human. Part II. Physiological observations on the human thalamus. Arch. Neurol. (Chicago), *3*:368–380, 1960.

72. Fields, H. L., Basbaum, A. I., Clanton, C. H., and Anderson, S. D.: Nucleus raphe magnus inhibition of spinal cord dorsal horn neurons. Brain Res., *126*:441–454, 1977.

73. Fitzgerald, M., and Lynn, B.: The sensitization of high threshold mechanoreceptors with myelinated axons by repeated heating. J. Physiol. (London), *365*:549–563, 1977.

74. Floyd, K., Koley, J., and Morrison, J. F. B.: Afferent discharges in the sacral ventral roots of cats. J. Physiol. (London), *259*:37P–38P, 1976.

75. Foerster, O., and Gagel, O.: Die Vorderseitenstrangdurchschneidung beim Menschen. Z. Ges. Neurol. Psychiat., *138*:1–92, 1932.

76. Foreman, R. D., Beall, J. E., Applebaum, A. E., Coulter, J. C., and Willis, W. D.: Inhibition of primate spinothalamic tract neurons by electrical stimulation of dorsal column or peripheral nerve. In Bonica, J. J., and Albe-Fessard, D., eds.: Advances in Pain Research and Therapy. Vol. I. New York, Raven Press, 1976, pp. 405–410.

77. Gent, J. P., and Wolstencroft, J. H.: Effects of methionine-enkephalin and leucine-enkephalin compared with those of morphine on brainstem neurones in cat. Nature, *261*:426–427, 1976.

78. Georgopoulos, A. P.: Functional properties of primary afferent units probably related to pain mechanisms in primate glabrous skin. J. Neurophysiol., *39*:71–83, 1976.

79. Gobel, S.: Synaptic organization of the substantia gelatinosa glomeruli in the spinal trigeminal nucleus of the adult cat. J. Neurocytol., *3*:219–243, 1974.

80. Gobel, S.: Golgi studies of the neurons in layer I of the dorsal horn of the medulla (trigeminal nucleus caudalis). J. Comp. Neurol., *180*:375–394, 1978.

81. Gobel, S.: Golgi studies of the neurons in layer II of the dorsal horn of the medulla (trigeminal nucleus caudalis). J. Comp. Neurol., *180*:395–414, 1978.

82. Gobel, S., and Hockfield, S.: An anatomical analysis of the synaptic circuitry of layers I, II, and III of trigeminal nucleus caudalis in the cat. In Anderson, D. J., and Matthews, B., eds.: Pain in the Trigeminal Region. Amsterdam, Elsevier–North Holland Publishing Co., 1977, pp. 203–211.

83. Goldstein, A., ed.: The Opiate Narcotics. New York, Pergamon Press, 1975.

84. Guilband, G., LeBars, D., and Besson, J. M.: Bradykinin as a tool in neurophysiological studies of pain mechanisms. In Bonica, J. J., and Albe-Fessard, D., eds.: Advances in Pain Research and Therapy. Vol. 1. New York, Raven Press, 1976, pp. 67–73.

85. Hallin, R. G. and Torebjörk, H. E.: Receptors with C fibers responding specifically to warmth in human skin. In Proceedings of the International Congress of Physiological Sciences, 27th, Paris, 1977, p. 301.

86. Handwerker, H. O.: Influences of algogenic substances and prostaglandins on the discharges of unmyelinated cutaneous nerve fibers identified as nociceptors. In Bonica, J. J., and Albe-Fessard, D., eds.: Advances in Pain Research and Therapy. Vol. 1. New York, Raven Press, 1976, pp. 41–45.

87. Handwerker, H. O., Iggo, A., and Zimmerman, M.: Segmental and supraspinal actions on dorsal horn neurons responding to noxious and non-noxious skin stimuli. Pain, *1*:147–165, 1975.

88. Hardy, J. D., Stokwijk, J. A. J., and Hoffman, D.: Pain following step increase in skin temperature. In Kenshalo, D. R., ed.: The Skin Senses. Springfield, Ill., Charles C Thomas, 1968, pp. 444–454.

89. Hardy, J. D., Wolff, H. G., and Goodell, H.: Pain Sensations and Reactions. Baltimore, Williams & Wilkins Co., 1952.

90. Hassler, R.: The division of pain conduction into systems of pain sensation and pain awareness. In Payne, J. P., Burt, R. A. P., Janzen, R., Keidel, W. D., Herz, A., and Steichele, C., eds.: Pain: Basic Principles, Pharmacology, Therapy. London, Churchill Livingstone, 1972, pp. 98–112.

91. Hassler, R., and Reichert, T.: Klinische und anatomische Befunde bei stereotaktischen Schmerzoperationen im Thalamus. Arch. Psychiat. Nervenk., *200*:93–122, 1959.

92. Heimer, L., and Wall, P. D.: The dorsal root distribution to the substantia gelatinosa of the rat with a note on the distribution in the cat. Exp. Brain Res., *6*:89–99, 1968.

93. Hekmatpanah, J.: Organization of tactile dermatomes C_1 through L_4 in the cat. J. Neurophysiol., *24*:129–140, 1961.

94. Hensel, H.: Cutaneous thermoreceptors. In Iggo, A., ed.: Handbook of Sensory Physiology. Vol. II. Somatosensory System. New York, Springer-Verlag, 1973, pp. 79–110.

95. Hensel, H., and Iggo, A.: Analysis of cutaneous warm and cold fibres in primates. Pfleuger. Arch., *329*:1–8, 1971.

96. Hentall, I. D.: Delayed off responses in substantia gelatinosa. Soc. Neurosci. Abst., 1977, no. 1607.

97. Hill, R. G., Pepper, C. M., and Mitchell, J. F.: Depression of nociceptive and other neurones in the brain by iontophoretically applied met-enkephalin. Nature, *262*:604–606, 1976.

98. Hiller, J. M., Pearson, J., and Simon, E. J.: Distribution of stereospecific binding of the potent narcotic analgesic etorphine in the human brain: Predominance in the limbic system. Res. Commun. Chem. Path. Pharmacol., *6*:1052–1061, 1973.

99. Hillman, P., and Wall, P. D.: Inhibitory and excitatory factors influencing the receptive fields of lamina 5 spinal cord cells. Exp. Brain Res., *9*:284–306, 1969.

100. Hinsey, J. C., and Gasser, H. S.: The component

of the dorsal root mediating vasodilation and the Sherrington contracture. Amer. J. Physiol. 92:679–689, 1930.

101. Hökfelt, T., Elde, R., Johansson, O., Luft, R., Nilsson, G., and Aremira, A.: Immunohistochemical evidence for separate populations of somatostatin-containing and substance P–containing primary afferent neurons in the rat. Neuroscience, 1:131–136, 1976.

101a. Hosobuchi, Y., Adams, J. E., and Linchitz, R.: Pain relief by electrical stimulation of the central gray matter in humans and its reversal by naloxone. Science, 197:183–186, 1977.

102. Hughes, J.: Isolation of an endogenous compound from the brain with pharmacological properties similar to morphine. Brain Res., 88:295–308, 1975.

103. Hughes, J., Smith, T., Morgan, B., and Fothergill, L.: Purification and properties of enkephalin—the possible ligand for the morphine receptor. In Goldstein, A., ed.: The Opiate Narcotics. New York, Pergamon Press, 1975, pp. 1–6.

104. Iggo, A., ed.: Pain and Itch: Nervous Mechanisms. CIBA Foundation Symposium. Boston, Little, Brown & Co., 1959.

105. Iggo, A., ed.: Handbook of Sensory Physiology. Vol. II. The Somatosensory System. New York, Springer-Verlag, 1973.

106. Iggo, A.: Activation of cutaneous nociceptors and their actions on dorsal horn neurons. Advances Neurol., 4:1–9, 1974.

107. Iggo, A.: Peripheral and spinal "pain" mechanisms and their modulation. In Bonica, J. J., and Albe-Fessard, D., eds.: Advances in Pain Research and Therapy. Vol. 1. New York, Raven Press, 1976, pp. 381–394.

108. Iggo, A., Ogawa, H., and Cervero, F.: Inhibition of nociceptor-driven dorsal horn neurons in the cat. In Bonica, J. J., and Albe-Fessard, D., eds.: Advances in Pain Research and Therapy. Vol. 1. New York, Raven Press, 1976, pp. 99–104.

109. Jansco, N., Jansco-Gabor, A., and Szolcsanyi, J.: Direct evidence for neurogenic inflammation and its prevention by denervation and by treatment with capsaicin. Brit. J. Pharmacol. Chemother., 31:138–151, 1967.

109a. Jessel, T. M., and Iversen, L. L.: Opiate analgesics inhibit substance P release from rat trigeminal nucleus. Nature, 268:549–551, 1977.

110. Jones, E. G., and Burton, H.: Cytoarchitecture and somatic sensory connectivity of thalamic nuclei other than the ventrobasal complex in the cat. J. Comp. Neurol., 154:395–432, 1974.

111. Jones, E. G., and Leavitt, R. Y.: Retrograde axonal transport and the demonstration of nonspecific projections to the cerebral cortex and striatum from the thalamic intralaminar nuclei in the rat, cat, and monkey. J. Comp. Neurol., 154:349–378, 1974.

112. Jones, E. G., and Powell, T. P. S.: The projection of the somatic sensory cortex upon the thalamus of the cat. Brain Res., 10:369–391, 1968.

113. Jones, E. G., and Powell, T. P. S.: Connexions of the rhesus monkey. I. Ipsilateral cortical connexions. Brain, 92:477–502, 1969.

114. Jones, E. G., and Powell, T. P. S.: Connections of the somatic sensory cortex of the rhesus monkey. II. Contralateral cortical connexions. Brain, 92:717–730, 1969.

115. Jones, E. G., and Powell, T. P. S.: Connections of the somatic sensory cortex of the rhesus monkey. III. Thalamic connexions. Brain, 93:37–56, 1970.

116. Kenshalo, D. R., ed.: The Skin Senses. Springfield, Ill., Charles C Thomas, 1968.

117. Kerr, F. W. L.: The organization of primary afferents in the subnucleus caudalis of the trigeminal: A light and electron microscope study of degeneration. Brain Res., 23:147–165, 1970.

118. Kerr, F. W. L.: Neuroanatomical substrates of nociception in the spinal cord. Pain, 1:325–356, 1975.

119. Kerr, F. W. L., and Lipman, H. H.: The primate spinothalamic tract as demonstrated by an anterolateral cordotomy and commissural myelotomy. Advances Neurol., 4:147–156, 1974.

120. Kitahata, L. M., Kosaka, Y., Taub, A., Bonikos, K., and Hoffert, M.: Lamina-specific suppression of dorsal-horn unit activity by morphine sulfate. Anesthesiology, 41:39–48, 1974.

121. Knighton, R. S., and Dumke, P. R., eds.: Pain. Boston, Little Brown & Co., 1966.

122. Konietzny, F., and Hensel, H.: Warm fiber activity in human skin nerves. Pfluger. Arch., 359:265–267, 1975.

123. Kornhuber, H. H., ed.: The Somatosensory System. Stuttgart, G.: Thieme, 1975.

124. Kreisman, N. R., and Zimmerman, I. D.: Representation of information about skin temperature in the discharge of single cortical neurons. Brain Res., 55:343–353, 1973.

125. Kuhar, M. J., Pert, C. B., and Snyder, S. H.: Regional distribution of opiate receptor binding in monkey and human brain. Nature, 245:447–450, 1973.

126. Kuhn, R. A.: Organization of tactile dermatomes in cat and monkey. J. Neurophysiol., 16:169–182, 1953.

127. Kumazawa, T., and Perl, E. R.: Excitation of marginal and substantia gelatinosa neurons in the primate spinal cord: Indications of their place in dorsal horn functional organization. J. Comp. Neurol., 177:417–434, 1978.

128. Kumazawa, T., Perl, E. R., Burgess, P. P., and Whitehorn, D.: Ascending projections from marginal zone (lamina I) neurons of the spinal dorsal horn. J. Comp. Neurol., 162:1–12, 1975.

129. Kuru, M.: Sensory paths in the spinal cord and brain stem of man. Tokyo, Sogensha Publishing Co., 1949.

130. LaMotte, C. C.: The Sensation of Warmth: Peripheral Neural Mechanisms (Ph.D. Thesis). Baltimore, Johns Hopkins University, 1972.

131. LaMotte, C.: Distribution of the tract of Lissauer and the dorsal root fibers in the primate spinal cord. J. Comp. Neurol., 172:529–561, 1977.

132. LaMotte, C.: Central projections of ventral root afferents and efferents diffusely labelled with HRP. Anat. Rec., 190:454, 1978.

132a. LaMotte, C., and de Lanerolle, N.: Human spinal neurons: Innervation by both substance P and enkephalin. Neuroscience, in press.

133. LaMotte, C., Pert, C. B., and Synder, S. H.:

Opiate receptor binding in primate spinal cord: Distribution and changes after dorsal root section. Brain Res., *112*:407–412, 1976.

134. LaMotte, C. C., Snowman, A., Pert, C. B., and Snyder, S. H.: Opiate receptor binding in rhesus monkey brain: Association with limbic structures. Brain Res., *155*:374–379, 1978.

135. LaMotte, R. H., and Campbell, J. N.: Comparison with the responses of "warm" and "nociceptive" C fiber afferents in monkey with human judgements of the thermal pain. J. Neurophysiol., *41*:509–528, 1978.

136. LaMotte, R. H., and Mountcastle, V. B.: Capacities of humans and monkeys to discriminate between vibratory stimuli of different frequency and amplitude: A correlation between neural events and psychophysical measurements. J. Neurophysiol., *38*:539–559, 1975.

137. Landon, D. N., ed.: The Peripheral Nerve. London, Chapman & Hall, 1976.

138. Lasek, R., Joseph, B. S., and Whitlock, D. G.: Evaluation of a radioautographic neuroanatomical tracing method. Brain Res., *8*:319–336, 1968.

139. LeBlanc, H. J., and Gatipon, G. B.: Medial bulboreticular response to peripherally applied noxious stimuli. Exp. Neurol., *42*:264–273, 1974.

140. Lende, R. A., Kirsch, W. M., and Druckman, R.: Relief of facial pain after combined removal of precentral and postcentral cortex. J. Neurosurg., *34*:537–543, 1971.

141. Lewin, W., and Phillips, C. G.: Observations on partial removal of the postcentral gyrus for pain. J. Neurol. Neurosurg. Psychiat., *15*:143–147, 1952.

142. Lewis, T.: Pain. New York, Macmillan Publishing Co., 1942.

143. Libet, B.: Electrical stimulation of cortex in human subjects, and conscious sensory aspects. *In* Iggo, A., ed.: Handbook of Sensory Physiology. Vol. II. The Somatosensory System. New York, Springer-Verlag, 1973, pp. 743–790.

144. Lieberman, A. R.: Sensory ganglia. *In* Landon, D. N., ed.: The Peripheral Nerve. London, Chapman & Hall, 1976, pp. 188–278.

145. Liebeskind, J. C.: Pain modulation by central nervous system stimulation. *In* Bonica, J. J., and Albe-Fessard D., eds.: Advances in Pain Research and Therapy. Vol. 1. New York, Raven Press, 1976, pp. 445–463.

146. Light, A. R., and Metz, C. B.: The morphology of the spinal cord efferent and afferent neurons contributing to the ventral roots of the cat. J. Comp. Neurol., *179*:501–516, 1978.

146a. Light, A. R., and Perl, E. R.: Reexamination of the dorsal root projection to the spinal dorsal horn including observations on the differential termination of coarse and fine fibers. J. Comp. Neurol., *186*:117–132, 1979.

146b. Light, A. R., and Perl, E. R.: Spinal termination of functionally identified primary afferent neurons with slowly conducting myelinated fibers. J. Comp. Neurol., *186*:133–150, 1979.

147. Loewenstein, W. R., ed.: Handbook of Sensory Physiology. Vol. 1. Principles of Receptor Physiology. New York, Springer-Verlag, 1971.

148. Long, R. R.: Sensitivity of cutaneous cold fibers to noxious heat: Paradoxical and cold discharge. J. Neurophysiol., *40*:489–502, 1977.

149. Marburg, D. L.: The effect on reaction to painful stimuli of lesions in the centromedian nucleus in the thalamus of the monkey. Int. J. Neurosci., *5*:153–158, 1973.

150. Maynard, C. W., Leonard, R. B., Coulter, J. D., and Coggeshall, R. E.: Central connections of ventral root afferents as demonstrated by the HRP method. J. Comp. Neurol., *172*:601–608, 1977.

151. Mehler, W. R.: Further notes on the centra median nucleus of Luys. *In* Purpura, D. P., and Yahr, M. D., eds.: The Thalamus. New York, Columbia University Press, 1966, pp. 109–217.

152. Mehler, W. R., Feferman, M. E., and Nauta, W. H. J.: Ascending axon degeneration following anterolateral cordotomy. Brain, *83*:718–750, 1960.

153. Melzack, M., and Wall, P. D.: On the nature of cutaneous sensory mechanisms. Brain, *85*:331–356, 1962.

154. Melzack, M., and Wall, P. D.: Pain mechanisms: A new theory. Science, *150*:971–979, 1965.

155. Miletic, V., Kovacs, M. S., and Randic, M.: Actions of somatostatin and methionine-enkephalin on cat dorsal horn neurons activated by noxious stimuli. Soc. Neurosci. Abst., *3*:488, 1977.

156. Moore, R. Y., and Goldberg, J. M.: Ascending projections of the inferior colliculus in the cat. J. Comp. Neurol., *121*:109–136, 1963.

157. Morin, F., Schwartz, H. G., and O'Leary, J. L.: Experimental study of the spinothalamic and related tracts. Acta Psychiat. Neurol. Scand., *26*:371–396, 1951.

158. Mountcastle, V. B.: Modality and topographic properties of single neurons of cat's somatic sensory cortex. J. Neurophysiol., *20*:408–434, 1957.

159. Mountcastle, V. B., and Powell, T. P. S.: Neural mechanisms subserving cutaneous sensibility, with special reference to the role of afferent inhibition in sensory perception and discrimination. Bull. Johns Hopk. Hosp., *105*:201–232, 1959.

160. Mountcastle, V. B., Talbot, W. H., Sakata, H., and Hyvarinen, J.: Cortical neuronal mechanisms in flutter-vibration studied in unanesthetized monkeys. Neuronal periodicity and frequency discrimination. J. Neurophysiol., *32*:452–484, 1969.

161. Munger, B. C.: Patterns of organization of peripheral sensory receptors. *In* Loewenstein, W. R., ed.: Handbook of Sensory Physiology. Vol. I. Principles of Receptor Physiology. New York, Springer-Verlag, 1971, pp. 524–553.

162. Nashold, B. S., Jr., Wilson, W. P., and Slaughter, G.: The midbrain and pain. Advances Neurol., *4*:191–196, 1974.

163. Nathan, P. W.: The gate-control theory of pain. Brain, *99*:123–158, 1976.

164. Nauta, W. J. H., and Kuypers, H. G. J. M.: Some ascending pathways in the brain stem reticular formation. *In* Jasper, H. H., ed.: Reticular Formation of the Brain. Henry Ford Hospital International Symposium. Boston, Little, Brown, & Co., 1958, pp. 3–30.

165. Oscarsson, O., Rosen, I., and Sulg, I.: Organiza-

tion of neurons in the cat cerebral cortex that are influenced from group I muscle afferents. J. Physiol. (London), *183*:189–210, 1966.

166. Osgood, C. P., Dujovny, M., and Faille, R.: Microsurgical lumbosacral ganglionectomy technique, anatomical rationale, and surgical results. *In* Bonica, J. J., and Albe-Fessard, D., eds.: Advances in Pain Research. Vol. 1. New York, Raven Press, 1976, pp. 99–104.

167. Pasternak, G. W., Goodman, R., and Snyder, S. H.: An endogenous morphine-like factor in mammalian brain. *In* Goldstein, A., ed.: The Opiate Narcotics. New York, Pergamon Press, 1975, pp. 13–17.

168. Payne, J. P., Burt, R. A. P., Janzen, R., Keidel, W. D., Herz, A., and Steichele, C., eds.: Pain: Basic Principles, Pharmacology, Therapy. London, Churchill Livingstone, 1972.

169. Pearl, G. S., and Anderson, K. V.: Effects of nociceptive and innocuous stimuli on the firing patterns of single neurons in the feline nucleus reticularis gigantocellularis. *In* Bonica, J. J., and Albe-Fessard, D., eds.: Advances in Pain Research and Therapy. Vol. I. New York, Raven Press, 1976, pp. 259–265.

170. Perl, E. R.: Myelinated afferent fibres innervating the primate skin and their response to noxious stimuli. J. Physiol. (London), *197*:593–615, 1968.

171. Perl, E. R., and Whitlock, D. G.: Somatic stimuli exciting spinothalamic projections to thalamic neurons in cat and monkey. Exp. Neurol., *3*:256–296, 1961.

172. Pert, A.: Analgesia produced by morphine microinjections in the primate brain. *In* Snyder, S. H., and Matthyssee, S., eds.: Opiate Receptor Mechanisms. Cambridge, MIT Press, 1975, pp. 87–91.

172a. Pickel, V. M., Reis, D. J., and Leeman, S. E.: Ultrastructural localization of substance P in neurons of rat spinal cord. Brain Res. *122*:534–540, 1977.

173. Poggio, G. F., and Mountcastle, V. B.: A study of the functional contributions of the lemniscal and spinothalamic systems to somatic sensibility. Bull. Johns Hopk. Hosp., *106*:266–316, 1960.

174. Poggio, G. F., and Mountcastle, V. B.: The functional properties of ventrobasal thalamic neurons studied in unanesthetized monkeys. J. Neurophysiol., *26*:775–806, 1963.

175. Pomeranz, B.: Specific nociceptive fibers projecting from spinal cord neurons to the brain: A possible pathway for pain. Brain Res., *50*:447–541, 1973.

176. Porter, L., and Semmes, J.: Preservation of cutaneous temperature sensitivity after ablation of sensory cortex in monkeys. Exp. Neurol., *42*:206–219, 1974.

177. Poulos, D. A., and Benjamin, R. M.: Response to thalamic neurons to thermal stimulation of the tongue. J. Neurophysiol., *31*:28–43, 1968.

178. Powell, T. P. S., and Mountcastle, V. B.: Some aspects of the functional organization of the cortex of the postcentral gyrus of the monkey: A correlation of findings obtained in a single unit analysis with cytoarchitecture. Bull. Johns Hopk. Hosp., *105*:133–163, 1959.

179. Price, D. D., and Browe, A. C.: Responses of spinal cord neurons to graded noxious and non-noxious stimuli. Brain Res., *64*:425–429, 1973.

180. Price, D. D., and Browe, A. C.: Spinal cord coding of graded nonnoxious and noxious temperature increases. Exp. Neurol., *48*:201–221, 1975.

181. Price, D. D., and Dubner, R.: Neurons that subserve the sensory-discriminative aspects of pain. Pain, *3*:307–338, 1977.

182. Price, D. D., Dubner, R., and Hu, J. W.: Trigeminothalamic neurons in nucleus caudalis responsive to tactile, thermal, and nociceptive stimulation of the monkey's face. J. Neurophysiol., *39*:936–953, 1976.

183. Price, D. D., Hu, J. W., Dubner, R., and Gracely, R. H.: Peripheral suppression of first pain and central summation of second pain evoked by noxious heat pulses. Pain, *3*:57–68, 1977.

184. Pubols, B. H., Jr., Welker, W. I., and Johnson, J. I., Jr.: Somatic sensory representation of forelimb in dorsal root fibers of racoon, coatimundi, and cat. J. Neurophysiol., *28*:312–341, 1965.

185. Pubols, L. M.: Somatic sensory representation in the thalamic ventrobasal complex of the spider monkey (Ateles). Brain Behav. Evol., *1*:305–323, 1968.

186. Ralston, H. J. III: The organization of substantia gelatinosa Rolandi in the cat lumbosacral spinal cord. Z. Zellforsch., *67*:1–23, 1965.

187. Ralston, H. J. III: Dorsal root projections to dorsal horn neurons in the cat spinal cord. J. Comp. Neurol., *132*:303–330, 1968.

188. Ralston, H. J. III: The fine structure of laminae I, II and III of the macaque spinal cord. J. Comp. Neurol., *184*:619–642, 1979.

189. Randic, M., and Miletic, V.: Actions of peptides on cat dorsal horn neurones activiated by noxious stimuli. *In* Ryall, R. W., and Kelley, J. S., eds.: Iontophoresis and Transmitter Mechanisms in the Mammalian CNS. Amsterdam, Elsevier–North Holland Publishing Co., 1977.

190. Randic, M., and Miletic, V.: Effect of substance P on cat dorsal horn neurons activated by noxious stimuli. Brain Res., *128*:164–169, 1977.

191. Ranson, S. W.: The tract of Lissauer and the substantia gelatinosa Rolandi. Amer. J. Anat., *16*:97–126, 1914.

192. Rethelyi, M.: Preterminal and terminal axon arborizations in the substantia gelatinosa of cat's spinal cord. J. Comp. Neurol., *172*:511–527, 1977.

193. Rethelyi, M., and Szentagothai, J.: The large synaptic complexes of the substantia gelatinosa. Exp. Brain. Res., *7*:258–274, 1969.

194. Rexed, B.: The cytoarchitectonic organization of the spinal cord in the cat. J. Comp. Neurol., *96*:416–496, 1952.

195. Richardson, D. E.: Thalamotomy for intractable pain. Confin. Neurol., *29*:139–145, 1967.

195a. Richardson, D. E., and Akil, H.: Pain reduction by electrical brain stimulation in man. I. Acute administration in periaqueductal and periventricular sites. J. Neurosurg., *47*:178–183, 1977.

195b. Richardson, E. E., and Akil, H.: Pain reduction by electrical brain stimulation in man. II.

Chronic self-administration in the periventricular gray matter. J. Neurosurg., *47*:184–194, 1977.

196. Roland, P. E.: Astereognosis. Arch. Neurol. (Chicago), *33*:543–550, 1976.

197. Rose, J. E., and Woolsey, C. N.: Cortical connections and functional organization of the thalamic auditory system of the cat. *In* Harlow, H. F., and Woolsey, C. N., eds.: Biological and Biochemical Bases of Behavior. Madison, Wis., University of Wisconsin Press, 1958, pp. 127–150.

197a. Sar, M., Stumpf, W. E., Miller, R. J., Chang, K. J., and Cuatrecasas P.: Immunohistochemical localization of enkephalin in rat brain and spinal cord. J. Comp. Neurol., *182*:17–38, 1978.

198. Satoh, M., Zieglgansberger, W., and Herz, A.: Interaction between morphine and putative excitatory neurotransmitters in cortical neurones in naive and tolerant rats. *In* Goldstein, A., ed.: The Opiate Narcotics. New York, Pergamon Press, 1975, pp. 229–234.

199. Scheibel, M. E., and Scheibel, A. B.: The organization of the nucleus reticularis thalami: A Golgi study. Brain Res., *1*:43–62, 1966.

200. Scheibel, M. E., and Scheibel, A. B.: Terminal axonal patterns in the cat spinal cord. II. The dorsal horn. Brain Res., *9*:32–58, 1968.

201. Schwartzman, R. J.: Thalamic sensory nuclear ablations in trained monkeys. Arch. Neurol. (Chicago), *23*:419–429, 1970.

202. Shealy, C. N., Mortimer, J. T., and Hagfors, N. R.: Dorsal column electroanalgesia. J. Neurosurg., *32*:560–564, 1970.

203. Shigenaga, Y., and Inoki, R.: Effect of morphine on single unit responses in ventrobasal complex (VB) and posterior nuclear group (PO) following tooth pulp stimulation. Brain Res., *103*:152–156, 1976.

204. Shigenaga, Y., Matano, S., Okada, K., and Sakai, A.: The effects of tooth pulp stimulation in the thalamus and hypothalamus of the rat. Brain Res., *63*:402–407, 1973.

204a. Simantov, R., Kuhar, M., Uhl, G., and Snyder, S.: Opioid peptide enkephalin: Immunohistochemical mapping in the rat central nervous system. Proc. Nat. Acad. Sci. (Wash.), *74*:2167–2171, 1977.

205. Sindou, M., Quoex, C., and Baleydier, C.: Fiber organization at the posterior spinal cord–rootlet junction in man. J. Comp. Neurol., *153*:15–26, 1974.

206. Smith, M. C.: Retrograde cell changes in human spinal cord after anterolateral cordotomies. Location and identification after different periods of survival. *In* Bonica, J. J., and Albe-Fessard, D., eds.: Advances in Pain Research and Therapy. Vol. I. New York, Raven Press, 1976, pp. 91–98.

207. Snyder, S. H.: Opiate receptors and internal opiates. Sci. Amer., *236*:44–56, 1977.

208. Snyder, S. H., and Matthysse, S.: Opiate Receptor Mechanisms. Cambridge, MIT Press, 1975.

209. Sprague, J. M., and Ha, H.: The terminal fields of dorsal root fibers in the lumbo-sacral spinal cords in the cat, and the dendritic organization of the motor nuclei. *In* Eccles, J. C. and

Schade, J. P., eds.: Progr. Brain Res., *2*:120–152, 1964.

210. Sterling, P., and Kuypers, H. G. J. M.: Anatomical organization of the brachial spinal cord of the cat. I. The distribution of dorsal root fibers. Brain Res., *4*:1–15, 1967.

211. Sumino, R., Dubner, R., and Starkman, S.: Responses of small myelinated "warm" fibers to noxious heat stimuli applied to the monkey's face. Brain Res., *62*:260–263, 1973.

212. Sweet, W. H., and Wepsic, J. G.: Stimulation of the posterior columns of the spinal cord for pain control: Indications, technique and results. Clin. Neurosurg., *21*:278–310, 1974.

213. Szentagothai, J.: Neuronal and synaptic arrangement in the substantia gelatinosa Rolandi. J. Comp. Neurol., *122*:219–240, 1964.

214. Takahashi, T., and Otsuka, M.: Regional distribution of substance P in the spinal cord and nerve roots of the cat and the effect of dorsal root section. Brain Res., *87*:1–11, 1975.

215. Tasker, R. R., Richardson, P., Reivcastle, B., and Emmers, R.: Anatomical correlation of detailed sensory mapping of the human thalamus. Confin. Neurol., *34*:184–196, 1972.

216. Taub, A., and Campbell, J. N.: Percutaneous local electrical analgesia: Peripheral mechanisms. Advances Neurol., *4*:727–732, 1974.

217. Terenius, L., and Wahlstrom, A.: Search for an endogenous ligand for the opiate receptor. Acta Physiol. Scand., *94*:74–81, 1975.

218. Terenius, L., and Wahlstrom, A.: Morphine-like ligand for opiate receptors in human CSF. *In* Goldstein, A., ed.: The Opiate Narcotics. New York, Pergamon Press, 1975, pp. 7–12.

219. Teschemacher, H., Opheim, K. E., Cox, B. M., and Goldstein, A.: A peptide-like substance from pituitary that acts like morphine. I. Isolation. *In* Goldstein, A., ed.: The Opiate Narcotics. New York, Pergamon Press, 1975, pp. 19–23.

220. Torebjörk, H. E.: Afferent C units responding to mechanical, thermal, and chemical stimuli in human non-glabrous skin. Acta Physiol. Scand., *92*:374–390, 1974.

221. Torebjörk, H. E., and Hallin, R. G.: Skin receptors supplied by unmyelinated (C) fibers in man. *In* Zotterman, Y., ed.: Sensory Functions of the Skin in Primates. Oxford, Pergamon Press, 1976, pp. 475–485.

222. Trevino, D. L., and Carstens, E.: Confirmation of the location of spinothalamic neurons in the cat and monkey by the retrograde transport of horseradish peroxidase. Brain Res., *98*:177–182, 1975.

223. Trevino, D. L., Coulter, J. P., and Willis, W. D.: Location of cells of origin of spinothalamic tract in lumbar enlargement of the monkey. J. Neurophysiol., *36*:750–761, 1973.

224. Van Hassel, H. J., Biedenbach, M. A., and Brown, A. C.: Cortical potentials evoked by tooth pulp stimulation in rhesus monkeys. Arch. Oral Biol., *17*:1059–1066, 1972.

225. Van Hees, J., and Gybels, J. M.: Pain related to single afferent C fibers from human skin. Brain Res., *48*:397–400, 1972.

226. Vyklicky, L., Keller, O. L., Brozek, G., and Butkhugr, S. M.: Cortical potentials evoked by

stimulation of tooth pulp afferents in the cat. Brain Res., *41*:211–213, 1972.

227. Wagman, I. H., and Price, D. D.: Responses of dorsal horn cells of M. mulatta to cutaneous and sural nerve A and C fiber stimuli. J. Neurophysiol., *32*:803–817, 1969.

228. Wallin, G., Torebjork, N. E., and Hallin, R. G.: Preliminary observations on the pathophysiology of hyperalgesia in the causalgic pain syndrome. *In* Zotterman, Y., ed.: Sensory Functions of the Skin in Primates. Oxford, Pergamon Press, 1976, pp. 489–499.

229. Westrum, L. E.: Early forms of terminal degeneration in the spinal trigeminal nucleus following rhizotomy. J. Neurocytol., *2*:189–215, 1973.

230. White, J. C., and Sweet, W. H.: Pain and the Neurosurgeon: A Forty Year Experience. Springfield, Ill., Charles C Thomas, 1969.

231. Whitsel, B. L., Petrucelli, L. M., and Werner, G.: Symmetry and connectivity in the map of the body surface in somatosensory area 11 of primates. J. Neurophysiol., *32*:170–183, 1969.

232. Wilcox, G. L., Luttges, M. W., and Mazer, D. J.:

Unit activity of substantia gelatinosa neurons. Soc. Neurosci. Abst. 1976, no. 1384.

233. Willis, W. D., Haber, L. H., and Martin, R. F.: Inhibition of spinothalamic tract cells and interneurons by brain-stem stimulation in the monkey. J. Neurophysiol., *40*:968–981, 1977.

234. Willis, W. D., Trevino, D. L., and Coulter, J. D.: Responses of primate spinothalamic tract neurons to natural stimulation of hindlimb. J. Neurophysiol., *37*:358–372, 1974.

235. Woda, A., Azerad, J., Guilbaud, G., and Besson, J. M.: Etude microphysiologique des projections de la pulpe dentaire chez le chat. Brain Res., *89*:193–213, 1975.

236. Yaksh, T. L.: Antinociceptive action of opiates in the spinal cords of cat and primate. Brain Res., *153*:205–210, 1978.

237. Yin, T. C. T., and Williams, W. J.: Dynamic response and transfer characteristics of joint neurons in somatosensory thalamus of the cat. J. Neurophysiol., *39*:582–600, 1976.

238. Zotterman, Y., ed.: Sensory Functions of the Skin in Primates. Oxford, Pergamon Press, 1976.

PSYCHIATRIC CONSIDERATIONS OF PAIN

Pain is a subjective experience. Most efforts to measure and understand it are woefully inadequate. In an attempt to define and quantify pain, Beecher cited some 850 references.[6] His conclusion was simple. Because pain is subjective, it cannot be described so that it is meaningful to another person. A quandary arises when a physician attempts to treat a patient with chronic pain. Many times the question becomes one of distinguishing real from imagined pain, which is a futile gesture.[102] Engel and Melzak and Chapman emphasize that the cortical perception of pain is essential for its verbalization.[26,64] It is this verbalization that is critical. Many tests designed to quantify and diagnose pain are themselves subjective. The physician asks, "How much does that hurt?" or, "Is this sharper or duller?" as the sensory portion of the neurological examination proceeds. Because of the difficulty in quantifying pain, a number of diagnostic tricks have evolved that are designed to obtain objective data from patients who say they are in pain.

Many articles concerning pain have been written by psychiatrists, psychologists, anesthesiologists, and neurosurgeons.* These specialists agree that the causes of this complaint are multifaceted and range from entirely neurophysiological to entirely psychiatric. Indeed, the diagnosis of pain in some respects resembles the diagnosis of schizophrenia: there are many potential causes, myriad subtypes within the broader classification, and overlapping features between the subtypes. This chapter delineates the subtypes of patients with chronic pain within categories that help to conceptualize them and will give insight into the best treatment modality for them and their natural course and prognosis.

The temporal component of chronic pain is an important and often overlooked factor. There is an obvious distinction between chronic and acute pain, both in its perception and in its treatment.[41,104] There are, however, many psychological factors associated with the acute pain process that may manifest themselves in patients with chronic pain, so a brief discussion of acute pain is in order.

Beecher reported that men who were wounded on the battlefield could experience severe pain and yet be far less likely to ask for morphine than a matched group of civilians undergoing major operations.[5] Only 32 per cent of the war-wounded patients requested narcotics, but 83 per cent of the operative patients asked for pain relief. Of course, the latter group was in a setting far different from that of the soldiers. To the civilians, an operation meant anxiety, illness, and possible disaster. Further, the civilian is removed from a comfortable home setting and placed in a frightening environment in the hospital. In contrast, an injury to the soldier meant his removal from combat, and getting out of combat reduced his anxiety. The difference in anxiety levels plus other factors in these two situations influenced the perception of acute pain. It is of interest that a double-blind investigation by Montilla and co-workers showed that 15 mg of a phenothiazine tranquilizer was as

---

* See references 10, 12, 30, 42, 57, 64, 72, 84, 86, 92, 104.

effective as 10 mg of morphine in reducing or relieving postoperative pain.[68]

Another cause of acute anxiety and pain is childbirth. The Lamaze technique is helpful in alleviating these adverse conditions. The technique employs two useful components, of which the first is called psychoprophylaxis.[13] It prepares the mother for the delivery by providing extensive instruction and thoroughly familiarizing her with the medical and practical aspects of pregnancy and delivery. The concept is simple. Anxiety is the result of an unrealistic fear of the unknown or a real fear based on misinformation. By making the delivery less of a mystery, less fearful, the Lamaze technique had good to excellent results in 65 per cent of the women who used it insofar as they requested little or no analgesics or anesthetics during delivery and reported less anxiety. If anxiety states that vary in intensity and fluctuate over time are carefully differentiated from anxiety as a personality disposition that remains relatively constant, there is a direct correlation between the degree of anxiety and the subjective appreciation of pain. Patients who have normal personality traits but are extremely anxious experience as much postoperative pain as patients who are anxiety-prone.[61] Thus, the anxiety-reducing predelivery education is one way in which the Lamaze technique works. The other useful component is the element of self-hypnosis. The self-hypnosis is similar to Hartland's ego-strengthening routine, or autogenic relaxation, which serves to distract the patient from the acute pain.[83] In these acute pain states narcotic analgesics, alone or in combination with hydroxyzine, are quite effective.[33] The nonnarcotic antianxiety drug hydroxyzine, however, is as effective as morphine, and a 100-mg intramuscular dose of hydroxyzine is as effective as an 8-mg intramuscular dose of morphine.[4,5]

The anticipation of pain produces anxiety, and the pain threshold is lowered by the anxiety.[15,20,21,25] This fact has led to the use of an antianxiety drug (diazepam) to reduce the fear-related components in the perception of acute pain. The tranquilizing drug allows the patient to tolerate pain for a longer period of time than can an untranquilized patient.[16] The anxiety-reducing properties of morphine may, in part, account for its analgesic effect in acute pain.[45] The setting in which the acute pain is experienced also does much to determine the perception of its intensity. Indeed, the setting or situation appears to have more of an influence on the perception of acute pain than does the personality of the patient.[56] This fact holds true for both the perception and the tolerance of acute pain, and creates the need to distinguish between traits that are personality types that are resistant to change over time and states that are immediate conditions surrounding the experience of acute pain.[61,70] In fact, even under hypnosis, it is possible to have two levels of acute pain perception. Thus, the state of a patient prior to and during acutely painful experiences is a most critical factor in determining subjective responses.[54]

From studies of acute pain, useful concepts regarding chronic pain have evolved. The first, almost obvious, conclusion is that the anticipation of the acute pain produces anxiety even in a normal individual.[21,61] Therefore one can imagine the anxiety a patient with chronic pain must experience upon arising every morning to face another day in the expectation of pain. Acute pain per se has a useful purpose. It warns the patient that something is amiss. Chronic pain merely reminds and nags. The chronic pain produces fears, anxiety, and depression, all of which can influence even the most well-adjusted individual.

If acute pain is examined from a psychiatric rather than a physiological viewpoint, the perspective is different. The acute pain may be the result of an event that was especially traumatic in terms of its psychiatric impact. Examples of this component are found in what are called post-traumatic neuroses.[52]

These neuroses may arise from car accidents in which a loved one was killed and the patient was only injured or from the death or severe wounding of a close friend while the patient suffered minimal damage but was forced to look on helplessly as the event took place. They may arise from injury suffered under frightening circumstances in which fear of death or paralysis was more intense than the actual injury itself. Additionally, persons with a psychiatric predisposition to utilize illness or injury may exaggerate the extent and severity of their injury. These patients often complain of chronic pain. The result may be influenced by or be due to their pathological condition, family reinforcement, iatrogenically induced narcotics addiction, or post-operative pain states.

In categorizing patients with chronic pain, many factors must be considered. The premorbid adjustment, or what the patient was like before he began to experience pain, is important. Another factor is the chronicity of the pain, i.e., at which stage in the entire experience of chronic pain is the patient situated? Is the pain acute, sub-acute, subchronic, or chronic? Another consideration is whether the pain was spontaneous or traumatic in origin.

The social setting is important, as is the health of the spouse or parents. Economic factors such as workmen's compensation, social security disability allowances, and unemployment payments also alter the situation, and the patient's present income and preinjury income levels need to be compared. The location of the pain, the description of the quality of the pain, and the degree of limitation reported and objectively determined are important factors. Finally, a thorough medical and psychiatric history is essential. After assembling these data, one can assign the patient with chronic pain to one of four groups.

The first group of patients with chronic pain are those with a good premorbid adjustment, both psychiatrically and sociologically, who have organically definable lesions with positive objective findings. Regardless of where the patient is in his "pain experience," it is apparent that pain has adversely affected his life. He has a definite basis for his chronic pain and may be experiencing psychiatric difficulties as the result of it.

The second broad category includes the patient with chronic pain who has a good psychiatric adjustment prior to his pain but whose pain has an undefinable or undetermined cause. He follows the same pattern as the patient with objective pain in that he experiences difficulties in his life as the result of the chronic pain.

The third group of patients with chronic pain have a mixed collection of psychiatric disorders involving abnormal personality types, neuroses, organic brain disease, and even psychosis. These patients have an organic cause for their chronic pain but have a premorbid, or prepain, adjustment that is suggestive of psychiatric problems. The disability of these patients is disproportion-ate to the degree of their organic impairment. The effect of chronic pain on their lives is overstated, and they may be considered to be patients with exaggerated pain. Pain from muscle tension and pain as the result of anxiety fall into this category. Since in these patients anxiety produces the effect of pain, they could be said to have "effected" pain.

The fourth group of patients with chronic pain is again a motley collection including those with psychoses, post-traumatic neuroses, depressive equivalents, and the like, and those who are malingering. They had psychiatric difficulties prior to the onset of their pain, but deny this fact and wish to attribute all problems to their pain. No organic basis can be found for their pain, and frequently, there is a disturbance of mood or thought processes.

The four categories are not rigidly drawn. In some cases a patient may overlap two or more categories. It is hoped that this introduction will serve as a framework to aid in the conceptualization of the types of patients with chronic pain and furnish guidelines for their treatment. The primary intent of this categorization is to establish homogeneous groups whose pain has a common etiology, follows a similar clinical course, and has a consistent response or lack of response to treatment. The four categories and the subtypes within them follow criteria outlined by Guze for establishing a valid psychiatric diagnosis that adheres to a medical model.[39] Although these categories are based for the most part on retrospective data, the necessity for a prospective confirmation is recognized.

PATIENTS WITH OBJECTIVE PAIN

Much has been written on the diagnosis and evaluation of psychiatric patients who present with the complaint of pain. Little information, however, can be found about, nor does there seem to be much attention paid to, the plight of the normal individual who is burdened by the disability of chronic pain. This situation may be due to the physician's frustration in providing adequate relief or to his sense of futility in even trying. The chronic pain discussed in this section specifically excludes that associated with terminal cancer. Even though there are many similarities between cancer pain and noncancer pain, the differences are so significant as to set apart the treatment of patients with cancer from that of the patients who are discussed in this section.

Pain of Identified Organic Origin

Etiology

There are many causes of organically produced chronic pain. They include sympathetic dystrophies, neuromas, peripheral neuropathies, postoperative complications of laminectomies, arachnoiditis, and central thalamic pain. Regardless of the cause, the common feature of chronicity is unrelenting intrusion of pain into a patient's life.

Pathology

In determining the validity of the complaint of chronic pain, it is necessary to rely more on objective tests, and to give less credence to tests that require a subjective interpretation. Positive findings in electromyographic and nerve conduction tests, deep tendon reflexes, muscle atrophy, and anatomical distribution all lend credence to the concept of a true organic basis for chronic pain. Recently, advances in thermography have made this a useful tool in accessing thermal involvement.[98] Of course, x-ray and computed tomography (CT), as well as bone scans, have enlarged the surgeon's diagnostic armamentarium. In recent years, biofeedback instruments, which measure muscle tension and temperature by means of surface electrodes, if of a sufficiently sensitive quality, can be used as recording devices for continuous monitoring of skin temperature and muscle tension. The more positive the objective test, the less one must rely on subjective examinations, which are always prone to faulty interpretation by the physician or adulteration by the patient.

Symptoms and Clinical Course

Since the causes vary so much, there are no pathognomonic symptoms of chronic pain due to an organic lesion. Patients with objective pain do have distinct similarities, however.

Premorbid Symptoms

Typically, the patient with objective pain has been married only once, has not been divorced or separated, has no financial difficulties, and has a good work record that shows steady advancement in pay and responsibility. There is no history of alcoholism or drug abuse in either the patient or his spouse. There has been no history of psychiatric problems in the patient or his family. Also, he has some hobbies, and his sexual relations are good. There is no evidence of dependent behavior, i.e., living at home with parents until the age of 30, or fear of not getting another job that causes him to remain in one even though he dislikes it. Usually there is no history of litigation.

Acute Pain (Up to Two Months)

During this period the patient with objective pain usually responds to acute pain by being more active than his physician recommended. He returns to work at an early date, shrugs off the disability, and expects the pain to subside in the near future. He may be somewhat "brave" about it, even stoical, kidding with both the doctor and members of the family. Typically, the score on the Minnesota Multiphasic Personality Inventory (MMPI) is normal. Also, the score on the Symptom Check List of 90 Questions (SCL-90), which correlates very well with the MMPI, is normal (Fig. 116–1). It should be noted that the SCL-90 takes only 20 minutes to complete and can measure changes in personality over given periods of time, which is not true for the MMPI.[24]

Subacute Pain (Two to Six Months)

By two to six months the pain is beginning to wear on the patient with objective pain, and the symptom check list begins to show signs of change. Scores on scales 1 and 3 on the MMPI are elevated, which indicates hypochondriasis and hysteria, the so-called "conversion V" seen in hysterical conversion reactions.[92] On the SCL-90, the score for the somatization scale is found to be elevated, while that for the depression scale is found to be normal, and this suggests that the patient with objective pain has not yet begun to experience the depression that chronic pain can bring. This

SCL-90-R

Name:_____   Technician:_____Ident. No._____

Location:_____   Visit No.:_____   Mode: S-R_____ Nar_____

Age:_____ Sex: M_____F_____Date:_____   Remarks:_____

INSTRUCTIONS

Below is a list of problems and complaints that people sometimes have. Read each one carefully, and select one of the numbered descriptors that best describes HOW MUCH DISCOMFORT THAT PROBLEM HAS CAUSED YOU DURING THE PAST_____INCLUDING TODAY. Place that number in the open block to the right of the problem. Do not skip any items, and print your number clearly. If you change your mind, erase your first number completely. Read the example below before beginning, and if you have any questions please ask the technician.

EXAMPLE

HOW MUCH WERE YOU DISTRESSED BY:

Descriptors
0 Not at all
1 A little bit
2 Moderately
3 Quite a bit
4 Extremely

Ex. Body Aches........... Ex. [3]   **Answer**

HOW MUCH WERE YOU DISTRESSED BY:

Descriptors
0 Not at all
1 A little bit
2 Moderately
3 Quite a bit
4 Extremely

1. Headaches.....................................☐
2. Nervousness or shakiness inside ....☐
3. Repeated unpleasant thoughts that won't leave your mind..☐
4. Faintness or dizziness..........................☐
5. Loss of sexual interest or pleasure..................☐
6. Feeling critical of others......................☐
7. The idea that someone else can control your thoughts ....☐
8. Feeling others are to blame for most of your troubles.....☐
9. Trouble remembering things ....☐
10. Worried about sloppiness or carelessness ....☐
11. Feeling easily annoyed or irritated ....☐
12. Pains in heart or chest ....☐
13. Feeling afraid in open spaces or on the streets ....☐
14. Feeling low in energy or slowed down ....☐
15. Thoughts of ending your life.....................☐
16. Hearing voices that other people do not hear ....☐
17. Trembling ....☐
18. Feeling that most people cannot be trusted ....☐
19. Poor appetite ....☐
20. Crying easily ....☐
21. Feeling shy or uneasy with the opposite sex..........☐
22. Feelings of being trapped or caught.................☐
23. Suddenly scared for no reason ....☐
24. Temper outbursts that you could not control..........☐
25. Feeling afraid to go out of your house alone..........☐
26. Blaming yourself for things ....☐
27. Pains in lower back ....☐

28. Feeling blocked in getting things done ....☐
29. Feeling lonely ....☐
30. Feeling blue ....☐
31. Worrying too much about things ....☐
32. Feeling no interest in things.....................☐
33. Feeling fearful ....☐
34. Your feelings being easily hurt ....☐
35. Other people being aware of your private thoughts .....☐
36. Feeling others do not understand you or are unsympathetic ....☐
37. Feeling that people are unfriendly or dislike you........☐
38. Having to do things very slowly to insure correctness ...☐
39. Heart pounding or racing........................☐
40. Nausea or upset stomach ....☐
41. Feeling inferior to others ....☐
42. Soreness of your muscles........................☐
43. Feeling that you are watched or talked about by others..☐
44. Trouble falling asleep ....☐
45. Having to check and doublecheck what you do ....☐
46. Difficulty making decisions ....☐
47. Feeling afraid to travel on buses, subways, or trains.....☐
48. Trouble getting your breath ....☐
49. Hot or cold spells ....☐
50. Having to avoid certain things, places, or activities because they frighten you ....☐
51. Your mind going blank ....☐
52. Numbness or tingling in parts of your body. ....☐

PAGE ONE

PLEASE CONTINUE ON THE FOLLOWING PAGE ▷

Figure 116–1   SCL-90-R psychological profile test—a 20-minute, 90-question personality inventory that is able to determine changes in objective ratings of anxiety, depression, somatic concern, phobias, and other psychological variables with as little as a five-day interval between test administration.

Illustration continued on opposite page

SCL-90-R

HOW MUCH WERE YOU DISTRESSED BY:	Descriptors 0 Not at all 1 A little bit 2 Moderately 3 Quite a bit 4 Extremely	HOW MUCH WERE YOU DISTRESSED BY:	Descriptors 0 Not at all 1 A little bit 2 Moderately 3 Quite a bit 4 Extremely
53. A lump in your throat	☐	71. Feeling everything is an effort	☐
54. Feeling hopeless about the future	☐	72. Spells of terror or panic	☐
55. Trouble concentrating	☐	73. Feeling uncomfortable about eating or drinking in public.	☐
56. Feeling weak in parts of your body	☐	74. Getting into frequent arguments	☐
57. Feeling tense or keyed up	☐	75. Feeling nervous when you are left alone.	☐
58. Heavy feelings in your arms or legs	☐	76. Others not giving you proper credit for your achievements	☐
59. Thoughts of death or dying	☐	77. Feeling lonely even when you are with people	☐
60. Overeating	☐	78. Feeling so restless you couldn't sit still	☐
61. Feeling uneasy when people are watching or talking about you	☐	79. Feelings of worthlessness	☐
62. Having thoughts that are not your own	☐	80. The feeling that something bad is going to happen to you	☐
63. Having urges to beat, injure, or harm someone	☐	81. Shouting or throwing things	☐
64. Awakening in the early morning	☐	82. Feeling afraid you will faint in public	☐
65. Having to repeat the same actions such as touching, counting, washing	☐	83. Feeling that people will take advantage of you if you let them	☐
66. Sleep that is restless or disturbed	☐	84. Having thoughts about sex that bother you a lot	☐
67. Having urges to break or smash things	☐	85. The idea that you should be punished for your sins	☐
68. Having ideas or beliefs that others do not share	☐	86. Thoughts and images of a frightening nature	☐
69. Feeling very self-conscious with others	☐	87. The idea that something serious is wrong with your body	☐
70. Feeling uneasy in crowds, such as shopping or at a movie	☐	88. Never feeling close to another person	☐
		89. Feelings of guilt	☐
		90. The idea that something is wrong with your mind.	☐

Figure 116-1 (*continued*)

Illustration continued on following page

stage occurs early in the entire chronic pain process and corresponds to the denial stage of the dying patient, as outlined by Kubler-Ross.[44,55] Since the patient with the objective pain is denying that he is going to face chronic disability, there is no evidence of depression. He still retains hope that the pain and disability, i.e., "loss of a loved object," will be resolved. Subtle changes in personality may begin to occur. The changes may be manifested as increased irritability, difficulty in going to sleep, being awakened from sleep by pain, social isolation, and the beginning of the use of analgesics and sleeping medication.

Chronic Pain
(Six Months to Eight Years)

Pain of this duration will cause even a previously stable patient with objective pain to begin to experience depression. His MMPI scores will begin to show the "neu-rotic triad," i.e., abnormally high scores for hypochrondriasis (scale 1), depression (scale 2), and hysteria (scale 3).[92] Using the SCL-90, one finds self-reports of somatization, obsessive-compulsiveness, interpersonal sensitivity, depression, anxiety, and hostility to be increased.[44] These changes indicate that the patient with objective pain may have begun to have suicidal thoughts, may have stopped or reduced work because of his pain, and recognizes the possibility that the pain may persist. The depression alternates with feelings of anger and attempts to bargain with physicians about pain relief, i.e., "just to get rid of 50 per cent of this pain . . ."; this stage corresponds to the advanced stages of a dying patient.[55] This comparison may seem extreme; however, it must be remembered that the patient with objective pain and the dying patient have experienced losses, either of function or of hope, and are trying to learn to cope with the loss.[44] Also, by this

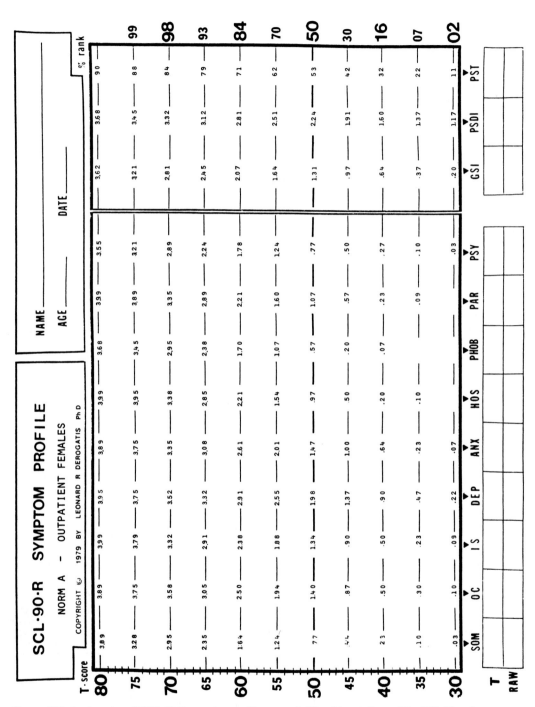

Figure 116–1 (*continued*) SCL-90-R symptom profile, norm A. The abbreviations of the SCL-90 scale represent: som, somatic concern; O-C., obsessive-compulsiveness; I-S., interpersonal sensitivity; dep., depression; anx., anxiety; hos., hostility; phob., phobia; par., paranoia; psy., psychoticism; GSI, general severity index; PSDI, positive symptom distress index; PST, positive symptom total.

Illustration continued on opposite page

SCL-90-R: COMPUTATION OF FACTOR SCORES

SOMATIZATION		OBSESSIVE-COMPULSIVE		INTERPERSONAL SENSITIVITY	
ITEM	SCORE	ITEM	SCORE	ITEM	SCORE
1. HEADACHES	1	3. REPEATED UNPLEASANT THOUGHTS THAT WON'T LEAVE YOUR MIND	3	6. FEELING CRITICAL OF OTHERS	6
4. FAINTNESS OR DIZZINESS	4	9. TROUBLE REMEMBERING THINGS	9	21. FEELING SHY OR UNEASY WITH THE OPPOSITE SEX	21
12. PAINS IN HEART OR CHEST	12	10. WORRIED ABOUT SLOPPINESS OR CARELESSNESS	10	34. YOUR FEELINGS BEING EASILY HURT	34
27. PAINS IN LOWER BACK	27	28. FEELING BLOCKED IN GETTING THINGS DONE	28	36. FEELING OTHERS DO NOT UNDERSTAND YOU OR ARE UNSYMPATHETIC	36
40. NAUSEA OR UPSET STOMACH	40	38. HAVING TO DO THINGS VERY SLOWLY TO INSURE CORRECTNESS	38	37. FEELING THAT PEOPLE ARE UNFRIENDLY OR DISLIKE YOU	37
42. SORENESS OF YOUR MUSCLES	42	45. HAVING TO CHECK AND DOUBLE CHECK WHAT YOU DO	45	41. FEELING INFERIOR TO OTHERS	41
48. TROUBLE GETTING YOUR BREATH	48	46. DIFFICULTY MAKING DECISIONS	46	61. FEELING UNEASY WHEN PEOPLE ARE WATCHING OR TALKING ABOUT YOU	61
49. HOT OR COLD SPELLS	49	51. YOUR MIND GOING BLANK	51	69. FEELING VERY SELF-CONSCIOUS WITH OTHERS	69
52. NUMBNESS OR TINGLING IN PARTS OF YOUR BODY	52	55. TROUBLE CONCENTRATING	55	73. FEELING UNCOMFORTABLE ABOUT EATING OR DRINKING IN PUBLIC	73
53. A LUMP IN YOUR THROAT	53	65. HAVING TO REPEAT THE SAME ACTIONS SUCH AS TOUCHING, COUNTING, WASHING	65		
56. FEELING WEAK IN PARTS OF YOUR BODY	56				
58. HEAVY FEELINGS IN YOUR ARMS OR LEGS	58				
TOTAL ITEM SCORE / 12		TOTAL ITEM SCORE / 10		TOTAL ITEM SCORE / 9	

DEPRESSION		ANXIETY		HOSTILITY	
5. LOSS OF SEXUAL INTEREST OR PLEASURE	5	2. NERVOUSNESS OR SHAKINESS INSIDE	2	11. FEELING EASILY ANNOYED OR IRRITATED	11
14. FEELING LOW IN ENERGY OR SLOWED DOWN	14	17. TREMBLING	17	24. TEMPER OUTBURSTS THAT YOU COULD NOT CONTROL	24
15. THOUGHTS OF ENDING YOUR LIFE	15	23. SUDDENLY SCARED FOR NO REASON	23	63. HAVING URGES TO BEAT, INJURE, OR HARM SOMEONE	63
20. CRYING EASILY	20	33. FEELING FEARFUL	33	67. HAVING URGES TO BREAK OR SMASH THINGS	67
22. FEELING OF BEING CAUGHT OR TRAPPED	22	39. HEART POUNDING OR RACING	39	74. GETTING INTO FREQUENT ARGUMENTS	74
26. BLAMING YOURSELF FOR THINGS	26	57. FEELING TENSE OR KEYED UP	57	81. SHOUTING OR THROWING THINGS	81
29. FEELING LONELY	29	72. SPELLS OF TERROR OR PANIC	72		
30. FEELING BLUE	30	78. FEELING SO RESTLESS YOU COULDN'T SIT STILL	78		
31. WORRYING TOO MUCH ABOUT THINGS	31	80. THE FEELING THAT SOMETHING BAD IS GOING TO HAPPEN TO YOU	80		
32. FEELING NO INTEREST IN THINGS	32	86. THOUGHTS AND IMAGES OF A FRIGHTENING NATURE	86		
54. FEELING HOPELESS ABOUT THE FUTURE	54				
71. FEELING EVERYTHING IS AN EFFORT	71				
79. FEELINGS OF WORTHLESSNESS	79				
TOTAL ITEM SCORE / 13		TOTAL ITEM SCORE / 10		TOTAL ITEM SCORE / 6	

PHOBIC ANXIETY		PARANOID IDEATION		PSYCHOTICISM	
13. FEELING AFRAID IN OPEN SPACES OR IN THE STREETS	13	8. FEELING OTHERS ARE TO BLAME FOR MOST OF YOUR TROUBLES	8	7. THE IDEA THAT SOMEONE ELSE CAN CONTROL YOUR THOUGHTS	7
25. FEELING AFRAID TO GO OUT OF YOUR HOUSE ALONE	25	18. FEELING THAT MOST PEOPLE CAN NOT BE TRUSTED	18	16. HEARING VOICES THAT OTHER PEOPLE DO NOT HEAR	16
47. FEELING AFRAID TO TRAVEL ON BUSES, SUBWAYS, OR TRAINS	47	43. FEELING THAT YOU ARE WATCHED OR TALKED ABOUT BY OTHERS	43	35. OTHER PEOPLE BEING AWARE OF YOUR PRIVATE THOUGHTS	35
50. HAVING TO AVOID CERTAIN THINGS, PLACES, OR ACTIVITIES BECAUSE THEY FRIGHTEN YOU	50	68. HAVING IDEAS OR BELIEFS THAT OTHERS DO NOT SHARE	68	62. HAVING THOUGHTS THAT ARE NOT YOUR OWN	62
70. FEELING UNEASY IN CROWDS, SUCH AS SHOPPING OR AT A MOVIE	70	76. OTHERS NOT GIVING YOU PROPER CREDIT FOR YOUR ACHIEVEMENTS	76	77. FEELING LONELY EVEN WHEN YOU ARE WITH PEOPLE	77
75. FEELING NERVOUS WHEN YOU ARE LEFT ALONE	75	83. FEELING THAT PEOPLE WILL TAKE ADVANTAGE OF YOU IF YOU LET THEM	83	84. HAVING THOUGHTS ABOUT SEX THAT BOTHER YOU A LOT	84
82. FEELING AFRAID YOU WILL FAINT IN PUBLIC	82			85. THE IDEA THAT YOU SHOULD BE PUNISHED FOR YOUR SINS	85
				87. THE IDEA THAT SOMETHING SERIOUS IS WRONG WITH YOUR BODY	87
				88. NEVER FEELING CLOSE TO OTHER PERSON	88
				90. THE IDEA THAT SOMETHING IS WRONG WITH YOUR MIND	90
TOTAL ITEM SCORE / 7		TOTAL ITEM SCORE / 6		TOTAL ITEM SCORE / 10	

ADDITIONAL ITEMS	
19. POOR APPETITE	19
60. OVEREATING	60
44. TROUBLE FALLING ASLEEP	44
64. AWAKENING IN THE EARLY MORNING	64
66. SLEEP THAT IS RESTLESS OR DISTURBED	66
59. THOUGHTS OF DEATH OR DYING	59
89. FEELINGS OF GUILT	89

SYMPTOM	TOTAL	N	RAW SCORES
SOMATIZATION			
OBSESS-COMPULSIVE			
INTER SENSITIVITY			
DEPRESSION			
ANXIETY			
HOSTILITY			
PHOBIC ANXIETY			
PARANOID IDEATION			
PSYCHOTICISM			
ADDITIONAL			

GLOBAL SCORES

GRAND TOTAL

1 GSI (GRAND TOTAL/90) 1 _____

2 PST 2 _____

3 PSDI (GT/PST) 3 _____

Figure 116–1 (*continued*) Computation of factor scores for SCL-90-R psychological profile test. (Copyright 1975, Leonard R. Derogatis, Ph.D., Clinical Psychometric Research. Reprinted by permission.)

stage the patient with chronic pain is experiencing trouble with his marriage, his sexual activity is reduced, and he begins to feel that he is a burden to his family and friends. He has lost some self-esteem, and questions, "Why me?" He may be abusing narcotics, have begun to "doctor shop," have had several additional operative procedures, and have feelings of guilt. His sleep pattern is disturbed, with difficulty falling asleep due as much to anxiety and depression as it is to pain, and awakening due to pain. Even depression may be reported. There may be weight loss due to reduced appetite secondary to depression, or weight gain due to reduced exercise secondary to limitation by pain. Usually the patient reports feeling hopeless and helpless, the classic manifestations of depression and anxiety. If he truly has objective pain, he is entitled to feel this way.[75,104]

Subchronic Pain
(Three to Twelve or More Years)

At this stage, the patient with objective pain has "learned to live with the pain," but still does not accept it. In fact, he never accepts either the pain or the attendant disability. In this way he differs from the dying patient, who appears peaceful in the final acceptance of death.[55] Unfortunately, the patient with objective pain has an indeterminate sentence and a more chronic, long-term course. By 3 to 12 years' time, he has discontinued narcotics, has changed his job or is functioning at his old job with almost the same degree of efficiency, and sexual activity has returned. His sleep is less disturbed, and the depression has been resolved. His marriage has either ended or has consolidated. The MMPI and SCL-90 scores show hypochondriasis or somatic concern (SOM). The depression scale scores are again low on the SCL-90, but because of the structure of the questions on the MMPI, it may not have returned to normal. At this time, the patient's faith in treatment is a lot less evangelical than in the earlier stages, and he is beginning to settle into a readjusted life style that demands coping with the chronic pain.

Diagnosis and Differential Diagnosis

In the subacute stage, the differential diagnosis of objective pain includes conversion of hysterical personality. The patient with objective pain is distinguished by a good premorbid (prepain) adjustment to life and a willingness to discard analgesics and sleeping medication. Findings on the physical examination are definitely positive, and objective and subjective evaluations coincide. One or more of the foregoing factors may be absent in conversion or in hysterical personalities. In the chronic stage, however, the patient with objective pain differs from the anxious and depressed patient in that he had a good premorbid adjustment, had no recent changes in life situations prior to the onset of the pain, and has objective physical findings. The patient with objective pain is more likely to be awakened from sleep by pain, which is unlike the anxious or depressed patient, who reports difficulty falling asleep and may attribute this not to pain per se but to worry about the pain or about something else. In the subchronic stage, the patient with objective pain is easily recognized. He can adequately describe the various stages of the chronic pain, starting with the good premorbid adjustment. Because of the absence of depression, the MMPI at this stage is not accurate, and reliance on only this diagnostic test will result in mistakenly confusing the patient with objective pain with the patient who has a psychosomatic problem. The inaccuracy of the MMPI is the result of the adjustment of the patient with objective pain to the chronic pain problem, not to a lack of concern or even to the hope of secondary gain seen in more obvious psychiatric disorders.

Since the MMPI has proved somewhat inadequate for the diagnosis of chronic pain, a 15-question screening test has been developed at the Chronic Pain Treatment Center at the Johns Hopkins Hospital (Table 116–1). A physician can administer the test in 10 minutes and be certain of his diagnosis approximately 85 per cent of the time. Nurses, physician's assistants, nurse practitioners, and psychologists can be trained to administer the test, thereby freeing the physician's time and providing him with an estimate of the validity of the patient's complaint and an approximation of the patient's psychological state. This test was designed not to replace the psychiatric evaluation but merely to allow a nonpsychiatric physician to assess quickly the degree of psychiatric overlay involved in the expression of chronic pain.

Treatment

Treatment of the patient with objective pain really begins in the subacute stage, at which time it is imperative to prevent iatrogenic addiction. The most commonly abused drugs during this stage, and during the subchronic stage, are oxycodone (Percodan), meperidine (Demerol), propoxyphene (Darvon), codeine, diazepam (Valium) and pentazocine (Talwin). Despite the natural inclination of a physician to help a patient, prescribing "pain relieving medications" is, in fact, not of much help. As patients with objective pain progress through the various stages of their chronic pain, many of them report that they find the narcotic analgesics of little or no value in relieving pain. Physicians are so conditioned to treat pain with analgesics that they rarely stop to think about the long-term effects on sleep, sexual activity, and mental alertness. Rather than treating the pain per se, it is best to treat the attendant anxiety, depression, and muscle spasm. Psychiatric intervention should begin at this stage.

In the subacute, subchronic, and chronic stages, it is important to aid the patient's sleep when it is altered by anxiety, depression, and pain. A tricyclic antidepressant given in a large dose at bedtime is most effective in helping the patient to sleep. The mechanism of action of the drugs in this category (amitriptyline [Elavil], doxepin [Sinequan], imipramine [Tofranil], and desipramine [Norpramin]) varies from sedation to stimulation. The degree of sedation is related to the ability of certain of these drugs to block the reuptake of serotonin presynaptically. The stimulant or antidepressant tricyclic drugs block the reuptake of norepinephrine.[67] To take advantage of the sedative side effects of doxepin and amitriptyline, it is best to prescribe 75 to 200 mg, all at bedtime, reserving the lower dosages for older or debilitated patients. Doxepin has fewer cardiovascular side effects than amitriptyline, and in small doses it is relatively safe to use in patients with mild electrocardiographic changes. All tricyclic antidepressants have some anticholinergic activity. As a result, they can create dry mouth, blurred vision, altered heart rate, and mild mental confusion in older patients. Used within existing guidelines, however, a large dose at night eliminates the need for any "sleeping medication" and provides a beneficial effect of both antidepressant and tranquilizing action on patients with objective pain.

Anxiety reduction in these patients may be accomplished by several means. Hydroxyzine (Vistaril) has a mild antianxiety property, even though its major mode of action is antihistaminic. For this reason, 50 mg three or four times a day is a useful antianxiety dose. The use of benzodiazepine derivatives, such as chlordiazeproxide (Librium), diazepam (Valium), oxazepam (Serax), clorazepate (Tranxene), and flurazepam (Dalmane), is to be avoided. These drugs work by blocking the release of serotonin, and although they do not interfere with REM sleep, they have been reported to interfere with stage IV sleep. Addiction, withdrawal, and tolerance have been reported with all these drugs and additionally, withdrawal from them can produce rebound insomnia. Also, depression has been reported to result from the administration of benzodiazepines. Small doses of phenothiazine tranquilizers such as chlorpromazine (Thorazine) or perphenazine (Trilafon) are useful in combating anxiety and the attendant muscle tension. These drugs may be used safely in combination with the tricyclic antidepressants.

Occasionally, the patient with objective pain experiences muscle tension and muscle spasms. The judicious use of a drug such as carisoprodol (Soma) or dantrolene (Dantrium) may help to ease the discomfort of this secondary effect of chronic pain.

The psychological and psychiatric support of the patient is most important throughout the entire chronic pain process. Group therapy, individual psychotherapy, vocational rehabilitation, family therapy, physical therapy, biofeedback, and an accepting attitude on the part of the physician will go a long way to reassure the patient with objective pain. In many cases, the patient will welcome psychological and psychiatric support if it is presented as an adjunct to therapy, not as therapy per se.

Any operative intervention to relieve pain is permissible. This ranges from facet denervations through thalamic stimulation, including epidural stimulation and specific nerve stimulation.[57] Since the patient has a relatively stable personality, he will accept failures in treatment appropriately even though such a failure may produce a temporary worsening of his depression.

TABLE 116–1 THE HENDLER TEN-MINUTE SCREENING TEST FOR PATIENTS

QUESTIONS

1. When did you first notice the pain that you now experience?
   - a. Sudden onset with accident or definable event — 0
   - b. Slow, progressive onset without acute exacerbation — 1
   - c. Slow, progressive onset with acute exacerbation without accident or event — 2
   - d. Sudden onset without an accident or definable event — 3

2. Where do you experience the pain?
   - a. One site, specific, well-defined, consistent with anatomical distribution — 0
   - b. Multiple sites, well-defined, consistent with anatomical distribution — 1
   - c. One site, inconsistent with anatomical considerations, not well defined — 2
   - d. Vague description, inconsistent or multiple sites, not well defined, not anatomically explainable — 3

3. Do you have trouble falling asleep at night, or are you ever awakened from sleep?
   (If answer is no, score three points and go on to question 4; If answer is yes, ask the following question.) What keeps you from falling asleep, or what awakens you from sleep?
   - a. Trouble falling asleep every night due to pain and awakened by pain every night — 0
   - b. Trouble falling asleep due to pain more than three times a week and awakened from sleep by pain more than three times a week — 1
   - c. Trouble falling asleep due to pain more than three times a week, but not awakened from sleep by pain more than twice a week — 2
   - d. No trouble falling asleep due to pain, not awakened from sleep by pain — 3
   - e. Trouble falling asleep or early morning awakening without being able to get back to sleep, both unrelated to pain — 4

4. Does weather have any effect on your pain?
   - a. Pain always worse in both cold and damp weather — 0
   - b. Pain always worse with damp or cold weather — 1
   - c. Pain occasionally worse with cold or damp weather — 2
   - d. Weather has no effect on the pain — 3

5. How would you describe the type of pain that you have?
   - a. Burning or sharp shooting pain, or pins and needles, or coldness, or numbness — 0
   - b. Dull aching pain with occasional sharp shooting pains, not helped by heat, hyperasthesias — 1
   - c. Spasm-type pain, tension-type pain, numbness over the area, helped by massage and heat — 2
   - d. Nagging or bothersome pain — 3
   - e. Excruciating or overwhelming pain, relieved by massage or heat — 4

6. How frequently do you have your pain?
   - a. Pain constant — 0
   - b. Pain nearly constant, 50% to 80% of the time — 1
   - c. Pain intermittent, 25% to 50% of the time — 2
   - d. Pain only occasionally present, less than 25% of the time — 3

7. Does movement or position have any effect on the pain?
   - a. Pain unrelieved by position change or disuse, with a history for previous operations for the pain — 0
   - b. Pain worsened by use or standing or walking, relieved by lying down or disuse — 1
   - c. Variable effects on the pain with position change and use — 2
   - d. No change in the pain with use or position change, no history of previous operations for the pain — 3

8. What medication have you used in the past month?
   - a. No medications at all — 0
   - b. Use of nonnarcotic pain relievers or non-benzodiazepam tranquilizers or antidepressants — 1
   - c. Less than three times a week use of narcotic or hypnotic or benzodiazepam — 2
   - d. Greater than four times a week use of narcotic or hypnotic or benzodiazepam — 3

9. What hobbies do you have, and can you still participate in them?
   - a. Unable to participate in any hobbies formerly enjoyed — 0
   - b. Reduced number of hobbies or activities relating to a hobby — 1
   - c. Still participates in hobbies but with some discomfort — 2
   - d. Participates in hobbies as before — 3

10. How frequently did you have sex and orgasms before the pain, and how frequently do you have sex and orgasms now?
    - a. Good sexual adjustment prior to pain (3 to 4 times a week) with no difficulty with orgasm, now sexual contact less than once a week and coitus interrupted by pain — 0
    - b. Good prepain adjustment (3 to 4 times a week) with no difficulty with orgasm, now loss of interest in sex (less than once a week), difficulty with orgasm or erection — 1
    - c. No change in sexual activity before versus after the pain — 2
    - d. Unable to have any sexual contact since the pain and difficulty with orgasm or erection prior to the pain — 3

11. Are you still working (doing your household chores)?
    - a. Works every day at same prepain job or same level of household duties — 0
    - b. Works every day, but job not the same as prepain job, with reduced responsibility or physical activity — 1
    - c. Works sporadically, reduced household chores — 2
    - d. Not at work or everyone else does household chores — 3

12. What is your income now compared to the time before your injury, the acquisition of pain, and what are the sources of your income?
    - a. Experiencing financial difficulty, family income 50% or less than prepain income — 0
    - b. Experiencing financial difficulty, family income 50% to 75% of the prepain income — 1

---

* Compiled in conjunction with Dr. Don Long.

WITH CHRONIC BACK PAIN

c. Patient unable to work and receives some compensation, spouse works, so family income at least 75% of prepain income   2
d. Patient's income 80% or more of gross pay prepain, spouse does not work   3

13. Are you suing anyone, or is anyone suing you, or do you have an attorney helping you with compensation or disability payments?
  a. No suit pending, does not have attorney   0
  b. Litigation pending but not related to the pain   1
  c. Patient is being sued as result of an accident   2
  d. Litigation pending or Workmen's Compensation case with a lawyer involved   3

14. If you had three wishes for anything in the world, what would you wish for?
  a. "Get rid of the pain" the only wish, ×3   0
  b. "Get rid of the pain" one of the three wishes   1
  c. Doesn't mention getting rid of the pain, but has specific wishes, usually of a personal nature, such as more money, a better relationship with spouse or children, etc.   2
  d. Does not mention pain, general nonpersonal-type wishes, i.e., "peace for the world"   3

15. Have you ever been depressed or thought of suicide?
  a. Admits to depression or history of depression secondary to pain, associated with crying episodes and thoughts of suicide   0
  b. Admits to depression, guilt, and anger secondary to pain   1
  c. History of depression before the pain or a financial or personal loss prior to the pain, now admits to some depression   2
  d. Denies depression, crying spells, or "feeling blue"   3
  e. History of a suicide attempt prior to the pain   4

Total

SCORING

A score of 17 points or less suggests that the patient has objective pain and is reporting a normal response to chronic pain. One may proceed with operative treatment of this patient if it is indicated. Usually this patient is willing to participate in all modalities of therapy, including exercise.

A score of 18 to 21 points suggests that the patient has exaggerated pain. Operative or interventional procedures may be performed with caution. This patient usually has a premorbid (prepain) personality type that utilizes the complaint of chronic pain. This patient may benefit from a chronic pain treatment center program with an emphasis on attitude change toward the chronic pain.

A score of 22 points or more suggests that a psychiatric consultation is needed. These patients freely admit to many premorbid (prepain) problems and great difficulty in coping with the chronic pain they now experience. Operative or interventional procedures should not be performed without prior psychiatric consultation.

Prognosis

When the patient with objective pain learns to live with his pain he usually can return to productive life. In many cases, he has returned to productive work even as early as the subacute stage. He may find a new job, or may function somewhat less actively at his old job. Familial and marital relationships may consolidate and eventually improve by the time the patient reaches the chronic stage. Even if pain-relieving procedures are unsuccessful, he remains in control of his life and is capable of functioning as a useful member of society.

Case History

R. M. is a 51-year-old white man. He is vice president of one of the largest companies in the United States and earns a large income. He has been married for 27 years, is the father of two children, and lives in an exclusive suburb of a major city. Three years ago, while he was working on his yacht, the engine slipped from a mounting and amputated his right thumb. Despite the painful injury, he returned to work the next day and continued to work, even though the pain increased to a nearly unbearable level.

The diagnosis of neuroma secondary to crush injury was made. Over the course of two years, he had six operations on the stump, hand, and forearm in the United States and in Europe. Finally, he received a thalamic electrode implant to reduce the pain, but even this had no effect. He was stoic and refused to submit to the distraction of his painful thumb. He continued to function as an executive for a year while undergoing the operations. Each new failure brought about mild depression, which was replaced by joyous anticipation of the next procedure that was finally to relieve his pain. After a year of operations, the patient became depressed, suicidal, unable to sleep, was awakened three or four times each night by the pain, and expressed hopelessness and helplessness as he recognized that no operative intervention would relieve the pain. He had refrained from taking pain medication for the first seven months of his ordeal, but then began taking oxycodone (Percodan), to which he finally became addicted. After taking this medication for six months he complained that he was no longer able to function at work and that the medication really did nothing to ease his pain and it "fogged" his mind. He noted that his concentration during the two-year period was markedly reduced, and his sexual activity, which had been very good prior to the onset of the pain, was reduced dramatically. By the end of the second year, the patient had made definite plans for suicide and had thought of scuttling his yacht in retaliation for it's having caused the loss of his thumb.

The large doses of Percodan were withdrawn, and antidepressant medication was instituted. Supportive psychotherapy and family counseling were started. By the end of the third year, the patient had begun to accept the fact that he would have to live with pain the rest of his life. Even though he experienced pain, he began to work more readily, his suicidal thoughts disappeared, and he reported that his sexual activity had increased.

His attitude regarding his pain has become one of expectant anticipation of new pain-relieving procedures. He reports that he will never accept his pain, but he is learning to live with it.

Pain of Undetermined Origin

Virtually the same pattern of behavior can be observed in patients with pain of undetermined origin as in patients with objective pain. Their only difference is the etiology of the pain. Many times occult cancer or formes frustes of known disorders may present as a pain of undetermined origin. The crucial factor in such cases is knowledge of the premorbid adjustment of the patient. If it is apparent that no real or secondary gain can be obtained by chronic pain and the psychological and psychiatric evaluations confirm the absence of pre-existing psychiatric conditions, one may proceed in a thorough evaluation of the cause of the pain. This type of patient taxes the clinical skills of any physician, and every effort must be made to resist the temptation to assign him a psychiatric diagnosis. Uematsu and Long have reported on the efficacy of thermography as a diagnostic aid in chronic pain.[99] Excellent discussions of difficult-to-diagnose cases can be found in the volumes edited by Hannington-Keff and Hart.[42,43]

Case History

K. G. is a 55-year-old white man who is a production manager at a machine tool company. He has been married for 32 years and has two children. For the past six years he has had pain in the left side of his chest at the level of the tenth rib. He has been evaluated for pancreatitis, intercostal neuralgia, radicular pain, and arthritis. He received epidural and intrathecal anesthesia for pain, which resulted in numbing of the skin but no relief of the pain. He could localize the pain, and his reports were consistent from one day to the next. The pain varied in intensity, but no objective findings were noted. The psychological premorbid adjustment had been good—a solid marriage, a good job, well-adjusted children, and an abiding interest in grouse hunting. He had had difficulty falling asleep for one year, and the pain had awakened him from sleep two or three times a week over the past three or four years. There was no history of drug addiction, but the patient reported reduced interest in sexual activity. He felt depressed and anxious, and his efficiency on his job was reduced. He reported an inability to participate in hunting or other hobbies. On examination, a raised, warm nodule was found along the tenth rib on the left side. The area was tender to palpation. X-rays and repeat laboratory studies were normal. The MMPI showed a "neurotic triad" with abnormally high levels in scales 1, 2, and 3. A thermographic evaluation revealed a 1.0° C increase in temperature over the affected area. The painful area was infiltrated with steroids and anesthetic agents, and the pain disappeared within two days. Three months after discharge the patient reported that his depression had resolved, that he experienced greater interest in sex and work, and that he was able to return to his hobbies. The relief of the pain had been most gratifying, but he was puzzled because he was somewhat anxious about readjusting his life back to the previous "prepain state." The final diagnosis was Tietze syndrome.

Intravenous Thiopental Test

Walters has made a useful suggestion on the differentiation between pain from a physiological cause and from a psychological cause.[102] It is the use of intravenous thiopental to place a patient in the state between heavy sedation and light sleep in which his conscious mechanisms and thought processes are removed. The following is Walters' description of the test.

In this test the pain and any physical signs are studied while perception and nocifensor mechanisms are altered by intraveous 2.5 per cent thiopental through stages of narcosis to corneal areflexia and surgical anesthesia. An anesthetist administers the thiopental to the patient who has had the usual preparation with an empty stomach and atropine injection. Injection of thiopental in 25- to 50-mg increments should be slow enough to observe the stages of hypoalgesia with the first 100 mg and of drowsy relaxation, least waking and light narcosis, midnarcosis with eyelash areflexia, and deep narcosis with corneal areflexia. The patient can be held at one level, or the level can be allowed to lighten, deepened, or taken again through a sequence as observation dictates. The clinician elicits pain reports and examines for tenderness, sensory deficits, motor signs, joint mobility, and any reflex or vegetative abnormality.

Sensory deficits in skin sensibility can be followed by observing the involuntary withdrawal and arousal responses to pinprick. Functional sensory deficits can persist into light narcosis and until the stage of eyelash areflexia. They vanish at levels at which pinprick of normal skin still evokes response.

Tenderness is tested under narcosis by estimating the amount of stimulation to the painful part required to arouse the patient compared with the amount needed to arouse him by stimulating a part of the body that has not been tender. Surface tenderness is tested by pinprick, lifting the skin by traction, and nipping the skin tangentially between thumb and forefinger. Muscles and tendons and peripheral nerve fibers can be stretched as well as palpated. Joints can be moved as well as palpated. When the part that has been tender requires just as much stimulation to arouse the patient as the comparable bodily part that has not been tender, the mechanism of tenderness can be considered to be extinct. Arousal is evidenced by a groan, grimace, withdrawal of a part, or an abrupt increase in the rate of breathing. Electroencephalographic recording during the test will show arousal patterns as well as the declines to the flat tracings of deep narcosis and surgical anesthesia.

Inspection of motor signs readily shows taut muscles. Muscular spasm and the degree of relaxation can be noted by palpation. Trigger areas and referred tenderness can be located. Power to move a limb freely, briskly, and powerfully may be seen in the withdrawal from pinprick. Functional motor weakness may be seen to recover. Apparently absent contact reflexes become active when a psychogenic inhibition is removed. Corneal reflexes that are absent on least waking may be present in light narcosis. Tendon reflexes that are inactivated by muscular tension or a psychogenic regional pain process usually reappear in light narcosis. Pilomotor reflexes in the painful region may become less active, while cold pale skin may warm up under narcosis.

Psychogenic pain mechanisms may be extinguished before sleep is reached, whereas major physiogenic pain usually persists into least waking. The signs of the physiogenic pain syndromes persist well into narcosis and the signs of physical lesions do not vary. In contrast, the psychogenic sensory deficits and motor weaknesses do not persist beyond the anesthesia level of eyelash areflexia.

Tenderness is a major sign to follow as one proceeds toward anesthetic levels. Psychogenic regional tenderness usually vanishes in light narcosis when the patient still can be readily roused by physiogenic pain from pinprick or pinch to normal skin or from squeezing a trapezius muscle. Occasionally, psychogenic regional tenderness has been found to survive until the stage of corneal areflexia and not to vanish until the patient can no longer be aroused by any skin pinch or trapezius squeeze.

The thiopental pain test is useful in the study of tender joints or nerve roots with limited movement and tight muscles. The involuntary local reflex muscle spasms persist into mid and deep narcosis, whereas the tight muscles of tension states and emotional postures rarely if ever survive beyond eyelash areflexia.

One useful fringe benefit of this pain test is in the diagnosis of malingering. No deliberate deceiver can hold his histrionic simulation of tenderness, sensory defects, weakness, or tight muscles when asleep. If these signs persist into light or deeper levels of the narcosis, then malingering pretense can be excluded.[102]

Youmans confirms that the intravenous thiopental test is useful in determining whether the patient's pain is on a physiological or a psychological basis.[107] For example, an emotionally unstable woman had symptoms and signs of a herniated intervertebral disc at the L4–L5 level. Her myelogram was normal. On intravenous thiopental testing, her straight-leg-raising sign persisted and she awakened and groaned even from the level of narcosis at which she had corneal areflexia. At laminectomy, a herniated fragment of disc was found far lateral in the root canal, which was not shown on the myelogram. Her operation and hospital course were uneventful, and she made a complete recovery.

PATIENTS WITH EXAGGERATED OR "EFFECTED" PAIN

These patients have a collection of psychiatric disorders. The only common features shared by them are that pain interferes with their lives and that they had poor premorbid (prepain) adjustment to life. This group of patients is complex and difficult to describe. In accordance with the new psychiatric classification system of Spitzer and Sheehy, called the Diagnostic and Statistical Manual, III, (DSM-III), most of the disorders that present as "effected" or exaggerated pain can be categorized.[89]

Any of the chronic mental disorders may present as pain, whether it be senile dementia, presenile dementia, or cerebrovascular dementia. The effects of pain are exaggerated in these types of patients. Abuse of drugs ranging from alcohol through cocaine or a mixture of drugs is found in the patient with exaggerated or "effected" pain. Occasionally, schizophrenia of the paranoid type or paranoid disorders may present as chronic pain, sometimes as exaggerated pain and sometimes as associated pain. Drug-induced dementias secondary to chronic pain may occur, since patients with pain are inclined to abuse barbiturates and opioids, alcohol and benzodiazepine. Chronic abuse of these drugs usually results in a moderate to large amount of 15- to 25-Hz low-voltage fast activity on electroencephalographic evaluation, which may be reversible upon withdrawal from the medication. The hysterical disorders, divided into somatization disorders (Briquet's syndrome), usually presenting as exaggerated pain, and hysterical conversion disorders, in which pain is used as the symptom, are discussed later as affected or associative pain problems. The personality disorders, if they can be considered to be diseases, present as exaggerated pain, and the patients are the compulsive, histrionic, narcissistic, and most importantly, the dependent type.[81] What Walters has called "psychogenic tissue tension pain," whether it be in smooth or striated muscle or in mucosa, or the edematous, distended tissue type of pain, can now be classified under "psychosomatic factors in physical conditions" in the DSM-III.[89,102] These categories could also apply to any of the patients with exaggerated pain, but then they would become meaningless because of the diversity of the patients' personality types. Generalized anxiety disorders and depression can result in psychogenic magnification.[102] As mentioned earlier, both the patient with objective pain and the patient with pain of undetermined origin could be grouped with those having the adjustment reaction with depressed, anxious, or mixed emotional features, since these emotions are admitted by them. Patients with adjustment reactions with physical symptoms however, easily fall into the category of those with affected pain, since they do not describe the normal emotional reaction but, rather, a physical equivalent of it. This problem is discussed in the next section, as is malingering, the malingerer being a most definite type of patient with affected pain.

In the following discussion, the format varies from subtype to subtype, but each group presented is a typical patient with "effected" or exaggerated pain.

Organic Mental Disorders Manifest in "Effected" Pain

Premorbid (Prepain) Adjustment

These patients may not give an accurate history. It is best to confirm information with a family member or friend. Usually, they will report decreased functioning and trouble with concentration, memory, and sleep in the early stages. Depression and a decline in intellectual powers and job ability will be evident, as will increased irritability. Overt psychosis and confusional states resulting from an organic brain syndrome can occur but rarely are misdiagnosed as the result of an exaggeration of pain, since the symptoms are so clear-cut by the time they reach this stage.

Symptoms and Clinical Course

The patient with exaggerated pain who has organic mental disease will ascribe all of his problems with sleep, depression, and concentration to the onset of pain. Not uncommonly, the pain began several years after the first clinical signs of the organic brain syndrome. This type of patient often reports that a pain that began or an injury that was sustained many years earlier is now beginning to be more bothersome. His speech pattern may be repetitive or concrete. The degree of disability seems disproportionate to the degree of physical injury or incapacitation. There usually is however, a real, definable organic cause of the pain, usually anatomically defined. As each new attempt to treat the pain meets with failure or success that is only short-lived, one begins to look for the true underlying pathological state.

Pathology and Etiology

Organic mental disorders have multiple causes, including arteriosclerotic cardiovascular disease, early degenerative cortical atrophy (Pick's disease, Alzheimer's dementia), senile degeneration, alcohol, barbiturates, diazepam, opioids, toxic solvents, and various infections ranging from syphilitic to viral.

Diagnosis and Clinical Tests

The most useful test is an electroencephalogram, which will show large amounts of diffuse, slow-wave activity (4 to 7 Hz) in a degenerative organic brain syndrome but will show 15- to 25-Hz diffuse fast activity in a toxic organic brain syndrome. The electroencephalogram may be followed by a computed tomographic scan, which will usually show diffuse cortical atrophy. If the electroencephalogram and the CT scan are not abnormal, it is useful to obtain a Bender-Gestalt test, which is an excellent way to determine the presence of an organic brain syndrome, especially when coupled with a memory quotient test and a Wechsler Adult Intelligence Scale (WAIS) to assess IQ. A difference of 15 points or more between verbal and performance IQ scores (with performance lower) lends substance to the diagnosis of organic brain syndrome. Another useful tool is the mini-mental status examination devised by Folstein and co-workers, which readily differentiates between organic and psychiatric disease.[31] The differential diagnosis includes a transient organic brain syndrome caused by excessive intake of analgesics, tranquilizers, or atropine-like substances. These substances need to be withdrawn for at least one week before it is possible to assess the degree of permanent organic impairment.

Treatment

Treatment is symptomatic at best. Sometimes merely confronting the patient and his family with the diagnosis of organic brain syndrome is enough to change the level of expectation of both the patient and the family, thereby providing more support and reducing anxiety. The patient no longer needs to exaggerate his pain, since the real problem is understood by everyone. Supportive psychotherapy and small doses of haloperidol (a butyrophenone), 1 mg three times a day up to 2 mg four times a day, are useful. Drugs with anticholinergic properties, such as the sedative phenothiazines (chlorpromazine) and all tricyclic antidepressants, except in small doses (10 to 25 mg at bedtime) should be avoided, since they can worsen the organic brain syndrome.

Prognosis

Once the patient with exaggerated pain is made aware of the diagnosis of the organic brain syndrome, the complaints about pain usually diminish. There is nothing to be done to prevent further deterioration except in cases in which the syndrome was transient and drug-induced. In these cases, abstinence from drugs to prevent further impairment is the only useful recommendation.

Case History

L. C. is a 56-year-old widowed white woman who is a self-employed insurance agent. She presented with low back, leg, neck, and shoulder pain. She said the pain had become progressively worse over the past three years. She had been treated with facet blocks of the lumbar region, which provided some pain relief. The patient then began to complain of neck, shoulder, and arm pain, although x-rays did not show any pathological changes in the cervical region. She responded to facet denervations in the cervical area, obtaining good relief of her neck, shoulder, and arm pain; she began, however, to complain of pain in her low back and legs as well as headache in the frontal region. At this time the electroencephalogram showed moderate amounts of diffuse slow activity (4 to 7 Hz); the Bender-Gestalt test showed a minimally abnormal record, and the Wechsler Adult Intelligence Scale showed an 18-point difference between the verbal and performance IQs. A more comprehensive history was obtained, at which time it was discovered the patient had begun to have difficulty with concentration and memory for approximately a year to a year and a half prior to the time that pain had become "debilitating." The patient believed that the pain had prevented her from more actively pursuing her insurance clients, and reported difficulty in driving long distances, owing to the discomfort of sitting in the car. She recognized that she was less effective in her office work, was depressed, less able to concentrate, and had impairment of memory. These developments caused her great concern. She was concerned and intimidated by the fact that she was forced to allow a younger agent to service her new accounts while she did more repetitive and mundane office work. When confronted with the diagnosis of an early organic brain syndrome, she was disturbed at first but later was relieved. She had thought her reduced mental function was due to psychological factors, and was relieved to find that in all likelihood it was the other way around. The patient responded quite well to small doses (1 mg three times a day) of haloperidol and returned to work with more realistic expectations about her abilities.

Paranoid Schizophrenia and Paranoid Disorders Manifest in "Effected" Pain

Few authors entertain the idea that a patient with schizophrenia may have organic ills.[10,84] Admittedly, the incidence is low, and one would expect to be able to diagnose a paranoid schizophrenic without much difficulty. Not all persons with a paranoid flavor, however, are schizophrenics. Indeed, the differential diagnosis for paranoid thoughts and delusions, i.e., feelings of persecution accompanied by delusions of grandeur (not merely suspiciousness), includes a very long list of disorders, among them amphetamine psychosis, mania, psychotic depression, true paranoid personality, neurotic life style, organic brain syndrome, alcoholic hallucinosis, and other stimulant abuse.[85] Therefore, it is best that the diagnosis of paranoid schizophrenia or paranoid states be left to a competent psychiatrist.

Premorbid Adjustment

Usually, a history of psychiatric difficulty, if not of psychiatric hospitalizations, can be obtained. The patient with exaggerated pain due to paranoia is usually single or has had a poor marital record, has a poor work record, and often has had difficulty with the law for assault or drug abuse.

Symptoms and Clinical Course

The patient with exaggerated pain and paranoid features considers pain as a personal assault on him. There may be a history of a traumatic onset of pain, or the pain symptoms may have developed slowly. The pain is usually anatomical in distribution and quality, but the cause may be ascribed to sources outside the body. These patients are usually demanding, insistant, somewhat hostile, and belligerent or overcontrolled in their manner. They persist in their requests for treatment and total relief.

Pathology and Etiology

Causes and pathological changes are the same as those mentioned earlier in the discussion of the differential diagnosis for paranoid schizophrenia.

Diagnosis and Clinical Tests

Patients with exaggerated pain and paranoid schizophrenia or paranoid disorders are best detected by a psychiatric evaluation, since the differential diagnosis is so extensive. Usually, the Minnesota Multiphasic Personality Index (MMPI) indicates psychotic or paranoid thinking. A history of auditory hallucinations of the persecutory type, i.e., "you are no good," or the hostile type, "you should kill yourself (or someone else)," as well as the extracorporeal explanation for pain, "God is punishing me" or "my husband has implanted a knife in my back," suggests a paranoid schizophrenic process. A litigious personality suggests a paranoid disorder when frank somatic delusions and hallucinations of the schizophrenic type may not be evident, and a more suspicious nature is noted.

Treatment

The drugs of choice are in the phenothiazine, butyrophenone, and thioxanthene categories. These medications usually diminish the complaints of pain. No operative intervention is indicated.

Prognosis

Adequate treatment with major neuroleptics as just outlined should reduce the complaints of pain. With adequate psychiatric care, the patient with exaggerated pain can be maintained at his usual level of functioning.

Case History

N. F. is a 27-year-old, unmarried, white man, a warehouse worker, who was injured while lifting a heavy box. He complained of low back and right leg pain, but a neurological examination was within normal limits, as was a myelogram. Thermography revealed a 0.5° C temperature increase in the area of the low back pain. The patient had had the pain for several years and was angry with all doctors for not treating it. He not only demanded a cure from a neurosurgeon but threatened to "come back and get" the neurosurgeon if a cure was not effected. Later he confided to the neurosurgeon that fellow workers were poisoning him and this had caused the back pain. Thorazine, 400 mg at bedtime and 100 mg three times daily, was prescribed, and the patient was able to return to work with minimal complaints about his leg and back pain.

Psychosomatic Factors in Physical Conditions Manifest in "Effected" Pain

Walters has described "psychogenic tissue tension pain" as the result of "psychic factors" causing "muscle tension."[102] The pain produced is not imagined and is measurable as increased electromyographic responses in the affected muscle group. This group of patients has "effected," not exaggerated, chronic pain, since anxiety produces the effect of pain.

Premorbid Adjustment

These patients report they have always been tense, anxious, nervous, or "highstrung," and they have marital difficulties, family disasters, sexual difficulties, and marginal or precarious financial conditions. They report that they are under a lot of pressure at home, or at work, have few outlets or hobbies, and little time to pursue relaxation.

Symptoms and Clinical Course

The usual complaint is muscle tension or tightness in the neck, arms, and shoulders, atypical facial pain, low back pain without involvement of the legs, and frontal or occipital "headache." The onset usually is slow and progressive, without a physically traumatic episode. Accidents, however, can trigger the onset of symptoms that remain far longer than the typical time course for resolution.[9] The patients report difficulty in falling asleep, which is due primarily to anxiety but in some cases to the pain itself. They report that sexual activity worsens the pain, and for that reason the patient engages in less sexual activity then he did prior to the pain.

Pathology and Etiology

The nervous tension that this type of patient feels is translated into a physical tension, much as a fist is tightened in anger.[46] This patient, however, tightens his neck, back, and shoulder muscles involuntarily and unconsciously. He becomes aware of stress only as it presents as muscle tension pain, thus the presenting symptom of "pain," in a particular muscle group. Posttraumatic events can progress to myofascial pain syndromes with trigger points.[9]

Diagnosis and Clinical Tests

The pain described by the patient follows anatomical boundaries for a specific muscle group. There are objective findings on thermographic evaluation, usually showing minimal (0.5° C) elevation of temperature over the affected muscle group. The neurological examination may show brisker than usual deep tendon reflexes, which suggests anxiety. Sweaty palms may also be noted on physical examination, as may tenderness, soreness, and palpable "knots" in the affected muscle groups. The Minnesota Multiphasic Personality Index (MMPI) usually shows elevated scores for scales 1 and 3 (a psychosomatic V). Using an electromyographic biofeedback machine as a recording instrument, one can detect severe muscle tension in the affected muscle group—10 to 250 μv. These patients report that the "pain" gets worse when they are under stress or tense, and better when they are relaxed. They report difficulty in going to sleep at night, but are not awakened by the pain. Heat or massage usually relieves the pain. Sexual activity usually is altered and is an excellent barometer of marital strife. In many cases, the sexual difficulties may be the cause of the conflict that resulted in the myofascial pain syndrome.

Treatment

Small doses of a phenothiazine neuroleptic (chlorpromazine [Thorazine], 50 mg four times a day, or perphenazine [Trilafon], 2 to 4 mg four times a day) are useful in reducing the perceived anxiety. This same concept has been found useful in reducing pain and anxiety by using Percogesic.[36] During the initial phase of treatment, carisoprodol (Soma), 350 mg four times daily, may also provide symptomatic relief from discomfort until the anxiety is controlled by phenothiazines. Electromyographic biofeedback is very helpful in retraining the affected muscle group and teaching the patient how to relax.[35] Many times, merely calling attention to the increased muscle tension by using the biofeedback device is useful. Instructing the patient to increase his muscle tension, which will demonstrate the association between increased tension and increased pain, is often the most effective initial training technique. After that, he learns to gain control over the particular muscle, and eventually can relax it at will, thereby reducing or eliminating the pain. Supportive and insight-oriented psychotherapy and family psychotherapy are useful.

Prognosis

This type of patient has a good recovery rate from "pain" per se. The environmental conditions that produce the stress, however, are the real culprit, and he may continue to experience "pain" of other sorts, either in a new muscle group or in a new fashion (sexual dysfunction, drinking alcohol, or the like).

Case History

M. F. is a 42-year-old white woman who presented with bilateral facial pain of four years' duration in the maxillary area. It radiated back to the ear and downward toward the mandible. Additionally, she had pain in the neck and shoulders. She reported financial difficulty and tension at home and on her job for the previous six to eight years. She was active sexually; however, the neck and shoulder pain diminished this activity. She was able to obtain relief from the pain with heat and massage. She had trouble falling asleep at night. Her family doctor had been treating her with propoxyphene (Darvon) and chlordiazepoxide (Librium), with minimal relief. The poor premorbid adjustment suggested an affective or associated pain problem, i.e., conversion pain, but the anatomical distribution was more suggestive of an organic pain of undetermined origin. A dental consultation provided the diagnosis of a temporomandibular joint syndrome, and electromyographic recordings using a biofeedback machine revealed muscle tension in excess of 250 μv in the masseter muscles.[88] Propoxyphene and chlordiazepoxide were discontinued, and perphenazine (Trilafon), 4 mg four times daily, and carisoprodol (Soma), 350 mg four times daily, were begun. Electromyographic biofeedback was used to try to treat the masseter muscle tension, and within two weeks the pain diminished to the point at which the carisoprodol could be discontinued and the per-

phenazine reduced to 2 mg three times a day.[35] The patient also had dental repositioning of her bite and left the hospital after a three-week stay, virtually pain-free. The neck and shoulder pain also diminished, and with repeated biofeedback treatments of the trapezius muscle, this pain also was eliminated.

Generalized Anxiety Disorder, Adjustment Reaction with Depressed or Anxious Mood or Mixed Emotional Features, or Affective Disorders of Depressive Type Manifest in "Effected" Pain

While the names may differ, these conditions are anxiety and depressive neuroses. They share the common feature of creating a patient who exaggerates his pain primarily because he has become more aware that the little nagging aches and pains do not set him apart (i.e., gain attention); everyone else has them too.

Premorbid Adjustment

Prior to presenting with pain, the patient in this category has experienced either depression or anxiety due to changes in life situation, such as the death of close relatives, divorce, financial difficulty, trouble with children, marital or sexual discord, legal problems, and myriad other situational upsets. Anything that creates stress and produces a loss can result in depression. In a situational or adjustment disorder, it is difficult, if not impossible, to separate depression from anxiety.[59] For this reason the drug manufacturers have marketed combination antidepressant and tranquilizing medicine (Etrafon and Triavil [combinations of amitriptyline and perphenazine]).

In the pure forms of the anxiety or affective disorders of the depressive type (the old neuroses), however, more severe symptoms are found. Much has been written about these patients; their pain complaints have been defined as "psychogenic magnifications" or "functional overlay," and they have been called "giving up–given up," "pain neurotic," "pain-prone," "low back losers," and "psychogenic pain patients." * Pilling and co-workers were able

---

* See references 10, 27, 80, 93, 102.

to separate this group into two subgroups.[72] The first, those with a "hysterical conversion V" (elevated scores on scale 1, hypochondriasis, and scale 3, hysteria with mild depression, on the Minnesota Multiphasic Personality Index [MMPI]), are discussed later. The second group, those patients with elevated scores on scales 1, 2, and 3 on the MMPI (hypochondriasis, depression, and hysteria), have exaggerated pain owing to anxiety or depression. This "neurotic triad" indicates that the patient admits to premorbid depression, that is, the depression preceded the onset of the pain. Pilling and co-workers, Blumer, and Sternback are careful to define the contrast between this type of patient and the hypochondriac. All three agree that a "pain neurotic" patient has characteristics that differ from those of a hypochondriac.[10,72,92] Pilling and others drew an excellent comparison between patients who presented with pain of questionable organic origin and patients who presented with a complaint other than pain.[72] Significant differences emerged rather dramatically. On direct questioning, only 12 to 14 per cent of the patients who presented with pain, compared with 35 per cent of the patients with other complaints, also admitted to depression and anxiety, which was significant at the $P < 0.001$ level. Additionally, of the men and women presenting with pain, significantly fewer had elevated depression scores on the MMPI (which provides an indirect measure for depression) than did patients without pain (65 per cent versus 77 per cent). Seventy-four per cent of the men with pain admitted to hypochondriasis on the MMPI, in comparison with 56 per cent of the matched control group. Thirty-six per cent of the women with pain had phobias, in comparison with 52 per cent of the group without pain. The patients with exaggerated pain complained more readily about their pain than did those with objective pain. They were reluctant to withdraw from narcotics. Usually a parent, child, or spouse had been chronically ill before the patient with exaggerated pain became ill. There were patients who presented with pain of ill-defined origin, and had significantly different premorbid and developmental histories from the patients who did not have pain. The patients with pain admitted to school phobias, fainting spells, and inability to form close relationships with one friend in childhood. They had psychiatric contacts significantly less often than their counterparts without pain. Pilling and others believe that these patients have substituted "pain" for anxiety and depression.[72] The patients share many features with the dependent personality types that are discussed later and often can have mixed disorders.

Symptoms and Clinical Course

The objective findings in this group may range from normal to moderate degrees of pathological change. Usually, an anatomical lesion is found, be it minimal degeneration or arthritic changes seen on x-ray, fusion site or donor site pain, or some degree of arachnoiditis. The clues, however, to classifying the pain these patients have as exaggerated rather than objective are their aberrant premorbid adjustment and their response to the pain. They become addicted to narcotics, either iatrogenically or through their own abuse. They cease to function at work and usually gain weight because of inactivity. They have trouble falling asleep at night, owing either to anxiety or to depression. They may be awakened at night by the pain. They may be overly anxious, as manifested by motor agitation, or depressed, as manifested by sad facies and slightly retarded motor activity, or may have a mixture of both. The patients with exaggerated pain complain more readily about their pain than those with objective pain. They resist withdrawal from narcotics. A sometimes subtle, sometimes overt, cause for anxiety or depression that existed prior to the onset of the pain can be found, and there is good evidence of secondary gain even at the sacrifice of primary goals. Sexual frequency may not be altered, but may have been altered prior to the onset of the pain. In general, these patients ascribe all their ills to the pain. A traumatic onset is possible, as is a slow progressive course.

Pathology and Etiology

The anxiety and depression are most often environmentally induced. Rarely does an endogenous depression present as pain (in that case the depressive symptoms are more evident). The premorbid adjustment is at the crux of the magnification of the pain, and emotional "pain" is denied. Chronic anxiety and situational anxiety can cause a patient to have exaggerated pain.

Diagnosis and Clinical Test

Electromyographic and nerve conduction studies may show slightly abnormal values, as may thermography (0.5° C differences). The pain is anatomically localized and compatible with clinically positive findings on x-ray. If there is attendant drug abuse, the electroencephalogram may show a moderate amount of 15- to 25-HZ diffuse activity. These patients with exaggerated pain are differentiated from patients with objective pain by their marginal premorbid adjustment and the total collapse they experience in response to pain, as well as their overconcern about the pain. The MMPI is useless as a diagnostic aid, since the profile in the group with exaggerated pain is exactly the same as in those with chronic objective pain. The treatment varies for each of them, and transient or "state" anxiety must be differentiated from chronic or "trait" anxiety.

Treatment

Accurate diagnosis is required in order to begin proper treatment. These patients can have external electrical stimulators, facet blocks and denervations, or even sympathectomies if indicated. Epidural wires and thalamic implants, however, and the stimulation of sciatic or brachial plexus by implanted devices are contraindicated. Perphenazine (Trilafon), 2 mg three times a day to 4 mg four times a day, can be used to relieve anxiety, be it either "state" (transient or reactive) or "trait" (chronic or neurotic), which needs psychotherapy as well. Amitriptyline (Elavil) or doxepin (Sinequan), 75 to 250 mg, at bedtime can be used for symptomatic treatment of the insomnia, and of the anxiety and depression if they are of the agitated type. A more stimulating type of tricyclic antidepressant can be used if there is a retarded or lethargic component to the depression that causes hypersomulence and difficulty arising in the morning. For this type of depression, desipramine (Norpramin) or imipramine (Tofranil) may be given in a dosage ranging from 25 mg three times a day to 50 mg four times a day. Psychotherapy is essential for these patients, either in a homogeneous group of patients with exaggerated pain and anxiety and depression, or as individual supportive and insight-oriented therapy. Couples therapy or sexual dysfunction therapy may be indicated if this is the cause of depression or anxiety or both, and vocational rehabilitation may be useful in some cases.

Prognosis

If the source of anxiety and depression can be identified and dealt with on a conscious level, the inability to cope with the pain disappears. It must be emphasized that medication is merely an adjunct to therapy, and the real "cure" comes with psychotherapy, which helps the patient to understand and confront the real conflicts in his life. Without adequate psychotherapy, this type of patient will continue to experience debilitating pain.

Case History

P. Z. is a 40-year-old white woman, an attorney who is married to another attorney. A fall led to a ruptured disc, which was operatively removed. Her back symptoms remitted, but over the course of three years she began to have pain in the neck, right arm, and shoulder. Thermography revealed a 0.5° C increase of temperature over the C4–C7 region on the right. Electromyographic studies were within normal limits, as were nerve conduction tests. X-ray examination revealed degenerative osteoarthritis of the cervical region. The patient obtained relief with facet denervations but was noticeably depressed when seen while in the hospital for the denervations. She claimed her depression was secondary to pain and that she was having trouble at work, since writing made the pain worse. She complained of difficulty falling asleep at night. Amitriptyline (Elavil), 100 mg at bedtime, was prescribed to relieve her depression and help her sleep. After one year of psychotherapy, it was learned that the husband was having an indiscreet extramarital affair, which the patient had denied but finally came to accept. Since they worked together, she really wanted to quit the office rather than be around him. Her sexual activity had been reduced to one or two times a month as the pain had progressed, and the reason given for abstinence was that the activity worsened her pain. After she was able to confront her husband about the affair and job situation, the husband decided he would abandon his mistress. Medication was discontinued, and the patient and her husband were seen as a couple for six months, after which they decided to remain married. It was, however, decided the wife should seek employment in another law office. She became less anxious and depressed, and eventually admitted that her pain was "uncomfortable" rather than "unbearable," as she had described it earlier. She recognized that she had become more aware of the pain during the situational stress and that when her situation was altered, she was far more able to cope with the existing pain.

Dependent Personality Manifest in "Effected" Pain

Many of the same features that are found in the anxious and depressed patient may be found in the patient with a dependent personality. Since dependency is a trait of an individual, however, it is most difficult to change, unlike transient reactive anxiety or depressive states, which can be resolved. Personality disorders "are characterized mainly by maladaptive patterns of behavior learned in childhood . . .", but ". . . persons with a personality disorder may also have a psychiatric illness with anxiety, depressive, or other psychiatric symptoms."[81] Admittedly, in diagnosing personality disorders ". . . the criteria used are more sociologic then medical in nature . . .", and treatment is usually directed at altering behavior.[81] The next group of patients with exaggerated pain, are those with personality disorders of dependent, compulsive, histrionic and narcissistic, and neurotic hysterical types called Briquet's syndrome, or somatization disorder, and are among the most frustrating to psychiatrists as well as to surgeons.

Premorbid Adjustment

The dependent patient with exaggerated pain has a long-standing history of reliance on other people. He may have relied on a parent and still maintain a frequent intimate contact, or may have been abandoned or rejected as a child. There usually is a family history of alcoholism. These patients may have been overprotected as children and have drifted toward a protective job situation, i.e., work in the civil service or the armed forces. They may have financial difficulties. Usually they have marital difficulties. They have a disproportionate distribution among families who have a patriarchial structure in which the mother serves as a

protector against an authoritarian father. They usually have been eager to please, outwardly compliant, yet demanding of attention in return. They have a higher incidence of peptic ulcer than the general population, and they masquerade as pseudoindependent types who disclaim any reliance on people.[28] They may also be aggressive in their passivity, by obstructing actions or being inefficient or procrastinating.[96] They have a "life style of invalidism."[93]

Symptoms and Clinical Course

Patients of this type may be characterized by their stated dependence on the doctors and their stated eagerness to comply. They usually are addicted to at least diazepam (Valium), if not harder narcotics, and not infrequently have excessive alcohol intake. They are of the lower socioeconomic class with financial trouble if they are men, or if women, regardless of socioeconomic class, they are married to dominantly aggressive men. They have been moderately to severely incapacitated by their pain and characteristically have become very inactive, relying heavily on family members to do their bidding. They appear to be in mild discomfort, concerned about remuneration from workmen's compensation or social security disability benefits, and are supplicative in their requests for doctors' certificates regarding their disability. They frequently ask what the doctor is going to do to help their pain, and are resistant to withdrawing from analgesics, sleeping medication, or benzodiazepines. They usually are not awakened by pain, but do have trouble falling asleep, although usually not because of pain. Their sexual activity is not diminished. Objective findings are minimal, but they resist participation in active physical exercise. Frequently, there has been at least a 20-lb weight gain since the onset of the pain.

Pathology and Etiology

Dependent personality types commonly have intermingled anxiety and depression.[72] A patient with exaggerated pain who has a pure dependent personality, however, is fearful of expressing aggressive tendencies. Pain, as a symptom, permits a passive-aggressive, passive-dependent way of functioning. These patients can demand and become hostile, then excuse themselves because they are in pain. Pain can also be used to punish themselves, as it is by depressed patients, for real or imagined transgressions, and thereby to resolve guilty feelings. Blumer confirms Pilling's findings and defines two subtypes of pain neurotics—those with and those without depression—and further clarifies the problem of the patient with exaggerated pain who is not depressed but is dependent. He found 26 of 27 such patients denied any emotional conflict, reporting that home life was wonderful, the job was fine, and if they could only be rid of the pain, everything would be restored to normality. Sixteen of the twenty-seven had close relatives or spouses who denied any conflicts at home, while 13 of the 27 had relatives who were crippled or deformed prior to the onset of pain in the dependent patient with exaggerated pain. The relative was usually found to have or to have had a significant role in the development of the patient. Twenty of the twenty-seven patients clearly requested an operation to "cure their pain." Blumer outlines this personality type as dependent, regressed, and in some cases covertly, if not overtly, sadomasochistic. They tend to conceal emotional conflicts.[10] Sternback confirms the findings of Blumer and Pilling, and reports a "neurotic triad" on the MMPI scores of these dependent patients who exaggerate their pain.[92]

Diagnosis and Clinical Tests

Unfortunately, no good psychological test to measure dependency is available. Minnesota Multiphasic Personality Index (MMPI) and Symptom Check List of 90 Questions (SCL-90) scores of the dependent patient with exaggerated pain usually show somatic concern or hypochondriasis, and some anxiety or depression. Objective physical tests reveal minimal abnormality. The diagnosis can be confirmed by observing a reluctance to take responsibility for their own care, a dependence instead on the doctor to fill out forms, call for appointments, and in general, "get them better." They are best characterized by their inertia, i.e., unwillingness to budge from "ground zero"—while at the same time they are protesting that they are trying but "just can't do anything." They have what Bonica

calls a lot of "down-time."[12] They are resistant to drug withdrawal and complain about their need for narcotic medication.

Treatment

Since there is no specific treatment for personality disorders per se, the dependent type of patient with exaggerated pain is best treated at a pain treatment center. Some authors have claimed success in treating personality disorders with psychotherapy, and while this may be so, the average person has neither the resources nor inclination to have "psychoanalytically oriented psychotherapy for 85 hours over two years."[47] By employing some of the techniques outlined by behavior therapists, new behavior can be taught to convert the "manipulative patterns learned in childhood."[60,81] Fordyce, one of the leading proponents of "operant conditioning" of patients with chronic pain, has outlined an inpatient program geared to retraining the patient by modifying the environment and rewarding the patient for new, more functional behavior.[32] Bonica has outlined an organizational scheme for a pain clinic.[12] Over 20 of these pain treatment centers are located in the United States.[63] Drug withdrawal is imperative, and hydroxyzine (Vistaril) may be used to assist the patient in the early stages of withdrawal. Fifty milligrams, orally, each four hours while awake, should be used for the first two days. The dose of hydroxyzine should be increased while the narcotics are withdrawn over a one-week period. As suggested for the treatment of the patient with exaggerated pain owing to generalized anxiety, tranquilizers and mood-elevating drugs may be used as indicated. Group therapy is the most efficient way to provide psychiatric support for dependent patients with exaggerated pain. Operative intervention should be limited to facet denervations. Physical therapy and exercise are imperative. All treatment is geared to attitudinal change.

Prognosis

Many times, two or three admissions to the pain treatment center are needed before any attitudinal change can be noted. The significant changes to be accomplished are acceptance of the chronic pain, abstinance from addictive medication, and increased activity. After three admissions, each one being approximately two weeks in length, the likelihood of any further alternation in attitude is very small.

Case History

C. V. is a 42-year-old white woman who formerly worked at a check-out stand in a supermarket. Since her injury three years prior to admission, she has not worked. She was injured when leaving her home to go to work, and no litigation is pending. She sustained bruises to her neck and midthoracic area as well as her low back, and was found to have a ruptured disc at L4–L5, which was successfully operated upon. Good relief was obtained. The pain in her low back, shoulder, and neck persisted, however. Prior to her injury, she had been married for 20 years to a truck driver who was "on the road a lot." Their sexual activity was good when he was home, but she resented his frequent stays away from home. She never told him of her resentment, however, because she feared his displeasure. She was raised in a protective, religious home, where she attended church every Sunday, and she had attended a parochial school through high school. She lived at home for four years after high school and then was married. She claimed her husband was a good provider who "took care" of her. Since the injury and recovery from the operation, she has been unable to work and has enlisted the aid of one of her sisters living close by to help her with housework and cooking for her family of five children and her husband. She states that she relies heavily upon the sister and older children for help. Her husband has become critical of her "laziness." She has found it difficult to function without her 30 mg of diazepam (Valium) and 4 to 7 tablets of oxycodone (Percodan) each day, and has gained 35 lb since her injury. Her sex life has been only mildly compromised, and she takes part in sexual intercourse to please her husband, even when it hurts her. When admitted to the pain treatment center, she was resistant to being withdrawn from drugs and tried various excuses to avoid the exercise program. She was congenial on the ward. In group therapy, she denied depression, but admitted to a longing need to have her husband take care of her, as she had "taken care of him all of these years." She admitted her reluctance to express her anger at him, however, since she feared he would leave her. Facet denervations helped her low back and shoulder and neck pain, and she was discharged free of drugs. Six months later she was readmitted for complaints of low back pain. She was taking the same amount of oxycodone (Percodan) and diazepam (Valium) as she had been on her previous hospitalization. This time, she very openly expressed fear of her husband's leaving her and her resentment at his traveling. She was willing to participate in the exercise program and

was withdrawn from narcotics. Facet denervations in the lumbar region gave her "50 per cent relief," which she "could live with." The couple was seen in couples therapy for three months, and at a nine-months follow-up, she was free of narcotics and had lost 20 lb, and her home life had improved considerably since her husband had switched from cross-country to local truck driving. It was this last change that probably was the most beneficial part of her treatment.

Compulsive Personality Manifest in "Effected" Pain

The obsessive-compulsive personality has been the subject of much psychiatric comment. "Wilhelm Reich described the compulsive character as 'living machines'."[85] While this may not be complimentary, it is an apt description.

Premorbid Adjustment

In almost every description, regardless of the source, the terms "rigidity" and "inhibition of emotional expression" arise. These styles of thinking mark an obsessive-compulsive personality from early childhood. Persons of this type have an overwhelming concern about rules, standards, and conformity. They are precise, meticulous, excessively neat, exact, dogmatic, and opinionated. They think things out thoroughly before making a decision, but in some cases are so obsessed with evaluating every conceivable option that they have trouble making a decision. They strive to be perfect. If they are not perfect, then they become self-punishing and guilty. Most authorities feel that there are underlying mechanisms of depression at work, because of the "punishing superego."[85] Their attitude toward sex is rather antiseptic, and control of any situation is important. The types of jobs they gravitate to involve precise work with repetitive patterns of behavior, such as tool and die making, watch making, and computer programming. These patients are steady workers and usually have no financial difficulty. Their marriages usually are intact.

Symptoms and Clinical Course

As could be expected, anything that makes the compulsive patient with exaggerated pain less than perfect is upsetting. Therefore, an injury or disability of any sort that impairs his control of the environment is untenable. These patients show excessive somatic concern for minor injuries. They have features that resemble hypochondriasis but differ in that the overconcern about pain usually has an anatomically defined basis and threatens disability or loss of function. They usually present with controlled anxiety, asking detailed and precise questions about their condition. They delight in submitting to objective test procedures in which something can be measured or seen. They adhere rigidly to schedules and to orders from a physician who is an authority figure. Sleep patterns indicate anxiety (trouble falling asleep), and sexual activity is reduced because of pain. Lack of ability to concentrate because of pain may be a chief complaint.

Pathology and Etiology

Basically, because of the need to control the environment and to be perfect, any pain that threatens long-term physical impairment produces an overconcern about the injury or disability, regardless of how slight.

Diagnosis and Clinical Tests

The SCL-90 can be useful in defining an obsessive-compulsive personality.[24] Scores for the somatic concern and obsessive-compulsive scales are elevated; the interpersonal sensitivity scale score is elevated and shows reduced awareness of personal relationships. The anxiety score is not elevated until the pain has become chronic (duration of six months or longer). By then, the hostility scale score is elevated as well, and to a lesser degree that of the depression scale. Physical findings and anatomical distribution are present, but usually to a lesser degree than in a patient with objective pain of undetermined origin. The exact diagnosis between some paranoid states and psychosis and exaggerated pain in a patient who has obsessive-compulsive features is difficult and, for that reason, is best left to a psychiatrist.[85]

Treatment

Any type of operative intervention that is indicated would be recommended in this group. However, a trial of tricyclic antidepressants of the sedative type (doxepin [Sinequan] or amitriplyline [Elavil]) may be the treatment of choice. The dose should be 75 to 200 mg at night. Additionally, a moderate dose of a phenothiazine tranquilizer (perphenazine [Trilfon], 3 to 4 mg four times a day) may help reduce anxiety about the pain. Exercise and a schedule of progressive increases in activity produce good results. If appropriate, reassurance that physical activity will not create additional anatomical and structural problems will go a long way toward helping the compulsive patient to learn to live with his pain. Also, if appropriate, reassurance that the patient will not suffer a disabling, crippling progression of the injury will help the obsessive-compulsive personality to accept the pain. Behavior modification, which is best conducted in an inpatient pain treatment center, probably is the most useful psychotherapeutic approach.[60]

Prognosis

With appropriate reassurance from a surgeon about the extent of the physical injury, proper medication, and behavior therapy, the patient with exaggerated pain due to an obsessive-compulsive personality most likely will steadily improve, and the complaint of pain will diminish. Only if the incapacitation due to the obsessive-compulsive features reaches the severity of a neurosis, with fixed thoughts and behavior, does the prognosis become guarded.

Case History

H. B. is a 41-year-old white man, a machinist, originally from the German-Swiss border. He has been in the United States 20 years. Three years ago he noticed a low back pain that occurred upon awakening. The pain was described as sharp at times and a dull aching type at other times. It was made worse by damp weather, and occasionally it went down the right leg. The patient also complained of moderate perirectal pain. Objective findings were minimal. Thermography revealed a 1.0° C increase in temperature over the lumbosacral area, and a 0.5° C increase over the right leg. Myelograms, x-rays, proctoscopic and neurological examinations all were within normal limits. The patient complained of trouble in sleeping at night, and in concentrating because of his pain. The pain interfered with work and sexual activity, and he was fearful that he would experience disability to the point of invalidism. External electrical stimulation gave some relief, and amitriplyline (Elavil), 200 mg at night, as well as perphenazine (Trilafon) 4 mg four times a day, helped the patient to sleep well and feel more relaxed during the day. Facet denervation gave good relief, but the patient was concerned about the etiology of the pain. Only repeated explanations and constant reassurance by the neurosurgeon about the anatomy of the pain reduced the patient's fear about a worsening process. After three weeks in a pain treatment center, with the full range of treatment approaches, he was able to return to a regular schedule of work.

Histrionic Personality Disorder Manifest in "Effected" Pain

Patients of this type are the classic hysterical personalities whose disorder has been called the "silver-slipper syndrome," while they have been dubbed "grand hysterics." Hysterical or histrionic personality disorders must be differentiated from conversion hysteria and Briquet hysteria.[17] The lack of clarity of this differential diagnosis is worsened by the misapplication of these terms by ill-informed psychiatrists and especially by the host of nonpsychiatrists who have written about patients with chronic pain. Three different disorders have been called "hysteria," and the criteria of diagnosis have been applied haphazardly. For the sake of an improved differential diagnosis, one must consider a hysterical or histrionic personality as a distinct subtype of patient with chronic pain of the exaggerating type. The Briquet hysterical syndrome is discussed later, as is conversion hysteria in patients who have an affected associative chronic pain problem.

Premorbid Adjustment

The histrionic personality disorder is just that, histrionic. Most frequently the patient is a woman. Her family will say that she has always been a bit theatrical and has overreacted in crisis situations. Since the ability to form deep, lasting, emotional ties is usually absent in this type of personality, most relationships are based on pathological mutual weakness of the partners. Usually the patient has a history of at least one broken engagement or divorce, and additionally, her family is more likely to have a history of alcoholism and divorce. These

patients are given to self-dramatization, seductiveness, vanity, and dependence on others for approval. While, as noted, the majority of people with histrionic personalities are women, the trait is found in men.[58] Frequent sexual encounters are not uncommon, nor are frequent abortive attempts at sexual encounters that are mostly flirtations and "near seductions." Financially, these patients may get by with help from friends or family, and despite a disruptive family life, they seem to be drawn to the family in a "moth-to-flame" self-destructive pattern. Sedative drugs and alcohol are frequently used and may impair intellectual function with continued heavy use. Marital discord is frequent, as is reported difficulty in dealing with family or job stresses. They may have made suicidal gestures in the past if circumstances have been extremely difficult.

Symptoms and Clinical Course

Histrionic patients with exaggerated pain are prone to use superlatives and extreme adjectives. Chodoff and Lyons list seven features of histrionic personalities: (1) vanity and egocentricity, (2) labile and excitable but shallow affectivity, (3) dramatic attention seeking and histrionic behavior, (4) exaggeration and falsification, (5) sexual seductiveness, (6) frigidity, and (7) dependent demanding behavior.[18] The pain these patients experience is always "excruciating" or "unbearable." They always have been to the best doctors and often tell the current physician, "you are so much better." They are labile in their affect, crying one moment and laughing the next. Often they compliment the doctor and act seductively. They rarely look ill and frequently wear "diaphanous" gowns, perfume, and make-up in the hospital. They may be manipulative and "dependently demanding."[17] One must be careful, however, not to use the term "histrionic" or "hysterical personality" in a pejorative sense, because to some degree, "these are features that occur in most women and they represent a characterization of feminity."[17] There are hysterical, histrionic personalities among men as well.[58] Elements of a dependent personality, as discussed earlier, may also apply.

There is a variation of the histrionic hysterical personality that usually makes excellent executive material.

The good hysteric is described as a woman with good native endowment and achievement, a stable life style, and well functioning obsessive defences, whose only psychopathology is that she has problems in heterosexual relationships.[17]

Her manner is businesslike and efficient, if not brusque. The histrionic personality may have variable, vague, or exaggerated pain; the "good hysteric" subtype precisely locates the pain and demands that it be treated. In that respect, some features of the compulsive personality with exaggerated pain might also apply. The patient with exaggerated pain due to histrionic personality usually does less work after the pain, but doesn't suffer any economic consequences. Sleep is rarely disturbed because of the pain. The pain never awakens the patient, but may cause trouble with anxiety or difficulty in falling asleep. Sexual function is usually not altered from the premorbid patterns, although in many cases, the pain may be utilized to avoid sexual contact.

Pathology and Etiology

To understand histrionic patients with exaggerated pain, one must focus on the essential need they have to be the center of attention. Their dress, their movements, their verbalizations, their facial grimacing, all are designed to attract notice. Therefore, any pain or disability is magnified, exaggerated, and "played for all it is worth" as an attention-getting mechanism as well as a means of manipulating family, friends, and others. There are common grounds for both histrionic and sociopathic personalities, and this should be borne in mind when dealing with the histrionic type of patient with exaggerated pain.[39]

Diagnosis and Clinical Tests

The need to distinguish between histrionic patients and patients with Briquet's syndrome who have exaggerated pain should be stressed. While some authors believe that the diagnosis of hysterical personality overlaps greatly (90 per cent) with the diagnosis of Briquet's syndrome, others believe there is a need to differentiate these two disorders.[17,53,89] The major difference lies in the absence of psychosomatic complaints per se and the exaggeration of any existing physical complaint by the histrionic personality. Thus, the focus is upon the symptom when dealing with histrionic personalities, and the onset of multiple physical complaints in addition to the pain suggests Briquet's syndrome. The MMPI scores usually are elevated in scales 1 (hypochondriasis) and 3 (hysteria), or possibly only in scale 3 (hysteria). The noticeable absence of depression suggests that the histrionic patient with exaggerated pain is not as incapacitated by the pain as she would lead one to believe. Minimal organic findings and marginal, if not normal, objective test results frequently are found. If there is an anatomical distribution to the complaint, the absence of clinical findings and positive objective tests does not make the diagnosis of conversion reaction, which is discussed later in the section on patients with affected pain. Also, true concern about the complaint militates against hysterical conversion reaction. Anxiety is also less likely to be evident than is irritability.[44] In comparison with patients with objective pain, this type of patient resists attempts to withdraw narcotics and benzodiazepines, and occasionally takes medication from hidden supplies while in the hospital.

Treatment

The histrionic patient with exaggerated pain requires the full-scale intervention available in a chronic pain treatment center. Every effort should be directed toward altering the patient's response to chronic pain by means of behavioral modification, family counseling and therapy, drug withdrawal, and exercise. Hydroxyzine (Vistaril), 50 mg, or small doses of perphenazine (Trilafon), 2 mg three times a day, may aid in withdrawal from drug usage. Since only a few histrionic personalities are good candidates for psychoanalysis, all efforts should be directed toward altering "current behavior."[69] No operative intervention is indicated beyond facet denervation and the use of implantable stimulating devices to relieve pain.[57] External electrical stimulating devices may make the pain "worse," and this type of histrionic patient is adept at manipulating. By observing the criteria for patient selection for implantation of stimulating devices, Erickson and his colleagues note, one can avoid the obvious pitfalls created by the patients with exaggerated pain who demand care. Out of desperation, these authors occasionally implanted stimulation devices in patients who did not meet the criteria; they were uniformly disappointed with the results.[29] In a six-month follow-up of patients receiving operations for intractable back pain, it was found that the patients who would not be improved by the operation had significantly higher MMPI scores for scales 1 and 3 (hypochondriasis and hysteria) than those who were improved.[11] This finding may not hold true, however, for certain populations of patients with chronic pain.[48] *Primum non nocere* (first, do not harm) is the watchword.

Prognosis

As mentioned in earlier sections, the treatment of personality disorders is difficult, and for that reason, the prognosis is guarded. The critical factor will be the response the family continues to have toward this type of patient with exaggerated pain. If the family reinforces pain behavior, no treatment can be helpful. If the pain is a device for manipulation that goes unchallenged, then the prognosis is poor. Only with the full cooperation of the family can this type of patient desist from making demands for pain treatment.

Case History

L. W. is a 33-year-old white housewife who is married for the third time. She complains of pain in her midthoracic area, radiating from her shoulder blades to her chest in the T7–T8 distribution on the right side. The onset was gradual over a three-year-period. She has had no operations on her back. The pain is worse when she moves her arms or lifts heavy objects. Point tenderness is apparent over T7 and T8, but on examination the area is normal. She had taken diazepam (Valium), 10 mg four times a day, and oxycodone (Percodan) three times a day for two years, which "eased the pain." She was told to see a psychiatrist because "the pain was all in her head." As a result, she greatly resented doctors because she knew the pain was "real." She described it as "so excruciating," "unbearable," and "disastrous." She had no difficulty falling asleep, nor was she awakened from sleep by the pain. There had been no alteration in the frequency of her sexual activity compared with the period of time before the pain. The patient denied depression, and her MMPI scores showed the classic elevations in scales 1 and 3. Thermographic evaluation, however, showed a 0.5° C higher temperature over the lower midthoracic region on the right than on the left.

While being seen in psychotherapy, the patient would arrive with heavy blue eye shadow, lipstick, at least three rings on one hand, perfume, low-cut revealing blouses, and short skirts. She used superlatives when describing situations or things. Her typical locutions were "the greatest," "divine," and the like. She complimented the treating physician on his appearance and skill, and she stated that she "knew he could help" get rid of her pain. Her husband was a hard-working, successful, and reserved businessman. He gave her jewels, a car, an expensive home, and a maid, but he spent too little time at home. When he rubbed her back, it would ease the pain. Occasionally, he would travel with her to various cities to see doctors about her pain. By his own report, he was upset when his wife was in pain and he tended to spend more time at home. He was, however, becoming annoyed with her complaints. Still, he was anxious to have her become pain-free.

Diazepam (Valium) was withdrawn. Carisoprodol (Soma), 350 mg four times a day, and perphenazine (Trilafon), 2 mg four times a day, were instituted. The patient refused to be withdrawn from oxycodone. Also, a transcutaneous stimulator was tried with some success. After one month, the patient complained that the medication was not helping and the stimulator caused an irritation. The patient had two periods of two weeks each in a pain treatment center over a course of nine months. During the first admission, she resisted attempts to withdraw her from oxycodone (Percodan), and was suspected of hoarding several illicit drugs. In the intervening months, she was seen in therapy once a week, and by the second admission, she began to comply with the program. Facet denervation gave 50 per cent relief from pain, and her husband reported a much improved attitude toward pain. She began to participate in more social activities, even though the pain "hurt like the devil." She regaled her friends with stories of her successful triumph over her pain, and began to use the new pain behavior as a manipulation technique to gain approval.

Briquet's Syndrome Manifest in "Effected" Pain

This type of patient with chronic pain has a hysterical neurosis accompanied by multiple somatic complaints. Pilowsky made note of the difficulty one experiences separating hypochondriasis, functional overlay, hysteria, and so-called somatization reactions or depressive anxiety equivalence.[74] Sternbach emphasizes this point, and hastens to add that the issue is not one of "imaginary" versus "real" pain, but one of "fascinated absorption" with the pain.[93] While one may argue whether to consider Briquet's syndrome hysterical neurosis or a personality type, hypochondriasis ("pseudoneurological conversion" or "dissociative phenomena") was known in ancient Greece and has remained enigmatic ever since.[76] Charcot and Janet viewed hysteria of the type described by Briquet as a heterodegenerative condition with organic-genetic origin.[17] This theory has fallen into disrepute, but the etiology of the condition is still not well understood.

Premorbid Adjustment

The patient with exaggerated pain and the Briquet syndrome usually is a woman who has a poor premorbid adjustment to life's stresses. Usually there is a long-standing history of feeling ill and having headaches, fatigue, anxiety, difficulty with menstruation, trouble with pregnancies, sexual maladjustment, and bowel problems. The criteria for diagnosis of this syndrome are covered later. There is a greater than normal incidence of marriage to delinquent or sociopathic partners and the presence of hyperactive children. Alcoholism and sociopathy are found more often in male relatives, while about 20 per cent of the patient's first-degree female relatives also suffer from Briquet's syndrome.[39] Marital maladjustment frequently is evident in the form of divorce or broken engagements.

Symptoms and Clinical Course

The patients with Briquet's syndrome, or hysterical neuroses and exaggerated pain, are concerned about the pain with which they present. Usually, the onset of their pain has been spontaneous, and they are ill-prepared to explain it. The pain is nonanatomical in distribution, and their complaints seem vague or changeable, the description of the intensity of pain varying from one day to the next. The quality of the pain, however, and its location remain relatively constant. There is usually an increase in invalidism due to the pain. No alteration in sleep patterns is noted. Sexual activity is usually diminished, ostensibly because of the pain but usually actually in response to pre-existing difficulties. Narcotic, hyp-

notic, and laxative drug abuse is found in a majority of the cases. These patients frequently report, "they have just gotten over" another debilitating disease. On occasion, Briquet's syndrome is found in males.[50]

Pathology and Etiology

Guze reports a higher incidence of sociopathy and delinquent behavior in association with Briquet's syndrome. A history of hyperactivity also may be found more frequently in patients with Briquet's syndrome, and these patients may use illness as a way to continue to excuse themselves from responsibility.[39] There are unsettled questions about their early sexual activity, but clinically it is well accepted that a history of sexual molestation by a family member or older man is not uncommon and is perhaps more frequent than in the general population. Probably, this finding relates to the higher incidence of alcoholism and sociopathy in the families of patients with Briquet's syndrome and exaggerated pain.

Diagnosis and Clinical Tests

In response to the suggestions by Spitzer and his colleagues, specific clinical criteria have been established for Briquet's syndrome.[89] No syndrome lends itself better to a comprehensive approach that takes into account not just the here and now of symptoms but also the circumstances surrounding the symptoms, the previous duration and course of the illness, the quality of the personal relationships, and the level of function at work.[94] The multivariant approach is well exemplified by the check list for the diagnosis of Briquet's syndrome. (Table 116–2).[71,76] In order to warrant the diagnosis of Briquet's syndrome, a patient must report 25 or more symptoms from a check list of 55 symptoms that are grouped into 10 categories. The reported symptoms must come from 9 of the 10 categories, and additionally, the patient must have a dramatic and complicated medical history before the age of 35 and have no medical diagnosis to explain the symptoms.[53]

The 10 symptom groups and the 55 symptoms are as follows: (1) feeling sickly for most of life, headache; (2) blindness, paralysis, anesthesia, aphonia, fits or convulsions, unconsciousness, amnesia, deafness,

TABLE 116–2 SYMPTOM ITEMS FOR RESEARCH CRITERIA FOR BRIQUET SYNDROME*

Group 1
  Headaches
  Sickly most of life
Group 2
  Blindness
  Paralysis
  Anesthesia
  Aphonia
  Fits or convulsions
  Unconsciousness
  Amnesia
  Deafness
  Hallucinations
  Urinary retention
  Ataxia
  Other conversion
    symptoms
Group 3
  Fatigue
  Lump in throat
  Fainting spells
  Visual blurring
  Weakness
  Dysuria
Group 4
  Breathing difficulty
  Palpitation
  Anxiety attacks
  Chest pain
  Dizziness
Group 5
  Anorexia
  Weight loss
  Marked fluctuations in
    weight
  Nausea
  Abdominal bloating
  Food intolerances
  Diarrhea
  Constipation

Group 6
  Abdominal pain
  Vomiting
Group 7
  Dysmenorrhea
  Menstrual irregularity
  Amenorrhea
  Excessive bleeding
Group 8
  Sexual indifference
  Frigidity
  Dyspareunia
  Other sexual difficulties
  Vomiting all nine months
    pregnancy or hospi-
    talized for hyperemesis
    gravidarum
Group 8
  Back pain
  Joint pain
  Extremity pain
  Burning pains of the
    sexual organs, mouth, or
    rectum
  Other bodily pains
Group 10
  Nervousness
  Fears
  Depressed feelings
  Need to quit working or
    inability to carry on
    regular duties because
    of feeling sick
  Crying easily
  Feeling life was hopeless
  Thinking a good deal
    about dying
  Wanting to die
  Thinking of suicide
  Suicide attempts

* From Reveley, M. A., Woodruff, R. A., Robins, L. N., Taibleson, M., Reich, T., and Helzer, J.: Evaluation of a screening interview for Briquet syndrome (hysteria) by the study of medically ill women. Arch. Gen. Psychiat., *34*:145–149, 1977. Copyright 1977, American Medical Association. Reprinted by permission.

hallucinations (the typical hysterical hallucinations, hearing someone call their name and seeing a vision of a decreased relative, do not indicate psychoses), or urinary retention; (3) fatigue, lump in the throat, fainting spells, visual blurring, weakness or dysuria; (4) breathing difficulty, palpitations, anxiety attacks, chest pain, dizziness: (5) anorexia, weight loss, marked fluctuations in weight, nausea, abdominal bloating, food intolerance, diarrhea, constipation; (6) abdominal pains or vomiting; (7) dysmenorrhea, menstrual irregularities (including amenorrhea for at least two months), or excessive menstrual bleeding; (8) sexual indifference, frigidity, dyspareunia, other sexual difficulties, vomiting all nine months of pregnancy; (9) back pain, joint pain, extremity pain, burning pains in the sexual organs or mouth or rectum, other bodily pains, (10) nervousness, fears, depressed feelings, the need to quit working or inability to carry on regular duties because of feeling sick, crying easily, feeling life is hopeless, thinking a good deal about dying, wanting to die, thinking of suicide, or attempting suicide.

For a symptom to be considered positive, one of the following conditions must be met. (1) The symptom must have caused the patient to see a physician. (2) The symptom must have been disabling over a period of time, i.e., have caused a change in life style or made a difference in functioning. (3) The symptom must have resulted in taking medication. (4) The scorer must believe the symptoms to be clinically significant, i.e., episodes of "paralysis" after a minor injury, without any of the previous three criteria being met. The tenacity of Briquet's syndrome is demonstrated by an eight-year follow-up study in which 25 of 28 patients whose problems were originally diagnosed as Briquet's syndrome continued to have the difficulty.[53] A simplified brief check list of 14 questions has been devised to aid in the rapid diagnosis of Briquet's syndrome (Table 116–3).[76] The screening test produced "false-positive" diagnoses at a rate of 8 per cent when applied to 50 medically hospitalized women, of whom only 1 was found to have Briquet's syndrome. This is in keeping with the estimated prevalence of the disorder in 1 to 2 per cent of the female population as a whole.[1] When the test was retrospectively applied to patients who were known to have Briquet syndrome, an 11 per cent "false-negative" record was obtained.[76] If the answer to question No. 1 of the screening interview is that the patient is less than 26 years old, then it is considered positive. As one proceeds through the questions, reaching a "stop" point suggests a diagnosis of Briquet's syndrome, and a fuller examination is needed. This simplified screening test could be used by an admissions worker or secretary, and could help direct the course of an interview as well as make clinical impressions or prejudices more objective.

Treatment

Before any treatment is begun, and only after the diagnosis is firmly established, the

TABLE 116–3 SCREENING INTERVIEW FOR BRIQUET SYNDROME*

QUESTIONS	BRIQUET SYNDROME		QUESTIONS	BRIQUET SYNDROME	
	Positive	Negative		Positive	Negative
1. "At what age did you first have a problem with bad health or with your nerves?"			12. "In general, has your sexual life been important to you, or could you have gotten along as well without it?"		
2. "Did you ever have a problem with vomiting (not of pregnancy alone)?"			If 12 is Yes, check box and stop. _____ □ Step 7		
3. "Did you ever have difficulty walking (not simply the result of leg or hip or back pain)?" If 2 and 3 are Yes, check box and stop. _____ □ Step 1			13. "Have you ever lost your voice so that you could not speak above a whisper for at least half an hour (not result of laryngitis)?"		
4. "Did you ever have back pain?"			If 13 is Yes, check box and stop. _____ □ Step 8		
5. "Have you ever had abdominal pain (not menstrual)?"					
6. "Have you ever felt so low that you thought of harming yourself?" If 1, 4, 5, and 6 are Yes, check box and stop. _____ □ Step 2			14. "Have you ever had any symptoms which seem quite strange to you, symptoms which might have taken you to a doctor, like double vision or unusual spells?" If 14 is Yes, check box. _____ □ Step 9		
7. "Have you ever had difficulty with your breathing (not associated with exercise)?"			If 14 is No, and 8 or 3 is No, check box. _____ □ Step 10		
8. "Have you ever had pain in your arms or legs (other than in your joints)?" If 2, 7, and 8 are Yes, check box and stop. _____ □ Step 3			If 14 is No, and 8 is Yes and 3 is Yes, check box. _____ □ Step 11		
9. "Have you ever experienced pain elsewhere in your body (not in chest, back, joints, arms, legs, or burning pain of mouth or rectum)?" If 2, 5, and 9 are No, check box and stop. _____ □ Step 4					
10. "Some women have very painful periods. Has that been your experience?" If 10 or 1 is No, check box and stop. _____ □ Step 5			**SCORING**		
11. "Do you remember a time when you lost your appetite?" If 11 and 4 are No, check box and stop. _____ □ Step 6			If the patient admits to both vomiting and ataxia, step 1 is positive, and she qualifies as eligible for a diagnosis of Briquet syndrome at step 1, regardless of subsequent answers. If she does not have both vomiting and ataxia, then step 2 is considered, and so on. In the study of Reveley and co-workers the questionnaires were scored in two ways: First, symptoms with medical explanation were counted as negative; second, the interview was rescored and medically explainable symptoms were counted as positive. Symptoms not medically explained were always scored positive.		

* From Reveley, M. A., Woodruff, R. A., Robins, L. N., Taibleson, M., Reich, T., and Helzer, J.: Evaluation of a screening interview for Briquet syndrome (hysteria) by the study of medically ill women. Arch. Gen. Psychiat., *34*:145–149, 1977. Copyright 1977, American Medical Association. Reprinted by permission.

treating physician should have an appropriate mental set. The author wishes to underscore a critical point made by Kaminsky and Slavney:

Treatment for patients with Briquet syndrome should avoid either challenging or ignoring medically unexplained symptoms and focus instead on vulnerabilities of the personality and ways to cope with stressful situations.[50]

Any attempt to challenge the reality and intensity of the pain will create antagonism and resentment on the part of the patient, and the remainder of the therapeutic association between the doctor and the patient will be spent in a struggle to convince the physician of the intensity and debilitating aspects of the pain.[52] In effect, a challenge about the intensity of the pain is exactly the reverse of therapeutic. Since the patient must now meet the insult to his personal integrity, he becomes more fixed in his symptoms.[40] The advice of Penfield and Cobb should be followed, and each patient who says he is in pain should be regarded as in pain unless there is proof that he is a malingerer.[40] To tell a patient "the pain is all in your head" creates a setting for therapeutic disaster. An excellent review of the various attempts to treat Briquet syndrome is found in an article by Scallet and his colleagues.[79]

Treatment modalities range from no treatment, placebos, and antianxiety drugs through psychotherapy, family therapy, group therapy, behavior therapy, and even include electroconvulsive and electrosleep therapy. If depression is a prominent feature of the Briquet syndrome, electroconvulsive therapy may be of some short-term help, but frequent relapses occur. Eclectic psychotherapy, dynamically oriented psychotherapy, and behavior therapy all seem to yield improvements in about two thirds of the patients, while combined autogenic training and electrosleep gives somewhat better results (80 per cent). It seems that a curative factor is really the autogenic relaxation.[79] Group therapy is effective in reducing anxiety and giving support to the patients while informing them about the various ways of adapting to their disease.[100] An excellent article on group therapy was offered by Ascher and is highly recommended for any practitioner interested in group therapy.[2] Treating patients with exaggerated pain and Briquet syndrome in a group strengthens the homogeneity of the group, since the common bond of pain, coupled with other somatic complaints, makes rich material for discussion. Homogeneous groups appear to become more cohesive than others, offer more immediate support, have better attendance, and provide more symptomatic relief; the participants tend, however, to remain superficial in their relationships.[106] With an experienced and skilled therapist, homogeneous groups are an efficient way to treat patients with Briquet's syndrome who have exagerated pain. Repeated hospitalization in a pain treatment center can prove therapeutic for patients who resist regular forms of therapy.

Prognosis

With short-term therapeutic techniques, rapid improvement can occur in 90 per cent of cases, but long-term benefits range from 45 to 80 per cent. These data, however, apply to the group of patients with Briquet

syndrome who agree to enter therapy of some sort. Only 25 per cent accept conventional therapy, so one must assume the high rate of improvement is due to a biased sample.[79] If a patient with Briquet's syndrome and exaggerated pain has been told "the pain is all in your head," all forms of therapy will fail until the patient is convinced that someone really believes that he has pain.

Case History

P. S. is a 53-year-old twice-married white woman who complained of pain in the cervical region, radiating to the trapezius muscles as well as the occipital area. Results of every objective study were normal except for indications of osteoporosis in the cervical area. The onset of the pain was gradual, i.e., the patient noted it had become worse over a one-month period. She had not been awakened from sleep by pain, but stated that she had trouble falling asleep and that the pain interfered with her work as a designer. Sexual activity already was virtually nonexistent, so the pain did not alter that aspect of her life. The past history included over 40 hospitalizations, including in retrospective order three face lifts, pulmonary embolism, laparotomy to remove adhesions, gallbladder removal, hysterectomy, multiple operations on the hand to replace arthritic joints, full dental extraction and a reconstructive procedure to her jaw, multiple crash diets, and frequent visits to the hospital emergency room for sprains and minor fractures sustained in falls. When first seen, she was taking almost every vitamin supplement available on the market, as well as thyroid medication, a diuretic, and methylphenidate (Ritalin). She had seen three doctors who, understandably, did not consider the pain a valid complaint and told her so. On the first visit, she was in tears, claiming no one believed her, including her son who is a physician on the staff of a major teaching hospital. The patient met the criteria for Briquet syndrome and was referred to an experienced psychotherapist. He reassured her that he believed she had pain, prescribed a transcutaneous stimulator, and discontinued her methylphenidate, thyroid medication, and all fat-soluble vitamins. Within three months, the pain was "under control" and the patient was less anxious and depressed. At the present time, she is attending a church devoted to holistic medicine, which claims not to supplant existing doctors but merely to provide the proper frame of mind for getting better. She reports that she feels better than she ever has in her life, and all the pains are gone. She attributes this directly to attending the faith-healing services at the church, since they believed she had pain and understood her problems.

PATIENTS WITH AFFECTED PAIN

This group contains the patients with affective or associative pain, patients *who do not have pain*. They may have had pain at one time. After the organic basis of pain was cured, however, the symptom of pain was so useful that it was retained. On the other hand, the symptom of pain may be retained unconsciously, with no malicious or devious intent. This distinction between conscious and unconscious motivation must be made, since determination of this factor decides the course and the outcome of treatment. Conversion is an unconscious defense mechanism that protects the individual from overwhelming and unacceptable psychic stress and must be distinguished from malingering, which is a conscious effort to deceive. Severe psychiatric disorders, such as psychosis or psychotic depression, may be manifest as pain, but in these the pain is neither unconscious nor conscious in origin but rather represents a delusional response. In these cases, the pain is incorrectly perceived. The distortions about the pain are due to disordered thinking and loss of the ability to express the perception coherently. It is imperative that a surgeon be able to recognize these patients, since any operative intervention could be disastrous and could delay proper treatment. Great care must be taken to make accurate diagnoses in this group of patients. It is important to avoid the mistake of confusing patients with exaggerated pain with those having an affected pain problem, or in other words, those who do not have actual pain.

Affected Pain in Malingering

To most physicians, the malingerer is probably the most offensive of all patients with chronic pain. It is difficult to maintain objectivity about these patients because they represent a collection of repugnant characteristics that are totally foreign to the sensibilities of most "respectable persons." The normal physician's response to them interferes with the needed objectivity and nonjudgmental understanding required for treatment, and this very fact more firmly entrenches the symptoms. As has been stated, "Nothing resembles malingering more than hysteria; nothing resem-bles hysteria more than malingering."[105] One note of caution is necessary. The malingerer may present with organically defined lesions, but he is likely to attribute these organic ills to a minor injury from which he may derive compensation, although in fact, they were present prior to the event. Usually, the malingerer consciously simulates disease to avoid responsibility, to evade difficult or dangerous duties, or to receive financial rewards.[105] As stated by Keiser, ". . . Money plays a notable role in this condition."[52]

Premorbid Adjustment

Since the key word to the definition of malingering is deceit, people prone to defraud or deceive must be considered with great skepticism.[52] People with previous arrest records or a history of illicit drug addiction can present as malingerers. Persons in financial stress are predisposed to seek compensation if the opportunity presents itself. The propensity toward malingering appears to be mostly situational, i.e., if it is expedient for an individual to feign illness, for either self-preservation or financial gain, he does. This fact may account for the finding by Flicker that 10 per cent of the military men seen because of poor family situations were predisposed to malingering.[22] Also, persons of low intelligence or from rural settings are more likely to present with the picture of malingering.[52] Of course, there is a great overlap between a low socioeconomic class and low level of intelligence, and this may contribute to the skewing of the incidence rates. Passive-aggressive and dependent persons tend to pick this form of disability.

Symptoms and Clinical Course

Symptoms can be as varied as the myriad ways one may injure himself, and can present as arm, neck, back, shoulder, or other pain. Since there are no objective ways to measure it, pain is an ideal symptom for a malingerer. The risk of detection is small. With low back pain, the Hoover's sign usually is present, i.e., the patient will "attempt to raise one leg without compensatory downward thrust of the other."[19] No muscle atrophy is found despite claims of disuse, and the patient is most concerned that the physician believe his pain.

The critical issue is whether possible financial or personal benefits can be derived from the injury, and a thorough sociological history is necessary if the symptoms are suspect. The malingerer does not get better over time, nor does his "disease" progress. Resistence to physical examinations, repeat evaluations, or objective testing suggests malingering. A careful sequential history is needed if an actual physical finding is present, since a malingerer who has had a previous (prepain) injury is less likely to be detected. Since the symptoms are consciously feigned, the conscious effort needed to maintain the symptoms should be noted. Traumatic onset of pain symptoms is common, but changes in life situations can precipitate malingering.

Pathology and Etiology

Avoidance of danger, financial gain, and a desire for sympathy are fairly common etiological bases for malingering.[22,52] It can be a defense against anxiety, dependence, or hostility.[52] Using pain as a symptom can make a malingering patient the center of attention, or can be used to retaliate for some real or imagined wrong perpetrated on the patient by an organization or individual.[22,52] Occasionally, pain can be used to avoid sexual contact with an objectionable partner or be the results of guilt for an extramarital affair.[14,78]

Diagnosis and Clinical Tests

Some authors believe it is useless to differentiate between malingering and conversion.[66] The treatment of the two is different, however, since malingering is conscious deceit, while conversion is an unconscious mechanism that serves to protect the individual from unbearable psychic distress. Conversion is amenable to psychotherapy and is discussed later. Keiser offers an excellent discussion of malingering and states that three factors are crucial to the establishment of a correct diagnosis of this disorder. The first is a meticulous physical examination, the second is freedom from bias on the part of the examiner, and the third is an understanding atmosphere "in which the patient feels free to discuss all of his fears associated with the accident and his treatment."[52] There are historical clues that a malingerer offers. Not uncommonly, he has seen his attorney before seeing a physician.

Several mechanisms are useful for arriving at the diagnosis of malingering. One is to record thoroughly, in writing, all symptoms mentioned during the initial interview, then ask the patient to repeat the symptoms on follow-up visits. Contradictions usually suggest malingering. If the patient is uncooperative, dislikes physical examinations or tries to avoid them, gives sullen or evasive answers, or in general has an adversary attitude, he may be malingering. Neurotics follow prescribed regimens faithfully, malingerers do not. The malingerer may depict himself in exclusively complimentary terms. Under narcosynthesis (with intravenous amobarbital), the malingerer usually insists that he has symptoms unlike conversion symptoms, which remit.[52]

Additional clues are offered by Davis and Weiss, who list 10 ways to differentiate psychoneurosis from malingering. The first clue is an inability to work coupled with retention of the capacity to play.[22] This author usually obtains such information by asking about hobbies and sex life at least five minutes after discussing the history of present illness. Usually a past history and family history take up a sufficient amount of time between questions about the disability on the job and those about the ability to engage in pleasurable experiences. Davis and Weiss confirm Keiser's observation regarding the adherence to medical regimens by neurotics, and the opposing unreliability of malingerers. They also suggest that a premorbid adjustment that has features of responsibility, honesty, and adequacy militates against the diagnosis of malingering.[22] If the patient admits to fears or dreams about the accident, he is probably neurotic. If he carries on allegedly lost functions when he thinks he is not being observed, he is malingering. Spying on a patient to determine whether he maintains his symptoms has been used by insurance companies and has been advocated by physicians.[105] Malingerers usually do not copy symptoms seen in others while in the hospital, but neurotics may do this. If a patient is willing to submit to operations and mental hospitalization, he probably is not malingering. If he refuses employment that utilizes skills that draw on unimpaired functions, he probably is malingering. Willingness to submit to examinations and objective tests suggests neurosis rather than malingering. Davis and Weiss suggest several psychological tests to diagnose malingering, but only the Minnesota Multiphasic Personality Index (MMPI) has any application to patients with chronic pain.[22] If the score of the F scale minus that of the K scale is greater than 9, then one may suspect malingering.

Apart from a psychiatric differential evaluation, the physical examination should include any tests indicated to rule out cholecystitis, cholelithiasis, pancreatitis, pancreatic tumor, penetrating ulcer, renal infection or infraction or tumor or calculi, ureteral calculi, menginitis, spinal cord tumor, or bladder infection or tumor, all of which can mimic the low back pain of spinal disorders. Additionally, benign prostatic hypertrophy and chronic prostatitis in males, and retroversion of the uterus, endometriosis, fibroids, ovarian cysts, pelvic inflammatory disease, and chronic cervicitis in females all can cause pain in the low back area.[51] Postcoital pain based on an organic disorder has been reported in both males and females, and is not always indicative of malingering.[50,97] Since patients who are malingering may have been coached by an unscrupulous lawyer, the history they give may include vague complaints about bowel, bladder, or sexual function, which requires a thorough rectal examination. A useful trick in the physical examination is to ask the patient to raise his arms over his head while prone or supine. Patients with back pain seldom have pain with this maneuver. When asked to kneel on a chair and try to touch the floor, malingerers will usually claim the pain is too great, but patients with severe disc and sciatic pain usually will be more willing to cooperate and will attempt to do this. Another excellent test is to straighten the patient's knee while he is sitting on the examining table, under the pretext of examining leg strength. If he can tolerate this, but does not permit straight-leg-raising in the supine position, he is malingering.[51] The Hoover test has already been mentioned. One additional maneuver is to use stethoscope pressure to evaluate the painful areas. The malingerer, not recognizing that the physician is really testing for pain, thinks that he is merely listening for something.

Treatment

Obviously, there is no indication for operative treatment, and psychiatric intervention is woefully inadequate. Confrontation produces resentment—and even lawsuits against the physician for libel and slander. The best approach is to be nonjudgmental and let the patient tell of the various conflicts in his life that prompted the malingering. Many times, merely having someone in whom he trusts and confides can allow the malingering patient a graceful way of exiting from the lie he has told himself and others. The physician should remember that malingering is not a pure blessing, since it carries components of fear, shame, and guilt.[52] The adversary role should be avoided, and the physician should carefully phrase his statements to reflect the absence of clinical findings in an objective fashion—without the use of the terms "fraud," "fakery," or "malingering." Compensation must be settled either by "outright rejection or by a lump-sum payment" to remove one variable in the etiology of malingering.[22] After the financial settlement, benign neglect can be instituted until the patient exhibits a willingness to enter psychotherapy. Family therapy may prove the best modality.

Prognosis

The award of a large sum of cash may not end the odyssey of the malingerer. If home conditions dictate, the patient may continue with the deception for the secondary gains afforded by family members. Only if the pattern is altered and interrupted can any benefit be derived from therapy, and if the family is unwilling to participte, then the physicians have lost their leverage against the malingerer.

Case Report

R. T. is a 35-year-old white male janitor who is married and has four children. The first onset of low back pain occurred after the patient lifted a heavy box at work. He reported that he felt a strain in his back, and he saw the company doctor, who discharged him to home and bed rest for three days. On the advice of the union shop steward, the patient consulted an attorney and began to gather information for his suit against the workmen's compensation insurance carrier. The patient complained of pain that prevented him from working and from having sex with his wife. Using compensation benefits, as well as social security disability payments, the patient began to take a course in appliance repair.

The physical examination was remarkable

only for the lack of signs to correlate with the expressed pain, a positive Hoover's sign, and ability to raise a bent leg while seated but not while supine. All test results were normal, and the psychiatric evaluation revealed a passive-dependent personality with anxiety and depression. The patient was made to return to work by the compensation board, until the case was settled. In the interim, the insurance carrier, using hidden cameras and private detectives, filmed the patient while he was lifting heavy objects at work when no one else was present and also while he was riding his son's motor scooter. In both circumstances, the patient did not seem to exhibit any sign of pain.

After a sympathetic re-evaluation, the patient broke into tears, claiming he really couldn't stand the work load on his job but was afraid to complain lest his fellow workers think he was weak and a "sissy." The reduction in sexual activity was due to a massive weight gain of 80 lb that his wife had experienced since her gallbladder removal. He now found her "fat and ugly," when before she had been "well-built." The patient agreed to undergo psychotherapy, which involved the wife and the intervention of a social worker to help the patient with vocational rehabilitation. After job retraining, and a 40-lb weight loss by the wife, the patient reported feeling less anxious and depressed. He is at present functioning well at his new place of employment, an appliance repair shop.

Aggravated Pain Due to Conversion

This group of patients with aggravated pain is constantly having its ranks swelled by inappropriate diagnosis. Very few patients with chronic pain fit into this category. Furthermore, a hysterical personality does not always precede conversion. In fact, Ziegler, Imboden, and Meyer found that only a minority of patients with conversion symptoms had "hysterical" personalities, while 30 per cent of the patients with conversion had depressive symptoms. Additionally, when they examined 100 depressive patients, they found conversion symptoms in 28 of them. They also found, however, that 75 of 134 patients with conversion had pain as the primary complaint.[108] Stephens and Kamp likewise found no predominance of hysterical personalities among persons with dissociative and conversion hysteria, but bid find the most common personality type with symptoms to be passive-dependent.[91] Slater followed up 85 patients with the diagnosis of

"hysteria" made at the Queen Square Hospital in London and found information that is disconcerting. After an average delay of nine years from the original diagnosis, only 19 of the 85 patients were symptom-free at the time of follow-up. Seven of the eighty-five had recurrent endogenous depression, two were schizophrenic, three had had neoplasms undetected at the time of original diagnosis, and four had committed suicide. One of those committing suicide had atypical myopathy and another had disseminated sclerosis. Twenty-four patients were thought to have organic disease coincident with their "hysteria," ranging from undiagnosed epilepsy to the residual of meningitis. Eight died of natural causes. Twenty-eight patients were believed to have simple "hysteria." All 28 were later found to have an organic basis for their complaints! Two persons with facial pain were later found to have trigeminal neuralgia. One young lady had pain in the neck that was subsequently diagnosed as thoracic inlet syndrome. One woman had pain in her right shoulder and arm that was later diagnosed as Takayasu's syndrome, and three persons had early, undetected dementia. The rest had a multiplicity of organic diseases including epilepsy, vestibular lesions, and total block of the spinal cord. Of the 85 patients with what was originally diagnosed as "hysteria" (meaning conversion symptoms), only 7 were found to have an acute psychogenic reaction resulting in the formation of a conversion symptom, while 14 were found to have Briquet syndrome.[87] In effect, one must use great caution before assigning the diagnosis of conversion neurosis or hysteria. In a psychiatric hospital, hysteria was found to account for 2 per cent of all psychiatric admissions, and this percentage has remained unchanged over a 50-year period.[91] The category of conversion, in patients with aggravated pain, must also include post-traumatic neurosis, incipient psychosis, and depression, all of which may be manifested with pain as the only symptom.

Premorbid Adjustment

As mentioned earlier, a hysterical personality, a histrionic personality, or the Briquet syndrome does not lie on a continuum with hysterical conversion symptoms. Entirely "normal" people, during overwhelming stress, may experience conversion symptoms, especially of the post-traumatic neurotic type described so well by Keiser.[52] The patient may have a passive-dependent life style, or have experienced extremely stressful events that have resulted in overwhelming anxiety or depression.[72,91] Unlike the histrionic hysterical personality, which usually is confined to women, the incidence of conversion is as high in men as it is in women.[17] Also, although persons with sociopathic personalities and hysterical neuroses frequently may experience conversion, reactions, Engel has found that hysterical histrionic personalities, depressed patients, hypochondriacal patients, and schizophrenics present with chronic pain.[26,39] Keiser has found that more intelligent and sophisticated people use pain as a conversion symptom rather than the gross paralysis that is found in a less sophisticated group. He attributes this difference in the groups to the social acceptability of chronic pain.[52] It is safe to say, however, that there is no typical premorbid personality, and the formation of conversion symptoms is more a function of the traumatic event (discussed under etiology) than of the personality of a patient, even though those with the previously mentioned personality disorders (dependent personality, sociopathic personality, histrionic personality, and patients with reactive depression) probably are more predisposed to conversion reactions.

Signs and Symptoms

Just as the premorbid adjustments and causes vary, so do the presenting signs and symptoms. The location of pain may be

. . . determined by the unconscious identification with a love object, the pain being either one suffered by the patient himself when in some conflict with the object, or a pain suffered by the object, in fact, or in the patient's fantasy.[26]

The patient with chronic pain who has had multiple operations may, on presentation, demand an operation. Often these patients have gastrointestinal or gynecological complaints compatible with both psychodynamic etiology and the need for an operation, i.e., women with sexual conflicts may experience pain in the genital area. If a close relative has died of stomach cancer, they may present with the complaint of pain in the abdomen. Back pain is commonly considered a classic conversion symptom of depression, the so-called "depressive equivalent" or "masked depression."[62] Atypical facial pain has been suggested to be purely a conversion reaction.[23] Headache could be included in this group. Also, post-traumatic neurosis can be manifest as chronic pain, with the location of the pain being determined by the circumstances surrounding its onset.[52] One might, however, take the stance that "conversion" should be a specific term, reserved for symptoms that mimic neurological disease, since the inclusion of unexplained pains—headaches, back aches, and abdominal pains—or other medical symptoms in the category of conversion would make the diagnosis meaningless and the differential diagnosis embrace a whole range of medical disorders.[39] This caution may be a bit too rigorous, since true conversion manifesting as pain responds as well to certain psychiatric treatments as conversion manifesting as neurological disease.

Pathology and Etiology

It must be recognized that a conversion reaction represents an unconscious resolution of a problem that allows the person to cope with an overwhelming stress.[52] Again, the emphasis here is on the unconscious formation of symptoms; therefore, the patient is convinced his pain is real. The significance of an accident or trauma to the patient is as important as the severity of the event. An especially repugnant event can produce conversion, even though it has merely been observed without the patient's participating in the action. Depression has been linked extensively to conversion, and the symptom most often expressed is low back pain.[62] This development occurs when pain is used as a symptom to replace grief, or as a response to a loss (death of a loved one) or to extreme stress.[38] Engel explains the unconscious selection of pain as the conversion symptom because it provides penitence, suffering, atonement, self-denial, and self-depreciation as a way to ease the feelings of guilt.[26,27] He found that, unconsciously, these patients do not believe they deserve success or happiness, and notes elements of sadomasochism in their sexual development as well as conflict over sexual impulses.[10,26] Pilowsky believes that pain may not be a conversion per se, but rather "serves a conversion function," which permits a physical symptom to block conscious awareness of a conflict that has overwhelming guilt associated with it.[74] Pilling and co-workers believe that, even when no trauma is involved, pain may substitute for anxiety as well.[72] As the symptoms become more difficult to understand, so do the causes. Patients who have had multiple operations for reasons of which they are not aware may request an operation to fulfill the primary gain of dealing with their fears of death, "cutting out" their guilt, being a "bloody sacrifice" to assuage guilt, or symbolically re-enacting sexual fantasies.[101] Pain may be a defense against an incipient psychosis due to situational stress or be a rare, bizarre manifestation of a schizophrenic process in which "pain" is a delusional representation of a conflict.[23,26] Whatever the source, one must take note of the unconscious use of pain.

Diagnosis and Clinical Tests

When pain is substituting for depression, there frequently is no suicidal ideation, no loss of appetite, no guilty feelings, but the presence of compensation. These patients usually make use of physical concerns and loss of social activity, but not of a depressed mode.[62] There are significant differences between patients with conversion and normal patients on a "face recognition test," which is designed to assess general vigilance or sustained attention.[8] It is not practical, however, for the usual physician to administer this test because of the time required and the need for special equipment. A simple "arm levitation" test does show significant differences between the suggestibility of patients with conversion hysteria and that of normal control patients. In this test, the patient is asked to close his eyes and to hold the nondominant arm extended horizontally as long as he can. For 30 seconds the patient is given the suggestion that the arm is weightless and moving upward. If the arm moves more than 13 cm upward (from the horizontal) during the 30 seconds of suggestion, then the patient is most likely prone to conversion, while a movement of 7 to 13 cm reveals some suggestibility.[8] An inconsistent pattern of pain distribution, as well as a nonanatomical distribution of pain, is most suggestive of conversion.[19] The most revealing diagnostic clue, however, is discovered by understanding the onset of the pain. The information is derived from a thorough, meticulous history. If there was a sudden onset with a loss of consciousness, no matter how brief, in a situation that was life-threatening to the patient or to others, with an "expansion of time" during the perception of the event, then the event was traumatic enough to produce conversion symptoms. A seemingly benign event may have great psychological impact on an individual if it reminds him of some previously unresolved conflict. This fact may not be readily discernible until after years of treatment, and it complicates the diagnosis. Events other than accidents that result in a loss can be severely traumatic psychologically and produce conversion symptoms. Examples of such events are the loss of a loved one through death, divorce, or other circumstances that the patient cannot control. It is this element of helplessness that primes an individual for a conversion reaction.

There are other useful tips in the diagnosis of conversion reactions. The presence of increased dreaming suggests an attempt to deal with the conflict. Patients with conversion differ from malingerers in their cooperative attitude, their honesty with the physician, their compliance with medical and testing regimens, a good employment record, and willingness to return to work. *La belle indifférence* may be present and manifest itself as a lack of intense concern about the symptoms and a feeling that everything will be all right.[52] *La belle indifférence*, however, was found in only 30 per cent of the patients with conversion reactions who were reviewed by Stephens and Kamp.[91] A good life style adjustment may be found in patients with conversion, because, to some degree, the conflict is resolved by the acquisition of the symptom. Conversion may be a defense against impending psychotic episodes, and conversion due to such an impending psychosis or delusions due to a schizophrenic process will become evident in a thorough mental status examination.[91]

Treatment

If the onset of pain and depression are coincident, even though the pain is masking or becoming the equivalent of the depression, an adequate trial of mood-elevating drugs is indicated. This trial would require 75 to 300 mg a day of amitriptyline (Elavil), doxepin (Sinequan), imipramine (Tofranil), or desipramine (Norpramin). The former two should be given all at night, but the latter two may be given in divided doses or all in the morning. If these antidepressants are given for at least one month without effect, tranylcypromine (Parnate, a monoamine oxidase inhibitor) may be added, beginning with 10 mg twice daily and increasing to 20 mg twice a day.[3] If antidepressant drugs fail, then electroconvulsive therapy has been reported to be useful for the treatment of the endogenous depression, usually with the resolution of the complaint of chronic pain.[59] Reactive depression, that is, depression that is the result of a loss such as chronic pain, death of a relative, or losing one's job does not respond to electroconvulsive therapy. Individual psychotherapy is indicated for this group of patients. For post-traumatic neurosis, a long-term analytically oriented psychotherapy situation is indicated, with the use of hypnosis or amobarbital or both to uncover the traumatic event.[52] The revelation about the event is not enough to effect a cure, and hypnosis and narcosynthesis are best left in the hands of an experienced psychiatrist, since there is a risk of precipitating a psychotic episode. For incipiently or frankly psychotic patients, phenothiazine tranquilizers should be used in adequate doses. Chlorpromazine (Thorazine), 500 to 1000 mg per day in divided doses, or perphenazine (Trilafon), 24 mg per day in divided doses, may be used. If needed, a butyrophenone such as haloperidol (Haldol), 20 to 40 mg per day in divided doses, may be used. The physician must be aware that butyrophenones, phenothiazines, and tricyclic mood-elevating drugs alone or together have been used successfully for postherpetic neuralgia and pain of disseminated visceral neoplasm.[95] For that reason, care must be taken in the interpretation of benefit from these drugs, since undiagnosed pain with a true organic cause may be misdiagnosed as hysterical conversion. Indeed, two of the three cases reported by Delaney as atypical facial pain appeared to be postherpetic in origin.[23] Therefore, it is difficult to determine whether the pain resolved as the result of treating a postherpetic neuralgia or an incipient psychotic episode.

Prognosis

If conversion is due to anxiety or depression, an adequate course of psychotherapy, medication, and if necessary, hospitalization will result in the resolution of the problem and an eventual cure. If the conversion is post-traumatic in nature, then psychotherapy directed at achieving a catharsis about the traumatic event will be beneficial. Early diagnosis and treatment of acute psychotic episodes manifesting as conversion will normally result in a brief hospital stay, in counter distinction to prolonged hospitalization if the synptom is prematurely or inappropriately removed, or remains undetected as a prepsychotic condition. Delusional pain due to a true schizophrenic psychosis may remit with the administration of psychotropic medication (phenothiazines, butyrophenones, thioxanthenes, dibenzoxazepines, and indolic compounds) but nothing can be done for the underlying process.

Case History

P. F. is a 45-year-old computer programmer who originally complained of a persistant occipital headache, loss of concentration, and inability to calculate figures since his automobile was hit from behind a month prior to his being seen. He had had a depressive episode after his divorce, which was five years prior to the accident. There was no history of other psychiatric problems.

The neurological examination, electroencephalogram, echoencephalogram, and brain scan were normal. Psychological testing revealed a 15-point discrepancy between verbal and performance IQ's, which suggested a difficulty with hand-eye coordination, and impaired concentration. The patient was an obsessive-compulsive individual who strove for perfection on his job and at home. He admitted to being somewhat depressed and had difficulty falling asleep. The working diagnosis was postconcussion syndrome versus post-traumatic neurosis. Amitriptyline (Elavil), 150 mg at bedtime, and perphenazine (Trilafon), 4 mg four times a day was instituted. He had not worked since the accident and stated that his difficulty in concentrating prevented him from running computer programs.

After three months of weekly therapy, the patient reported that his concentration had improved. He hesitated to return to full-time employment because of his fear of making mistakes. Nevertheless, he did return and performed satisfactorily. The lawsuit against the driver who struck his car was not settled because the driver was uninsured and had left the country. The patient felt cheated. As therapy progressed, he became less anxious and depressed, and at six months had no symptoms other than the occipital headache. A psychodrama was done in which the patient re-experienced the accident and his fear of dying at the time he was struck, and additional analytically oriented therapy was instituted. The headaches still persisted.

After one year of therapy, the patient recalled an incident in which his mother struck him in the back of the head when he was 5 years old, because he had refused to tie his shoes. He immediately jumped up from the couch after recalling the incident and explained that the blow to the back of the head in the accident was exactly like the blow he had experienced when he was 5 years old. He remembered, however, how frustrated he felt when he was young, because he was not able to retaliate against his mother for the punishment, and how angry he felt toward her, just as he had felt toward the driver of the car that struck him and sped away. He stated that he wanted to kill both the driver and his mother, at which point he burst into tears. The next week the occipital headaches were gone.

SUMMARY

Chronic pain is a most difficult complaint to diagnose accurately. The physician must have a nonjudgmental approach. Patients with chronic pain may be divided into two broad categories: (1) those who have a good prepain adjustment to life and, because of pain, develop psychiatric problems; and (2) those who have a psychiatrically definable problem prior to the onset of pain and either exaggerate or use the pain to their benefit in a conscious or unconscious fashion. Diagnosis and treatment of the first group is straightforward, and the greatest curative factor is time. As the patient learns to deal with his pain, he functions better. Since chronic pain can mean different things to each of the psychiatrically definable personalities that experience it, diagnosis and treatment of the second group is as varied as the field of psychiatry itself. There is no such entity as "imagined pain," but there is exaggerated or faked pain, or "pain" that represents a psychodynamic conflict, that is perceived as pain even though there may not be any organic basis. To tell a patient "the pain is all in your head" is to invite a therapeutic disaster, since the judgment

placed against the patient makes him all the more determined to convince his physician that "the pain is real." Not challenging a patient about the intensity or reality of his pain is the first step toward the appropriate treatment of chronic pain. Accurate diagnosis is the key to accurate treatment, and no physician should proceed with any treatment unless he, in good conscience, can justify the approach, whether it be operative or psychiatric.

REFERENCES

1. Arkonac, O., and Guze, S.: A family study of hysteria. New Eng. J. Med., 268:239–242, 1963.
2. Ascher, E.: Group psychotherapy. In Practice of Medicine. Vol. X. Hagerstown, Md., Harper & Row, 1971.
3. Ayd, F. J.: Int. Drug Ther. Newsletter, 11:29–32, 1976.
4. Beaver, W. T.: Comparison of morphine, hydroxyzine, and morphine plus hydroxyzine in postoperative pain. In Recent studies on the nature and management of acute pain. A special report, Hosp. Pract., pp. 8–13, Jan., 1976.
5. Beecher, H. K.: Relationship of significance of wound to pain experienced. J.A.M.A., 161: 1609–1613, 1956.
6. Beecher, H. K., Review of pain. Pharmacol. Rev., 9:59–97, 1957.
7. Belkin, S. C., and Quigley, T. B.: Finding the causes of low back pain. Res. Staff Physician, 23:58–63, 1977.
8. Bendefeldt, F., Miller, L. L., and Ludwig, A. M.: Cognitive performance in conversion hysteria. Arch. Gen. Psychiat., 33:1250–1254, 1976.
9. Berges, P. V.: Myofascial pain syndromes. Postgrad. Med., 53:161–168, 1973.
10. Blumer, D., Psychiatric considerations in pain. In Rothman, R., and Simeone, R., eds.: The Spine. Philadelphia, W. B. Saunders Co., 1975.
11. Blumetti, A. E., and Modesti, L. M.: Psychological predictors of success or failure of surgical intervention for intractable back pain. In Bonica, J. J. and Albe-Fessard, D., eds.: Advances in Pain Research and Therapy. Vol. 1. New York, Raven Press, 1976, pp. 323–325.
12. Bonica, J. J., Fundamental considerations of chronic pain therapy. Postgrad. Med., 53:81–85, 1973.
13. Bornstein, I.: Psychoprophylactic Preparation for Painless Childbirth. New York, Grune & Stratton, Inc., 1958.
14. Broderick, C. B.: The case for sexual fidelity. Med. Aspects Human Sexuality, 10:16–25, 1976.
15. Bronzo, A., and Powers, G.: Relationship of anxiety with pain threshold. J. Psychol., 66:181–183, 1967.
16. Chapman, C. R., and Feather, B. W.: Effects of diazepam on human pain tolerance and pain

sensitivity. Psychosom. Med., *35*:330–339, 1973.

17. Chodoff, P.: The diagnosis of hysteria: An overview. Amer. J. Psychiat., *131*:1073–1078, 1974.

18. Chodoff, P., and Lyons, A.: Hysteria: The hysterical personality and hysterical conversion. Amer. J. Psychiat., *114*:734–740, 1958.

19. Collins, R. D.: Illustrated Manual of Neurologic Diagnosis. Philadelphia, J. B. Lippincott Co., 1962.

20. Conn, J. H.: The inter-relationship between anxiety and pain. J. Amer. Soc. Psychosom. Dent. Med., *8*:40–52, 1961.

21. Davidson, P. O., and Neufeld, R. W. J.: Response to pain and stress: A multivariate analysis. J. Psychosom. Res., *18*:25–32, 1974.

22. Davis, D., and Weiss, J. M. A.: Malingering and associated syndromes. In Arieti, S., and Brody, E., eds.: American Handbook of Psychiatry. 2nd Ed. Vol. 3, Adult Clinical Psychiatry. New York, Basic Books, 1974.

23. Delaney, J. F.: Atypical facial pain as a defense against psychosis. Amer. J. Psychiat., *133*:1151–1154, 1976.

24. Derogatis, L. R., Rickels, K., and Rock, A.: The SCL 90 and the MMPI: A step in the validation of a new self reporting scale. Brit. J. Psychiat., *128*:280–289, 1976.

25. Drew, F. J., Moriarty, R. W., and Shapiro, A. P., An approach to the measurement of the pain and anxiety responses of surgical patients. Psychosom. Med., *30*:826–836, 1968.

26. Engel, G. L.: Psychogenic pain and the pain prone patient. Amer. J. Med., *26*:899–918, 1959.

27. Engel, G. L.: A life setting conducive to illness— the giving-up-given-up complex. Ann. Intern. Med., *69*:293–300, 1968.

28. Engel, G.: Chapter 26.3 *in* Freedman, A., Kaplan, H., and Sadock, B., eds.: Comprehensive Textbook of Psychiatry. 2nd Ed. Vol. 2. Williams & Wilkins Co., Baltimore, 1975, pp. 1638–42.

29. Erickson, D. L., Michaelson, M. A., and Acharya, A.: Pain patient selection for implantable stimulating devices. *In* Bonica, J. J., and Albe-Fessard, D., eds.: Advances in Pain Research and Therapy. Vol. 1. New York, Raven Press, 1976, pp. 479–482.

30. Finneson, B. E.: Diagnosis and Management of Pain Syndromes. 2nd Ed. Philadelphia, W. B. Saunders Co., 1969.

31. Folstein, M., Folstein, S., and McHugh, P.: Mini-mental state: A practical method for grading the cognitive state of patients for the clinician. J. Psychiat. Res., *12*:189–198, 1975.

32. Fordyce, W. E.: The operant conditioning method for managing chronic pain. Postgrad. Med., *53*:123–128, 1973.

33. Forrest, W. H.: Bioassay of morphine and morphine plus hydroxyzine in postoperative pain, *In* Recent studies on the nature and management of acute pain, a special report. Hosp. Pract., pp. 19–22, Jan. 1976.

34. Frank, J. D.: Persuasion and Healing: A Comparative Study of Psychotherapy. Baltimore, Johns Hopkins University Press, 1973.

35. Gessel, A.: Biofeedback in Pain Management.

Audiocassette, T-11. Biomonitoring Application Inc., 270 Madison Ave., New York, 1975.

36. Gilbert, M. M.: The efficacy of Percogesic in relief of musculoskeletal pain associated with anxiety. Psychosomatics, *17*:190–193, 1976.

37. Gough, H.: The F minus K dissimulation index for MMPI. J. Consult. Psychol., *14*:403–413, 1950.

38. Greene, W. A.: Role of a vicarious object in the adaptation to object loss. Psychosom. Med., *20–21*:344–350, 1958–1959.

39. Guze, S.: The validity and significance of the clinical diagnosis of hysteria (Briquet syndrome). Amer. J. Psychiat., *132*:138–141, 1975.

40. Hackett, T. P.: Pain and prejudice. Why do we doubt that the patient is in pain? Med. Times, *99*:130–139, 1971.

41. Halpern, L. M.: Theories of pain transmission and perception. *In* Recent studies on the nature and management of pain, a special report. Hosp. Pract., pp. 41–44, Jan., 1976.

42. Hannington-Kiff, J. G., Pain Relief. Philadelphia, J. B. Lippincott Co., 1974.

43. Hart, F. D.: The Treatment of Chronic Pain. Philadelphia, F. A. Davis Co., 1974.

44. Hendler, N., Derogatis, L., Avella, J., and Long, D. M.: EMG biofeedback in patients with chronic pain. Dis. Nerv. Syst., *38*:505–509, 1977.

45. Hill, H. E., Kornetsky, C. H., Flanary, H. G., and Wikler, A.: Effects of anxiety and morphine on discrimination of intensities of painful stimuli. J. Clin. Invest., *31*:473–480, 1952.

46. Holmes, T. H., and Wolff, A. G.: Life situations, emotions and backache. Res. Publ. Ass. Res. Nerv. Ment. Dis., *29*:750–772, 1949.

47. Horton, P. C.: The psychological treatment of personality disorders. Amer. J. Psychiat., *133*:262–265, 1976.

48. Jamison, K., Ferrer-Brechner, M. T., Brechner, V. L., and McCreary, C. P.: Correlation of personality profile with pain syndrome. *In* Bonica, J. J., and Albe-Fessard, D., eds.: Advances in Pain Research and Therapy. Vol. 1. Raven Press, New York, 1976, pp. 317–321.

49. Kaminetzky, H. A.: Postcoital pelvic pain. Med. Aspects Human Sexuality, *11*:93, 1977.

50. Kaminsky, M. J., and Slavney, P. R.: Methodology and personality in Briquet's syndrome: A reappraisal. Amer. J. Psychiat., *133*:85–88, 1976.

51. Keim, H. A.: Low Back Pain. Ciba Clinical Symposium 25, No. 3, 1973.

52. Keiser, L.: The Traumatic Neurosis. Philadelphia, J. B. Lippincott Co., 1968.

53. Kimble, R., Williams, J. G., and Agras, S.: A comparison of two methods of diagnosing hysteria. Amer. J. Psychiat., *132*:1197–1199, 1975.

54. Knox, V. J., Morgan, A. H., and Hilgard, E. R.: Pain and suffering in ischemia. Arch. Gen. Psychiat., *30*:840–847, 1974.

55. Kubler-Ross, E.: On Death and Dying. New York, Macmillan Co., 1969.

56. Liberman, R.: An experimental study of the placebo response under three different situations of pain. J. Psychiat. Res., *2*:233–246, 1964.

57. Long, D. M.: Use of peripheral and spinal cord stimulation in the relief of chronic pain. *In*

Bonica, J. J., and Albe-Fessard, D., eds.: Advances in Pain Research and Therapy. Vol. 1. Raven Press, New York, 1976, pp. 395–403.

58. Luisada, P., Peeley, R., and Pittard, E.: The hysterical personality in men. Amer. J. Psychiat., 131:518–522, 1974.

59. Mandel, M. R.: Electroconvulsive therapy for chronic pain associated with depression. Amer. J. Psychiat., 132:632–636, 1975.

60. Marks, I.: The current status of behavioral psychotherapy: Theory and practice. Amer. J. Psychiat., 133:253–261, 1976.

61. Martinez-Urrutia, A.: Anxiety and pain in surgical patients. J. Consult. Clin. Psychol., 43:437–442, 1975.

62. Maruta, T., Swanson, D., and Swanson, W.: Pain as a psychiatric symptom: Comparison between low back pain and depression. Psychosomatics, 17:123–127, 1976.

63. Medical World News: Management of chronic pain; medicine's new growth industry. pp. 54–77, Oct. 18, 1976.

64. Melzack, R., and Chapman, C. R.: Psychological aspects of pain. Postgrad. Med., 53:69–75, 1973.

65. Mendels, J., Weinstein, N., and Cochrane, C.: The relationship between depression and anxiety. Arch. Gen. Psychiat., 27:649–653, 1972.

66. Miller, H.: Accident neurosis. Brit. Med. J., 1:992–998, 1961.

67. Modigh, K.: Effects of clomipramine (Anafranil) on neuro-transmission in brain monoamine neurones. J. Int. Med. Res., 1:274–290, 1973.

68. Montilla, E., Frederik, W. S., and Cass, L. J.: Analgesic effect of methotrimeprazine and morphine: A clinical comparison. Arch. Intern. Med. (Chicago), 111:275–278, 1963.

69. Moskowitz, R. A.: Epithelializing an epithet: Therapies of the hysterical personality disorder. Dis. Nerv. Syst., 37:65–67, 1976.

70. Mumford, J. M., Newton, A. V., and Ley, P.: Personality, pain in perception and pain tolerance. Brit. J. Psychol., 64:105–107, 1973.

71. Perley, M., and Guze, S.: Hysteria: The stability and usefulness of clinical criteria. New Eng. J. Med., 266:421–426, 1962.

72. Pilling, L., Brannick, T. L., and Swenson, W. M.: Psychologic characteristics of psychiatric patients having pain as a presenting symptom. Canad. Med. Ass. J., 97:387–394, 1967.

73. Pilowsky, I.: Abnormal illness behavior. Brit. J. Med. Psychol., 42:347–351, 1969.

74. Pilowsky, I.: The psychiatrist and the pain clinic. Amer. J. Psychiat., 133:752–756, 1976.

75. Pinsky, J. J.: Psychodynamics and psychotherapy in the treatment of patients with chronic intractable pain. In Crue, B., Jr., ed.: Pain: Research and Treatment. New York, Academic Press, 1975.

76. Reveley, M. A., Woodruff, R. A., Robins, L. N., Taibleson, M., Reich, T., and Helzer, J.: Evaluation of a screening interview for Briquet syndrome (hysteria) by the study of medically ill women. Arch. Gen. Psychiat., 34:145–149, 1977.

77. Robins, E.: Categories versus dimensions in psychiatric classification. Psychiat. Ann., 6:368–374, 1976.

78. Sarno, J. E.: Psychosomatic back ache to avoid

79. Scallet, A., Cloninger, R. C., and Ekkehard, O.: The management of chronic hysteria: A review and double-blind trial of electrosleep and other relaxation methods. Dis. Nerv. Syst., 37:347–353, 1976.

80. Schmale, A. H.: Giving up as a final common pathway to changes in health. Advances Psychosom. Med., 8:20–40, 1972.

81. Schwartz, R. A., and Schwartz, I. K.: Are personality disorders diseases? Dis. Nerv. Syst., 37:613–617, 1976.

82. Scobie, B. A.: Costochondral pain in gastroenterologic practice. Letter to Editor. New Eng. J. Med., 295:1261, 1976.

83. Scott, D. L.: Modern Hospital Hypnosis Especially for Anaesthetists. Chicago, Year Book Medical Publishers, Inc., 1974.

84. Shanfield, S. B., and Killingsworth, R. N.: The psychiatric aspects of pain. Psychiat. Ann., 7:24–35, 1977.

85. Shapiro, D.: Neurotic Styles. New York, Basic Books, 1965.

86. Shealy, C. N.: The pain patient. Amer. Fam. Physician, 9:130–136, 1974.

87. Slater, E.: Diagnosis of "hysteria." Brit. Med. J., 1:1395–1399, 1965.

88. Small, E. W.: An investigation into the psychogenic basis of the temporomanidibular joint myofascial pain dysfunction syndrome. In Bonica, J. J., and Albe-Fessard, D., eds.: Advances in Pain Research and Therapy. Vol. 1. New York, Raven Press, 1976, pp. 889–894.

89. Spitzer, R., and Sheehy, M.: DSM III: A classification system in development. Psychiat. Ann., 6:102–109, 1976.

90. Spitzer, R. L., Endicott, J., and Robins, E.: Clinical criteria for psychiatric diagnosis and DMS-III. Amer. J. Psychiat., 132:1187–1192, 1975.

91. Stephens, J., and Kamp, M.: On some aspects of hysteria: A clinical study. J. Nerv. Ment. Dis., 134:305–315, 1962.

92. Sternbach, R. A.: Pain Patients: Traits and Treatment. New York, Academic Press, 1974.

93. Sternbach, R. A., Murphy, R. W., Akeson, W. H., and Wolf, S. R.: Chronic low back pain: Characteristics and management of the "low back loser." Postgrad. Med., 53:135–138, 1973.

94. Strauss, J. S.: A comprehensive approach to psychiatric diagnosis. Amer. J. Psychiat., 132:1193–1197, 1975.

95. Taub, A.: The use of psychotropic drugs alone and adjunctively in the treatment of otherwise intractable pain: Postherpetic neuralgia; Disseminated visceral neoplasm. In Voris, H. C., and Whisler, W. W., eds.: Treatment of Pain. Springfield, Ill., Charles C Thomas, 1975.

96. Teicher, S.: In Freedman, A., Kaplan, H., and Sadock, B., eds.: Comprehensive Textbook of Psychiatry. 2nd Ed. Vol. 2. Baltimore, Williams & Wilkins Co., 1975, pp. 2176–2182.

97. Tolia, B. M.: Postcoital pain and testicular torsion. Med. Aspects Human Sexuality, 11:98–99, 1977.

98. Uematsu, S.: Medical Thermography; Theory and Clinical Application. Los Angeles, Brentwood Publishing Corp., 1976.

sex. Med. Aspects Human Sexuality, 11:90, 1977.

99. Uematsu, S., and Long, D. M.: Thermography in chronic pain. *In* Uematsu, S., ed.: Medical Thermography Theory and Clinical Applications. Los Angeles, Brentwood Publishing Corp., 1976.

100. Valko, R. J.: Group therapy for patients with hysteria (Briquet's disorder). Dis. Nerv. Syst., *37*:484–487, 1976.

101. Wahl, C., and Golden, J.: The psychodynamics of the polysurgical patient: Report of sixteen patients. Psychosomatics, *7*:65–72, 1966.

102. Walters, A.: Psychiatric considerations of pain. *In* Youmans, J. R., ed.: Neurological Surgery. Vol. 3. Philadelphia, W. B. Saunders Co., 1973, pp. 1615–1645.

103. Weiner, A., Liss, J. L., and Robins, E.: A sys-tematic approach for making a psychiatric diagnosis. Arch. Gen. Psychiat., *31*:193–196, 1974.

104. Wilson, W. P., Blazer, D. G., and Nashold, B. S.: Observations on pain and suffering. Psychosomatics, *17*:73–76, 1976.

105. Woolsey, R. M.: Hysteria: 1875–1975. Dis. Nerv. Syst., *37*:379–386, 1976.

106. Yalom, I.: The Theory and Practice of Group Psychotherapy. New York, Basic Books, 1970.

107. Youmans, J. R.: Personal communication, 1978.

108. Ziegler, F., Imboden, J., and Meyer, E., Contemporary conversion reactions: A clinical study. Amer. J. Psychiat., *116*:901–909, 1960.

GENERAL CONSIDERATIONS IN THE MANAGEMENT OF CHRONIC PAIN

Acute pain of somatic origin is relatively well understood in the simplest psychological and anatomical terms. The thresholds for the sensation of human pain have been accurately measured.[6] The pathways by which it is perceived in the periphery and transmitted to consciousness can be traced, at least in their simplest form. The complex interactions that may occur at the spinal cord, brain stem, thalamic, and even cortical levels are not well understood, but the general pathway is well defined.[4] Pain and suffering as human experiences, however, are much more complex phenomena involving the pain itself, the patient's previous experiences with pain, and the underlying personality as well as personal, social, and ethnic factors. These aspects are only beginning to be elucidated. Pain as a manifestation of psychiatric disease is an even more complicated problem. The relationships between pain as a psychiatric symptom and the psychiatric effects of chronic pain in the human have only recently been appreciated and certainly have not been well defined.[5] In order to understand the interactions of these processes with the simple perception of pain by any individual, it is necessary to examine the many factors that influence the expression of pain in our society. A complaint of pain may reflect a straightforward organic problem. It may be a symptom of a purely psychiatric condition. A minor pain may be intensified consciously or subconsciously by a desire for financial gain. Pain may be a powerful tool with which to manipulate the environment and escape from unpleasant tasks. Pain may be used as an excuse for decreased ability that is actually the result of failing mental function. It is important to recognize the effects of pain upon the individual and to separate its psychosocial effects from its physical effects. Only when all the multiple factors that may influence pain in the human can be carefully analyzed and controlled is it likely that an adequate treatment of any pain problem will be possible.[1]

CLASSIFICATION

In order to compartmentalize pain problems, it is convenient to divide the human pain experience into two general categories, acute and chronic.

Acute Pain

Acute pain can be subdivided into two forms. The first of these may occur in the course of any disease that has the potential for producing pain and is self-limited. Either the disease runs its course or correct diagnosis and adequate treatment eliminate the disease and the symptom of pain. Acute pain may also be of a second type characterized by exacerbations with long remissions between. An example of such a problem is trigeminal neuralgia. Usually it is possible to diagnose the pain and to provide therapy that either is curative or, at least, relieves the pain. Alleviation of acute pain with narcotics is usually completely satisfactory. Furthermore, the short-term use of narcotic drugs for the management of acute pain has few complications, and addiction rarely occurs. Except in the highly addictive personality, narcotics may be used with safety for several weeks without fear of addiction. When they are used beyond one month, however, it is wise to proceed on a limited withdrawal schedule when they are discontinued. The longer the drugs are used, the more difficult it is to withdraw them. The severity of the patient's withdrawal symptoms will relate both to the length of time drugs are used and to the amount of drug used. Symptoms of tolerance usually do not become apparent for approximately three months, and maximum tolerance appears to occur after approximately six months of use. While the newer techniques of neuromodulation for pain eventually may be found to have broad application in acute pain as well as in chronic pain, the bulwark of the therapeutic armamentarium in acute pain is still the administration of narcotics.

Chronic Pain

Chronic pain is the second major category of pain experience. It can be defined as significant pain persisting for more than a few weeks for which there is no adequate therapy available to treat the underlying problem, which might be expected to relieve the pain. In neurosurgical thought it is common to further subdivide chronic pain into that caused by a malignant process and that caused by a benign process. It is semantically incorrect to speak of benign or malignant pain; it is the cause of the pain that may be benign or malignant. Further, the effect of the pain may be benign or malignant to the patient's well-being. All chronic pain is malignant in its effect upon the sufferer. The pain of malignant disease, especially those lesions associated with a short life expectancy, may be handled appropriately by destructive operative procedures within the central nervous system,

TABLE 117–1 PHASES OF BEHAVIOR IN CHRONIC PAIN

PHASE	PATIENT'S BEHAVIOR
I	Denial
	Search for therapy
	Vulnerable to quackery
II	Hostile, aggressive, litigious
	Drug misuse
III	Depression, despair, insomnia
	Search for therapy
	No attempt at self-help
	Drug misuse
IV	Acceptance of disability
	Realistic approach to therapy
	Can be helped

whereas pain of benign origin usually is better treated without operations that destroy some part of the nervous system.[7] There is, however, increasing awareness that the differentiation between pain of benign and malignant origin is artificial and that the principles of the management of chronic pain remain the same irrespective of the cause of the process. This chapter defines the effects of chronic pain and its therapy upon the individual and discusses the principles of its management. The specific details of management are the subjects of other chapters in this book.

One of the most important goals of the evaluation of a patient with chronic pain is to understand the effects of the pain upon the patient. The effects appear to be similar to those described for chronic disease in general and for the approach of death and dying in particular. Patients with chronic pain may be said to pass through four evolutionary phases (Table 117–1). It is very important for the examining and treating physician to recognize the phase in which the patient presents, for there are obvious connotations that affect any reasonable treatment plan.

Phase I

The first phase is a period in which the patient and usually the family deny the presence of a disability. During this period patients usually refuse to accept restrictions, behave inappropriately, and often do things that are detrimental to the treatment program. Often they desperately rush from physician to physician searching for an easy answer or a cure. They are particularly prone to seek operative answers to problems for which an operation is not appropriate and to seek out physicians whose treatment plans agree with their own concept of the problem.

Phase II

The second phase of chronic pain is easier to define. It is characterized by marked anger and hostility. Interestingly enough, it is common for the anger and hostility to be directed at the most recent physician involved in the patient's care rather than at the original precipitating incident or the physicians who have undertaken treatment plans that were ineffectual. It is extremely important to recognize this anger and hostility, for it has been the experience of many that it is during this phase that litigation is likely to occur. Patients in this phase have unrealistic expectations of therapy. They frequently demand to be cured without risk or complication and will become unjustifiably angry at the physician who offers them an honest assessment of their disease, the possibilities for therapy, and the eventual outcome of a successful treatment plan.

Phase III

The third phase of chronic pain is the one in which the usual patient presents to a chronic pain treatment program. It is characterized by despair and depression inappropriate to the magnitude of the problem. Patients in this phase may still naively be searching for the ultimate cure and may still have inappropriate life goals. Their approach to the problem, however, is one of profound despair, exaggerating the magnitude of the disability, their inability to function, and the severity of the pain. Insomnia is a common problem, and severe depression with all that it connotes is the rule. It is important to understand that treatments employed for patients who are profoundly depressed are unlikely to be effective, and their efficacy cannot even be accurately assessed until the depression is satisfactorily treated.

Phase IV

The fourth phase in the attitude of the patient incapacitated by chronic pain is one of acceptance. During this phase, the patient comes to have a rational understanding of the pain process and clearly recognizes and accepts the disability that the disease entails. Patients in this phase will accept treatment plans, evaluating and accepting the risks and complications as well as the limitations on eventual success. It is possible to deal with them in terms of the use of harmful medications and rehabilitation programs, and it is possible to have them accept the realities of the situation in terms of function. The aim of any comprehensive pain treatment program is primarily to bring the patients to phase IV, irrespective of the cause of their pain and irrespective of the amenability of the pain to treatment.

SPECIFIC EFFECTS

In addition to these general manifestations that are characteristic of all patients with chronic pain, the specific effects of the chronic pain experience are important. They fall into several broad categories that require separate discussion.

Psychiatric Effects

The first of these categories is the psychiatric effects of chronic pain. Virtually all patients with chronic pain become seriously depressed, have symptoms of chronic anxiety, are subject to insomnia and feelings of despair. It is possible that these effects are all situational, but it is increasingly thought that the diffuse reticular connections of the pain pathways in the brain stem, hypothalamus, thalamus, limbic system, and frontal lobes may produce depression, anxiety, and insomnia directly.[4]

Physical Effects of Inactivity

Another very important effect of chronic pain is upon the physical well being of the patient. It is standard practice to limit a patient's activities when pain results from those activities. In our society, patients with chronic pain routinely abandon all forms of physical activity and become sedentary. There are a general loss of body strength, muscle weakness that often intensifies the underlying pain problem, joint stiffness, and unwillingness on the part of the patient to participate in exercise programs that would be beneficial. Obesity often complicates this situation and is often intensified by the patient's anxiety and chronic physical inactivity.

Drugs

Routinely, the drug utilization of patients with chronic pain is inappropriate.[3] In a survey of 100 consecutive patients admitted to The Johns Hopkins Pain Treatment Program, it was found that 90 per cent were addicted to narcotics, and 90 per cent were misusing or abusing other kinds of medications (Table 117–2). The majority of patients with chronic pain have been given diazepam (Valium), which is an excellent antianxiety agent but which causes depression with long-term use and certainly may markedly accentuate an underlying depression. Barbiturates have their own habituating properties, and their long-term use may lead to accentuation of muscular and skeletal pain problems. Short-acting barbiturates in small doses can be taken for many weeks before habituation occurs, but in doses above 0.4 gm per day, they have been seen to cause profound withdrawal symptoms in as little as three weeks.

The detrimental effects of the misuse of most psychoactive drugs upon higher mental function are well known. It is necessary to eliminate addiction to narcotics, barbiturates, and related drugs. It is of equal importance to eliminate the abuse or misuse of nonnarcotic analgesics. Propoxyphene (Darvon) and pentazocine (Talwin) are both liable to misuse and have deleterious side effects when taken in the large dosage so commonly employed by patients with chronic pain. In large doses, both drugs are capable of producing depression of brain function and hallucinations. Typical withdrawal symptoms that might be expected from narcotics are seen with both but are usually less serious. The side effects of pentazocine are much more pronounced than those of propoxyphene. Before psychotropic drugs are given to a patient complaining of chronic pain, the psychiatric status of this patient must be carefully identified. Chronic anxiety should be treated with antianxiety agents. Depression must be treated with antidepressants. An appropriate psychiatric diagnosis is necessary before these drugs should be prescribed.

In addition to dealing with the specific problems that drug abuse and misuse present, it is also necessary to modify the patient's thinking concerning the use of drugs. Most patients with chronic pain believe that medications exist that will relieve their pain effectively. They do not recognize the evils of narcotic addiction, and most are unwilling to accept the fact that no nonnarcotic analgesics stronger than aspirin can be utilized without the possibility of unfortunate side effects. Also it is extremely important to impress upon these patients that the proper use of psychotropic medication will result in improvement in their symptoms, whereas the improper use is likely to cause unpleasant side effects and may actually worsen the situation. The general belief of patients in the efficacy of drug therapy requires that the use of drugs in the treatment of chronic pain follow specific guidelines and that those guidelines be carefully explained to them. Psychotropic drugs must be directly applicable to the symptoms that should be treated, and drugs must be chosen that have no long-term side effects that would be deleterious. Nonnarcotic analgesics are employed, but narcotics are not utilized on a long-term basis for the treatment of chronic pain. There may be an occasional patient in whom the long-term use of narcotics for chronic pain of benign origin is warranted, but these patients are very rare and must be carefully selected by some process other than trial and error. The adequate treatment of pain cannot proceed in the face of serious psychiatric and addictive problems. On the other hand, the use of narcotics in terminal stages of malignant disease may be entirely appropriate. Even here, however, there is increasing evidence that the patient's tolerance for narcotics escalates while their efficacy in pain relief decreases, and at that point in the patient's course, when pain relief is most necessary,

TABLE 117–2 DRUG MISUSE AND ABUSE IN CHRONIC PAIN*

	PER CENT
Addicted to narcotics	90
Misusing/abusing narcotics	90
Misusing/abusing psychotropics	80
Prescriptions from multiple physicians	over 50
Withdrawal symptoms	90
Inappropriate combinations of drugs or inappropriate ingestion	97

* One hundred patients admitted to The Johns Hopkins Pain Treatment Program.

the narcotics are least able to provide it. Narcotic addiction is a serious problem for most patients, and of these drugs should be considered in the treatment of chronic pain only when the situation is desperate and only when the patient's life expectancy is less than three to six months so that tolerance and decrease in efficacy will not become major problems. Exceptions to this rule certainly exist, but they are rare, and if long-term narcotic maintenance is to be utilized, the patients must be carefully chosen.

The major aspects of drug misuse and abuse in patients with chronic pain fall into several general categories. The high-low syndrome of narcotic addiction is probably the most important. The patient has pain and requires a narcotic. A euphoric high then exists for several hours. The effects of the narcotic decline, and the need for the narcotic signals itself by a return or accentuation of pain. The drug is administered, a second high results, which gradually falls to a low signaled again by worsening of pain, and this process repeats interminably. Sooner or later the patient's signal for drug need becomes pain, and it then becomes impossible to ascertain whether or not the increasing pain is simply a need for the narcotic.

The second major category is the accentuation of pain problems by the inappropriate choice of drugs or the accentuation of psychotropic symptoms by the inappropriate choice of psychoactive drugs. Diazepam (Valium) is a good example of a drug that should not be used in chronic pain. Although an excellent antianxiety agent for short-term use and a good muscle relaxant, in long-term use it accentuates depression. Barbiturates should not be employed, because pain or its accentuation is an idiosyncratic response to administration of these drugs. Meprobamate is another antianxiety agent that should not be used in chronic pain; one of the side effects of meprobamate withdrawal is accentuation of pain. Another major drug effect is sleep deprivation due to the employment of barbiturates or other hypnotics that do not provide normal sleep. This simply intensifies the insomnia of the usual patient with chronic pain. In summary, it is virtually impossible to assess the efficacy of pain therapy without strict control of the drug profile.

Iatrogenic Problems

Patients with chronic pain are confronted with the potential for iatrogenic problems that go well beyond drug administration. Such patients invite inappropriate or unnecessary therapy. The treatment is well intentioned and often is precipitated by the patient's insistence upon additional therapy. Such patients often undergo multiple operative procedures with an increasingly small chance of gaining relief by any one of them. Each of these procedures has the potential for neurological catastrophe and for worsening the underlying situation. The patients may undergo extensive diagnostic studies. Six to ten myelograms are not unusual in the history of a patient with chronic low back pain who is admitted to a pain treatment center. The cost and potential harm of these repetitious studies are both important. One of the major aims of the accurate evaluation of a patient with chronic pain should be to establish a diagnosis clearly so that additional diagnostic studies are unnecessary.

Operative procedures should be utilized only when there are a specific problem to be corrected and a reasonable chance of success. If a specific procedure cannot be chosen that has a reasonable chance of relieving the patient's pain or correcting the underlying problem, then it is unlikely that any procedure is warranted. Patients with chronic pain will search for additional operative procedures, although the majority of them have already undergone a multiplicity of ineffectual procedures. Just as they believe in the efficacy of medicine for treating their problems, they also believe in the efficacy of an operation to correct virtually any kind of difficulty. Nerve blocks and related procedures are viewed in a less favorable light—but still are more acceptable than noninterventional treatment. It is important that the physician choose the most appropriate treatments and employ interventional procedures only when they are clearly indicated and only in the context of the overall management of the patient. It is obvious that it is not always possible to choose those patients who will respond to a given procedure, and certainly all operative procedures have a percentage of failure. Again, it is extremely important that the treating physician choose an operation as a method of therapy only when it is clearly indicated. It must not be used in a desperate attempt to treat an insoluble problem without clear-cut indications.

Effects of the Legal System

The legal system may be a major problem in the management of the patient with chronic pain. In the United States, patients are rewarded for the presence of pain as a symptom. Judgments involving large sums of money often are predicated upon the presence of pain, a subjective sensation on the part of the patient, or suffering, a subjective response on the part of the observers. It is difficult to assess the degree of pain a patient has or his response to therapy when major financial considerations are involved. This is true not only for litigation involving an accident but is equally true for industrial commission claims and for claims of disability for the purpose of obtaining social security or other benefits. If the patient is unable to work solely because of pain, and if relieving the pain means that the patient must return to work, then it is unlikely that therapy will be effective unless the patient is well motivated and clearly wishes to return to work irrespective of underlying disability. While no data allow a blanket statement on the matter, it is the experience of many working in the field that a large number of patients with industrial commission claims are not well motivated for return to work and that satisfactory pain relief in these patients is unlikely.[2] Reports of the effectiveness of therapy tend to be unreliable and are often colored by the status of the disability claim. This is equally true for the acquisition of social security benefits or other retirement claims. If the patient seriously wishes to retire, then no therapy will be of value. In these situations treatment should be predicated upon a careful analysis of the vocational status of the patient and a review of the possible solutions with him. Appropriate goals may be set for each patient, and vigorous criteria kept for decisions about disability.

The problems often are compounded by employers, insurance carriers, and members of the legal profession. Frequently it is difficult for a well-motivated individual to return to work following an accident that has left him with a minor disability. Insurance carriers often thrust themselves into the physician-patient relationship and seem to be interested only in the cost of therapy, not its aims. It is unreasonable to assume that a patient who is addicted to narcotics, is seriously depressed, and has undergone multiple low back operations can be expected to function satisfactorily without attention to all his problems. Yet this is often the expectation of the insurance carrier of such a patient's industrial commission claim. There is a tendency in both the medical profession and society in general to assume that a patient who has major psychiatric problems associated with chronic pain is, in fact, primarily a psychiatric patient or is malingering. The situation often is that both the insurance carrier and the patient, as well as the employer, have unreasonable expectations concerning therapy. Relief of pain and return to a worthwhile existence are likely to occur only when the patient's problem is considered in its entirety and treatment of all aspects of the chronic pain is implemented. As long as the patient is rewarded for having pain, it is unlikely that any therapy will be of value in restoring him to a useful function in society.

The adversary system in which many patients with chronic pain find themselves is extremely harmful to their care. A legal proceeding in the courts or with the industrial commission is often necessary for the patient to achieve the reimbursement that he may or may not deserve. In such a situation, any person who ventures an opinion that is detrimental to the patient's financial aims immediately becomes an adversary. This means that a physician who makes an honest assessment of the situation, concludes that the patient is much more functional than the patient believes, and plans a reasonable treatment program to return him to a functional existence is angrily viewed by the patient and often by his lawyer as an adversary and the treatment program as detrimental to the patient's cause. It is not difficult to see how ineffective such a treatment program is likely to be. On the other hand, a physician who suggests an inappropriate treatment program or operative procedure that is almost certain to be ineffectual will probably be viewed by both parties as supportive, and it is likely that this treatment program will be followed. As long as the treatment of chronic pain is intimately associated with the legal process and as long as the patient and physician are placed in an adversary position by this process, it is unlikely that an effective program for evaluation and treatment of chronic pain can be formulated when any legal entanglement exists. Indeed, it is highly desirable that there be settlement of legal claims before definitive therapy is undertaken. An attempt should be made to bring the patient to a rational understanding of his problem and to get him to make a reasonable legal settlement. If the patient refuses to follow this advice, it is unwise to perform operative procedures or to initiate an involved treatment program unless the pain problem is a very straightforward one with a clear etiology.

Social Aspects

Closely allied to these aspects of the problem are the social effects of chronic pain. Such patients often achieve gratification through the behavior they demonstrate in response to chronic pain. The occurrence of pain may be associated with attention from family and friends, visits to a physician or a hospital, and solicitude from all those who observe the suffering. By this kind of behavior, the patient may also acquire money and drugs that have a pleasant effect. In order to treat pain satisfactorily and to treat the behavior associated with chronic pain, it is necessary to investigate all the social facets that have brought the patient to the state of chronic pain and to acquaint the immediate family or those responsible for the patient with the psychological effects of chronic pain, the effects of drugs, and the possible effects of treatment upon the situation. Most individuals are sympathetic to patients who are obviously suffering, and often this sympathetic behavior is the worst response to give these patients. Instead of encouraging maximum function within the framework of the disability, it encourages the worst aspects of chronic pain behavior. Patients receive attention, drugs, and care in proportion to their complaints of chronic pain, and it is obvious what the outcome of such a social situation will be. The patient's function at work and in activities not related to employment will be equally adversely effected. At a time when he should be planning for maximum employment, for maximum vocational and nonvocational activity, and for maximum self-care, encouragement is given from all sides to become less functional.

EVALUATION AND TREATMENT

The basic plan for evaluation and treatment of pain is no different from that for any other disease state. Acute pain may be a symptom, but chronic pain can be called a disease just as correctly as epilepsy, for example. The first step is careful diagnosis. The diagnosis should be followed by treatment of the underlying disease process whenever possible. Symptomatic treatment of the pain is satisfactory for the first few weeks while the treatment process is undertaken. The most important considerations at this stage for the physician involved in the treatment of pain are those aspects that, unless handled wisely, will eventually cause the development of chronic pain behavior.

There is controversy concerning the ability of individuals to function adequately during the long-term use of narcotics. Certainly, persons who are addicted appear to function adequately in their work and family as long as they receive adequate supplies of their narcotic. Some physicians specializing in the treatment of pain allow a patient to use a small amount of narcotic on a regular basis. It is the experience of the author, however, that it is unacceptable for a patient who is being treated for a pain problem to continue to use narcotics. Further, all patients whose maintenance on methadone has been attempted have abused the drug, and all have returned for further treatment. In the author's experience of treating almost 1000 patients over a ten-year period, no patient who continued to take narcotics during the time that he was being treated has had successful control of his pain problem. The patients may state that their pain is under better control during the treatment, but they all continue to take drugs, and none improve their life style. As a result of this experience, the author does not perform operative procedures in a patient who cannot be successfully withdrawn from narcotics.

Inappropriate or harmful medications such as diazepam, barbiturates, other sleep medications, and psychotropic drugs prescribed without a specific diagnosis must be avoided. The earliest signs of anger, hostility, chronic anxiety, depression, and insomnia should be appreciated and treated appropriately. The psychiatric aspects of pain should be appreciated early, separated from the physical problem, and treated appropriately. The deleterious effects of prolonged inactivity must be realized and the patient returned to function as rapidly as possible. Prompt and direct dealing with the patient's social and vocational problems will greatly reduce the possibility of the later development of chronic pain behavior. An early honest assessment of disability and vocational potential may not be to the liking of the patient, the lawyer, or the insurance company, but will be helpful in allowing a realistic appraisal of the patient's condition.

It is important to make plans for the future with the patient and to avoid potentially harmful or ineffectual treatments, particularly those involving operative procedures. This is of major importance in problems involving the low back and neck. Application of these principles will avoid production of a patient suffering from a chronic pain neurosis (Table 117–3). When the chronic pain neurosis already exists,

however, its prompt recognition and attention to all facets of the problem will still allow the successful treatment of pain in a significant percentage of patients and the improvement of an even larger group.

In summary, there is no panacea for pain. The physician's efforts should be directed to the accurate diagnosis and treatment of the painful process, and when this is impossible, to the application of the most appropriate pain relieving procedures. When no procedure can be realistically expected to relieve the pain, it is especially important that this be recognized and inappropriate and ineffectual therapies avoided. Nowhere is the dictum of "physician do no harm" more important than in the therapy of chronic pain. Recognition of the effects of chronic pain upon the patient and the application of these principles of management will greatly reduce the number of patients developing a chronic pain neurosis and will facilitate the management of all patients with chronic pain.

TABLE 117–3 THE PAIN NEUROSIS

Physical disability
Depression
Anxiety
Multiple physician visits
Drug utilization and abuse
Narcotic addiction
Ineffectual, potentially harmful therapy
Social-vocational disability
Legal entanglements
Enforced retirement, loss of income
Destruction of personal relationships
Rejection from the health care system

REFERENCES

1. Blumer, D.: Psychiatric considerations in pain. *In* Rothman, R., and Simeone, F., eds.: The Spine. Philadelphia, W. B. Saunders Co., 1975.
2. Finneson, B. E.: Low Back Pain. Philadelphia, J. B. Lippincott Co., 1973.
3. Long, D. M.: Use and misuse of drug therapy in chronic pain. *In* Abstracts. First World Congress on Pain, Florence, 1975.
4. Mayer, D. J., and Price, D. D.: Central nervous system mechanisms of analgesia. Pain, 2:379–405, 1976.
5. Melzack, R.: The Puzzle of Pain. New York, Basic Books, Inc., 1973.
6. Mountcastle, V. B.: Medical Physiology. Vol. 2. Chapter 63. St. Louis, C. V. Mosby Co., 1974.
7. White, J. C., and Sweet, W. H.: Pain and the Neurosurgeon. Springfield, Ill., Charles C Thomas, 1969.

118

CEPHALIC PAIN

Beginning a discussion of head or face pain with a diagnosis and then defining the characteristics of the pain to justify the diagnosis makes of it (can be) a self-fulfilling prophecy. When treating patients, one must proceed in the reverse order. The patient's complaints generate in the physician's mind a series of conjectures or possible diagnoses. Next come further inquiry and investigative measures to refute the least likely diagnosis, and finally a tentative diagnosis that appears to be the most correct one is accepted. Textualized information is useful largely in presenting data that may define patterns of information for recall and comparison by the physician as a patient's problem unfolds itself to him. The patient cannot identify the significance of his pain. The physician must make this interpretation.

Caution must be exercised when considering the problem of a patient with head and face pain. The physician must avoid focusing unduly on his specialty interest and asking questions related to it. For instance, with the same set of complaints the dentist might ask about the symptoms of pulpitis, the otologist might ask about the symptoms of chronic otitis media, the orthopedist might ask about the symptoms of cervical arthritis and the internist might ask about the symptoms of arteritis. This practice, common to all physicians, may fail to develop the full scope and balance of available information required for a proper diagnosis.

Patterns of referred or diffuse discomfort, so common in the head and face, may pre-empt a primary position in the patient's mind. Sometimes they must be readjusted to secondary priority by the physician despite the patient's protestations. The "source" pain may be minor but may trigger severe secondary pain patterns. For instance, cervical spondylosis with severe occipital neuralgia, occult pulpitis, or sinusitis may trigger exacerbations of migraine in a previously asymptomatic but susceptible patient.

Before beginning a discussion of the clinical aspects of cephalic pain a brief review of the anatomy and physiology of cephalic pain mechanisms seems necessary.

ANATOMY AND PHYSIOLOGY OF PAIN-SENSITIVE STRUCTURES IN THE HEAD

Nerve Supply*

All pain-sensitive intracranial structures in the supratentorial compartment are supplied by branches of the trigeminal nerve. These structures include: the basal dura of the anterior and middle fossae, the arteries of the circle of Willis and the proximal portions of the major intracranial arteries, the meningeal arteries, the superior surface of the tentorium, and the walls of the major dural venous sinuses. The dural structures are supplied mainly by branches of the ophthalmic division of cranial nerve V. The middle meningeal artery is accompanied by small unnamed branches of the maxillary and mandibular divisions of the fifth nerve and small unnamed branches of all three divisions. The superior surface of the tentorium is supplied by the nervus tentorii, a branch of the ophthalmic division. The exact innervation of the proximal portions of the main branches of the circle of Willis are unknown but probably arise from the ophthalmic division.

---

* See references 23, 29, 32, 49, 50.

R. B. KING AND R. F. YOUNG

The infratentorial basal dura, the inferior tentorial surface, and the proximal major arteries and veins of the posterior fossa are innervated by the ninth and tenth cranial nerves and the upper cervical nerves, primarily C2 and C3. The ninth and tenth cranial nerves primarily supply the inferior tentorial surface, the region of the torcular herophili and straight sinus, and the dura in the region of the sigmoid sinus. The major arteries of the posterior fossa, including the posterior meningeal artery, and the dura of the floor of the posterior fossa near the rim of the foramen magnum are supplied by cervical nerve roots two and three.

Nearly all extracranial structures of the head that cause cephalic pain are supplied by the trigeminal nerve and its branches. These include the extracranial arteries, pericranium and periosteum, paranasal air sinuses, teeth, periodontal structures, and orbital contents. In contrast, the pharynx, tonsils, tonsillar fossa, and eustachian tube are supplied by the glossopharyngeal and vagus nerves. The tympanic membrane itself and the external auditory canal are supplied by the facial nerve. General somatic afferent portions of the seventh, ninth, and tenth cranial nerves enter the descending trigeminal tract and synapse in the rostral spinal trigeminal nucleus. General visceral afferent portions of nerves VII, IX, and X descend in the tractus solitarius and synapse in the nucleus solitarius. Thus, although general somatic afferent information from the head is carried centrally by the fifth, sixth, seventh, and tenth cranial nerves, all of this information is processed centrally in the trigeminal system.

Pain Referral Patterns

Information concerning pain referral from structures in the head comes from three major sources: (1) patients with well localized pathological processes producing pain, (2) stimulation of various structures in awake patients undergoing operative procedures, and (3) patients who have undergone section of various cranial nerves for the relief of intractable pain.

Such studies reveal that pain from pathological processes in the supratentorial compartment is referred primarily to the orbital, retro-orbital, or frontal region ipsilateral to the lesion. The pain results from traction or distortion of the proximal portions of the major intracranial arteries or basal dura primarily at the point of attachment of the major arteries and veins to the dura. Displacement of the middle meningeal artery may refer pain to the subtemporal area or jaw.

Pain from pathological processes in the posterior fossa is referred to the occipital or suboccipital region or the upper cervical region. Because of the dual innervation that cranial nerves IX and X give to the posterior fossa dura and to the ear and retroauricular region, pain from posterior fossa lesions, particularly in the cerebellopontine angle, is often referred to the ipsilateral ear or periauricular area.

DENTAL DISORDERS

Pain of dental origin may occur in the distribution of the mandibular or maxillary nerves or may virtually suffuse one side of the head. The area of major ache and discomfort is often migratory and poorly localized. Pain and paresthesias may be intermittent and last a few seconds or persist for days. The discomfort may range from a mild dull ache or intense deep boring ache to a sharp lancinating and pulsating pain requiring differentiation from classic tic douloureux. There may be no discernible precipitating factors, but frequently the pain is intensified or altered by thermal stimuli such as hot or cold liquids, by cold air drawn into the mouth, or by pressure on a tooth or its adjacent structures.

If the pain is provoked by hot or cold stimulation of a tooth, the abnormality is likely to be found in or connected to the tooth pulp. If the pain is caused by pressure on the tooth, the dentin is the most likely site of disease. Touch, pressure, or thermal stimuli at the cervical portion of the tooth (junction of enamel and root) provoke pain from exposed dentin at this site. Pain of periodontal origin is usually provoked by firm tooth pressure, with jaw clenching or chewing or by direct pressure contact with periodontal structures.

Patterns of referred pain from one tooth to others may be a source of confusion. Testing with stimuli applied to one tooth may provoke symptoms in a tooth some distance away. Such patterns of referred pain usually remain ipsilateral and in the same jaw. Occasionally, however, pain in an upper molar or premolar may abate following appropriate treatment of a lower molar or even a lower incisor tooth. Occasionally many teeth may be carious with associated pulpitis or periodontal disease, yet the patient may categorically deny a history of toothache. This apparent paradox has no clear explanation.

Dental pain may also be referred to the neck and suboccipital region because of sustained contraction of cervical musculature. Such pain may be indistinguishable from muscle contraction (tension) headache of any origin.

Pain that persists following dental procedures is often related to trauma of the inferior alveolar nerve during the administration of local anesthetic or during the extraction of mandibular third molars, the roots of which commonly encroach upon or encircle the alveolar canal that contains the inferior alveolar nerve. Occult alveolar osteitis may be symptomatic for weeks or months. Zealous and repeated procedures at the site of the initial manipulation may serve only to accentuate or perpetuate the patient's pain. As a rule, the symptoms subside as the post-traumatic inflammatory process diminishes during conservative management.

Following the loss of teeth, alveolar resorption may extend to the mental foramen, allowing direct pressure on the mental nerve by dentures or by chewing. Persistent sharp pain provoked by pressure is then referred to the chin and mandible. While digital pressure at the site of the mental foramen may identify the local source of the pain, correction by adjustment of prostheses may be complicated and difficult. Further manipulation and local blocks must be avoided to allow the inflammatory process secondary to trauma to subside. In most instances the symptoms will gradually abate. Rarely are local denervation procedures warranted.

Occult pulpitis is often difficult to demonstrate even with excellent dental radiographic examinations or temperature and pressure testing of individual teeth. Commonly it is associated with pain that spreads from the region of the affected tooth. Only after months of persistent examination and reevaluation may the specific tooth responsible for severe and persistent discomfort be identified.[43] It is important to realize that simple skull x-rays may not reveal evidence of dental disease and that specific dental x-rays may be required. Figure 118–1 illustrates a tiny periapical abscess that was the cause of severe lower jaw pain initially thought to be due to trigeminal neuralgia. Plain skull x-rays had been normal, but dental films confirmed the pathological process, which was easily treated. Primary dental disorders are a common cause of "atypical facial pain" and commonly require multidisciplinary care and management.[14,40]

The case reported by Rubach in 1963 is particularly instructive in this respect:

A 21-year-old woman complained of extreme pain spreading over the right side of the face from behind the ear to the orbit, down the side of the nose, and along the lower border of the mandible. "Shooting pains" extended into the cervical region. A generalized dental-type pain affected equally all teeth from the cuspids posteriorly on the right side. Lateral head tilt exaggerated pain in the cuspid region. Severe pain extended to the vertex. Her daily symptoms had persisted for a year to a year and a half with sporadic exacerbations at three-month intervals. She had seen many physicians and dentists, and had undergone contrast studies of her sinuses. Cardiac and arterial problems had been considered in the differential diagnosis. Electroencephalograms and electrocardiograms were normal. Migraine had been considered, as had psychosomatic disorders. Tranquilizers were of no avail.

When she was seen, it was "obvious that she was extremely nervous," which she denied, save for fear of dentists. She had insisted on general anesthesia for dental extractions and would be treated by only one oral surgeon at a distance from her home. A thorough oral and dental examination including x-rays revealed only a "peculiar large radiolucent area in the crown of the maxillary right third molar." Pulp testing with electric current, ethyl chloride, and heat failed to identify the source of her complaints. On the basis of the radiographic evidence and "contrary to clinical findings," the right upper third molar was excavated under local anesthesia. The patient complained bitterly that the anesthetic was not effective and believed that none had been given. When a small opening was achieved in the occlusal portion of the tooth and local anesthetic was applied directly through the then visible carious cavity, her pain was relieved. The tooth was extracted with a diagnosis of quiescent painful pulpitis. She remained free of symptoms of

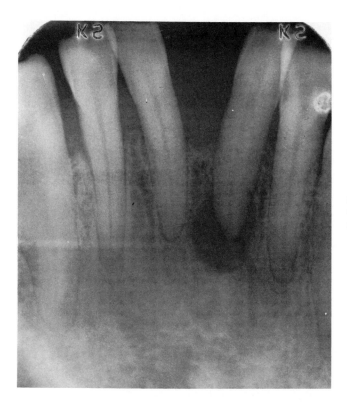

Figure 118–1 Periapical dental abscess in a mandibular tooth. Such lesions will be missed by plain skull x-rays and require special dental films.

facial pain during a three-month reported follow-up.[35]

SINUSITIS

Occult sinusitis, particularly of the ethmoid and sphenoid cells, may be associated with cephalgia ranging from a sense of fullness to local pressure or a dull to severe ache. Usually these symptoms are periodic and accentuated during sleep. Frequently pain of ethmoid sinusitis is referred to the inner canthus of the eye and the upper and lateral side of the nose in the distribution of the infratrochlear nerve, which courses along the lateral wall of the ethmoids. There is occasional unilateral frontal and orbital or ocular radiation associated with inflammatory disease of a lateral ethmoid cell adjacent to the orbit. The headache is usually accentuated by straining and exertion. In sphenoid sinusitis, persistent deep boring and at times sharp painful ache is referred to the bitemporal, occipital, glabellar, mastoid, or mandibular ramus regions. The pressure pain may be poorly localized but promptly relieved by decongestants as long as they are appropriately administered high in the nasal passage. This may require packing with cocaine at the air cell stoma in order to achieve sufficient drainage of the high-pressure sinus. Patients often describe a sense of stuffiness high in the nasal passages that does not obstruct air passage through the lower airways. They frequently have a mild postnasal drip, but it is rarely copious and often is negligible. Their pain tends to diminish by afternoon. X-rays obtained under these circumstances may show a fluid level in the brow-up lateral projection but more commonly show only a slightly cloudy air cell that the radiologist would think inconsequential except for its clear clinical correlation with the patient's complaints.

Frontal sinusitis rarely provokes pain other than in the supraorbital region or high in the anterior orbital region and is most often associated with local tenderness over the frontal sinuses and mild edema of the forehead. Transillumination and percussion over the affected sinus may give clear evidence of the process underlying the complaint.

An infection in the maxillary antrum often produces a sense of fullness or deep ache in the upper teeth and occasionally hypesthesia or hyperpathia in the distribution of the infraorbital nerve. Opacity on transillumination, tenderness to pressure over the antrum, progressive pain during the day, and abnormal x-rays should clearly identify the problem. Figure 118–2 illustrates typical radiological findings in maxillary sinusitis. With chronic disease, the pain may extend far beyond the second division or the infraorbital nerve and be referred as soreness, tenderness, and diffuse deep aching pain throughout one side of the face, including the upper teeth.[48]

Pain associated with chronic pansinusitis is bilateral and associated with diffuse severe deep face and head pain in the anterior half of the cranial vault and face, often with a preponderance of bifrontal and orbital pain. Occlusion of a sinus stoma, osteomyelitis, or pyocele may herald the onset of pain late in the course of chronic disease. Acute pansinusitis is seldom overlooked, for multiple local signs and clear evidence of systemic illness accompany the pain. Sinusitis is rarely, if ever, limited to a single air cell. It is, in essence, an inflammatory process of all air cells with preponderance at times in one or another or multiple loci. Patterns of pain, therefore, are usually widespread and often migratory. Referred pain patterns may predominate over pain as a localizing complaint.

Pain due to the "vacuum sinus" is usually sudden and severe at the time of onset. It may be associated with rapid atmospheric pressure changes or changes in altitude.[39] Occasionally it occurs when the mucous membrane of the stoma swells and occludes the sinus. The air in the sinus absorbs slowly and causes intense pain that may begin rather abruptly. Often, in this circumstance, the patient will describe the feeling of a sucking sensation high behind the nose with pain that is promptly relieved as a patent stoma is re-established with topical decongestants. Repeated administration of the decongestants may be necessary over a period of time.

Although sinus disease has long been considered a common cause of headache and face pain, it probably accounts for no more than 5 to 10 per cent of patients with these complaints.[4]

The basis for pain related to occult sinusitis may be persistent, but it may be difficult to identify. This is especially true in remote areas of the ethmoid and sphenoid systems. The early diagnosis usually is not made because of facial or head pain, but because of complaints of nasal obstruction or postnasal discharge and the demonstration of local tenderness, persistent purulent rhinorrhea, and confirmatory x-ray findings. The alleviation of symptoms depends upon appropriate management of the underlying local process. Denervation procedures play no role in the management or resolution of pain of chronic sinusitis.

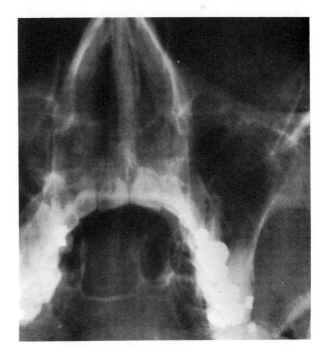

Figure 118–2 Caldwell view of the sinuses demonstrates thickening of the mucosa of the left maxillary antrum. Similar but less apparent changes are also present on the right. These changes are due to chronic maxillary sinusitis.

Encephaloceles within the sinus system and inclusion cysts of the antrum or frontal sinuses rarely, if ever, cause pain although they may show striking changes on x-rays.

CARCINOMA OF THE HEAD AND NECK

The early diagnosis of these lesions usually does not depend upon an analysis of pain patterns except for those tumors that arise within the bones of the nasopharyngeal area, such as the mandible or antrum. Even then, hypesthesia, anesthesia, loose teeth, proptosis, diplopia, nasal obstruction with bleeding or discharge, stuffy ear, or localized tenderness, swelling, and masses usually precede the onset of pain.

Pain induced by carcinoma of the face, sinuses, nasopharynx, cervical lymph nodes, scalp, and cranium is most often a deep, boring, heavy ache, debilitating in its progressive persistence, regional or diffuse in its distribution, and a late sign of the primary disorder. Pain may be bilateral early in the course of the disease if deep structures of the nasopharynx or midline sinuses are affected. Sharp stabbing pains remote from the region of the primary neoplasm, referred to the suboccipital region, ear,

temporal region, and into the distribution of the three divisions of the trigeminal nerve (often with hypesthesia) are commonly superimposed. As a rule no particular factor provokes or relieves the persistent pain. Resection of the primary lesion with antecedent or postoperative x-ray therapy will often control the pain.

The following case report illustrates the necessity for pursuing a definite diagnosis for pain complaints and also the difficulty with definitive treatment.

A 46-year-old woman was seen two years after the onset of an ''abnormal sensation'' in the left side of her oral cavity. Two months prior to evaluation she had onset of a deep, boring pain with occasional sharp exacerbations located in the left maxillary antrum and the retro-orbital and periauricular regions. Occasional feeling of formication was noted over the left frontal scalp. Sharp darts of pain into the left eye occurred rarely. Hot fluids were tolerated poorly because they felt excessively hot. Initially neurological examination was unremarkable. Plain skull x-rays and sinus x-rays were normal. Pain persisted in spite of medical management. Onset of analgesia in the left V_2 and V_3 divisions eight months later led to repeat radiological investigation. Plain skull x-rays including the submentovertex view, while suspicious owing to indistinctness of the sella, were read as normal (Fig. 118-3). Tomograms, however, disclosed a very

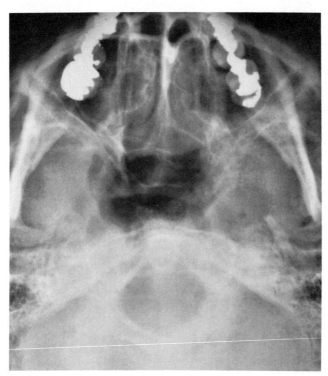

Figure 118-3 Submentovertex radiograph. No definite pathological change is identified. Projection of the anterior arches of C1 and C2 and the odontoid over the upper end of the clivus makes evaluation of the latter structure impossible.

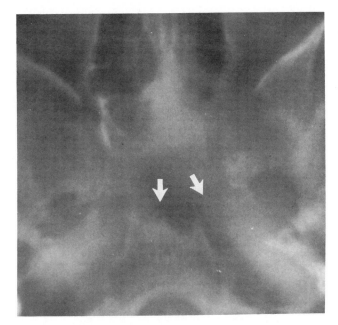

Figure 118–4 Basal tomogram from the same patient as the roentgenogram in Figure 118–3. Massive destruction of the skull base including the upper clivus and medial petrous ridges (*arrows*), especially the left, is identified.

large osteolytic lesion with likely origin in the sphenoid sinus producing massive destruction of the clivus, sellar floor, and base of the skull (Figs. 118–4 and 118–5). Biopsy of the associated soft-tissue mass revealed a poorly differentiated squamous cell carcinoma. Radiotherapy of the primary lesion produced significant improvement in her facial pain.

In many instances, multiple operations with reconstructive procedures have re-solved the primary issue and with it the patient's distress until terminal events became evident. When, however, scarring in the region of previously successful operation, x-ray therapy, or residual occult carcinoma is associated with severe pain, the selection of appropriate operative procedures for relief is difficult.

Peripheral nerve blocks with lidocaine and at times alcohol may help plot an oper-

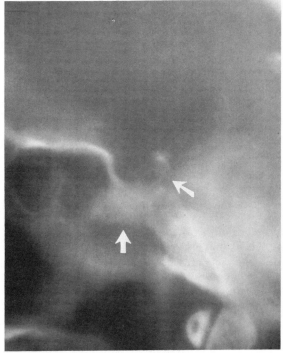

Figure 118–5 Lateral tomogram of the same patient as in Figures 118–3 and 118–4. Destruction of the upper end of the clivus (*slanted arrow*) and dorsum sellae is seen. In addition the posterior portion of the sphenoid sinus contains a soft-tissue mass (*vertical arrow*) and the posterior sinus wall cannot be identified. Biopsy confirmed a squamous cell carcinoma.

ative stratagem for denervation of the region. Pain referred deep into the ear, however, may remain despite all measures. Spinal trigeminal tractotomy at or below the level of the obex has been recommended as the one procedure most likely to give satisfactory relief for unilateral pain. It may be combined with section of rootlets of cranial nerves IX and X for pain in the throat and pharynx, with high cervical (C1, C2, C3, C4) dorsal rhizotomy when pain extends into the cervical region, and with section of the nervus intermedius for pain in the auditory canal. Theoretically such a procedure should interrupt virtually all known pain afferents for that side of the head and neck, but even though total analgesia in this area has been apparently achieved, some patients will still complain of a persistent, deep, boring ache referred to the base of the skull or auditory canal. These procedures should be reserved for patients whose life expectancy clearly extends beyond a period of convalescence lasting six to eight weeks and in whom hemorrhage or respiratory obstruction are not threatening.

Individuals whose pain is well circumscribed to a region of the face, mandible, or antrum may gain significant relief following trigeminal rhizotomy.[46]

When the pain is bilateral the problem is compounded and its resolution is rarely achieved. Instances have been reported in which satisfactory rhizotomy or tractotomy has given rewarding pain relief despite some difficulty in maintaining head posture. Thalamotomy, either unilaterally or bilaterally, with lesions at the caudal inferior portion of the centrum medianum medial to the posterior ventromedial nucleus and rostral to the red nucleus has been considered recently as the probable procedure of choice. Some surgeons have extended the thalamic lesion more laterally. The ultimately most appropriate positioning for such a destructive lesion cannot yet be categorically defined. Nevertheless, long-term survivals with alleviation of pain without analgesia or other disability have been reported and are gradually increasing in number. If morphine can achieve satisfactory relief without compromising the patient's mental resources, and if the patient is not expected to live more than three months, there is little reason to perform a thalamotomy or an extensive denervation procedure. On the other hand, it is probable that in a highly selected group of patients with a reasonable expectation of prolonged survival, thalamotomy may significantly alleviate pain.

TEMPORAL ARTERITIS

Characteristically this problem occurs in patients over 70 years of age. Although the disease was once thought to be a localized inflammation of the superficial temporal or superficial temporal and ophthalmic arteries, this is now known to be incorrect. Hollenhorst and co-workers have indicated that the condition is a systemic disease associated with inflammation of many large and medium-sized arteries and should be regarded as a "collagen" disease affecting the elderly.[16] The distribution of the pain may vary greatly from patient to patient and, indeed, from time to time in the same individual.[17,34] Although it is common for the patient to experience very short, fleeting, mild, sharp, pin-sticking–like pains in the distribution of the temporal artery with spots of tenderness here and there along its course, similar symptoms may be found in only the distribution of the postauricular arteries or the occipital arteries, or at times in all three. Pain in the temporal muscles and masseters with "anginal" characteristics may occur with chewing. The symptoms are rarely bilateral at the same time. Eye pain, though not common, may be severe and is usually retro-ocular and orbital. A low-grade fever may occur in early days or weeks of the illness, but rapid loss of vision on the side of the symptoms may develop suddenly within the first 24 to 48 hours. Tender nodules along the course of the temporal, postauricular, or occipital arteries are commonly found.

Local procaine (Novocaine) blocks of the temporal artery as a temporizing procedure may relieve the symptoms until massive steroid therapy can take effect. The response to steroids may be dramatic, and symptoms may resolve in a matter of hours.[3] Prolonged delay of treatment in order to establish a definitive diagnosis is unjustified. Steroids should be started promptly on the basis of clinical suspicion, after appropriate laboratory studies have been obtained, in order to avoid sudden irreversible visual loss. Laboratory studies should include blood count, sedimentation rate, and serum protein electrophoresis. These may demonstrate leukocytosis, mild hypochromic anemia, and elevated sedimentation rate. Changes in serum proteins may include an increase in alpha-2 globulin, a reduction in serum albumin and occasionally an increase in gamma globulin. If vision is compromised, treatment must be undertaken on an emergency basis to preserve sight.

Biopsy of an affected scalp vessel will establish the diagnosis. As large a segment of artery as possible should be removed, since the pathological changes may be segmental and may be missed if only a limited biopsy is performed. The giant cell periarteritis that can be found in the biopsy of the temporal artery is characteristic of the disease.[38] It is a necrotizing granulomatous panarteritis particularly affecting the tunica media of large and medium-sized arteries in the distribution of the external carotid artery but also of vertebral-basilar arteries, coronary arteries, and at times arteries of the aortic arch. The marked inflammatory reaction with lymphocytic and polymorphonuclear leukocytic infiltration of the adventitia is characteristic. There is segmental necrosis of the media adjacent to the internal elastic lamina, which may be interrupted. The large multinucleated giant cells lie primarily at the junction of the media and the intima with masses of extracellular fibrillary substance staining heavily with phosphotungstic acid. There is no evidence of bacteria or virus particles in such specimens. The histological characteristics are probably specific and suggest a systemic arterial disorder unlike other forms of arteritis.

Prodromal symptoms may last as long as two years before the acute onset of amaurosis and temporal artery pain.[10,24] This syndrome has been called polymyalgia rheumatica and is associated with migratory rheumatoid and muscular pain, a low-grade fever, fatigability, a rising sedimentation rate, and a gradual increase in serum gamma globulins. It is thought by some that the primary cause of death in this disorder is coronary artery occlusion, which ultimately occurs in a third of these patients. The characteristic amaurosis occurs in 15 to 20 per cent of this group but has been reported in 50 per cent of patients in whom the diagnosis has been based on more specific symptoms. Long-term steroid therapy may control the angina associated with the coronary artery disease and hold the remaining elements of the syndrome in abeyance.

TEMPOROMANDIBULAR JOINT PAIN

This problem occurs most commonly in middle-aged women. Usually it is provoked by chewing or jaw clenching. It is characterized by deep pain in the region of the temporomandibular joint radiating toward the temple, the anterior wall of the external auditory canal, occasionally to the postauricular region, and commonly into the distribution of the third division of the trigeminal nerve. If the history and physical findings have not been precisely documented it may be confused with facial pain from other causes.[1,7,8] Although sharp pains, occasionally lancinating, may override the associated ache and be provoked by chewing, paroxysmal flashes of pain are not usually a major feature of this syndrome. Cutaneous trigger points are not evident, although hyperpathia may be demonstrable.

Associated symptoms of fullness in the ear, occasional and intermittent sensation of impaired unilateral hearing, mild dizziness, or tinnitus secondary to disturbance of eustachian tube patency may mask other symptoms characteristic of the primary disorder.[1] On rare occasions these symptoms herald metastatic carcinoma, abscess, osteomyelitis, or occult fractures of the joint elements or supporting structures.

While there is no evidence of peripheral sensory deficit or other neurological findings despite occasional subjective complaints of numbness and tingling of the earlobe or external canal, commonly there is tenderness at the anterior wall of the external auditory canal that is easily elicited by mild digital pressure against this surface. It is accentuated by jaw opening and closing. Often the pterygoid muscles are exquisitely tender on palpation. It is less common to have tenderness directly over the temporomandibular joint that can be noted by digital pressure or jaw motion. Commonly the pain can be aggravated or provoked by jaw movement and can almost invariably be accentuated by forced jaw closure. Gross malocclusion of the teeth often is apparent on visual inspection. Frequently there is an associated overbite or underbite, occlusal gap, or limited range of jaw opening. Occluding surfaces of the teeth may show flattening at their sites of abutment. Lateral deviation of the jaw and occasionally a click that can be heard with a stethoscope or felt with the examining finger placed in the ear canal adjacent to the affected joint are associated with jaw movements. Secondary trismus of masseter and pterygoid muscles often accompanies the syndrome, adding diffuse tenderness and pain as secondary manifestations of the primary disorder. The pain is almost invariably unilateral. X-rays of the temporomandibular joint may not prove to be helpful, though occasionally flattening, asymmetry, or destruction of the mandibular condyle and temporal fossa in full opening and occlusion can be visualized. Tomography can be especially helpful in defining alterations in the joint structure.

Although discontinuity of the cartilaginous plates has sometimes been suggested as one underlying process, it would seem that tension and stress on the supporting ligaments and tendons associated with secondary muscle spasm are the major sources of the pain.[5] Treatment involves prevention of tooth grinding and jaw clenching, especially at night, and correction of any malocclusion that contributes to the asymmetrical stress imposed upon the temporomandibular joints. A mandibular sling, cork bite pads, and muscle relaxant drugs are useful to help relieve the acute pain. Usually the combination of these measures achieves satisfactory resolution of the pain.

OCCIPITAL NEURALGIA

Occipital neuralgia or neuritis is rarely a herald of serious primary disease. It more commonly is a secondary manifestation of a benign process affecting the second cervical dorsal roots or the occipital nerves.[46]

Chronic cervical strain associated with a vague sensation of tightness and deep ache in the suboccipital region and taut or tender suboccipital muscles following flexion or extension injury of the cervical spine may become associated with overriding periodic lancinating pain from the occipital region to the vertex. Referred temporal and retro-orbital pain on the ipsilateral side may de-velop concomitantly with increasing neck pain that extends also to the shoulders. Tenderness of the greater occipital nerve as it emerges through the deep fascia along the occipital line and a Tinel sign readily elicited by tapping the nerve at this site presumably indicate associated partial demyelination or regeneration in this sensory nerve. Direct trauma such as a blow by a blunt instrument or a penetrating wound may be followed by sharp, severe, radiating occipital pain and a diffuse suboccipital ache. The greater occipital or postauricular nerve is occasionally entrapped by a suture during repair of lacerations of the scalp. Hypalgesia or hypesthesia in the second cervical nerve distribution often can be demonstrated.

Heat, massage, muscle relaxants, and analgesics may suffice in symptomatic management. An alcohol block following a test procaine block may be required to break the persistent cycle of muscle spasm, suboccipital pain, and further tension in the cervical muscles. The relief obtained from the alcohol block may persist for many months. Cervical braces frequently aggravate the symptoms because of direct pressure on the occipital nerves.

Should the symptoms be more persistent or associated with progressive sensory loss, consideration should be given to identifying underlying pathological processes that may contribute to its persistence.[37] Entrapment of the occipital nerve in scar tissue or sutures may follow direct injuries. Uncommonly it has been the sole symptom of an otherwise occult Arnold-Chiari syndrome, cerebellar tumor, spinal tumor, arachnoiditis, bony anomaly of the atlas or axis, or unusual artery loop in which the second and third cervical dorsal roots may be stretched or tethered by the local lesion. In instances in which persistent sensory deficit of radicular distribution, rather than sensory changes in the distribution of the greater occipital nerve alone, can be demonstrated on clinical testing, early consideration should be given to a subarachnoid origin for the symptom. In any event, should the symptoms persist despite all conservative measures, contrast studies including cervical air and iophendylate (Pantopaque) myelography and posterior fossa pneumography may be required to identify the unusual case in which uncommon but more serious causes may be associated with radiculopathy of the second cervical nerve.

Occipital tic douloureux has occasionally been suggested as an appropriate diagnostic term for an apparently idiopathic severe form of occipital neuritis often associated with hyperpathia in the receptive field of the occipital nerve. Only in rarest instances has it been suggested that a trigger point was found in association with paroxysmal pain in this distribution without sensory deficit or hyperpathia. Although medication otherwise reserved for the management of patients with tic douloureux may be tried in these instances, it has seldom proved useful.

An occipital neurectomy may be indicated in those patients in whom local nerve blocks gave relief initially but through repetition have lost their effectiveness. Of course, a spinal or subarachnoid lesion must be excluded as a cause of the symptoms. Care must be taken to avulse the distal, but not the proximal portion of the occipital nerve—serious damage to the spinal cord may be caused by avulsion of the proximal portion. Avulsion of the nerve may give long-lasting or permanent relief. Occasionally interruption of the postauricular nerve is also necessary. Patients to undergo occipital neurectomy must be carefully selected in the absence of a specific etiological process for the occipital neuralgia. Psychological testing should be considered preoperatively, since the neuralgia may be a manifestation of underlying anxiety. In some cases the neuralgia may be associated with persistent muscle contraction (tension) headaches, and both may have their origin in unresolved psychological conflicts. Rhizotomy is rarely, if ever, indicated in the absence of symptoms that can be related to a subarachnoid lesion.

POST-TRAUMATIC CEPHALGIA

When pain occurs as a persistent and occasionally progressive and localized symptom following head trauma with an onset often many months after the accident, it may relate to a local process wherein a peripheral branch of a cutaneous nerve has become entrapped as a consequence of the injury. A neuroma of the supraorbital nerve underlying a laceration of the brow, the entrapment of the infraorbital nerve at the site of a fractured antrum, or the mandibular nerve trapped at the site of an old mandibular fracture may well be identified and corrected by local measures. A test block with lidocaine will frequently and precisely identify the source of the difficulty. Neuromas of the postauricular nerve or greater occipital nerve due to lacerations or occipital injuries are less common.

Extensive basilar skull fractures often associated with injuries of the middle third of the face may entrap dura and arachnoid in multiple fracture sites of the floor of the middle or frontal fossae. Such a process may at a late date be associated with severe but intermittent exacerbations of steady ache with superimposed sharp pains in the temporal, retro-orbital, or auricular-occipital regions. They are often exacerbated by cough, strain, or exertion. Stripping the dura from the floor of the middle fossa or releasing arachnoidal-dural adhesions may give temporary or lasting relief in very selected cases.[30]

Following diastatic linear fractures of the cranial vault (particularly common in children) the dura may be torn and a false dural membrane incorporating arachnoid and cerebral vessels re-established within the line of fracture. Severe sharp pain occurring at the site of the fracture, often with referred retro-orbital pain on the ipsilateral side, exacerbated by cough, straining and exertion, and augmented in the erect position as opposed to the prone position, may be readily corrected by exploration of the fracture site with debridement of arachnoidal adhesions and primary closure or grafting of the dural defect to restore disrupted anatomical planes.[22] An illustrative case follows:

A 46-year-old woman was seen because of an increasingly severe left frontal headache of several years' duration. The pain was aggravated by straining, which also caused local left frontal swelling. The pain was severe enough to limit her physical activity seriously. She had been struck in the left side of the forehead by the heel of a shoe at age 12, but had suffered neither laceration nor unconsciousness. She was then asymptomatic for 15 to 20 years before gradual onset of headache, which become incapacitating because of its severity with exertion. A palpable skull defect in the left frontal region and soft underlying bulge accentuated by Valsalva maneuver were noted on physical examination. Skull roentgenograms are shown in Figures 118–6 and 7. At operation a shell of outer skull table

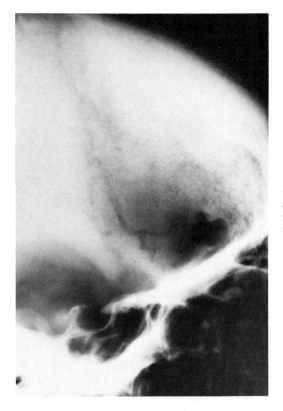

Figure 118-6   Lateral plain skull x-ray in a woman with right frontal headache. A multilobular, smoothly demarcated lytic lesion is apparent low in the right frontal region. Minimal sclerosis of the anterior superior margin of the defect is noted.

was encountered in which bluish arachnoid membrane was visible through multiple perforations in the bone. Uncapping this lesion revealed a dural defect and small underlying leptomeningeal cyst. In addition, evidence of an old fracture was visible with magnification. The dural defect was repaired, and a Silastic button was inserted to obliterate the skull opening. The patient has been free of headache since.

More diffuse and bizarre forms of persistent facial pain following fracture of the zygoma, mandible, maxilla, and elements of the base of the skull have been at times so severe and unremitting that trigeminal rhizotomy and rarely trigeminal tractotomy have been attempted in their alleviation.[46] While many reports of such efforts have indicated a degree of success, others suggest that persistent paresthesia and dysesthesia recur and herald recrudescence of a portion or all of the original complaint. Only in extreme circumstances are such major procedures undertaken for the alleviation of posttraumatic head and neck pain.

POSTHERPETIC NEURALGIA

A persistent burning ache overridden by stabs of severe, sharp, and at times lancinating pains associated with hyperpathia

and dysesthesia may persist for a few weeks or many months following an attack of herpes zoster. Ordinarily the diagnosis is not difficult, since the initial vesicles usually are large and visible and the patchy scarring in the skin that follows as the vesicles subside is characteristic in its appearance. Only in circumstances in which the vesicular eruption has not been identified and the gradual onset and persistence of pain cannot therefore be related to the initial infection is the diagnosis sometimes difficult.[9,44] Characteristically the viral infection affects the ophthalmic division of the trigeminal nerve and less commonly the maxillary division. Fortunately, this painful state gradually subsides in the majority of patients. Over a period of many months it will diminish to such an extent that medical management is quite reasonable. Although the cutaneous manifestations usually are prominent, frequently there is an associated aching sensation that is referred to the orbit or sinuses, that may be persistent, and that suggests involvement of dura and orbital elements innervated by the trigeminal nerve.

Many drugs have been used in attempts to alleviate this distressing problem. Those that have been helpful in the management

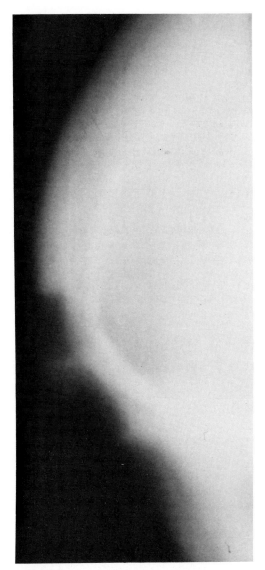

Figure 118-7 Tangential view of the same patient as illustrated in Figure 118-6. The inner table is beveled more than the outer table, suggesting that the lesion arose intracranially, although a lesion arising within the diploic space cannot be excluded. Differential diagnosis based on both physical examination and x-rays might include sinus pericranii or leptomeningeal cyst. Operative exploration confirmed the latter diagnosis.

of tic douloureux are useless in this circumstance. Steroids offer little in the way of relief, though they may be useful in the acute phase to minimize the inflammatory phenomenon. Codeine may suffice, particularly when augmented by chlorpromazine, during the daytime. At night, when the pain tends to be more evident, stronger medication may be required. In severe cases meperidine (Demerol) or morphine and aspirin taken before retiring (a second dose kept at the bedside for use if necessary during the night) usually allows the patient a reasonable night's sleep and thereby helps to prevent the exhaustion that gradually overwhelms many of these elderly patients.[11,25] Most of these patients easily abandon the use of narcotics as the pain gradually subsides. Recently a combination of the psychotropic drugs amitriptyline and fluphenazine has been suggested as medical treatment for patients in whom the pain does not subside. The suggested initial dosages are 75 mg amitriptyline at bedtime and 1 mg fluphenazine three times a day. The dosage of the latter may be increased to as much as 3 or 4 mg three times a day. If successful pain control is not achieved at this dosage level it is unlikely that larger doses will be effective and further increases in dosage are not recommended.[42]

Only in rare instances are operative procedures required in the management of this problem. In those unfortunate few, the results of operative intervention have been uncertain. Excision or undermining of skin and isolation of skin flaps have at times afforded relief that lasted many months or years. If local denervation by procaine affords temporary relief, then denervation by section of the posterior root of the trigeminal nerve or spinal trigeminal tractotomy may be effective. These measures, however, should not be undertaken unless clear and marked improvement has followed the local procaine infiltration of the affected area and temporary peripheral denervation procedures have given relief. Thalamotomy, even in these elderly patients, has sometimes satisfactorily alleviated their pain, though at times it has been associated with some intellectual impairment other unfavorable sequelae.

Electrical massage and percussion of the affected area may give periods of relative relief, although usually some ache, dysesthesia, and hyperpathia persists. Patients with severe dysesthesia and hyperpathia are particularly difficult to relieve with either drugs or denervation procedures.

ATYPICAL FACIAL NEURALGIA

This group of patients has diminished as physicians have become more skilled in the search for the cause of the pain. Still, after one has assiduously sought a demonstrable organic cause for their misery, there remains a perplexing group of patients for whom no clear organic or psychiatric basis for their complaint can be discerned. They frequently describe their symptoms in unusual terms with such adjectives as pressing, gnawing, crawling, boring, bursting, twisting, and drawing. In addition, there may be an ache or sharply painful component that may periodically be superimposed on the more persistent base of bizarre perceptions. Usually they relate their symptoms to deep structures and less commonly to cutaneous elements. Their complaints spread beyond known borders of somatosensory and autonomic neural pathways; factors that provoke or aggravate the pain are seldom identified. The patients often appear neurotic; many are middle-aged women. Analgesics give little or brief relief. Indeed, the use of narcotics frequently compounds the problem not only for the patient but for the physician.

The care of these patients is difficult and seldom rewarding. Relief has characteristically been transient or negligible despite the many modes of management that have been attempted. Many appear chronically ill, some become emaciated, and most are, or become, depressed.[21] In the course of time they drift in despair from one physician to another, leaving a line of frustrated practitioners behind. One can attempt supportive measures directed toward mood stabilization and elevation of depression, and can be alert to the development of new signs whereby an occult organic basis for their discomfort may become revealed at a later date. Psychiatric support with a realistic discussion of their difficulty and analysis of psychological factors that may contribute to their suffering seldom is sufficient to satisfy the patient. Long-term psychiatric care may be more useful. Standard operative procedures such as retrogasserian rhizotomy, alcohol injection, or nerve avulsion are to be avoided. Only in unusual instances has temporary alleviation been achieved by operation. Following operative intervention, many patients complain bitterly that their pain is even more severe.

The following case report illustrates some of the difficulties in the diagnosis and treatment of patients with atypical facial pain as well as the necessity for thorough evaluation in an effort to reduce the number of those left in the "idiopathic" group.

A 56-year-old woman had had the onset of left facial pain nine years prior to her referral. The pain was located in the maxillary trigeminal division and was described as "tic like." Over the next year, pain spread to include the mandibular division, and a retrogasserian rhizotomy was performed. For the next three years the patient was relatively pain-free. Subsequently, she described a feeling as if her left eye were being "pulled out" and an associated vague drawing discomfort of the entire left side of her face. Because of associated trouble with mastication and depression, her weight decreased to 76 lb. A course of 12 electroshock treatments were administered, which produced improvement in the depression although her pain persisted accompanied by a moderate deficit in recent memory. Her situation was fairly stable until one day prior to her referral, when she became drowsy, vomited several times, and was mute. Lumbar puncture confirmed a subarachnoid hemorrhage. Angiography revealed three intracranial aneurysms (Figs. 118–8 and 118–9). Most pertinent was a large left middle cerebral artery aneurysm that appeared unruptured. The patients neurological state never improved to a level that would have permitted operative treatment. The possibility is strong, although not unequivocal, that this aneurysm was the etiological agent underlying her facial pain.

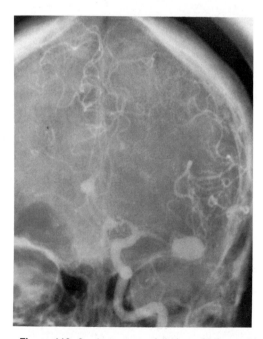

Figure 118–8 Anteroposterior view of left carotid angiogram in a woman with atypical facial pain for nine years and recent subarachnoid hemorrhage. Intracranial aneurysms are demonstrated arising from the left middle cerebral artery, the anterior communicating artery, and the anterior cerebral artery. Marked vasospasm is also present.

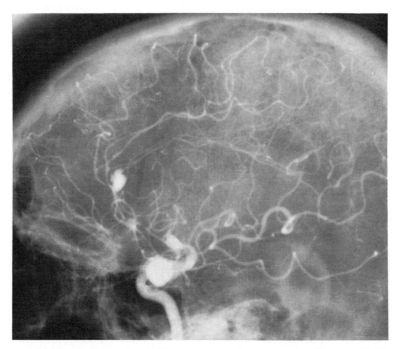

Figure 118-9 Lateral view of the left carotid angiogram for the same patient illustrated in Figure 118-8. The three aneurysms are again visualized. It was felt that the middle cerebral artery lesion might have been the cause of the patient's atypical left facial pain.

Fortunately the number of patients remaining in this group gradually diminishes as skills are developed to find primary organic and behavioral causes that underly their unusual complaints. Recently Janetta suggested that many cases of facial pain may be due to compression of the trigeminal sensory root by contiguous arterial loops. Posterior fossa exposure of the posterior root under the operating microscope has usually allowed the vessel to be dissected free of the root and a cushion to be interposed between the two.[19] A larger experience and sufficient follow-up will allow full evaluation of this procedure. We can hope that some day there will no longer be a need for this unsatisfactory classification.

CEPHALGIA OF PSYCHOLOGICAL ORIGIN

A discussion of pain of psychosomatic origin is fraught with the danger of generating incredulity, doubt, or even disgust on the part of the neurosurgeon. It is unfortunate that this is the case. Such a reaction is hazardous; when confronted by a patient with bizarre, extravagant, circumstantial, often paradoxical, and profuse complaints

of pain, the surgeon may stop short of a thorough search for an underlying organic basis for the complaint. Too often, the premature conclusion is reached that the patient's behavior substantiates the impression that he is neurotic or depressed. At the other extreme, the surgeon may overlook the bizarre pattern and complaint of pain that is a dire "request" for psychiatric help. If the surgeon fails to recognize this problem he cannot even help by directing the patient to a psychiatrist.

It is odd perhaps that so many patients with pain, apparently of psychosomatic origin, refer the pain to the head, face, and neck. Such, however, probably is true of nearly two thirds of these patients. Females clearly predominate over males. Many are anxious, depressed, and in emotional conflict. They tend not to speak in terms of their emotional state but try rather to establish communication with a physician through a discussion of their discomfort and pain. These patients have most often been described as having psychoneurotic reactions of the conversion or obsessive compulsive types. They are often aggressive, critical people, usually conscientious and prone to push themselves at maximum capacity over protracted periods of time.

They are often depressed out of proportion to their physical discomfort.

The patterns of psychosomatic behavior that appear concomitantly with symptoms of severe pain fall into a relatively limited number of categories.[31] Most commonly the patients are depressed. Although well-masked, the hallmark symptoms of depression can usually be elicited quickly. These patients suffer from lack of interest in life's activities, sleeplessness (beginning often at progressively earlier hours in the morning), anorexia, weight loss, relative impotence, unexplained fatigue, pessimism, difficulty in concentrating and memory difficulties that do not follow a usual organic pattern. Many consider, but few attempt, suicide.

Conversion reaction related to hysteria is usually marked by a lack of anxiety or depression. There is no stereotyped personality, although many such patients are egocentric, dramatic, dependent, immature, and vain. This combination of circumstances is most commonly seen in women in association with conversion hysteria, which has often been investigated as though it were of organic origin.

The hypochondriac with exaggerated concern and worry at times may manifest psychosomatic head and neck pain frequently associated with increased tension in the musculoskeletal systems of head support. It varies greatly from time to time and in degree. It may be difficult to extricate, in these patients, the symptoms that otherwise would lead to an earlier diagnosis of organic disease.

Probably one of the most common forms of psychosomatic pain is tension headache associated with spasm in the cervical musculature that is usually occipital and frequently seen in anxiety states. Pain is usually suboccipital, bitemporal, or bifrontal, spreading gradually in that sequence. It rarely affects facial structures. Alleviation of the primary anxiety and symptomatic care will often suffice in the patient's management.

Occasionally patients with impending psychotic breakdowns may complain of somatic delusions manifested as head and face pain. Most commonly their reports are extravagant, relating such phenomena as maggots, objects piercing through a portion of the cranial vault or face, exploding fire-crackers, or bursting bubbles in the head, or bizarre feelings of exaggerated and distorted growth patterns of the nose and eye, teeth, lips, or ears. Because of their extraordinary patterns, these somatic delusions are clear warnings of psychotic delusions. Usually psychiatric care with hospitalization is urgently required.

The diagnosis and management of these patients is extremely complex. It is important to remember that inappropriate management may fix, perpetuate, or indeed, acutely exaggerate their basic problems.

MIGRAINE OR VASCULAR HEADACHES

An extraordinarily expansive literature with a wide variety of terms has developed surrounding headache and faciocephalgic pain of vascular origin. Friedman has reviewed this material with admirable clarity.[12]

The variety of pain, the array of theories proposed to explain the clinical symptoms, and the variety of names given to subgroups that appear definable have been confusing. The Ad Hoc Committee of the National Institute of Neurological Diseases and Blindness, however, proposed a useful classification for vascular headaches of the migraine type.[13]

1. Classic migraine. Headache is recurrent and periodic; familial and personality factors appear frequently as contributing elements; prodromata are definite and well described; contralateral neurological deficit, visual, motor, or sensory, is common. The pain is unilateral, throbbing, aching, and at times sharp in character, lasting from four to six hours, spreading frequently to the opposite side of the head, beginning occasionally on alternating sides of the head, and associated with nausea and vomiting in the full-blown attack.

2. Common migraine. Prodromata are rare, although a vague sense of awareness of a pending headache may precede the actual event for several hours or even days. This prodroma may include vague psychic disturbances such as difficulties with continuous thought, mild nausea, and anorexia. The headache may last many hours or several days. It is steady, unilateral, aching and throbbing, often associated with

chills, feverishness, fatigue, depression, nausea, vomiting, and nasal congestion on the side of the headache.

3. Cluster headache. Prodromata are uncommon; the pain often occurs suddenly and may awaken the patient from sleep. It recurs in closely related series of attacks followed by remissions of months or even many years. Autonomic manifestations are common with conjunctival congestion, lacrimation, stuffiness in the nasal passages, and occasionally ptosis or myosis associated with unilateral or bilateral sweating and reddening of the face on the side of the pain. The acute attack usually ceases after half an hour to an hour and a half, terminating as suddenly as it began. Familial tendencies are rare. Attacks are most common in older men.

4. Hemiplegic or ophthalmoplegic migraine. This rare form may occur frequently in the young adult. Pain is moderate in degree, occurs on the same side as the ophthalmoplegia, and may be accompanied by transient paralysis of extraocular muscles. The latter may occur as the headache diminishes, the former having persisted for several days. Hemiparesis and sensory deficit are not uncommon accompaniments of the headache. The neurological deficits may persist for days after the termination of the headache, and occasionally a persistent third nerve paralysis, usually mild in degree and often limited to only a large pupil, may remain as a permanent deficit. This symptom complex clearly simulates the attacks of pain that may accompany aneurysm of the internal carotid artery at its junction with the posterior communicating artery, though the latter usually gives more severe pain that is sharper in quality, briefer in duration, unassociated with autonomic findings, and commonly associated with intermittent nuchal rigidity following the headache.

5. Lower-half headache. Although relatively uncommon and easily confused with atypical facial neuralgia, it has been described by some as periodic migrainous neuralgia and by others as basilar artery migraine.[2] Occurring commonly in young women, it is frequently related to menstruation, often associated with visual prodromata, vertigo, dysarthria, ataxia, tinnitus, and tingling of the fingers and toes. The order, of course, may vary. A disturbance

of consciousness and awareness may make the patient appear dazed during its onset. Symptoms usually do not last more than 45 minutes and may be followed by a severe throbbing headache in the occipital region or even by vomiting. The facial pain extending from the retro-orbital and frontal region may extend into the region of the second and third divisions of the trigeminal nerve and is usually of an aching or burning quality. Angiomas and other vascular lesions of the posterior fossa may simulate this condition, but as a rule persistent and progressive deficits develop in such patients.

Although the vascular nature of these headaches is generally accepted, the incidence of cerebral vascular accidents occurring concomitantly with the headache is extraordinarly low. Patients with "hemiplegic migraine" may fully recover from their neurological deficit following innumerable attacks over many years. Despite these truisms, it is nevertheless evident that permanent damage to neurological structures, particularly the occipital lobe cortex, may follow a series of severe migraine headaches.

To speak of migraine without headache seems paradoxical. Yet there are gradually accumulating references to transient episodes of fully reversible neural deficit in patients with a personal or strong family history of migraine.[47] Of special interest to neurological surgeons is a group of such patients, usually children, with transient focal neural deficits and depressed states of consciousness following minor head trauma. The onset of the neurological deficit or depression of conscious level occurs 5 to 30 minutes after the injury and clears up in from several hours to two to three days. In many, this sequence has been seen after each of several minor head injuries. It has been suggested that this clinical sequence is in consequence of cerebral arterial spasm induced by trauma causing a temporary stretching of major cerebral vessels in susceptible patients who often have a strong family and occasionally a personal history of migraine.[15]

It is now generally accepted that an initial vasoconstriction followed by dilatation accompanies the headache in its sequential development. Whether the release of toxic agents from the cerebral vascular tree or scalp vessels is related to the onset of this sequence is under investigation. Many such agents have been considered, including acetylcholine, neurokinin, bradykinin, histamine and 5-hydroxytryptamine. Although, judging by published reports, neurokinin appears to be a likely candidate, its relationship to these vascular headaches has not been clearly established.

Abnormal arteriovenous shunts producing vascular and cerebral anoxia with secondary increase in blood flow have also been suggested as underlying mechanisms for migraine headache. These two hypotheses, abnormal shunting versus the release of chemical agents that alter vascular tone and cerebral blood flow, are not necessarily mutually exclusive.[18]

Several authors have confirmed the presence of a low plasma level of serotonin with increased excretion of 5-hydroxyindoleacetic acid following an attack. Catecholamine metabolism, therefore, may also be affected in this sequence of events. These biochemical studies, of course, seek to establish a metabolic basis for a change in microcirculation, the latter being the immediate precursor to the migraine sequence.

Systemic physiological changes have long been known to accompany the headache cycle. These include changes in fluid balance with local or general edema, electrolyte retention, and diuresis. Manipulation of these symptoms, however, has consistently failed to provoke headache in normal subjects.

No correlation of neurophysiological changes in the central nervous system accompanying these events has been observed. Electroencephalography has thrown little light on any underlying mechanisms, although from 26 to 75 per cent are found to have abnormal electroencephalograms.

Although some authors have doubted the significance of behavior characteristics in patients predisposed to migraine, most agree that "they tended to come from families that take great pride in attainment and adhere to rigid norms of behavior that deny expression of aggressive or demonstrative feelings. Such families punish those members who defy their standards in various ways, so that resentment or hostility toward a parent or other respected or beloved person tends to be deeply suppressed. The conflict, with its associated anxiety over an inevitably emerging hostility, along with the pressure to conform to family standards in order to continue desired relations, triggers the headache."[12] In general, these patients are compulsive, perfectionistic, and poorly adaptive under stress.

Treatment

The treatment of migraine headache on a symptomatic basis associated with a particular attack has been almost entirely confined to the use of ergot preparations. Some authors, indeed, have expressed the opinion that they would just as soon abandon any general classification or subclassification of migraine and related headache patterns and rely entirely on a therapeutic trial with ergotamine tartrate to determine whether a particular patient's headache, particularly that which is bizarre and not easily classified, is related to the migraine sequence. Ergotamine tartrate combined with caffeine, sedation, and at times an antinauseant are most effective in the initial treatment of these attacks. It is very important that the medication be taken early in the course of the attack, preferably during the prodroma. While ergotism is a rare side effect of this treatment, particularly in patients who have persistent headache requiring daily medication, it is extremely serious. It usually occurs only when the drug is taken in large and continued doses or when there are pre-existing contraindications.

Many patients find, however, that 20 grains of aspirin, followed by an additional 10 grains at hourly intervals until the attack subsides, will adequately suppress their symptoms, allowing them to continue in their daily activities until they are able to seek rest or the symptoms subside. At these dose levels, however, many patients require antacids and they may experience some mental clouding, depression, and intolerance to confusion and multiple simultaneous challenges during this period of time.

More recently, methysergide maleate (Sansert) has been used in an attempt to treat these headaches prophylactically. It may often reduce their number and severity, but it is totally ineffective during an attack. Adverse, and at times serious, side effects have been experienced by patients who are estimated to number between 10 and 25 per cent. Reduction of the dose may limit the side effects of nausea, cramps, vomiting, and restlessness, but frequently the medication will have to be discontinued as peripheral vascular effects begin to make themselves evident. Retroperitoneal fibrosis and inflammatory or fibrotic reactions in the heart, mediastinum, lungs, and pleura have been reported.

Several other agents have also been used very recently for prophylaxis of migraine headache. The two most widely used are propranolol (Inderal) and cyproheptadine (Periactin). Propranolol is an adrenergic sympathetic blocking agent. The initial dosage of 10 mg four times a day may be increased gradually to 40 mg four times a day if necessary. The drug cannot be used in patients exhibiting bradycardia, congestive heart failure, asthma, or hypoglycemia. Cyproheptadine is an antagonist of both serotonin and histamine and may be used successfully for migraine prophylaxis. The usual dosage of 4 mg four times a day may produce slight drowsiness, but other side effects are rare.[45] Clonidine, an antihypertensive agent, may also be useful in migraine prophylaxis. The main pharmacological action of this imidazoline derivative is to decrease significantly the responsiveness of blood vessels to vasoconstrictor or vasodilator substances. Total daily doses of 25 to 50 mg have been recommended, and side effects are reportedly rare.[6]

In any form of persistent, protracted headache related to the migraine syndromes, it may become necessary to consider hospitalization for full medical workup. Operative intervention for this problem is rarely indicated. Only in those cases that are most refractory to medical management or in which side effects on standard medications are intolerable should the possibility even be considered. Though such a move may at times seem indicated because of the patient's great distress, one should recognize that the operative literature catalogs the use of a wide range of procedures of which the results have been erratic and are not predictive of a high level of probable success.

Very commonly psychological matters may well contribute to the patient's symptoms to an extraordinary degree and remain masked for protracted periods, even throughout a series of exceptional operative procedures. The following case report is instructive in this context.

A 41-year-old man of dapper attire, precise manner, and well-modulated speech came several hundred miles seeking operative relief of his right-sided head pain. Attacks of pain came in clusters, were severe in degree with a feeling of searing heat, followed by sharp throbbing pains surging on that side of the head, and accompanied by tearing, lacrimation, conjunctival congestion, and stuffiness on that side of his nose. The pain spread from the upper two thirds of his face behind his ear into his suboccipital region and vertex. Only heavy analgesics relieved the pain during the period of an attack, which would last characteristically for several hours, coming on frequently at night, but also occurring during the daytime. Clusters would last three to four weeks and then disappear for one to six months. He had had several previous operative procedures, including biopsy of the right temporal artery, ligation of the right external carotid artery, alcohol blocks, and excision of the post-auricular and occipital nerves and occipital artery, a cervical sympathectomy on the right, interruption of the right middle meningeal artery and greater superficial petrosal nerve, and a rhizotomy of C2 on the right. A gasserian gangliolysis had been performed six months before. After most of these procedures his relief had lasted for one-month to six-month intervals similar to his spontaneous remissions.

Because of concern for his uncommonly compulsive demeanor and behavior, he was sent to a psychiatrically oriented neurologist who promptly elicited the history that up to the age of 20 this man had been a roustabout in the oil fields of the midwest, involved in many weekend brawls, and a heavy drinker. At the age of 20 he was thoroughly beaten by one of his victims and spent three weeks in the hospital convalescing. During that three-week interval he determined that he would change his way of life and from that time forward, as he clearly admitted, he had never sworn nor raised his voice in anger, far less struck another person nor moved as though to do so. He had risen to a position of major executive responsibility in the oil industry. The neurologist described to him and helped him to develop techniques for expressing his frustration and rancor in more or less socially acceptable ways. He was not heard of for the next two and a half years. At that time a telephone call from the midwest revealed that he had his first recurrence of headache. At that time he had been "trapped" in a marital triangle between his immediate superior and his next superior and the wife of one of them. He was not involved, but in the office confrontation between these two, was trapped as a witness and accused wrongly of being a party to the developments. Realizing he was in an impossible situation from which he could not readily extricate himself, but still exercising his own internal constraints, he developed an extraordinarily severe unilateral headache of the kind he had previously experienced and called for further counsel.

It may be appropriate to ask whether any of his operative procedures had been of avail in alleviating his primary problem.

HEADACHES RELATED TO TUMORS

Many have attempted to construct constellations of headache symptoms that will correlate with an intracranial mass lesion. Only in rare instances has the correlation been successful in the absence of additional clinical and laboratory data. Headache as a sign of intracranial disease is essentially referred pain. It may arise by three primary mechanisms having their effect either at the site of or remote from the primary lesion: (1) altered tension on major veins and dural sinuses, meningeal vessels, large intracranial arteries, and extracranial vessels; (2) inflammatory processes of scalp, bone, or dural structures; and (3) direct invasion or compression of somatosensory cranial nerves or sympathetic afferent pathways.[26,32,50] It is little wonder then that organic cranial and intracranial disorders are difficult to identify or localize by the characteristics of the headaches they provoke.

Patients with intracranial tumors frequently report headache as a primary symptom.[26,36,50] It is commonly unilateral at onset, frontal or occipital, steady or throbbing, increased by exertion, and progressive. Headache beginning with these characteristics in patients over the age of 40 years commonly is found to have been the first sign of tumor. Headache may, however, be generalized or entirely wanting even in the presence of severely increased intracranial pressure. Infratentorial tumors as contrasted to supratentorial tumors may more commonly cause headache as a first symptom, although this would be extremely rare with eighth nerve tumors and brain stem gliomas. It is common with intraventricular masses in which the headache may be of sudden onset, explosive in intensity, bitemporal or frontal in distribution, and followed soon by coma without localizing deficit.

Wolff summarized his observations of headache as an aid in localization of brain tumors as follows: (1) Although the headache of brain tumor is often referred from a distant intracranial source, it approximately overlies the tumor in about one third of all patients. (2) Brain tumor headache in the absence of papilledema is of great localizing value. In about two thirds of such patients the headache immediately overlies or is near the tumor; when unilateral, it is on the same side as the tumor. (3) Headache is usually present with posterior fossa tumor and is initially in the back of the head. (4) Headache may be absent with any of the common types of supratentorial tumors, but it is the first symptom in one third and is usually in the front of the head. (5) Headache is usually the first symptom of posterior fossa tumor except in cerebellopontine angle tumors. (6) The headache of posterior fossa tumor is almost always over the back of the head, although it may occur elsewhere as well. (7) The headache of cerebellopontine angle tumors is frequently and sometimes solely postauricular on the side of the tumor. (8) Headache from supratentorial tumors is rarely in the back of the head unless associated with papilledema. (9) When supratentorial tumors cause headache in the back of the head, headache in the front of the head is usually also present. (10) When headache is both frontal and occipital it indicates extensive displacement of the brain and has little localizing value. The history of the headache, whether it was initially on the left or the right, frontal or occipital, may indicate the site of the lesion. (11) Brain tumor headache is usually intermittent, but when it is continuous its value in localization is greatly enhanced.[24]

While such retrospective generalities may at times be helpful when other signs are lacking, they have little to offer prospectively in most patients.

A ''cough'' or ''exertional'' headache may be the sole sign of an intracranial mass lesion.[33,41]

A 53-year-old used car auctioneer with serious domestic difficulties and a business that was verging on bankruptcy complained that for six months he had had ''twinges'' or ''pulses'' of brief pain deep in his head near the midline, lasting seconds only but recurring from two to three to several times a day—with few exceptions while he was working in the auction ring. They were accentuated with physical activity and

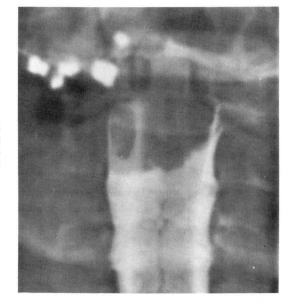

Figure 118–10 Posteroanterior view of cervical myelogram in a man with "cough" headache of six months' duration. A large multilobulated lesion is identified and is producing a complete subarachnoid block.

were at times "real sharp" when evoked by a violent cough or sneeze. He described "rusty cords" pulling in his neck when he turned his head. His family and past history were not remarkable. He had not had headaches before the onset of his chief complaint. No additional neurological complaints could be elicited. Findings of a detailed neurological examination were normal. He continued under the care of his family physician and was treated on a symptomatic basis until he was seen again three years later. His symptoms were unchanged although his head pains were somewhat more easily provoked by exertion. Neurological examination still revealed no abnormality. Because of the persistent "cough headache" a spinal puncture was performed. The cerebrospinal fluid protein was 204 mg per 100 ml. A total block at the C1 level was found on Pantopaque myelography (Figs. 118–10 and 118–11). Subtotal resection of a fourth ventricle ependymoma was followed by deep x-ray therapy. He has remained asymptomatic for four years.

Although cough headache or exertional headache may, over a period of years gradually subside and seem unrelated to a mass lesion, it must be considered a cardinal indicator of an intracranial mass lesion when it occurs with no antecedent headache history in an almost "pure form" and persists or is progressive—whether it is focal, lateralized, or midline, as in this instance.

The headache associated with brain tumor may at times be bizarre. An example is given in the following case history.

A distraught young woman with seven young children and with a husband who was not well was working desperately to maintain a rented marginal farm. She had complained of a "crown" headache at the vertex for several months and particularly of a feeling of maggots or ants gnawing through her scalp at the vertex. At first the feeling was intermittent and mild but had gradually become more constant and for several weeks had been severe and unremitting. Nothing relieved or aggravated her distress. A

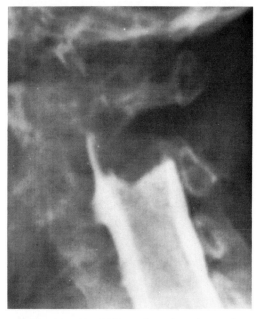

Figure 118–11 Oblique view of myelogram from same patient as illustrated in Figure 118–10. The lesion is mainly dorsal in location and has the characteristics of an intradural extramedullary lesion. An exophytic ependymoma arising in the fourth ventricle was identified and subtotally removed at operation.

carefully documented neurological examination and history gave no clue to organic disease. One month later her family physician found papilledema. Neurological examination again was negative for other findings. She had a large right temporal lobe glioma. After temporal lobectomy she returned to her home and former duties—the scalp symptoms that she had so vividly described did not recur.

HEADACHES RELATED TO ANEURYSMS AND VASCULAR ANOMALIES

Headache may occur as a warning sign in up to 60 per cent of patients who will subsequently suffer a subarachnoid hemorrhage as a result of a ruptured intracranial aneurysm.[20,27] Review of such patients indicates that the headache that occurs as a forwarning of a major subarachnoid hemorrhage presents a fairly characteristic clinical picture. The headache is often described as "unusual" and unlike any other the patient has ever experienced. The pain is usually sudden in onset and severe or disabling in intensity. King and Saba found that in 26 per cent of warning headaches the pain was frontal, in 14 per cent it was retroorbital, and in 31 per cent it was biooccipital at onset.[20] Often the headache became bifrontal and occipital within an hour or two after onset. Recurrent acute and intense headaches were reported for more than six months by 40 per cent of the patients, for one to six months by 21 per cent, and for one to four weeks by 33 per cent. Symptoms associated with warning headaches include nausea and vomiting, neck pains or stiffness, syncopal attack or brief coma, visual disturbances, motor or sensory symptoms, and seizures. It is suggested that warning headache may be due to expansion of the aneurysmal sac and adjacent artery, minor subarachnoid hemorrhage, or ischemic cerebral lesions possibly secondary to arterial spasm or embolization from the aneurysmal orifice. Warning signs including headache are most common with aneurysms of the anterior circulation and distinctly rare with posterior fossa lesions. When forewarning signs, particularly the characteristic headache, are identified, lumbar puncture should be carried out for confirmation of the diagnosis. This should be done promptly, since the interval between onset of minor warning aneurysmal leak and major hemorrhage is about 10 days. Not every headache with the characteristics just described heralds a major subarachnoid hemorrhage or the presence of an unruptured aneurysm. Considering the very small risk of lumbar puncture, properly performed, and the significant mortality rate and morbidity associated with major subarachnoid hemorrhage, more liberal use of lumbar puncture is suggested to evaluate suspicious headaches.

Congential berry aneurysms of the internal carotid artery or posterior communicating artery may also cause severe, sharp pains in the retro-orbital region, radiating in the distribution of the ophthalmic division of the trigeminal nerve and simulating migraine attacks. These head pains are uniformly unilateral and are often associated with ipsilateral anisocoria, paresis of extraocular muscles innervated by the third cranial nerve, and mildly diminished perception of somatosensory stimuli in the brow and forehead. Similar lesions of the middle cerebral artery butting the dura of the lesser wing of the sphenoid may cause short, sharp stabs of lightning-quick pain referred to the eye or orbit, but these are not usually associated with radiation of pain to the forehead with sensory change or other cranial nerve deficits. The patient whose angiograms are shown in Figures 118–8 and 118–9 is an example of facial pain related to an unsuspected intracranial aneurysm. Aneurysms in other locations, except for giant aneurysms in the parasellar region, seldom provoke pain in a pattern sufficiently common to lead to suspicion or a diagnosis.

Occasionally arteriovenous malformations of the dura or extracranial cervical region may be associated with unilateral localized headache that waxes and wanes with exertion and remains localized to the side of the lesion. These patterns of cephalgia are presumably independent of subarachnoid bleeding and related primarily to the distention of the vascular tree and dural structures adjacent to the lesion.

REFERENCES

1. Alderman, M. M.: Disorders of the temporomandibular joint and related structures. *In* Burket, L. W., ed.: Oral Medicine: Diagnosis and Treatment. 6th Ed. Philadelphia, J. B. Lippincott Co., 1971.
2. Bickerstaff, E. R.: Basilar artery migraine. Lancet, *1*:15–17, 1961.

3. Birkhead, N. C., Wagener, H. P., and Schick, R. M.: Treatment of temporal arteritis with adrenal corticosteroids; Results in fifty-five cases in which lesion was proved by biopsy. J.A.M.A., 163:821–827, 1957.

4. Boles, R.: Paranasal sinuses and face pain. In Alling. C. C., et al., eds.: Facial Pain. Philadelphia, Lea & Febiger, 1968, p. 135.

5. Carlson, G. E., Oberg, T., Bergman, F., and Fajers, C. M.: Morphological changes in the mandibular joint disk in temporomandibular joint pain dysfunction syndrome. Acta Odont. Scand., 25:163–181, 1967.

6. Carroll, J. D.: Migraine—general management. Brit. Med. J., 2:756–757, 1971.

7. Costen, J. B.: A syndrome of ear and sinus symptoms dependent upon disturbed function of the temporomandibular joint. Ann. Otol., 43:1–15, 1934.

8. Costen, J. B.: Neuralgias and ear symptoms. J.A.M.A., 107:252–255, 1936.

9. Easton, H. G.: Zoster sine herpete causing acute trigeminal neuralgia. Lancet, 2:1065–1066, 1970.

10. Fessel, W. J., and Pearson, C. M.: Polymyalgia rheumatica and blindness. New Eng. J. Med., 276:1403, 1967.

11. Foster, J. B.: Facial pain. Brit. Med. J., 4:667–669, 1969.

12. Friedman, A. P.: The migraine syndrome. Bull. N.Y. Acad. Med., 44:45–60, 1968.

13. Friedman, A. P., Finley, K. H., Grahan, J. R., Kunkle, E. C., Ostfeld, A. M., and Wolff, H. G.: Ad hoc committee on classification of headache. J.A.M.A., 179:127–128, 1962.

14. Gibilisco, J. A., Goldstein, N. P., and Rushton, J. G.: The differential diagnosis of atypical facial pain. J. Lancet, 85:450–454, October, 1965.

15. Haas, D. C.: Migrane attacks triggered by mild head trauma and their relation to certain post traumatic disorders of childhood. J. Neurol. Neurosurg. Psychiat., 32:548–554, 1969.

16. Hollenhorst, R. W., Brown, J. R., Wagener, H. P., and Schiek, R. M.: Neurologic aspects of temporal arteritis. Neurology (Minneap.), 10:490–498, 1960.

17. Horton, B. T., and Magath, T. B.: Arteritis of the temporal vessels; report of seven cases. Proc. Staff Meet. Mayo Clin., 12:548–553, 1937.

18. Hutchinson, J. H.: Migraine. (Annotations.) Lancet, 2:1122, 1966.

19. Janetta, P. J.: Arterial compression of the trigeminal nerve at the pons in patients with trigeminal neuralgia. J. Neurosurg., 26:159–162, 1967.

20. King, R. B., and Saba, M. I.: Forewarnings of major subarachnoid hemorrhage. N.Y. State J. Med., 74:638–639, 1974.

21. Lascelles, R. G.: A typical facial pain and depression. Brit. J. Psychiat., 112:651–659, 1966.

22. Low, N. L., and Correll, J. W.: Head pain due to leptomeningel cysts. Brit. J. Surg., 53:791–793, 1966.

23. McNaughton, F. L.: The innervation of the intracranial blood vessels and dural sinuses. Ass. Res. Nerv. Ment. Dis. Proc., 18:178–200, 1938.

24. Meadows, S. P.: Temporal or giant cell arteritis—ophthalmic aspects. In Smith, J. L., ed.: Neuro-ophthalmology. Vol. IV. St. Louis, C. V. Mosby Co., 1968, p. 148, 157.

25. Miller, H.: Pain in the face. Brit. Med. J., 2:577–580, 1968.

26. Northfield, D. W. C.: Some observations on headache. Brain, 61:133–162, 1938.

27. Okaware, S.: Warning signs prior to rupture of an intracranial aneurysm. J. Neurosurg., 38:575–580, 1973.

28. Penfield, W.: A contribution to the mechanism of intracranial pain. Ass. Res. Nerve. Ment. Dis. Proc., 15:399–416, 1935.

29. Penfield, W., and McNaughton, F.: Dural headache and innervation of the dura mater, Arch. Neurol. Psychiat., 44:43, 1940.

30. Penfield, W., and Norcross, N. D.: Subdural traction and post-traumatic headache. Arch. Neurol. Psychiat., 36:75–78, 1936.

31. Pilling, L. F.: Psychosomatic aspects of facial pain. In Alling, C. C., et al., eds.: Facial Pain. Philadelphia, Lea & Febiger, 1968, p. 107.

32. Ray, B. S., and Wolff, H. G.: Experimental studies on headache-pain-sensitive structures of the head and their significance in headache. Arch. Surg., 41:813–956, 1940.

33. Rooke, E. D.: Benign exertional headache. Med. Clin. N. Amer., 52:801–808, 1968.

34. Reiner, M., and Wyss, J.: Giant cell arteritis. Praxis, 58:1524–1533, 1969.

35. Rubach, W. C.: "Atypical facial neuralgia" due to pulpitis. Oral Surg., 16:1039–1041, 1963.

36. Rushton, J. G., and Rooke, E. D.: Brain tumor headache. Headache, 2:147–152, 1962.

37. Scott, M.: Occipital neuralgia. Penn. Med., 71:85–88, 1968.

38. Smith, K. R., Jr.: Electron microscopy of giant-cell (temporal) arteritis. J. Neurol. Neurosurg. Psychiat., 32:348–353, 1969.

39. Stagman, J.: Sphenoid vacuum cephalalgia. Headache, 3:30–32, 1967.

40. Sutcher, H. D.: The dentist in research, diagnosis, and treatment of head pain. Headache, 8:16–22, 1968.

41. Symonds, C.: Cough headache. Brain, 19:557–568, 1956.

42. Taub, A.: Relief of postherpetic neuralgia with psychotropic drugs. J. Neurosurg., 39:235–239, 1973.

43. Thoma, K. H., and Robinson, H. B. G.: Oral and Dental Diagnosis. 5th Ed. Philadelphia and London, W. B. Saunders Co., 1960.

44. Verbin, R. S., Heineman, H. S., and Stiff, R. H.: Localized odontalgia occurring during herpes zoster of the maxillary division of the fith cranial nerve. Oral Surg., 26:441–445, 1968.

45. Weber, R. B., and Reinmuth, O. M.: The treatment of migraine with propranolol. Neurology (Minneap.), 22:366–369, 1972.

46. White, J. D., and Sweet, W. H.: Pain and the Neurosurgeon. Springfield, Ill., Charles C Thomas, 1969.

47. Whitty, C. W. M.: Migraine without headache. Lancet, 2:283–285, 1967.

48. Williams, H. L.: Vasoatonic headache associated with chronic maxillary sinusitis. Arch. Otolaryng. (Chicago), 88:95–97, 1968.

49. Wolff, H. G.: Experimental studies on headache: Pain sensitive structures of the head and their significance in headache. Arch. Surg., 41:813–856, 1940.

50. Wolff, H. G.: Headache and other head pain. 3rd ed. Rev. by D'Alessio, D. J. New York, Oxford University Press, 1972.

119

GENERAL CONSIDERATIONS, MEDICAL THERAPY, AND MINOR OPERATIVE PROCEDURES FOR TRIGEMINAL NEURALGIA

HISTORICAL BACKGROUND

Trigeminal neuralgia is a painful affliction of the peripheral branches of the trigeminal nerve, the etiology of which is uncertain. Among its many synonyms are tic douloureux, trifacial neuralgia, major trigeminal neuralgia, and idiopathic trigeminal neuralgia. Early descriptions of painful conditions of the face extend as far back as the first century A.D.[72] It was not until 1776, however, that trigeminal neuralgia was described as a clinical entity. Nicolas André reported five cases, and struck by the clinical manifestations of this disorder, called it tic douloureux.[1] Only sporadic case reports appeared in the late eighteenth and early nineteenth centuries, and it was obvious from these that the disorder was not understood.[20] It remained for Charles Bell to demonstrate the anatomical basis for sensation in the face. In a series of studies reported first in 1821 and again in 1829, he clearly described motor and sensory components of the trigeminal nerve.[3,4] He also determined the function of the facial nerve and thus was able to distinguish between the two. An anatomical background for trigeminal neuralgia was defined therefore, and the groundwork laid for a logical approach to treatment.

The severe pain of trigeminal neuralgia has caused many forms of treatment to be used in an effort to give relief. Among them are purging, extract of hemlock, ferrous carbonate, and trichlorethylene.[15,18,40,57,67] André considered a direct approach to the problem, advocating caustics to expose and destroy the offending nerve. However, most attempts to cut the peripheral branches of the fifth nerve were failures.[14] Thus, surgical treatment of trigeminal neuralgia had an inauspicious beginning. Limitations to peripheral neurectomy were soon realized.[21]

In 1891 Sir Victor Horsley and his associates reported an intradural approach to the gasserian ganglion through the temporal bone whereby the sensory root could be exposed and sectioned.[39] In the United States, one year later, Hartley described the extradural approach to the ganglion that he excised.[37] Shortly afterward a similar approach was described by Krause in Germany, and the procedure became known as the Hartley-Krause method.[51] The advantages of root section in contrast to ganglion excision became apparent, but it was postulated that the loss of sensation to the face following root section would be permanent.[2,16,45,71] In discussing trigeminal root section, Tiffany, in 1896, advocated sparing of the first division to protect the eye.[75] Two years earlier he had suggested that the motor root could be preserved, but it was not until 24 years later that this was actually done.[74] In 1918, Peet reported sparing of the motor root in five of eight trigeminal root sections.[65] Frazier, however, deserves much of the credit for developing the tech-

---

nique of differential root section.[22,23] His is a classic operation still employed today.

ETIOLOGY

The underlying mechanism responsible for trigeminal neuralgia is obscure. Most agree that it is an afferent reflex phenomenon of some sort. Its location is still debated. Some believe that it originates centrally within the brain stem. Others postulate a more peripheral location within the sensory root of the trigeminal nerve.

Lewy and Grant conceived of trigeminal neuralgia as a partial thalamic syndrome and demonstrated small lesions in the ipsilateral thalamus and in the thalamocortical radiations in some of their patients.[54] Wilson considered the paroxysms of pain to be sensory epileptiform discharges originating in some efferent sensory inhibitory mechanism, presumably within the central trigeminal apparatus.[77] Others noted the frequency of trigeminal neuralgia in patients with multiple sclerosis in whom, at autopsy, plaques had been found in the central trigeminal pathways.[17,35,63] Dott believed the mechanism to be in the brain stem and thought it analogous to an electrical short circuit deflecting benign stimuli into the pain pathway.[15]

In a series of brilliant studies, King and his associates were able to evoke activity in small pain fibers in the caudal region of the spinal tract of the fifth cranial nerve by electrically stimulating large touch fibers in the peripheral branches.[48-50] Delayed responses were also recorded in the third division after stimulation of a peripheral branch of the second division. By irritating the descending tract and nucleus of the fifth nerve with alumina gel and later with strychnine, they evoked responses to electrical stimulation in its peripheral divisions that were increased both in amplitude and duration. Such an overreaction was never observed when the focus of irritation was applied anywhere else along the course of the trigeminal apparatus. On the basis of these observations they suggested a mechanism underlying trigeminal neuralgia within the spinal trigeminal pathways in the brain stem.

Kugelberg and Lindblom studied 50 patients with trigeminal neuralgia.[53] By varying the amplitude or frequency of the cutaneous stimulus, they found a definite refractory phase during which the threshold for a subsequent paroxysm was raised. Noting frequently a latency of 15 to 30 seconds between stimulus and response, they also postulated a central origin of trigeminal neuralgia. They conceded that occasional short jabs of pain might result from interaction or short-circuiting of touch and pain fibers.

After a thorough review of the subject, List and Williams concluded that the best explanation of the pathogenesis of trigeminal neuralgia was based on neurophysiological grounds.[56] They suggested that the paroxysms of pain represent a "pathologic multineuronal reflex in the trigeminal system of the brain stem." They believed that pathological changes frequently found in the trigeminal system might produce abnormal electrical potentials resulting in an abnormal central excitatory state.

Dandy believed that the mechanism responsible for trigeminal neuralgia lay in the sensory root.[11-13] He advocated the posterior approach to the fifth nerve and concluded that, in nearly 11 per cent of his patients, gross lesions, tumors, aneurysms, and angiomas were responsible for "trigeminal neuralgia." Later reviews of his 205 cerebellopontine angle tumors disclosed 31 patients with trigeminal neuralgia.[28,29] Dandy also incriminated structural abnormalities in relation to the sensory root in an additional 49 per cent of his series. Others have related trigeminal neuralgia to posterior fossa tumors, middle fossa tumors, and subclinoid aneurysms.[25,33,61,69]

Taarnhøj obtained relief in a young man with trigeminal neuralgia by removing a cholesteatoma that was compressing the sensory root.[78] The root itself was left intact. In considering the etiology of this disorder, he reasoned that compression of the trigeminal root would most likely occur where it extends from the ganglion "posteriorly, through the narrow channel formed by the dura to the upper sharp margin of the petrous bone." He reported 10 patients with trigeminal neuralgia who were relieved by decompressing this portion of the root.

Gardner noted Taarnhøj's success and followed the example in 20 cases of his own.[26] In 1953 he reported good results in this series and theorized that trigeminal neuralgia results from the short-circuiting of nerve impulses within the sensory root where it crosses the apex of the petrous bone. To evoke such a pathological process, he believed, loss of insulating myelin sheath was essential.

In a symposium concerning the structural aspects of trigeminal neuralgia, most of the contributors implicated the sensory root.[52] The following is a summary of their findings.

Progressive demyelination of "normal" trigeminal roots and ganglia occurs in association with aging. This demyelination, however, is more pronounced in patients with trigeminal neuralgia and may result from a mechanical factor, a dural band crossing the sensory root at the petrous apex, or a mild to severe compression of the root by small tortuous arteries. In an earlier report, Kerr found a significant incidence of dehiscence of the bone forming the roof of the carotid canal.[46] He suggested that the resulting proximity of the ganglion to the pulsating carotid artery might be an etiological factor in trigeminal neuralgia. King was the only contributor favoring the brain stem as the source of the disorder.

Gardner has a theory that he bases on the hypothetical presence of parasympathetic fibers in the sensory root of the fifth nerve.[27] The existence of these fibers is inferred from the studies of Lewy, Groff, and Grant and has been demonstrated by Hering and others.[30,38,55,58] Gardner concludes that compression of the sensory root (by an aberrant branch of the superior cerebellar artery or by angulation over the petrous apex) results in approximation of intact axis cylinders devoid of their insulating myelin sheath. An artificial synapse from transaxonal excitation of pain fibers results in the paroxysms of pain characterizing trigeminal neuralgia. In such a reflex, "the evoked efferent discharge is short-circuited into the afferent pain fibers." Although it has not been proved, the efferent arc of this reflex is thought to be parasympathetic.

Jannetta believes that trigeminal neuralgia may be an entrapment syndrome, a consequence of arteriosclerotic stretching, or rarely, of congenital abnormalities of branches of the superior cerebellar artery, which compress and distort the trigeminal root in the vicinity of its entrance into the pons.[43] He along with Rand first described this abnormality in 1966.[44] Subsequently, he reported his results following vascular decompression in 43 patients with trigeminal neuralgia. Although four patients required reoperation, the procedure was successful ultimately in all of them.[43]

CHARACTERISTICS

Pain alone, confined to the distribution of one of more branches of the trigeminal nerve, is the outstanding feature of this disorder. Objective findings as determined by the routine neurological examination are absent.

This disorder is more common in women in a ratio of 3:2, usually beginning in the fifth and sixth decades.[36] The second and third divisions of the trigeminal nerve are about equally affected. Involvement of the first division is uncommon—approximately 2 to 5 per cent. Occasionally the disorder is bilateral, but rarely is such involvement simultaneous.

Pain occurs in paroxysms "likened to a thousand burning needles pricking and stabbing, to knives cutting and piercing, to something searing the flesh, to wires that tingle with electrical pain, to a crescendo agony finishing by a burst or explosion as of a firework."[77] Such attacks last only a minute or two although rarely in long-standing cases they may go on longer. Attacks may be precipitated by touching the face—even by a breeze on the face—or by such movements as talking, eating, or smiling or by hot or cold fluids. Pain is not evident between attacks. It occurs less frequently at night.

The patient may talk out of the opposite side of his mouth in an attempt to immobilize the affected side. One side of the face may be unwashed or unshaved. When the third division is involved, that side of the tongue may be coated. Often the involved side is protected by a scarf or shawl.

In most cases, trigger points will be found within the terminal distribution of the involved division. Even the lightest touch to the area may evoke an attack. Such a finding may establish the diagnosis.

Occasionally patients with trigeminal neuralgia associated with multiple sclerosis have noted numbness of the face that usually preceded the onset of pain.[70] Such paresthesias have been bilateral, occurring even on the side opposite the pain.

Remissions are characteristic. They may

last for weeks or years. Usually such intervals become progressively shorter and each recurrence more severe. Factors responsible for these remissions are unclear.

In long-standing cases, pain confined to one division may extend secondarily to involve another. The trigger point remains in the primary division, however, which continues to be most severely involved. Treatment directed to the primary division usually will relieve the secondary division as well.

DIFFERENTIAL DIAGNOSIS

Atypical Facial Neuralgia

This disorder commonly affects high-strung middle-aged women, not the elderly.[32] Most often, pain is confined to the central portions of the face, the cheek, or the orbit, but may extend on to the back of the head and neck. Usually it is vaguely described as dull-aching, nagging, or boring, and such patients insist that it is unbearable. Paroxysms of lancinating pain are not characteristic nor are there specific trigger points. There seems to be a large psychiatric component to this condition. Attacks upon the trigeminal nerve are ineffective and actually may worsen the condition.

Vasomotor Neuralgia

The differentiation of vasomotor neuralgia from trigeminal neuralgia should pose no problem. It is found predominantly in 30- to 50-year-old men. Attacks occur regularly, usually at night. Pain begins in one side of the face, usually in the infraorbital region. Gradually it increases in severity and extends to the same side of the head and neck. Often there is flushing of the face, injection of the cornea with tearing of the eye, or stuffiness of the ipsilateral nostril. Rarely there is an ipsilateral Horner's syndrome.[76] Usually the pain disappears completely within one to three hours and the patient feels entirely well.

Postherpetic Neuralgia

Herpetic involvement of the trigeminal nerve most frequently affects the ophthalmic division. The initial pain is confusing until the characteristic erythema and vesicle formations appear.[32] It is, however, constant, burning or aching in nature, not paroxysmal. The pain that persists as postherpetic neuralgia is unremitting and described as burning or crawling. Sensory root section is of no benefit, since the disease process extends into the trigeminal nucleus.[72]

Nasopharyngeal Tumors

These tumors, most often squamous cell carcinomas, are usually in the fossa of Rosenmüller and may invade the base of the skull. Pain in the face is common. It is constant, dull-aching in nature, and may be accompanied by sensory changes within the distribution of the trigeminal nerve. Often there is palsy of other cranial nerves as well. Skull x-rays may show erosion of the base, erosion of the floor of the sella turcica, or a mass in the nasopharynx.

Intracranial Tumors

Pain indistinguishable from that of trigeminal neuralgia has been reported as the only manifestation of certain tumors arising within or close to the fifth nerve.[27] These include neuromas, meningiomas, and cholesteatomas in the cerebellopontine angle as well as neuromas and meningiomas originating within the gasserian ganglion. Cases have been reported in which tumors of the cerebellum have displaced the pons against the opposite sensory root, producing "trigeminal neuralgia" contralaterally.[34,64]

Usually, however, such tumors produce neurological changes. There may be a diminished corneal reflex or loss of sensation over one or more branches of the fifth nerve, along with signs of motor root impairment. Often, involvement of adjacent cranial nerves is evident.

Pain in the face is uncommon in patients with cerebellopontine angle tumors. It is more apt to occur with those rare tumors involving the gasserian ganglion and, initially, may be paroxysmal. Eventually the pain becomes more constant and is accompanied by sensory changes. In most cases then, a careful history and objective examination should distinguish intracranial tumors from trigeminal neuralgia. When necessary, further diagnostic studies should dispel any doubt.

Dental Pain

Initially pain is localized to the tooth involved and may be accompanied by swelling. The pain may extend to the upper or lower jaw and may be referred to the ear or temporomandibular region. Usually it is constant, dull-aching—often worse at night.

TREATMENT

Medical Management

Diphenylhydantoin

The beneficial effects of diphenylhydantoin (Dilantin) in trigeminal neuralgia have been known since 1942.[5] Rationale for the use of this drug has been the possible relationship suggested by the similarity of the paroxysmal afferent discharge to epilepsy. Experimentally induced hyperexcitability states within the trigeminal apparatus and in peripheral nerves have been depressed by diphenylhydantoin.[48,60] The reported clinical experience with this drug in trigeminal neuralgia attests to its efficacy.[8,41] Often, however, control is incomplete and unsustained. In some patients toxicity of the high dosages necessary to obtain relief limits its usefulness. The usual dose is 100 mg three to four times a day, but this may be extended to as much as 100 mg six times a day if necessary.

Mephenesin Carbamate

King found mephenesin (Tolserol) more effective than diphenylhydantoin in depressing experimentally induced overreactions to tactile facial stimuli.[47] In a clinical trial of mephenesin and later of mephenesin carbamate (Tolseram) alone or in conjunction with diphenylhydantoin, he obtained satisfactory relief in 86 per cent of patients with trigeminal neuralgia. Although the drug has not been used extensively, it should be considered in patients refractory to diphenylhydantoin. The dose of mephenesin carbamate (Tolseram) varies between 5 and 15 ml from five times a day to as often as every three hours.

Carbamazepine

Carbamazepine (Tegretol) has received enthusiastic support since its introduction by Bloom in 1962.[7] Although unrelated to the hydantoins, its action is similar to that of diphenylhydantoin in that both drugs suppress synaptic transmission in the spinal trigeminal nucleus. Depression by carbamazepine is more prolonged.

In 1968 Birchfield reported a series of 41 patients with tic douloureux in whom carbamazepine was tried. Thirty of them experienced good to complete relief, and eight others had partial relief. In 12 patients the drug was discontinued because of toxic reactions—skin reactions, leukopenia, and liver damage. He concluded that carbamazepine had a practical efficacy of 66 per cent in providing adequate pain relief without toxicity.[6]

Treatment with carbamazepine (Tegretol) usually is begun with 200 mg three times a day. Often dosages must be adjusted, and in some patients, 200 mg five to six times a day may be necessary. The drug should not be used in patients with liver disease or blood dyscrasias. The signs of intoxication should be monitored initially by a complete blood count, urinalysis, and liver function tests, and by blood counts weekly during the first month of treatment and monthly thereafter. Liver function should be assessed monthly. Skin reactions are not uncommon with Tegretol, and in severe cases, the drug must be stopped.

Chlorphenesin Carbamate

Clorphenesin carbamate (Maolate) is a recent addition to the medical management of trigeminal neuralgia.[9,10] Apparently its action is similar to that of mephenesin, although its duration of action is considerably longer. This drug has been effective particularly when added to a regimen of carbamazepine or diphenylhydantoin, or both, in patients whose pain has been controlled incompletely by these measures. The suggested dose is 400 mg in the morning, 400 mg at noon, and 800 mg at bedtime. Once pain has been relieved, the dosage is gradually reduced to the lowest possible maintenance level.

Alcohol Block*

Blocking the peripheral branches of the fifth nerve with alcohol may be effective, but since nerve destruction is postganglionic, sensation returns in from $8^1/_2$ to 16 months. Blocking the gasserian ganglion results in more permanent relief, but the hazards of this procedure—palsy of other cranial nerves owing to escape of the alcohol under the basal subarachnoid space and the inability to achieve differential destruction of ganglion cells—are such that this technique is rarely employed. Jaeger has reported pain relief in 96 of 100 patients after injecting the gasserian ganglion with boiling distilled water.[42]

Rationale of Alcohol Block

The rationale for alcohol block of the peripheral division of the trigeminal nerve is as follows:

1. The outcome of operative section can be predicted with virtual certainty. If a satisfactory injection affords no relief, operation may not be indicated.

2. Prolonged numbness of the face allows the patient time to weigh permanent numbness of his face against his original pain.

3. In long-standing cases of trigeminal neuralgia, some patients are unable to eat and may be debilitated. In such cases, temporary relief of a year or so permits them to restore their nutritional status, and they become better operative risks.

4. Alcohol block may allow very old patients to complete their life span without operation.

5. Occasionally patients may obtain permanent relief. Examples of pain-free periods of as long as 30 years have been recorded.

Precautions

The following precautions minimize the problems attending alcohol block:

1. Supraorbital and supratrochlear nerve blocks are rarely performed, since avulsion of these nerves is readily accomplished and more adequate pain control is assured. Attempts to block the ophthalmic nerve itself

may lead to damage of the eye or the oculomotor nerve or its branches.

2. Twenty-four hours prior to blocking with alcohol, a block with long-acting agent such as tetracaine (Pontocaine) should be employed. Patients can thus preview the long-term results of alcohol injection, and the physician can detect possible complications from his technique and avoid prolonged, perhaps permanent, complications after alcohol injection. He can also determine the exact amount of alcohol necessary to accomplish the desired result. A small measured amount of local anesthetic solution comparable to the amount of alcohol advocated should be used first as a test dose.

3. Never more than 1.5 ml of alcohol is injected at any one time in any of the divisions of the trigeminal nerve. It is seldom necessary to use more than 0.5 ml of alcohol in blocking any of the branches of the fifth nerve.

4. Blocking of another division or repeated blocking of the same division should not be done until at least 24 hours have elapsed. In spite of an adequate block, some patients experience sensations resembling their previous pain for 24 to 72 hours. After this period, such sensation usually subsides and the patient is pain-free. If pain persists and sensation has returned, repeat block is indicated. If pain persists after adequate analgesia has been achieved over one division, blocking of another division may be indicated.

5. Alcohol block should not be attempted until the technique has been mastered. While complications from local anesthetic agents are usually transient, complications from alcohol may be permanent.

Preparation of Patient

Alcohol injection on an outpatient basis is satisfactory. The patient should take nothing by mouth for six hours prior to the procedure and should arrange to remain at bed rest nearby for two hours following block. The incidence of nausea and vomiting following alcohol injection is approximately 10 per cent.

The indications for alcohol block as well as the technique to be employed should be explained in detail to the patient. He should be thoroughly briefed in all possible complications of this procedure. He should be

---

* Written in conjunction with L. Donald Bridenbaugh, M.D.

warned of the transient but severe pain attending injection of the alcohol.

Technique

The technique for the infiltration of the individual branches of the trigeminal nerve is detailed by Moore.[59] If block with a local anesthetic solution has produced relief of pain, one can proceed with alcohol injection.

Local anesthesia is employed in making the skin wheal and for superficial infiltration only. The nerve itself should not be blocked with a local anesthetic agent. If, in this manner, the pain of the alcohol injection is eliminated, one cannot be assured of proper placement of the needle. Furthermore, the volume of the local anesthetic solution will dilute the alcohol and may render the block ineffective.

The needle is placed with careful attention to appropriate landmarks. Prior to injection, paresthesias of the nerve must be elicited. X-ray control is not routine. This prolongs the block procedure time and is inconvenient; also, the information obtained is not always accurate. On the other hand, x-rays to determine the needle's position may be helpful when learning the technique, when paresthesias are difficult to elicit, or if correct placement of the needle is questioned. Additional advantages are that, when obtained during preliminary block with a short-acting anesthetic agent, x-rays serve as guidelines for subsequent films taken at the time of alcohol block, and that x-rays establish a permanent record of the position of the needle in case the alcohol block must be repeated.

Thirty-five per cent iodopyracet (Diodrast) may be employed as a solvent for the crystals of local anesthetic agent. In this manner x-rays within 5 to 10 minutes following injection will show the exact spread of the solution. In 10 to 15 per cent of cases, however, Diodrast may intensify the discomfort after the intended anesthesia has dissipated.

The quantity of alcohol is carefully measured and injected. A 2- or 3-ml Luer-Lok syringe or a tuberculin syringe should always be included in the regional block tray so that the alcohol may be accurately measured. The syringe to be used for the injection of alcohol should not be used to measure any other solution. It should be used only to measure and inject the alcohol.

Small sterile ampules (2-ml size) should be used and should never be opened until the time of injection. If highly concentrated alcohol is loosely stoppered or allowed to stand open for any length of time, it will absorb moisture from the air and may become contaminated with spores. The exact amount of alcohol used should be recorded on the patient's chart.

After injection, 2 cc of air is blown through the needle before it is removed. This maneuver prevents sinus tracts from forming between the alcohol deposit and the site of injection. It also prevents residual alcohol from being deposited upon other nerve fibers, particularly the motor division, as the needle is withdrawn.

Complications

Paresthesias are not uncommon following alcohol block. Patients may complain of a "woody" sensation or of "worms crawling over the face." This complication is not mentioned in two large series, but in that of Peet and Schneider some degree of paresthesia persisted in 48 per cent.[66,69,72] Permanent facial weakness may occur as well as permanent lateral rectus palsy.[69]

Other complications following alcohol block usually result from interference with the blood supply to this area and are not due to the effects of alcohol per se. They may vary from small hematomas to ulcerations, sloughs, or gangrene of the area supplied by the terminal branches of the injected division. These complications are infrequent and should not pose a contraindication to the procedure.

The treatment of such cases includes antibiotic drugs, hot wet packs, incision and drainage, and, if necessary, debridement and skin grafting. Stellate ganglion block may improve circulation to the involved area.

Minor Operative Procedures

Postganglionic Section

Avulsion of the peripheral branches of the fifth nerve may be worthwhile palliation in selected patients with trigeminal neuralgia.[31] This is especially true when pain is confined to the first division, as the corneal anesthesia attending preganglionic section is avoided. As already mentioned, supraorbital alcohol block is dangerous and may be ineffective.

Relief of pain following supraorbital and infraorbital nerve avulsion persists for an average period of 33 months, which compares favorably to the duration of relief following the alcohol block. It is the procedure of choice in patients too ill to withstand an intracranial procedure or those patients in whom the pain is confined to the first, or the first and second, divisions. Avulsion also may be worthwhile in patients in whom the diagnosis is uncertain. Persistent pain in the presence of adequate anesthesia rules out trigeminal neuralgia, and a major procedure with permanent consequences will have been avoided.

When the third division is involved, avulsion of the submental nerve usually is ineffective since its cutaneous supply is so limited. Avulsion of the inferior dental nerve in the mandible spares the lingual branch of the third division, a matter of little consequence since the painful paroxysms rarely involve the tongue. It entails a burr hole through the midportion of the mandible, however, and avulsion rarely extends beyond the confines of the bony opening. Alcohol block of the third division is probably more effective.

Supraorbital Nerve Avulsion

Operative technique for this and the following procedure is as described by Poppen.[68]

Local anesthesia after adequate preoperative sedation is satisfactory. The eyebrow should not be shaved. The incision can be made within it, centered over the supraorbital notch, and the dissection carried to the orbit so that all branches are exposed. The supraorbital nerve should be sectioned at a point somewhat distant to its exit through the foramen, with the proximal end carefully wrapped around the end of a hemostat so that, with firm traction, as much nerve as possible is removed. Other branches, including the supratrochlear nerve, should be dealt with similarly. The peripheral branches should also be avulsed. Infiltrating the nerve with local anesthetic beforehand minimizes the pain of avulsion.

Infraorbital Nerve Avulsion

Again local anesthesia is employed. An intraoral incision is preferable in the soft tissue over the maxilla just above the gingival mucous membrane. Exposure of the maxillary bone is extended up to the infraorbital foramen cautiously to avoid opening the maxillary sinus. Avulsion of the infraorbital nerve may be augmented by applying electrocoagulation with a needle or wire inserted into the infraorbital foramen.

REFERENCES

1. André, N. A.: Observations Pratiques Sur Les Maladies de L'Urétre. Paris, Chez Delaguette, Imprimeur de College et de L'Acad. Roy. de Chir., 1756, pp. 318–382.
2. Barker, L. F.: Protocols of microscopic examination of several gasserian ganglia. J.A.M.A., 34:1093–1098, 1900.
3. Bell, C.: On the nerves. Giving an account of some experiments on their structure and functions which lead to a new arrangement of the system. Phil. Trans. Roy. Soc., London, 398–424, 1821.
4. Bell, C.: On the nerves of the face. Being a second paper on the subject. Phil. Trans. Roy. Soc., London, 1:317–335, 1829.
5. Bergouignan, M.: Cures heureuses de névralgies faciales essentielles par le diphenylhydantoinate de soude. J. Méd. Bordeaux, 119:146–147, 1942.
6. Birchfield, R. I.: Tegretol in the treatment of tic douloureux: Experience with its use and the guidelines for therapy. Bull. Mason Clin., 22:58–67, 1968.
7. Bloom, S.: Trigeminal neuralgia: Its treatment with a new anticonvulsant drug (G-3288). Lancet, 1:839–841, 1962.
8. Braham, J., and Saia, A.: Phenytoin in the treatment of trigeminal and other neuralgias. Lancet, 2:892–893, 1960.
9. Dalessio, D. J., ed: Wolff's Headache and Other Head Pain. 3rd Ed. New York, Oxford University Press, 1972, pp. 585–589.
10. Dalessio, D. J.: Chlorphenesin for trigeminal neuralgia. J.A.M.A., 225:1659, 1973.
11. Dandy, W. E.: The treatment of trigeminal neuralgia by the cerebellar root. Ann. Surg., 96:787–795, 1932.
12. Dandy, W. E.: Concerning the cause of trigeminal neuralgia. Amer. J. Surg., 24:447–455, 1934.
13. Dandy, W. E.: The Brain. Lesions of the Cranial Nerves. In Lewis, D., ed.: Practice of Surgery. Hagerstown, Md., W. J. Prior Co., 1934, pp. 167–202.
14. Davis, L., and Haven, H. A.: Surgical anatomy of the sensory root of the trigeminal nerve. Arch. Neurol. Psychiat., 29:1–15, 1933.
15. Dott, N. M.: Facial pain. Proc. Roy. Soc. Med., 44:1034–1037, 1951.

16. Ferrier, D.: Removal of the gasserian ganglion for severe neuralgia. Lancet, 2:925–926, 1890.

17. Finesilver, B.: Trigeminal neuralgia in multiple sclerosis. J. Nerv. Ment. Dis., 90:757–764, 1939.

18. Fothergill, J.: Observations on the use of hemlock. Medical Observations and Inquiries, London, 3:409–411, 1769.

19. Fothergill, J.: Of a painful affection of the face. Medical Observations and Inquiries, London, 5:129–142, 1776.

20. Fothergill, S.: A Concise and Systematic Account of Painful Affection of the Nerves of the Face: Commonly Called Tic Douloureux. London, Murray, 1804.

21. Fowler, G. R.: The operative treatment of facial neuralgias; A comparison of methods and results. Ann. Surg., 3:269–320, 1886.

22. Frazier, C. H.: Trigeminal neuralgia; fourteen years experience with fractional section of the sensory root as the major operation. J.A.M.A., 89:1742–1744, 1927.

23. Frazier, C. H.: Operation for the radical cure of trigeminal neuralgia: Analysis of 500 cases. Ann. Surg., 88:534–547, 1928.

24. Fromm, G. H., and Killian, J. N.: Effect of some anticonvulsant drugs on the spinal trigeminal nucleus. Neurology (Minneap.), 17:275–280, 1967.

25. Gardner, W. J.: Cerebral angiomas and aneurysms. Surg. Clin. N. Amer., 16:1019–1030, 1936.

26. Gardner, W. J.: The mechanism of tic douloureux. Trans. Amer. Neurol. Ass., 78:158–173, 1953.

27. Gardner, W. J.: Trigeminal neuralgia. Clin. Neurosurg. (Proc. Cong. Neurol. Surg.), 15:1–56, 1968.

28. Gonzales Revilla, A.: Neurinomas of the cerebellopontile recess; clinical study of 160 cases including operative mortality and end results. Bull. Johns Hopk. Hosp., 80:254–296, 1947.

29. Gonzales Revilla, A.: Differential diagnosis of tumors at the cerebellopontile recess. Bull. Johns Hopk. Hosp., 83:187–212, 1948.

30. Granit, R., Leksell, L., and Scoglund, C. R.: Fibre interaction in injured or compressed region of nerve. Brain, 67:125–140, 1944.

31. Grantham, E. G., and Segerberg, L. H.: An evaluation of palliative surgical procedures in trigeminal neuralgia. J. Neurosurg., 9:390–394, 1952.

32. Grinker, R. R., Bucy, P. C., and Sahs, A. L.: Neurology. 5th Ed. Springfield, Ill., Charles C Thomas, 1960, pp. 289–291.

33. Hamby, W. B.: Trigeminal neuralgia due to radicular lesions. Arch. Surg., 46:555–563, 1943.

34. Hamby, W. B.: Trigeminal neuralgia due to contralateral tumors of the posterior cranial fossa. Report of two cases. J. Neurosurg., 4:178–182, 1947.

35. Harris, W.: Bilateral trigeminal tic: Its association with heredity and disseminated sclerosis. Ann. Surg., 103:161–172, 1936.

36. Harris, W.: An analysis of 1433 cases of paroxysmal trigeminal neuralgia (trigeminal tic) and the end results of gasserian alcohol injection. Brain, 63:209–224, 1940.

37. Hartley, F.: Intracranial neurectomy of second and third divisions of the fifth nerve. A new method. New York J. Med., 55:317–319, 1892.

38. Hering, E.: Cited by Gardner, W., ref. 27.

39. Horsley, V., Taylor, J., and Coleman, W. S.: Remarks on the various surgical procedures devised for the relief or cure of trigeminal neuralgia (tic douloureux). Brit. Med. J., 2:1139–1143, 1191–1193, 1249–1252, 1891.

40. Hutchinson, B.: Cases of Tic Douloureux Successfully Treated. London, Longmans, 1820.

41. Iannone, A., Baker, A. B., and Morrell, F.: Dilantin in the treatment of trigeminal neuralgia. Neurology (Minneap.), 8:126–128, 1958.

42. Jaeger, R.: Permanent relief of tic douloureux by gasserian injection of hot water. Arch. Neurol. Psychiat., 77:1–7, 1957.

43. Jannetta, P. J.: Trigeminal neuralgia and hemifacial spasm—etiology and definitive treatment. Trans. Amer. Neurol. Ass., 100:89–91, 1975.

44. Jannetta, P. J., and Rand. R. W.: Transtentorial retrogasserian rhizotomy in trigeminal neuralgia by microneurosurgical technique. Bull. Los Angeles Neurol. Soc., 31:93–99, 1966.

45. Keen, W., and Spiller, W. G.: Remarks on resection of the gasserian ganglion. Amer. J. Med. Sci., 116:503–532, 1898.

46. Kerr, F. W. L.: Etiology of trigeminal neuralgia. Arch. Neurol., 89:15–25, 1963.

47. King, R. B.: The medical control of tic douloureux: Preliminary report on the effect of mephenesin on facial pain. J. Neurosurg., 15:290–298, 1958.

48. King, R. B., and Barnett, J. C.: Studies of trigeminal nerve potentials. Overreaction to tactile facial stimulation in acute laboratory preparations. J. Neurosurg., 14:617–627, 1957.

49. King, R. B., and Meagher, J. N.: Studies of trigeminal nerve potentials. J. Neurosurg., 12:393–402, 1955.

50. King, R. B., Meagher, J. N., and Barnett, J. C.: Studies of trigeminal nerve potentials in normal compared to abnormal experimental preparations. J. Neurosurg., 13:176–183, 1956.

51. Krause, F.: Resection des Trigeminus Innerhalb der Schädelhole. Arch. Klin. Chir., 44:821–832, 1892.

52. Kruger, L., ed.: Structural aspects of trigeminal neuralgia: A summary of current findings and concepts. J. Neurosurg., 26:109–190, 1967.

53. Kugelberg, E., and Lindblom, U.: The mechanism of pain in trigeminal neuralgia. J. Neurol. Neurosurg. Psychiat., 22:36–43, 1959.

54. Lewy, F. H., and Grant, F. C.: Physiopathologic and pathoanatomic aspects of major trigeminal neuralgia. Arch. Neurol. Psychiat., 40:1126–1134, 1938.

55. Lewy, F. H., Groff, R. A., and Grant, F. C.: Autonomic innervation of the face. II. An experimental study. Arch. Neurol. Psychiat., 39:1238–1249, 1938.

56. List, C. F., and Williams, J. R.: Pathogenesis of trigeminal neuralgia. A review. Arch. Neurol. Psychiat., 77:36–43, 1957.

57. Locke, J.: Letters to Doctor Mapletoft: Letters IX and X, Paris, 4 December 1677. European Magazine, March, 185–186, 1789.

58. Marrazzi, A. S., and Lorente de No, R.: Interaction of neighboring fibres in myelinated nerve. J. Neurophysiol., 7:83–101, 1944.

59. Moore, D. C.: Regional Block. 4th Ed. Springfield, Ill., Charles C Thomas, 1967, pp. 71–111.

60. Morrell, F., Bradley, W., and Ptashne, M.: Effect of diphenylhydantoin on peripheral nerve. Neurology (Minneap.), 8:140–144, 1958.

61. Olivecrona, H.: Cholesteatomas of the cerebellopontine angle. Acta Psychiat. Neurol., 24:639–643, 1949.

62. Oppenheim, H.: Cited by Stookey, B., and Ransohoff, J., ref. 72.

63. Parker, H. L.: Trigeminal pain associated with multiple sclerosis. Brain, 51:46–61, 1928.

64. Parker, H. L.: Paroxysmal trigeminal pain with tumors of the nervus acusticus. J. Neurol. Psychopath., 17:256–261, 1937.

65. Peet, M. M.: Tic douloureux and its treatment with review of the cases operated upon at the University Hospital in 1917. J. Mich. Med. Soc., 17:91–99, 1918.

66. Peet, M. H., and Schneider, R. C.: Trigeminal neuralgia. A review of 689 cases with a follow-up study of 65 per cent of the group. J. Neurosurg., 9:367–377, 1952.

67. Plessner, W.: Uber Behandlungsversuche der Trigeminus Neuralgie mit Trichloräthylen. Mschr. Psychiat. Neurol., 44:374–386, 1918.

68. Poppen, J. L.: An Atlas of Neurosurgical Techniques. Philadelphia, W. B. Saunders Co., 1960, pp. 16–25.

69. Ruge, D., Brochner, R., and Davis, L.: A study of the treatment of 637 patients with trigeminal neuralgia. J. Neurosurg., 15:528–536, 1958.

70. Rushton, J. G., and Olafson, R. A.: Trigeminal neuralgia associated with multiple sclerosis, report of 35 cases. Arch. Neurol. 13:383–386, 1965.

71. Spiller, W. G., and Frazier, C. H.: The division of the sensory root of the trigeminus for relief of tic douloureux, an experimental, pathological and clinical study with a preliminary report of one surgically successful case. Philadelphia Med. J., 8:1039–1049, 1901.

72. Stookey, B. P., and Ransohoff, J.: Trigeminal Neuralgia: Its History and Treatment. Springfield, Ill., Charles C Thomas, 1959.

73. Taarnhøj, P.: Decompression of the trigeminal root and posterior part of ganglion as treatment in trigeminal neuralgia. Preliminary communication. J. Neurosurg., 9:288–290, 1952.

74. Tiffany, L. McL.: Intracranial neurectomy and removal of the gasserian ganglion. Ann. Surg., 19:47–57, 1894.

75. Tiffany, L. McL.: Intracranial operations for the cure of facial neuralgia. Trans. Amer. Surg. Ass., 14:1–52, 1896.

76. White, J. C., and Sweet, W. H.: Pain, Its Mechanism and Neurosurgical Control. Springfield, Ill., Charles C Thomas, 1955, p. 496.

77. Wilson, S. A. K.: Neurology. Baltimore, Williams & Wilkins Co., 1940, vol. 1, pp. 385–386.

120

TREATMENT OF TRIGEMINAL NEURALGIA BY PERCUTANEOUS RHIZOTOMY

Cephalea, a painful affliction of the face, resembling migraine and trigeminal neuralgia, was first described by Aretaeus in the first century A.D.[2] Since antiquity there have been references to the condition. Facial pain terrified man for centuries before Locke first recorded the medical description of the disorder, since known as trigeminal neuralgia. Locke, as reported by Dewhurst, described the condition as observed in the Countess of Northumberland in 1677. He commented on the etiology of this malady as follows:

If I durst interpose my opinion in a case so extraordinary as this, I should ask whether you did not think this to proceed from the same affections in the nerves in the place where the tooth was drawn, which draws all the rest into consent and convulsive motions on this side of the face.[8]

The recognition of trigeminal neuralgia as a definite clinical entity is credited to Nicolas André in 1756.[1] He recommended applying caustics to the exposed nerve over days until it was laid bare and destroyed. Seventeen years later, in 1773, Forthergill, unaware of André's account, presented a description of 14 cases that has not been surpassed in subsequent writings.[10] A totally satisfactory method of treating trigeminal neuralgia has never been described. Patients should not be subjected to inconsequential drug therapy, for example, vitamins and vasodilators, nor should they be submitted to procedures on the mouth, teeth, sinuses, or nerves at a distance (acu-puncture). The initial treatment for all cases of trigeminal neuralgia should be medical. Carbamazepine (Tegretol) is the drug most likely to succeed. Over 90 per cent of patients in the series on which this report is based achieved at least partial relief, and the dangerous side effects have been decidedly few. When failure occurs it is due in most circumstances to increasing severity of the pain or intolerable side effects as a consequence of toxic drug levels. Other anticonvulsants, diphenylhydantoin (Dilantin) and clonazepam (Clonopin), have been of considerably less value.

When an operative procedure is necessary, the simplest and least hazardous method should be chosen. Partial destruction of the sensory pathway to eliminate painful input has been the major goal of operative therapy. Injection of sclerosing agents such as alcohol or phenol, and peripheral section or avulsion of nerve trunks may provide short-term relief (three months to three years) and can be performed safely under most circumstances. These procedures, however, are rarely effective for recurrent pain or pain involving multiple divisions of the nerve. The goals of modern surgical therapy are long-term control, minimal neurological deficit, and negligible morbidity.

Jannetta has challenged the need for the destructive procedures and has cited the observations of Dandy and of Gardner that trigeminal neuralgia is caused in most instances by vascular compression at the

J. M. TEW, JR.

brain stem locale.[7,12,21] This hypothesis provides an attractive rationale for a method of treatment whose results are still being analyzed.

The concept of electrocoagulation of the gasserian ganglion for trigeminal neuralgia was proposed by Kirschner in 1932.[22] Except for placement of the needle under radiographic control, the technique of Kirschner employed none of the techniques of stereotaxy. The speed and simplicity of the method led to its widespread popularity in Europe. Unfortunately, many complications were reported.[4,17,40,43] Several deaths were attributed to carotid artery injury and meningitis. Although Thiry continued to use much the same crude technique as Kirschner, he was able virtually to eliminate the serious complications by reducing the intensity of the electrocautery.[39] Shürman and Butz accomplished further improvement in the results by controlled partial coagulation under neuroleptic analgesia.[29] Sweet advanced the hypothesis that the differential sensitivity of pain-conducting fibers of the trigeminal nerve to heat could be exploited to achieve lasting pain control.[33] Experimental studies by Letcher and Goldring and by Frigyesi and co-workers have confirmed Sweet's premise.[11,23] Blockade of conduction in A delta and C fibers by a temperature level less than that required to abolish transmission in A fibers accounts for the clinically observed preservation of touch perception with superimposed analgesia (Fig. 120–1).

The success of the percutaneous radio-frequency technique in operating on the trigeminal nerve is due to the application of neuroanatomical and neurophysiological principles. A number of changes have been made in technique, and the following points have proved to be of value.

1. *Short-term anesthesia.* Reversible anesthesia is induced by the ultra–short acting barbiturate methohexital (Brevital) administered by intravenous injection.

2. *Radiographic localization.* Precise placement of the electrode tip in the midst of the posterior rootlets is made under radiological control (cineradiography) according to three-dimensional internal landmarks.

3. *Physiological localization.* Isolated electrical stimulation at 50 to 75 Hz with a 100- to 400-mv square-wave pulse of 1 msec duration evokes sensory responses that localize the electrode tip in the posterior rootlets. The provocation of ticlike paroxysms of pain further confirms the proper needle placement.

4. *Controlled lesion production with temperature monitoring.* The extent of the lesion is controlled by the volume of the uninsulated electrode tip, the duration of current, and the temperature level. The temperature monitor provides an additional degree of safety, which virtually eliminates uncontrollable spread of current or sudden unexpected overheating.

5. *Physiological testing.* Rapid reversibility of the anesthetic agent permits testing of cutaneous and oral perception of pain and touch in an alert, cooperative patient.

Figure 120–1 Postoperative sensory chart of a patient with neuralgia involving the maxillary and mandibular divisions. Analgesia to painful stimulation is present in the maxillary zone and hypalgia in the mandibular zone. Touch perception was normal (200 to 300 mg) in each area of the face and mouth.

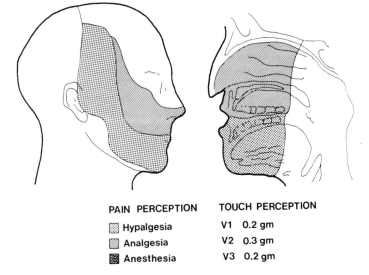

PAIN PERCEPTION

▨ Hypalgesia
▧ Analgesia
▨ Anesthesia

TOUCH PERCEPTION

V1 0.2 gm
V2 0.3 gm
V3 0.2 gm

Electrocoagulation can be applied repetitively until the desired result is achieved.

TECHNIQUE OF PERCUTANEOUS TRIGEMINAL RHIZOTOMY

Selection and Preparation of Patients

All patients with intractable trigeminal neuralgia who have failed to achieve long-standing control with medical therapy are candidates for percutaneous rhizotomy. If a person is less than 50 years of age or has any indication of pain of an atypical nature, additional diagnostic studies should be performed; these include tomography of the temporal bone, computed tomography, and selective angiography of vertebral and carotid systems.

Patients should be carefully screened by history and physical examination. Both the patient and family should read and listen to an explanation of the operative procedures available for the control of trigeminal neuralgia. The risks and expected results should be explained. Often, it is wise to have the patients discuss the procedure with others who have undergone major trigeminal procedures. This reinforces the patient's understanding and appreciation of the possibility of undesirable sensory loss. If the patient expresses concern about sensory deficit, electrocoagulation should not be performed. Rather, a differential lidocaine block can be done to enable the patient to experience the effects of sensory deprivation. The latter procedure may also be helpful in deciding whether an atypical form of facial pain will respond to partial root destruction.

Patients under 50 years of age should be encouraged to undergo posterior fossa exploration if they do not wish to be subjected to a facial sensory deficit or if their pain is of an atypical nature that suggests the possibility of tumor, vascular anomaly, or other kinds of compression of the trigeminal root. All of the author's patients with trigeminal neuralgia are exposed to a discussion of the various forms of medical and surgical therapy. Eight patients have elected to undergo primary posterior fossa exploration during the same period that five hundred have undergone a percutaneous procedure. Obviously, many patients come to the author's clinic with a pre-existing bias for a percutaneous procedure, but whenever appropriate, they have been urged to consider a direct exploration and operative decompression.

The patient must be informed about disagreeable side effects such as facial dysesthesia. Careful instruction of the patient leads to better acceptance of side effects and greatly reduces the incidence of disappointing postoperative results. The informed patient should assist in making the decision regarding the mode of treatment. If the patient elects a destructive procedure such as electrocoagulation, he should be encouraged to indicate the degree of sensory deficit he believes he can tolerate. Partial sensory loss is associated with a higher incidence of recurrence, though patients are usually not reluctant to undergo repeated percutaneous rhizotomy should it prove to be necessary.

Needle Placement

The procedure should be done in the radiography suite (Fig. 120–2). The patient is anesthetized with an intravenous injection of 30 to 50 mg of methohexital (Brevital). A hollow 19-gauge needle with a terminus bare for 5, 7.5, or 10 mm is selected. In general a 5-mm electrode is selected for single division neuralgia, a 7.5-mm one for two divisions, and a 10-mm one for selected cases requiring total destruction of the posterior rootlets. The electrode is placed stereotaxically by freehand manipulation, although a guiding apparatus may be used.[37] Three landmarks are placed on the skin of the face (Fig. 120–3A). The anterior approach to the foramen ovale, as advocated by Härtel is utilized (Fig. 120–3B and C).[16] Cineradiographic control in the lateral plane is used and the needle electrode is aimed toward the intersection of planes extending from two external landmarks: (1) a point 3 cm anterior to the external auditory meatus, and (2) a point corresponding to the medial aspect of the pupil. The needle is directed toward a point as viewed on the lateral plane radiographic image 5 to 10 mm below the floor of the sella turcica along a line corresponding to the profile of the clivus (Fig. 120–4). Entrance of the needle into the foramen ovale is signaled by a wince and a

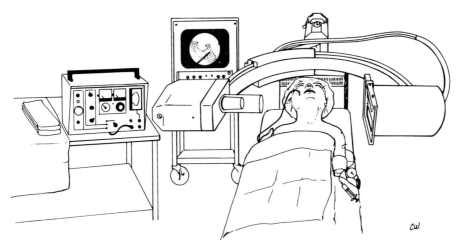

Figure 120–2 The procedure is accomplished under image intensification. A lateral view of the final needle placement is projected on the television monitor.

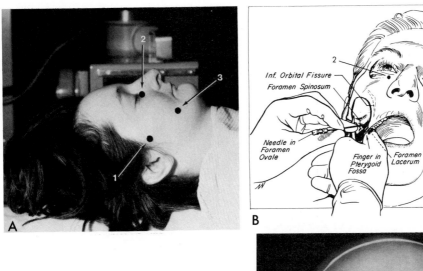

A

B

Inf. Orbital Fissure
Foramen Spinosum

Needle in
Foramen
Ovale

Finger in
Pterygoid
Fossa

Foramen
Lacerum

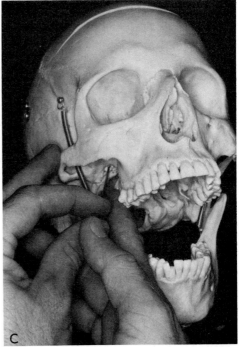

C

Figure 120–3 *A.* External landmarks for electrode placement: (1) 3 cm anterior to the external auditory meatus; (2) the medial aspect of the pupil; and (3) the site of needle penetration 2.5 to 3 cm lateral to the oral commissure. *B.* Needle placement according to the technique of Härtel. *C.* Freehand placement of the needle electrode. The guiding finger of the right hand touches the lateral wing of the pterygoid bone.

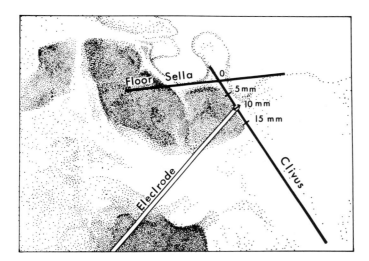

Figure 120–4 The needle trajectory is monitored on the image intensifier by aiming for a point 5 to 10 mm below the floor of the sella turcica.

brief contraction of the masseter muscle, indicating contact with the mandibular sensory and motor fibers. The stylet is withdrawn to elicit a flow of cerebrospinal fluid and to exclude penetration of the carotid artery. The needle is then advanced until the tip reaches the vicinity of the clival line (Fig. 120–5).

The results of anatomical studies have been confirmed by physiological stimulation and clinical observation. These findings have greatly increased the safety and ease with which this procedure can be performed.[38] The more important of these observations are as follows.

Definition of Internal Landmarks

The relationship of the trigeminal rootlets to the profile of the clivus and the distance from the foramen ovale to the retrogasserian fibers are such that the rootlets of the third, second, and first divisions can be successively stimulated, with consistent relia-

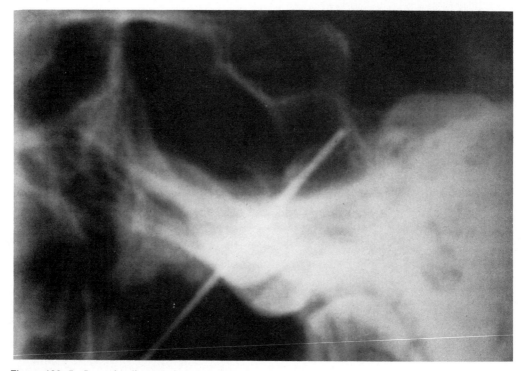

Figure 120–5   Lateral radiograph demonstrating proper placement of the electrode for a maxillary root lesion.

bility by using a small electrode tip (5 mm) and advancing the electrode in calibrated steps (Fig. 120–6A and B). The maxillary rootlets can be most reliably isolated with the tip of the electrode projected at the clival line. Cisternal fluid can be aspirated in nearly all circumstances except when operative exploration or alcohol injection has been conducted. The relationship of the rootlets to the clival line is important, since cisternal injection studies have indicated that the pia-arachnoid membrane may be reflected off the peripheral nerve (Fig. 120–6C). Therefore, aspiration of cerebrospinal fluid does not invariably indicate that the needle tip has reached the retrogasserian fibers.

Definition of Neurovascular Relations

The relationship of the carotid artery to the mandibular nerve, trigeminal ganglion, and retrogasserian fibers is demonstrated in Figure 120–7. The carotid artery is vulnerable to injury at three sites: first, at the foramen lacerum, where posteromedial deviation of the needle may penetrate the cartilaginous covering of the foramen lacerum. Second, immediately upon entrance into the cranial cavity (middle fossa), the carotid artery lies directly behind the mandibular nerve. The carotid canal is devoid of bony covering in 85 per cent of cases studied anatomically.[15] An inferior and medial deviation of the penetrating electrode may therefore pierce the nerve and the carotid artery at the same site. Such an occurrence probably took place in the case reported by Rish.[28] Third, the artery may be penetrated within the cavernous sinus if the electrode is directed too far cephalad along the clival line. Carotid cavernous fistula development has been reported.[42] Attention to the trajectory of the electrode has virtually eliminated vascular complications.

Relationship of Cranial Nerves III, IV, and VI to Trigeminal Rootlets

Penetration of the foramen ovale by the proper trajectory and avoidance of excessive penetration (5 mm beyond the profile of the clivus) have eliminated ocular nerve complications in the last 200 patients of the author's series. The abducens, the most frequently injured nerve, can be avoided if the electrode trajectory is maintained between the 5- and 10-mm planes and the electrode does not penetrate more than 5 mm deep beyond the clival line. Oculomotor and trochlear palsies rarely occur unless the needle penetrates the cavernous sinus (Fig. 120–8).

Lesion Localization

Final placement of the electrode tip is determined by the response to electrical stimulation. An isolated square-wave pulse of 1 msec duration, 100 to 400 mv, and 5 to 75 Hz is used to localize the tip of the electrode. Reproduction of a characteristic burst of ticlike pain provoked by the low-voltage stimulation is the best evidence for appropriate localization of the electrode tip. Paresthesias in the distribution of the involved nerve or trigger zone should occur at a still lower current level. Stimulation should be performed immediately on entering the foramen ovale and prior to advancing the electrode to a deeper level. The needle should be advanced in 5-mm increments until the appropriate stimulation effect is achieved or the needle tip reaches a point 5 mm deep to the profile of the clivus (Fig. 120–9). If the trajectory of the electrode is directed too caudad, only mandibular stimulation will be obtained; whereas if the trajectory is too much toward the cephalad, or superior, aspect of the clival line, only ophthalmic stimulation may be noted (cf. Figs. 120–5 and 120–8). In the former position, the needle may puncture the carotid artery in a site deep and medial to the ganglion. In the latter trajectory, the cavernous sinus may be penetrated, with resultant hemorrhage or neurovascular injury if a lesion is produced (Fig. 120–10). It should be emphasized that these two extremes of needle placement are to be avoided. When the needle has been so placed, it must be withdrawn and repositioned, and the stimulation trials must be repeated.

Observation of cerebrospinal fluid flow gives a helpful clue to appropriate localization of the electrode. There are, however, many other foramina at the base of the skull that permit access to the subarachnoid space, and should there be any concern, a basal view x-ray should be obained (Fig. 120–11). Furthermore, failure to obtain a flow of cerebrospinal fluid does not preclude the production of a satisfactory retro-

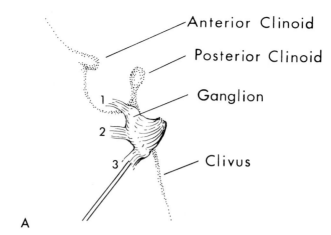

Anterior Clinoid

Posterior Clinoid

Ganglion

Clivus

A

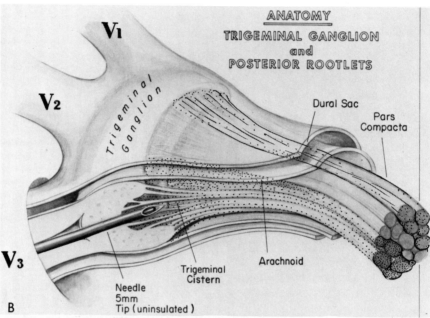

V₁

V₂

V₃

ANATOMY
TRIGEMINAL GANGLION
and
POSTERIOR ROOTLETS

Trigeminal Ganglion

Dural Sac

Pars Compacta

Arachnoid

Trigeminal Cistern

Needle
5mm
Tip (uninsulated)

B

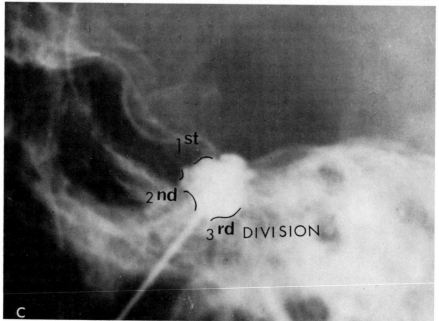

1st

2nd

3rd DIVISION

C

Figure 120-6 *See legend on opposite page*

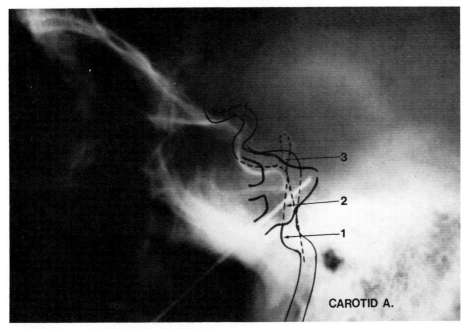

Figure 120–7 A lateral composite illustration of the electrode tip and its trajectory to the mandibular nerve (1), the carotid artery in Meckel's cave (2), and the cavernous carotid artery (3).

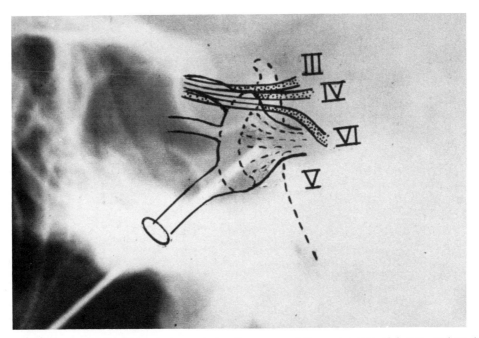

Figure 120–8 A lateral radiograph demonstrates the course of the oculomotor, abducens, and trochlear nerves and their relationship to the electrode trajectory. The electrode tip should not extend more than 5 mm deep to the clival line (*dashed line*).

Figure 120–6 *A*. Composite illustration of the relationship of the trigeminal rootlets to the profile of the clivus. *B*. The lamination of the trigeminal rootlets and the relationship of the trigeminal cistern to the ganglia. *C*. A contrast (Pantopaque) cisternogram of the trigeminal cistern demonstrating the reflection of the cerebrospinal fluid space at the peripheral nerve.

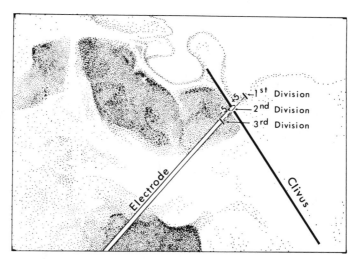

Figure 120–9   The relationship of the electrode tip to the clival line and the sites of stimulation of each trigeminal root segment.

gasserian lesion. In patients who have had previous intracranial procedures and sclerosing injections (even those limited to the peripheral nerve) the normal retrocisternal space may be obliterated by arachnoid scar.

If movement of the eye or the facial or masseter-pterygoid muscles occurs with stimulation testing, the position of the electrode may need to be changed. These phenomena seldom occur unless the electrode is in an aberrant position or the level of stimulation is too high. Frequently, a strong masseter contraction is a sign that the needle should be inclined more cephalad and laterally. Despite these precautions, partial muscle weakness is an inevitable side effect of the procedure in 15 to 20 per cent of patients.

Production of the Lesion

Sodium methohexital anesthesia is administered, and the first lesion is made at 60° centigrade for 60 seconds. A lesion of

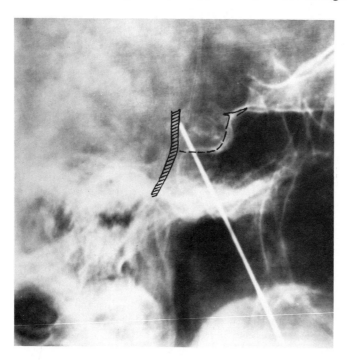

Figure 120–10 A lateral radiograph demonstrating the needle position in the posterior margin of the cavernous sinus where stimulation not only provoked ophthalmic paresthesia but eye movements indicating stimulation of the oculomotor and trochlear nerves were also observed.

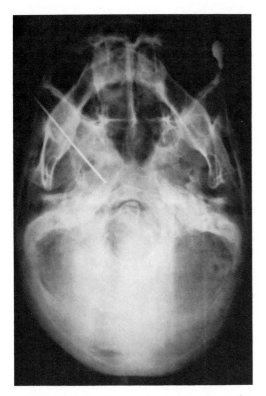

Figure 120–11 Basal radiograph confirms electrode placement in the foramen ovale.

higher temperature and longer duration may be chosen if stimulation has suggested that the arachnoid space and nerve are encased in scar, if a dense sensory lesion is desired, if the patient does not relish repeated coagulation of the nerve and a short operative time is required.

A facial blush usually appears during coagulation of the nerve and aids further in localizing the trigeminal zone. According to studies by Gonzalez and co-workers, this phenomenon is a result of stimulation of a vasodilator system emerging from the brain stem and passing to the facial vasculature with the trigeminal nerve.[13] While the observation of facial blush is not entirely reliable for localization, it is of considerable value in preventing unexpected spread of a lesion to an undesired trigeminal zone. On several occasions, the author has seen the forehead begin to flush, although the stimulation had not suggested that an ophthalmic lesion might result. In each case prompt retraction of the electrode averted unwanted denervation of the cornea.

The lesion can be tailored by carefully altering the electrode position, controlling the temperature, and monitoring the location and degree of sensory deficit. A curved electrode to provide alternatives for exploring the root anatomy and refining the lesion has been developed.

Intraoperative Testing

When the patient has awakened fully, careful sensory testing of his face is done. Repeated lesions are made until the desired effect is achieved. The goal of sensory impairment in trigeminal neuralgia (mandibular and maxillary divisions) is demonstrated in Figure 120–1. A less dense sensory loss may be advisable if the patient is concerned about the consequences of paresthesia. Most patients tolerate this type of sensory impairment well, however, and are gratified that the risk of recurrent tic pain is slight.

After a partial lesion has been produced, it may be extended without further anesthesic agent. Perception of pain is minimal, and the cooperation of a conscious patient is critical when partial preservation of nociceptive sensation of the cornea or other radicular zones is desired.

Once the desired sensory deficit has been achieved, the patient is observed for an additional 15 minutes to determine whether a fixed lesion has been produced. If the examination indicates a stable level of analgesia, careful sensory testing and plotting of the distribution and degree of deficit are performed. Observations concerning masseter, pterygoid, facial, and ocular muscle function are recorded. The patient is returned to his room and observed for 24 hours.

Prior to discharge, the patient and his family are informed by the medical and nursing staff of possible complications, the means of preventing them or detecting them if they should occur, and precautions and actions to be taken by the patient. These instructions are both verbal and written. They specify that if there is substantial loss of corneal sensation, the patient should place artificial tears on the cornea every four hours. If blurring of vision or injection of the cornea occurs, the patient should communicate with the surgeon, and the eye should be inspected. The diet should be restricted to soft foods for two weeks, and jaw opening exercises practiced for two additional weeks. Care should be exercised to avoid biting the lip, tongue, or buccal mucosa. Should maceration occur, irrigation of the mouth with warm saline solution every four hours is practiced. Abstinence from scratching or irritating the analgesic skin is stressed.

If patients have consumed large amounts of carbamazepine (Tegretol) they may display early signs of drug withdrawal and should be started on tranquilizing drugs prior to discharge from the hospital.

RESULTS

In eight years, the author has treated 500 patients with typical trigeminal neuralgia by percutaneous rhizotomy. A careful follow-up record has been maintained on all of them. The duration of follow-up extends from one to eight years for 400 patients in this group. The results in these 400 patients are reported for the incidence of recurrent pain and long-term results, while the entire group is analyzed for early results and occurrence of operative side effects.

The average age of the group was 63 years, and women made up 61 per cent of the patients. The painful condition had been present for eight years, during which time 91 per cent of the group had been treated with carbamazepine. All others had received some form of appropriate medical therapy. Neurectomy or injection (32 per cent) and rhizotomy (12 per cent) had been performed in an attempt to control the pain. The pain was localized on the right in 61 per cent and bilaterally in 5 per cent of patients (Table 120–1).

The results of treatment by the percutaneous rhizotomy were analyzed on the basis of short-term (less than one year) and

TABLE 120–1 ELECTROCOAGULATION TREATMENT OF 500 PATIENTS

	PER CENT
Average age 63 years	
Female	62
Side of pain	
Right	61
Left	39
Bilateral	5
Division of trigeminal nerve involved	
V1	2
V2	18
V3	18
V1, V2	15
V2, V3	40
V1, V2, V3	7

TABLE 120–2 FOLLOW-UP OF ELECTROCOAGULATION TREATMENT OF 500 PATIENTS

DURATION OF FOLLOW-UP (YEARS)	NUMBER OF CASES
9	3
8	5
7	25
6	44
5	74
4	89
3	101
2	88
1	46
<1	25

long-term (one to eight years) follow-up evaluation (Table 120–2).

The short-term evaluation demonstrated that 92 per cent of patients judged their result as excellent (no side effects) or good (minor side effects); 7 per cent had only fair results (major side effects or poor relief of pain; 1 per cent of patients had a failing result (no pain relief). The grading was performed by the patients. A major side effect is defined as a permanent disabling side effect such as facial palsy, diplopia, blindness, or paralysis (there was no such occurrence in this experience), or a side effect that was permanently disabling in the patient's opinion, such as painful dysesthesia, sensory deprivation, keratitis, or difficulty with mastication. Since nearly all side effects were subjective in nature, the author relied heavily on the patient's interpretation of the severity of his complaints. The deterioration of results in the long-term follow-up related in most instances to a worsening of sensory complaints rather than to recurrent trigeminal neuralgia. Of the patients followed for longer periods of time, the group with excellent or good results decreased to 85 per cent and the group with fair results increased to 14 per cent, a change largely attributable to recurrence of pain or apparent worsening of the side effects. Recurrent pain required that the operation be repeated in 12 per cent. In most circumstances a second operation resulted in satisfactory control of the pain.

SIDE EFFECTS

The undesirable side effects tabulated for all cases in the author's series are listed in

TABLE 120–3 SIDE EFFECTS OF PERCUTANEOUS RHIZOTOMY IN 500 CASES OF TRIGEMINAL NEURALGIA

SIDE EFFECTS	PER CENT
Masseter-pterygoid weakness	22
Sensory disturbance	26
Dysesthesia (major)	3
Painful analgesia-anesthesia (minor)	12
Sensory deprivation	
Major	3.5
Minor	7.5
Ocular complications	
Absence of corneal reflex	11
Transient blurred vision	6
Keratitis	4
Diplopia	3
Herpes simplex	3
Arteriovenous fistula	0.2
Carotid puncture	0.2
Meningitis	0.2

order of occurrence in Table 120–3. Complaints related to sensory side effects are the most consistent adverse effect of the procedure.

Sensory Disturbance

Some sensory deficit was created in all patients by the thermocoagulation lesion. The occurrence of disturbing side effects could not be entirely related to the degree of sensory deficit. All patients reported some paresthesias or were conscious of sensory deprivation. Most, however, reported that they readily adjusted to the sensory aberration and did not mention any complaint in subsequent questionnaires. Twenty-six per cent of the patients reported sensory deficits of major or minor degree at the time of the examination for this follow-up. The majority of sensory complaints were related to sensory deprivation (7.5 per cent) or painful paresthesias in the analgesic or anesthetic zone (12 per cent) and were minor in nature. Residual sensory complaints of a major nature persisted in 32 patients (6.5 per cent), 17 patients complained severely of sensory loss, but dysesthesia was an even more distressing disturbance in 15 individuals. Complaints of drooling, loss of taste, and loss of ability to localize food effectively related to diminution of sensory perception were seldom as objectionable as sensations of swelling, crawling, itching, burning, and other dysesthetic sensations.

Eight of the fifteen patients were so disabled that they were considered to be suffering from "anesthesia dolorosa." Most patients with similar histories as regards their neuralgia had minimal complaints related to their postoperative neurological disturbance. "Anesthesia dolorosa," a painful anesthesia, is characterized by the constant presence of burning, aching, crawling, itching, and boring sensations. The condition is usually present in an anesthesic zone, but surprisingly, three patients were never anesthetic in any trigeminal zone, a finding that suggests that the disorder is not confined to persons with anesthesia. The major part of the discomfort is retro-orbital, regardless of the site of the original pain. The full degree of the pain may not develop for months or longer after the lesion has been made.

This regrettable condition is most likely to occur in patients with sensory loss involving the ophthalmic and maxillary division. The deficit is always major, that is, either analgesia or anesthesia. The patients seldom have had a trial period of sensory deficit by neurectomy or injection prior to the creation of the provoking lesion. The author has observed that these patients may have a premorbid personality that tolerates aggressive treatment poorly. They have few interests, have had other long-term problems, and promptly forget the painful condition for which the lesion was created, focusing their attention on the newest disorder.[3,9] The latest woe in life is the worst! Five of the author's patients were elderly women who became reclusive as their symptoms became more and more disagreeable. Excoriations of the face developed about the nostrils and scalp in four of these five patients. Uncontrollable scratching and maceration of the skin was suspected as the reason.

There is no uniformly effective treatment for anesthesia dolorosa. All types of tranquilizing drugs, analgesics, sedatives and antidepressants have been tried with little effect.[3,35] Psychotherapy may be helpful when combined with drug therapy. Various forms of operative treatment have been suggested, but the results have been rather disappointing. Cutting the remainder of the roots, cervical sympathectomy, bulbar tractotomy, vascular decompression of the posterior roots, frontal leucotomy, and thalamic electrical stimulation have been recommended with varying success.* In the author's opinion, the results of all these procedures are poor when applied to true anesthesia dolorosa. All of them have been discarded except deep electrical stimulation, which is an innovative procedure that is under evaluation.

Ocular Complications

Eye complications occurred in 7 per cent of the patients in the author's series. Four per cent developed neurolytic keratitis. Thirty per cent of this group had preservation of corneal touch perception, suggesting that the loss of pain sensation is the major factor predisposing to corneal ulceration. The corneal lesion was reversible in each of these patients in response to early ophthalmological care. Meticulous eye care is required; the use of a soft contact lens and occasional tarsorrhaphy have been successful in preventing permanent visual loss. Intermittent blurring of vision was a complaint in 29 patients (6 per cent) even though corneal touch perception was preserved in a high percentage of them. The corneal reflex, however, was markedly reduced, and corneal pain perception was absent in over 90 per cent of this group. This finding suggests that nociception is critical in the prevention of minor corneal injuries. Conversely, experience indicates that persons with residual sensory perception of the cornea adjust more rapidly to the deficit and rarely develop ulceration. Patients with anesthesia of the cornea rarely develop keratitis in the late postoperative period. Meticulous instruction concerning all features of eye care is mandatory for the patient and the family. Careful adherence to this policy has prevented the serious eye complications sometimes seen following this procedure. One hundred and nineteen patients in the group had neuralgia involving or limited to the ophthalmic division. Of these patients, 22 per cent achieved pain relief without losing corneal sensation, and only 6 per cent developed neurolytic keratitis.

---

* See references: Cutting remainder of roots, 26; cervical sympathectomy, 25; bulbar tractotomy, 31; vascular decompression, 19; frontal leucotomy, 41; electrical stimulation, 18.

Transient diplopia occurred in 13 patients (2.6 per cent); the condition was caused by temporary abducens palsy in most instances. The diplopia was self-limiting and seldom persisted longer than two months. This complication developed more readily in patients undergoing coagulation of the ophthalmic division. Abducens palsy may be produced if the thermal lesion is created with the tip of the electrode extending more than 10 mm past the profile of the clivus as observed on the lateral radiograph of the skull (see Fig. 120–9). Trochlear and oculomotor palsy may occur if the electrode trajectory brings the tip too cephalad, where the cavernous sinus may be encountered (see Fig. 120–10).

The incidence of loss of corneal sensation and paresis of ocular nerves has been greatly reduced in recent years by performing electrocoagulation with the patient alert and cooperating during the final stages of the production of the lesion. In addition, understanding of the anatomical relationship of the cranial nerves to the trigeminal rootlets and the radiographic landmarks is of extreme importance in diminishing undesirable eye complications.

Motor Paresis

Paresis of the muscles innervated by the motor root of the trigeminal nerve occurred in 22 per cent of the author's patients. In most instances the deficit was partial and transient.

Weakness of the masseter, temporalis, and pterygoid muscles causes a mild degree of disability due to jaw deviation and loss of chewing power. Trismus was a more troublesome problem but could be avoided or diminished by avoidance of strain to the muscles postoperatively and the use of jaw exercises.

Difficulty in hearing, with tinnitus, inconstant roaring, and popping sounds, was reported by a few patients. These symptoms are attributable to paresis of the small muscles about the eustachain tube (tensor veli palatini) and tympanic membrane (tensor tympani). Difficulty with mastication was reported by several patients who had no motor paresis. They related their difficulty to loss of sensation in the mouth.

Herpes Simplex

The lesions of herpes simplex were noted in 3 per cent of patients. Since many patients were not examined more than 48 hours postoperatively, this figure is probably unduly low.

RECURRENCE OF TRIGEMINAL PAIN

During the follow-up period, which covered eight years, 15 per cent of the author's patients had pain of sufficient severity to require reoperation or resumption of drug therapy. Forty-nine (10 per cent) underwent repeat electrocoagulation, ten (2 per cent) were treated by posterior rhizotomy performed through a suboccipital approach. This latter group of patients was unique in that either they had unusually intractable pain that could not be controlled by the percutaneous approach or a direct approach was made to investigate the possibility of a causative lesion.

Recurrence of pain following percutaneous rhizotomy of the trigeminal nerve occurred more frequently during the early years following the procedure. Recurrence of pain was seen during the first year in nearly half the patients. In most of these persons lesions of minimal nature were made to limit the degree of sensory deficit. It was determined that the recurrence rate was high in patients with minimal sensory deficit, a finding also recorded with other procedures. Subsequently, patients have been advised to have lesions inducing analgesia in zones that were painful and hypalgesia in adjacent areas. The result has been a significant reduction in recurrence of pain, but as was to be expected, more patients have complained of troublesome numbness.

The lesion should be developed, as nearly as possible, to suit the patient. A temporary period of relief associated with mild sensory deprivation may provide a trial period for the apprehensive patient who is concerned about tolerating the effects. When recurrence of pain occurs, a more analgesic lesion frequently is requested. Occasionally the patient may request a reduplication of the previous procedure, noting that the two or three years of relief was appreciated and an increase of numbness could not be toler-ated. Most patients do not express concern about repeating the procedure when it is necessary to control recurrence of tic pain.

COMPARISON OF PERCUTANEOUS RHIZOTOMY WITH OTHER MAJOR OPERATIVE PROCEDURES

Comparisons of percutaneous rhizotomy with other major operative procedures are based mainly on the complications and the incidence of recurrent pain. Percutaneous rhizotomy has not been performed for as long as intracranial rhizotomy; therefore the recurrence figures may not be entirely comparable. The figures for mortality and morbidity rates are, however, significant (Table 120–4).

The percutaneous approach has the fewest deaths and a lower incidence of morbidity. The recurrence rate compares favorably with intracranial rhizotomy if analogous portions of the root are destroyed in both operations. Facial palsy has been eliminated by percutaneous rhizotomy, but ocular palsy occurs with a frequency equal to that of other major operative procedures. The incidence of troublesome numbness ranks with that of other forms of posterior rhizotomy. This major side effect should, however, be eliminated by the decompression procedures. Temporal decompression is associated with a prohibitive recurrence rate, but vascular decompression as described by Jannetta appears to provide an attractive alternative to percutaneous rhizotomy, particularly in the young patient.[20] As more experience accumulates with this method, the incidence of successful pain relief and freedom from recurrence can be better defined. The author bases the following observation on experience gained during examination and exploration of the trigeminal root through a retromastoid approach in 18 patients with primary or recurrent trigeminal neuralgia: (1) vessels touching or distorting the trigeminal root near the brain stem is an inconstant finding. (2) Angiography is of little value in predicting the relationship of the vessels to the nerve and discerning the site of deranged anatomy. (3) Decompression or separation of the vascular structures from the nerve is associated with a high de-

TABLE 120-4   ANALYSIS OF COMPARATIVE TECHNIQUES IN 2446 CASES OF TRIGEMINAL NEURALGIA

TECHNIQUE	RECURRENCE OF PAIN (PER CENT)	POSTOPERATIVE FOLLOW-UP YEARS (AVERAGE)	RELIEF OF PAIN (PER CENT)	MORTALITY RATE (PER CENT)	SIDE EFFECTS (PER CENT)						
					ATAXIA	CORNEAL ULCER	FACIAL PALSY	OCULAR PALSY	MASSETER PALSY	PARESTHESIA	ANESTHESIA DOLOROSA
Percutaneous rhizotomy											
Tew (500 cases)	15	4	99	0	0	4	0	2.5	22	26	2
Sweet and Wepsic (274 cases)*	22	4	91	0	0	+[b]	0	0	43	2	1
Menzel et al. (315 cases)†	80	12	97	0	0	0	0	—[a]	50	93	2
Siegfried (416 cases)‡	5	2	96	0	0	2	0	2	30	4	
Decompression											
Svien and Love (100 cases)§	84	4	24	1	0	0	—[a]	0	0	0	0
Transtemporal rhizotomy											
Peet and Schneider (553 cases)‖	14	8	95	1.6	—[a]	15	6[a]	—[a]	—[a]	55	4
Posterior fossa rhizotomy											
Dandy (88 cases)¶	—[a]	2	100	2		0	1	2	0	0	0
Vascular decompression											
Jannetta (200 cases)**	4.5	4	98	0.5	2	0	0	1	0	0	0

[a] Not reported.
[b] One patient blind.

* Controlled thermocoagulation of trigeminal ganglion and results for differential destruction of pain fibers. Part I. Trigeminal neuralgia. J. Neurosurg., 40:143–156, 1974.
† Long-term results of gasserian ganglion electrocoagulation. J. Neurosurg., 42:140–143, 1975.
‡ 500 percutaneous thermocoagulations of the gasserian ganglion for trigeminal pain. Surg. Neurol., 8:126–131, 1977.
§ Results of decompression operation for trigeminal neuralgia four years plus after operation. J. Neurosurg., 16:653–663, 1959.
‖ Trigeminal neuralgia. J. Neurosurg., 9:367–377, 1952.
¶ An operation for the cure of tic douloureux: Partial section of the sensory root at the pons. Arch. Surg. (Chicago), 18:687–734, 1929.
** Microsurgical approach to the trigeminal nerve for tic douloureux. Progr. Neurol. Surg., 7:180–200, 1976.

gree of mild facial sensory deficit. (4) In the absence of facial sensory deficit or subsequent to the return of normal sensation, a remarkable occurrence of recurrent pain was observed. (5) Unless a definite compressive lesion is found, partial section of the root should be performed.

CONCLUSIONS

Percutaneous rhizotomy of the trigeminal nerve is a procedure capable of producing long-lasting relief from trigeminal neuralgia and has a quite low incidence of complications. Extratrigeminal complications are rare and reversible in most instances. The incidence of recurrent pain is no greater than with intracranial partial section of the posterior rootlets, but the lesser morbidity associated with a percutaneous procedure makes it a more attractive alternative for most patients. The occurrence of postoperative sensory disturbances is similar to that associated with intracranial rhizotomy. This disturbing side effect can be nearly eliminated by meticulous attention to patient selection and by the creation of a minimal sensory deficit in patients who express fear of sensory aberrations. The reliability and control inherent in the stereotaxic approach makes the percutaneous operation preferable to all other major destructive procedures.

Percutaneous trigeminal rhizotomy is, however, a destructive procedure. It is not considered the ideal treatment of facial pain. A continued search for more acceptable nondestructive therapy is necessary.

REFERENCES

1. André, N.: Cited in Stookey, B., and Ransohoff, J.: Trigeminal Neuralgia: Its History and Treat-

ment. Springfield, Ill., Charles C Thomas, 1964, pp. 13–23.

2. Aretaeus, the Cappadocian. Edited and translated by Francis Adams, London, Sydenham Society, 1956.

3. Aring, C. D.: Personal communication, 1978.

4. Bauer, K. H.: Die elektrokoagulation des Ganglion Gasseri. Chirug., 16:1–5, 1944.

5. Dalessio, D. J.: Chronic pain syndromes and disordered cortical inhibition: Effects of tricyclic compounds. Dis. Nerv. Syst., 28:325–328, 1967.

6. Dandy, W. E.: An operation for the cure of tic douloureux: Partial section of the sensory root at the pons. Arch. Surg. (Chicago), 18:687–734, 1929.

7. Dandy, W. E.: Concerning the cause of trigeminal neuralgia. Amer. J. Surg., 24:447–455, 1934.

8. Dewhurst, K.: A symposium on trigeminal neuralgia. J. Hist. Med., 12:21–36, 1957.

9. Engle, G. L.: "Psychogenic" pain and the pain prone patient. Amer. J. Med., 26:899–918, 1959.

10. Fothergill, J.: Of a painful affection of the face. Medical Observations and Inquiries, London, 5:129–142, 1776.

11. Frigyesi, T., Siegfried, J., and Brozzi, G.: The selective vulnerability of evoked potentials in the trigeminal sensory root to graded thermocoagulation. Exp. Neurol., 49:11–21, 1975.

12. Gardner, W. J.: Concerning the mechanisms of trigeminal neuralgia and hemifacial spasm. J. Neurosurg., 19:947–958, 1962.

13. Gonzalez, G., Onofrio, B., and Kerr, F.: Vasodilator system for the face. J. Neurosurg., 42:696–703, 1975.

14. Goodman, L. S., and Gilman, A., eds.: The Pharmacological Basis of Therapeutics. Macmillan, 5th Ed., New York, 1975, pp. 152–200.

15. Harris, F. S., and Rhoton, A. L.: Anatomy of the cavernous sinus: A microsurgical study. J. Neurosurg., 45:169–180, 1976.

16. Härtel, F.: Ueber die intracranielle Injektionsbehandlung der Trigeminusneuralgie. Med. Klin., 10:582–584, 1914.

17. Hensell, V.: Ist die Elektrokoagulation des Ganglion Gasseri auch heute noch kerechtigt? Chirurg., 28:544–548, 1957.

18. Hosobuchi, Y., Adams, J. E., and Rothkin, B.: Chronic thalamic stimulation for the control of facial anesthesia dolorosa. Arch. Neurol. (Chicago), 29:158–161, 1973.

19. Jannetta, P.: Personal communication, 1977.

20. Jannetta, P.: Microsurgical approach to the trigeminal nerve for tic douloureux. Progr. Neurol. Surg., 7:180–200, 1976.

21. Jannetta, P.: Treatment of trigeminal neuralgia by suboccipital and transtentorial cranial operations. Clin. Neurosurg., 24:538–549, 1976.

22. Kirschner, M.: Electrocoagulation des Ganglion gasseri. Zbl. Chir., 47:2841–2843, 1932.

23. Letcher, F. S., and Goldring, S.: The effect of radiofrequency current and heat on peripheral nerve action potential in the cat. J. Neurosurg., 29:42–47, 1968.

24. Menzel, J., Piotroswki, W., and Penholz, H.: Long-term results of gasserian ganglion electrocoagulation. J. Neurosurg., 42:140–143, 1975.

25. Olivecrona, H.: The syndrome of painful anesthesia following section of the sensory root of the fifth nerve in tic douloureux. Acta Chir. Scand., 82:99–106, 1939.

26. Olivecrona, H.: Trigeminal neuralgia. Triangle, 5:60–69, 1961.

27. Peet, M. M., and Schneider, R. C.: Trigeminal neuralgia. J. Neurosurg., 9:367–377, 1952.

28. Rish, B. L.: Cerebrovascular accident after percutaneous rf thermocoagulation of the trigeminal ganglion. J. Neurosurg., 44:376–377, 1976.

29. Shürman, M., and Butz, M.: Temporal retrogasserian resection of trigeminal root versus controlled elective percutaneous electrocoagulation of the ganglion of Gasser in the treatment of trigeminal neuralgia. Report on a series of 531 cases. Acta Neurochir. (Wien), 26:33–35, 1972.

30. Siegfried, J.: 500 percutaneous thermocoagulations of the gasserian ganglion for trigeminal pain. Surg. Neurol., 8:126–131, 1977.

31. Sjöqvist, O.: Ten year's experience with trigeminal tractotomy. Brasil Med. Cir., 10:259–274, 1948.

32. Svien, H. S., and Love, J. G.: Results of decompression operation for trigeminal neuralgia four years plus after operation. J. Neurosurg., 16:653–663, 1959.

33. Sweet, W. H.: Controlled thermocoagulation of trigeminal rootlets in man. In Morley, T. P., ed.: Current Controversies in Neurosurgery. Philadelphia, W. B. Saunders Co., 1976.

34. Sweet, W. H., and Wepsic, S. G.: Controlled thermocoagulation of trigeminal ganglion and results for differential destruction of pain fibers. Part I. Trigeminal neuralgia. J. Neurosurg., 39:143–156, 1974.

35. Szasz, S.: The nature of pain. Arch. Neurol. (Chicago), 74:174–181, 1955.

36. Taub, A.: Relief of postherpetic neuralgia with psychotropic drugs. J. Neurosurg., 39:235–239, 1973.

37. Tew, J. M., Keller, J. T., and Williams, D. S.: Application of stereotaxic principles to the treatment of trigeminal neuralgia. J. Appl. Neurophysiol., 41:146–156, 1978.

38. Tew, J. M., Keller, J. T., and Williams, D. S.: Functional surgery of the trigeminal nerve: Treatment of trigeminal neuralgia. In Rasmussen, T. B., and Marino, R.: Raven Press, Functional Neurosurgery. New York, 1979, pp. 129–141.

39. Thiry, M. S.: Expérience personnelle basée sur 225 cas de neuralgie essentielle du trijumean traités par électrocoagulation stéréotaxique du ganglion de Gasser entre 1950 et 1960. Neurochirurgie, 8:86–92, 1962.

40. Tonnis, W., and Kreissel, H.: Die Bedeutung einer sog. faltigen Differentialdiagnose für die chirurgische Behandlung der Trigeminusneuralgie. Deutsch. Med. Wschr., 12:1202–1205, 1951.

41. White, J. C., and Sweet, W. H.: Pain and the Neurosurgeon, a 40 Year Experience. Springfield, Ill., Charles C Thomas, 1969, pp. 218–219.

42. Williams, P.: Personal communication.

43. Zenker, R.: Die Behandlung der Trigeminusneuralgie unter besonderer Berücksichtigung der Grundlagen, der Ausführung und der Ergebnisse der Punktion und Elektrokoagulation des Ganglion Gasseri nach Kirschner. Ergebn. Chir. Orthop., 31:1–82, 1939.

121

TREATMENT OF TRIGEMINAL NEURALGIA THROUGH TEMPORAL CRANIOTOMY

EXTRADURAL SENSORY ROOT SECTION

Temporal extradural trigeminal root section as developed by Frazier is the classic operation for trigeminal neuralgia. Usually, the motor root can be spared. The cosmetic implications of temporal and masseter muscle atrophy and the intolerable sequelae of bilateral motor paralysis should pain occur on the opposite side make it important to spare the motor root. If sensory root section is done close to the gasserian ganglion, the first division usually can be identified and preserved, thus leaving corneal sensation intact.

Operative Technique

The procedure discussed here follows the technique described by Peet and Echols and amplified by Kahn.[3,6]

General anesthesia is preferable, although some, considering the risk in old and debilitated patients, prefer using local infiltration. The patient is placed in the sitting position. Elevating and wrapping the legs with Ace bandages combats sudden drops in blood pressure and, it is hoped, decreases the chance of air embolism. Pressure suits are preferable. The legs are slightly flexed to prevent the sequelae of prolonged stretching of the sciatic nerve.

The position of the head is important, since minor variations may distort landmarks to such an extent that even the skilled operator becomes lost (Fig. 121–1). The head should be straight in the lateral plane or tilted slightly away from the operator.[8] Its position in the anteroposterior plane is such that the zygoma is parallel to the floor or tilted slightly so that its anterior end extends slightly above the horizontal plane.

A vertical incision approximately 8 cm in length is made 2 cm in front of the external auditory meatus, extending superiorly from the lower border of the zygoma (Fig. 121–2). Carrying the incision below this point endangers the upper branches of the facial nerve. The temporal muscle is split to a point below the zygoma. A burr hole is made in the temporal bone and enlarged to about 4 cm in diameter. It must extend well forward and to the floor of the temporal fossa.

To facilitate elevation of the temporal lobe, the dura is separated along the entire perimeter of the bony defect for a distance of about 1 cm. Careful dissection at this point will avoid splitting the dura and leaving its outer layer adherent to the floor of the temporal fossa, a real hazard in the elderly. Should this occur, one can only retreat and start the extradural dissection over again. By gradually elevating the temporal lobe, the extradural dissection is extended medially and slightly anteriorly to the foramen spinosum. If the middle meningeal artery is torn prior to its exposure at the foramen spinosum, the bleeding point should be exposed immediately and coagulated. As one proceeds medially in the ex-

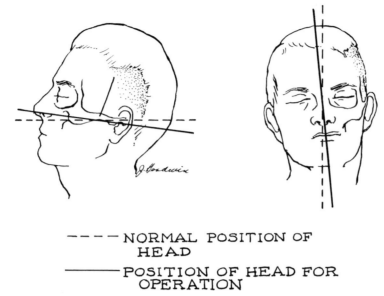

– – – – NORMAL POSITION OF
HEAD

———— POSITION OF HEAD FOR
OPERATION

Figure 121–1   Correct position of the head for optimal exposure of gasserian ganglion and sensory root in the extradural approach to sensory root section. The zygoma should be tilted slightly so its anterior end extends slightly above the horizontal plane. The head can be tilted slightly away from the operator.

tradural dissection, venous oozing will be encountered from tributaries to the inferior petrosal sinus posteriorly and to the cavernous sinus medially. This can be controlled by packing with small pledgets of Gelfoam.

Pitfalls at this stage of the procedure are dissecting too far posteriorly or anteriorly. A posterior dissection can go over the petrous bone into the posterior fossa. Less hazardous but very confusing is dissecting anteriorly and encountering the second division of the fifth nerve at the foramen rotundum instead of the middle meningeal artery at the foramen spinosum.

The foramen spinosum is plugged with cotton, and the middle meningeal artery coagulated or clipped and cut. The third division at its foramen ovale will be found 2 to 3 mm anterior and slightly medial to the foramen spinosum. One must proceed anteriorly at this point to avoid getting lost beneath the gasserian ganglion. With identification of the third division begins the most critical phase of the operation—separating the dura from the dura propria of the gasserian ganglion. Injecting the third division with Ringer's solution may be helpful. Blunt dissection is begun at the foramen ovale and extended superiorly to expose the third and second divisions (Fig. 121–3). The first division should not be exposed. One then continues superiorly and pos-

teriorly to expose the gasserian ganglion and sensory root. The temporal dura and dura propria are densely adherent at two points: the posterior border of the gasserian ganglion near the exit of the third division, and 10 to 15 mm further posterior on the floor of the middle fossa. Sharp dissection should be used at these points to avoid traction on the underlying greater superficial petrosal nerve. Traction may destroy the greater superficial petrosal nerve, producing a dry nasal mucous membrane, or may be transmitted to the facial nerve, causing paralysis of the face. The sensory root is bathed in cerebrospinal fluid, which imparts a blueness to the overlying dura propria. Continuing the dissection to "where the blue begins" completes the exposure.

An incision is made in the dura propria just posterior to the ganglion in line with the second division. The ganglion itself should not be exposed since the destruction of ganglion cells may produce trophic changes within the distribution of their fibers. The constant gush of cerebrospinal fluid resulting from opening the dura propria must be cleared by suction to maintain exposure of the sensory root.

The rootlets constituting the sensory root can be avulsed piecemeal with a dull right-angled hook. Fibers of the first division may be separated from those of the second and third divisions by a small space. This

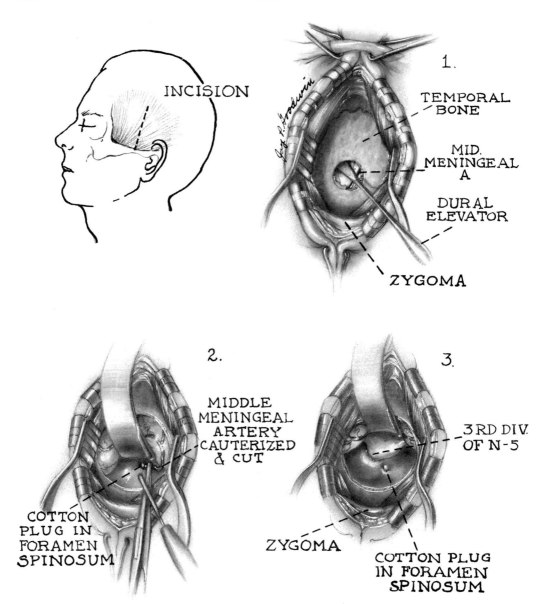

Figure 121–2 The incision should be approximately 8 cm in length, approximately 2 cm in front of the external auditory meatus. It should not extend below the lower border of the zygoma. *1.* Separating the dura along the perimeter of the burr hole prior to enlarging the bony defect helps to avoid splitting the dura. *2.* When the foramen spinosum is encountered it should be plugged with cotton to avoid troublesome bleeding from the middle meningeal artery. The distal artery can then be cauterized and cut. *3.* The third division will be encountered exiting through its foramen ovale 2 to 3 mm anterior and slightly medial to the foramen spinosum.

should be identified if possible and every effort made to spare the superior fibers. As the avulsion of sensory fibers extends medially, care must be taken to identify and spare the motor root. This lies medial to the sensory fibers, is somewhat larger, and extends diagonally downward and forward in a slightly different direction from the sensory root. A tug on the ganglion will dis-

place the sensory fibers laterally, separating them from the motor root, which remains medial. It is well to remember at this point that there may be a dehiscence of the thin lamina of bone separating the gasserian ganglion from the internal carotid artery lying behind it. A tear in the artery at this point can be catastrophic.

After the sensory root section is com-

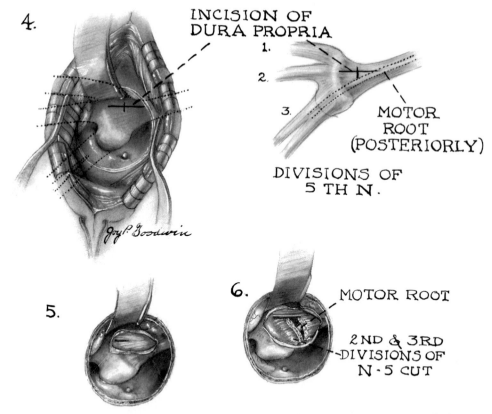

Figure 121–3 *4.* The second division and the distal portion of the sensory root are exposed. A transverse incision is made in the dura propria over the sensory root and should not extend to the ganglion itself. *5.* If the sensory root is exposed close to the ganglion, a small space will often be seen between the first and second divisions. *6.* Fibers of the second and third divisions are avulsed piecemeal with a blunt nerve hook. The motor root can be identified medially, running at a slightly different angle from the smaller sensory fibers.

pleted, the temporal dura is allowed to fall back, and the wound is closed in layers. Usually drainage is not necessary.

Complications

The following statistics are derived from the larger series reported by Peet and Schneider and by Stookey and Ransohoff.[7,11]

The operative mortality rates attending sensory root section were 0.82 and 1.6 per cent. This seems low considering the average age of these patients at the time of operation.

Facial weakness of some degree has been noted in 6.5 and 7.8 per cent of patients. In most instances such weakness is temporary.

Paresthesias were significant in 56 per cent of Peet and Schneider's series. Five per cent of these patients considered the paresthesias to be as troublesome as the preoperative pain.[3] In most instances, however, patients are willing to accept such symptoms if they have been warned of them before the operation.

Herpes simplex was evident in 14 per cent of the patients reported by Stookey and Ransohoff. This is not a serious complication, but, if unexpected, its appearance may be a source of concern.

Interstitial keratitis was noted in 15 per cent of Peet and Schneider's series. Such a complication may result from section of, or damage to, the first division but may occur even when it is spared. It may be serious if untreated, especially if accompanied by facial paralysis. In such instances, tarsorrhaphy is required.

Recurrence of pain can be anticipated in 15 per cent of patients who undergo sensory root section. In half of them, recurrence will be in the division involved preoperatively. In the others, pain will have extended into a division left intact at the time of operation.

INTRADURAL SENSORY ROOT SECTION

The intradural approach to the gasserian ganglion avoids the sometimes troublesome bleeding attending the extradural exposure and lessens considerably the chances of damaging the greater superficial petrosal nerve and secondarily the facial nerve.[15] The consequences of trauma to the exposed temporal lobe and its vessels, however, appear to outweigh the advantages of this technique, and it has not been widely accepted in the United States. If the temporal dura is friable and densely adherent to bone, it may be the procedure of choice.

Operative Technique

After exposing the temporal dura in the manner already described, adequate exposure of the temporal lobe can be accomplished by making a T-shaped dural incision, reflecting the wings of cut dura with stay sutures to the temporal muscles. Wilkins prefers utilizing a curved dural flap with its base superior to protect the temporal lobe.[15] The exposed temporal lobe is elevated with care. When necessary, veins extending from the temporal lobe to the dura are coagulated and cut. The superior petrosal sinus is identified on the superior surface of the petrous ridge. The ganglion can be found by palpating the medial floor of the temporal fossa just anterior to the sinus with an instrument such as a ganglion knife. Here the overlying dura is soft and yielding. The ganglion is exposed by a stellate dural opening. The technique from this point on has already been detailed.

DECOMPRESSION AND COMPRESSION OF SENSORY ROOT

Reasoning that trigeminal neuralgia resulted from pressure on the sensory root as it crosses over the apex of the petrous bone, Taarnhøj decompressed the root in this area by cutting the overlying dural sheath and obtained relief in 10 consecutive patients with this disorder.[13] Later he described his results in 70 patients with trigeminal neuralgia followed for up to three years, and noted recurrences in seven cases.[14] Other observations extending over longer periods indicated a recurrence rate of 60 per cent and 85 per cent.[2,12]

Between 1951 and 1953, Shelden, Pudenz, Freshwater, and Crue obtained relief in 10 patients with trigeminal neuralgia by decompressing the peripheral branches of the fifth nerve at the foramen ovale and foramen rotundum. Noting Taarnhøj's results following decompression of the sensory root, they found it difficult to explain the mechanism of relief from decompression at such divergent parts of the trigeminal nerve, other than by the fact that both procedures entailed some degree of trauma to the nerve. In 1955 they reported relief in 29 patients in whom the sensory root was "compressed" by a small dental roll and later by a blunt dissector.[9] Hamby, employing a similar technique in 86 patients followed for as long as five years, found recurrences in only 8 per cent.[2] Graf noted recurrences in 24 per cent of 100 patients who were treated by this method and followed for as long as eight years.[1] Of these 100 patients, 70 had been included in Hamby's report. Seventy-six per cent of them described facial paresthesias, and in 11 patients the discomfort was greater than after alcohol block. Stender reported relief in 16 patients with trigeminal neuralgia after merely opening the dura propria.[10] In two others, temporary relief was obtained by exposing the gasserian ganglion without opening the dura propria.

Operative Technique

Although Taarnhøj performed his decompression operation via the intradural route, the extradural approach advocated by Norlene and by Love seems preferable.[4,5] Exposure of the gasserian ganglion may be accomplished in the manner already described. The incision in the dura propria, however, is continued posteriorly above the sensory root through the superior petrosal sinus, which is clipped and cut. Electrocoagulation in this area may injure the facial nerve. The trochlear nerve should be identified along the free edge of the tentorium before it extends behind the superior petrosal sinus. The incision in the tentorium should be then extended to its free edge, carefully avoiding any tension on the trochlear nerve.

In the compression procedure of Schelden, Pudenz, Freshwater, and Crue, a vertical incision is made in the dura propria just behind the ganglion to expose the sensory root, which is gently compressed with the back of a blunt dissector.[9]

REFERENCES

1. Graf, C. J.: Trigeminal compression for tic douloureux, an evaluation. J. Neurosurg., 20: 1029–1032, 1963.
2. Hamby, W. B.: Effectiveness of various operations for trigeminal neuralgia. J. Neurosurg., 17:1039–1044, 1960.
3. Kahn, E. A., Crosby, E. C., Schneider, R. C., and Taren, J. A.: Correlative Neurosurgery. 2nd Ed. Springfield, Ill., Charles C Thomas, 1969, pp. 492–498.
4. Love, J. G.: The surgical treatment of trigeminal and glossopharyngeal neuralgia: Decompression of gasserian ganglion and its root for trigeminal pain. J. Int. Coll. Surg., 21:1–14, 1954.
5. Norlene: Cited by Hamby, W. B., ref. 2.
6. Peet, M. M., and Echols, D. H.: Surgery of disorders of cranial nerves. In Bancroft, F. W., and Pilcher, C., eds.: Surgical Treatment of the Nervous System. Philadelphia, J. B. Lippincott Co., 1946, pp. 258–262.
7. Peet, M. H., and Schneider, R. C.: Trigeminal neuralgia. A review of 689 cases with a follow-up study of 65 per cent of the group. J. Neurosurg., 9:367–377, 1952.
8. Shelden, C. H.: Compression procedure for trigeminal neuralgia. J. Neurosurg., 25:374–381, 1966.
9. Shelden, C. H., Pudenz, R. H., Freshwater, D. B., and Crue, B. L.: Compression rather than decompression for trigeminal neuralgia. J. Neurosurg., 12:123–126, 1955.
10. Stender, A.: "Gangliolysis" for the surgical treatment of trigeminal neuralgia. J. Neurosurg., 11:333–336, 1964.
11. Stookey, B. P., and Ransohoff, J.: Trigeminal Neuralgia: Its History and Treatment. Springfield, Ill., Charles C Thomas, 1959.
12. Svien, H. J., and Love, J. G.: Results of decompression operation for trigeminal neuralgia four years plus after operation. J. Neurosurg., 16:653–655, 1959.
13. Taarnhøj, P.: Decompression of the trigeminal root and posterior part of ganglion as treatment in trigeminal neuralgia. Preliminary communication. J. Neurosurg., 9:288–290, 1952.
14. Taarnhøj, P.: Decompression of trigeminal root, J. Neurosurg., 11:299–305, 1954.
15. Wilkins, H.: The treatment of trigeminal neuralgia by section of the posterior sensory fibers using the transdural temporal approach. J. Neurosurg., 25:370–373, 1966.

122

TREATMENT OF TRIGEMINAL NEURALGIA BY SECTION OF THE SENSORY ROOT IN THE POSTERIOR FOSSA

The operation for division of the sensory root of the trigeminal nerve as it traverses the lateral cistern adjacent to the pons was introduced and developed by Dr. Walter Dandy.[2-4] Much of the controversy that surrounded the operation earlier has been dissipated by time, experience, the introduction and improvement of other techniques, and the refinement of methods for the diagnosis of tumors of the cerebellopontine angle. Among the controversial points were the ease and safety of the method, the physiological implications, uncertainty about the uniqueness of the result, and concern about the incidence of tumors unrecognizable except at the time of operation.

The ideal result of any treatment for trigeminal neuralgia is permanent relief of pain with preservation of function. In terms of surgical treatment these are antithetical. Permanent relief can be assured only by total division of the sensory root while integrity of function can only be assured when there is no operation at all. Nonoperative treatment is preferable, and operation should be considered only when there is failure of or intolerance to medical therapy. When operative treatment is necessary, the procedure should be the minimal one that will give an excellent chance of lasting relief and the least impairment. It is in pursuit of this goal that a number of conservative operations have been devised.[8,9,11] Open operative procedures are being abandoned now in favor of effective and less hazardous percuraneous methods,

the development of which has been reviewed by Sweet and Wepsic.[10]

SPECIAL INDICATIONS FOR THE POSTERIOR APPROACH

Bilateral Trigeminal Neuralgia

Practically speaking this means neuralgia on the second side, that on the first side having been treated earlier by a method that has given dense sensory impairment in one or several divisions or paralysis of the motor root on that side. Because the need is clear for an operation that produces minimal functional impairment, the subtotal suboccipital operation is preferred.

Trigeminal Neuralgia with Signs

Although it is almost universally accepted that there are no neurological signs in tic douloureux, it is, in fact, not uncommon to find some depression of the corneal reflex and nasal tickle with mild hypalgesia on the affected side. These findings arouse the suspicion of tumor and may lead to further investigations, usually without a tumor being found. If surgical treatment is necessary and the operator would like to exclude a tumor or find it early, the posterior approach is preferable. Olivecrona has called attention to the occurrence of trigeminal neuralgia in the third division in younger

---

K. WELCH

persons, with or without minimal signs, as a result of epidermoid tumors in the angle.[7] The incidence of silent tumors was given by Walker and co-workers as 1.2 per cent.[13]

Combined Trigeminal and Glossopharyngeal Neuralgia

The two are sometimes clearly combined and at other times not distinguishable. The suboccipital operation is a necessity in those instances.

CONTRAINDICATIONS

These include local lesions of the scalp or bone, and deafness on the side contralateral to the proposed rhizotomy.

The operation is not effective in the treatment of painful dysesthesia of the face following a rhizotomy by the temporal route, and if total section is contemplated for the relief of pain in cancer it must be remembered that division of the major trunk of the root may be complete while facial sensation is not abolished.

TECHNIQUE

The hair need be shaved only posteriorly on the one side. The lateral position with the head of the operating table tilted upward offers advantages over others in that the exposure is aided by gravity.[12] Osmotic agents are not necessary. The scalp and muscle flap advocated by Dandy or a paramedian linear incision is satisfactory for access to the cerebellopontine angle.

If the Dandy exposure is used the vertical limb of the skin incision begins just medial to the tip of the mastoid process and extends superiorly and slightly laterally for about 5 cm before curving medially and inferiorly. Care should be exercised in incising the deep cervical fascia and muscles so that a sufficient cuff is left superiorly for the closure. It is important to the exposure that the bony opening extend to the asterion and that the opening be large enough (about 3.5 cm along its lateral extent) to permit binocular vision to the depth of the wound. After the dura is opened cerebrospinal fluid is released from the cisterna magna by inserting a spatula toward the cistern and rupturing

its arachnoid. If the arachnoid of the cistern is not seen, fluid will escape slowly anyway and only a little patience is required.

Next, a spatula is inserted beneath the cerebellum and retraction is made upward and mediad to expose the exit of the ninth and tenth cranial nerves and then the eighth, hiding the seventh. The arachnoid above the seventh and eighth nerves may be thin and transparent or may disintegrate so that the sensory root of the trigeminal may be seen at once. If it is opaque and thicker, a hole is made in it and this is dilated to expose the upper part of the angle. The relationships between the sensory root, the superior petrosal vein and occasional arterial branches, especially the anterior inferior cerebellar artery, are determined. It is rarely necessary to divide the superior petrosal vein even when it is in the direct line of sight to the sensory root, as the root may be teased a bit laterally to bring it from in front of the vein and into view. There is an ebb and flow of cerebrospinal fluid with controlled ventilation. During the few moments required to section the root the patient should be allowed to remain apneic. The fraction of the root to be sectioned is lifted away from the remainder with a nerve hook and cauterized or divided.

The dura is sewn, and the remainder of the closure is quite standard. A local dressing is to be preferred to one that encircles the head.

COMPLICATIONS

Postoperative hemorrhage, infection, and thromboembolic complications occur occasionally. Other untoward results arise from injury to cranial nerves. Deafness on the side operated on, undoubtedly the result of traction on the auditory nerve, is the most common. Complications of facial and corneal insensitivity, including unpleasant dysesthesia of the face, seem proportional to the density of sensory impairment and unrelated to the route by which the operation has been accomplished. If the cornea is insensitive, a lateral tarsorrhaphy may be indicated.

Craigmile lists the complications in 39 cases as follows: epidural hematoma, 1, recovered; supratentorial subdural hematoma, 1, died; oculomotor paresis, 2; persistant hearing loss, 2; transient hearing loss, 2; factitious ulceration of the nose, 1.[1] Olivecrona found facial paralyses in 3.1 per cent of patients undergoing this operation.[6]

RESULTS

When the posterior third or approximately half of the major trunk of the root is divided, there results mild to moderate hypalgesia and hypesthesia in the distribution of the third division, spilling over into the second and occasionally into the first. The degree and extent are quite variable. The pain of trigeminal neuralgia is relieved, but may recur in approximately one tenth to one fifth of the patients.[5,6,13,14]

REFERENCES

1. Craigmile, T. K.: Complications of the posterior fossa section of the trigeminal sensory root. Presentation to the Western Neurosurgical Society, Pebble Beach, California, November 5, 1969.
2. Dandy, W. E.: Section of the sensory root of the trigeminal nerve at the pons. Preliminary report of the operative procedure. Bull. Johns Hopk. Hosp., 36:105–106, 1925.
3. Dandy, W. E.: An operation for the cure of tic douloureux. Partial section of the sensory root at the pons. Arch. Surg., 18:687–734, 1929.
4. Dandy, W. E.: The treatment of trigeminal neuralgia by the cerebellar route. Ann. Surg., 96:787–795, 1932.
5. Hamby, W.B.: Effectiveness of various operations for trigeminal neuralgia. J. Neurosurg., 17:1039–1044, 1960.
6. Olivecrona, H.: The surgery of pain. Acta Psychiat. Kbh., 46:suppl.:268–280, 1947.
7. Olivecrona, H.: Cholesteatomas of the cerebellopontine angle. Acta Psychiat. Kbh., 24:639–643, 1949.
8. Shelden, C. H., Pudenz, R. H., Freshwater, D. B., and Crue, B. L.: Compression rather than decompression for trigeminal neuralgia. J. Neurosurg., 12:123–126, 1955.
9. Stender, A.: "Gangliolysis" for the surgical treatment of trigeminal neuralgia. J. Neurosurg., 11:333–336, 1954.
10. Sweet, W. H., and Wepsic, J. G.: Controlled thermocoagulation of trigeminal ganglion and rootlets for differential destruction of pain fibers. J. Neurosurg., 40:143–156, 1974.
11. Taarnhøj, P.: Decompression of the trigeminal root and the posterior part of the ganglion as treatment in trigeminal neuralgia. Preliminary communication. J. Neurosurg., 9:288–290, 1952.
12. Walker, E.: A simplified suboccipital technique for trigeminal, acoustic or glossopharyngeal rhizotomy. J. Neurol. Neurosurg. Psychiat., 13:127–129, 1950.
13. Walker, E., Miles, C. F., and Simpson, J. R.: Partial trigeminal rhizotomy using suboccipital approach. Arch. Neurol. Psychiat., 75:514–521, 1956.
14. White, J. E., and Sweet, W. H.: Pain: Its Mechanism and Neurosurgical Control. Springfield, Ill., Charles C Thomas, 1955.

123

TREATMENT OF TRIGEMINAL NEURALGIA BY MICRO-OPERATIVE DECOMPRESSION

Trigeminal neuralgia is a painful condition caused by an abnormality of the root entry zone of the trigeminal nerve.[12,13] While the abnormality usually is associated with cross-compression by an arterial loop that has impinged upon the nerve as a result of vascular elongation due to the aging process, it is also possible for a cross-compressing vein to be the cause.[7–11,15–21] A number of independent neurosurgical investigators have now verified these abnormalities.* Recently it has been established that extra-axial benign cerebellopontine tumors associated with trigeminal neuralgia appear to cause vascular cross-compression of the root entry zone, which causes the pain just as it does in patients without tumors.[22] Given these recent findings, it is the authors' belief that the differentiation between "idiopathic" trigeminal neuralgia and "symptomatic" trigeminal neuralgia can be consigned to the annals of medical history. Trigeminal neuralgia is common in multiple sclerosis and, concordant with the foregoing findings, is due to a multiple sclerosis plaque at the root entry zone of the nerve, as has been verified at both postmortem examination and operation.[18,19]

The following discussion deals with (1) some of the findings in the history and on physical examination in patients with trigeminal neuralgia, (2) the anatomy of the trigeminal nerve in the cerebellopontine angle, (3) the technique of retromastoid craniectomy and microvascular decompression of the trigeminal nerve, and (4) the operative findings and results in a large series of patients.

CLINICAL FINDINGS IN TRIGEMINAL NEURALGIA

History

In an analysis of the first 100 patients who had a micro-operative decompression, it was found that the first medical person to see 80 of them was a dentist.[20] The patient thought he had a toothache, and the dentist frequently removed one or more teeth—sometimes at the insistence of the patient, who would almost force the dentist to remove the tooth. More frequently, however, the dentist was not aware of the diagnosis, and one or more teeth were removed on his advice. Removal of teeth rarely helped the patient. Nevertheless, some dentists are currently treating patients with facial pain, including trigeminal neuralgia, with extensive periodontal procedures, describing foci of inflammation, infection, and osteomyelitis in these patients. Disordered trigeminal sensation may be a real factor in the development of trigeminal facial pain.

---

* See references 1, 2, 5, 14a, 29, 37–39, 41.

P. J. JANNETTA

PAIN

For this reason, an open-minded interest should be maintained regarding these efforts.

The onset of the trigeminal neuralgia usually is remembered well by the patient, regardless of how much earlier it occurred. This is in sharp contrast to other facial pain problems, in which the onset is mild, gradual, and not memorable. Occasionally a patient has a prodrome of paresthesias and dysesthesias in the area of a future tic. These episodes are mild and brief and may be separated from a first bout of true tic by some time. Some patients may have a relatively long pain-free interval, up to many months or a year, after the first attack before the pain becomes more frequent.

Most tic patients give an extracted history of present illness in which it can be considered that positional changes have an influence upon the pain. It has long been known that tic patients usually do not have many attacks at night. The hypothesis has been advanced that this is because the sleeping brain is not susceptible to the tic, and those attacks that do occur have usually been considered the result of stimulation of a trigger point by bed clothing. The author has observed at operation that the vessels of the brain and the brain stem appear to move differentially with changes in the position of the head. This is so whether the arachnoid has been opened or not, but of course the presence of a craniectomy, no matter how small, may exert some distorting influence. In the sitting position, the artery or vein is universally seen to be cross-compressing, notching, and grooving the root entry zone of the nerve. But when the patient lies in the lateral position with the ipsilateral side up, the artery may be a millimeter or two away from the root entry zone. The groove in the nerve is usually seen, however, and the vessel can be moved back to the point of the groove very easily. The converse should be true, i.e., with a patient lying on the ipsilateral side, differential movement may impact the vessel against the root entry zone more significantly. Questioning will reveal that the patient frequently gets into a certain routine position of comfort when going to bed at night so that his pain stops before he goes to sleep. The patient usually lies supine or in the contralateral-lateral decubitus position, but not in the ipsilateral-lateral decubitus position. At the request of the author, five patients, all of whom were having severe tic, were asked to go to bed, lie in their position of comfort, and stay that way through the night without going to sleep. In doing this the patients found that the tic quieted down, only to recur if they got out of bed. It may be of significance that many patients with hyperactive disorders of the other cranial nerves (i.e., the facial, vestibulocochlear, and glossopharyngeal nerves) that are due to neurovascular compression may also have a history of change in symptoms with a change in position, but except for those with vertigo and tinnitus, not as frequently as in the fifth nerve problems.

Patients with tumors as the cause of the tic have a history of present illness that is no different from the classic tic history. Indeed, the only patients with tumors as the cause who were included in the series were those who did have a classic history.

Trigger points are found in the area of the nose and around the eyes, which is the area of pure distribution of the trigeminal nerve. Trigger points are evanescent and move about over time, implying a dynamic changing process, which is reasonable if one considers the electron microscopic changes noted in trigeminal neuralgia.[4]

Physical Findings

Patients with trigeminal neuralgia frequently have mild sensory loss in the pure trigeminal distribution. This was first noted by Lewy and Grant in 25 per cent of their patients with trigeminal neuralgia.[27] On careful testing, the author noted hypalgesia or hypesthesia or both in 15 of 46 consecutive patients who had not had a prior operative procedure.[19] It must be emphasized that these are mild changes. One of these 46 patients had a tumor as the cause of the neurovascular compression but had no sensory abnormality. Two principles must be adhered to if one is to find these abnormalities: the first is that the pure trigeminal distribution must be tested, i.e., the nose and the area around the eyes, and also the corneal reflex; the second is that the examiner must follow routine neurological practice for tracing sensory abnormality by starting from the abnormal and going toward the normal. The abnormal area is usually around the nasolabial fold region over the upper lip, and the abnormality consists of mild hypalgesia, frequently with associated hypesthesia. Mild repetitive pinprick stimulus is used, starting in this area and going in every direction from it, and the response is then evaluated against the opposite side. The corneal reflex may be decreased, especially in first division trigeminal neuralgia, and may be decreased in only part of the cornea, especially the upper half. These changes will revert to normal gradually after microvascular decompression of the nerve.

Jaw opening is frequently uneven in patients with trigeminal neuralgia as though there is some lag on the side of the pain. This may be because the patient guards himself from an attack of tic, but since the motor-proprioceptive fascicles are frequently denervated in trigeminal neuralgia, it is possible that some of this abnormal movement may be due to unilateral motor trigeminal denervation or lack of proprioception.[43] These changes of denervation in the temporalis and masseter muscles also gradually revert to normal after microvascular decompression.[19,20]

The patient, if he is having severe attacks of pain, will hold his face quite still, keeping the muscles of facial expression as immobile as possible, and will talk with a "stiff upper (and lower) lip." When observed during an attack, although it occurs rapidly, the patient quite commonly clenches his jaws. It is not known whether this is the subject's response to the pain or something automatic that happens in the disordered function of the trigeminal nerve that precipitates the attack or one of the sequence of the same abnormal impulses that are extant at the time of the attack. Neurophysiological studies may clarify this point. The unshaved, unwashed face, the unbrushed teeth, and the unmade-up face are not seen as frequently as previously by the author, for newer medications have certainly helped to diminish acute exacerbations of pain. Periodontitis and dental caries are common, however, by the time a patient has been suffering for a long time, because he cannot tolerate dental care. Patients should be reassured that they may go to the dentist soon after discharge from the hospital.

ANATOMY OF THE TRIGEMINAL NERVE IN THE POSTERIOR FOSSA

Nerve Roots

The trigeminal nerve is located high and anteromedially in the posterior fossa. It arises from the lateral pons just inferomedial to the ala of the cerebellum and courses in a generally horizontal anterolateral direction between the pons and Meckel's cave. The diameter of the nerve is surprisingly variable, and there is some variability in relationships of the roots. But in general, the 100 or more fascicles making up the dorsal root in Meckel's cave ramify widely and decrease in number so that as the nerve approaches the brain stem there are usually about 65 fascicles that can be counted. Fascicles coalesce into a somewhat gelatinous area surrounded by tough pia mater within 1 cm to 0.5 cm of the brain stem. This is the so-called "fibrous cone" described by Dandy. Two motor-proprioceptive fascicles exit from the pons on the superomedial side of the sensory portio major. They arise as a spray of fascicles that fuse within a few millimeters into two distinctly separate but contiguous structures. Some connections are seen between motor-proprioceptive and sensory roots, variable in number, with connections all the way to and including the gasserian ganglion. The motor-proprioceptive fascicles, after fusing, course on the medial side of the sensory root. They then cross under the gasserian ganglion and exit from the intracranial cavity under the third division at the foramen ovale.

The "fibrous cone" region is truly an internal as well as external cone, as seen in multiple serial histological sections of the trigeminal nerve. In such tissue sections, it is seen that the entry zone of the various fascicles of the dorsal root enter a truncated area of tissue that is widest at the brain stem and contains central nervous system myelin. Each axis cylinder peripheral to this point in the dorsal root is covered by Schwann cell myelin. A goodly percentage, perhaps 20 per cent, of the fascicles do not enter this "fibrous cone" but instead separately enter the pons between the motor-proprioceptive fascicles and the portio major. Physiological studies in Lende's laboratory, verified in the author's laboratory, have shown that the "motor" fascicles are indeed both motor and proprioceptive.[6,35,40] The coalescent portio major at the brain stem, or so-called "fibrous cone," is surrounded by pia-arachnoid, separate from all other fascicles. This can be transected in entirety, preserving not only the motor-proprioceptive fibers but also the other "accessory" fascicles (intermediate fascicles) that have arisen from the dorsal root at variable distances from the brain stem.[7–11,15] The latter fascicles have a separate pial covering to the brain stem. If selective section of the portio major truly at the brain stem is accomplished, considerable light touch perception is preserved, as is the corneal reflex, although it may be somewhat diminished. Histological studies of the trigeminal nerve in several species by Vidic and Stefanotas have verified the presence of three groups of fascicles at the brain stem.[49] Electrophysiological studies in humans, done by Ley and Bacci after selective portio major section, have verified such a realignment of function distribution involving concentration of pain pathways in the portio major.[28]

Some variations do exist in the relationships of the various fascicles of the trigeminal nerve root entry zone.[14] It has been shown that the entry zone may be more or less obliquely horizontal or vertical. The relationships remain the same with the exception of an occasional aberrant fascicle, as found in large cadaver series. Such fascicles and such variations have not caused any difficulty in aligning oneself to the nerve properly at operations. Provost and Hardy have verified the presence of "accessory" or "intermediate" fascicles of the trigeminal nerve and have described three variations in their anatomy. They stated: "As the intermediate fibers mediate the tactile sensations, . . . [section of] the major portion resulted in a complete relief of trigeminal pain with preservation of normal tactile sensations."[41] Pertuiset and associates have, however, been able to identify intermediate fascicles at operation in only one out of two cases.[36] Maspes and coworkers, again in an operative study, were under the impression that they could appreciate the "accessory" fascicles in only half of their cases but stated also that they might have sectioned intermediate fascicles in some of their patients.[32]

Relationships of the Trigeminal Nerve in the Posterior Fossa

As mentioned earlier, the trigeminal nerve is located high, anteriorly, and medially in the posterior fossa. Considerable dissection is necessary to elevate the cerebellum from the lower cranial nerves to visualize the trigeminal nerve clearly from a low suboccipital craniectomy. It is very difficult to see the trigeminal nerve root entry zone from this approach unless the cerebellum has already been hollowed out by a cerebellopontine angle tumor such as an acoustic neuroma or a cholesteatoma. In Dandy's approach to the nerve, dissection is carried around the cerebellum, rather like opening the pages of a book with the anterior surface of the cerebellum acting as one page and the petrous bone as the other.[7–11] In this approach, the trigeminal nerve is seen well at Meckel's cave and posteriorly, but visualization of the true root entry zone may be difficult, although much easier than from underneath the cerebellum and easier with the patient in the lateral position than sitting. If the superior surface of the cerebellum is exposed and the lateral sinus and adjacent tentorium are elevated slightly with stay sutures, however, one can achieve an excellent appreciation of the trigeminal nerve in situ and the anatomy of the root entry zone.

One must appreciate that the angle of the entry zone of the trigeminal nerve in relationship to the plane of the surface of the pons is acute. Indeed, the nerve may be nearly parallel to the plane of the pons. The portio major side of the entry zone thus spreads posteriorly for a considerable distance. Minimal to essentially no cerebellar retraction is necessary to expose the nerve except in the area covered by the ala of the cerebellum. The superior petrosal vein, which usually blocks the view, takes origin from cerebellar transcortical venous structures over the anterior-superior and anterior surface of the cerebellum, generally with two major branches coalescing to form an inverted Y of variable length that enters the superior petrosal sinus. The structure is encased in archnoid, often all the way up to the superior petrosal sinus. The trigeminal nerve is seen just medial and anterior to this vein, usually, at 10 times magnification, in the same field as the trochlear nerve coursing around the brain stem.

In the normal situation, the horizontal loop of the superior cerebellar artery parallels the trochlear nerve just below it. This vessel usually bifurcates quite proximally so that there are two and rarely three loops coming around the midbrain-pons junction to course posteromedially to the superior cerebellar surface and adjacent brain stem. In elderly patients, this loop is often quite elongated, but it still remains generally horizontal at the brain stem. Meckel's cave is anterolateral to the root entry zone but at the same level in younger people, in whom the nerve has a generally horizontal course. In the elderly patients, however, the brain may sag, and the trigeminal nerve may course cephalad at a fairly steep angle before entering Meckel's cave.

In dolichocephalic patients, the angle between the two petrous ridges is quite acute, and the nerve may not enter Meckel's cave at a right angle to the petrous bone. In more brachycephalic patients, the angle between the petrous bones is closer to 90 degrees, and the trigeminal nerve enters Meckel's cave at more of a right angle to the petrous bone. The nerve runs in a more directly anteroposterior direction and is more nearly parallel to and directly adjacent to the pons in the dolichocephalic group. Exposure of the nerve and vascular micromanipulation may be more difficult in dolichocephalic patients because superolateral exposure is limited.

If the surgeon is to view these structures with ease and clarity, several considerations must be observed. First, the patient must be positioned so that the superior surface of the cerebellum is essentially in the horizontal plane. Second, the bony dissection of the suboccipital craniectomy should be carried well over the lateral sinus and should be lateral enough to clear the initial portion of the descending limb of the sigmoid sinus. Third, high magnification is necessary to see both the normal structures and the abnormalities in the trigeminal root entry zone.

Etiology of Tic Douloureux

Various theories, frequently speculative, have been proposed regarding the etiology of tic douloureux. The literature is vast. The ideas of many serious investigators who have considered aspects of the etiology cannot be included in this brief review. Until recently, no one other than Dandy had demonstrated a reasonably consistent abnormality in tic douloureux. He described abnormalities, usually vascular, about the dorsal root of the trigeminal nerve in the posterior fossa in over 40 per cent of patients and other questionable abnormalities in another 18 per cent.[7-11] Others, however, could not confirm these abnormalities. Dandy apparently never attempted to move vessels away from the nerve, but avulsed the nerve with a hook or electrocautery or both. He, therefore, could not state to the satisfaction of others that the vessels were causative, but he did treat tic douloureux effectively by tumor removal in 5.6 per cent of his 215 cases. In 2.8 per cent of them, he found that aneurysms of the basilar artery pressed upon the sensory root. He found cavernous angiomas in 2.3 per cent of the cases; an artery compressing the root in 30.7 per cent; and in another 14 per cent, a branch of the petrosal vein crossing the sensory root or passing directly through it. He was less convinced about the etiological relationship of the veins. In another 1 per cent of the cases, he found congenital malformations at the base of the skull, and in seven cases the sensory root was tightly adherent to the brain stem. The percentage of patients in whom he observed abnormalities increased significantly with further experience.[10]

Revilla studied 473 patients from the Johns Hopkins Hospital, who were operated upon by a cerebellar approach from 1925 to 1945. Twenty-four had tumors of the posterior fossa producing tic douloureux, among which 11 were neuromas, 9 were epidermoid cysts, and 4 were meningiomas.[42] Gardner explored the trigeminal nerve in the posterior fossa in 18 patients with recurrent trigeminal neuralgia. He found an arterial loop compressing the nerve in six, an acoustic tumor in two, a crowded posterior fossa owing to basilar impression in one, a cirsoid aneurysm of the basilar artery in one, and a homolateral dislocation of the pons that was compressing the nerve in two. He found no explanation for the tic douloureux in the remaining six cases.[12]

Knight, in 1954, studied the incidence of herpes simplex virus in patients with tic douloureux, but although all his patients had high antibody titers for herpes simplex, no control group unaffected with tic douloureux was similarly studied.[24] Recent studies of herpes simplex virus cultures from the trigeminal ganglion would appear to corroborate other impressions that the virus is endemic to ganglia in general.[3] Vesicles may appear with any nonspecific trauma. Such would appear to be the case in the author's series of retromastoid craniectomies in which the incidence of postoperative perioral herpes simplex has been higher in the patients who had section of the trigeminal nerve for pain due to malignant metastases than in the patients who had tic douloureux. Lee, Taarnhøj, and Olivecrona described sagging of the hindbrain in elderly patients and suggested that this would cause traction on the trigeminal nerve at the petrous ridge.[26,34,47,48] Gardner and co-workers stated that the demineralization of the base of the skull in aging results in an upward tilt of the petrous pyramid and the consequent angulation of the sensory root over the petrous ridge would produce "short circuiting" and cause tic douloureux. They noted that tic douloureux was three times as common on the side of the higher petrous ridge, if asymmetry of the ridges was noted radiographically, than on the side of the lower ridge.[13] Malis modified Taarnhøj's technique of middle fossa decompression by opening the dura propria and crossing band of fibers to mobilize the trigeminal nerve. Forty-four operations were done in 43 patients, achieving delayed relief after four to five days in 8 of the patients, the only procedure other than the present series with this sequence of pain relief.[30] It is of interest in the author's cadaver studies that opening the dura propria allows considerable lateral mobility of the trigeminal roots in the posterior fossa.

Lewy and Grant noted in patients with tic douloureux that there was a 50 per cent incidence of cardiomegaly, angina pectoris, and heart murmurs, and an extremely high incidence of arteriosclerotic vascular disease; they built a superb case for arteriosclerosis as a cause of tic douloureux, but then concluded that the tic was a manifestation of a thalamic dysfunction, limited to the face in general but associated with other somatic complaints.[27] It is of interest that 80 per cent of their patients had signs of pyramidal or extrapyramidal disease. Sixty per cent had evidence of renal dysfunction, and there were twenty per cent who had a family or personal history of migraine.

Kerr proposed that there may be a defect in the floor of the middle fossa, under the gasserian ganglion, especially in elderly patients. The carotid artery may thus pulsate against the ganglion. He suggested that: "The carotid acts as a traumatic agent impinging on the ganglion root, thus promoting a more severe breakdown of myelin sheath in older individuals . . . or the carotid pulsation may act simply as an additional irritative factor in a primarily degenerate disease of the nerve."[23] Kerr proposed this as a theory; he clearly affirmed that he had no evidence that the bony defect was pertinent to the clinical situation.

Abnormality of the Root Entry Zone as Cause of Tic

Until recently, the operative procedures for trigeminal neuralgia were done without magnification. In many instances, a gross abnormality was noted in the posterior fossa at operation for trigeminal neuralgia, e.g., an acoustic neuroma, arteriovenous malformation, or aneurysm. In such cases the clinical diagnoses of trigeminal neuralgia, "idiopathic" or "cryptogenic," were quickly changed to the primary diagnosis of "acoustic neuroma," and the trigeminal neuralgia was, therefore called "symptomatic trigeminal neuralgia." With the magnification and lighting afforded by the binocular operating microscope, in concert with an operative procedure directed at the brain stem area of the trigeminal nerve, it has become apparent that all trigeminal neuralgia is "symptomatic." Only gross lesions could be appreciated in the past, but now subtle abnormalities causing disordered and hyperactive sensory function can be seen and treated.

Primary first division trigeminal neuralgia is rare. In the present series, correlation of the location of the facial pain with the direction from which neurovascular compression takes place shows that the 4 per cent of patients with primary first division tic douloureux all had trigeminal root entry zone compression and distortion by an arterial loop compressing the inferolateral portio major. The loop appeared to be the anterior inferior cerebellar artery or a branch of it. The direct correlation of superomedial compression by the superior cerebellar artery in lower facial tic has been such that the operative exposure can be planned rather precisely.

Trigeminal neuralgia predominates in middle and old age. The correlation of tic with arteriosclerosis was nicely described by Lewy and Grant in 1938.[27] This correlates well with arteriosclerotic tortuous elongation of arteries such that a vascular loop may impinge upon cranial nerves. The reasons for the predominance in women is not clear. It may be explained by the fact that the posterior fossa is smaller in women than in men and a horizontal looping of the superior cerebellar artery may not be able to continue to develop laterally but instead slides along the belly of the pons rather than out into the cerebellopontine angle. This is conjecture, and better information is needed. Several observers of demineralized soft bone and sagging of the brain in the elderly consider that these may also be contributory. The rarity of a combination of first and third division tic douloureux may be explained by the fact that a "scissors-type" pinch of two vessels upon the nerve should be rare. This too is conjectural, as the author has not operated upon such a patient. The presence of mild but real sensory deficit and electromyographic changes in the motor portion of the trigeminal nerve after prolonged tic douloureux, all of which are reversible after neurovascular decompression, belies other impressions that there is no neurological deficit with tic douloureux.

The tendency of the episodes to become more frequent and more severe may correlate with progressive elongation of a vascular loop. Waning of pain may be explained by neural accommodation and also by electron microscopic evidence, which has shown simultaneous denervation and reinnervation, suggesting that "short circuits" may be obliterated only for others to form. Treatment with some antiepileptic drugs does help patients with trigeminal neuralgia. These are drugs that cut down neuronal transmission, normal or abnormal. It would

appear from electron microscopic studies that there must be abnormal neuronal transmission in the trigeminal nerve of a patient with tic douloureux.

The occasional bilateral cases would appear to be more than just coincidence. The author relieved bilateral neurovascular compression by the superior cerebellar arteries in a recent case. A 67-year-old man developed unilateral right-sided second and third division trigeminal tic and was successfully operated upon six years later. Six months after the operation, pain began in the opposite side of the face in the left third division distribution. Operation one year later gave relief of this pain also.

Multiple sclerosis patients have been shown by postmortem examination to have a demyelinated plaque at the root entry zone.[33] The author has seen this abnormality in operative patients, and the clinical correlation is agreeable with the thesis of root entry zone abnormality. Operative findings of abnormality, usually vascular, of the trigeminal nerve root entry zone in trigeminal neuralgia serves as key evidence that such abnormality is the etiological agent. These findings are reviewed later in this chapter and are collated in Table 123–1. The postoperative course following decompression of the nerve at the pons is also illuminating in that mobilization of a vessel off the nerve without nerve manipulation

TABLE 123–1 OPERATIVE FINDINGS IN TRIGEMINAL NEURALGIA

OFFENDING STRUCTURE OR DISEASE	NUMBER OF PATIENTS	
Arterial		103
Superior cerebellar artery	82	
Anterior inferior cerebellar artery	9	
Posterior inferior cerebellar artery	1	
Superior cerebellar and anterior inferior cerebellar arteries	3	
Superior cerebellar artery and unnamed artery	4	
Unnamed artery	4	
Venous		19
Arterial and venous		22
Superior cerebellar artery and vein	16	
Anterior inferior cerebellar artery and vein	1	
Anterior inferior cerebellar artery, superior cerebellar artery, and vein	1	
Vein and unnamed artery	4	
Tumor		13
Multiple sclerosis		4
Atrophic nerve		2
Total		163*

* Cases from the author's series.

generally leaves the patient with some pain in the immediate postoperative period. The pain gradually occurs less frequently, becomes less severe, and then disappears. This temporary pain is usually relieved by diphenylhydantoin even when this same medication did not help preoperatively. The subtle sensory abnormalities found in long-standing tic douloureux revert to normal, with improvement usually beginning immediately postoperatively. The area of facial numbness following recurrence after other operative procedures may shrink significantly after vascular decompression, and mild numbness may disappear entirely.

Vascular compression-distortion of the nerve root entry zone has been noted in two brains at postmortem examination. Such specific changes have not been noted in many brains, at operation or at postmortem examination, in those without trigeminal neuralgia. It is, however, conceivable that such changes will be found some time, as the duration and degree of vascular compression-distortion necessary to cause trigeminal neuralgia is not known.

MICRO-OPERATIVE DECOMPRESSION IN TRIGEMINAL NEURALGIA

Indication for Operation

The procedure to be described appears to be indicated in patients with trigeminal neuralgia that is intractable to good medical therapy (diphenylhydantoin, carbamazepine, or both), or who have had toxic reactions to these drugs, if they have an estimated survival time of five years or more. The author uses 70 years as the usual cutoff age but has operated on older people who were vigorous, who were in excellent condition, and who came from long-lived families. Alksne, using an ingenious supine position for retromastoid exposure, has performed the procedure safely in a number of older patients.[1] A contralateral position or Alksne's supine position is best for most of these older patients.

Many patients seek treatment for recurrent trigeminal neuralgia following another operative procedure. A prior unsuccessful procedure or a recurrence is not a contraindication to operation.

Plain roentgenography of the skull in-

cluding a basal view, a CT scan with contrast (particular attention is paid to the posterior fossa), and complete otovestibular testing are obtained in all patients. Despite the complete special otovestibular testing, the author missed 11 of 14 tumors preoperatively in his first 161 patients. Better computed tomography is increasing the yield. Selective vertebral angiograms have been performed in younger patients. An arteriovenous malformation was found preoperatively in a 28-year-old woman early in the series. In patients with lower facial tic douloureux, angiograms may show a downward sweep of the ipsilateral superior cerebellar artery as it comes around the pons. This finding on the angiogram may be helpful in suggesting the etiological factor preoperatively, but otherwise it is not of much help. As a result, routine angiography is not indicated; however, a unilateral vertebral angiogram may be indicated to rule out a pontocerebellar arteriovenous malformation. Routine lumbar puncture is not useful.

Operative Technique

The patient is prepared 12 hours before operation with dexamethasone, 10 mg intramuscularly. This drug is continued postoperatively in a dose of 4 mg every 6 hours for 48 hours and then discontinued. A central venous pressure line and an indwelling bladder catheter are placed before operation. The legs are wrapped with Ace bandages, and the patient is anesthetized, intubated, and placed in a lateral decubitus position with the head fixed in a pin headholder. A Doppler ultrasonic flowmeter is then positioned over the right atrium, and cardiac sounds are monitored throughout the operation for air embolism and changes in cardiac rate and rhythm.[31] Some traction is exerted on the neck with the headholder, the neck is flexed to the point at which the chin is about one fingerbreadth from the sternum, and the head is rotated slightly to the ipsilateral side. The patient is placed high on the table on bolsters so that the surgeon's forearm will be vertical when working in the cerebellopontine angle with elbows resting on the headboard of the table. Fifty grams of mannitol is given intravenously as a bolus over a 15- to 20-minute period, starting soon after intubation. The bolus of mannitol is necessary for easy exposure without excessive cerebellar retraction. In older patients, the cerebellum appears to be comparatively smaller in the posterior fossa than in younger patients, perhaps because the brain has "sagged."

The ipsilateral posterior side of the head from midline to the ear and from just below the vertex to the hairline is shaved in the operating room. The headpiece of the operating table, with the pad taped into place, is left on the table in a horizontal position as an elbow rest in all the author's posterior fossa cases. A vertical incision approximately 7 cm long is made 2 cm medial to the mastoid process with about one third of the incision above the nuchal line. The incision is placed far enough laterally to avoid the greater occipital nerve and tilted laterally following the hairline. It is carried directly to the calvarium except caudally, where further dissection of the deeper muscles is performed with the electrocautery. Periosteal elevators are used to separate the nuchal muscles, fascia, and pericranium away from the calvarium. A self-retaining angulated retractor with posts for the micro-operative retractor is placed. The posteromedial aspect of the mastoid eminence is cleared. The electrocautery blade on cutting current is helpful in separating the attachments of the nuchal line to the calvarium. A piece of cervical muscle is taken for the implant.

A craniectomy about 3 by 3 cm in size is then performed high and laterally in the posterior fossa, exposing the horizontal portion of the lateral sinus and extending into the mastoid air cells laterally if necessary. The open cells are waxed heavily. An incision is made in the dura mater well under the lateral sinus and extending caudally. The superolateral dural flap is incised to the lateral sinus and the dura is sutured to the galea, tenting the lateral sinus up and away. More bone may be rongeured superolaterally at this point if exposure is not adequate. It is important to achieve this superolateral exposure, and the short time necessary to obtain it is well worthwhile (Fig. 123–1). The micro-operative retractor is then put into place over a rubber dam fashioned from a piece of rubber glove that is cut to size. A relatively narrow blade is used, and no cerebellar retraction is used at this point. The retractor is placed superficially over the lateral aspect of the superior surface of the cerebellum.

The operating binocular microscope with a 250-mm focal length objective is then used for the remainder of the procedure. Minimal retraction is necessary to find the superior petrosal vein, which is usually shaped like an inverted Y. With sharp dissection, the arachnoid is opened over the vein, which is then coagulated with bipolar coagulation. A set of micro-operative instruments with bayonet-shaped handles is used for this and the remainder of the intra-

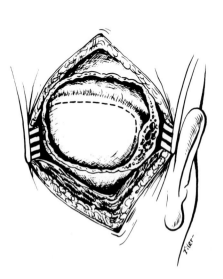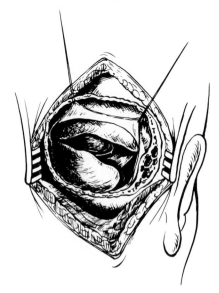

Figure 123–1   Right retromastoid craniectomy. Neck is placed on the stretch with chin flexed and head turned slightly to the ipsilateral side. Craniectomy must clear the lateral sinus to facilitate exposure without undue retractor pressure on the cerebellum.

cranial dissection. The Valsalva maneuver is performed after partial and after complete section of the vein, as it is easy to miss some of the anterior limb of the Y in coagulating.

After the superior petrosal vein is divided, the retractor is placed more deeply, again over the rubber dam. The arachnoid is opened anteromedial to the vein, exposing the trigeminal nerve. The trochlear nerve is usually seen before the trigeminal nerve is clearly visualized and is easily avoided; if it is in the center of the field, the dissection is too far cephalad. The trigeminal nerve courses obliquely from Meckel's cave to the pons just anteromedial to the superior petrosal vein. A variable degree of forward or backward tilt of the operating table may be necessary at this point and subsequently to give a good horizontal line of sight to the trigeminal nerve and allow cerebrospinal fluid to run out of the arachnoidal defect and around the cerebellum. The retractor, with joints only partially tightened, can be moved about gently and gradually as dissection continues. It must not be allowed to slip down over the side of the cerebellum onto the seventh and eighth cranial nerves or to compress the cerebellum significantly. The arachnoid is next dissected from the trigeminal nerve. It may be adherent both to the nerve and to the artery, compressing and distorting the nerve. The arachnoid must be separated from the trigeminal nerve for most of the length of the posterior roots. After some experience, the relationship of the artery to the trigeminal nerve can usually be appreciated before the arachnoid is opened.

The usual situation in lower facial tic douloureux is that the superior cerebellar artery is found coursing cephalad around the pons and then bifurcating, with the medial and lateral branches impinging upon the anterosuperior aspect of the entry zone of the nerve, the motor-proprioceptive fascicle side, as it loops back to the brain stem and cerebellum (Fig. 123–2). After sharp and blunt dissection of the widely opened arachnoid from the nerve and the visible part of the artery, the arterial loops are gently teased out from between the trigeminal nerve and the pons (Fig. 123–3). The loops are usually longer in older patients and especially in those with long-standing tic douloureux. They must be manipulated carefully. The arterial loops may be quite adherent to the nerve or easily separable from it. Perforating branches to the pons have accommodated in length to the loop and will not tear with gentle manipulation of the vessel over the trigeminal nerve. The vascular loops may, however, be too long to move safely, especially in older patients. In this case, selective section of the portio major is preferable.

In first division tic douloureux it is the anterior inferior cerebellar artery that is seen compressing the inferolateral portion of the trigeminal nerve entry zone at the pons at the portio major side (Fig. 123–4). The superior cerebellar artery has a normal horizontal loop in this case.

A small piece of muscle from the cervical incision, Teflon felt, silicone sponge, or polyvinyl chloride sponge (Ivalon) is carved to fit between the brain stem and nerve on one side and the artery on the other. A groove is cut for the artery and if necessary for the nerve. The implant is placed between the artery and the nerve at the brain stem. The Valsalva maneuver is performed

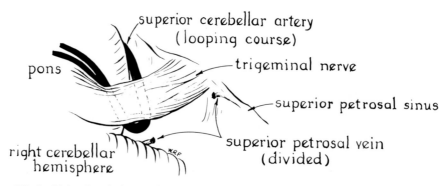

Figure 123–2   Right trigeminal nerve, lower facial tic douloureux, supracerebellar route. Diagrammatic representation of the view through the microscope *after* dissection of arachnoid and *before* mobilization of superior cerebellar artery.

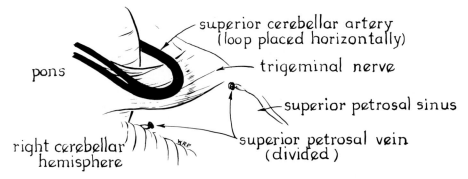

Figure 123–3   Right trigeminal nerve, lower facial tic douloureux after decompression, supracerebellar route. Diagrammatic representation of the view through the microscope after arterial loop has been mobilized by changing the axis of the loop.

several times under control of the anesthetist to see if the relationships are stable.

If the patient has multiple sclerosis or if the vessel cannot be safely moved, a rare situation, selective section of the portio major is performed by entering the coalescent inferolateral portio major at the brain stem and not distal to it. The section should be proximal to the multiple sclerosis plaque. With a small 45-degree micro-nerve hook (and rarely needing a 90-degree hook, which is felt to be dangerous in the posterior fossa), the soft white material inside the portio major is transected easily. If one stays inside the arachnoid, the motor-proprioceptive fascicles and "accessory fascicles" (intermediate fascicles), which are compressed by the vessel between the artery and the kidney bean–shaped portio major, may be preserved, thus preserving relative light touch sensation.

A piece of Gelfoam is placed over the arachnoid opening. This appears to decrease postoperative headache. The retractor is removed, and the dura is closed with interrupted and running sutures of silk. The incision is closed in layers, and a small dry dressing is applied. Postoperatively, the head of the bed is kept elevated about 10 degrees. The patient is usually able to return from the neurosurgical intensive care unit to the floor on the morning of the first postoperative day. Postoperative care is routine, as for any intracranial procedure.

POSTOPERATIVE COURSE AND OPERATIVE RESULTS

If the trigeminal nerve is manipulated during the operation, the patient awakens without any pain. If the nerve is not manipulated during the dissection, the patient will frequently have some trigeminal neuralgia for periods ranging from the immediate postoperative period up to several weeks after operation. The pain usually responds quite well to small doses of diphenylhydantoin and gradually disappears over a six- to eight-week period of time. Such a course of gradually decreasing postoperative tic douloureux has been seen in approximately 40 per cent of the author's patients.

There have been four postoperative

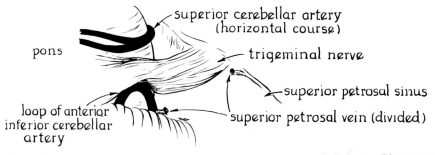

Figure 123–4   Right trigeminal nerve, upper facial tic douloureux, supracerebellar route. Diagrammatic representation of the view through the microscope before caudal-lateral vascular cross-compression of trigeminal nerve root entry zone is relieved.

deaths in 417 retromastoid procedures for classic and atypical trigeminal neuralgia from January 1972 through April 1978. One case was that of a 79-year-old woman who was operated upon in a seated position rather than in the usual lateral position for the elderly; she had reported that she was 59 years of age. She died from an ischemic cerebral infarction on her ninth postoperative day. The second patient was a 69-year-old woman who had a history of leukemia-in-arrest but who, on work-up, was found to have an acoustic neuroma with trigeminal neuralgia. She was operated upon in the lateral position. She suffered a cerebral hemispheric stroke postoperatively and died on her third postoperative day. The third patient developed a cerebellar brain stem infarction, presumably due to arterial kinking by the implant. The fourth death was that of a 54-year-old man who underwent an exploration for trigeminal neuralgia. At operation a large arteriovenous malformation involving the superior cerebellar artery at the brain stem was discovered. It had been undetected prior to operation despite CT scan. Bleeding developed during the procedure, and the superior cerebellar artery was clipped to control it. The patient developed a cerebellar infarction in the immediate postoperative period and died on the third postoperative day.

Of 274 patients with classic trigeminal neuralgia, 15 had decreased hearing subsequent to their operative procedure. This is believed to be due either to stretching of the eighth cranial nerve or the development of a hemotympanum during the operation. In these patients, the hearing deficit usually resolves within six weeks to three months postoperatively. Hearing impairment persisted in three patients. Complications are collated in Table 123–2.

A complete follow-up on 274 patients (279 nerves with tic douloureux, five cases bilateral) treated with microvascular decompression from January 1971 through June 1977 indicates that 32 patients had recurrence or never had relief of their pain postoperatively. Most recurrences occurred early (under six months postoperatively). Only two late recurrences were noted (over one year). Repeat retromastoid craniectomy with microvascular decompression was performed in 18 patients, 12 of whom were relieved of their pain. Nerve section or radiofrequency rhizotomy was

TABLE 123–2   COMPLICATIONS IN 274 PATIENTS*

COMPLICATION	NUMBER OF PATIENTS
Air embolism (rarely serious)	29
Herpes simplex (postoperative)	21
Decreased hearing	
Temporary	15
Persistent	3
Serous otitis media	7
Aseptic meningitis	6
Stitch granuloma/abscess	6
Hematoma	
Cerebellar	1
Posterior fossa subdural	1
Hemispheric subdural (5 and 9 weeks postoperative, one following head trauma)	2
Cerebellar infarction (both well)	2
Pneumonia	2
Pseudomeningocele	2
Bacterial meningitis	2
Death	1

* The author's series.

performed in five patients and was successful in three. It was found, in early recurrences, that the surgeon had usually missed a blood vessel or that the implant was inadequate in size, configuration, or position (Table 123–3). Experience shows that more than one vessel is commonly involved in tic, and it is suggested that the nerve be decompressed from every vessel that may compress it anywhere in the region.

In both instances of late recurrences (at four and four and one half years), continued arterial elongation was found. In the first such recurrence an arterial loop from the cerebellum was found to be cross-compressing the trigeminal nerve from the side. Review of the prior operative photographs disclosed that this vessel had been nowhere

TABLE 123–3   TYPICAL TRIGEMINAL NEURALGIA RECURRENCES*

OFFENDING STRUCTURE (SECOND OPERATION)	NUMBER OF PATIENTS
Superior cerebellar artery	5
Anterior inferior cerebellar artery	2
Vein	2
Superior cerebellar artery and vein	3
Superior cerebellar and anterior inferior cerebellar arteries	1
Anterior inferior cerebellar artery and vein	1
Vein and arachnoid cyst	1
Prosthesis causing distortion	1
Slipped prosthesis	1
Reactive prosthesis	1

* Findings at reoperation in 18 cases from the author's series.

near the nerve at the first operation. Microvascular decompression was successful in relieving symptoms. In the second patient, review of the first procedure revealed that the two distal branches of the already bifurcated superior cerebellar artery were causing the cross-compression. The nerve had been decompressed by inserting a small implant of plastic sponge. At reoperation, it was found that the proximal superior cerebellar artery had continued to elongate, pushing the distal branches and the implant right off the nerve so that the proximal artery was now cross-compressing the nerve. This situation developed because at the first operation, the surgeons were afraid to dissect too vigorously in this somewhat frail, aging woman and settled for a decompression without extensive arterial mobilization and a modest inferolateral section of the portio major. Postoperatively her pain remained for two months and then disappeared again. In retrospect, a larger implant covering the side of the trigeminal root entry zone would have prevented recurrence in the first patient. Better mobilization of the artery, truly changing the axis of the loop from vertical to horizontal, and using a large implant might have been beneficial in the second patient.

In the six patients who were not relieved of their pain at the second procedure, extensive scarring was noted around the nerve in three. In one other, vascular compression was not particularly striking at either the first or second operation. Of the remaining patients with recurrences, 12 in number, 1 committed suicide, and 1 is lost to follow-up (the recurrence is presumed to be persistent). Two of these patients had equivocal vascular compression noted at their operation (making three in all without striking vascular compression out of 279 trigeminal nerves). In all but five patients, pain is well controlled with diphenylhydantoin or carbamazepine.

Other significant morbidity included two patients with bacterial meningitis, both now well. Two patients had postoperative temporary facial weakness, one of them being one of those who had meningitis, which occurred three weeks after discharge from the hospital. The other case occurred in the immediate postoperative period.

The early time of recurrence as well as the operative findings in those who had a second retromastoid procedure tend to indicate that the major reason for recurrence was inadequacy of the initial operative procedure. The failure rate for microvascular decompression is 32 of 279 cases or 11.6 per cent for the first operation. If one includes patients who obtained relief of pain with repeat exploration, the failure rate drops to 7.6 per cent. There was no hypalgesia or anesthesia dolorosa resulting from the micro-operative decompression procedure. Consequently, the author believes that the retromastoid approach and microvascular decompression operation is the procedure of choice for classic trigeminal neuralgia in patients with five years or more of life expectancy, since it produces relief of pain without nerve damage and with minimal morbidity and few deaths. The older destructive procedures have been generally replaced by radiofrequency rhizotomy, which is an excellent procedure with respect to early morbidity and relief of pain.[46–48,50] It is still an operative procedure that entails some deaths and significant morbidity (anesthesia dolorosa and other problems of disordered sensation loom as the major long-term problems). Quality of survival should be of some significance in this regard. The incidence of anesthesia dolorosa after radiofrequency rhizotomy is higher than the mortality rate for retromastoid craniectomy. People who are not made numb *forget* their pain and are truly normal. These procedures complement each other. The neurosurgeon faced with a choice of operative treatment should probably do the procedure that he can do best. If both types of procedures are available, then the decision should be tailored to the individual patient.

REFERENCES

1. Alksne, J.: The lateral decubitis position for 5th nerve decompression in the treatment of trigeminal neuralgia. Neurosurgical Society of America, Colorado Springs, 1977.
2. Apflebaum, R. I.: A comparison of percutaneous radio-frequency trigeminal neurolysis and microvascular decompression of the trigeminal nerve for the treatment of tic douloureux. Neurosurgery, *1*:16, 1977.
3. Baringer, J. R., and Swoveland, P.: Recovery of herpes-simplex virus from human trigeminal ganglions. New Eng. J. Med., *288*:648–650, 1973.
4. Beaver, D. L., Moses, H. L., and Ganote, C. E.: Electron microscopy of the trigeminal ganglion.

III. Trigeminal neuralgia. Arch. Path. (Chicago), *79*:571–582, 1965.

5. Becker, D. B.: What's new in neurological surgery. Bull. Amer. Coll. Surg., *63*:23–27, 1978.

6. Bennett, M. H., and Jannetta, P. J.: Unpublished data.

7. Dandy, W. E.: Section of the sensory root of the trigeminal nerve at the pons. Bull. Johns Hopk. Hosp., *36*:105–106, 1925.

8. Dandy, W. E.: Operation for cure of tic douloureux; partial section of the sensory root at the pons. Arch. Surg. (Chicago), *18*:687–734, 1929.

9. Dandy, W. E.: Treatment of trigeminal neuralgia by the cerebellar route. Ann. Surg., *96*:787–795, 1932.

10. Dandy, W. E.: Concerning the cause of trigeminal neuralgia. Amer. J. Surg., *24*:447–455, 1934.

11. Dandy, W. E.: Surgery of the brain. *In* Lewis' Practice of Surgery. Vol. 12. Hagerstown, Md., W. F. Prior Co., 1945, pp. 167–187.

12. Gardner, W. J.: Concerning the mechanism of trigeminal neuralgia and hemifacial spasm. J. Neurosurg., *19*:947–958, 1962.

13. Gardner, W. J., Todd, E. M., and Pinto, J. P.: Roentgenographic findings in trigeminal neuralgia. Amer. J. Roentgen., *76*:346–350, 1956.

14. Gudmundsson, K., Rhoton, A. L., and Rushton, J. G.: Detailed anatomy of the intracranial portion of the trigeminal nerve. J. Neurosurg., *35*:592–600, 1971.

14a. Hankinson, H. L., and Wilson, C. B.: Microsurgical treatment of hemifacial spasm. Western J. Med., *124*:191–193, 1976.

15. Jannetta, P. J.: Gross (mesoscopic) description of the human trigeminal nerve and ganglion. J. Neurosurg., *26*:109–111, 1967.

16. Jannetta, P. J.: Arterial compression of the trigeminal nerve at the pons in patients with trigeminal neuralgia. J. Neurosurg., *26*:159–162, 1967.

17. Jannetta, P. J.: Letter: complications from microsurgical treatment of tic douloureux. J. Neurosurg., *40*:675, 1974.

18. Jannetta, P. J.: Microsurgical approach to the trigeminal nerve for tic douloureux. Progr. Neurol. Surg., *7*:180–200, 1976.

19. Jannetta, P. J.: Treatment of trigeminal neuralgia by suboccipital and transtentorial cranial operations. Clin. Neurosurg., *24*:538–549, 1977.

20. Janetta, P. J.: Unpublished data.

21. Jannetta, P. J., and Rand, R. W.: Transtentorial subtemporal retrogasserian neurectomy in trigeminal neuralgia by microsurgical technique. Bull. Los Angeles Neurol. Soc., *31*:93–99, 1966.

22. Jannetta, P. J., and Wilkins, R. H.: Trigeminal neuralgia caused by benign tumors Report of 14 cases. Submitted to Neurosurgery, 1980.

23. Kerr, F. W. L.: Evidence for a peripheral etiology of trigeminal neuralgia. J. Neurosurg., *26*:168–174, 1967.

24. Knight, G.: Herpes simplex and trigeminal neuralgia. Proc. Roy. Soc. Med., *47*:788–790, 1954.

25. Laha, R. K., and Jannetta, P. J.: Atypical trigeminal neuralgia. Submitted to J. Neurosurg., 1980.

26. Lee, F. C.: Trigeminal neuralgia. J. Med. Ass. Georgia, *26*:431, 1937.

27. Lewy, F. G., and Grant, F. C.: Physiopathologic and pathoanatomic aspects of major trigeminal neuralgia. Arch. Neurol. Psychiat., *40*:1126–1134, 1938.

28. Ley, A., and Bacci, F.: Trigeminal neuralgia; sensory defects and clinical results after selective division of the fifth nerve root by the suboccipital approach, using microsurgical technique. Excerpta Medica Fifth International Congress of Neurological Surgery, Tokyo, 1973, p. 171.

29. Loeser, J. D.: What to do about tic douloureux. J.A.M.A., *239*:1153–1155, 1978.

30. Malis, L. I.: Petrous ridge compression and its surgical correction. J. Neurosurg., *26*:163–167, 1967.

31. Maroon, J. C., and Albin, M. S.: Air embolism diagnosed by Doppler ultrasound. Anesth. Analg. (Cleveland), *53*:399–402, 1974.

32. Maspes, P. E., Nicola, G. C., Pagni, C. A., and Villani, R.: Results of transtentorial juxtapontine selective trigeminal rhizotomy in tic douloureux. Presented at Microsurgery Symposium, Vienna, 1972.

33. Olafson, R. A., Rushton, J. G., and Sayre, G. P.: Trigeminal neuralgia in a patient with multiple sclerosis. An autopsy report. J. Neurosurg., *24*:755–759, 1966.

34. Olivecrona, H.: La cirugia del dolor, Arch. Neurocir. (Buenos Aires), *4*:1–10, 1947.

35. Pelletier, V. A., Poulos, D. A., and Lende, R. A.: Functional localization in the trigeminal root. J. Neurosurg., *40*:504–513, 1974.

36. Pertuiset, B., Philippon, J., Fohanno, D., and Khalil, M.: Traitement microchirurgical de la névralgie faciale essentielle par neurotomie rétrogassérienne sélective transtentorielle. Rev. Neurol. (Paris), *126*:97–106, 1972.

37. Personal communications to the authors.

38. Petty, P. G.: Arterial compression of the trigeminal nerve at the pons as a cause of trigeminal neuralgia. Inst. Neurol. Madras, Proc., *6*:93–95, 1976.

39. Petty, P. G., and Southby, R.: Vascular compression of the lower cranial nerves: Observations using microsurgery, with particular reference to trigeminal neuralgia. Aust. New Zeal. J. Surg., *47*:317–320, 1977.

40. Poulos, D. A., and Lende, R. A.: Functional localization in the trigeminal ganglion in the monkey. J. Neurosurg., *32*:336–343, 1970.

41. Provost, J., and Hardy, J.: Microchirurgie du trijumeau; anatomie fonctionnelle. Neurochirurgie, *16*:459–470, 1970.

42. Revilla, A. G.: Tic douloureux and its relationship to tumors of the posterior fossa. J. Neurosurg., *4*:233–239, 1947.

43. Saunders, R. L., Krout, R., and Sachs, E., Jr.: Masticator electromyography in trigeminal neuralgia. Neurology (Minneap.), *21*:1221–1225, 1971.

44. Sjoqvist, O.: Eine neue Operationsmethode bei Trigeminuseuralgie, Durchschneidung des Tractus spinalis trigemini. Zbl. Neurochir., *2*:247–281, 1938.

45. Sjoqvist, O.: Ten years experience with trigeminal tractotomy. Brasil Med. Cir., *10*:259–274, 1948.

46. Spiller, W. G., and Frazier, C. H.: The division of the sensory root of the trigeminus for relief of tic douloureux; an experimental, pathological and

clinical study with a preliminary report of one surgically successful case. Philadelphia Med. J., *8*:1039–1049, 1901.

47. Taarnhøj, P.: Decompression of the trigeminal root and the posterior part of the ganglion as a treatment in trigeminal neuralgia; preliminary communication. J. Neurosurg., *9*:288–290, 1952.

48. Taarnhøj, P.: Decompression of the trigeminal root. J. Neurosurg., *11*:299–305, 1954.

49. Vidic, B., and Stefanotas, J.: The roots of the trigeminal nerves and their fiber components. Anat. Rec., *163*:330, 1969.

50. Wepsic, J. G.: Tic douloureux; etiology, refined treatment. New Eng. J. Med., *288*:680–681, 1973.

51. Wilkins, R. H., and Albin, M. S.: Unusual entrance site of venous air embolism during operation in the sitting position. Surg. Neurol., *7*:71–72, 1977.

124

GLOSSOPHARYNGEAL AND GENICULATE NEURALGIAS

GLOSSOPHARYNGEAL NEURALGIA

Historical Background

It was not until 1921 that glossopharyngeal neuralgia was defined as a clinical entity by Harris.[11] After unsuccessful mandibular alcohol blocks in two patients with pain in the throat, he deduced quite correctly that the pain was in the glossopharyngeal nerve. Eleven years earlier, Weisenberg had described a patient with pharyngeal pain due to pressure on the ninth nerve from a cerebellopontine angle tumor that was not relieved by partial section of the gasserian ganglion.[40] Sicard and Robineau had sectioned the ninth, tenth, and in one case the twelfth cranial nerves as well as a portion of the sympathetic chain in three patients with probable glossopharyngeal neuralgia, which they reported in 1920.[35] They failed to relate this disorder solely to the ninth nerve.

The syndrome as such was documented in subsequent reports, and in 1924 Adson described three cases in which temporary relief was obtained by extracranial avulsion of the glossopharyngeal nerve.[1,8,36] He suggested that intracranial section of the ninth nerve would be necessary for permanent relief and, indeed, first carried this out in 1925.[23] It remained for Dandy to describe the intracranial approach to the ninth nerve and to report success in two patients with glossopharyngeal neuralgia.[6] His technique, described in 1927, is the one at present employed in the surgical treatment of this disorder.

The occurrence of syncope and cardiac arrest in association with glossopharyngeal neuralgia was first described in 1942.[30] Soon other examples of such an association were reported; in these cases relief was obtained by intracranial section of the ninth nerve and filaments of the vagus nerve as well.[27,29,32,39]

Etiology

As in trigeminal neuralgia, the mechanism underlying glossopharyngeal neuralgia is unknown. In some cases the disorder may be related to pressure on the ninth nerve. Dandy stressed the incidence of cerebellopontine and nasopharyngeal tumors in patients who have glossopharyngeal neuralgia, possibly as high as 25 per cent.[6] Other causes cited are shrapnel wounds in the neck, vascular lesions, and ossification of the stylohyoid ligament.[3,10,22,26]

Characteristics

Glossopharyngeal neuralgia is not common, there being 1 case for every 70 cases of trigeminal neuralgia.[37] In its entirety, the area of involvement lies within the sensory distribution of the glossopharyngeal nerve and the auricular and the pharyngeal branches of the vagus nerve.[4] Typically pain occurs in severe lancinating paroxysms, but it may be continuous and of varying intensity, and, in some, too mild to be of any serious consequence.[2,38] The throat and base of the tongue are most commonly involved. Often pain extends to the ear and may extend to the base of the jaw and into the neck. The pain may be confined to the throat. Occasionally the ear alone is in-

J. S. TYTUS

volved, incriminating the tympanic branch of the glossopharyngeal nerve.[28]

Attacks may be induced by swallowing, chewing, and even talking. They may be accompanied by salivation and repeated coughing as if to clear the throat.[43] During an attack a patient may exert pressure with a finger deep within the ear.[7] Trigger zones are not common. They are occasionally found in the tonsillar fossa, but may lie in the region of the ear. In rare instances, syncope, cardiac arrest, and convulsions may accompany an attack.

When the symptoms are classic there should be little doubt in the diagnosis. It may be exceedingly difficult, however, to differentiate from trigeminal neuralgia if the pain is confined to the root of the zygoma.[20] Differentiation from geniculate neuralgia also may be difficult when pain is confined to the ear alone. It is helpful if one can reproduce the pain by stimulating the throat in the region of the tonsillar fossa. Cocainization of the tonsillar fossa may bring relief. If pain in the ear persists following this procedure, it may be relieved by tetracaine (Pontocaine) block of the jugular foramen, which suggests a contribution from the posterior auricular branch of the vagus nerve.[31]

Treatment

Patients with glossopharyngeal neuralgia may benefit from a trial of the medical regimen already discussed for trigeminal neuralgia. In some the pain will never be severe enough to warrant operative intervention. In most cases, however, operative intervention is the treatment of choice.

Operative Technique

Extracranial Approach

The glossopharyngeal nerve may be sectioned where it passes between the external and internal carotid arteries anterior to the hypoglossal nerve. This approach was introduced by Adson and, since then, has been advocated by others.[1,34]

Wilson and McAlpine have described sectioning the glossopharyngeal nerve in the pharynx, an approach amplified by Ishii.[19,42] A tonsillectomy is performed and the nerve is exposed where it courses beneath the inferior tonsillar pole at the junction of the posterior and lateral walls of the tonsillar fossa.

Intracranial Approach

To achieve permanent relief of glossopharyngeal neuralgia, intracranial preganglionic section of the nerve is necessary. Section of the upper two fibers of the vagus nerve as well has been advocated, since its posterior auricular branch may be involved.[4,6,21,37,39]

Suboccipital craniectomy is best accomplished with the patient in the sitting position under general anesthesia. A curved incision is made from just below the occipital protuberance to a point over and just below the mastoid process.[25] A generous suboccipital craniectomy is carried out and the dura opened in a stellate fashion with the edges sutured to the subcutaneous tissue for retraction (Fig. 124–1). The cerebellar hemisphere is elevated, and the lateral cistern over the lower cranial nerves is opened. The jugular foramen is exposed. The ninth nerve, lying most anteriorly, is distinctly separated from the vagus nerve by a dural septum and should be easy to identify. It is grasped with a blunt nerve hook and cut. The two most anterior fibers of the vagus nerve are isolated with the nerve hook and then cut. Magnification greatly facilitates this procedure. The dura is closed and the incision reapproximated in layers.

The sensory loss resulting from ninth nerve section presents no problem. There may be difficulty in swallowing initially, but this soon disappears. Cardiovascular complications have been reported following section of the upper vagal roots.[24] It would seem prudent, then, to monitor the cardiac status closely during the operation and for 24 hours afterwards.

GENICULATE NEURALGIA

Historical Background

After a thorough investigation of herpetic inflammation of the geniculate ganglion, Ramsey Hunt accurately described the sensory component of the facial nerve, the nervus intermedius, and outlined both its somatic and visceral distribution.[12–18] He also defined the clinical entity that bears his

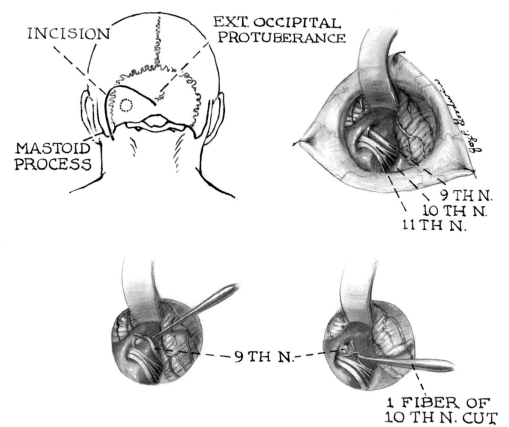

Figure 124–1 The curved incision should begin just below the external occipital protuberance medially and extend laterally to include the lambdoidal suture down to a point just below the mastoid process. Suturing the edges of the cut dura to the subcutaneous tissue facilitates exposure. The ninth nerve can be seen lying anteriorly, separated from the vagus nerve by a dural septum. It can be mobilized with a dull nerve hook and cut. In most cases the upper two fibers of the vagus nerve also should be sectioned.

name and a pain syndrome that he called "geniculate neuralgia."

In 1909 Clark and Taylor reported obtaining relief in a patient with geniculate neuralgia by sectioning the pars intermedia or sensory portion of the facial nerve. In this patient, as well as in two others described later, pain was severe and involved chiefly the ear.[9,41] There are few subsequent reports of this nature.

Sachs recently reported relief of pain after sectioning the nervus intermedius in four patients with pain primarily confined to the face followed for as long as 10 years after operation.[33] The findings strongly suggested histamine cephalalgia in two patients, and atypical facial neuralgia in the others. Sachs suggested the term "nervus intermedius neuralgia," but cautioned against overenthusiasm for nervus intermedius section in such cases until this condition was more thoroughly investigated.

Characteristics

Hunt described two forms of geniculate neuralgia: otological, in which pain is centered within the ear with secondary radiation into the deeper structures of the face, and prosopalgic, in which pain involves primarily the deeper structures of the face—the posterior orbit and the posterior nasal, malar, and palatal regions.

The otological form constitutes a fairly definite clinical entity with severe, often excruciating, pain beginning within the ear or just in front of it. The pain may occur intermittently, even in paroxysms, or it may be constant. Extension into the face occurs, but is not particularly severe. There may be trigger points in front of or within the ear. Periods of remission are reported. Glossopharyngeal neuralgia poses the greatest problems in differential diagnosis, which in some cases can be resolved only by performing the operation with the patient awake and stimulating the nerve.[28]

Hunt's prosopalgic form is considerably more indefinite and is difficult to distinguish from atypical facial neuralgia and, in some instances, even histamine cephalalgia. The pain is diffuse, constant rather than intermittent, and may be accompanied by lacrimation or other signs of parasympathetic overactivity.

Treatment

The otological variety is very painful, and every effort should be made to obtain relief. The primary therapy to be considered is operation, although a preliminary trial with Dilantin, Tolseram, and Tegretol may be warranted.

The prosopalgic type, on the other hand,

seems so indefinite that it would be difficult to justify a radical approach to the problem except under extreme circumstances. Indications for section of the nervus intermedius in such cases must await a more precise definition of the condition as a clinical entity.

Operative Technique

Local anesthesia seems preferable in these cases since one should reproduce the patient's symptoms by stimulating the nervus intermedius before cutting it. The head should be firmly fixed with the patient in the sitting position.

The lateral posterior fossa approach already outlined is satisfactory. The internal auditory meatus is exposed and the seventh nerve, lying most anteriorly, is identified (Fig. 124–2). The nervus intermedius will be found just behind it in front of the acoustic nerve. Depressing the eighth nerve and separating the nervus intermedius from above is usually satisfactory, although in some cases elevating the eighth nerve and exposing the nervus intermedius from below may be easier.[25] Again, the use of the operating microscope will greatly facilitate the dissection. If stimulation of the nervus intermedius reproduces the patient's symptoms, the nerve is cut. Closure is carried out in the manner already described.

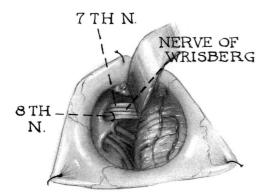

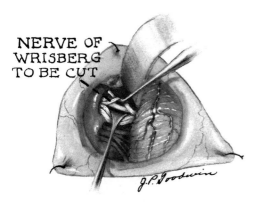

Figure 124–2 The seventh and eighth cranial nerves can be readily identified at their exit through the internal auditory meatus. The nervus intermedius (nerve of Wrisberg) will be found lying behind and slightly inferior to the seventh nerve. Gently depressing the eighth nerve facilitates exposure. Once the nervus intermedius is identified, it is carefully separated from the seventh nerve with a blunt nerve hook and cut.

REFERENCES

1. Adson, A. W.: The surgical treatment of glossopharyngeal neuralgia. Arch. Neurol. Psychiat., *12*:487–506, 1924.
2. Bohm, E., and Strang, R. R.: Glossopharyngeal neuralgia. Brain, *85*:371–388, 1962.
3. Brihaye, J., Perier, O., Smulders, J., and Franken, L.: Glossopharyngeal neuralgia caused by compression of the nerve by atheromatous vertebral artery. J. Neurosurg., *13*:299–302, 1956.
4. Chawla, J. C., and Falconer, M. A.: Glossopharyngeal and vagal neuralgia. Brit. Med. J., *3*:529–531, 1967.
5. Clark, L. P., and Taylor, A. S.: True tic douloureux of the sensory filaments of the facial nerve. I. Clinical report of case in which cure was effected by physiologic extirpation of the geniculate ganglion. II. Report of surgical treatment. J.A.M.A., *53*:2144–2146, 1909.
6. Dandy, W. E.: Glossopharyngeal neuralgia (tic douloureux): Its diagnosis and treatment. Arch. Surg., *15*:198–214, 1927.
7. Davenport, G.: Cited by Bailey, P.: Neuralgias of the cranial nerves. Surg. Clin. N. Amer., *11*:61–77, 1931.

8. Doyle, J. B.: A study of four cases of glossopharyngeal neuralgia. Arch. Neurol. Psychiat., 9:34–36, 1923.

9. Furlow, L. T.: Tic douloureux of the nervus intermedius (so-called idiopathic geniculate neuralgia). J.A.M.A., 119:255–259, 1942.

10. Graf, C. J.: Glossopharyngeal neuralgia and ossification of the stylohyoid ligament. J. Neurosurg., 16:448–453, 1959.

11. Harris, W.: Persistent pain in lesions of the peripheral and central nervous system. Brain, 44:557–571, 1921.

12. Hunt, J. R.: On herpetic inflammations of the geniculate ganglion. A new syndrome and its complications. J. Nerv. Ment. Dis., 34:73–96, 1907.

13. Hunt, J. R.: Otalgia considered as an affection of the sensory system of the seventh cranial nerve. Arch. Otol. N.Y., 36:543–556, 1907.

14. Hunt, J. R.: A further contribution to the herpetic inflammations of the geniculate ganglion. A syndrome characterized by herpes zoster oticus, facialis, or occipitocollaris, with facial palsy and auditory symptoms. Amer. J. Med. Sci., N.S. 136:226–241, 1908.

15. Hunt, J. R.: The sensory system of the facial nerve and its symptomatology. J. Nerv. Ment. Dis., 36:321–350, 1909.

16. Hunt, J. R.: The symptom-complex of the acute posterior poliomyelitis of the geniculate, auditory, glossopharyngeal, and pneumogastric ganglia. Arch. Intern. Med., 5:631–675, 1910.

17. Hunt, J. R.: The sensory field of the facial nerve: A further contribution to the symptomatology of the geniculate ganglion. Brain, 38:418–446, 1915.

18. Hunt, J. R.: Geniculate neuralgia (neuralgia of the nervus facialis). A further contribution to the sensory system of the facial nerve and its neurologic conditions. Arch. Neurol. Psychiat., 37:253–285, 1937.

19. Ishii, T.: Glossopharyngeal neuralgia: Surgical treatment and electron microscopic findings. Laryngoscope, 86:577–583, 1976.

20. Kahn, E. A., Crosby, E. C., Schneider, R. D., and Taren, J. A.: Correlative Neurosurgery, 2nd Ed. Springfield, Ill., Charles C Thomas, 1969, p. 492.

21. Karnosh, L. J., Gardner, W. J., and Stowell, A. Glossopharyngeal neuralgia: Physiologic considerations of the role of the ninth and tenth cranial nerves. Report of cases. Trans. Amer. Neurol. Ass., 72:205–207, 1947.

22. Lillie, H. I., and Craig, W. McK.: Anomalous vascular lesions in cerebellopontile angle. Severe neuralgic pain in ear and profound nervous disturbance; operation and recovery. Arch. Otolaryng., 23:642–645, 1936.

23. Love, J. G.: Diagnosis and surgical treatment of glossopharyngeal neuralgia. Surg. Clin. N. Amer., 24:959–962, 1944.

24. Nagashima, C., Sakaguchi, A., Kamisasa, A., and Kawanuma, S.: Cardiovascular complications on upper vagal root section for glossopharyngeal neuralgia. J. Neurosurg., 44:248–253, 1976.

25. Poppen, J. L.: An Atlas of Neurosurgical Techniques. Philadelphia, W. B. Saunders Co., 1960, pp. 78–285.

26. Pudenz, R. H., and Shelden, C. H.: Cited by Graf, C. J. ref. 10.

27. Ray, B. S., and Stewart, H. J.: Glossopharyngeal neuralgia: A cause of cardiac arrest. Amer. Heart J., 35:458–462, 1948.

28. Reichert, S. L.: Tympanic plexus neuralgia: True tic douloureux of the ear or so-called geniculate neuralgia: Cure effected by intracranial section of the glossopharyngeal nerve. J.A.M.A., 100:1744–1746, 1933.

29. Richburg, P. L., and Kern, C. E.: Glossopharyngeal neuralgia with syncope and convulsions. J.A.M.A., 152:703–704, 1953.

30. Riley, H. A., German, W. J., Wortis, H., Herbert, C., Zahn, D., and Eichna, L.: Glossopharyngeal neuralgia initiating or associated with cardiac arrest. Trans. Amer. Neurol. Ass., 68:28–29, 1942.

31. Robson, J. T., and Bonica, J.: The vagus nerve in surgical consideration of glossopharyngeal neuralgia. J. Neurosurg., 7:482–484, 1950.

32. Roulhac, G. E., and Levy, I.: Glossopharyngeal neuralgia associated with cardiac arrest and convulsions. Arch. Neurol. Psychiat., 63:133–139, 1950.

33. Sachs, E., Jr.: The role of the nervus intermedius in facial neuralgia. Report of four cases with observations on the pathways for taste, lacrimation and pain in the face. J. Neurosurg., 28:54–60, 1968.

34. Shaheen, O. H.: A surgical technique for the relief of glossopharyngeal neuralgia. Ann. Otol., 72:873–884, 1963.

35. Sicard, R., and Robineau: Algie velo-pharyngee essentielle. Traitment chirurgical. Rev. Neurol., 36:256–257, 1920.

36. Siebert, H.: Über Erkrankungen Peripherischer Nerven. Mschr. Psychiat. Neurol., 49:364–370, 1921.

37. Spurling, R. G., and Grantham, E. G.: Glossopharyngeal neuralgia. Southern Med. J., 35:509–512, 1942.

38. Stookey, B. B., and Ransohoff, J.: Trigeminal Neuralgia, Its History and Treatment. Springfield, Ill., Charles C Thomas, 1959, pp. 111–119.

39. Svien, H. J., Hill, N. C., and Daly, D. D.: Partial glossopharyngeal neuralgia associated with syncope. J. Neurosurg., 14:452–457, 1957.

40. Weisenberg, T. H.: Cerebellopontile tumor diagnosed for six years as tic douloureux. The symptoms of irritation of ninth and twelfth cranial nerves. J.A.M.A., 54:1600–1604, 1910.

41. Wilson, A. A.: Geniculate neuralgia. Report of a case relieved by intracranial section of the nerve of Wrisberg. J. Neurosurg., 7:473–481, 1950.

42. Wilson, C. P., and McAlpine, D.: Glossopharyngeal neuralgia treated by trans-tonsillar section of the nerve. Proc. Roy. Soc. Med., 40:82–83, 1946.

43. Wilson, S. A. K.: Neurology. Baltimore, Md., Williams & Wilkins Co., 1940, Vol. I, pp. 412–413.

125

TREATMENT OF PAIN OF GLOSSOPHARYNGEAL AND VAGUS NERVES BY PERCUTANEOUS RHIZOTOMY

Perhaps the most difficult decision in dealing with painful conditions that involve the lower face and oropharyngeal regions is determining the cause of the pain and the neural pathways involved. Diverse lesions of the intracranial and oropharyngeal structures give rise to painful states that resemble neuralgia of the glossopharyngeal and vagus nerves. Such lesions as neoplastic invasion, postoperative scarring, vascular lesions, and elongation of the styloid process are examples of the protean causes that must be considered prior to undertaking an operative procedure for pain control. Therefore, a comprehensive evaluation of the nervous, vascular, and upper respiratory systems is mandatory when a procedure for pain relief is being chosen. The application of selective blocking of trigger zones and nerves will usually help to develop a clearer understanding of the specific pathways involved in the pain problem. In cancer of the tongue, antrum, or floor of the mouth, pain frequently is referred through trigeminal, glossopharyngeal, and vagal nerve fibers.

A new approach to the treatment of these complex pain problems was developed as a result of experiences with percutaneous trigeminal rhizotomy. It became known, inadvertently, that an electrode could be placed in the neural compartment of the jugular foramen with considerable ease. A discussion of six cases treated by this technique has been published.[3]

TECHNIQUE OF PERCUTANEOUS VAGOGLOSSOPHARYNGEAL RHIZOTOMY

The technique of placing an electrode in the neural portion of the jugular foramen was learned serendipitously while operating on patients with trigeminal neuralgia. During the early years of the author's experience with trigeminal rhizotomy the electrode was placed blindly, and after the needle had penetrated the foramen at the base of the skull, x-rays were obtained to determine its precise placement. On several occasions these radiographs demonstrated passage of the needle into the posterior fossa by way of the jugular foramen (Fig. 125–1).

Subsequent anatomical studies indicated that this procedure could be done with the same reliability associated with percutaneous rhizotomy of the trigeminal nerve.[4,5] A

J. M. TEW, JR.

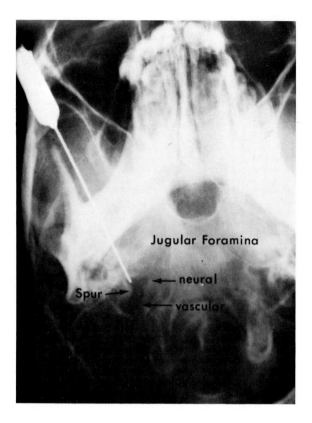

Figure 125–1 Electrode penetrating the neural portion of the jugular foramen. Note the bony spur that divides the neural from the vascular portion of the foramen.

basal view of the skull demonstrates that the nervous portion of the jugular foramen is in a direct line with and inferior to the foramen ovale (Fig. 125–2). Therefore, a technique similar to that for needle placement in the foramen ovale can achieve penetration of the jugular foramen (Fig. 125–3). Caudal inclination of the electrode, 14 degrees from the trajectory used to penetrate the foramen ovale, is required (Fig. 125–4). Special care must be exercised to avoid penetration of the carotid artery as the needle passes just medial to the orifice of the carotid canal. The sagittal projection of the needle toward the medial aspect of the pupil is the same as that used for penetration of the foramen ovale.

The location of the electrode must be confirmed by lateral and basal radiographs of the skull. Aspiration of cerebrospinal fluid and electrical stimulation provide further evidence of proper localization of the needle electrode.

Stimulation with 100- to 300-mv square-wave current for 1 msec at 10 to 75 Hz will provoke pain in the ear and throat. Coughing and contraction of the sternocleidomas-

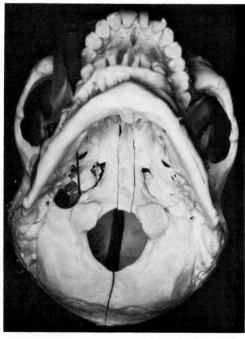

Figure 125–2 A basal view of the skull demonstrates the electrode placement in the medial and cephalad portion of the jugular foramen (pars nervosa). Note the alignment relative to the foramen ovale and the entrance to the carotid canal.

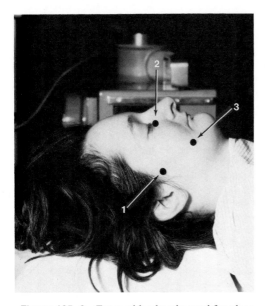

Figure 125–3 External landmarks used for placement of an electrode in the jugular foramen: (1) 3 cm anterior to the external auditory meatus, (2) medial aspect of the pupil, and (3) 2.5 cm lateral to the oral commissure (point of needle entry).

toid muscles will be evoked at slightly higher levels of current.

Thermocoagulation of the rootlets of the nerves should be performed after small amounts of methohexital (Brevital), 30 to 40 mg, have been injected intravenously. Monitoring of the temperature provides a method for gradual progressive destruction of the sensory nerve fibers. Sparing of the motor nerve fibers has not been possible; however, the author's experience with patients who had intact motor function preoperatively has been limited. The procedure is ideally suited for patients with invasive cancer of the head and neck, since commonly they have already lost vocal cord function on the affected side.

One should be experienced with both the technique of percutaneous rhizotomy and the physiological principles outlined in Chapter 120 prior to undertaking this procedure. The radiological and physiological steps must be followed carefully in each procedure. The techniques differ only in

Figure 125–4 Trajectory for electrode entering the foramen ovale or foramen jugulare. Note that one should change the vertical trajectory 14 degrees caudad while maintaining a similar inclination in the sagittal plane (aim for the medial aspect of the pupil) when penetrating the foramen jugulare. The image intensifier is used to monitor the electrode position. A complete technical description is given in Chapter 120.

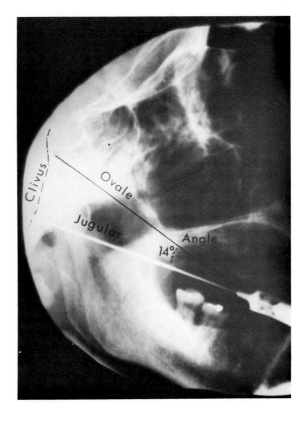

the variations in anatomy that concern the jugular foramen and the predominantly motor nature of the ninth, tenth, and eleventh cranial nerves.

Percutaneous rhizotomy is not advisable for the patient with idiopathic glossopharyngeal neuralgia whose vocal cord function is intact. Such a patient should undergo root section if his medical condition permits.[2]

RESULTS OF PERCUTANEOUS VAGOGLOSSPHARYNGEAL RHIZOTOMY

Using this technique, the author has operated on 11 patients, 9 of whom suffered excruciating pain due to invasive neoplasms of the head, neck, and oropharynx. Two patients had idiopathic neuralgia. Five of nine patients suffering intractable pain due to cancer were completely relieved until their deaths 4 to 18 months later. The other four patients were inadequately relieved because of insufficient nerve destruction or the spread of tumor to structures innervated by the trigeminal nerve or upper cervical nerve roots. These four patients with carcinoma required trigeminal rhizotomy, and three underwent section of the upper cervical roots to denervate adjacent areas involved by tumor.

Two debilitated patients with idiopathic pain that was intractable to medical therapy were completely relieved by percutaneous rhizotomy.[1] Vocal cord paralysis developed in both, however, and one developed aspiration pneumonia.

In conclusion, percutaneous rhizotomy of the vagus and glossopharyngeal nerves is a safe and effective procedure for patients with invasive cancer of the base of the skull. The procedure should not be performed when preservation of vocal cord function is desired.

REFERENCES

1. Bohm, E., and Strang, R. B.: Glossopharyngeal neuralgia. Brain, *85*:371–388, 1962.
2. Chawla, J. C., and Falconer, M. A.: Glossopharyngeal and vagal neuralgia. Brit. Med. J., *3*:529–531, 1967.
3. Tew, J. M.: Percutaneous rhizotomy in the treatment of intractable facial pain. (Trigeminal, glossopharyngeal and vagal nerves.) *In* Schmidek. H. H., and Sweet, W. H. eds.: Current Techniques in Operative Neurosurgery. New York, Grune & Stratton, 1977, pp. 409–426.
4. Tew, J. M., and Keller, J. T.: The treatment of trigeminal neuralgia by percutaneous radiofrequency technique. Clin. Neurosurg., *24*:557–578, 1976.
5. Tew, J. M., Keller, J. T., and Williams, D. S.: Application of stereotaxic principles to the treatment of trigeminal neuralgia by the percutaneous radiofrequency technique. J. Appl. Neurophysiol., *41*:146–156, 1978.

126

PAIN OF
SPINAL ORIGIN

Many of the aspects of pain of spinal origin are discussed in other chapters. The treatment of pain originating from metastatic malignant disease is discussed in Chapters 127, 129, 131, and 132. Specific problems such as pain following brachial plexus avulsion, postherpetic neuralgia, and the postincisional syndromes are discussed in Chapter 128. There remain two major areas in pain of spinal origin that require separate discussion. One of these is the chronic back pain complained of by that group of patients characterized by the general appellation "the chronic low back cripple," and the other is the so-called pain of paraplegia. The more straightforward aspects of disc disease are discussed in Chapters 78, 79, and 80. The patients included in the category of "chronic low back cripple" and those with the failed discectomy syndrome are much more complicated. This review presupposes that no further definitive neurosurgical or orthopedic therapy is available and deals with the symptomatic alleviation of pain only.

THE CHRONIC LOW
BACK CRIPPLE

The usual patient who presents with incapacitating back and leg pain has initially suffered a spinal injury or herniated intervertebral disc in the lumbar or cervical region. These patients continue to complain of pain following extensive therapy programs.[2,36] The causes of this type of pain are many, and each must be considered separately. There may be recurrent disc disease, root injury either by disc herniation or as a result of an operation, epidural fibrosis with compression of a nerve root, arachnoiditis, pain generated from a pseudarthrosis or a fusion mass or a bone graft donor site, a facet syndrome secondary to instability in the spine, or coccydynia. It is important to assess the contribution of each of these possible factors to the pain syndrome so that therapy may be directed specifically at the painful area whenever possible. Evaluation should include both plain films of the painful area and motion films to determine instability. Repeat myelography or computed tomography of the spine is indicated if there is a question concerning the origin of the pain. Electromyography can be helpful in determining nerve root injury, and thermography often will show a decrease in temperature in the distribution of an injured root, thereby giving a clue to the anatomical lesion. The history is most important in determining the origin of pain in the chronic low back cripple. In order to substantiate the impressions gained through the history, the examination, and the diagnostic studies, differential blocks of possible sites of origin of the pain usually are indicated.[12,19]

Recurrent Disc Herniation

Recurrent disc herniation or a secondary disc herniation at a level above a previously herniated disc always is possible. The syndrome is usually clear-cut and suggests disc herniation. Because new symptoms are superimposed upon old symptoms and signs, however, it may be difficult to separate them from the effects of previous disc her-

D. M. LONG

niation and operation. Myelography should be diagnostic, and removal of the disc with decompression of the nerve root usually is adequate therapy.

Nerve Root Injury

Injury to one or more nerve roots may occur as a result of disc herniation or as a consequence of operative manipulation. Again, the pain syndrome is typical. Usually there is little back pain associated with it unless there is a separate back problem that is generating pain. Typically, the pain is burning in character. It traverses the course of the sciatic nerve in the distribution of the injured root. Usually there is an associated neurological deficit, but this is not always the case. The skin temperature is reduced in the distribution of the nerve, and electromyography indicates denervation.

Blockade of the root in the neural foramen relieves the pain and substantiates the diagnosis. Because the results of operative rhizotomy have not been good, the open procedure is rarely indicated.[11,38] Radiofrequency neurotomy in the neural foramen as close to the posterior root ganglion as possible is a simpler technique and has a somewhat higher success rate. Operative rhizotomy has a 25 to 35 per cent success rate, whereas the rate of success of radiofrequency neurotomy is approximately 50 per cent.[15] Long-term evaluations of patients who have had radiofrequency neurotomy are not yet available, and the procedure requires continued evaluation.

Epidural Fibrosis

The signs and symptoms of nerve root compression secondary to epidural fibrosis cannot be differentiated from those of recurrent disc herniation or nerve root injury. The diagnosis is generally made by myelography or at the time of operation. The signs and symptoms are simply suggestive of nerve root compression (Fig. 126-1). Blockade of the involved root relieves the pain. When the syndrome is present after a single disc herniation, it usually is possible to reoperate carefully, meticulously dissect scar from the root, eliminate bony com-

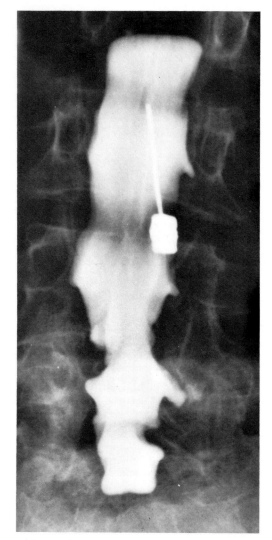

Figure 126-1 Myelogram in a 68-year-old white woman who had undergone five previous operations on the lower part of the back. The marked irregularities at L4–L5 and L5–S1 at the site of the previous operations are typical of epidural fibrosis. The patient suffered from intractable back and bilateral sciatic pain.

pression, and remove additional degenerated disc material. The reoperation may be very helpful. When pain has recurred after such an attempt, however, it is unlikely that further decompressive procedures will be of any value. In this case, radiofrequency neurotomy may be done. If the fibrosis has spread or multiple roots are involved, it is more likely that one of the techniques of neuromodulation or the general approach of conservative management will be indicated.[22,25]

Arachnoiditis

The pain of arachnoiditis is one of the most difficult problems in all of pain management (Figs. 126–2 and 126–3). The syndrome usually is characterized by burning

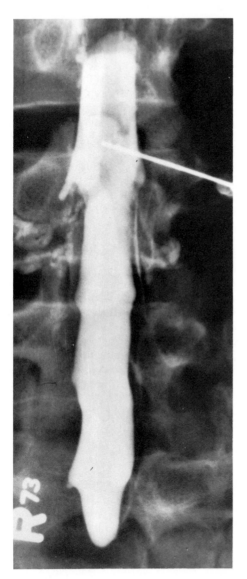

Figure 126–2 Lumbar myelogram demonstrating the typical tubular form of arachnoiditis. The lumbar sac is filled, but no nerve roots are visible in the dye column. The mass of the cauda equina can be seen as a shadow immediately beneath the needle. The patient was a 38-year-old white man who had undergone five operations upon the low back. He complained of intractable back and leg pain. At the time of operation, the roots of the cauda equina were found to be circumferentially adherent to the dural sac. Microdissection of the roots provided excellent pain relief. The lumbar myelogram demonstrates severe arachnoiditis and complete block at L3–L4.

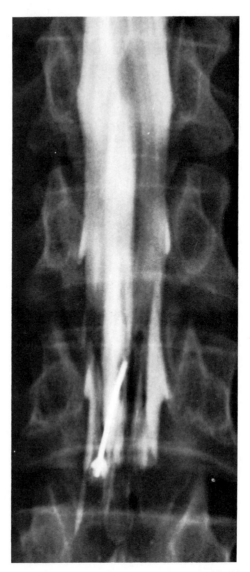

Figure 126–3 The patient was a 36-year-old white man who had had one previous operation. He complained of intractable bilateral leg pain and back pain. The nerve roots can be seen as negative shadows in the dye column, and all the roots of the cauda equina are adherent. At the time of operation the block was found to be a combination of intradural and extradural scar. Decompression and microdissection of the nerve roots has provided reasonable pain relief.

pain in both lower extremities. The pain may be isolated to a single root when the involvement is local, or may be widespread, involving many roots. There often may be a progressive neurological deficit with loss of bowel and bladder control and a syndrome similar to intermittent claudication in the lower extremities. In the absence of progressive neurological deficit, pain is the major consideration. The pain usually will have to be treated symptomatically. When progressive neurological deficit is present, reoperation with careful microdissection of the arachnoiditis from the elements of the cauda equina is warranted. The risks of this procedure are great, and it is a tedious and difficult operation. Its success in stopping progressive neurological deficit is excellent, however. Long-term pain relief is less satisfactory. Approximately 50 per cent of such patients achieve excellent relief of pain, but it is rare that the procedure is warranted for pain alone except when all other measures have failed. The pain of arachnoiditis will sometimes respond to intrathecal steroid administration. In this circumstance, 40 to 100 mg of methylprednisolone is injected into the lumbar subarachnoid space. These injections often cause severe pain and remarkable muscle spasms in patients suffering from arachnoiditis. A significant percentage, however, will receive months to years of relief from a single injection. When intrathecal steroids are not warranted or are not effective, the neuromodulation techniques are the best procedures currently available. Some of these patients will respond to transcutaneous stimulation, and many will respond to implantation of spinal cord stimulators. A trial of temporary spinal cord stimulation is warranted after conservative care has been given a thorough trial. Twenty-four hours of stimulation with good pain relief is sufficient to predict success of an implantable stimulator. Forty-eight to seventy-two hours is, however, more desirable and should be utilized if possible. In questionable situations, it may be necessary to leave the electrode in place for some time, and stimulation periods of as long as several weeks can be maintained. Longer use of the electrode requires that the patient be educated in maintaining its cleanliness and redressing it. Some neurosurgeons send these patients home and allow them to utilize the stimulator in their home environment. This practice usually is not necessary, but in some cases it may be advantageous when the patient cannot tell, from a few days of stimulation, whether the pain is relieved.[22,25,29]

Spinal Fusions

There are several reasons why fusions of the spine may cause pain. A pseudarthrosis may be present, and such areas of abnormal movement are often painful. Injection of local anesthetic into the region will relieve this pain and establish the diagnosis after the pseudarthrosis has been identified by x-ray. It is not unusual for pain to occur at a level above or below a fusion, owing to the abnormal strain placed on the joints at those levels. This situation can usually be readily appreciated from the history. The patient characteristically has pain in a localized area and can point to exactly where it occurs. The pain is aggravated by activity, particularly flexion and extension, and is usually relieved by rest. Again, blockade of the facets immediately above or below the area of fusion is diagnostic, and radiofrequency denervation of the facets is an excellent procedure.

The donor site in the ilium is also a frequent source of pain to patients with fusions. The diagnosis can be verified by infiltrating the area with local anesthetic. Injection of a dilute phenol solution or radiofrequency denervation throughout the area of the fusion donor site is usually sufficient to solve the pain problem.

Another group of patients appear to have pain originating from the fusion mass. Of patients undergoing facet blockade for continued back pain following discectomy and fusion, only 10 per cent were found to have responded favorably. However, 87 per cent had excellent relief of pain following infusion of local anesthetic on the posterior aspect of the fusion mass. Clinical application of this finding has not yet been possible.[27]

Coccydynia

Coccydynia is a perplexing syndrome in which there is burning pain in the coccyx. It may be unilateral or bilateral, characteristically occurs in middle-aged and elderly women, and has no known cause. It often appears as a symptom of psychiatric disturbance, and these patients must be carefully evaluated for possible psychiatric disease. Electrical stimulation done in the course of facet denervation has, however, elicited the fact that a common referral site for pain from L5–S1, and to a lesser extent from L4–L5, is into the region of the coccyx. A certain percentage of the patients with coccydynia, when appropriately chosen, can be relieved by facet denervation. Facet blocks in the lumbar region are performed in patients in whom a psychiatric diagnosis can be eliminated. Relief of pain following multiple facet blocks suggests that facet denervation will be effective. While it is still not certain how many patients with coccydynia fall into this category, it is definite that, in some patients with this complaint, instability of the spine is the likely cause and can be helped by facet denervation.[1,27]

Peripheral Blockade in Evaluation of the Chronic Low Back Cripple

By judicious use of differential blocks, it usually is possible to decipher the origins of pain in many of these patients. There is little evidence in the literature, however, that peripheral blocks of this kind are therapeutic for the chronic low back cripple. Their usual purpose is to delineate the source of the pain. It may be necessary to block individually such structures as facets, the posterior primary ramus, an injured root, a pseudarthrosis, a painful donor site, a fusion mass, or the disc itself. Individual blockade of these structures will often allow the site from which the pain originates to be identified accurately. These remarks presuppose that the patient had been managed according to the general principles of low back care and that the usual conservative means of treatment have been ineffective. It also is assumed that the patients have been thoroughly evaluated for the psychiatric aspects of the problem and subjected to the general management programs that should be employed in all patients with chronic pain as outlined in Chapter 116.

When the patient is a candidate for interventional procedures after successful implementation of the initial phases of a comprehensive pain program, properly chosen nerve blocks will usually delineate the source of the pain. An injection of a local anesthetic into the disc will distinguish those patients whose pain is secondary to disc degeneration and compression. Individual root blocks may be utilized to single out those patients with pain from root injury or compression. Facet blocks will identify those patients with pain originating in facet instability. Blockade of a pseudarthrosis in a fusion, the donor site, or the

fusion mass will identify patients with pain originating within these areas of abnormality. Arachnoiditis does not respond to these measures and is diagnosed more by exclusion than by response to any block. Sympathetic blocks may be used to identify patients suffering from reflex sympathetic dystrophies, and epidural blockade is often useful when pain is diffuse and multisegmental. This will delineate the exact extent of the pain and, at least, identify the spinal levels involved.[12]

The Facet Syndrome

Recently it has been re-emphasized that many patients suffering from the chronic low back syndrome have pain secondary to abnormal movement of the facet or involvement of structures innervated by the medial branch of the posterior primary ramus.[1,32] A so-called facet denervation has been devised in which an attempt was made to destroy the innervation of the facets by an open operation or by radiofrequency denervation.[27,32] It now appears likely that these procedures are effective in some patients because they involve the medial branch of the posterior primary ramus and provide generalized denervation of the back. This point is not yet certain, but it seems likely that any success the so-called facet denervation may have derives from far more than the partial destruction of the multiple sensory branches that enter the facet.[3]

These patients have a typical history. The pain is located primarily in the back, is aggravated by activity and totally relieved by bed rest. Usually it is improved by bracing. Leg pain is not a major part of the syndrome and, when it occurs, it usually is nonradicular. Radiation into the hip and upper leg in a diffuse fashion, however, is common. The diagnosis is made by temporary blockade of the involved facets. Since the majority of problems occur at C4–C5, C5–C6, C6–C7, and C7–T1 in the cervical region, and L3–L4, L4–L5, and L5–S1 in the lumbar region, these areas are blocked first. Bilateral blocks are usually employed, but unilateral blocks may be used if the pain is limited to one side. Relief of pain by the facet blocks is suggestive of the facet syndrome. Facet denervation usually is effective and approximately 70 per cent of patients who have not had spinal operations and who are chosen because of successful facet blockade will achieve relief with radiofrequency facet denervation that may last for several years. The procedure probably is better termed a medial branch neurotomy, however. It seems likely that the effect of the lesion is nonspecific. It is primarily of value in patients who have not undergone operation and has little effect upon any of the postoperative pain syndromes except instability.[27]

Facet and Root Blocks

The techniques for individual root blocks are well accepted and are not described further here. The technique for facet block, however, requires accurate description. In the lumbar region, the patient is readied in the prone position, and the location of the facets is carefully identified by fluoroscopy. A needle is passed from approximately 6 cm lateral to the midline to a point where the transverse process joins the root of the facet beneath the anteriormost margin of the inferior facet. One milliliter of 1 per cent lidocaine or its equivalent is injected at each facet level to be blocked. In the cervical region the approach is directly posterior and about 2 cm from the midline. The needles are placed directly on the facets under fluoroscopic control, and 0.5 ml of 1 per cent lidocaine is injected at each level to be blocked. L3–L4, L4–L5, and L5–S1 are routinely blocked in the lumbar region. In the cervical region, it is usual to block C4–C5, C5–C6, C6–C7, and C7–T1.

Radiofrequency Neurotomy

Radiofrequency neurotomies are either directed at specific nerves or utilized as a part of the so-called facet denervation and are employed in a similar fashion. In the lumbar region, the facet denervation needles are inserted at the level of each transverse process about 6 cm from the midline and, under fluoroscopic control, are directed at the same target point, which is the junction of the superiormost margin of the transverse process with the root of the facet at the caudal end of the neural foramen. Stimulation is then applied. Any commercial stimulator may be used. In general,

frequencies of 75 to 100 Hz, a 1-msec pulse, and voltages of 0 to 1 will be sufficient to stimulate the sensory nerves. Stimulation assures that the electrode has not moved too near the anterior root, and the spread of stimulation should mimic the patient's pain for optimum results to be obtained. A radiofrequency lesion is created with commercially available equipment. The parameters of lesion production should be carefully assessed for each radiofrequency generator, and the combination of parameters chosen that will destroy the maximum amount of tissue in this situation. In the cervical region, the electrodes are positioned as for a block, directly on the facet. Because of the proximity to the spinal cord and the vertebral artery, it is necessary to make lesions here at a lower temperature. In general, temperatures above 65° C should be avoided, and temperatures of 55° to 60° C often are satisfactory. The results of facet denervation in 149 patients with the chronic low back pain syndrome are given in Table 126–1.

Identical techniques are employed when a nerve root or a peripheral nerve is the target. The guide needle is placed as close to the target nerve as possible. Electrical stimulation is applied (1 msec, 60 to 100 Hz, 0.1 to 1.0 v) to be certain of the proximity to the nerve. The nerve is then carefully anesthetized. Otherwise, the lesion production will be very painful. Progressive lesions are produced until the desired loss of function and relief of pain are obtained. It is possible to produce analgesia with only minimal neurological deficit by carefully titrating current flow. These techniques may be very valuable for any pain syndrome involving nerve roots or peripheral nerves whose function is not critical. Pain relief is long lasting in 50 per cent of patients.[15]

TABLE 126–1 RESULTS OF FACET DENERVATION IN CHRONIC LOW BACK PAIN SYNDROME (149 PATIENTS)

HISTORY	RESULTS (PER CENT)		
	Excellent	*Fair*	*Failed*
No previous operation	61	18	21
1 operation	27	35	38
2 operations	0	35	65
More than 2 operations	0	26	74
Previous fusion	0	7.5	92.5
Drug addiction	0	0	100
Arachnoiditis	0	0	100

Adjunctive Measures To Avoid Reoperation

There are several other techniques that may occasionally be valuable in treating the chronic low back cripple before reoperation. The infusion of epidural local anesthetic with large doses of steroids is reputed to be successful in relieving pain of spinal origin.[4,12] The technique is probably not successful in more than one third of patients, even for a short time, but may give prolonged symptomatic relief to a small number of them. The use of intrathecal steroids has been mentioned. They may be of real value in arachnoiditis, but success is temporary, and permanent relief is rarely obtained. Some patients may be maintained by occasional blocks of this type, though eventually these simple local procedures will usually fail.[4] A small percentage of patients with a chronic low back syndrome will be dramatically helped by a trial of body casting. This does not seem to be directly related to instability, and it should not be inferred that lumbosacral fusion is indicated when this kind of favorable response to body casting is obtained. Rather it appears to be a nonspecific effect of decreasing total sensory input from the back. When body casting is satisfactory, then immobilization in a lightweight plastic laminate jacket may be of real value. It should be remembered when a body cast or brace is utilized that it is extremely important to have the patient in a meaningful exercise program.[12]

The efficacy of intradiscal injection of agents to dissolve an offending disc is not yet proved. Many patients have been treated. Results are equivocal, and controlled studies will be necessary before decisions can be made about the value of this therapy.[34]

Reoperation

As the last resort, reoperation may sometimes be necessary (Figs. 126–4, 126–5, and 126–6). It may be necessary to take down a fusion because of compression of spinal fluid pathways or neural structures, to perform a widespread laminectomy for decompression of the cauda equina and individual roots, or to dissect free arachnoidal adhesions to stop progressive neurolog-

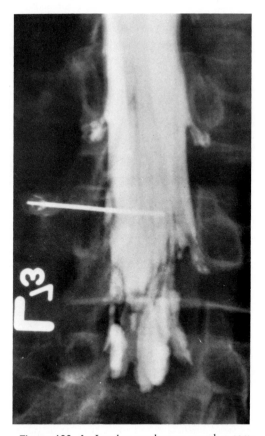

Figure 126–4 Lumbar myelogram reveals a complete block of spinal fluid flow over the body of L4 and severe intradural and extradural scarring. Nerve roots of the cauda equina can be seen matted together in the dural sheath. There are large extradural defects on the right side at L3–L4 and obvious intradural scarring as well. The patient is a 45-year-old white man who complained of severe back and leg pain. At the time of exploration, a large free fragment of disc was found at L3–L4 in combination with marked intradural and extradural scarring that had produced a complete block. Operation consisted of removal of the disc and extradural and intradural dissection of the scar. Pain relief has been satisfactory.

ical deficit or in an attempt to relieve pain. These are difficult procedures and should be undertaken only by individuals skilled in their performance and with broad experience in reoperative neurological procedures in the lower part of the back. This is particularly true of microdissection for arachnoiditis, which is a tedious procedure that requires an individual skilled in the use of the microscope, bipolar dissection, and micro-operative tools. Individual nerve roots must be teased free from arachnoidal reaction over long distances. With anything less than the most meticulous dissection, the possibility of serious nerve root injury

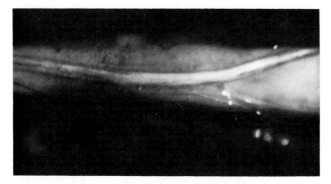

Figure 126–5 The condition found at operation in the patient whose myelogram is shown in Figure 126–2. The dense opaque arachnoid can be seen throughout the length of the L3 through L5 decompression. One large and several small nerve roots are seen coursing in the thickened arachnoid.

exists. Even in the most careful hands, injuries to small sacral roots are not uncommon. These procedures should be undertaken only as a last resort or with the clear-cut indication that there is a pathological process to be treated. They rarely are indicated as a treatment for pain alone and in general are not very successful as pain-relieving procedures.[12]

Neuromodulation of Pain

The techniques of neuromodulation have been found to be of considerable value in patients with chronic pain for whom none of the standard techniques are useful. Neuroaugmentation techniques have received their greatest application in the chronic low back cripple group of patients.

Transcutaneous Electrical Stimulation

The simplest form of neuromodulation is transcutaneous electrical stimulation, which grew out of the attempts to utilize implantable stimulators for pain relief. First conceived as a method for predicting success or failure of implantable stimulators,

transcutaneous stimulation was soon accepted as a treatment modality in its own right. It has been explored carefully during the development of neuromodulation as an effective pain relieving technique, and a great deal has been written concerning the syndromes to be treated and the techniques of stimulation to be used.[8–10,23,30] There are now a multiplicity of stimulating devices available on the market (Fig. 126–7). Most are battery-powered devices with approximately the same range of stimulus parameters. The majority utilize a spike or modified rectangular wave with variable pulse width, frequency, and amplitude.

The development of techniques for application of transcutaneous electrical stimulation has been largely empiric.[23] Experience dictates that the most effective electrode placements are those that cover or capture the area of pain—usually over painful areas or immediately proximal to them. Electrodes may also be placed over major peripheral nerves that supply the painful area or over major plexuses. Stimulation is applied initially at levels easily tolerable to the patient. It has also been suggested that high-level stimulation for short periods of time may provide pain relief that lasts for an extended period. In most in-

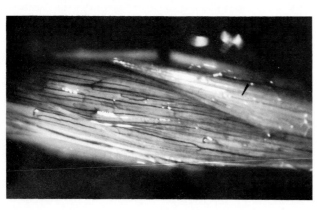

Figure 126–6 Less severe arachnoiditis. Normal nerve roots of the cauda equina are seen coursing throughout the operative photograph. In the area indicated by the arrow, the roots of the cauda equina on the right side are densely adherent to each other and bound together by typical intradural arachnoiditis. Careful microdissection produced adequate relief of intractable right leg pain.

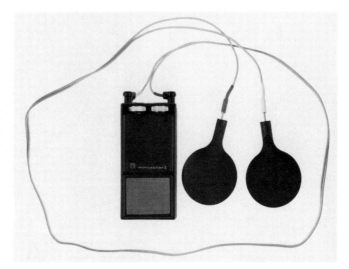

Figure 126–7 A transcutaneous stimulating device. The electrodes may be placed over or proximal to the painful area. The patient has to experiment with various placements to determine the most beneficial one.

stances. patients are taught to use the electrical stimulator and then allowed to carry out an extensive home trial, utilizing the device as much or as little as necessary. The amount of time required for electrical stimulation to be effective and the length of pain relief following use of the electrical stimulators are extremely variable. Many patients require hours of use of the device each day. Some patients, particularly those with peripheral nerve injuries, are able to use the device for only a short time to obtain excellent long-lasting relief after stimulation. If patients are felt to have had a satisfactory experience with the stimulator, then purchase is recommended after a one- or two-month trial. The device can be utilized for long periods of time, and the only serious side effect at present has been the development of a skin rash in a percentage of these patients.

Transcutaneous electrical stimulation may be employed in many painful states. It is effective in a significant percentage of patients with otherwise intractable pain and will be the only therapy required for those who are carefully chosen.[23] The stimulation may be employed over a major plexus or over the course of the major peripheral nerves in painful extremities.[23]

Implantable Peripheral Nerve Stimulators

Implantable peripheral nerve stimulators rarely are employed except in peripheral nerve injury.[21] They have been utilized in an attempt to treat the pain of chronic nerve root injury origin. Short-term results of sciatic stimulators for chronic low back pain usually are good, but the long-term results are not good and the procedure is not utilized frequently (Fig. 126–8).[6,21,30]

Spinal Cord Stimulation

Spinal cord stimulation is more satisfactory for pain of diverse origin. Approximately 50 per cent of such patients, otherwise untreatable, may be benefited significantly by this technique.[21] Percutaneously inserted epidural spinal cord stimulators may be more effective than operatively implanted devices. The simplicity of this procedure is attractive, and the short-term success rate appears to be approximately 70 per cent. Patients can be carefully chosen by trials of temporary epidural stimulation utilizing externalized electrodes. Patients who achieve good success with these techniques are candidates for implantation of permanently indwelling electrode systems (Figs. 126–9 and 126–10).[26]

The majority of patients treated with stimulators implanted in the spinal cord have suffered from chronic low back pain syndromes secondary to degenerative disc disease, multiple operations, and the complications of these procedures. The original spinal cord stimulators (so-called dorsal column stimulators) were implanted via laminectomy.[25]

Review of the data concerning their implantation indicates that approximately 50 per cent of patients treated with these devices achieve satisfactory pain relief. This

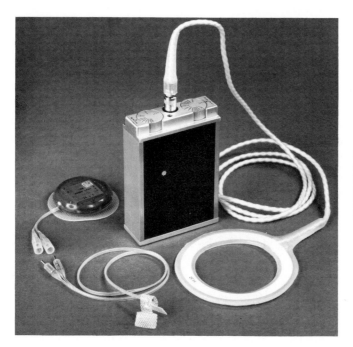

Figure 126-8 A peripheral nerve stimulator. The radiofrequency device and the cuff electrode are seen on the left. These represent the implantable portion of the device. The external battery power supply and the antenna are shown in continuity on the right.

figure is reasonable when one considers that these are patients for whom no other therapy is available. Because of the potential complications and technical difficulties of the procedure, however, the standard spinal cord stimulators implanted by lami-nectomy are now utilized only for specific groups of patients.*

The most commonly used spinal cord stimulators are those that utilize wire elec-

---

* See references 5, 13, 20, 24, 25, 28, 31, 35, 37.

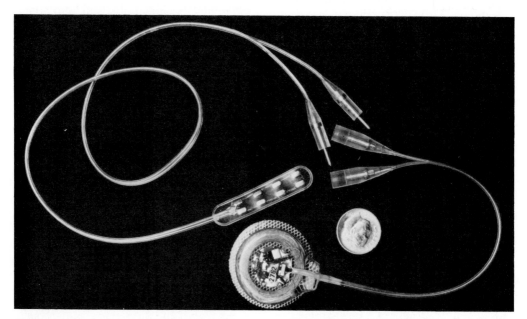

Figure 126-9 One type of implantable stimulator demonstrated in detail. The radio receiver and its output lead are compared with a dime to indicate size. The electrode shown here is devised for cerebellar stimulation. Similar types of electrodes with slightly different configurations are used routinely for spinal cord stimulation utilizing the same system.

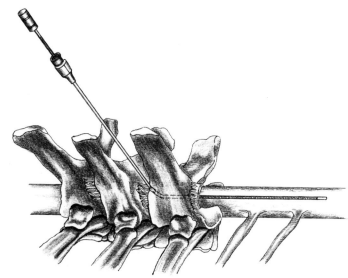

Figure 126–10 Artist's schematic drawing of the implantation of a percutaneously implanted epidural electrical stimulator. The 17-gauge thin-wall needle has been placed in the epidural space in the midline. A flexible wire electrode is now being threaded in the epidural space on the dorsal surface of the cord to the appropriate spinal level. The procedure is performed under fluoroscopy.

trodes that can be implanted percutaneously through needles. The technique for the use of these devices is very simple. The standard procedure is to test their efficacy by temporary stimulation with an epidural electrode. A standard epidural puncture is made, and a thin, flexible insulated wire is threaded into the epidural space under fluoroscopic control. The electrode is brought out through the skin, and stimulation is performed for several days. The relief of pain that is achieved is of real predictive value in determining the success of an implantable stimulator. The temporary electrodes are withdrawn after a thorough trial, and permanent electrodes are put in place if it appears the patient will benefit from spinal cord stimulation. The permanent electrodes can also be inserted through epidural needles. In this way, accurate electrode placement can guarantee good stimulation. If there is any question concerning electrode placement, the current models are fitted with temporary connectors that can be brought out through the skin after implantation of the entire device. Once it has been determined that the device can be implanted, the electrodes are attached to a radio receiver that is identical to those employed for all other human tissue stimulators. The external controls are the same for all these nervous system stimulators. The short-term success rates with this technique approach 70 per cent. The most serious problem is movement of the elec-

trode, requiring reoperation for replacement.

Brain Stimulation

Whether in the posterior medial thalamus, the sensory nuclei of the thalamus, or the posterior limb of the internal capsule, brain stimulation has been found effective for patients with pain of somatic and central nervous system origin. The majority of patients treated with this technique have suffered from thalamic pain, anesthesia dolorosa, and pain of spinal injury. As experience with it expands, this technique may very well prove to be valid therapy for the chronic low back cripple. At this time it is reserved for patients with severe nervous system injury sustained in the course of an operation upon the lower part of the back and those with severe arachnoiditis who do not respond to spinal cord stimulation.[16–18]

The treatment of the chronic low back cripple is a complicated process. The foregoing measures should be superimposed upon a comprehensive pain program and are unlikely to be successful if employed separately. These treatments are employed with the understanding that the general measures for low back care, which are important, are the responsibility of the patient. These always include weight loss, a meaningful exercise program, a functional activity program, and compliance with a comprehensive pain treatment program.

Anything less than this is unlikely to produce a long-term satisfactory result.[6,20,31]

POSTINCISIONAL SYNDROMES

There is a small group of patients who suffer characteristic pain following specific types of operative procedures. The most common of these is the so-called postthoracotomy syndrome, which consists of burning neuritic pain that follows the course of the thoracotomy and is related to injury of an intercostal nerve. The same kind of pain may occur with flank and abdominal incisions, but this is much less frequent. The diagnosis is made by the characteristic burning dysesthetic quality of the pain, its relationship to the previous incision, and its relief by blockade near the neural foramen. Posterior rhizotomy can be performed but rarely is necessary. Postincisional syndromes can usually be treated effectively by radiofrequency neurotomy. It is well to remember that, in general, at least three roots must be destroyed to obtain adequate pain relief.[14]

PAIN OF PARAPLEGIA

There are basically two mechanisms by which the paraplegic suffers pain. The first is mechanical in origin and relates to local abnormalities at the site of the fracture. The second pain problem originates in the spinal cord and represents one of the most difficult pain management problems.[14]

Pain of Mechanical Origin

The most likely cause of pain in the region of the fracture is instability. This is sometimes secondary to a poorly healed fracture. In this case fusion usually is indicated. More commonly, it is secondary to abnormal strain placed upon facets above and below the fracture site or above and below a fusion, or facets that have been injured at the time of the primary spinal trauma. Local facet blocks will usually relieve this kind of pain, and facet denervation frequently is successful. A second cause for local pain of this type is localized compression of nerve roots at the site of fracture. Root blocks will make the diagnosis, and radiofrequency neurotomy usually is curative. Patients often complain of a third type of generalized problem—a diffuse muscular aching in the region of the fracture. This pain has no specific treatment, but may respond to transcutaneous electrical stimulation.[7]

Spinal Cord Injury

The pain of spinal cord injury is a characteristic phenomenon.[14] It is diffuse below the level of the injury and corresponds to the area of sensory loss. It usually is burning and dysesthetic in character, often brought on by light touch, even though the patient has no perception of sensation. It often is related to motor movement, but more commonly it is spontaneous. The pain is constant but exacerbated by emotional disturbance. Careful questioning of these patients will indicate that much of the complaint relates to disordered sensation and not specifically to pain. Nevertheless, there is a major burning painful component that is distressing. No local measures have been of value. Cordotomy is in general ineffective, though destruction of the spinal cord above the level of the injury will usually relieve the pain.[33] Unfortunately, pain may recur after months to years even with resection of the spinal cord above the level of injury.[14] Transcutaneous electrical stimulation usually has little value in the treatment of pain of spinal origin but infrequently will bring relief. The medication regimen of amitriptylene (Elavil), 75 to 100 mg at bedtime, and fluphenazine (Prolixin), 1 mg three times a day, has been utilized empirically in these patients and will occasionally bring excellent results. Carbamazepine (Tegretol) and diphenylhydantoin (Dilantin) have been ineffective generally.

Stimulation of the spinal cord is more satisfactory for pain of diverse origin, and the percutaneously inserted epidural spinal cord stimulators may be effective. The simplicity of this procedure is attractive, and patients can be carefully chosen by trials of temporary epidural stimulation utilizing externalized electrodes. Patients achieving good success with these techniques are candidates for implantation of permanently indwelling electrode systems. Deep brain stimulation has been utilized in a small number of patients and is a promising avenue of therapy, but remains to be investigated.

It is especially important to recognize that these patients are often depressed, seriously addicted to narcotics, and without motivation. A comprehensive rehabilitation pain treatment program including elimination of harmful drugs and establishment of meaningful life goals may be very effective, and many patients thought to be suffering from hopeless pain of spinal injury origin can be satisfactorily rehabilitated by these measures alone.[2]

PAIN OF UNKNOWN ORIGIN

There remains a group of spinal pain problems for which no definitive cause can be found. As with virtually all other painful syndromes without a known cause, it is wise to avoid interventional procedures in this situation. Such patients should be carefully examined psychiatrically, and every effort should be made to discover the origin of the pain. When no underlying cause can be found, however, it is well to limit procedures to diagnostic blocks, simple procedures without risk, and the usual conservative measures for chronic low back problems.[2,12]

REFERENCES

1. Badgley, C. E.: The articular facets in relation to low back pain and sciatic radiation. J. Bone Joint Surg., 23:481–496, 1941.
2. Blumer, D.: Psychiatric considerations in pain. In Rothman, R., and Simeone, F., eds.: The Spine. Philadelphia, W. B. Saunders Co., 1975.
3. Bogduk, N., and Long, D. M.: The anatomy of the so-called articular nerves and their relationship to facet denervation in the treatment of low back pain. J. Neurosurg., 51:172–177, 1979.
4. Breivik, H., Hesta, P., Molner, I., and Lind, B.: Treatment of chronic low back pain and sciatica: Comparison of caudal epidural injections of bupivacaine and methyl prednisolone with bupivacaine followed by saline. In Bonica, J. J., and Albe-Fessard, D., eds.: Advances in Pain Research and Therapy. Vol. 1. New York, Raven Press, 1976, pp. 927–931.
5. Burton, C.: Dorsal column stimulation. Surg. Neurol., 4:171–180, 1975.
6. Campbell, J. N., and Long, D. M.: Peripheral nerve stimulation in the treatment of intractable pain. J. Neurosurg., 45:692–699, 1976.
7. Campbell, J. N., and Long, D. M.: Transcutaneous electrical stimulation for pain, efficacy and mechanism of action. In preparation.
8. Clark, K.: Electrical stimulation of the nervous system for control of pain. Surg. Neurol., 4:164–167, 1975.
9. Davis, R., and Lentini, R.: Transcutaneous nerve stimulation for treatment of pain in patients with spinal cord injury. Surg. Neurol., 4:100–102, 1975.
10. Ebersold, M. J., Laws, E., Stonnington, H., and Stillwell, G.: Transcutaneous electrical stimulation for treatment of chronic pain. Surg. Neurol., 4:96–100, 1975.
11. Echols, D. H.: Sensory rhizotomy following operation for ruptured intervertebral disc: Review of 62 cases. J. Neurosurg., 31:35–338, 1969.
12. Finneson, B. E.: Low Back Pain. Philadelphia, J. B. Lippincott Co., 1973.
13. Fox, J. L.: Problems encountered with neuropacemakers. Surg. Neurol., 2:59–64, 1974.
14. Freeman, L. W., and Heinburgery, R. F.: Surgical relief of pain in paraplegic patients. Arch. Surg., 55:433–440, 1947.
15. Gucer, G., Uematsu, S., and Long, D. M.: Radiofrequency differential neurotomy for pain of chronic nerve root injury. In preparation.
16. Hosobuchi, Y., Adams, J. E., and Rutkin, B.: Chronic thalamic stimulation for the control of facial anesthesia dolorosa. Arch. Neurol. (Chicago), 29:158–161, 1973.
17. Hosobuchi, Y., Adams, J., and Rutkin, B.: Chronic thalamic and internal capsule stimulation for control of central pain. Surg. Neurol., 4:91–93, 1975.
18. Hosobuchi, Y., Adams, J. E., and Weinstein, P. R.: Preliminary percutaneous dorsal column stimulation prior to permanent implantation. Technical note. J. Neurosurg., 37:242–245, 1972.
19. Hubbard, J. H.: The management of chronic pain of spinal origin. In Rothman, R., and Simeone, F., eds.: The Spine. Philadelphia, W. B. Saunders Co., 1975.
20. Hunt, W. E., Goodman, J. H., and Bingham, W. G.: Stimulation of the dorsal spinal cord for treatment of intractable pain. Surg. Neurol., 4:153–157, 1975.
21. Long, D. M.: Electrical stimulation for relief of pain from chronic nerve injury. J. Neurosurg., 39:718–722, 1973.
22. Long, D. M.: Use of peripheral and spinal cord stimulation in the relief of chronic pain. In Bonica, J. J., and Albe-Fessard, D., eds.: Advances in Pain Research and Therapy. Vol. 1. New York, Raven Press, 1976, pp. 395–403.
23. Long, D. M., and Carolan, M. T.: Cutaneous afferent stimulation in the treatment of chronic pain. Advances Neurol., 4:755–759, 1974.
24. Long, D. M., and Erickson, D.: Stimulation of the posterior columns of the spinal cord for relief of intractable pain. Surg. Neurol., 4:134–142, 1975.
25. Long, D. M., and Hagfors, N.: Electrical stimulation in the nervous system: The current status of electrical stimulation of the nervous system for relief of pain. Pain, 1:109–123, 1975.
26. Long, D. M., North, R., and Fischell, R.: A clinical study of spinal epidural stimulation for the

treatment of intractable pain. Submitted for publication.

27. Lora, J., and Long, D. M.: So-called facet denervation in the management of intractable back pain. Spine, *1*:121–126, 1976.

28. Nashold, B. S., and Friedman, H.: Dorsal column stimulation for control of pain. Preliminary report on 30 patients. J. Neurosurg., *36*:590–597, 1972.

29. North, R. B., Fischell, T. A., and Long, D. M.: Chronic dorsal column stimulation via percutaneously inserted epidural electrodes. Preliminary results in 31 patients. Appl. Neurophysiol. *40*:184–191, 1977–1978.

30. Picaza, J. A., Cannon, B., Hunter, S., Boyd, A., Guma, J., and Naurer, D.: Pain suppression by peripheral nerve stimulation. Part II. Observations with implanted devices. Surg. Neurol., *4*:115–127, 1975.

31. Pineda, A.: Dorsal column stimulation and its prospects. Surg. Neurol., *4*:157–164, 1975.

32. Rees, W. E. S.: Multiple bilateral subcutaneous rhizolysis of segmental nerves in the treatment

of the intervertebral disc syndrome. Ann. Gen. Proc. (Australia), *16*:126–127, 1971.

33. Rosomoff, H. L.: Bilateral percutaneous cervical radiofrequency cordotomy. J. Neurosurg., *31*:41–45, 1969.

34. Schwetschenau, P., Ramirez, A., Johnston, J., Barnes, E., Wiggs, C., and Martins, A.: Double blind evaluation of intradiscal chymopapain for herniated lumbar discs: Early results. J. Neurosurg., *45*:622–628, 1976.

35. Shealy, C. N.: Dorsal column stimulation. Surg. Neurol., *4*:142–146, 1975.

36. Sterbach, R. A., Wolfe, S. R., Murphy, R. W., and Akeson, W. H.: Traits of pain patients: The low back loser. Psychosomatics, *14*:226–229, 1973.

37. Sweet, W. H., and Wepsic, J. G.: Stimulation of the posterior columns of the spinal cord for pain control: Indications, technique, and results. Clin. Neurosurg., *21*:278–310, 1974.

38. White, J. C.: Posterior rhizotomy. Clin. Neurosurg., *13*:20–41, 1966.

127

PAIN OF
VISCERAL ORIGIN

Pain of visceral origin is conveniently divided into that caused by malignant disease and that which results from benign disease. Visceral pain from malignant disease is one of the most common problems faced by the neurosurgeon and one of the painful conditions that responds most readily to neurosurgical destructive procedures. There has been a significant discussion of the pathways by which visceral pain is carried to consciousness.[16] The most likely possibility appears to be via afferent fibers in association with the autonomic nervous system. It is also known that a significant number of small unmyelinated fibers enter the spinal cord by way of the anterior root, and it is possible that visceral afferent fibers join with somatic nerves for transmission of visceral pain.[13,16]

MALIGNANT VISCERAL DISEASE

Because the anatomical localization is important in decisions about the management of visceral pain of malignant origin, it is best to divide this pain problem according to anatomical localization rather than tumor type. Lung cancer, breast cancer, prostatic cancer, and cervical cancer are the most likely neoplasms to cause pain that requires specific treatment. Pain is commonly associated with direct involvement of adjacent tissues, spread to bone, involvement of an adjacent nerve plexus, and pathological fractures.[16]

Chest Wall Infiltration

Chest wall infiltration is most like to occur with lung cancer or breast cancer. The involvement is almost always unilateral, and extensive chest wall involvement may be surprisingly painless. Percutaneous cordotomy is a satisfactory method of relieving pain of this type.[9] The level must be raised well above the highest painful level in order to assure permanent pain relief. Adequacy of pulmonary function must be ascertained prior to the decision for cordotomy. Pulmonary reserve may have been reduced by the resection of lung tissue, lung infiltration, pleural effusion, or diaphragmatic paralysis. In percutaneous cordotomy, the lesion may extend far enough medially to injure respiratory fibers on the same side, which is usually the side of the normal lung. This situation may represent a serious problem for the patient whose respiratory function is impaired.[12]

Posterior rhizotomy is an alternative method of treatment. It may be accomplished by radiofrequency neurotomy performed percutaneously or by operative posterior rhizotomy.[2,4,13] The debilitated state of most of these patients usually makes the simpler percutaneous cordotomy the treatment of choice.[9]

Brachial Plexus Infiltration

The pain of brachial plexus infiltration often is excruciating. It usually is burning in character and involves the entire upper extremity with diffuse spread of pain into the chest wall. In addition, the patients complain of the lack of sensation and of the feeling of heaviness that the weakness in the extremity brings. Posterior rhizotomy rarely is indicated, since it leaves a functionless denervated extremity. Percutaneous cordotomy is the treatment of

---

D. M. LONG

choice. The respiratory function of the patient must be assessed prior to cordotomy, and if it is marginal, great care must be taken to not injure respiratory fibers. A high level of analgesia on the body is necessary to assure total relief of pain. A C2 level usually is required. Percutaneous cordotomy gives satisfactory relief of pain, but most patients continue to find the lack of sensation and motor function unpleasant.[9,12]

A related problem occurs with brachial plexus involvement secondary to scarring and the effects of radiation. In this instance, the same progressive loss of function may be present, and the pain often is excruciating. The pain tends to be of a burning dysesthetic character and is associated with autonomic manifestations such as changes in sweating and skin temperature or abnormal reactivity to cold. It is important to determine whether the pain is actually caused by tumor invasion or by the postirradiation syndrome. Exploration of the brachial plexus may be necessary to determine this fact. It is most important to make this decision, for with infiltration of the plexus with tumor, percutaneous cordotomy is the best treatment. When the problem is secondary to scarring and irradiation change, however, then other approaches must be sought. Such patients may live for extended periods and have late complications from destructive procedures.

Fortunately, these patients respond well to one of several forms of neuromodulation, as described in Chapter 126.[1] Transcutaneous electrical stimulation applied across the brachial plexus will relieve many of them.[7] Also, the implantation of a brachial plexus stimulator usually is successful. The brachial plexus stimulator is implanted via a supraclavicular approach. A 5- to 6-cm incision parallel to the clavicle is usually satisfactory. The entire brachial plexus is exposed, and the anterior scalene muscle is divided. The cuff electrode of the brachial plexus stimulator is wrapped around the entire plexus and sutured in place. The radio receiver of the stimulator is left on the same side on the anterior chest wall over the pectorals. Usually it is important to obtain stimulation in the entire plexus area. If an individual area is to be stimulated, then a smaller electrode may be placed around on individual trunk, division, or branch.[1]

Bone Pain and Pathological Fracture

Widespread bony metastases are often extremely painful. The most common tumors to present in this way are carcinoma of the breast and carcinoma of the prostate. Usually more definitive therapy—radiotherapy, chemotherapy, or endocrine therapy—should be utilized prior to any decision for a pain-relieving procedure. When the malignant metastasis is from breast or prostate, ablation of the pituitary may be considered. Hypophysectomy is extremely effective in relieving bone pain in carcinoma of the breast when the tumor is hormonally sensitive, and a significant number of patients with carcinoma of the prostate with intractable bone pain will be helped.[10] If the bone pain is from well-localized metastatic disease (often associated with pathological fracture), then percutaneous cordotomy is the procedure of choice. Widespread bone pain not amenable to therapy by other means may be relieved by one of the techniques of neuromodulation. Surprisingly, transcutaneous electrical stimulation is often very helpful in the management of such patients and may provide relief that is quite satisfactory. The results with spinal cord stimulation can be spectacular in this problem. Some of the author's most gratifying experiences have been with patients with widespread bony metastases treated by this method. Brain stimulation, discussed in Chapter 126, has not been used extensively, but is a promising technique for the relief of patients with bone pain.[8]

A less common cause of pain with bony metastases is compression of one or more nerve roots secondary to direct compression by tumor or collapse of an involved vertebral body. Local decompression with or without section of the involved nerve root usually is indicated in such cases.

Pelvic Infiltration

Pain located in the pelvis usually is bilateral. Most commonly it is associated with uterine cervical cancer or rectal cancer. When pain is unilateral, percutaneous cordotomy is the procedure of choice. When the pain is bilateral, however, a bilateral cordotomy is required. If the pain is midline or even on one side of the pelvis, a bilateral cordotomy will be required in almost every case. In the situation in which the pain is in the pelvis and appears to be unilateral, it will be found that the more severe pain is on one side and masking the lesser pain in the midline or on the other side. As soon as the more severe pain is relieved, the lesser pain will become symptomatic. In performing an open cordotomy in the dorsal area, both spinothalamic tracts should be cut at one operation. If a radiofrequency cordotomy is done, it is appropriate to wait until a second procedure for the second one to be sure that it is necessary. Likewise, if an open cordotomy is done in the high cervical area, it is wise to do the opposite side in the dorsal area as a second procedure.

It is possible to perform bilateral cordotomy safely if there is no attempt to achieve high levels. Bilateral cordotomy carries greater risk than the unilateral procedure, however. There is a significant risk of impairment of bladder and sexual function, and the risk of serious respiratory difficulty is greater. Percutaneous cervical cordotomy combined with open thoracic cordotomy under local anesthesia minimizes the risk of respiratory insufficiency, but has the same risk of impairing bladder and sexual function. Most commonly, however, such patients already have impaired bladder and sexual function. Often colostomy has been performed, so the side effects of the cordotomy are less important than the desired pain relief. In this case, bilateral cordotomy can be done, but the patient still must be warned of the possibility of requiring permanent catheter drainage of the bladder.[9,12]

When bowel and bladder function have been lost, it may be possible to divide all of the sacral fibers by a simple procedure. The caudal end of the dural sac is exposed by a small sacral laminectomy. The S1 roots are identified, and the sac is ligated and cut below the S1 roots.[2] It is said that preservation of a single S2 root will preserve bladder function. The variability of innervation of the human bladder is great enough, however, to make it wise to perform differential sacral root blocks prior to making this decision.[11] These blocks will allow adequate assessment of which roots are important in bladder control and will also assure that the procedure will be successful. If block of the sacral root relieves pain, then it is virtually certain that division of the root would eliminate the pain problem. When one sacral root is spared in order to preserve bladder function, the possibility of pain recurrence always exists.[2,11]

Involvement of the *lumbosacral plexus* may be bilateral or unilateral. Percutaneous cordotomy is the procedure of choice. The same syndrome of postirradiation neuritis may occur in the lumbosacral plexus. Although the techniques of neuromodulation are much more difficult to use here, spinal cord stimulation is useful and will relieve many such patients (Table 127–1).[6,8]

In patients with far advanced malignant disease in whom preservation of bowel and bladder function is not a consideration, the subarachnoid injection of absolute alcohol or phenol may be a useful technique. These neurolytic agents are injected into the subarachnoid space, and destruction of the appropriate nerves can be carefully controlled by pooling the material around the nerves to be destroyed. The control of the procedure is not sufficiently precise, however, to allow its use in patients with intact neurological function, except in the hands of skilled individuals. The technique is capricious, and only an experienced operator is able to obtain pain relief consistently without excessive neurological deficit. For this reason, these intrathecal procedures have never achieved great popularity and are relegated for the most part to the treatment of patients who already have serious neurological deficits or are in the terminal stages of the disease.[3]

Another technique for the management of midline perineal pain is midline myelotomy. In this procedure, the spinal cord is split in longitudinal fashion in the midline over the areas to be denervated. The procedure has been utilized primarily in the lower lumbar and sacral segments. Pain relief is reasonable, but the procedure has a

TABLE 127–1 RESULTS OF DORSAL COLUMN STIMULATION FOR CANCER PAIN*

RELIEF OBTAINED	NUMBER OF PATIENTS (59 TOTAL)	PER CENT
Excellent	19	32
Satisfactory	<u>13</u>	<u>22</u>
	32	54

* Data from Long, D. M., and Hagfors, N.: Electrical stimulation in the nervous system; The current status of electrical stimulation of the nervous system for the relief of pain. Pain, 1:109–123, 1975.

distressing incidence of dysesthesias and has received limited application to date. Usually a neurological deficit can be avoided.[5]

Neuromodulation techniques may be valuable in pelvic or abdominal pain. Transcutaneous electrical stimulation applied over the appropriate lumbar or sacral roots will benefit some of these patients. Spinal cord stimulation has been valuable and a success rate greater than 50 per cent has been reported.[6] The most difficult problems, however, those of midline perineal pain, are equally difficult to treat with spinal cord stimulation, for it is not uncommon for these devices to fail to produce stimulation in the pelvis and so fail to provide pain relief.[8]

Abdominal Cancer

When abdominal pain secondary to malignant disease is unilateral, percutaneous cordotomy is the treatment of choice. When the pain is bilateral it is very frequently secondary to axial involvement. This is particularly true of carcinoma of the pancreas, which is the most serious of these pain-producing lesions. Bilateral cordotomy carries the same risk as it does when used for treatment of the pain of chest or pelvic neoplasms. It is much easier, however, to achieve adequate pain relief at adequate levels than with either of the other two groups. Care must be taken to bring the levels only as high as required for pain relief, but in general, this is simpler to control than when bilateral high levels are required or when pelvic pain must be relieved.[9]

Neuromodulation techniques are also effective (Table 127–2). Transcutaneous electrodes applied over the splanchnic bed, or in the appropriate area of thoracic outflow for the pain involved, may often give excellent pain relief. Fortunately, this is particularly true with carcinoma of the pancreas, which is an extremely difficult pain problem to manage. Spinal cord stimulation may be effective and certainly can be tried on a temporary basis before resorting to bilateral percutaneous cordotomy.[6,7,8]

Pain of pancreatic carcinoma or that caused by infiltration of the abdominal wall in the region of the pancreas is often re-

TABLE 127–2 DORSAL COLUMN STIMULATION FOR CANCER PAIN AS REPORTED IN LITERATURE

REPORT	NUMBER OF PATIENTS	RESULTS	
		Excellent	Good
Shelden et al.*	17	5	3
Long and Erickson†	6	2	1
Nashold‡	1	—	—
Nielson et al.§	16	8	2
Hunt et al.‖	1	—	—
Pineda¶	4	2	2
Clark**	4	—	2
Burton††	1	—	—
Hoppenstein‡‡	9	2	3
	59		

* Electrical stimulation of the nervous system. Surg. Neurol., 4:127–133, 1975.

† Stimulation of the posterior columns of the spinal cord for relief of intractable pain. Surg. Neurol. 4:134–142, 1975.

‡ Dorsal column stimulation for control of pain: A three year follow-up. Surg. Neurol., 4:146–148, 1975.

§ Experience with dorsal column stimulation for relief of chronic intractable pain, 1968–73. Surg. Neurol., 4:148–153, 1975.

‖ Stimulation of the dorsal spinal cord for treatment of intractable pain. Surg. Neurol., 4:153–157, 1975.

** Electrical stimulation of the nervous system for control of pain. Surg. Neurol., 4:164–167, 1975.

†† Dorsal column stimulation. Surg. Neurol., 4:171–180, 1975.

‡‡ Electrical stimulation of the ventral and dorsal columns for relief of chronic intractable pain. Surg. Neurol., 4:187–199, 1975.

lieved by celiac blocks. The block is first performed with local anesthetic, and if that is successful, alcohol or phenol blockade of the celiac ganglion is done. Pain relief usually is satisfactory, though the procedure is dangerous because of the proximity of great vessels. Occasionally posterior rhizotomy may be indicated, but it rarely is useful in abdominal pain.

NONMALIGNANT VISCERAL DISEASE

The pain of nonmalignant visceral disease is usually treated most adequately by direct attention to the disease process itself. Operative procedures are rarely indicated, except in a few very specific situations. The advent of neuromodulation techniques and the possibility of carrying out percutaneous radiofrequency neurotomy with safety have altered this indication in certain specific nonmalignant visceral problems.

Pancreatic Pain

The pain of pancreatitis is one of the most difficult to manage. This pain may respond to transcutaneous electrical stimulation applied over the T5 through T10 area or over the T12 region posteriorly.[7] When transcutaneous stimulation is ineffective, the use of percutaneously implanted spinal cord stimulating electrodes in the same area may be effective. Celiac axis block is also useful, but its danger makes it more attractive in treating cancer pain. Bilateral dorsal root section, T5 through T10, has been advocated, but it is a major procedure and involves a significant risk of paraplegia. It should be employed only as a last resort after failure of neuromodulation techniques.[16]

Cardiac Pain

The two pain problems that may become important in the management of a patient with cardiac disease are pericarditis and intractable angina. Both have been treated by operative means, usually bilateral thoracic sympathectomy at the appropriate levels (T1–T4). The treatment has not found widespread usage.[14,15] Neuromodulation techniques may prove to be useful in these patients. Transcutaneous stimulation has been used for the treatment of both pericarditis and angina, though its safety and efficacy have not yet been proved. Spinal cord stimulation with the electrodes placed in the upper thoracic area has been used for the treatment of otherwise intractable angina, but the number of patients treated to date is too small to allow any judgment concerning the usefulness of these techniques.

Pleuritic Pain

If the pain of pleuritis is widespread, then no operative procedure except cordotomy is likely to be of value. In more localized pain, particularly that which follows operation, it usually is possible to denervate the area by peripheral neurotomy or posterior rhizotomy. The appropriate nerves should be chosen by differential local anesthetic blocks, and then radiofrequency lesions of these nerves, or their operative division, can be performed to achieve excellent relief of the pain.[4]

Gallbladder and Stomach Pain

These two organs rarely present pain syndromes that require neurosurgical intervention. When chronic ulcer pain is not relieved by the usual means, or when gallbladder outlet stricture produces a chronic pain problem, it may be possible to treat them satisfactorily by the use of transcutaneous electrical stimulation over the splanchnic bed. Stimulation of the spinal cord is an alternative method of therapy that can be used if transcutaneous electrical stimulation is ineffective. A trial of stimulation is always warranted before a permanent implant is performed. These disease states are difficult to assess. Brief favorable responses to therapy are common, and it is important to be as certain as possible that the procedure will be effective by a prolonged trial of temporary stimulation.

Splanchnicectomy also may be considered. The magnitude of the operation required is significant, however, and the diagnosis of organic disease must be made carefully. Simpler measures should be exhausted before any major interventional procedures are employed.[16]

Intra-Abdominal Pain of Unknown Cause

One of the most common presentations in a gastroenterological practice is undiagnosable abdominal pain. Many of these patients are referred to the chronic pain treatment center or to the physician interested in pain. It is rare that any interventional procedure is warranted in an abdominal pain problem in which a definitive diagnosis cannot be reached.

A second problem, and one that is even more complicated, is the undiagnosable postoperative abdominal pain. Again, unless there appears to be a clear-cut reason for the pain, it is unwise to do interventional procedures. The more operations the patient has undergone, the less likely there is to be a treatable cause. Of course, if the symptoms are suggestive of a neuroma, then diagnostic nerve blocks and radiofrequency or operative neurotomy may be employed. The response of these undiagnosable pains to nerve blocks is variable, and the fact that a block has been effective in relieving pain does not mean that division of the appropriate nerve will be equally effective.

Renal and Vesical Pain

There are few nonmalignant renal processes that require therapy for pain. When it is certain that the pain is of renal or ureteral origin, however, then sympathectomy of the splanchnic trunks and T10–L1–L2 rhizotomy usually will relieve it. Posterior rhizotomy by the radiofrequency approach in the general area of T10 through L1 or L2 may also be effective. Diagnostic nerve blocks should be performed to be certain of the level of neurotomy that is required.[4,11,14]

Bladder pain is one of the most serious problems for which there is no satisfactory neurosurgical answer. Cordotomy has been employed, but it must be bilateral and carries a risk that usually is unjustified by the level of pain.[9,12] Differential sacral blocks may be effective if the pain is mediated from one or two sacral roots. Operative or radiofrequency lesions may then be performed on the appropriate roots. It is important to control these lesions carefully with cystometry so that no impairment of bladder control occurs. The possibility of loss of sexual function in such procedures is always present. Transcutaneous electrical stimulation applied over the sacral area may be very valuable in controlling bladder pain. Percutaneously inserted spinal cord or cauda equina stimulating electrodes can be used. Electrodes have been placed in the sacral region with good relief of bladder pain, and higher electrodes in the low thoracic region have also been utilized effectively in ureteral pain.[11]

Dysmenorrhea

Pelvic neurectomy or presacral neurectomy has been advocated for relief of dysmenorrhea.[14,15] Success is variable and the procedure is rarely employed now. Transcutaneous electrical stimulation has been reported to be of benefit in treating such patients.[7] No extensive controlled studies have been reported that would allow assessment of the efficacy of the technique, however. Spinal cord stimulation should be effective, but its use has not been reported.

Pain of Vascular Origin

The pain of vascular ischemic disease, the shoulder-hand syndrome, and severe vasospastic conditions can be considered under the general heading of pain of vascular origin. The pain of all these conditions appears to be mediated largely through afferents with the sympathetic system, though this is still unproved. Sympathetic blockade is the most reliable way of relieving this pain. Temporary sympathetic blockade is carried out at the appropriate levels in the sympathetic chain to obtain temporary chemical sympathectomy for the painful part. When repeated sympathetic blocks are effective in relieving the pain but do not permanent relief, then sympathectomy can be relied upon to relieve the pain.[16] Transcutaneous electrical stimulation has been reported to be of great value in the treatment of pain of vascular origin. Increases in blood flow have been reported, and significant pain relief has been described. Implantable stimulators have not been used in a sufficient number of patients to assess their efficacy.[1]

GENERAL CONSIDERATIONS

The most common, and the most serious, visceral pain problems are those that complicate malignant disease. All too often, the neurosurgeon is asked to see a patient in the terminal stages of disease, no longer able to tolerate procedures that would have relieved the pain, hopelessly addicted to narcotics, and with profound neurological loss. Such a patient can rarely be benefited by any procedure, and the risks and complications of intervention are much greater than they would have been earlier. It is important, if interventional procedures are to be used, that they be applied early when their beneficial effects can give the patient a significant period of freedom from pain and from the risks of long-term narcotic addiction. It is equally important, however, for the neurosurgeon to be certain that the pain that the patient suffers warrants a destructive procedure. Pain requiring the regular use of narcotics should be present before cordotomy is done. While there are no fixed guidelines, in general, the patients should at least require codeine three to four times a day on a regular basis before consideration of an interventional procedure is warranted.

In late stages of the disease, narcotic addiction may be an acceptable complication of the only means of treating otherwise intractable pain, but the problem of tolerance makes narcotics less than satisfactory even in this situation. Cordotomy is the procedure of choice in most patients with malignant disease when the pain is unilateral. Bilateral cordotomy can be successfully employed, but the risks are significantly greater. Transcutaneous electrical stimulation is surprisingly effective in malignant disease and may be employed to relieve pain, especially in the early stages of the pain process. Spinal cord stimulation may be very valuable. More than 50 per cent of patients with cancer pain can be improved significantly by the use of an implantable spinal stimulator.[6] The advent of the percutaneous techniques for implantation of spinal cord stimulators has made this low percentage much more attractive. The use of spinal cord stimulation for the treatment of cancer pain is steadily increasing. Deep brain stimulation, particularly that applied to the reticular areas of the thalamus, is most attractive in theory. An insufficient number of patients have been treated to allow a judgment about the value of this technique, and deep brain stimulation must be considered to be still in the assessment phase. It is important to remember the general principles of chronic pain management when dealing with patients with pain of visceral origin, even when the underlying process is malignant. Control of the general effects of pain upon the patient is still important. Many patients suffering from intractable pain of cancer will prove not to need an interventional procedure after treatment of depression, elimination of harmful drugs and narcotic addiction, and the use of transcutaneous electrical stimulation.

Patients with visceral pain problems of nonmalignant origin should be treated as comprehensively as possible. Interventional procedures should be avoided; neuromodulation techniques are more attractive than destructive procedures in such patients. Any interventional procedures should follow accurate diagnosis of the cause of the pain.

REFERENCES

1. Campbell, J., and Long, D. M.: Peripheral nerve stimulation in the treatment of intractable pain. J. Neurosurg., 45:692–699, 1976.
2. Felsoory, A., and Crue, B. L.: Results of 19 years experience with sacral rhizotomy for perineal and perianal cancer. Pain, 2:431–434, 1976.
3. Flanigan, S., and Boop, W. C.: Spinal intrathecal injection procedures in the management of pain. Clin. Neurosurg., 21:229–238, 1974.
4. Gucer, G., Uematsu, S., and Long, D. M.: Radiofrequency differential neurotomy for relief of pain of chronic nerve root injury origin. In preparation.
5. Hosobuchi, Y.: Midline myelotomy for relief of perineal pain. Presented to American College of Surgeons, Miami, 1975.
6. Long, D. M.: Spinal cord stimulation for pain of cancer. Presented to the First World Congress, International Society for the Study of Pain, Florence, 1975.
7. Long, D. M., and Carolan, M. I.: Cutaneous afferent stimulation in the treatment of chronic pain. Advances Neurol., 4:755–759, 1974.
8. Long, D. M., and Hagfors, H.: Electrical stimulation of the nervous system: The current status of electrical stimulation of the nervous system for relief of pain. Pain, 1:109–123, 1975.
9. Mullan, S.: Percutaneous cordotomy (RF). Advances Neurol., 4:677–682, 1974.
10. Ray, B. S.: Hypophysectomy by craniotomy. In Youmans, J. R., ed.: Neurological Surgery. Philadelphia, W. B. Saunders Co., 1973, pp. 1915–1927.
11. Rockswold, G., Bradley, W. E., and Timm, G. W.: Electrophysiological Technique for Evaluating Lesions of the Conus Medullaris and Cauda Equina. J. Neurosurg., 45:321–326, 1976.
12. Rosomoff, H. L.: Percutaneous radiofrequency cervical cordotomy for intractable pain. Advances Neurol., 4:683–688, 1974.
13. White, J. C.: Sensory innervation of the viscera: Studies of visceral afferent neurones in man based on neurosurgical procedures for the relief of intractable pain. Res. Publ. Ass. Nerv. Ment. Dis., 23:373–390, 1943.
14. White, J. C.: Role of sympathectomy in relief of pain. Progr. Neurol. Surg., 7:131–152, 1975.
15. White, J. C., and Bland, E. F.: The surgical relief of severe angina pectoris: Methods employed and end results in 83 patients. Medicine (Balt.), 27:1–42, 1948.
16. White, J. C., and Sweet, W. H.: Pain, Springfield, Ill., Charles C Thomas, 1969.

128

PAIN OF PERIPHERAL NERVE INJURY

The pain that follows an injury to a peripheral nerve or major plexus is a rare syndrome, but a rewarding one to treat. Usually it is secondary to neuroma formation, but other interesting problems arise. There may be phantom limb pain, causalgia and related sympathetic dystrophy syndromes, and related vascular insufficiency syndromes. All are responsible for pain following nerve injury.[15] The causes of pain after peripheral nerve injury often are multiple. Neuroma formation is associated with abnormally sensitive receptors, spontaneous firing in small unmyelinated fibers, and prolonged inappropriate activity following stimulation.[13] The injured fibers may be deficient in myelin, and it has been suggested that ephapsis from non–pain-carrying to pain-carrying fibers may occur.[14] In some problems of pain following nerve injury, it has been discovered, there is a greater loss of large myelinated fibers than of small unmyelinated fibers. The preponderance of unmyelinated C-fibers, which can be activated by nonpainful stimulation, is thought to be responsible for the dysesthetic pain that occurs in these syndromes. The gate theory of pain perception offers a further explanation for pain occurring in situations of sensory imbalance.[12] The loss of large myelinated fibers removes an inhibitory effect upon the activity of small fibers so that the normal modulation of painful input does not occur. Central effects of nerve injury are largely unstudied. The predominant thought has been that the pain is secondary to peripheral mechanisms of abnormal sensation. It is, however, possible that abnormalities may occur within the spinal cord and at higher levels, but these have not been explored in any significant way.

A multiplicity of treatments for neuralgias of peripheral nerves have been employed. These have included excision of neuromas, proximal neurotomy, neurotomy with suture, internal and external neurolysis, posterior rhizotomy, subarachnoid injection of neurolytic agents, cordotomy, and sympathectomy (Fig. 128–1, Table 128–1).[14] White and Sweet report a success rate of slightly over 50 per cent with these numerous procedures.[15] Fortunately, many of these diverse syndromes respond predictably to the new techniques of neuromodulation. The results with electrical stimulation in pain of peripheral nerve injury origin have been the most gratifying of all those achieved in treating all types of pain by neuromodulation.[2,3,5,6]

NEUROMODULATION TECHNIQUES IN PERIPHERAL NERVE INJURY

Percutaneous Stimulation

Transcutaneous electrical stimulation is discussed at greater length in Chapter 126. It is a valuable tool in pain treatment in general, but particularly useful in neuralgias from injury to peripheral nerves. Aside from the metabolic peripheral neuropathies, virtually all the painful states resulting from peripheral nerve injury can be managed by transcutaneous electrical stimulation, and interventional procedures are

D. M. LONG

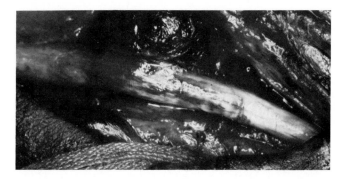

Figure 128-1 Severe brachial plexus compression by false aneurysm secondary to gunshot wound in a 28-year-old man. The patient presented with acute loss of function that was progressive. Resection of the aneurysm and vascular repair was accomplished with good return of function. The patient suffered from severe pain during the recovery phase, but the pain spontaneously relented and has not required further treatment.

less commonly indicated than was previously the case.

Percutaneous stimulation of peripheral nerves via needle electrodes is performed in order to assess the possible value of an implantable peripheral nerve stimulator. The technique is straightforward. The patient is prepared as for any peripheral nerve block. An insulated needle electrode is then inserted in the general vicinity of the nerve to be blocked. The same system that is used for percutaneous cordotomy is quite effective. Stimulation is begun at a low level (1 msec or less, 75 to 100 Hz, less than 1 volt) until the nerve is found. The electrode is then left in place and a current sufficient to elicit paresthesias, but not strong enough to be unpleasant, is then continued. After 10 to 15 minutes of this current, definite hypesthesia will develop in the distribution of the nerve. Stimulations lasting longer than 45 minutes are to be avoided, for this hypesthesia and loss of motor function may then persist for several hours or longer. It is not necessary to obtain hypesthesia or loss of motor function in order to obtain pain relief. Pain is often relieved immediately. One or two repeat stimulations should be sufficient to determine whether an implantable stimulator will, in fact, be successful. If

there is any question concerning the adequacy of pain relief, it is always wise to repeat the stimulation until both surgeon and patient can be certain that it is satisfactory. The best predictor for a highly successful stimulator implantation is prolonged pain relief following such a stimulation. A single stimulation is often followed by relief that lasts several hours or even days.

Implantation of Peripheral Nerve Stimulators

When patients are carefully chosen by their response to a successful percutaneous stimulation, it is usual to achieve excellent pain relief with these implantable nerve stimulators (Fig. 128-2). They currently enjoy the best success rates of all of the implanted nervous system stimulators. This is true, however, only when their use is limited to pain of peripheral nerve injury origin that responds well to temporary stimulation proximal to the site of injury. The success of these devices in relieving pain remote from a site of injury or proximal to the site of implantation is much less good, and they are not recommended for these purposes. Infection and operative injury to the nerve being dissected are the only serious short-term complications. Long-term complications have been few, but scarring around nerves resulting in progressive dysfunction remains a possibility.

The implantable peripheral nerve stimulating devices are all similar in design. They consist of cuff electrodes attached to passive receivers. Energy is supplied by an external power source coupled through the intact skin. The electrodes are placed around the appropriate nerve or plexus proximal to the site of injury. The receiver is placed in a convenient subcutaneous location; usually

TABLE 128-1 SUCCESS OF STANDARD TREATMENTS FOR NERVE INJURY PAIN*

PROCEDURE	SUCCESS RATE (PER CENT)
Resection of single neuroma	30–50
Neurotomy	25
Neurotomy with suture	20–25
Neurolysis (with or without transposition)	50
Posterior rhizotomy	75
Cordotomy	50
Mechanical percussion	25 or less

* Estimates of success are based upon a review of reported series.

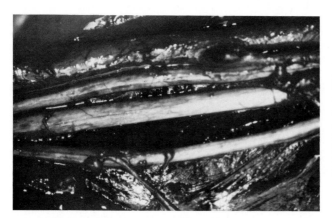

Figure 128–2 Severe stretch injury of the brachial plexus. Note the avascular appearance of the injured nerves. The patient was a 22-year-old man who suffered a stretch injury to the plexus and laceration of the axillary artery in a motorcycle accident. External and internal neurolysis with repair of the axillary artery failed to relieve the pain. Implantation of a brachial plexus stimulator at a second procedure gave excellent relief of pain.

subclavicular for upper extremity and posterior gluteal for lower (see Fig. 126–2 in Chapter 126).

CAUSES OF NERVE INJURY PAIN

Neuroma

A painful neuroma that has developed on a transected nerve can be excised directly. This is effective when the neuroma is exposed and when excision can lead to formation of a new neuroma in an area less likely to be traumatized. A single neuroma excision is warranted if blockade of the nerve proximal to the neuroma gives total relief of pain. Multiple neuroma removals are rarely warranted, and if pain recurs after a single resection, it is unlikely that further attempts will be successful.[14] A number of methods have been tried to prevent re-formation of neuromas. The cut end of the nerve has been drilled into adjacent bone, capped with tantalum or Silastic, and placed in Silastic tubes. None of these techniques is effective in preventing neuroma formation in all cases.

Another technique that has been employed successfully is proximal neurotomy with or without suture. The nerve is cut as far back from the neuroma as is practical without sacrificing important neurological function. Two or three transections have been employed with resuture of each on the theory that some of the fibers would regenerate through each suture line but none through all, thus making neuroma re-formation less likely.

The neuroma in continuity is a more difficult problem (Fig. 128–3). This is particularly true when there is retained nerve function that makes it unwise to sacrifice the nerve. Neurolysis with careful division of the epineurium may be valuable.[1] It is worthwhile considering when there is partial loss of nerve function associated with pain. The neurolysis may improve nerve function and relieve pain simultaneously. In some instances, excision of an neuroma in continuity and resuture of the nerve are indicated. This would most likely occur when nerve function has been largely disrupted and when a large neuroma is present. Intraneural lysis of adhesions may also be of considerable value. In this in-

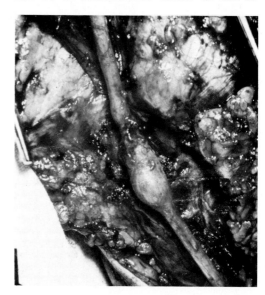

Figure 128–3 Neuroma in continuity in a 26-year-old woman who had a penetrating injury to the ulnar groove two years prior to the present admission. The neuroma is clearly seen. The patient had total loss of ulnar nerve function and severe pain in the distribution of the nerve. Resection of the neuroma and reanastomosis of the nerve eliminated the pain, but provided no return of sensory or motor function.

stance, the nerve is explored and an extraneural lysis of adhesions is performed. The epineurium is then opened, and under the operating microscope, the intraneural adhesions are meticulously dissected until the fascicles of the nerve are free and no longer scarred. This procedure is more effective in restoring neural function than in relieving pain, but both may follow it.

The new techniques of neuromodulation are much more effective in relieving pain of neuromas and intraneural scarring. Transcutaneous electrical stimulation applied proximal to the area of nerve injury relieves the majority of such patients.[8] A thorough trial of transcutaneous electrical stimulation is warranted in most cases of peripheral nerve injury. When transcutaneous stimulation is not effective, then an implantable device, placed proximal to the area of nerve injury, usually will relieve the pain satisfactorily. When it is not possible to place the device proximal to the lesion, short-term relief of pain often is obtained, but long-term success is poor.[3,5,6] Patients can be chosen for implantation of a stimulating device by percutaneous trials of electrical stimulation delivered to the nerve through an electrode. Patients who respond with good pain relief to this kind of electrical stimulation will regularly respond to an implantable stimulating device.

Pain of Amputation

In addition to the pain of neuromas, amputations present two other major pain syndromes. The first may be characterized as simply a tender *painful stump*. Localized pain in a stump is usually the result of a sensitive neuroma, but some patients develop hyperesthesia and pain in the entire stump that is refractory to removal of end-bulb neuromas. When there is a major autonomic component to the painful syndrome, sympathectomy may be helpful. The results of temporary sympathectic blockade are not reliable in predicting long-term relief from sympathectomy, and the over-all results from sympathectomy are not good.[15] Anterolateral cordotomy has been very effective, but the prolonged survival of these patients may often lead to late recurrence of the pain.[7] Fortunately, the neuromodulation techniques have been effective with

these patients as well. Transcutaneous electrical stimulation or a stimulator implanted upon major nerves proximal to any possible injury by the amputation have been very effective.[3]

The second major pain syndrome that follows amputation is the so-called *phantom limb pain*. In this syndrome, the usual phantom appears to be painful, and often seems to be distorted. These patients are extremely distressed by the abnormal sensations. A similar syndrome may occur with avulsion injury in the brachial plexus without loss of an extremity. No local measures have been effective (Table 128–2). Sympathectomy and posterior rhizotomy have failed to relieve the pain. Anterolateral cordotomy has been the most effective method of treating it, but the rate of late recurrence of pain is probably as high as one third of the patients.[15] In the patients who have late recurrence, an increase in the dysesthesias often is reported. Frontal leucotomy and stereotaxic procedures in the thalamus and brain stem are effective in some cases. These procedures have never become popular with surgeons who perform stereotaxic procedures, and the number of patients treated by any of these techniques is small. Again, the new techniques of neuromodulation are promising. Many patients with phantom limb pain can be relieved by transcutaneous electrical stimulation applied over the course of major nerves previously innervating the extremity. When this technique is not successful, implantation of stimulators on these major nerves may be. Patients can be chosen by temporary percutaneous stimulation of the appropriate plexus or major nerves. In some patients, spinal cord stimulation has been effective. This has been particularly true in a small number of patients with pain after avulsion of the brachial plexus. Unfortunately, when neuromodulation techniques fail, other measures are equally likely to prove ineffective and there remains a small group of these patients whose

**TABLE 128–2 INEFFECTIVE
TREATMENT OF PHANTOM LIMB PAIN**

Repeated resection of neuromas
Neurectomy
Reamputation
Periarterial sympathectomy
Posterior rhizotomy
Resection of sensory cortex

pain is completely intractable. Deep brain stimulation is a promising technique, but one that as yet has not been widely enough applied to be fully assessed.

Causalgia and Causalgia-Like Syndromes

The term "causalgia" was originally utilized to describe a painful syndrome that occurred following partial injury to major mixed nerves by low-velocity missiles. True causalgia is a clear-cut, easily diagnosable, syndrome.[14] The patients develop trophic changes in the distribution of the injured nerve and extreme hypersensitivity. Light touch or emotional irritation are particularly potent stimuli for intensifying the pain. The pain is diffuse and burning, and is associated with significant psychological changes in the patient. The patient will often sit for hours at a time with the affected part wrapped in a cool cloth, protecting it from the environment. There are a number of causalgia-like syndromes that have been described as minor causalgia or mistaken for the primary syndrome. Probably it is better to consider causalgia as a spectrum of related pain and dysautonomic syndromes following nerve injury. The semantic division of these patients would not be important except for the fact that true causalgia virtually always responds to sympathectomy, whereas the causalgia-like syndromes do not display this gratifying response (Table 128–3).[14,15] Patients with burning pain without the trophic changes and distinctive emotional aspects of true causalgia are unlikely to respond to sympathectomy. In any patient thought to have causalgia or a causalgia-like syndrome, however, sympathectic blockade is warranted. Several blocks should be performed, usually at least three. Often a causalgia-like syndrome may be interrupted

permanently by repeated blocks. This is particularly true early in the first stages of the painful process. Success with this technique usually is heralded by gradually increasing periods of relief following each block. When this occurs, it is wise to continue performing blocks daily for at least several weeks. If after this period of time, prolonged relief is not obtained, then operative sympathectomy is the procedure of choice. The long-term success of sympathectomy in these pain syndromes is excellent, and recurrence of pain is rare. The causalgia-like syndromes do not respond as well, and favorable response to sympathetic block is not as predictable as in true causalgia. Further discussion of sympathectomy and its applications is given in Chapter 134.

Neuromodulation techniques appear to have some value in these syndromes. Transcutaneous electrical stimulation, proximal to the nerve injury, may be of significant value. If the electrical stimulation is applied in the area of hyperesthesia, the pain is worsened to an almost unbearable level. Implantable nerve stimulators appear to be of value in treating the causalgia-like syndromes and, at this time, are more successful than sympathectomy. They constitute the best procedure currently available for those causalgia-like syndromes that do not respond well to sympathectic block or to sympathectomy.[3,5,6] Before resorting to any operative procedure, a trial of transcutaneous electrical stimulation in any of these syndromes is warranted. These syndromes are so debilitating, however, that it is wise to proceed immediately to an operative procedure as soon as it is obvious that it will be necessary. There is no reason to leave such a patient seriously incapacitated for a long time, hoping for remission or a cure with conservative measures.

The mechanism of causalgia and its related syndromes is not well understood. It is possible that this represents the appreciation of pain transmitted through the viscerosensory system that runs with the sympathectics.[11] It has also been suggested that sympathectomy eliminates short circuiting of efferent sympathectic impulses through injured sensory axons.[14] Neither of these suggestions has been substantiated, and the central effects of these types of injuries are virtually unknown.

TABLE 128–3 SYMPATHECTOMY IN PERIPHERAL NEURALGIAS*

SYNDROME	SUCCESS RATE (PER CENT)
Causalgia	62.5–100
Post-traumatic dystrophy	50–100
Shoulder-hand syndrome	100, early; less than 50, late

* Estimates are based upon a review of the literature.

Reflex Sympathetic Dystrophy

A related problem that remains largely unexplained is variously termed post-traumatic dystrophy, reflex sympathetic dystrophy, or Sudeck's atrophy. The syndrome is characteristically brought on by a relatively minor injury (Fig. 128–4). The original injury may not have involved a major peripheral nerve (Fig. 128–5). Distal joints are frequently the site of primary injury. The most common location for injury appears to be the wrist. Following the injury, there slowly develops a chronically cool, cyanotic, sweaty extremity. Characteristically, the pain is increased on exposure to cold but is not affected by emotional stimuli in the same way as is causalgia. Usually there is remarkable dysesthesia, rapid demineralization with fibrosis of tendon sheaths and muscles, and fixation of joints. There are striking trophic changes in the skin, and with time peripheral nerve injury becomes apparent with obvious steadily decreasing nerve function. Progressively declining conduction times in the affected nerves can be measured. If the

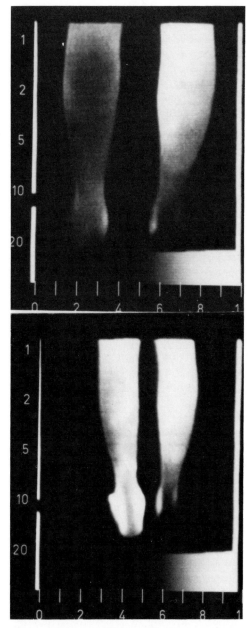

Figure 128–5 Reflex sympathetic dystrophy secondary to minor peripheral nerve injury in the left foot of a 24-year-old white woman. The upper thermogram reveals a 2° difference in temperature in the distribution of the sciatic nerve on the left side. The lower thermogram demonstrates an increase in temperature of 2.5° following left lumbar sympathectomy that was successful in relieving the patient's pain.

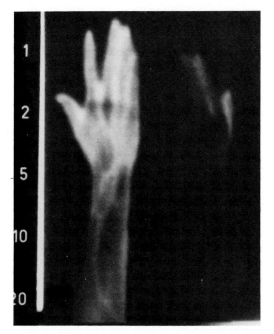

Figure 128–4 Typical reflex sympathetic dystrophy secondary to intraoperative blunt injury to the left ulnar nerve in a 41-year-old white woman. Thermography reveals a 3° decrease in temperature of the ulnar distribution of the left arm. Stellate ganglion blocks effectively relieved the pain and restored normal temperature.

syndrome is not treated effectively, the changes become irreversible and may gradually extend to involve the entire extremity.

Temporary sympathetic blockade usually

will affect these symptoms favorably. Unfortunately, operative sympathectomy is not as highly successful as it is with causalgia, but still the majority of such patients will be relieved. Such patients respond, at least partially, to transcutaneous electrical stimulation, and this technique often will be of great benefit in their management. Some of these patients will respond to implantable electrical stimulators, but the long-term effect of these devices has not been as good as one would like. Pain relief remains adequate as long as the patient is not using the extremity, but the progressive neurological deficits are not always stopped or reversed.

These patients must be carefully differentiated from a group of poorly motivated individuals who cease using an extremity after a minor injury. Quite often these latter patients have undergone a sprain or fracture and claim to have a useless extremity after removal of the cast or bandage. Pain, muscle atrophy, and osteoporosis all may develop. The autonomic symptoms are usually much less marked than in true reflex sympathetic dystrophy, and psychiatric disturbances are much more obvious. It is important to differentiate these patients from those who really need urgent intervention, because they require motivation, psychiatric assistance, and rehabilitation only. Operative intervention may worsen the situation.[9]

The Shoulder-Hand Syndrome

A related syndrome is the unusual problem that develops in the shoulder following coronary artery disease. A pain in the shoulder, arm, and hand develops, with muscular atrophy, osteoporosis, and fixation of joints, particularly the shoulder joint. While most common after coronary insufficiency, this syndrome may occur with cervical osteoarthritis or localized shoulder disease, or after any prolonged illness that requires the patient to remain in bed. In the early course of the problem, sympathetic block usually is adequate if coupled with active physical therapy during the time that the pain is relieved by sympathetic blockade. A few shoulder manipulations following blocks are usually sufficient to end the syndrome. In those few patients in whom this does not prove cura-

tive, it may be necessary to perform cervical sympathectomy. Cervical sympathectomy is virtually always successful, but is rarely necessary, except in the late stages of a neglected disease.[14]

Pain of Vascular Disease

Occlusive Vascular Disease

Pain in occlusive vascular disease usually is caused by ischemia and the metabolites that are produced in skin and muscle with inadequate blood supply. Small-vessel disease may also occur in peripheral nerves, and an ischemic polyneuropathy result. The pain that these patients suffer is extremely severe and often leads to amputation. A trial of sympathetic blockade usually is warranted. A favorable response to sympathetic blocks means that sympathectomy usually will relieve the pain. There is no good evidence that sympathectomy improves circulation to muscle, but it may be helpful in relieving symptoms in a patient who is not a candidate for arterial reconstruction. Sympathectomy will increase walking tolerance in the patient with intermittent claudication, but is rarely employed as a treatment. White has described open peripheral neurotomy for pain in gangrenous toes. In this procedure, the appropriate sensory nerves are crushed well above the ankle to denervate the painful toes.[10] Complete regeneration of the nerve will eventually occur. Pain relief was adequate in a significant number of these patients, however, thereby avoiding amputation.

Neuromodulation techniques have recently been described as of value in treating the pain of occlusive vascular disease. Increases in blood flow to the ischemic extremity were reported, and pain relief by transcutaneous electrical stimulation was said to be good.[4] The use of neuromodulation is still in a phase of evaluation, and it is not possible to assign these techniques a place in the management of pain of vascular disease as yet.[3]

Raynaud's Phenomenon

Digital ischemia with blanching of the fingertips upon exposure to cold as an isolated event and as a complication of peripheral nerve injury is well known. The spontaneous problem most often afflicts young women and can be severe enough to produce gangrene. While the vasomotor and sudomotor disturbances are the most common symptoms, pain may be a factor in extreme cases and is particularly likely to be important in the vasoconstrictive syndrome that follows minor peripheral nerve injury. Sympathectomy is usually successful in the treatment of these syndromes. More recently, transcutaneous electrical stimulation has been employed effectively.[3] At present, it appears that a trial of transcutaneous electrical stimulation applied over the major nerves of the extremity should certainly precede sympathectomy. A few patients with this syndrome have undergone implantation of stimulators upon peripheral nerves, but the results are still not certain over the long term. Fortunately, the combination of transcutaneous electrical stimulation and sympathectomy appears to be successful in relieving the majority of such patients.

Peripheral Neuropathy

One of the most frustrating pain problems in the general category of peripheral neuralgia is the pain of peripheral neuropathy. Usually this pain is in the lower extremities and virtually always is more or less symmetrical, is burning in character, is associated with trophic and autonomic changes, and is most distressing to the patients. The most common causes are diabetes, alcoholism, and occlusive vascular disease. The diagnosis is readily made from the clinical examination and by electromyography. There are virtually no procedures that are of value. The disease is too extensive for posterior rhizotomy or peripheral nerve section to be helpful. Sympathectomy rarely is effective, though sympathetic block may bring short-term relief.[14] Transcutaneous electrical stimulation routinely worsens the patient's condition, and the process is too widespread to allow implantation of peripheral nerve stimulators.[3] Spinal cord stimulators have been employed in a small number of patients, but no significant success has yet been obtained. Deep brain stimulation has not been utilized. Cordotomy rarely is indicated. In general, there are no interventional procedures that are of value in the peripheral neuropathies. Treatment of the underlying disease whenever possible is the best form of therapy. Unfortunately, control of diabetes, reduction of alcohol intake, correction of dietary deficiencies, and similar symptomatic treatments do not always bring about any improvement in the pain of the peripheral neuropathy. This pain remains one of the most difficult management problems. Some patients will respond to the arbitrary use of a combination of antidepressant and antianxiety agents. Amitriptyline, 75 to 100 mg at bedtime, with fluphenazine, 1 mg three times a day, is effective in many of them. The reasons for pain relief by this medication regimen are unknown.

Postherpetic Neuralgia

Previously postherpetic neuralgia was one of the most intractable of chronic pain problems. The patients suffering this excruciatingly painful process often were elderly, had debilitating diseases, and were not suitable candidates for major interventional procedures. The diagnosis is readily made by the appearance of the healed lesions of herpes and by the history (Fig. 128–6). The pain is intense and emotionally distressing. It may be associated with a remarkable hyperesthesia. It is possible for postherpetic neuralgia to exist without there having been a skin eruption, in which case the diagnosis is usually made by the characteristics of the pain and the radicular distribution. It is most common in the thorax. The second most common distribution is in the first division of the trigeminal nerve and the upper cervical roots. Postherpetic neuralgia may, however, occur in any area. Peripheral neurotomy, dorsal root section, and sympathectomy are all ineffective. Many local procedures such as ethyl chloride spray, injection of subcutaneous steroids, and undermining of involved skin, have been employed.[14] The only one of these that has been useful is resection of the hyperesthetic area. This is rarely possible because of the large areas of skin involved. Cordotomy has been utilized for this problem, but the results are not uniformly good, and many of the patients who suffer from this problem are not good candidates for an interventional procedure because of age or intercurrent disease.[7] Fortunately, in the recent

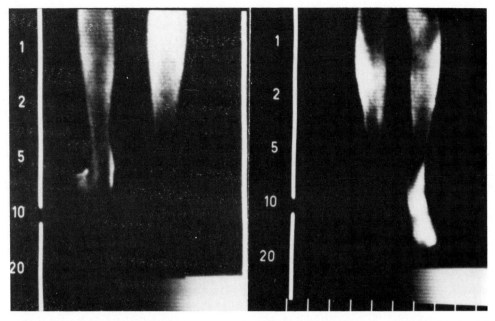

Figure 128-6 Thermogram indicating 5° decrease in temperature of left foot as compared with the right in a 68-year-old white man with sciatic neuropathy secondary to painful herpes zoster. Transcutaneous electrical stimulation was utilized for symptomatic pain relief. The thermogram was repeated 14 months after the onset of the disease and was normal at that time. The pain had relented following symptomatic therapy.

past, two potential modes of therapy have become available. In patients with postherpetic neuralgia who do not have severe hyperesthesia, transcutaneous electrical stimulation will give relief in a very significant percentage. The stimulating electrodes should be placed above and below the area of pain. Care must be taken not to place them over hyperesthetic areas, or the pain will be made worse. Excellent long-term pain relief is obtained in a significant percentage of patients with this method, and usually it is the simplest and most effective way of treating this frustrating problem.[3] The effectiveness of the psychotropic drug combination of amytriptyline (Elavil, 75 to 100 mg at bedtime) and fluphenazine (Prolixin, 1 mg three times a day) is equal to that of neuromodulation. Many of the elderly patients suffering from this problem cannot tolerate large doses of these drugs, however, which is unfortunate, since an excellent response is obtained routinely. It requires two to four weeks to get maximum pain relief with these drugs, and the patients must be encouraged to continue using the medication for several weeks until maximum clinical benefit can be obtained.

SUMMARY

Only a short time ago, direct operations and sympathectomy, posterior rhizotomy, or cordotomy, were the most common treatments for peripheral nerve pain. The advent of neuromodulation techniques has changed this picture significantly. The neuralgias of peripheral nerves respond more favorably to neuromodulation than do any other of the painful syndromes. As a general rule, it is wise to perform local procedures when there is a possibility that nerve function can be improved, when the exact status of the nerve is unknown, or when there is some obvious anatomical problem that needs correction. In other situations, the neuromodulation techniques are much superior to any of the destructive interventional procedures previously used to treat the pain caused by nerve injury.[2,3,5,14] The transcutaneous stimulating techniques should be applied first. Neuromodulation devices must be employed proximal to the site of injury to be effective. Transcutaneous electrical stimulation will prove beneficial in the majority of such patients, and it is not common that they require additional treatment. When transcutaneous electrical stimulation is not effective, the implantable stimulating devices are extremely valuable. These are placed in the most specific place, preferably upon the injured nerve proximal to its area of injury. Less effective, but also acceptable placement is on the appropriate plexus or a parent nerve. The implantable stimulating devices are nearly always effective in relieving pain when temporary percutaneous stimulation or transcutaneous electrical stimulation has been effective.

REFERENCES

1. Brown, H. A.: Internal neurolysis in the treatment of peripheral nerve injuries. Clin. Neurosurg., *17*:99–111, 1969.
2. Campbell, J., and Long, D. M.: Peripheral nerve stimulation in the treatment of intractable pain. J. Neurosurg., *45*:692–699, 1976.
3. Campbell, J., and Long, D. M.: Transcutaneous electrical stimulation for pain: Efficacy and mechanism of action. In preparation.
4. Dooley, D.: Unpublished data.
5. Long, D. M.: Electrical stimulation for relief of pain from chronic nerve injury. J. Neurosurg., *39*:718–722, 1974.
6. Long, D. M.: Cutaneous afferent stimulation for the relief of pain. Progr. Neurol. Surg., *7*:35–51, 1976.
7. Mullan, S.: Percutaneous cordotomy for pain. Surg. Clin. N. Amer., *46*:3–12, 1966.
8. Picaza, J., Cannon, B. W., Hunter, S., Boyd, A., Guma, J., and Maurer, D.: Pain suppression by peripheral nerve stimulation. Part 2. Surg. Neurol., *4*:115–124, 1975.
9. Shaw, R. S.: Pathologic malingering: The painful extremity. New Eng. J. Med., *271*:22–26, 1964.
10. Smithwick, W. H., and White, J. C.: Peripheral nerve block in obliterative vascular disease of the lower extremity. Further experiences with alcohol injection or crushing of sensory nerves of lower leg. Surg. Gynec. Obstet., *60*:1106–1114, 1955.
11. Threadgill, F. D.: Personal communication, 1974.
12. Wall, P. D., and Sweet, W. H.: Temporary abolition of pain in man. Science, *155*:103–104, 1967.
13. Wall, P. D., and Gutnick, M.: Ongoing activity in peripheral nerves: The physiology and pharmacology of impulses originating from a neuron. Exp. Neurol., *43*:580–593, 1974.
14. White, J. C.: Painful injuries of nerves and their surgical treatment. Amer. J. Surg., *72*:468–488, 1946.
15. White, J. C., and Sweet, W. H.: Pain and the Neurosurgeon. Springfield, Ill., Charles C Thomas, 1969.

129

MANAGEMENT OF PAIN BY CONDUCTION ANESTHESIA TECHNIQUES

Certain types of pain may be managed with conduction or block anesthesia. In some instances it is desirable to use reversible local anesthetics. In other circumstances, an agent lytic to nervous tissue is purposely injected.

REVERSIBLE LOCAL ANESTHETIC AGENTS

Reversible local anesthetics may be used in the diagnosis of pain or as therapy for it. The site of origin of pain may be identified. Central pain may be distinguished from peripheral pain, or visceral from somatic pain. The pathway by which peripheral pain is conducted to the central neuraxis can be determined, as well as the dermatomes that are involved. A number of diseases can be diagnosed, and the participation of the sympathetic nervous system in painful or vasospastic conditions can be recognized.

Diagnostic Uses

Central Versus Peripheral Pain

Under certain circumstances, pain felt in the periphery may have its site of origin in the central neuraxis. Pain from a thalamic lesion is an example of this phenomenon. Chronic pain from a peripheral disease or lesion may eventually be perpetuated by a central mechanism. In both these circumstances, the only information sought through use of a nerve block is whether the pain originates peripheral to the central neuraxis or centrally above the level of the cervical cord. The only requisite of such a block is that it involve all the sensory input from the peripheral area. Although this type of block may be achieved with conduction anesthesia, for instance a sciatic or popliteal nerve block for the lower extremities, a more convenient method is diagnostic spinal anesthesia, which can be used to differentiate central from peripheral pain and also to determine the dermatome level of the highest pathway of peripheral pain to the spinal cord.

A spinal anesthetic is administered for differential diagnosis only if the suspected peripheral origin of pain is caudad to the fourth thoracic dermatome. An intrathecal puncture is done with a styletted No. 25 needle in a convenient lumbar interspace, preferably below L2, with the patient in a lateral position and the painful side uppermost. If the pain is bilateral, the procedure is done in the prone position. The table is flexed to flatten the lumbar curve and adjusted to make the vertebral column horizontal. The head of the table should be angulated so that the patient's head and cervical spine are lower than the rest of the vertebral column (Fig. 129–1).

When free flow of spinal fluid is demonstrated, a hypobaric mixture of tetracaine (Pontocaine) and distilled water is injected. The mixture is prepared by dissolving 20 mg of Pontocaine Niphanoid crystals in 10 ml of sterile, triple-distilled water. Care is taken to use distilled water prepared for intrathecal injection and supplied in autoclaved ampules. (Sterile distilled water available for mixing drugs in hospital phar-

---

V. L. BRECHNER

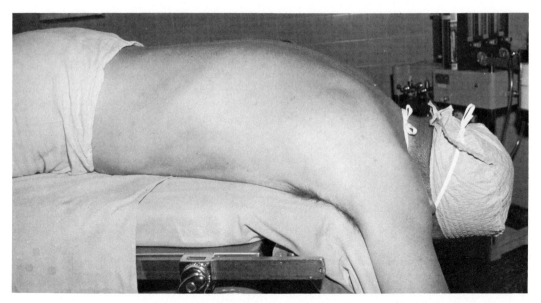

Figure 129-1 Proper position for differential diagnostic spinal anesthesia using hypobaric anesthetic agent. Notice that the table has been flexed to flatten the lumbar curve. The spinal canal from the sacrum to the midthoracic region is approximately horizontal, and the head and cervical area of the spine are lower than the midthoracic area.

macies is not suitable for this technique because a preservative, benzyl alcohol, has usually been added.) A syringe containing the hypobaric mixture is attached to the needle and the solution is injected in 2-ml increments, each followed by a 10-minute observation period. Following each injection, the patient is closely questioned about the persistence of pain. Ten minutes after an injection, the resulting areas of hypalgesia are carefully recorded, and it is noted whether the pain has been relieved. If pain persists, the next 2-ml dose is injected. Each subsequent injection increases the level of anesthesia toward the thoracic area. The first injection of 2 ml of hypobaric tetracaine seldom provides analgesia above the mid-lumbar area. The dermatomic level of anesthesia achieved at the time the patient's pain is relieved is recorded. If pain has not been relieved by the time the dermatomic level of T4 has been reached, the test is discontinued and it is assumed that the origin of pain is in the central neuraxis above the level of T4.

Diagnostic spinal anesthesia is sometimes employed when a patient continues to complain of chronic low back pain after surgical correction has been attempted. These patients frequently have chronic arachnoiditis as a result of the previous operations. It is possible under such circumstances to produce ''spotty'' spinal anes-thesia. Nerve roots and portions of the cord that are densely bound by fibrous tissue are poorly penetrated by local anesthetics. It is important in managing such a patient to search carefully for areas of retained sensation below the level of the spinal anesthesia. Nerve roots unpenetrated by the local anesthetic continue to conduct pain after other roots have been anesthetized. Thus, pain of peripheral origin may persist even though hypalgesia from the spinal anesthesia can be demonstrated at a level considerably cephalad to the site of pain.

Somatic Pain and Segmental Dermatomal Involvement

There are circumstances in which it is desirable to identify the specific dermatomes involved in a painful process. They may be determined, depending upon the area being investigated, by using intercostal, paravertebral somatic lumbar, trans-sacral, paravertebral cervical, or epidural nerve blocks.

An epidural nerve block is perhaps the easiest to achieve. It has the disadvantage, however, of producing bilateral anesthesia. Also, dermatomic involvement is determined by the quantity of anesthetic injected through a single needle rather than by the precise placement of a needle at each intervertebral foramen.

Intercostal Nerve Block

The intercostal nerve block is probably the simplest of all peripheral nerve blocks. It is well to remember the extensive overlapping of adjacent sensory dermatomes demonstrated by Foerster.[12] To block a segment effectively, it is necessary to anesthetize the dermatome above and the one below, as well as the suspected segment. The nerve block must be accomplished central to the lateral cutaneous branch of the intercostal nerve for effective anesthesia of the chest wall.

The procedure is accomplished most conveniently at the level of the dorsal angles of the ribs. This area can be located by drawing a line parallel to the vertebral spines and 3 inches lateral to them. The patient should be either sitting and bending forward with the scapulae retracted laterally by clasping the opposite elbow in each hand, or he should be positioned prone on a narrow table with the arms hanging over the side (Fig. 129–2). The ribs can usually be palpated at the dorsal angle. A skin wheal is made at the lower border of each palpated rib, and a No. 25 needle is inserted through the skin wheal directly down to the lower border of the rib. The needle is then withdrawn $1/16$ inch and displaced downward by moving the loose overlying skin in a caudal direction. The needle is reinserted to a depth that previously contacted bone and then inserted an additional $1/8$ inch. After careful aspiration, 1 to 3 ml of 1 per cent lidocaine (Xylocaine) without epinephrine is injected. Following an intercostal nerve block, it is imperative that the lungs be ausculated to exclude the possibility of an iatrogenic pneumothorax (Fig. 129–3). Under no circumstances should an intercostal block be attempted if the ribs are not easily palpable at the site of needle insertion.

Lumbar Paravertebral Somatic Nerve Block

Although many textbooks map osseous landmarks for this block, such landmarks are misleading.[3,20] The needle can be deflected by fascial planes and tendinous insertions of muscles as well as by spasm of the strong paravertebral muscle masses. The trajectory of the needle point through these tissues has little relationship to the attitude of the shaft of the needle prior to its entry through the skin. Therefore, for paravertebral somatic lumbar nerve block, x-ray and fluoroscopic assistance should be used in all cases (Fig. 129–4).

The block is done with the patient in the prone position, and an initial posteroan-

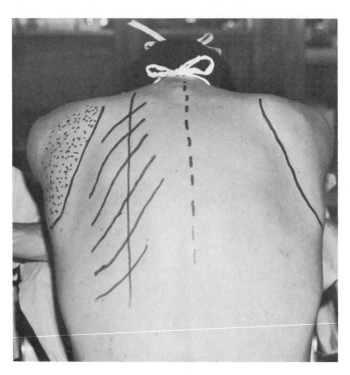

Figure 129–2 Position for intercostal nerve block by posterior approach. The patient is sitting. The scapulae have been displaced laterally by having the patient bend forward and bring his elbows together. The posterior angle or ribs can be palpated in most patients. The lower margins of the ribs have been marked, and a line parallel to the spine has been drawn midway between the upper angle of the scapula and the thoracic spines. The intersection of this line with the lower border of each rib marks the site where the needle is to be inserted.

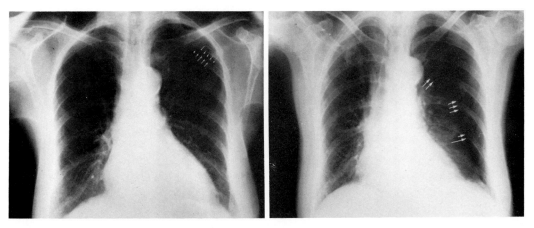

Figure 129–3 Pneumothorax following intercostal nerve block. Note in the film to the left, pneumothorax with 20 per cent collapse. Patient was hospitalized and observed; three hours later repeat film shows 60 per cent collapse. There was prompt re-expansion after the insertion of chest tubes.

terior view is observed with the fluoroscope. With the tip of a 25-gauge needle, a site directly over the lateral margin of the intervertebral foramen is selected and marked by an intradermal injection of local anesthetic. A No. 22 styletted needle approximately 4 inches long is then inserted through this skin wheal and is advanced

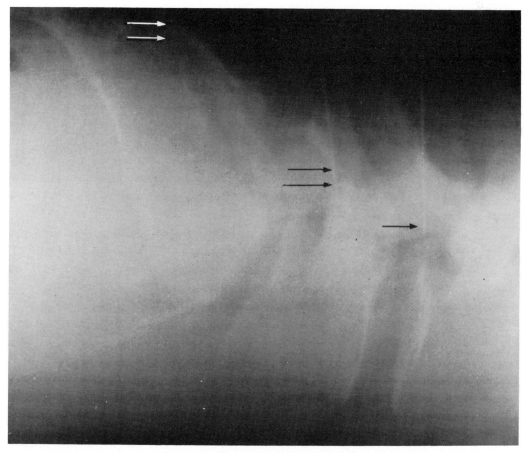

Figure 129–4 Lateral film of lumbar vertebrae 4 and 5 showing placement of needles at the intervertebral foramen. The needle has been placed through the S2 hiatus also. An anteroposterior fluoroscopic view is necessary to be certain that the needle point has not been deflected laterally or medially.

slowly to a depth of approximately 3 cm, when a lateral film is taken. This usually localizes the needle point at or near the intervertebral foramen. Final adjustments are then made, and 3 to 5 ml of a 1 per cent solution of lidocaine without epinephrine is injected after careful aspiration.

Trans-Sacral Injections

Fluoroscopy and roentgenography are also employed during trans-sacral needle placement. Because of the dense ligaments located on the dorsum of the sacrum and the possibility that a needle point may be deflected and change its trajectory, it is possible to confuse the sensation of a needle popping through a ligament with that of one entering a sacral foramen.

The patient is placed in the prone position. A posteroanterior view is taken under fluoroscopic control, and the dorsal sacral foramen is identified. A skin wheal is placed directly above the foramen with a No. 25 needle. A 2-inch No. 22 needle is then inserted through this skin wheal and directed down to the foramen. A lateral film is taken to confirm correct needle placement.

Cervical Paravertebral Somatic Block

The transverse processes of the cervical vertebrae usually can be palpated laterally without difficulty. There are neither overlying tendinous or ligamentous bands nor a powerful muscle mass that may deflect the needle point. For these reasons, paravertebral somatic nerve block in this area may be done without guidance of the fluoroscope.

The block is done with the patient lying supine and with his head turned to the side opposite the one to be blocked. Chassaignac's tubercle, which is the anterior prominence of the transverse process of the sixth cervical vertebra, is palpated and the tip of the mastoid process is located. A line connecting these two points usually lies a short distance anterior to the lateral aspect of the transverse processes. By careful palpation approximately half a fingerbreadth below this line, the C2, C3, C4, and C5 transverse processes can usually be distinguished. A skin wheal is made over each transverse process to be blocked. A No. 22 3-inch needle is inserted carefully through the skin

wheal to the transverse process, and after careful aspiration, 3 to 5 ml of 1 per cent lidocaine is injected at each process.

In performing this nerve block, it is important to recall the configuration of the transverse processes. They form a cuplike bony trough through which the nerve root emerges. A sleeve of dura frequently envelops the emerging nerve root. A needle advanced to the paravertebral area may enter such a dural sleeve, and the anesthetic then be injected intrathecally instead of paravertebrally. For this reason, careful aspiration is done and a test dose of 1 ml of local anesthetic is injected before the total quantity of agent is administered. Because the vertebral artery traverses the cervical transverse processes and a needle inserted into the vertebral artery would allow local anesthetic to be injected almost directly to the midbrain, aspiration must also exclude intravascular placement of the needle.

Epidural Anesthesia

The somatic nerve block of epidural anesthesia is accompanied by a sympathetic nerve block in the involved areas.

The epidural space may be entered by the needle in the lumbar, the cervical, and the upper and lower thoracic areas. In the midthoracic area between T3 and T9, the configuration of the dorsal spine makes epidural placement of a needle very difficult. In using epidural anesthesia as a diagnostic segmental block, one must rely upon demonstration of a postblock area of hypalgesia to differentiate the dermatomes involved instead of relying upon the position of the needle point at the intervertebral foramen as with paravertebral somatic block.

Epidural placement of a needle is predicated upon the observation that intraspinous ligaments and ligamentum flavum are dense fibrous structures into which it is impossible to inject fluid or air. A No. 20 to No. 22 styletted 3-inch short-bevel needle is inserted into the intraspinous ligament in a manner similar to that employed for an intrathecal anesthesia. The stylus is removed and a 2-ml syringe containing either air or normal saline is firmly attached to the needle hub. Pressure upon the plunger of the syringe will be met with resistance, and it will be impossible to inject the syringe contents as long as the needle point lies within the ligament. As the needle is advanced slowly with firm pressure continuously applied to the plunger of the syringe, the careful observer will notice increased resistance to its passage when it enters the ligamentum flavum. Shortly after this the needle will pop into the epidural space and the pressure exerted upon the syringe plunger will suddenly find release as either air or liquid, whichever is employed, is injected. The stream of liquid has a tendency to push the dura ahead of the needle and create a small space in the epidural area.

After careful aspiration, approximately 2 ml of 1 per cent lidocaine is injected as a test dose. If hypotension and other signs of spinal anesthesia do not appear, 2 ml of anesthetic for each dermatome to be anesthetized is injected. By injecting the anesthetic slowly and maintaining the patient in the lateral position for 30 minutes following the injection, the ensuing hypalgesia can be confined largely to the dependent side.

Any person performing such a block must be capable of managing all the sequelae of total spinal anesthesia.

Sympathetic System Syndromes

The sympathetic nervous system becomes anatomically separate from the somatic nervous system at the paravertebral sympathetic ganglia. In the lumbar and thoracic region, ganglia lie anterolateral to the vertebral bodies. In the cervical area, the three sympathetic ganglia lie just anterior to the transverse processes of the cervical vertebrae. Because in all these localities the ganglia are separated by a centimeter or so from the somatic nerve root, it is possible to achieve sympathetic nerve block without involving somatic nerves. Although a "differential diagnostic" spinal nerve block has been described, in which different concentrations of local anesthetic injected intrathecally are relied upon to block the more susceptible sympathetic fibers, experience shows that anatomical separation is far more reliable in any differential diagnostic procedure.[2]

In general, paravertebral sympathetic nerve block of the thoracic ganglia is not done because of the danger of iatrogenic pneumothorax.

Sympathetic nerve block is useful in diagnosing the minor and major causalgias.[9,11] The sudden relief of burning pain following the blockade while the somatic innervation of the area remains demonstrably intact is diagnostic of the causalgic syndromes.

These types of nerve blocks may also be employed to differentiate between mechanical obstruction of circulation and vasospastic obstruction. With the proper sympathetic blockade, improvement in vasospastic obstruction is pronounced, but mechanical obstruction is not altered.

Vasodilatation after a sympathetic nerve block is evidence that the nerve block is effective and that the condition is vasospastic. If the vasodilatation of sympathetic denervation does not occur after needles are inserted and local anesthetic is injected, it could be because of one of two reasons. First, a vasospastic phenomenon does not exist and the poor circulation is a result of mechanical obstruction. Second, the nerve block has been improperly performed and blockade of the sympathetic ganglia has not occurred. In the latter circumstance, if the negative results were interpreted as meaning that the circulatory disorder was mechanical, the patient would be subjected to inappropriate operation and denied appropriate therapy. In circumstances in which vasospastic phenomena are suspected, positive evidence of proper needle placement must be secured. For this reason, it is the author's practice in diagnostic sympathetic nerve blocks to use fluoroscopy and radiography to confirm needle placement.

Aside from x-ray evidence of proper needle placement, there are other confirming signs of sympathetic nerve blockade not associated with vasodilatation. One of the most convenient is suppression of the galvanic skin reflex (Fig. 129–5).[7,25] This reflex involves alterations in skin electrical resistance associated with sympathetic nerve discharge. If a galvanic skin response is present prior to sympathetic nerve block and disappears after the injection of local anesthetic, this is evidence that sympathetic nerve block has occurred. Persistence of circulatory obstruction under these conditions would indicate mechanical blockade.

Paravertebral Lumbar Sympathetic Nerve Block

After emerging from the intervertebral foramen, the somatic nerves course laterally and caudad so that at the level of the

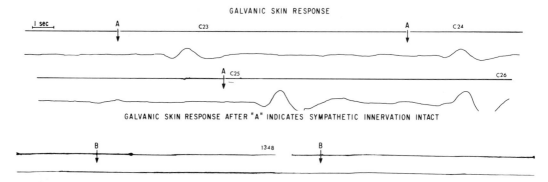

Figure 129-5   Galvanic skin response. This record was obtained using the electroencephalographic amplification of the GME cardioencephalograph (Middleton, Wisconsin). One of the bipolar electrodes was applied to the volar surface of a hand and the other was applied to the dorsal surface of the hand. Johnson and Johnson Telectrodes No. 1801 were used as electrodes. A pinprick was administered as a stimulus to the patient at A and B on the record. The tracings following the letters A were done prior to a stellate ganglion block of the involved extremity. The tracings after B were taken following the stellate ganglion block. Note that following A there is a biphasic alteration in electrical resistance of the extremity and that following B there is no delayed response. This record is graphic evidence that a sympathetic nerve block has been achieved.

tips of the transverse processes of the lumbar vertebrae, the major nerve trunks are more closely applied to the cephalolateral edge. As stated before, the paravertebral sympathetic ganglia lie anterolateral to the vertebral bodies. The procedure is done with x-ray and fluoroscopic assistance. The caudolateral angle of the transverse process involved is identified fluoroscopically and a skin wheal is placed directly above it. A styletted No. 22 6-inch needle with a small adjustable rubber marker on the shaft is inserted through the skin wheal to the transverse process. Depth of penetration is marked at the shaft. The needle is then withdrawn to subcutaneous tissue and redirected medially at an angle of approximately 10 degrees from the vertical. Without altering the attitude of the needle, it is displaced caudally by traction on the skin and is then reinserted 3 to 4 cm deeper than the transverse process or until bony obstruction is met. Fluoroscopic or anteroposterior and lateral films are taken, and appropriate adjustment of depth and angle of the needle are made. Final films should confirm that the needle point is adjacent to the anterolateral aspect of the vertebral body (Fig. 129-6). If a single needle is properly placed at the L2 or L3 area, injection of 10 to 20 ml of 1 per cent lidocaine without epinephrine will effectively block all the lumbar sympathetic ganglia. It is not necessary to place a needle at each of the lumbar vertebrae.

Epidural Anesthesia for Differential Sympathetic Nerve Block of Lower Extremity

Although an epidural block may not necessarily distinguish sympathetic from somatic pain, there are circumstances in which such a differentiation can be made. All the sympathetic fibers to the lower extremities leave the intervertebral foramen cephalad to the L3 interspace. Injection of 3 to 5 ml of local anesthetic epidurally at the L2 interspace will produce sympathetic blockade involving the entire lower extremity and somatic anesthesia involving only the area of the anterior portion of the thigh. If such anesthesia produces relief of severe pain in the foot or toes, it can properly be assumed that the sympathetic blockade was responsible.

Stellate Ganglion Block

The stellate ganglion is located anterior to the transverse processes of the seventh cervical and first thoracic vertebrae. It can conveniently be approached anteriorly to achieve sympathetic blockade of the upper extremity and ipsilateral side of the face and head. The patient lies in the supine position, and Chassaignac's tubercle on the anterior surface of C6 is palpated. The C7 transverse process is approximately 1.5 cm caudad to Chassaignac's tubercle. The great vessels of the neck underlying the sternocleidomastoid muscles are displaced

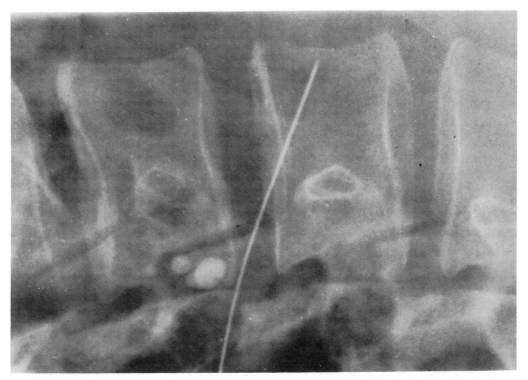

Figure 129–6 A lateral film of the lumbar area showing the needle placed for lumbar sympathetic nerve block. Note the tip of the needle is near the anterior portion of the vertebral body. Anteroposterior views observed under image intensification fluoroscopy showed the tip of the needle to be approaching the midline.

laterally by the operator's left index finger. A skin wheal is made over the C7 transverse process, and a No. 25 1½-inch needle is inserted through the skin wheal and directed to the anterior surface of the transverse process. The needle is then withdrawn approximately ¹⁄₁₆ inch. After careful aspiration, 10 ml of 0.5 per cent lidocaine without epinephrine is injected.

It is important to remember the vital structures that are closely adjacent to the ganglia. Injection of the vertebral artery, which lies just dorsal to the stellate ganglion, would be catastrophic. The mixed nerve roots of C6, C7, and T1 are close to the ganglion and, as noted before, the dural sleeves of the roots may extend far enough laterally to allow inadvertent intrathecal injection. The recurrent laryngeal nerve is closely related to the stellate ganglion; if the injection is made medial to the transverse processes, paralysis of the nerve may result with transient hoarseness. Bilateral stellate ganglion blocks should never be done because of the possible complication of bilateral recurrent laryngeal nerve paralysis. The dome of the pleura extends into the neck in this area. Pneumothorax can be

a troublesome complication of this block. The phrenic nerve is also close to the stellate ganglion, lying lateral to the transverse process. If an injection is made too far laterally, therefore, phrenic nerve paralysis may result. Although stellate ganglion block is a relatively simple procedure, it is, of all the nerve blocks, the most liable to complication because of adjacent anatomical structures.

Visceral Versus Somatic Pain

There are certain circumstances in which it is important to differentiate visceral from somatic pain. The occurrence of pain associated with chronic pancreatitis and carcinoma of the pancreas is an example of visceral pain that may be confused with peripheral somatic pain. This differentiation can be made by comparing the results of somatic nerve block of the involved areas with the relief associated with celiac plexus block.

Celiac Plexus Block

The patient is placed in the prone position and the twelfth rib is palpated and identified. The identification of the lateral tip of the twelfth rib is best accomplished fluoroscopically. The dorsal spines of the twelfth thoracic and the first lumbar vertebrae are palpated. A skin wheal is made over the twelfth rib approximately 7 cm on either side of the first lumbar dorsal spine. A No. 20 styletted needle, approximately 6 inches long, is inserted through this skin wheal at an angle of 45 degrees to the skin, in the direction of the vertebral body of the twelfth dorsal vertebra, until it impinges on the body of the vertebra. It is withdrawn to subcutaneous tissue, redirected at a lesser angle, and reinserted until it touches the body of the vertebra. It is again withdrawn and reinserted at a still lesser angle until the tip is felt to pass along the side of the body of the vertebra and anterior to it. At this point, lateral and posteroanterior films are taken to confirm that the point is anterior to the vertebral body. Ten milliliters of 0.5 per cent lidocaine may then be injected on each side to achieve a reversible celiac plexus block that will block all visceral pain impulses arising from the abdomen with the exception of those arising from the viscera of the pelvis.

Celiac plexus block may be complicated by intrathecal injection unless care is taken. During insertion of the needle it is possible for the trajectory of the point to differ from that expected by observation of the shaft of the needle. The point may be deflected to enter the intervertebral foramen and intrathecal space. It is absolutely necessary that, on x-ray, the needle point be visualized anterior to the vertebral body. It is particularly important that the left first lumbar artery, which supplies the lower portion of the spinal cord, be avoided. For this reason, careful aspiration is mandatory.

Paravertebral sympathetic block of the first lumbar ganglion may result on relief of visceral pain similar to that achieved by injection of the celiac plexus. This may result from spread of the injected material to the celiac plexus or be because fibers passing from the celiac plexus are involved in the first lumbar sympathetic ganglion.

Myofascial Pain Syndromes

Myofascial pain syndromes are a major source of discomfort to patients in the later years of life. These syndromes, as yet poorly understood by physicians, are dramatically relieved by local anesthetics injected into appropriate muscular trigger points.[19,29] They are characterized by a painful trigger point in muscle or fascia. Stimulation of this trigger point provokes local pain and also causes radiation of pain to other areas. The radiation of the pain does not follow usual dermatomal pathways. The syndromes are reproducible, however, in that a trigger point identified in a certain area of muscle or fascia will consistently provoke radiation of pain to a typical area.

These syndromes are diagnosed by exploring for trigger zones in certain muscle and fascial areas. Particularly susceptible are the muscles supporting the shoulder girdle and neck. The palpating finger carefully goes over these muscles until it encounters an area of firmness that is tender. Pressure on this point causes local and radiating pain as just described. Injection of this area of muscle with 1 or 2 ml of local anesthetic precipitates a brief exacerbation of pain and radiation followed by complete relief. Such a sequence is diagnostic of myofascial pain syndrome.

Therapeutic Uses for Temporary Relief of Pain

Painful conditions resulting from trauma, may, under certain circumstances, be more advantageously treated by reversible nerve block than by the administration of narcotics. The pain relief can be achieved by blocking peripheral nerves (as in intercostal nerve block), by blocking paravertebral somatic nerves, or by using epidural anesthesia.

Continuous epidural anesthesia is perhaps the easiest and most effective method. A polyethylene catheter can be inserted through a No. 16 Hueber point needle into the epidural space and can remain in the space after the needle has been withdrawn. The anesthetic is injected at will through the catheter. The duration of this type of anesthesia, however, is limited. If epidural anesthesia is employed continuously for longer than 48 hours, the duration of pain relief from any single injection becomes shorter and the concentration of anesthetic injected must be increased. Each subsequent injection produces discomfort that lasts until the anesthetic has taken effect.

These observations have been interpreted by some as evidence of tachyphylaxis to the local anesthetic. An alternate explanation would be that the injections produce tissue edema in the epidural space, which retards penetration of anesthetics to neural elements. The concentration needed for anesthesia would thus be increased. Also, since the space within the epidural area would be reduced by edematous tissue, the pressure attended by injection of 10 or 15 ml of fluid would provoke discomfort. In spite of the fact that these developments terminate the usefulness of epidural anesthesia after several days, it may be of value during the initial treatment of certain conditions.

Traumatic Somatic Pain

Common traumatic conditions in which local anesthesia is of use are rib fractures, postoperative incisional pain, and compression fracture of a vertebra (frequently a consequence of metastatic carcinoma).

Rib Fracture

The pain and splinting of respiration associated with fracture of ribs may be temporarily alleviated by intercostal nerve block of the involved segments. Some local anesthetics now available (0.75 per cent bupivacaine or 2 per cent etidocaine) have a duration of effect of six to eight hours. Patients with such fractures may develop a pulmonary disability from failure to cough and clear mucus and other debris from the airway. Under such circumstances, an intercostal nerve block may allow many hours free from pain for proper tracheal toilet.

If extensive trauma to the chest has occurred and pain relief from narcotics is inadequate, a more prolonged period of pain relief may be achieved without intermittent blocking by using an epidurally placed catheter. The tip of the catheter is advanced to the dermatomal area located centrally in the painful process. Local anesthetics can then be injected repeatedly through this catheter to provide relief for several days. It is important to select a concentration of anesthetic that will block painful sensory fibers but will not interrupt motor conduction. For this reason, it is best to commence with 0.5 per cent lidocaine or 0.25 per cent bupivacaine. As was discussed previously, it may be necessary to increase the concentration of local anesthetic used later in the course of treatment. This will not necessarily be attended by muscle paralysis, however, as long as the most dilute concentration that is effective is used.

Postoperative Incisional Pain

Following incision in the upper abdomen and thorax, postoperative pain may prevent some patients, particularly the obese, from effectively clearing the airway of mucus and debris. As in rib fracture, an intercostal block may allow an interlude of several hours during which the patient may cough and clear his airway without associated somatic pain. It must be emphasized to such a patient that a vigorous tracheal toilet is the major purpose for the temporary local anesthesia.

Compression Fracture

Compression fracture of vertebrae occurs in certain types of metastatic carcinoma. It produces sudden excruciating pain that frequently cannot be controlled with narcotics and is an indication for the epidural insertion of a catheter and injection of local anesthetic. Because of the intense pain associated with a compression fracture and the possibility of neurological damage due to improper position, this procedure can be technically more difficult than the usual epidural anesthesia. A patient must be adequately sedated prior to the insertion of a catheter, and a compromise in his position that does not jeopardize the integrity of the spinal column but is less than optimal for insertion of the needle must be accepted.

When percutaneous cordotomy is subsequently undertaken in such a patient, the continuous epidural anesthesia may provide comfort during the procedure and allow the patient to be awake and cooperative.

Syndromes of the Sympathetic Nervous System

Major and Minor Causalgia

Reversible nerve block of the paravertebral sympathetic ganglia may be employed diagnostically or therapeutically in the causalgic types of syndromes. Minor causalgias, if treated early and repeatedly with sympathetic ganglion block, may respond with complete remission and cure. The observation is made that with each injection, the duration of pain relief is longer than would be expected from the duration of action of the specific local anesthetic. It is also observed that when the pain does return, it returns at a lesser intensity than prior to the injection. This progress continues until the pain is reduced to acceptable levels or entirely eliminated.

Major causalgias are usually more stubborn than minor ones and are not as readily treated with therapeutic sympathetic nerve blocks. They usually require total continuous denervation rather than the partial intermittent denervation of repeated blocks. Sympathetic nerve block is mainly a diagnostic procedure, and except under unusual circumstances, the patient should be referred for preganglionic sympathectomy once the diagnosis is established.

There is, however, a close association of conversion hysteria with causalgia. For this reason, any causalgic patient thought to be a candidate for sympathectomy should be evaluated carefully both psychologically and psychiatrically prior to any operative intervention.

Vasospastic Conditions

In general, sympathetic nerve blocks are employed in these conditions as a diagnostic measure or as a temporary means of providing enhanced collateral circulation in preparation for operation.

There are certain circumstances, however, in which sympathetic nerve block may be the only treatment prescribed. Occasionally after instrumentation, as in angiography, a major artery may go into intense spasm. A stellate ganglion block in the upper extremity or a paravertebral lumbar sympathetic block in the lower extremity may bring immediate and dramatic relief of the spasm and return of adequate circulation to the limb.

After peripheral embolism has occurred in an extremity, it may be desirable to enhance collateral circulation as quickly as possible while the patient is being prepared for operative intervention. Sympathetic nerve block may be employed to increase collateral circulation around the mechanical obstruction.

Other Medical Conditions Treated by Reversible Nerve Block

Myofascial Pain

As stated before, myofascial pain in muscle and supportive tissue is characterized by a painful trigger area and a typical area of radiation of pain that does not follow dermatomal references. One of the common myofascial syndromes is the splenius capitis syndrome with a trigger point near the insertion of the splenius muscle into the occiput. Pain is radiated over the back of the head into the forehead and sometimes into the eye. The Sternocleidomastoid syndrome is associated with a trigger point in the upper portion of the sternocleidomastoid muscle with pain radiating into the zygoma, temporal area, and eye. Trigger points within the levator scapulae muscle may cause pain radiating to the anterior portion of the chest wall and the neck or down the ipsilateral arm.

Myofascial syndromes are provoked by conditions associated with wasting muscle, unusual posture, and formation of fibrous tissue. Because of this, patients who have resectional operations for carcinoma, or x-ray therapy and perhaps perfusion procedures with anticarcinogenic agents (all of which are associated with a prolonged period of convalescence and with generalized muscle wasting) are often subject to myofascial pain syndromes. When a myofascial syndrome occurs in such a patient, however, it is frequently misdiagnosed as peripheral metastasis from the carcinoma, even if such metastasis cannot be demonstrated. Failure to recognize a myofascial syndrome may limit efforts to relieve the patient's pain.

The myofascial pain can be dramatically relieved by injection into trigger points of any local anesthetic. The duration of the pain relief exceeds the duration of action of the local anesthetic. Repeated treatment results in disappearance of the pain syndrome.

Pulmonary Embolus

Pulmonary embolism is a medical emergency that may be attended by considerable chest pain and intercostal muscle splinting. As the pain is usually aggravated by deep breathing and coughing, the persistence of the pain may interfere with the normal tracheal toilet that is necessary for survival. Under these circumstances, an intercostal nerve block to the involved dermatomes may provide a brief pain-free period in which the patient's tracheal toilet may be performed without discomfort.

Acute Herpes Zoster

Herpes zoster is a classic situation in which a peripheral somatic nerve block not only provides temporary relief, but at times seems to enhance remission of symptoms.

Acute Pancreatitis or Carcinoma of the Pancreas

Acute pancreatitis and carcinoma of the pancreas can be attended by exquisite pain in the upper abdomen. After demonstration that the pain may be relieved by reversible celiac plexus block, several courses of action are possible. The pain can be treated by insertion of an epidural catheter to the lower thoracic vertebrae, thus providing a blockade of visceral fibers from the celiac plexus as they enter the vertebral column. In the case of pancreatic cancer, the celiac plexus may be blocked with 50 ml of 50 per cent alcohol.

Painful Therapeutic Procedures

Certain types of cystitis are sometimes treated by the instillation of a bleaching agent, oxychlorosene (Clorpactin). With this treatment, the bladder goes into an intense spasm that may last for hours. The pain cannot be alleviated by narcotics. Continuous caudal or epidural anesthesia will allow treatment to proceed with comfort for the patient.

Trigeminal Neuralgia

The use of local anesthetics in the management of trigeminal neuralgia is discussed in Chapter 119.

INTRATHECAL NEUROLYTIC AGENTS IN TREATMENT OF PAIN

Although neurospastic conditions may be treated by chemical rhizotomy, somatic pain of advanced malignant disease is the condition for which the procedure is used most frequently.

The results of such injections are at times unpredictable, and complications can be serious. It follows that proper selection of candidates and careful attention to details of technique and patient care must be observed.

Selection of Patients

The selection of candidates for this type of treatment depends upon the extent of the patient's disease, his refractory response to narcotics, and achievement of relief following a trial injection with reversible local anesthetic, as well as his acceptance of what can reasonably be expected and the complications that may occur.

Type of Disease

Use of intrathecal neurolytic injections should be limited to patients with incurable carcinoma who are suffering from somatic pain. This type of pain is described as dull or cutting or tearing in nature. Although it is constant, the intensity may wax and wane. The pain has a dermatomal distribution, and any referred pain is along the involved dermatome. A site of origin can usually be demonstrated. Narcotics have some effect although they may not adequately control the pain.

The patient's condition must be unresponsive to other rational therapeutic procedures directed toward the cause of pain such as additional x-ray and anticarcinogenic or hormonal therapy that could cause a regression of metastasis and control the pain.

Trial with Narcotics

The patient must be obviously unresponsive to properly managed and carefully selected analgesic, narcotic, and tranquilizing medication.

Trial with Reversible Local Anesthetic

It must be established upon repeated occasions that conduction anesthesia involving the segments to be included in the neurolytic injection will relieve the pain. The patient must also have the experience of sensing numbness or lack of sensation and have some opportunity to evaluate the degree of muscle weakness that may accompany such a block.

A convenient method of providing a trial period of conduction anesthesia is to insert an epidural catheter to the involved segment and administer a local anesthetic repeatedly over a period of several days. It can then be demonstrated that the pain is relieved with the onset of anesthesia and that it returns with the return of sensation (Fig. 129–7).

Motor Evaluation

Motor power must be evaluated prior to and following the injection of an intrathecal neurolytic agent. This can be accomplished by measuring and recording strength of motion and muscle contraction with biomechanical recorders such as the spring force scale and goniometer.

Agents

The two neurolytic agents commonly employed intrathecally are absolute alcohol and phenol 5 to 7.5 per cent in glycerol or iophendylate (Pantopaque).[4,28] Because these agents differ widely in specific gravity, the site of action and the positioning of the patient differ with the agent. The site of action of absolute alcohol is at the emergence of the dorsal root from the spinal cord, whereas phenol in glycerol acts at the dorsal ganglion.

Phenol in Glycerol

A mixture of phenol and glycerol is extremely hyperbaric compared with spinal fluid, having a specific gravity of 1.25. All positioning of the patient, therefore, is oriented toward placing the dorsal ganglia of the painful dermatomes in the most dependent position. The involved side is lowermost and the patient is rotated backward at an angle of approximately 40 degrees.

The solutions that have been employed previously with success are either a 5 per cent or 7.5 per cent mixture of phenol in glycerol or in Pantopaque.[17,18,22] In general, although the Pantopaque mixture allows x-ray visualization during an injection, these solutions seem to have less neurolytic activity than phenol in glycerol. The 5 per cent solution has less neurolytic activity than the 7.5 per cent and is, therefore, less likely to involve motor fibers. Successful sensory lysis, however, is less frequent with the 5 per cent than with the 7.5 per cent solution, and the author prefers to use the stronger solution, relying upon proper positioning to prevent anterior root involvement. Either solution injected intrathecally behaves clinically as a reversible anesthetic within the first 10 minutes of its

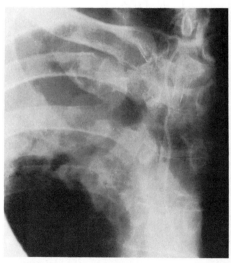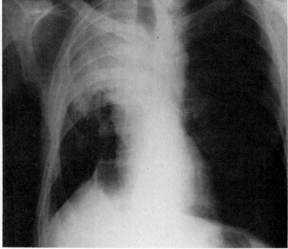

Figure 129–7   The patient has a tumor of the lung extending into the right supraclavicular area. An epidural catheter has been inserted through the T9–T10 interspace and advanced cephalad to the T5 vertebra. Intermittent injections of local anesthesic through this catheter completely relieved the patient's pain, which involved the upper portion of the right side of the chest. Eventually, the patient was treated with intrathecal phenol, injected as described in the text, to involve the T2, T3, T4, and T5 dermatomes.

application to a dorsal ganglion. If, by misadventure, the injection involves dermatomes other than those intended, the patient may be repositioned during the first 10 minutes after application without permanent neurolysis. As the solution comes in contact with the dorsal ganglia, the patient experiences a feeling of warmth and tingling in the involved dermatomes. There is never a sharp or painful paresthesia. The feeling of warmth indicates which dermatomes are involved by the injection. The patient should be alert and cooperative and under only mild sedation so that he can describe his feelings as they occur.

Absolute Alcohol

Absolute alcohol, in contrast to phenolglycerol mixtures, is extremely hypobaric. Its site of action is at the dorsal root at its emergence from the spinal cord. All positioning of the patient, therefore, is determined by the hypobaric characteristics of the agent and the site of action.[13,24] The patient is positioned in the manner that places the emergence of the dorsal root from the cord in the uppermost portion of the vertebral canal. Alcohol is a rapid and irreversible neurolytic agent. As it is injected, the neurolytic effect is virtually instantaneous. Unlike phenol, alcohol causes painful paresthesias during the injection. The distribution of the paresthesia indicated the dermatomes involved in the neurolysis.

Anatomy

The dorsal roots emerge from the cord as small filaments that combine to form a root. Because of these filamentous origins, this point is more susceptible to neurolytic action than the remainder of the root. An incorrect impression shared by many is that the dorsal ganglion is consistently located close to the spinal cord level from which the ventral and dorsal roots originate. Figure 129–8 illustrates that, although close approximation of the dorsal ganglion to the origin of the dorsal root occurs in the cervical and upper thoracic areas, there is wide separation between the root origin and the dorsal ganglion in the sacral, lumbar, and lower thoracic areas. The dorsal ganglion is located in the intervertebral foramen through which the mixed nerve formed by

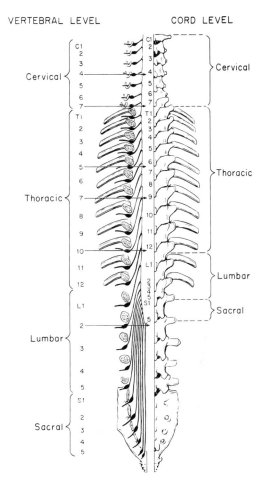

Figure 129–8 Diagramatic view of the spinal cord and vertebral column. Note that in the cervical and upper thoracic area the dorsal ganglia are close to the level at which the dorsal root emerges from the spinal cord. In the lower thoracic lumbar and sacral areas there is increasing separation of the dorsal ganglia from the site on the spinal cord from which the dorsal root emerges.

the union of the dorsal and ventral roots emerges. Since the spinal cord ends approximately at the first or second lumbar vertebra, the dorsal root origin and the location of the dorsal ganglion are widely separated in the lower area of the spinal column. With hyperbaric phenol, the needle is placed at the interspace from which the mixed nerve emerges. With alcohol, the needle is inserted at a more cephalad vertebral level.

The configuration of the dural sleeve investing the nerve roots as they emerge through the intervertebral foramen and the volume contained in the sleeve differ in various areas of the spinal column. In the cervical and upper thoracic areas the cuff is long, chalice-shaped, and contains a larger volume than in the lower thoracic and lumbar areas, at which levels the cuff is quite shallow. The dural cuff enlarges again in the sacral area. Because of the anatomical difference, a larger volume of hyperbaric phenol in glycerol may be injected in the cervical and upper thoracic region than in the lumbar.

Technique

Hypobaric Alcohol

Figure 129–9 illustrates the proper position of the patient for injection of absolute alcohol intrathecally in an effort to lyse the posterior roots of the L1, L2, and L3 dermatomes on the right. The procedure is done with the patient in the prone position. The operating table is flexed to place the lower thoracic area at the apex of the bow in the spinal column and is rotated to the left so that the patient's right side is uppermost. A short-bevel No. 22 needle is inserted intrathecally at each interspace, and 0.25 ml of absolute alcohol is slowly injected through each needle. Each injection is timed to consume at least three minutes. The position is maintained for 45 minutes after injection to assure dilution of the alcohol by cerebrospinal fluid to a concentration that cannot be neurolytic.

Hyperbaric Phenol and Glycerol

Figure 129–10 shows proper positioning for the injection of hyperbaric phenol and glycerol. Two metal upright poles are padded and securely fastened to the side of an operating table. The patient is placed in a lateral position, involved side downward, and positioned so that he leans back against these uprights at approximately a 20-degree angle. The operating table itself can be tilted to the side for an additional 20 degrees. This will allow backward tilting of the patient's spinal column at an angle of 40 degrees. The agent is injected through a single needle inserted at an interspace in the middle of the involved segments and is timed to take three minutes for each 0.75 ml injected.

The volume injected varies with the site of the injection. If cervical or upper thoracic segments are involved, a total of 3 ml may be used if necessary. In the lumbar region, the maximum allowable is 0.75 ml. A volume of 0.75 ml will disperse itself over four to five interspaces in the lumbar area. Sacral segments may be treated by injection of a volume of 0.75 to 1 ml through a needle placed in the L5-S1 interspace with the patient in a sitting position and then tilted backward and leaning to the involved side during the injection.

During the injection, the patient can confirm the actual site of neurolytic activity by

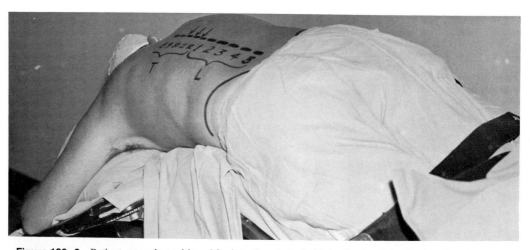

Figure 129–9 Patient properly positioned for intrathecal alcohol injection involving lumbar dorsal roots. The needles are to be inserted at the interspaces marked with arrows. There are T9–T10, T10–T11, and T11–T12 for injection of the lumbar dorsal roots. Note that the site of injection is the highest area in the thoracic curve and that the side to be injected is uppermost.

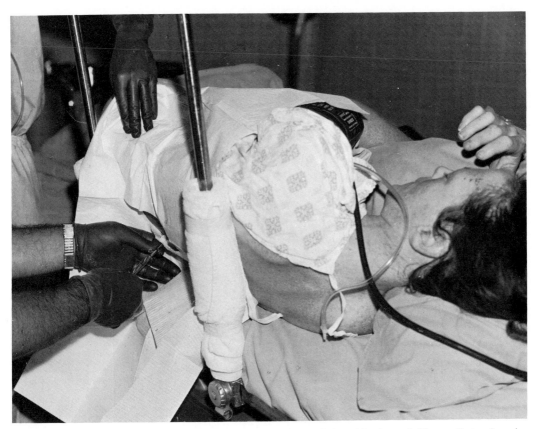

Figure 129–10 A patient is receiving an intrathecal injection of phenol in glycerol. The needle has been inserted in the L2–L3 interspace. This is to involve dermatomes comparable to those that would have been involved in the alcohol injection illustrated in Figure 129–9. Note that the patient is leaning backward on the uprights at an angle of 20 degrees and the table has been tilted backward 20 degrees, making the sum of backward tilt 40 degrees.

describing the dermatomes that feel warm and "tingling." During the first 10 minutes, the tilt of the table may be altered to spread the hyperbaric phenol into desired areas if the initial feeling of warmth described by the patient is in the wrong dermatomes. Once the proper dermatomes are involved, the patient's position remains unaltered for 45 minutes.

Complications

Certain anatomical characteristics are responsible for the occurrence of complications with these nerve blocks. The first is that the ventral or motor root is closely related to the sites of injection and may be involved in any neurolytic procedure. Motor weakness or paralysis may result.

The pelvic nerve receives its sensory as well as motor innervation from S2, S3, and S4. Any sclerotic injection that involves the pelvic nerve will affect the detrusor muscle and internal sphincter of the bladder, which will result in some degree of bladder dysfunction. S1 and S2 are likewise involved with the pudendal nerve, so that sclerotic injection of these segments can be expected to affect the external sphincter. Neurolytic injections involving sacral segments will therefore be complicated by bladder dysfunction.

The innervation of the descending and the sigmoid colon is from the lumbar region on the left. Any injection of a neurolytic agent in the left lumbar area will interrupt the afferent impulses from the descending colon and sigmoid and will cause severe constipation.

Neurolysis of the lower caudal outflow will also cause rectal incontinence. Fortunately, most patients requiring sacral chemical neurolysis have had a previous colostomy as treatment of their disease, and also have a denervated bladder from the sacral metastases causing the pain.

Postinjection Management

Management following an intrathecal neurolytic block deserves special consideration. The keynote is a hopeful attitude on the part of the physician. If the first block is unsuccessful, the patient must be reassured that additional injections will be made until pain relief is achieved or until it becomes quite obvious that success is impossible. A repeated attempt may be made within 24 hours. If motor weakness occurs, the patient must be reassured that function may return within days or weeks. The aid of a skilled physiatrist should be enlisted to facilitate such recovery.

These patients must be supported with narcotics during the period following an intrathecal neurolytic injection. Under no circumstances should an attempt be made to withdraw narcotics—for several reasons. First, withdrawal symptoms may occur if the narcotic is withheld, and the symptoms of withdrawal may be interpreted as failure of the block to relieve pain. Also, an unrecognized acute withdrawal syndrome can be lethal. Second, patients who have far-advanced carcinoma usually have more than one site of pain or discomfort. Even though a neurolytic injection may control a major cause of pain, other sites of pain may become distressing. Finally, muscle cramps occur following blocks with phenol in glycerol, and intermittent paresthesia may follow intrathecal alcohol. For these reasons, analgesics and narcotics should be continued in appropriate dosage.

During the first 24 to 48 hours following the block, motor function and bladder and bowel function must be re-evaluated. During the entire management of the patient, great care must be taken to be certain that a decubitus ulcer does not develop in a blocked area.

Results

Fifteen cases are summarized in Table 129–1. This is too small a number to discuss the percentage of good or bad results. Of the 15 cases, however, 12 have had good results.

The results of intrathecal sclerotic injection can be summarized as follows. For intrathecal alcohol: Dogliotti reported 100 cases with good results in 59 per cent.[10] Stern reported 50 cases with good results in 63 per cent, and more recently, Kuzucu reported a series of 322 cases in which his good results are listed at 58 per cent.[15,30] It is reasonable to expect, therefore, that 58 per cent to 60 per cent good results will be observed in the use of intrathecal alcohol.

The results with intrathecal phenol are comparable to those with alcohol. Mayer reported 32 cases with good results in 50 per cent; three years later he reported 106 cases with good results in 68 per cent.[17,18] In 1966 Caine reported a small series with good results in only 47 per cent, and more recently Bracht presented a series of 60 cases with good results in 90 per cent.[4,6]

Present Indications

The advent of percutaneous cordotomy has greatly altered the management of intractable pain. The procedure is easily accomplished in the awake patient and does not involve a laminectomy. Many patients previously considered as too poor a risk for classic cordotomy are excellent candidates for the percutaneous technique. By old standards, these patients would have received intrathecal neurolytic agents in preference to cordotomy.

Rosomoff reported the results of percutaneous cordotomy in 100 patients.[26,27] In his immediate results, 92 of the 100 patients had total improvement and all were alive. Four weeks later, of his original 100 patients, only 77 were living, and of those, 67 had good results. Twelve weeks later there were 66 still living of whom 46 had good results, and 24 weeks later 39 were still living with 32 good results.

Because of these excellent results with percutaneous cordotomy, the use of intrathecal neurolytics in present practice should be limited to special circumstances. The patient shown in Figure 129–10 is illustrative of such a special circumstance. She was emotionally incapable of cooperating to the extent necessary to accomplish a percutaneous cordotomy.

The frequency of respiratory complications following bilateral high cervical percutaneous cordotomy may be an indication

TABLE 129–1 SUMMARY OF 15 PATIENTS RECEIVING INTRATHECAL PHENOL AND GLYCERIN

PATIENT	AREA OF PAIN	DIAGNOSIS	AREA BLOCKED	METHOD AND NUMBER	COMPLI-CATIONS	RESULTS
L.R.	Right hand	Carcinoma	C5–C7; T1–T2	1 ml 7.5% phenol; 2 blocks	0	Good
W.J.	Left upper quadrant	Fibrosarcoma	T8–T12	Alcohol, 3 blocks; 0.75 ml 7.5% phenol, 4 blocks	Bladder, leg weakness Constipation	Initially fair; finally good
W.M.	Right side of chest	Carcinoma	T7–T8	1 ml 5% phenol, 1 block	0	Good
J.P.	Leg spasms	Transverse myelitis	T12–L3	1 ml 7.5% phenol, 5 blocks	0	Good
E.E.	Loins and sacrum	Carcinoma	L1–L2	0.75 ml 7.5% phenol, 1 block	0	Good
S.M.	Upper part of chest	Carcinoma	T4–T6	0.5 ml 7.5% phenol, 1 block	Tingle of hand for 1 hour	Good
J.W.	Pelvis	Carcinoma	T11–L2	0.4 ml 7.5% phenol, 2 blocks	Constipation, temporary Weakness of legs	Good
R.R.	Loins and sacrum	Carcinoma	T10–T12	0.5 ml 7.5% phenol, 1 block	0	Fair
B.J.	Pelvis	Carcinoma	S2–S4	0.1 ml 5% phenol, 1 block	0	Poor
E.Z.	Arm and chest	Carcinoma	C3–T3	1 ml 7.5% phenol, 1 block	0	Good
E.A.	Chest	Herpes and depression	T5–T7	0.75 ml 7.5% phenol	0	Fair
K.K.	Leg and foot	Carcinoma	L2–S3	0.75 ml 7.5% phenol, 1 block	Bladder	Good
H.W.	Chest	Intercostal neuralgia	T3–T4	0.5 ml 7.5% phenol, 1 block	0	Good
I.M.	Chest	Carcinoma	T8–T9	0.5 ml 5% phenol, 5 ml 7.5% phenol, 2 blocks	Bladder	Good
C.L.	Leg and foot	Carcinoma	L1–S3	0.5 ml 5% phenol	Bladder, leg weakness	Good

for using intrathecal neurolytics instead in some patients.

Following bilateral cervical percutaneous cordotomy, a syndrome identified as Oden's syndrome has been reported.[31] The patient is able to breathe adequately while awake but becomes apneic when normal sleep occurs. It would seem therefore that another indication for intrathecal neurolytics would be bilateral pain involving cervical areas such as the brachial or cervical plexus. A percutaneous cordotomy could be done on the side of major involvement and intrathecal phenol employed on the other side.

Neurolytic Injections of Sympathetic Ganglion and Celiac Ganglia

Visceral pain originating within the abdominal cavity may be controlled by injection of the of neurolytic agents into the celiac plexus.[5] It has also been reported that paravertebral sympathetic ganglion block at the level of L1 will relieve abdominal visceral pain, although the effectiveness could possible be due to involvement of the celiac plexus by paravertebral injections into the loose areolar tissue at this site. Neurolytic injections into lumbar paravertebral sympathetic ganglia 2-3-4 are also employed in treatment of vasospastic occlusive disease of the lower extremity.[8] Twenty milliliters of 50 per cent alcohol or 10 ml of 5 per cent phenol in water may be used for paravertebral sympathetic block. A total of 50 ml of 50 per cent alcohol is used for celiac plexus block.

The technique of needle placement is not difficult. Perhaps because of this, most of the literature does not emphasize the critical importance of radiographic control to confirm needle location. Needles employed for these blocks should be 6 inches long, styletted, and 20 to 22 gauge. Such a needle can be deflected by fascial planes so that the trajectory of the point has no relationship to the direction of the shaft of the needle before entering the skin.

If the needle point is deflected so as to

enter the intervertebral foramen and pierce a dural sleeve, catastrophe can result from the injection. The accidental entry into a lumbar artery, particularly the first on the left, can cause a grave complication, anterior spinal artery thrombosis, if the injection is completed. It is mandatory, therefore, that films be obtained demonstrating that the needle point lies along the anterolateral surface of the vertebral body during a lumbar paravertebral sympathetic block and anterior to the T12 vertebral body during celiac plexus block. It is imperative to aspirate the needle carefully prior to injection.

Neurolytic Agents in Nonpainful Conditions

Neurolytic agents have been employed in the management of spastic conditions that accompany some types of paralysis.[14,16,21,23] Following spinal cord transection, violent muscle spasms may so contort the extremities as to make impossible the use of braces or even serene repose in a wheelchair. Persistent spasm may contribute to development of decubitus ulcers.

The previously described technique of intrathecal injection of phenol in glycerol may be altered to involve the motor root: the patient is positioned so that anterior roots come in contact with the injected mixture, and a concentration of phenol that is lytic to large motor fibers is used. The patient is placed in the lateral position with a 20- to 40-degree tilt forward instead of backward. A solution of 7.5 to 10 per cent phenol in glycerol is employed. The volume of material injected is as described for a sensory block.

It can be anticipated that intrathecal insertion of a needle will be difficult in such cases. The long supporting paravertebral muscles are frequently involved in the spastic conditions, contorting the lumbar vertebral column in various degrees of rotation, lordosis, and scoliosis. Frequently, the simplest method is to perform the lumbar puncture under general anesthesia with a proper endotracheal airway. Relaxation of the paraspinal muscles is then obtained with adequate quantities of muscle relaxant. Insertion of the needle is facilitated, and the possibility of a sudden spasm distorting the position at a critical time is eliminated.

REFERENCES

1. Adriani, J.: Labat's Regional Anesthesia. Philadelphia, W. B. Saunders Co., 1967.
2. Ahlgren, G. W., Stephen, C. R., Lloyd, A. C., and McCollum, D. E.: Diagnosis of pain with a graduated spinal block technique. J.A.M.A., 195:125, 1966.
3. Bonica, J.: The Management of Pain. Philadelphia, Lea & Febiger, 1953.
4. Bracht, E. A., DeKrey, J. A., and Buechel, D. R.: Permanent intradural blocks. Presented at West Coast Anesthesia Residents Conference, April 20 and 21, 1968, UCLA.
5. Bridenbaugh, L. D., Moore, D. C., Campbell, R. D., Management of upper abdominal cancer pain. J.A.M.A., 190:877, 1964.
6. Caine, H. D.: Subarachnoid phenol block in the treatment of pain and spasticity. Paraplegia, 3:152, 1966.
7. Collins, V. J.: Principles of Anesthesiology. Philadelphia, Lea & Febiger, 1966, pp. 814–816.
8. DeKrey, J. A., Schroeder, C. F., and Buechel, D. R.: Selective chemical sympathectomy. Anesth. Analg. (Cleveland), 47:633, 1968.
9. DeTakats, G.: Causalgia state in peace and war. J.A.M.A., 128:699, 1945.
10. Dogliotti, A. M.: Traitement des syndromes douloureux de la périphérie par l'alcoolisation subarachnoid. Presse Méd., 39:1249, 1931.
11. Evans, J. A.: Reflex sympathetic dystrophy. Ann. Intern. Med., 26:417, 1947.
12. Foerster, O.: The dermatomes in man. Brain, 56:1, 1933.
13. Gallager, H. S., Yonezawa, T., Hay, R. C., and Derrick, W. W.: Subarachnoid alcohol block. II. Histologic changes in the central nervous system. Amer. J. Path., 38:679, 1961.
14. Kelly, R. E., and Gautier-Smith, P. C.: Intrathecal phenol in the treatment of reflex spasms and spasticity. Lancet, 2:1102, 1959.
15. Kuzucu, E. Y., Derrick, W. W., and Wilber, S. A.: Control of intractable pain with subarachnoid alcohol block. J.A.M.A., 195:541, 1966.
16. Liversedge, L. A., and Maher, R. M.: Use of phenol in relief of spasticity. Brit. Med. J., 2:31, 1960.
17. Maher, R. M.: Relief of pain in incurable cancer. Lancet, 1:18, 1955.
18. Maher, R. M.: Neurone selection in relief of pain: Further experiences with intrathecal injections. Lancet, 1:16, 1957.
19. Michele, A. A., Davies, J. J., Krueger, F. J., and Lichtor, J. M.: Scapulocostal syndrome (fatigue-postural paradox). New York J. Med., 50:1353, 1950.
20. Moore, D. C.: Regional Block. Springfield, Ill., Charles C Thomas, 1965.
21. Nathan, P. W.: Intrathecal phenol to relieve spasticity in paraplegia. Lancet, 2:1099, 1959.
22. Nathan, P. W., and Scott, T. G.: Intrathecal phenol for intractable pain: Safety and dangers of method. Lancet, 1:76, 1958.
23. Persen, R., and Juul, J. P.: Intrathecal phenol in treatment of spasticity. Acta Neurol. Scand., 38:69, 1962.
24. Peyton, W. T., Semansky, E. K., and Baker, A. B.: Subarachnoid injection of alcohol for relief of intractable pain with discussion of cord

changes found at autopsy. Amer. J. Cancer, *30*:709, 1937.

25. Richter, C. P.: Instruction for using the cutaneous resistance recorder in peripheral nerve injuries, sympathectomies and paravertebral block. J. Neurosurg., *3*:181, 1946.

26. Rosomoff, H. L., Brown, C. J., and Sheptak, P.: Percutaneous radiofrequency cervical cordotomy: Technique. J. Neurosurg., *23*:639, 1965.

27. Rosomoff, H. L., Sheptak, P., and Carrol, F.: Modern pain relief: Percutaneous cordotomy. J.A.M.A., *196*:482, 1966.

28. Saltzstein, H. C.: Intraspinal injection of absolute alcohol for the control of pain in far advanced malignant growth. J.A.M.A., *103*:242, 1934.

29. Sola, A. E., and Williams, R. L.: Myofacial pain syndromes. Neurology (Minneap.), *6*:91, 1956.

30. Stern, E. L.: Relief of intractable pain by intraspinal injection of alcohol. Amer. J. Surg., *25*:217, 1934.

31. Tenicola, R., Rosomoff, H. L., Ferst, J., and Safer, P.: Pulmonary function following percutaneous cervical cordotomy. Anesthesiology, *29*:7, 1968.

130

DORSAL RHIZOTOMY

Dorsal rhizotomy for the relief of pain was first performed in 1888 by both Bennett in England and Abbe in the United States.[1,3] Although this operation was seen to have great theoretical potential for the alleviation of pain, reports throughout the twentieth century have shown that many patients did not obtain the planned analgesia or relief of their symptoms.[7,12,14] During the period between World War I and World War II, dorsal rhizotomy was employed to alleviate angina pectoris as well as pain from other visceral structures. In recent years, developments in pharmacology and surgery have almost eliminated these applications of rhizotomy. More recently, however, dorsal rhizotomy has been utilized to relieve pain due to malignant diseases and injuries to nerves. Despite the long experience with this procedure, it is not well established.

One of the major problems in an analysis of the applicability and efficacy of dorsal rhizotomy is the paucity of reported cases. Although many thousands of patients have had this operation, data are available on only a few hundred. Many surgeons have failed to report long-term follow-up. As is well known, immediate relief is no guarantee that pain will not recur in a few weeks or months. Table 130–1 contains the data on the long-term success of dorsal rhizotomy reported in the literature. Success is defined as pain relief present at least three months postoperatively or until death in a patient with cancer if survival did not last three months. Success rates vary from 25 to 75 per cent in the larger series. Clearly, the theoretical advantages of dorsal rhizotomy have not been reflected in the long-term results. The analysis of this problem will help place dorsal rhizotomy in its proper position among other pain-relieving operative procedures.

ADVANTAGES AND DISADVANTAGES

Like all other operative measures to alleviate pain, dorsal rhizotomy has its advantages and disadvantages. In theory and in practice dorsal rhizotomy is superior to peripheral neurectomy in the treatment of chronic pain. The primary advantage is the sparing of motor fibers and the absence, therefore, of paralysis. The complete transection of all the dorsal roots to an extremity will, however, in man, lead to both anesthesia and functional paralysis, the latter probably based on the loss of gamma afferents and other proprioceptive fibers. Total dorsal rhizotomy of a limb is rarely a satisfactory operative procedure. Resection of sacral dorsal roots may interfere with both sphincters and sexual function, and must therefore be highly selective. In contrast, extensive areas of the cervical, thoracic, and upper lumbar regions may be denervated without significant deficits of function. In these areas motor loss is rarely a problem and proprioceptive information does not appear to be important for most activities.

Selective dorsal rhizotomies may be utilized in the extremity to alleviate pain. Some advocate resection of portions of several roots. Others have shown that preservation of a single root to an extremity will suffice for proprioception and leave motor function reasonably intact. The area of cutaneous anesthesia produced by resection of a single root or adjacent pair of roots is not identical in every patient. Furthermore,

---

J. D. LOESER

TABLE 130-1 RESULTS OF SPINAL DORSAL RHIZOTOMY

		REASON FOR OPERATION			
		Malignant Disease		Benign Process	
AUTHOR	YEAR	Number	Per Cent Success*	Number	Per Cent Success*
Groves[8]	1911	—	—	22	27
Haven and King[9]	1942	—	—	5	100 (angina pectoris) (1 postoperative death)
Ray[16]	1943	?	?	?	?
Lindgren and Olivecrona[11]	1946	—	—	7	16 (angina pectoris) (1 postoperative death)
Bohm and Franksson[4]	1958	7	100	8	88
Sicard[18]	1963	0	—	195	75
Scoville[17]	1966	2	100	10	40
Echols[5]	1969	0	—	62	60
White and Sweet[22]	1969	33	58	51	70
Smith[20]	1970	1	100	9	100
Echols[6]	1970	—	—	19	63
Loeser[12]	1972	7	43	29	25
Onofrio and Campa[14]	1972	18	28	211	37
Paillas and Pellet[15]	1972	6	0	42	76
White and Kjelberg[21]	1973	—	—	62	65
Barrash and Leavens[2]	1973	71	70	—	—
Sindou et al.[19]	1974	20	65	—	—

* Success is defined as pain relief at least three months after operation.

cutaneous sensory loss may not be coterminous with underlying osseous or joint anesthesia. Resection of a pair of roots may lead to surprisingly little sensory loss if adjacent roots are normal. This is well illustrated by Figures 130–1 and 130–2, taken from the classic studies of White and Sweet.[22] There is little question that overlapping of dermatomes is prominent in man. The sensory loss produced by rhizotomy always has a hypesthetic region surrounding the anesthetic zone. Finally, the study by Hodge and King has shown that the regions of relative and absolute sensory loss are not anatomically stable and are influenced by pharmacological agents.[10] This fascinating observation may explain why pain relief and analgesia are sometimes transient after dorsal rhizotomy.

Another advantage of dorsal rhizotomy is the ability to render anesthetic a circumscribed region of the body. The area of sensory loss can be determined preoperatively by selective somatic nerve blocks at the neural foramina. Intraoperative testing can be carried out by applying a cotton pledget soaked in local anesthetic to the isolated intradural dorsal root if the operation is performed under local anesthesia. Unfortunately, the region of sensory loss several months after rhizotomy is not always as extensive as that produced by nerve blocks. Dorsal rhizotomy can be used to denervate

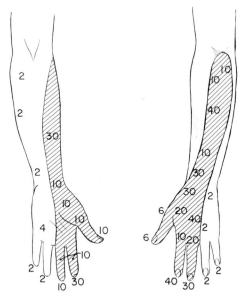

Figure 130–1 Extent of sensory loss after posterior rhizotomy of C6 and C7. Pain threshold to pinprick is marked in grams (40 gm represents complete analgesia). This woman retained light touch to 2.4-gm hair and experienced only slight reduction in position sense. At one year after operation she was able to identify coins and button up her dress without difficulty. Pain following C5–C6 vertebral fracture-dislocation was well relieved. (From White, J. C., and Sweet, W. H.: Pain and the Neurosurgeon: A Forty-Year Experience. Springfield, Ill., Charles C Thomas, 1969. Reprinted by permission.)

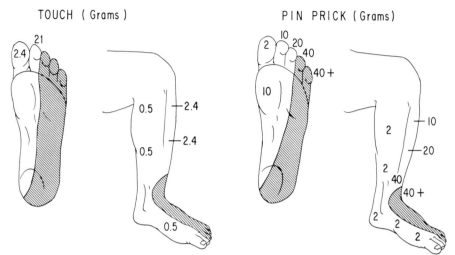

Figure 130–2 Extent of sensory loss of posterior rhizotomy of L5 and S1. Pain and touch thresholds are marked in grams: 40-gm pinprick and 21-gm hair represent full anesthesia. Sense of position was lost in last two toes; vibration sense was lost below ankle. Graphesthesia is present only in big toe. (From White, J. C., and Sweet W. H.: Pain and the Neurosurgeon: A Forty-Year Experience. Springfield, Ill., Charles C Thomas 1969. Reprinted by permission.)

a section of the body without impairing sensation in more distal segments. In contrast, cordotomy results in loss of pain and temperature sensation over the entire side of the body up to three segments below the level of the lesion. The region of sensory loss produced by rhizotomy is, however, much more stable than that produced by cordotomy. Unlike cordotomy, the rhizotomy is not followed significantly often by return of pain 3 months to 10 years after operation.

Dorsal rhizotomy has disadvantages, too. Complete denervation of an extremity is rarely acceptable. Midline or bilateral pain requires bilateral rhizotomies for its relief. If the patient has normal anal and urinary sphincters and sexual function, sacral rhizotomies must be undertaken with great caution to avoid the production of incontinence or impotence. When the sphincters are already inoperative, sacral rhizotomy can be extremely effective in the relief of perineal pain.[3]

Another disadvantage is the loss of all modalities of sensation following dorsal rhizotomy. This contrasts with cordotomy, which produces loss of only pain and temperature sensation. While the loss of all sensation may be of little consequence over the torso, it is a major drawback to rhizotomies that affect the extremities. Annoying dysesthesias are less common after dorsal rhizotomy than after cordotomy. Intraoperative neurological complications due to

damage of the spinal cord are also less common after dorsal rhizotomy than after cordotomy. Although the operative incision may be uncomfortable for some patients long after the wound has healed, rhizotomy never leads to the problems of neuroma formation that so frequently plague peripheral neurectomies.

By far the major disadvantage of dorsal rhizotomy has been the failure to obtain adequate long-term pain relief in 25 to 75 per cent of patients. Causes of less-than-optimal results can be divided into four categories: technical errors, sensory overlap, sprouting, and dynamic changes. Technical errors include failure to transact all the fascicles of a root, failure to cut the desired root, and incorrect identification of the roots that must be cut to produce anesthesia in a specified region. There may rarely be intradural or extradural anastamoses between roots, which can lead to unexpected results from dorsal rhizotomy.

Sensory overlap as shown in Figure 130–3 has been studied carefully in man since the pioneering work of Foerster.[7] Not only do adjacent dorsal roots have common cutaneous fields, but underlying muscle, bone, and joint afferents may be part of quite different sclerotomes or myotomes. These are not identical in every patient. This means, obviously, that dorsal rhizotomy for pain relief cannot be based upon textbook diagrams of sensory fields, but must be based upon evaluation of the indi-

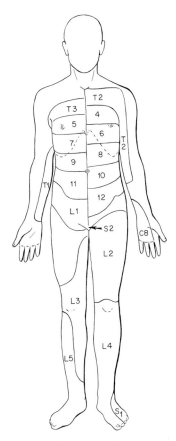

Figure 130-3 The spinal dermatomes: This diagram, modified from Foerster's photograph of a male model, shows the extent and degree of overlap of the spinal sensory nerves from C8 through S1.

From our own experience there is good evidence to add that the occipital portion of the scalp to the vertex, most of the auricle, and skin of the upper neck are supplied by C2 and C3, with an occasional contribution from an inconstant posterior rootlet of C1. C3 and C4 supply the sensory innervation to the tip of the shoulder, supraclavicular fossa, upper three ribs in front, and spine of the scapula behind, overlapping the upper intercostal nerves. C5 supplies the skin covering the deltoid muscle; C6 supplies the lateral and posterior aspect of the upper arm, forearm, thenar eminence, and thumb; and C7 supplies the thumb and first three fingers, overlapping the area of C6 and C8, shown in the diagram. S1, in addition to supplying the outer half of the foot, also supplies the lateral side of the calf and posterior thigh. S2 innervates the posterior upper thigh, side of the penis, vagina, and labium minor. S3, with the two lower sacral and coccygeal nerves, innervates the perineum and the perianal and coccygeal areas. (From White, J. C.: Dolor, 1969. Courtesy of Revista del Instituto Nacional de Neurología. Mexico.)

vidual's neurological status and response to nerve blocks.

Sprouting is also given as a reason why dorsal rhizotomies may fail to maintain pain relief. It has been demonstrated both histo-

logically and physiologically that branches of intact cutaneous nerves will grow into adjacent denervated skin. The sensory loss following neurectomy or rhizotomy will always decrease slightly in a circumferential mode. This is why it is important to cut enough dorsal roots to render anesthetic a wider region than just the source of the pain. Sprouting within the spinal cord has also been proposed as one of the causes of failure. Although histological evidence for intraspinal axonal sprouting in animal models exists, functional central sprouting has not been proved.

Dynamic changes do occur after rhizotomy and may be responsible for some of the failures. The studies of Hodge and King and Miller and co-workers have shown that cutaneous sensory fields are not solidly "wired in" to the nervous system but are capable of modification by drugs or transection of adjacent roots.[10,13] These phenomena may explain why pain relief is present in the immediate postoperative period but disappears in a few weeks.

Dorsal rhizotomy has remained a commonly performed operation for pain for over 75 years. It is clearly superior to peripheral neurectomy: pain relief is more likely, motor deficits can be avoided, and painful neuromas do not occur. For pain originating from the upper cervical, thoracic, and upper lumbar regions it is probably more effective than cordotomy, although when the pain originates in an extremity or over an extensive area, a cordotomy may be preferred. Since the beneficial effects of a cordotomy may fade over several years, the patient with a long life expectancy might be better served by dorsal rhizotomy, which rarely loses its effectiveness after three to six months. If the source of the pain is likely to spread, a cordotomy may be the wiser choice. Certainly, a major feature of the choice of an operation for pain relief will always be the surgeon's personal skill and prior experience.

INDICATIONS AND CONTRAINDICATIONS FOR DORSAL RHIZOTOMY

Dorsal rhizotomy for pain relief should not be offered to a patient until the surgeon has full knowledge of the pathological condition leading to the chronic pain, the patient's overall health status, and the availability and practicality of alternative modes of therapy. It is essential that the surgeon determine that alternative therapy directed at the cause of the patient's pain is unlikely to succeed before performing any destructive procedure. Dorsal rhizotomy is not the treatment to utilize if the patient's life expectancy is less than 30 to 60 days. Preterminal patients often have problems with wound-healing and infections, and postoperative recuperation in a hospital that occupies more than 25 per cent of a patient's remaining life seems unacceptable. Pharmacological methods or percutaneous cordotomy are more applicable to patients with less than 60 days' life expectancy. The presence of iatrogenic drug addiction in a patient with chronic pain should not be a contraindication to dorsal rhizotomy. When pain relief follows operation, it will be even easier to gradually reduce the narcotic dosage. The presence of local infection adjacent to the operative site or significant systemic infection is, of course, an absolute contraindication to dorsal rhizotomy.

Dorsal rhizotomy seems more effective for pain originating in certain regions and due to specific disease processes. When pain due to cancer originates in the upper cervical region, cervical rhizotomy alone rarely suffices. The trigeminal and glossopharyngeal, the nervus intermedius, and upper fibers of the vagus nerves or the descending trigeminal tract often must be sectioned in addition. When a neoplasm is causing pain by invasion of viscera and body wall, dorsal rhizotomy is not as satisfactory as cordotomy. Dorsal rhizotomy can be employed to treat pain secondary to the peripheral neuropathies that occasionally follow thoracic or abdominal operative procedures. Two roots above and two roots below the injured nerves should be resected; consistently good results have not been reported, however. Pain due to coronary ischemia can be relieved by bilateral T1 through T4 dorsal rhizotomies. Pain from other viscera may also be relieved by appropriate rhizotomies. In the patient who has perineal pain due to malignant disease or the treatment thereof by operation or radiation, selective dorsal rhizotomies can be very effective. The patient who has had urinary and anal diversionary procedures and who has persistent perineal pain is an especially good candidate for bilateral S3 through Co1 rhizotomies. The place of dorsal rhizotomy in the treatment of the patient with the "failed lumbar disc" is uncertain. Good long-term results vary from 15 to 63 per cent. Diffuse arachnoiditis rarely responds to dorsal rhizotomy; focal scarring about a single nerve root may offer a much better prognosis.

Nerve blocks should be used to evaluate a candidate for dorsal rhizotomy. The data from a single block should not be relied upon; rather, the block must be repeated on several occasions to delineate which roots are involved in the patient's pain and rule out a placebo response to the block. Nerve blocks also give the patient a preview of the effects of operation. Some patients will be found who prefer pain to numbness. Radiographic control of needle placement is required to pinpoint the level of the nerve block. Although nerve blocks will indicate the region of anesthesia produced by a subsequent dorsal rhizotomy, they do not predict a successful long-term operative result.[12,14]

TECHNIQUES FOR PERFORMING DORSAL RHIZOTOMY

The technical aspects of performing a dorsal rhizotomy are well known among neurosurgeons. The operation is facilitated by utilization of the operating microscope and microdissection tools but does not require any unique operating equipment. Most surgeons prefer the intradural approach, but Scoville and Smith have both described extradural approaches and ganglionectomy in the thoracic region.[17,20] These latter techniques have not found widespread acceptance.

Although dorsal rhizotomy is usually performed under general endotracheal anesthesia, it can also be done with local or regional nerve blocks. The choice of anesthesia is a function of the technical expertise available, the preoperative evaluation of the patient, the patient's personality, and the surgeon's preference. The position of the patient during the operation is dictated by several factors. It is unwise to perform a dorsal rhizotomy in the sitting position under local or regional anesthesia because of the headache, nausea, and vomiting produced by the loss of cerebrospinal fluid. The sitting position is, however, useful for cervical rhizotomies under general anesthesia; a venous catheter situated in the right atrium should be employed to monitor and treat potential air embolism. The prone, oblique, and lateral decubitus positions may be employed for thoracic, lumbar, or sacral rhizotomies. Segmental epidural anesthesia is effective but should be undertaken only by those thoroughly familiar with the technique. Operation under local anesthesia permits the surgeon to block each root temporarily with a cotton pledget soaked in lidocaine (Xylocaine) and ascertain the sensory loss prior to transecting the root and to be certain that the entire painful area has been denervated by the rhizotomies. A technically perfect initial operative result can be thereby guaranteed; many patients, however, will not accept a major operation under local anesthesia. Well-controlled preoperative selective nerve blocks with radiological localization do reduce the need for operation under local anesthesia.

It is obviously essential to know the exact level of the laminectomy. In the upper cervical and lower lumbar regions it is usually sufficient to count the spinous processes. In the lower cervical, thoracic, and upper lumbar regions it is helpful to utilize adjunctive measures. A short needle can be driven into a spinous process under local anesthesia and broken off flush with the skin. The region is x-rayed to localize the needle, which is readily identified at the time of operation. Alternatively, a needle can be placed in the interspinous ligament immediately prior to the procedure and x-rayed to prove its location. Methylene blue (0.25 to 0.50 ml) is then injected, and the needle is removed. After the skin incision has been made, the location of the dye can be ascertained. Finally, ambiguities that become apparent during the operation can sometimes be resolved by an intraoperative x-ray.

Unilateral dorsal rhizotomies are easily performed in the lateral decubitus position with the operative side uppermost. This permits the spinal cord to fall away from the dural foramina and exposes a major portion of the intradural root. The midline incision in the skin should extend one spinous process above and one below the planned laminectomy. After subperiosteal

dissection of the paravertebral muscles on the side of the rhizotomies, hemilaminectomies are performed. It is usually necessary to remove one or two more laminae than the number of roots to be sectioned to achieve adequate exposure. The dura is opened in the middle of the bony defect and held by stay sutures to maximize visualization of the subjacent roots. The arachnoid is incised as far laterally as possibly so that the dural incision does not overlie that in the arachnoid. This appears to reduce the risk of postoperative cerebrospinal fluid leakage. At this stage an operating microscope is employed for inspection of each of the roots and careful dissection of major blood vessels away from the roots themselves (Fig. 130–4). Compromise of a major feeding vessel can lead to ischemic myelitis and must be avoided. Each root is then destroyed by bipolar coagulation and transection with microscissors. It is prudent to mark with silver clips the most rostral and caudal roots that have been divided.

Bilateral dorsal rhizotomies are best performed with the patient prone or in the sitting position if the cervical roots are to be sectioned. The prone position requires careful support of the chest and abdomen to prevent increased venous pressure and excessive epidural bleeding. Bilateral subperiosteal muscle dissection and laminectomy and a midline dural incision are utilized. Local wound pain and muscle

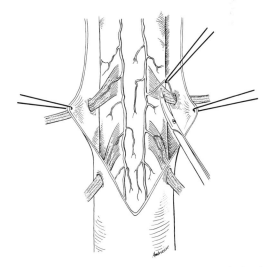

Figure 130–4 Posterior rhizotomy. Method of sparing important feeding arteries that accompany some of the posterior roots. (From White, J. C.: Dolor, 1969. Courtesy of Revista del Instituto Nacional de Neurología, Mexico.)

spasm are significantly greater than after a unilateral approach.

Dorsal rhizotomies in the upper cervical and sacral segments require special attention. The surgeon should not overlook the fact that the first cervical root may have some sensory fibers. If denervation in the occipital region is required, these fibers must be diligently searched for and transected. Individual roots leaving the conus medullaris cannot be identified with clarity. Size of the roots and location of major vessels are not reliable indicators. It is wisest to perform lower lumbar and sacral rhizotomies by identifying the nerve roots as they pass through their dural sleeves. Usually this passage occurs over the body of the vertebra above the bony foramen of each root. For example, transection of the L5 dorsal root requires a laminectomy of L4. Identification of the sacral roots is best made by electrically stimulating the isolated root prior to its transection. Stimulation of S1 produces only leg muscle contraction; that of S2 and S3 produces contraction of bladder and anal musculature and less muscular activity in the leg. Lower sacral and coccygeal roots do not produce an easily testable muscular activity when stimulated. Patients who have had fecal and urinary diversionary procedures and have chronic perineal pain may be candidates for transection of all the fibers of S3 through Co1. This operation is readily performed through an L5–S1 laminectomy and midline incision of the distal end of the dural sac. Root identification is confirmed by electrical stimulation prior to transection.

The importance of a watertight closure of the dura cannot be overemphasized. A small dural leak can lead to a cerebrospinal fluid fistula that requires secondary closure. Muscle and fascial planes also must be appropriately closed. The typical patient is kept at bed rest for three to five days until his postoperative headache abates. Progressive activities are encouraged until discharge, which is usually 7 to 10 days after operation. Strenuous activities are curtailed until fascial healing has occurred approximately a month later.

Failure to achieve anesthesia in the desired area is a complication that should be dealt with by prompt reoperation and sectioning of the correct dorsal roots. Lack of pain relief in spite of anesthesia in the region of the pain is usually not an indication for further dorsal rhizotomies. One of the most dreaded complications of dorsal rhizotomy is the development of an epidural clot. Careful hemostasis is obviously the best preventive measure; mutliple layer closure of muscle and fascia is also helpful. Frequent postoperative assessment of neurological function will allow the early detection of progressive neurological deficit and prompt evacuation of a clot should it occur.

CONCLUSION

Dorsal rhizotomy has a place in the treatment of chronic pain. Careful assessment of the patient preoperatively, attention to detail intraoperatively, and follow-up during the postoperative period are required to make this operation as beneficial as possible. Patient selection remains the most important single predictor of a successful outcome.

REFERENCES

1. Abbe, R.: A contribution to the surgery of the spine. Med. Rec., *35*:149–152, 1889.
2. Barrash, J. M., and Leavens, M. E.: Dorsal rhizotomy for the relief of intractable pain of malignant tumor origin. J. Neurosurg., *38*:755–757, 1973.
3. Bennet, W. H.: Subdural division of posterior roots of spinal nerves. Lancet, *1*:839–840, 1889.
4. Bohm, E., and Franksson, C.: Coccygodynia and sacral rhizotomy. Acta Chir. Scand., *116*:268–274, 1958–1959.
5. Echols, D. H.: Sensory rhizotomy following operation for ruptured intervertebral disc. A review of 62 cases. J. Neurosurg., *31*:335–338, 1969.
6. Echols, D. H.: The effectiveness of thoracic rhizotomy for chronic pain. Neurochirurgia, *13*:69–74, 1970.
7. Foerster, O.: Resection of the posterior spinal nerve-roots in the treatment of gastric crises and spastic paralysis. Proc. Roy. Soc. Med., *4*:226–254, 1911.
8. Groves, E. W. H.: On the division of the posterior spinal nerve roots: (I) for pain, (II) for visceral crises, (III) for spasm. Proc. Roy. Soc. Med., *4*:119–225, 1911.
9. Haven, H., and King, R.: Section of the posterior roots for the relief of pain in angina pectoris. Surg. Gynec. Obstet., *75*:208–219, 1942.
10. Hodge, C. J., and King, R. B.: Medical modification of sensation. J. Neurosurg., *44*:21–28, 1976.
11. Lindgren, L., and Olivecrona, H.: Surgical treatment of angina pectoris. J. Neurosurg., *4*:19–39, 1946.
12. Loeser, J. D.: Dorsal rhizotomy for the relief of chronic pain. J. Neurosurg., *36*:745–750, 1972.

13. Miller, J., Basbaum, A. I., and Wall, P. D.: Restructuring of the somatotopic map and appearance of abnormal neuronal activity in the gracile nucleus after partial deafferentation. Exp. Neurol., *50*:658–672, 1976.

14. Onofrio, B. M., and Campa, H. K.: Evaluation of rhizotomy. Review of 12 years experience. J. Neurosurg., *36*:751–755, 1972.

15. Paillas, J. W., and Pellet, W.: Dorsal nerve root section in the treatment of refractory peripheral pain. *In* Janzen, R., et al., eds.: Pain. Baltimore, Williams & Wilkins, 1972, pp. 209–213.

16. Ray, B. S.: The management of intractable pain by posterior rhizotomy. Res. Publ. Ass. Res. Nerv. Ment. Dis., *23*:319–407, 1943.

17. Scoville, W. B.: Extradural spinal sensory rhizotomy. J. Neurosurg., *25*:94–95, 1966.

18. Sicard, A.: Resultats du traitment chirugical des sciatiques. Bull. Acad. Nat. Med. (Paris), *147*:469–474, 1963.

19. Sindou, M., Fischer, G., Goutelle, A., and Mansuy, L.: La radicellotomie postérieure sélective. Neurochirurgie (Paris), *20*:391–408, 1974.

20. Smith, F. P.: Trans-spinal ganglionectomy for relief of intercostal pain. J. Neurosurg., *32*:574–577, 1970.

21. White, J. C., and Kjellberg, R. N.: Posterior spinal rhizotomy: A substitute for cordotomy in the relief of localized pain in patients with normal life expectancy. Neurochirurgia (Stuttgart), *16*:141–170, 1973.

22. White, J. C., and Sweet, W. H.: Pain and the Neurosurgeon. Springfield, Ill., Charles C Thomas, 1969, pp. 633–660.

131

STEREOTAXIC CORDOTOMY

Although percutaneous cordotomy is a natural extension of stereotaxic technology, its basic anatomical goal is no different from that of all older historical methods of spinal tractomy by open operation. In 1910, Schuller first suggested the deliberate section of the anterolateral tracts of the spinal cord for the relief of pain.[32] But it was not until two years later that Martin, at the urging of Spiller, performed the initial dorsal cordotomy in man.[35] Foerster and Gagel were the first to utilize the cervical route for access.[6] The literature contains a large number of reports concerning technique, results, and complications of open cordotomy, all of which conclude that it is a useful short-term method for the alleviation of pain in patients with malignant disease but one attended by substantial risk, and the duration of its effect is variable in those fortunate enough to survive for longer periods of time. Therefore, the concept of a percutaneous, stereotaxic procedure, accomplished under local anesthesia, simply, easily, and with low rates of morbidity in patients who, otherwise, might not be acceptable for a major open operation was most attractive. Mullan and his associates deserve recognition for this visionary innovation.[21]

The initial method of percutaneous cordotomy utilized a needle with a radioactive tip, inserted into the spine at C1–C2 laterally, coming to lie anterolaterally in the subarachnoid space adjacent to the ventral quadrant of the spinal cord.[21] Although some success could be claimed for this procedure, it was abandoned because of the unpredictable immediate and long-term effects of radiation on spinal cord and the limited and uncertain supply of isotopic needles for general use. The next approach introduced a wire electrode into the parenchyma of the spinal cord and used a direct current source for lesion-making in the ventral quadrant.[20] This method, also, proved insufficient insofar as the configuration of the lesion was erratic, the duration of current flow to produce a satisfactory lesion was often longer than the patient could tolerate lying on the operating table without dislodging the electrode, and the results were equally unpredictable over time. Rosomoff and his associates proposed a technique using radiofrequency current to produce the lesion, which allowed for rapid, solid lesion-making, equipment that was available commercially or easily built, and portable instrumentation.[31] This technique became the basic standard, although there have been a number of modifications of access route (i.e., anterior, posterior, medullary, low cervical), methods of target localization, electrode design, and radiofrequency lesion makers (with respect to current flow time or configurations).* The operation presented here is that utilized by the author, as first described in 1965 and modified through the years of experience to date. Other methods are mentioned briefly at the end of this segment to acquaint the reader with variations of technique and modifications for potential improvement or prevention of inherent liability.

INDICATIONS

The technique of percutaneous cordotomy may be considered for any patient with somatic pain below the level of the mandible. Percutaneous cordotomy is indicated for patients with pain from cancer, including those who previously could not be

---

* See references 5, 7–10, 15, 36–38.

H. L. ROSOMOFF

subjected to the major operation of laminectomy and spinothalamic section because of debilitation or a preterminal state. It is indicated, also, for those individuals with painful conditions that are intractable and nonmalignant in nature. In the selection of patients, it is necessary to differentiate pain with a lancinating or toothache-like quality from distressing dysesthesias, such as burning, prickling, pressure, crawling, and the like. The former is mediated by the lateral spinothalamic tract, and ventrolateral cordotomy will alleviate pain in more than 90 per cent of cases. The latter is not transmitted entirely through the ventral quadrant, and these discomforts will be relieved imperfectly or not at all. In the patient with a mixed pain picture, i.e., lancinating pain and dysesthesias, the initial response to a successful cordotomy may be relief of all types of discomfort. Within a few days to weeks, however, the dysesthesias return to conscious perception. Their perception, sometimes, seems to be heightened by the absence of the lancinating component, which previously had been the overriding sensation. It will still be possible to demonstrate dense analgesia to pinprick, confirming ablation of the anterolateral ascending pain system. It therefore follows that dysesthetic ''pain'' is transmitted elsewhere, but possibly in closely approximate structures in which conduction is interrupted temporarily by the trauma of operation, only to return to function with resolution of the post-traumatic operative effects. One exception to this statement is the relief of tabetic or pseudo-tabetic pain, which does have a dysesthetic quality, but in which cordotomy is an effective means of producing relief.

When bilateral cordotomy is required, the contralateral procedure is performed as a second stage no less than one week later.

CONTRAINDICATIONS

Severe pulmonary dysfunction is the major contraindication to cordotomy. The absence of a lung, per se, does not interdict the procedure, however, provided that remaining pulmonary function is satisfactory. Recently incurred neurological deficits, such as paresis or rectal-bladder disturbance, may be aggravated or their recovery delayed by the superimposition of cordotomy; when this is so, the effect is usually temporary.

PREOPERATIVE PREPARATION

In addition to the correction of blood volume deficits and fluid and electrolyte disturbances, an estimation of pulmonary function should be obtained. This should include determinations of forced vital capacity, forced expiratory volume and flow rate, minute volume breathing room air, and minute volume in response to breathing 5 per cent carbon dioxide. Values less than 50 per cent of predicted represent a calculated risk relative to the potential complication of sleep-induced apnea.

ANESTHESIA

Local anesthesia is used, 1.5 per cent lidocaine, as for intrathecal instillation, being the agent of choice. The patient should be maintained in as alert and cooperative a state as is possible. Premedication therefore consists only of his usual dosage of analgesic with a suitable supplement of a tranquilizing drug. Hydroxyzine (Vistaril), 25 to 50 mg intramuscularly, has been used most extensively, but the agent preferred by the individual surgeon can be substituted. The goal is for the patient to be alert and cooperative so that modifications of the procedure can be made as needed. Confusion of the patient must be avoided, otherwise accurate testing of his responses in respect to level of analgesia or the early onset of untoward effects such as paresis will not be possible. No food or fluids are allowed for four hours prior to the procedure.

POSITION OF PATIENT

The position of the patient is critical. The patient is supine with an adjustable inflatable pad beneath the shoulders. The head is immobilized in an opposing grip cup headholder with padding over the eyes. The pad is inflated to extend the neck at the shoulders and the headholder is closed so as to flex the head upon the cervical spine. Both maneuvers are accomplished in order to place the top of a special sighting device at a level opposite the junction of the ear lobe

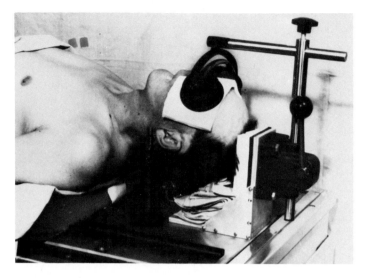

Figure 131–1 Position of patient with sighting device.

and the face. This assures maintenance of the air, to be instilled later in the procedure, in the proper position for visualization of the spinal cord; and the sighting device provides a guide for the introduction of the cordotomy needle, since external soft-tissue landmarks are too inconstant to be serviceable (Fig. 131–1).

EQUIPMENT

The percutaneous cordotomy tray consists of an 18-gauge, thin-walled, 3.5-inch (9-cm), short-beveled spinal needle, 19- and 25-gauge needles, a two-way stopcock, a glass for the anesthetic, a cup, forceps, sponges and towels for skin preparation, two 10-ml syringes, a polyethylene insulated electrode and holder, a coaxial radio-

frequency cable, and a micromanipulator. Figure 131–2 pictures one commercially available unit (Radionics RFG-5 generator); however, others are manufactured or the components can be made by personal design. Radiological visualization may be accomplished with conventional equipment using standard or Polaroid film, or an omnidirectional cinefluorographic unit may be employed to expedite the procedure. The spinal cord lesion is made with a radiofrequency generator, which must be standardized to produce a 5-mm ellipsoid after 30 seconds of exposure. This standardization may be accomplished by inserting the electrode with its connections from the lesion generator of choice into egg white or red meat and then observing the quantity of substance that is coagulated as to function of current and time. The usual parameter to

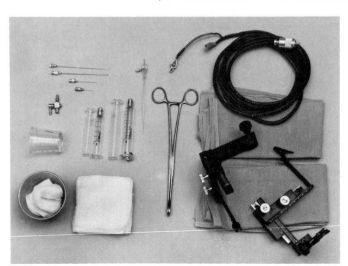

Figure 131–2 Cordotomy equipment tray.

effect this lesion with the Radionics RFG-2A generator is an output of 2.2 w at 110 ma and 20 v. This generator supplies a constant current source. The voltage will rise to compensate for an increase of impedance (see the section on corroboration of electrode position), so an excessive temperature level may be reached, creating a gas bubble and unwanted destruction of spinal cord by explosion. For this reason, if the voltage increases suddenly during lesion making and amperage decreases responsively, do not increase the wattage. Withdraw, replace the electrode, and begin anew. Constant voltage generators are also available that are designed to avert this problem (Radionics RFG-3AV). If impedance rises rapidly, as it would with gas formation, the radiofrequency current will fall rapidly. This automatically reduces the power and tissue heating. This mode of operation is safe when a thermal sensing electrode is not used. Each operator must know the characteristics of his equipment, which vary from manufacturer to manufacturer, instrument to instrument, and one operative set-up to another (i.e., cable length and loops, electrode size, tip exposure, and the like). The cordotomy electrode consists of 0.51-mm steel insulated with No. 50 polyethylene. The electrode is prepared to extend 4 mm beyond the tip of the 18-gauge needle with the distal 2 mm bared and the proximal 2 mm insulated.

STEREOTAXIC CORDOTOMY TECHNIQUE

Introduction of Needle

The patient is positioned on the table as described previously. The cervical spine is visualized radiographically in the anteroposterior view so as to delineate the odontoid process and the pedicles of the second cervical vertebra. The lateral view of the same area is obtained, and the skin is then prepared with an antiseptic. The sighting device is placed opposite the C1–C2 interspace in the lateral view, and a point in the spinal canal one third of the distance dorsal to the vertebral body is sighted on the device for the insertion of a lidocaine wheal in the skin (Fig. 131–3). After the wheal is raised, the skin is punctured with the 19-gauge needle, and the 18-gauge cordotomy

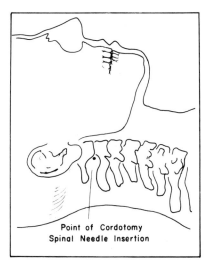

Figure 131–3 Point of insertion of needle.

needle is introduced through the hole in the wheal parallel to the table and perpendicular to the axis of the spinal column. Additional lidocaine is injected for analgesia along the route of insertion. When the needle meets resistance, the field is visualized radiographically in the lateral view. If the needle is found to be against a lamina, its course must be corrected. When inserted properly, it should be seen in the interspace against the ligamentum flavum (Fig. 131–4).

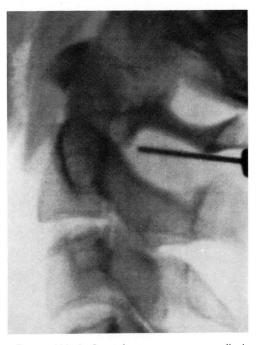

Figure 131–4 Lateral roentgenogram, needle in situ.

Epidural Block and Entry into Spinal Canal

It is important to penetrate slowly through the ligamentum flavum so as to enter the epidural space before puncturing the dura mater. Two milliliters of lidocaine is introduced to produce an epidural block. This will lessen or abolish any pain generated later by the radiofrequency current. Occasionally, venous blood is encountered if an epidural vein is punctured. It has not been a problem, and the slow injection of lidocaine will help to tamponade the bleeding. A total of 8 to 10 ml of lidocaine will have been used for analgesia at this point. The next resistance to be met is the dura mater; it is punctured and the subarachnoid space is entered. The patient should be warned beforehand that this may be painful owing to contact with or traction on the C2 root by the needle. The stylet is removed, and a free flow of cerebrospinal fluid should occur. If no flow is obtained, the needle may have entered the spinal cord, but no harm has been observed to occur as a result. In either circumstance, the spinal canal should now be visualized in the anteroposterior view. The needle may often be found to have penetrated too deeply. The micromanipulator is attached to the hub of the needle, and the needle is withdrawn until spinal fluid flows and the needle tip is in the gutter between the projected lateral edge of the odontoid process and the wall of the spinal canal, as shown in Figure 131–5.

Air Myelogram

The stopcock is attached and 10 cc of air is injected to outline the spinal cord; an additional 0.1 ml of lidocaine is introduced to reinforce the epidural block. Mullan prefers emulsified Pantopaque to outline the dentate ligament, which he uses as his identifying landmark for the insertion of the electrode.[18] The author used the air myelogram to outline the ventral edge of the spinal cord for his point of reference. A lateral roentgenogram is taken to see the position of the needle. It may be necessary to raise the hub of the needle with the micromanipulator, thus directing the tip of the needle posteriorly in order to aim it toward the spinothalamic tract in the anterior quadrant of

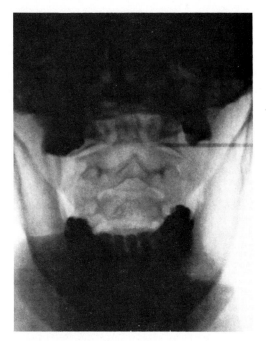

Figure 131–5 Anteroposterior roentgenogram, needle in situ.

the spinal cord (Fig. 131–6). It is preferable to introduce the electrode more anteriorly rather than posteriorly where it is in the vicinity of the corticospinal tract. When an image intensifier is used to visualize the spi-

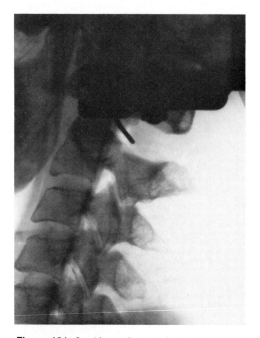

Figure 131–6 Air myelogram, lateral view, needle in situ.

nal contents, the pulsating shadow is *not* the spinal cord—it is the air–cerebrospinal fluid level. Spinal cord movement is not seen under these circumstances. The cord appears stationary, as a shadow in the middle third of the canal and parallel to the floor.

Introduction of Electrode

When a satisfactory position has been attained in the lateral view, the electrode is inserted into the anterior quadrant of the spinal cord. Its location is confirmed in both the anteroposterior and lateral views before the radiofrequency current is applied (Fig. 131–7). As a rough guide, on the lateral exposure, the electrode is seen 2 to 3 mm behind the anterior shadow representing the ventral surface of the cord. In the anteroposterior view, assuming that the cord is not displaced and that it is approximately the same width as the odontoid process itself, the tip of the needle should be just lateral to a line projected downward from the odontoid; the electrode should protrude 4 mm beyond this. Occasionally, the spinal cord is quite mobile and the parenchyma may not be punctured until the electrode has pushed the spinal cord to the contralateral wall of the canal.

Corroboration of Electrode Position

Corroboration of the electrode position may be obtained in three ways: by measurement of impedance, by electrical stimulation, and by incremental enlargement of the lesion with concomitant clinical testing. Although the author recognizes impedance measurements and electrical stimulation as adjunct methods of establishing electrode placement, it has been his custom to utilize incremental enlargement of the lesion with concomitant clinical testing as the sole technique for establishing electrode position. This has proved highly successful, and there has been no difficulty in penetrating the anterior quadrant of the spinal cord and establishing a lesion with the appropriate effect. The method is described under the heading Generation of Lesion, which follows. If desired, however, a more quantitative corroboration of electrode penetration can be obtained by measuring impedance or stimulating the spinal cord. The impedance measurement method makes use of the fact that cerebrospinal fluid and spinal cord tissue have different electrical resistances to flow of current from the electrode tip.[9] Technically, impedance is the ratio of voltage to current in an alternating current circuit. By measuring impedance at

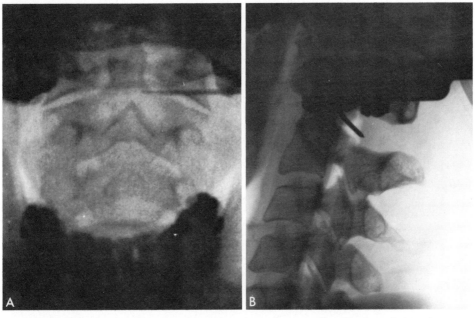

Figure 131–7 Anteroposterior, *A*, and lateral, *B*, views, needle with electrode insertion.

the tip of the electrode as it is advanced toward the spinal cord, the impedance monitor will register a reading indicative of the location of the electrode in tissue, fluid, or air. As the electrode tip is advanced toward the spinal cord, transitional values, read in ohms, are observed. These are: infinity if the tip is in air, 150 to 250 ohms if the tip is immersed in cerebrospinal fluid, 250 to 350 ohms if it is in contact with the spinal cord, and 350 to 750 ohms when it is solidly embedded in spinal cord substance. These values are only average numbers for the electrode previously described. Smaller electrodes give higher impedance values, and each electrode type should be standardized for appropriate value recognition. Once the electrode has been determined to be embedded in spinal cord, electrical stimulation, if it is to be utilized, can be performed with a needle in the contralateral deltoid muscle as the indifferent electrode and the cordotomy electrode as the cathode. At low frequencies, 1 to 6 cps, stimuli of 1 msec duration and 0.3 to 1.5 v, will elicit ipsilateral motor responses if the electrode is in the anterior gray matter. If the electrode is in proximity to the more posterior and laterally placed corticospinal descending motor fibers, the threshold is somewhat higher, ranging from 0.8 to 2.0 v with 1 msec duration pulses. In order to elicit a sensory response, a higher frequency range of 50 to 60 cps is utilized with which tingling on the contralateral side of the body can be evoked with stimuli of 0.4 to 4.0 v of 1 msec duration. The responses are usually regional and not somatotopic, and presumably reflect electrode proximity to the anterolateral ascending system for pain of the spinal cord.[37,38]

Generation of Lesion

The coaxial cable is attached to the electrode, with the shank of the needle serving as the ground (Fig. 131–8). The radiofrequency current is applied in increments of 2.5 sec. The patient is warned that the current is being passed, because the lidocaine blocks may not be completely effective and some pain may be perceived. The patient is tested after each increment of current, on the contralateral side for analgesia, on the ipsilateral side for evidence of weakness. As the increments of current are lengthened, the level of analgesia will rise from the foot, to leg, to thigh, to abdomen, and upward as high as the C3 dermatome, if desired. The level of analgesia may be elected according to the need of the patient. When this level is reached, no further increments are given, but the time of current passage producing the desired level of analgesia is repeated three times to assure solid necrosis. A 30-second wait between applications of current is advised in order to allow interim cooling of the tissue. A maximum size lesion producing a C3 level of analgesia

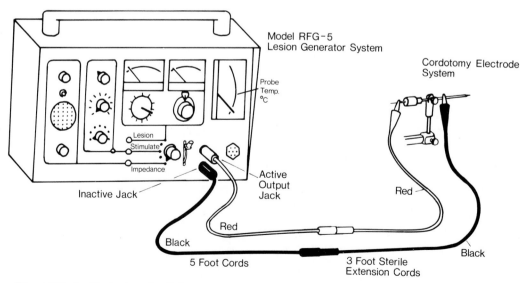

Figure 131–8 Electrode and radiofrequency current generator system. (Courtesy of Radionics, Inc., Burlington, Massachusetts).

should be obtained with an eventual current of 30 seconds' duration. If the higher levels have not been rendered analgesic, the electrode is moved medially 1 mm at a time, and the current is reapplied until the desired result is attained. If weakness should develop during the procedure, the operation is discontinued immediately. The paresis will usually become undetectable within a few minutes, and another attempt at cordotomy may be made at a later date.

POSTOPERATIVE CARE

The patient is returned to his room with the same orders postoperatively as were in force preoperatively. Analgesics are continued in the immediate postoperative phase for headache from the air myelogram or for pain on the side not rendered analgesic. He may eat and drink at will, but he should remain in bed overnight to minimize his headache. Ambulation to the bathroom is permitted, but only with assistance, as ataxia due to coincident spinocerebellar tract dysfunction may appear several hours postoperatively. This, and other complications, are described in the results of a series of 1279 cordotomies in 789 patients that were reported by Rosomoff in 1974.[26]

OTHER METHODS AND MODIFICATIONS

In 1966, Lin and associates described an anterior approach to percutaneous lower cervical cordotomy.[15] They evolved this approach primarily to avoid respiratory complications potential to high cervical cordotomy. In fact, this is a valid consideration, if high cervical levels of analgesia are not required. The procedure is technically more difficult to perform, however, since it is a transdiscal needle insertion, which limits mobility for positioning of the electrode. When bilateral lesions are required, the basic lateral C1–C2 method may be used for the initial operation. The anterior approach can then be utilized for the contralateral side, so as to minimize the risk of sleep-induced apnea.

Crue and his co-workers described a posterior approach through C1–C2 or the atlanto-occipital junction for high cervical percutaneous radiofrequency cordotomy in 1968, as did Hitchcock a year later.[5,10] This approach has the disadvantage of traversing the spinal cord from behind forward, although these authors did not report complications relative to the structures that were transgressed. They thought, perhaps, that lesion siting was easier and higher levels of analgesia could be achieved. The experience reported was, however, too small to justify definitive conclusions. One further application of this method was to the relief of facial pain for trigeminal tractotomy by positioning the needle rostrally in the medulla rather than in the cervical spinal cord.[39]

Other than these different access routes, most modifications of the Rosomoff technique relate to target localization and lesion making. Mullan has long been the advocate of electrical stimulation of the spinal cord to identify the target area.[18] Several investigators have also reported the physiological characteristics of spinal cord target sites.[8,36-38] Impedance measurements for detection of spinal cord penetration have been routine for Gildenberg and others who do not consider the "feel" of needle insertion, as advocated by Mullan, to be reliable.[9,18] The relationship of radiofrequency electrical current and lesion size has been studied by Fox.[7] Radiofrequency generator characteristics are detailed by the major producers of these units, who include instructions on methods of standardization for each operator to follow.

RESULTS

In a series of 1279 cordotomies reported by the author, there was a slight preponderance of males, but in essence, the distribution was symmetrical.[26] Old age and infirmity were not contraindications, as long as a patient could be placed on the operating table for the introduction of a spinal needle. There were more than 20 patients over the age of 80 years and one over age 90 years at the time of operation.

An analysis of the disease states for which the procedures were performed indicates a preponderance of malignant disease among the initial 300 patients (Table 131–1). Once the value of the procedure had become established, however, patients with benign conditions were referred more often for pain relief, until there was almost an

TABLE 131–1 CONDITIONS FOR WHICH
PERCUTANEOUS CORDOTOMY WAS PERFORMED*

MALIGNANT	NO. OF PATIENTS	BENIGN	NO. OF PATIENTS
Lung	61	Radiculopathy	22
Gastrointestinal	56	Neuropathy	12
Genitourinary	25	Vascular	11
Uterus	24	Amputation	8
Breast	19	Herpetic	4
Pancreas	12	Fracture	4
Sarcoma	8	Post-thoracotomy	3
Undifferentiated	4	Tumor	3
Melanoma	3	Arthritis	2
Myeloma	3	Miscellaneous	9
Miscellaneous	7		
Total	222 (74%)	Total	78 (26%)

* Initial 300 patients.

equal number of both types of referrals. Cancer of the lung, followed by gastrointestinal neoplasia, was the most common diagnosis among the malignant diseases. Lumbar radiculopathy, as found in the back that has been unsuccessfully operated on more than once, and peripheral neuropathies were the most common indications for intervention in benign states. During the last five years, lumbar radiculopathy has become an infrequent cause for the use of cordotomy. The multidisciplinary pain team approach and the advent of transaxial and computed tomography have provided successful approaches to management that avoid ablative intervention. Parenthetically, it should be noted that where axial tomography has demonstrated bony encroachment as the cause of continuing symptoms, e.g., spinal stenosis, facetal hypertrophy, or the like, removal of the offending bony elements has resulted in improvement or resolution of the painful state.[29,30] For the remainder, the pain team has achieved acceptable control of pain by liberal and aggressive application of physical medicine and psychological-psychiatric techniques together with drug detoxification and pharmacological manipulation, or, unhappily, patients have been identified in whom no intervention, including cordotomy, is indicated.[28] Rhizotomy, as an alternative procedure, is not utilized, as the author has found this method to be eminently unsuccessful and attended by a high incidence of postoperative deafferentation syndrome, for which no treatment is at present available.

A total of 531 patients underwent unilateral cordotomy for pain relief. There was an early slight preponderance of male pa-

tients, but, again, the statistics indicate an almost equal distribution between males and females later in the series.

One third, 258 patients, had bilateral cordotomies. Here, too, the distribution of males and females was equal. It is important to point out that the author had little or no hesitation in performing bilateral procedures when pain relief demanded such treatment. These were staged operations, at least one week apart.

An analysis of the unilateral and bilateral procedures in respect to disease states indicates that malignant disease was the most common cause of the painful condition requiring relief, whether unilateral or bilateral. An interesting finding in respect to bilateral interventions is that, although the previous clinical impression was that bilateral procedures were needed most frequently in individuals with benign disease such as the lumbar radiculopathies, 35 per cent of the patients with malignant disease required bilateral intervention. The corollary to this analysis is that the majority of individuals with benign disease required only unilateral procedures. Only 30 per cent went on to bilateral intervention. In malignant disease involving viscera, anatomically, pain representation is bilateral. When open cordotomy is utilized, bilateral section is recommended. The experience with percutaneous cordotomy, however, particularly when pain reference has been strongly lateralized, is that unilateral cordotomy will be effective. Since bilateral percutaneous cordotomy is a staged procedure anyhow, the contralateral side is done only when pain becomes significant on the opposite side and it is the opposite side that becomes painfully projected, not reappearance of pain on the ipsilateral side. Should the latter occur, it is due to failure of the ipsilateral cordotomy, which must then be repeated.

Repeat cordotomies were necessary following 18 per cent of the procedures, that is, 24 per cent of the patients experiencing pain relief. In the majority of instances, this was because an imperfect lesion was placed at the first sitting because of excess caution exercised by the surgeon performing the procedure. The less common reasons for repetition were the loss of analgesia at a later date or return of islands of pain perception.

Approximately 30 per cent of the patients had pain in the neck, upper extremities, or thorax. They would have required high levels of analgesia for control of their symptoms. The remaining patients had pain in the abdomen, perineum, back, or lower extremities.

Although it is possible to control the level of analgesia by marching the level up the side of the body as the increments of current are increased, it was found that 60 per cent of the cordotomy procedures achieved levels in the cervical or high thoracic areas. Only 30 per cent of the patients had pain problems that would have required such levels. It was the surgeon's preference, however, to aim for higher levels of analgesia in order to offer better pain control and protection against dropping of the level postoperatively, rather than to produce a level that was too low, necessitating reoperation for pain that had been relieved completely. At follow-up, analgesic levels were found to be the same or higher in 54 per cent of the cordotomies, the 19 per cent that were higher offering additional protection. Thirty-two per cent were lower, usually within the accepted criterion of two to four dermatome segments. This group usually defined itself within 72 hours and

tended to maintain the lower level throughout follow-up. When further decrease was seen, it was remote in time and no particular pattern was observed. Thirteen per cent of the cordotomies proved to be inadequate, requiring repetition if the patient was willing. Interestingly, 9 per cent of the levels of analgesia disappeared, a still unsolved problem of cordotomy by whatever technique employed. Repeat of the cordotomy invariably reproduced an acceptable level of analgesia, however. The remaining 4 per cent with no level of analgesia or spotty analgesia were technically inadequate, and they, too, were repeated.

These follow-up data were obtained by questionnaire. The patients examined themselves and reported the historical and physical results. Because of the preponderance of malignant diseases, almost two thirds of the patients were dead or lost from follow-up within three months of operation. Only 25 per cent were available for analysis of the results after one year, and their numbers rapidly decreased thereafter into the eighth year.

The complication rate was low (Table 131–2). Ipsilateral hemiparesis appeared temporarily in 5 per cent of the patients undergoing cordotomy, lasting usually only 2 to 14 days. The 3 per cent of cases listed as permanent occurred in patients who died early and who did not survive long enough to recover from their deficit. Weakness was rarely severe, only to be identified sometimes by hyperreflexia or a Babinski sign. These data are to be compared with the risk of paresis of up to 45 per cent with an open operative procedure.[3,4,17,33,41] It was the most common complication, but it had to be searched for in the postoperative examination. It sometimes was present for only a few hours and was associated with decreased deep tendon reflexes, muscular hypotonia, especially in the ipsilateral lower

TABLE 131–2 COMPLICATIONS OCCURRING IN 1279 PERCUTANEOUS CERVICAL CORDOTOMIES

COMPLICATION	TEMPORARY		PERMANENT	
	Number	Per Cent	Number	Per Cent
Paresis	63	5	34	3
Ataxia	252	20	44	3
Urinary dysfunction	123	10	29	2
Sexual dysfunction	—		54	4
Postcordotomy dysesthesia syndromes	—		10	1
Dysesthesias			199	16

extremity, and no Babinski sign. Often, permanent ataxia, 3 per cent, was difficult to distinguish from a mild paresis. Catheterization was required following 10 per cent of the procedures, usually in patients whose bladder mechanism was already disturbed by disease. Two per cent of patients were left with permanent catheters, mostly for nursing convenience. Again, the figures are to be compared with bladder failure of up to 100 per cent in some open cordotomy series. Information relative to sexual function was difficult to obtain. The 4 per cent incidence of difficulty was described usually as a decrease in voluptuous sensation about the genitals on the side rendered analgesic. Impotence was reported only occasionally, even with bilateral cordotomies, but these data may be unreliable, since the history of sexual performance was often poor, particularly in the elderly and infirm. The incidence was so small as to not even record a percentage. Postcordotomy dysesthetic syndromes, i.e., burning distress throughout the entire area made analgesic, was uncommon, less than 1 per cent, and usually not severe. Its pathophysiological mechanism is still unknown. Dysesthesias, 16 per cent, are listed separately. These sensations, such as tingling, burning, prickling in the area of pathological implication, are not complications per se. They are uncomfortable feelings that were usually present preoperatively but were not conspicuous because of the overriding pain. Once the pain was ablated by the cordotomy, the dysesthesias became discernible and prominent. Often, patients referred to the dysesthesias by calling them pain. This confusion of terms causes difficulty later in the analysis of the success of cordotomy for pain relief.

Respiratory complications deserve special consideration, as they represent the only life-threatening risk.[1,2,11,19,29] Two distinct but related physiological functions may be affected; namely, the respiratory motor function and the control of ventilation. Either or both may be impaired by cordotomy. Respiratory motor function, as assessed by the vital capacity, breathing capacity, and maximum thoracic pressure, does not undergo a definitive change. Failure of these parameters to demonstrate more significant motor dysfunction may, however, be due to limitation of respiratory movements by pain on the initial study. Thus, potentially, cordotomy-induced changes may be masked. For example, some patients with initial predicted vital capacities of 40 to 50 per cent have increased their capacities to 70 to 80 per cent after being rendered pain-free by unilateral cordotomy. Moreover, fluoroscopy failed to reveal any evidence of diaphragmatic paresis in this group of patients. Thus, it is evident that the concept of pure motor dysfunction, as the proposed mechanism of respiratory failure in open cordotomy, is insufficient to explain the observed clinical phenomena.[23]

Ventilatory control mechanisms, however, appear to be affected both selectively and independently. There is a reduction of tidal volume on breathing air and carbon dioxide, and an increase of the respiratory rate. With more extensive lesions, the tidal volume reduction is greater, and the respiratory rate fails to increase adequately, so that the minute ventilation on breathing air and carbon dioxide decreases. There is nothing to suggest that the reduction of responsiveness to carbon dioxide is due to interruption of a specific receptor pathway for carbon dioxide. Rather, it seems that this is a manifestation of a general reduction of the respiratory system's responsiveness and that the carbon dioxide response test is a simple clinical tool for its recognition.

In the author's experience, patients who developed overt clinical syndromes all have undergone bilateral procedures and had high levels of analgesia.[13,29] The functional changes they sustained were qualitatively the same as those seen in the other groups. They had, however, a greater reduction in vital capacity, resting ventilation, and carbon dioxide response, and developed a more irregular pattern of breathing than the patients who remained asymptomatic. The most notable feature of the symptomatic group was the marked reduction of the tidal volume and minute ventilation response to carbon dioxide.

The pattern of respiratory dysfunction observed in these patients was similar to that seen with lesions of the lateral reticular formation of the medulla resulting from poliomyelitis. In a series of 20 cases reported by Plum and Swanson, 13 had irregular breathing, variable periods of apnea, and a reduced carbon dioxide response.[24] These patients also had spinal poliomyelitis with reduced vital and maximal breathing capacities, however, and the decreased response to carbon dioxide was ascribed to the increased work of breathing. Linderholm and Werneman, in a study of 71 patients convalescing from poliomyelitis, noted a similar decrease in carbon dioxide response in patients with predominantly cerebral symptoms in whom, presumably, the reticular formation was involved extensively.[16] They were able to identify a group with decreased vital capacity and maximum breathing capacity but with a normal response to carbon dioxide; this demonstrated that motor impairment does not necessarily result in an impaired carbon dioxide response, and that the two effects are independent of each other.

Damage to reticular ascending or descending tracts during cordotomy would explain the great similarity in the alteration of respiratory function seen in postcordotomy subjects and those with reticular formation lesions.[22] It might be postulated that the initial impairment of respiratory function is a decrease in tidal volume that is compensated for by an increase in respiratory rate; as the lesion increases in extent, this compensatory increase in rate might fail to occur and the result would be a significant reduction in minute ventilation.

These observations parallel closely the observations made in cats by Hugelin and Cohen.[12] When the reticular formation was stimulated, they noted, an increasing stimulus caused successively an increased rate, followed by increased flow, and then an increased tidal volume. Therefore, ablative lesions of the reticular formation might be expected to produce changes in the reverse order, namely, an initial reduction in tidal volume followed by failure of rate compensation. This was the common pattern observed. Factors that depress reticular formation activity, such as sleep, barbiturates, and narcotics, aggravate the clinical manifestations of the postcordotomy respiratory syndrome. Indeed, sleep- or drug-induced apnea has been characteristic of the most severely affected patients.[34] Specifically, ablation of the ascending reticular pathways during cervical cordotomy can result in impairment of respiratory control mechanisms as manifested clinically by an irregular breathing pattern, hypoventilation, and drug- or sleep-induced apnea.[13,14] The incidence of this major complication, the only life-threatening consequence of cordotomy,

was 3 per cent. It is delayed in onset and can be predicted by testing the patient's response to breathing carbon dioxide. Ablation of the response, which normally is a two- to threefold increase in minute volume, presages the appearance of the syndrome. Not all patients do go on to apnea, but such individuals are candidates for apnea and must be observed carefully. They may require intubation and supportive artificial ventilation, should respiration fail. The process is usually self-limiting, lasting a few days to three weeks. Minor changes in respiration, such as shortness of breath intermittently, without embarrassing blood-gas levels, may occur in another 3 per cent of patients. They pass without event. The only deaths in this series were attributable to sleep-induced apnea that went undiscovered or was treated inadequately. This was early in the experience when little was known about the problem.

Although bilateral open cordotomy in the thoracic area was a routine procedure in many medical centers, bilateral open cervical cordotomy was performed less frequently because of the alleged greater risks.[23,33,41] Mortality rates for the bilateral cervical operation have ranged from 20 to 36 per cent; death has almost always been attributed to respiratory failure, although debilitation and advanced state of disease undoubtedly have been contributory factors. Morbidity in the form of permanent bladder dysfunction has been recorded in 11 to 92 per cent, and paresis less frequently, 2 to 12 per cent.

In a series of 100 patients undergoing bilateral percutaneous cervical cordotomy the mortality rate was 2 per cent if the deaths included are limited to those in which the cordotomy procedure was clearly implicated, or 12 per cent including those who died soon after operation but in whom autopsy proved primary disease as a cause of death.[25] The cause of death was sleep-induced apnea. Here, therefore, the assessment of pulmonary function is important, but unfortunately not prognostic.[29] The chance of permanent paresis is 3 per cent; if motor disability includes ataxia, the risk is 5 per cent. Permanent bladder dysfunction occurs in only 2 per cent, and autonomic disturbances are not a problem. Although it has been said that bilateral cordotomy leads to impotence and loss of erotic sensation, this has not been invariable.[40]

It does not occur in all patients; so, perhaps, the psychological implication of disability and the primary disease are more important factors than the suprasegmental interruption of spinal cord pathways.

Immediately following both unilateral and bilateral cordotomy, patients considered themselves to be pain-free or so comfortable that no analgesics were necessary in more than 90 per cent of cases. By the end of three months, however, these measures of success had decreased to 84 per cent. Dysesthesias, which had become prominent and which could not be distinguished from lancinating, toothache-like pain, were one reason for failure. Incomplete analgesia, originally or because fibers that were blocked temporarily by the radiofrequency current became conductive again at this later time, was another cause. By the end of one year, almost 40 per cent were classed as failures. This does not mean that these patients did not benefit by the procedure, but only that they did not have absolute pain relief. It is estimated that more than half of these patients believed they had received major help, could return to normal activities, and did not have problems of drug usage or distress severe enough to warrant repeat cordotomy. By two years and thereafter, an average 60 per cent no longer had complete pain relief and, therefore, were classified technically as failures. As before, half of this group still considered themselves to have benefited. These data could be interpreted as disappointing. They probably are not, however, in that some 70 per cent continue to have beneficial effects and are satisfied with their results. It is a testimony to the viability and tenacity of the nervous system that the best efforts devised by man cannot totally and irrevocably destroy pain, which is a primary, basic protective mechanism. The ease of the operation, however, the drastic reduction of risk, and the additional advantage of being able to repeat it, literally ad infinitum, recommend the percutaneous method as the best yet devised.

REFERENCES

1. Belmusto, L., Brown, E., and Owens, G.: Clinical observations on respiratory and vasomotor disturbance as related to cervical cordotomies. J. Neurosurg., 20:225–232, 1963.
2. Belmusto, L., Woldring, S., and Owens, G.: Localization and patterns of potentials of the respiratory pathway in the cervical spinal cord in the dog. J. Neurosurg., 22:277–283, 1965.
3. Bischof, W., and Schütte, W.: Complications after cordotomies. Zbl. Neurochir., 25:233–245, 1965.
4. Brihaye, J., and Rétif, J.: Comparison des résultats obtenus par la cordotomie antérolatérale au niveau dorsal et au niveau cervical. Neurochirurgie, 7:258–277, 1961.
5. Crue, B. L., Todd, E. M., and Carregal, E. J. A.: Posterior approach for high cervical percutaneous radiofrequency cordotomy. Confin. Neurol., 30:11–52, 1968.
6. Foerster, O., and Gagel, O.: Die Vorderseitenstrangdurchschneidung beim Menschen. Eine klinisch-pathophysiologisch-anatomische Studie. Z. Ges. Neurol. Psychiat., 138:1–92, 1932.
7. Fox, J. L.: Experimental relationship of radiofrequency electrical current and lesion size for application to percutaneous cordotomy. J. Neurosurg., 33:415–421, 1970.
8. Gildenberg, P. L., Lin, P. M., Polakoff, P. P., and Flitter, M. A.: Anterior percutaneous cervical cordotomy. Determination of target point and calculation of angle of insertion. Technical note. J. Neurosurg., 28:173–177, 1968.
9. Gildenberg, P. L., Zanes, C., Flitter, M. A., Lin, P. M., Lautsch, E. F., and Truex, R. C.: Impedance measuring device for detection of penetration of the spinal cord in anterior percutaneous cervical cordotomy. Technical note. J. Neurosurg., 30:87–92, 1969.
10. Hitchcock, E.: Stereotaxic spinal surgery. A preliminary report. J. Neurosurg., 31:386–392, 1969.
11. Hitchcock, E., and Leece, B.: Somatotopic representation of the respiratory pathways in the cervical cord of man. J. Neurosurg., 27:320–329, 1967.
12. Hugelin, A., and Cohen, M. I.: The reticular activating system and respiratory regulation in the cat. Ann. N.Y. Acad. Sci., 109:586–603, 1963.
13. Krieger, A. J., and Rosomoff, H. L.: Sleep-induced apnea. Part 1: A respiratory and autonomic syndrome following bilateral percutaneous cervical cordotomy. J. Neurosurg., 39:168–180, 1974.
14. Krieger, A. J., Christensen, H. D., Sapru, H. N., and Wang, S. C.: Changes in ventilatory patterns after ablation of various respiratory feedback mechanisms. J. Appl. Physiol., 33:431–435, 1972.
15. Lin, P. M., Gildenberg, P. L., and Polakoff, P. P.: An anterior approach to percutaneous lower cervical cordotomy. J. Neurosurg., 25:553–560, 1966.
16. Linderholm, H., and Werneman, H.: On respiratory regulation in poliomyelitis convalescents. Acta Med. Scand., 154:suppl. 316:135–157, 1956.
17. McKissock, W.: Spinothalamic cordotomy: Reassessment of effectiveness and limitations. Excerpta Med., 36:27, 1961.
18. Mullan, J.: Percutaneous cordotomy. J. Neurosurg., 35:360–366, 1971.
19. Mullan, S., and Hosobuchi, Y.: Respiratory hazards of high cervical percutaneous cordotomy. J. Neurosurg., 28:291–297, 1968.
20. Mullan, S., Hekmatpanah, J., Dobben, G., and

Beckman, E.: Percutaneous intramedullary cordotomy utilizing the unipolar anodal electrolytic lesion. J. Neurosurg., *22*:548–553, 1965.

21. Mullan, S., Harper, P. V., Hekmatpanah, J., Torres, H., and Dobben, G.: Percutaneous interruption of spinal-pain tracts by means of a strontium-90 needle. J. Neurosurg., *20*:931–939, 1963.

22. Nathan, P. W.: The descending respiratory pathway in man. J. Neurol. Neurosurg. Psychiat., *13*:81–87, 1956.

23. Ogle, W. S., French, L. A., and Peyton, W.: Experiences with high cervical cordotomy. J. Neurosurg., *13*:81–87, 1956.

24. Plum, F., and Swanson, A. G.: Abnormalities in central regulation of respiration in acute and convalescent poliomyelitis. Arch. Neurol. Psychiat. (Chicago), *80*:267–285, 1958.

25. Rosomoff, H. L.: Bilateral percutaneous cervical radiofrequency cordotomy. J. Neurosurg., *31*:41–46, 1969.

26. Rosomoff, H. L.: Percutaneous radiofrequency cervical cordotomy for intractable pain. Advances Neurol., *4*:683–688, 1974.

27. Rosomoff, H. L.: Bony encroachment of the lumbar spine: A cause of low back surgery failure. Florida Med. Ass., *63*:884–888, 1976.

28. Rosomoff, H. L., Green, C. J., and Silbret, M.: The multidisciplinary team approach to the diagnosis and treatment of chronic low back pain. Post, J. D., ed.: Radiographic Evaluation of the Spine. New York, Masson Publishing Inc., U.S.A., 1980, pp. 672–679.

29. Rosomoff, H. L., Krieger, A. J., and Kuperman, A. S.: Effects of percutaneous cervical cordotomy on pulmonary function. J. Neurosurg., *31*:620–627, 1969.

30. Rosomoff, H. L., Post, M. J. D., and Quencer, R. M.: Axial radiology of the lumbar spine. Clin. Neurosurg., *25*:251–265, 1978.

31. Rosomoff, H. L., Carroll, F., Brown, J., and Sheptak, P.: Percutaneous radiofrequency cervical cordotomy: Technique. J. Neurosurg., *23*:639–644, 1965.

32. Schuller, A.: Uber operative Durchtrennung der Ruckenmarksstrange (chordotomie) Wien. Med. Wschr., *60*:2292–2296, 1910.

33. Schwartz, H. G.: High cervical cordotomy: Technique and results. Clin. Neurosurg., *8*:282–293, 1962.

34. Severinghaus, J. W., and Mitchell, R. A.: Ondine's curse—failure of respiratory center automaticity while awake. Clin. Res., *10*:122, 1962.

35. Spiller, W. G., and Martin, E.: The treatment of persistent pain of organic origin in the lower part of the body by division of the anterolateral column of the spinal cord. J.A.M.A., *58*:1489–1490, 1912.

36. Taren, J. A., Davis, R., and Crosby, E. C.: Target physiologic correlation in stereotaxic cervical cordotomy. J. Neurosurg., *30*:569–584, 1969.

37. Tasker, R. R., and Organ. L. W.: Percutaneous cordotomy. Physiologic identification of target site. Confin. Neurol., *35*:110–117, 1973.

38. Tasker, R. R., Organ, L. W., and Smith, K. C.: Physiologic guidelines for the localization of lesions by percutaneous cordotomy. Acta Neurochir., *210*:111–117, 1974.

39. Todd, E. M., Crue, B. L., and Carregal, E. J. A.: Posterior percutaneous tractomy and cordotomy. Confin. Neurol., *31*:106–115, 1969.

40. White, J. C.: Cordotomy: Assessment of its effectiveness and suggestions for improvement. Clin. Neurosurg., *13*:1–19, 1966.

41. White, J. C., and Sweet, W. H.: Pain and the Neurosurgeon. A Forty-Year Experience. Springfield, Ill., Charles C Thomas, 1969.

132

CORDOTOMY BY OPEN OPERATIVE TECHNIQUES

HISTORICAL BACKGROUND

In 1850, Brown-Séquard published the first outline of the conduction of sensation in the spinal cord.[8] Müller, in 1871, and Gowers, in 1878, described injuries to the spinal cord associated with loss of pain sensation that suggested that the anterolateral part of the spinal cord carried pain impulses.[33,62] In 1889, Edinger described the spinothalamic tract in kittens and amphibians; in 1902, Petren indicated its possible clinical function.[19,20,74] In 1905, Spiller performed a critical autopsy on an individual who had lost only pain and temperature sensation in the lower half of the body without loss of other sensation. The finding of small tuberculomas bilaterally in the anterolateral quadrants of the cord furnished the first conclusive proof that it was the anterolateral quadrant of the spinal cord that carried pain and temperature sensation in man.[87] In 1910, Schüller performed a section of the anterolateral quadrant in monkeys, which he named chordotomie, and suggested the procedure for the relief of the pain of gastric crises.[83] In 1911, at Spiller's direction, Martin performed the first anterolateral cordotomy in man for pain.[88] Foerster, in 1913, without knowledge of Spiller and Martin's work, performed with Tietze an anterolateral cordotomy for gastric crisis; and at the same time Beer, in New York, reported cordotomy for the relief of nerve plexus pain secondary to carcinoma.[4,22] In the ensuing 50 years high thoracic cordotomy, unilateral or bilateral, became the standard procedure for the operative relief of intractable pain; a number of neurosurgeons contributed improvements in technique.* In 1929 and 1931 respectively, Foerster and Gagel in Germany and Stookey in the United States performed high cervical cordotomy, and further improvements in the procedure were made by Schwartz, French, and others.† In 1939, Hyndman and Van Epps proposed differential section of the spinothalamic tract to produce restricted areas of analgesia.[40] In 1954, Hamby recommended section at C4–C6 from the posterior approach.[35] The early contributions to the procedure of open cordotomy are reviewed by Stookey and by White and Sweet.[90,102]

In 1963, Collis published a case report, and in 1964 Cloward described in detail the anterior cervical approach to the lateral spinothalamic tract.[11,13] Recently, Hardy and his associates have renewed interest in this approach used with the operating microscope.[36]

In 1926, at Greenfield's suggestion, Armour first performed midline commissural myelotomy to sever the crossing spinothalamic fibers to relieve the pain of gastric crises.[1] According to White and Sweet, the operation was done by Leriche in 1929 and published in 1936.[102] The subsequent development of this procedure is reviewed by Cook and Kawakami, by King, and by White and Sweet.[14,44,102]

In 1963, Mullan and co-workers revolutionized the field of pain relief by introducing percutaneous lateral cervical cordotomy executed with a strontium needle.[65]

---

* See references 9, 21, 26, 41, 90, 92, 98, 101–103.
† See references 21, 27, 28, 60, 84, 85, 89.

C. E. BRACKETT

This advance was soon followed by their proposal to use a direct current electrolytic lesion and, in 1965, by Rosomoff and associates' introduction of the radiofrequency lesion and other refinements of technique.[64,81] To avoid sleep apnea, Lin, Gildenberg, and others introduced the anterior percutaneous approach at lower cervical levels; Crue and co-workers, Fox, Hitchcock, and others pioneered the stereotaxic posterior percutaneous approach.* Since then improvements in localization with contrast material, in stimulation and recording techniques for physiological as opposed to anatomical localization, and in lesion making techniques have served to increase accuracy, to avoid complications, and to extend the usefulness of the percutaneous procedure (see Chapter 131).† A survey by Gildenberg in 1973 revealed that of 552 neurosurgeons responding, 275 performed percutaneous cordotomy and 300 performed open cordotomy, a number performing both.[32]

Although at present percutaneous cordotomy has replaced the open procedures in many clinics, there remain definite indications for anterolateral cordotomy by the open method. This chapter reviews the pertinent anatomy, indications, operative technique, and complications for open cordotomy by the posterior approach in the thoracic and cervical regions, the anterior cervical approach, and midline myelotomy for the relief of intractable pain.

ANATOMY AND PHYSIOLOGY

Our understanding of the anatomy and physiology of central pain pathways has been extensively revised in recent years in the light of new anatomical and physiological techniques.‡ Figure 132–1 shows in elementary diagrammatic form the anatomy of the pain pathways in the spinal cord as understood at present. They are discussed in greater detail in Chapter 115.

Crue's group, Kerr, Mansuy and Sindou, and Willis have recently reviewed segmental and spinal cord pain mechanisms.[16,42,52,104] Finely myelinated beta and delta fibers and poorly myelinated or unmyelinated C fibers carry pain in the dorsal root, where they are interspersed with other sensory fibers. Just proximal to entry into the pia, the pain-carrying A delta and C fibers separate from other sensory fibers to

---

* See references 18, 23, 31, 38, 50, 97.

† See references 18, 24, 25, 32, 39, 45, 46, 55, 56, 59, 63, 66, 73, 78–80, 82, 92–94, 96.

‡ See references 3, 15–17, 29, 30, 34, 41–43, 52, 54–61, 70, 71, 82, 86, 92–94, 96, 98–100, 102, 104, 105.

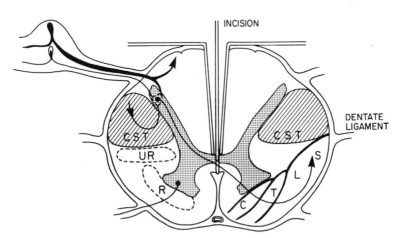

Figure 132–1 Diagrammatic representation of the spinal cord pathways. The anatomy indicated is entirely diagrammatic and approximate, since the volume and location of the tracts change from segment to segment, and their exact distribution is not completely known and is subject to considerable anatomical variation. No attempt has been made to indicate the complicated interneuronal anatomy of the dorsal horn. The collaterals of the entering dorsal column fibers and descending fibers ending on the dorsal horn fibers, both of which modulate cellular activity, are indicated. The incision for midline anterior commissure myelotomy is also shown. CST, cortical spinal tract; UR, urinary and rectal fibers; R, respiratory fibers (phrenic fibers medial to C and intercostal fibers medial to T of spinal thalamic tract) in the cervical area. C, cervical; T, thoracic; L, lumbar; S, sacral fibers of the spinal thalamic tract.

form the lateral division of the dorsal root.[42] Collaterals are given off that ascend and descend several segments along with collaterals from neurons in the substantia gelatinosa. Recent studies have shown that the substantia gelatinosa neurons project to cervical cord, brain stem, and thalamus, usually centrally.[30,105] Synaptic connection is made with the cell bodies of secondary neurons in laminae I, V, and VI, whose axons cross via the anterior commissure to form the contralateral spinothalamic tract. Extensive modulation of dorsal horn synaptic activity is achieved via collaterals to laminae II and III of large primary afferents going to the dorsal column, and descending inhibitory and excitatory fibers from the cortex passing via the corticospinal tract to end on cells in the dorsal horn. The interneurons of laminae II and III of the substantia gelatinosa provide an extensive network for activation of spinothalamic cells of origin of laminae I, V, and VI. Pain stimuli activate marginal cells of lamina I, while other sensation activates large collaterals playing on gelatinosa cells of II and III with extensive interneuronal inhibition of lamina I and nonnoxious discharge in the spinothalamic tract.

The lateral spinothalamic tract extends from the dentate ligament nearly to the ventral midline. It occupies much of the anterolateral quadrants, approaching the gray matter, being mixed with fasciculi propria and autonomic fibers. The tract is thought to be more compact and dorsally located in the high cervical region.[60] The topographical arrangement of fibers within the anterolateral quadrant have been the basis of a number of anatomical and physiological studies in man and animal.* It is currently believed that the arrangement of fibers as outlined by Walker on the basis of two human autopsy studies and his studies with Weaver of cordotomy and myelotomy in the monkey most closely coincides with clinical findings following open cordotomy and stimulation data in awake man.[98,100] Although there appears to be a general topographic relationship with the most dorsal and lateral sacral fibers and the most ventral and medial cervical fibers, there is considerable variation and overlap.

Willis, by stimulation studies, found a similar distribution in monkeys.[104] He found spinothalamic neurons responding to heat, cold, pain, and mechanical pressure applied to the skin, and a general intermixing of touch, pain, and temperature fibers in the spinothalamic tract. He doubts there is a separate ventral spinothalamic tract for touch. Furthermore, as Sweet has stressed, there may be extensive variation in the size and location of the descending motor tracts, even to the extent of there being entirely unilateral pathways, and these may give rise to variation in the location of pain pathways in the anterolateral quadrant.[61,92] Furthermore, examples of purely ipsilateral analgesia after cordotomy have been described.[29,92,102] Taken in conjunction with the variation in results following what appears to be anatomically technically satisfactory cordotomy, data derived from stimulation studies and autopsies, and the scattered focal high-frequency lesions seen during the development of the procedure of percutaneous cordotomy, these findings have led to the conclusion that there is considerable variation in the location and arrangement of ascending pain fibers in the anterolateral quadrant.† This circumstance has made it clear in recent years that identification of pain-carrying fibers by electrophysiological means in the awake patient is needed to obtain routinely satisfactory levels, and that reliance on anatomical landmarks exclusively may not be adequate.[92] In addition, Sweet has pointed out the disastrous results that may follow when the dentate ligament is located in an abnormal position.[92] A number of cases have been reported in which section along the line of a far-posteriorly located dentate ligament has resulted in paralysis due to section of the cortical spinal pathways. Furthermore, the anterior roots may exit more laterally than usual, and incision carried to the anterior root may result in inadequate levels of analgesia, or the ventral root may be more medial than usual with increased risk of damage to the anterior spinal artery. The performance of a technically satisfactory section of the anterior lateral quadrant is not difficult, but the problem of anatomical variability cannot be overcome unless stimulation at the time of operation is included in the protocol. Although some have advised routine use of such stimulation (Sweet, Schwartz), other authors have

---

* See references 38–41, 60, 82, 96, 98, 100, 102.

† See references 34, 38, 43, 55, 59, 91–94, 96, 102, 103.

found it to be unreliable and unsatisfactory.*

Mehler has shown that the minority of spinothalamic tract fibers ascend directly in the tract to end in the ventral posterior sensory nuclear complex of the thalamus.[57,58] These fibers are thought to carry sharply localized bright epicritic surface pain, such as pinprick. As the spinothalamic tract ascends through the brain stem, most of its volume is given off as collaterals to the reticular formation, where a medial multisynaptic pathway ascends in the periaqueductal gray matter, ending in the internal medullary lamina and medial nuclei of the thalamus. Extensive connections are made to hypothalamus and limbic lobe. This medial pathway is thought to carry slowly conducted, poorly localized, diffuse deep pain, called protopathic by Head, and thought to be related to the opioid system of the brain.

The location of other ascending pathways for pain are speculative at present. Diffuse deep poorly localized pain may be carried multisynaptically via collaterals of substantia gelatinosa cells spanning five or six segments in the tract of Lissauer and the substantia gelatinosa.[30,105] Whether the spinocervical, spinoreticular, spinotectal, or ventral spinothalamic pathways are clinically important for pain transmission is not known, nor is the role of the diffuse fibers in the fasciculi propria.

Thus, stereotaxic lesions of the medial thalamus may relieve severe pain without loss of dermal perception of pinprick, whereas lesions of the ventral posterolateral sensory nuclei may produce dermal analgesia to pinprick without loss of pain sensation.

Since there appear to be a general intermixing of touch, temperature, and pain fibers and considerable diffusion and variation of location of pain fibers from specific parts of the body, it may be preferable to speak of anterolateral quadrant cordotomy rather than spinothalamic tractotomy.

INDICATIONS

The neurosurgeon trained in percutaneous cordotomy and operating in a well-equipped clinic with adequate radiological and neurophysiological methods of localization may find few indications for open

cordotomy. The patient who, for various reasons, is unable to tolerate the testing procedures while awake, or the patient with anatomical changes in the cervical spine, such as severe arthritis, which make the procedure impossible, may be a candidate for open cordotomy under general anesthesia. Occasionally patients are encountered in whom an adequate cordotomy cannot be obtained by the percutaneous method. Some physicians prefer, when bilateral cordotomy is needed, to employ a percutaneous lesion at C1–C2 contralateral to the side of the most or highest pain, and then proceed with an open cordotomy at a lower level on the opposite side. Thus, although most skilled percutaneous cordotomists prefer to perform bilateral percutaneous cordotomies, Gildenberg found that more than 50 per cent of neurosurgeons questioned still did open cordotomy, more than those doing percutaneous procedures.[32]

The physician who does not have access to the necessary equipment or for geographical reasons cannot transfer his patient to a center so equipped may prefer to perform cordotomy by the open method. Hitchcock saw 3000 patients in his pain clinic in 10 years: 66 required open high cervical cordotomy, and 106 had posterior stereotaxic procedure.[38] Rosomoff, Tasker, and others show clear preference for percutaneous technique because, although overall end-results may be the same as for the open procedure, the percutaneous method is easier, safer, and more precise.[79,95]

OPERATIVE TECHNIQUE

In the following pages the author's technique for open cordotomy at the various levels is described. These techniques have been learned from a number of others and in most instances represent variations from the techniques of others. They have been evolved to reduce the magnitude of the procedure, to reduce postoperative symptoms and complications, and to give good cord visualization.

Posterior Thoracic Cordotomy

The posterior thoracic and high cervical cordotomies may be done with the patient in the prone or sitting position and under local or general anesthesia. The advantage

---

* See references 10, 27, 28, 84, 85, 92.

of the sitting position is a bloodless field; the disadvantage is the risk of hypotension and air embolism. The author has preferred to utilize the prone position and general anesthesia. Sweet, however, admitting the inconsistencies of responses, has pointed out the importance of stimulation and testing of the patient in order to achieve an optimal lesion at minimal risk, and a similar plea has been made by Schwartz and by others.[85,92] Contrariwise, French, Chou and his co-workers, and others have felt that testing is difficult and unreliable under local anesthesia in these critically ill patients.[10,28]

Under endotracheal anesthesia the patient is positioned on chest rolls in the prone position with the head of the table only slightly elevated to avoid air embolism. A right atrial catheter should be placed, and cardiac Doppler monitoring is used to deal with air embolism should it occur. After suitable preparation, a midline incision is made extending one spine above and below the interspace in which the cordotomy is to be done. If unilateral cordotomy is to be performed, incision of the fascia and separation of the muscles from the spines and laminae is sharply limited to T1–T2 on the side contralateral to the pain. If the cordotomy is to be bilateral, the muscles and fascia are separated from the spines and laminae of T1–T2 on the side opposite the worst pain and T3–T4 on the opposite side. A small portion of the inferior margin of the T1 and the superior margin of the T2 hemilaminae are removed laterally along with the ligamentum flavum in the same manner as one would approach a lumbar or cervical disc. It is important that the bony removal be carried laterally to the facet in order to gain the most lateral possible exposure to the cord. The bone edges are waxed and an inverted longitudinal semilunar incision is made in the dura (Fig. 132–2). This modified flap is sewn to the muscle mass laterally. At this juncture one is looking at the posterior lateral aspect of the cord. The arachnoid is opened and the dentate ligament identified. The lateral dentate attachment to the dura may be left intact or it may be sectioned. A fine clamp is placed flush with the edge of the dentate ligament against the cord and rotated gently posteriorly. An avascular area is chosen or, if one cannot be found, the pia may be lightly cauterized with a fine-tip bipolar cautery down to the level of the anterior

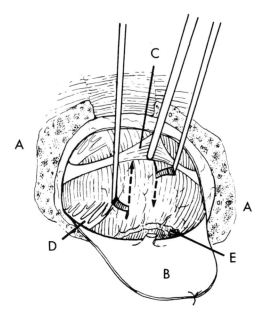

Figure 132–2 Operative approach for posterior thoracic and high cervical open cordotomy. A, partial hemilaminectomy of superior and inferior hemilamina; B, semilunar dural flap reflected laterally and then tied to the muscle; C, dentate ligament sectioned and held at its attachment to the cord with a fine hemostat; D, anterior roots; E, anterior spinal artery. After the pia has been opened with microscissors, the downcutting knife is inserted at the level of the dentate ligament and swept downward to emerge at the line of the anterior roots; the upcutting knife is inserted in the pial opening midway between the anterior roots and anterior spinal artery and brought up to the line of the dentate ligament. Rotation of the cord and anterior spinal artery is exaggerated in this diagram to show the extent of the upcutting incision between the line of the anterior roots and the anterior spinal artery.

root. A small incision is made into the pia with a No. 11 knife at the ventral edge of the dentate ligament, and by using the microscissors the pia is opened down to an area 1 to 2 mm anterior to the anterior root. Care must be taken to avoid the midline anterior spinal artery, which is on the surface. It is essential to open the pia with either a knife or scissors, as it is very tough. The cord will be markedly distorted if the pia is not opened prior to cordotomy. At this juncture a downcutting cordotomy knife or the tip of a razor blade cracked to make a fine blade is inserted parallel to the dentate ligament with the cord minimally rotated. The depth of the incision should be 5 mm. The blade is then swept downward to emerge at the level of the anterior root. An upcutting knife or the razor blade turned in the holder is then inserted into the cord 2 mm anterior to the ventral roots and brought upward to just below the level of the dentate ligament to complete the section. It is desirable to complete the cordotomy the first time with these two cuts, since repeated minimal cuts will simply cause edema and dislodge fibers from their normal position rather than sectioning them, causing later reduction in the effective level of analgesia. Bleeding is minimal and easily controlled with Gelfoam. The dural flap is then closed with fine sutures, and the laminectomy wound is closed in the usual way. If a bilateral procedure is to be performed, one simply goes to the opposite side and repeats the procedure at T3–T4. This type of staggered fascial and muscle approach limited to two laminae has minimized postoperative pain, which was a frequent accompaniment of complete bilateral laminectomy involving several vertebrae as they were commonly done in the past. Further, the posterior roots are not disturbed, avoiding postoperative radicular pain.

Posterior High Cervical Cordotomy

In an effort to obtain the high levels of analgesia needed to cope with pain in the chest, arm, and brachial plexus, Foerster and Gagel, and later Stookey introduced the high cervical cordotomy.[21,89] On the basis of their anatomical studies. Morin, Schwartz, and co-workers presented evidence that the spinothalamic tract was more dorsal and compact at the high cervical area, and because of this advocated high cervical cordotomy as the procedure of choice.[60,84,85] The operations were done with the patients in the prone position and under local anesthesia in order to allow intraoperative sensory testing for adjustment of the incision.[84,85] French, on the other hand, reporting an extensive series, felt that testing under local anesthesia was unreliable and preferred using the sitting position and general anesthesia for bilateral procedures.[28] The risk of hypotension is present, however, and is combated by having the patient wear a G suit and by careful monitoring of arterial and central venous pressure. Air embolism is monitored by cardiac Doppler technique and treated by placing the patient in the right lateral position, aspirating air from the right atrial catheter, and using vasopressor drugs when appropriate.

In the Schwartz procedure, by having the patient voluntarily flex the neck and placing a spreader between the spine of C2 and the base of the skull, adequate room is developed so that bone removal is unnecessary. Others have preferred doing a modified hemilaminectomy of C1–C2.

The patient is intubated and is placed prone on chest rolls with the head in the Mayfield headholder and the neck slightly flexed. Severe flexion should be avoided, particularly in older patients, because of the risk of cord or vertebral artery compression in the event that cervical arthritis is present. The head of the bed is elevated somewhat to provide for good venous drainage. A right atrial catheter and Doppler detector are in place to monitor for air embolism. A midline incision from the inion to C4 is made very much as in the thoracic procedure, and if bilateral cordotomy is intended, bilateral exposure can be made, separating the muscles from the skull and the spines and laminae of C1–C2. If necessary a small portion of the hemilaminae of C1 and C2 may be removed, or C1 and C2 may be spread apart with a Gelpie retractor. The ligamentum flavum is removed, and the dura is opened in exactly the same fashion as in the thoracic procedure and sutured to the muscle. The dentate ligament is grasped, and the cordotomy is carried to a depth of 5 mm in similar fashion to that previously described for the thoracic cordotomy. The incision needs to be carried medial to the anterior root just short of the anterior spinal artery. If a bilateral procedure is to be done at the same procedure, the cord incisions should be staggered as far as possible longitudinally. The incisions should not be deeper than 4 mm, and care should be taken to avoid the area just lateral to the anterior horn in an effort to avoid the respiratory fibers. Closure is performed in the same way as described previously.

Anterior Cervical Cordotomy

In 1964 Cloward reported a series of cervical cordotomies performed via the anterior approach that he had previously introduced for the treatment of cervical disc disease. Agreeing with Hamby, who had selected the C4–C5 segment as most suitable for posterior cordotomy, Cloward selected the C4–C5 space as most suitable for the anterior approach, since the incision would be below the phrenic outflow and above the anterior horns subserving the fine muscles of the hand, so that if the anterior horn was involved in the incision the weakness should involve the upper arm.[11,35] A standard Cloward midline approach to the anterior cervical vertebrae was made. The disc was removed and an 18-mm drill centered at the C4–C5 interspace in the midline. The opening was then squared up with the Kerrison punch, and the posterior longitudinal ligament was removed. Venous bleeding was stopped with Gelfoam or, if necessary, dural tack-ups, and the dura was opened in a cruciate fashion, giving excellent access to the anterior aspect of the cord. Section was done with a razor blade or special knife, and the dura was closed with sutures.[11] Cloward has not reported subsequently on his experience with this procedure, although in a personal communication he states that it has been extremely satisfactory and that bilateral procedures have been accomplished with negligible leg and sphincteric motor involvement.[12] It is Dr. Cloward's feeling that the procedure is safer, especially for bilateral cordotomies, and gives uniformly high levels of analgesia. More recently, Hardy and co-workers revived interest in the procedure by utilizing the operating microscope and essentially following Cloward's technique.[36] They emphasized the possibility of selective cordotomy through this approach and reported on 10 cases with no long-term follow-up. Although the procedure can be done under local anesthesia so that testing would be possible, most of Cloward's patients were operated on under general anesthesia, since he felt that the patient's cooperation for testing was unnecessary. Hardy experienced difficulty with the cruciate dural incision and recommended closure of the dura with silver clips.

With the patient supine and the head slightly extended and turned to the opposite side, under satisfactory endotracheal anesthesia, a transverse oblique incision is made following the skin lines at the approximate level of C4–C5 or C5–C6, usually on the right side. Although there is less risk of injury to the recurrent laryngeal nerve on the left, it is less convenient for the right-handed surgeon, and no difficulties with the recurrent nerve have been encountered as long as care has been taken with the dissection.

Following application of skin drapes, a standard Cloward approach is made to the anterior vertebral surface. It is important that the fascial planes be opened adequately to allow easy retraction and give access to the midline. The prevertebral fascia is opened, and the medial borders of the colli muscles are cauterized and the muscles lifted laterally for the insertion of the Cloward retractor blades. For brachial plexus lesions, the C2–C3 or C3–C4 space

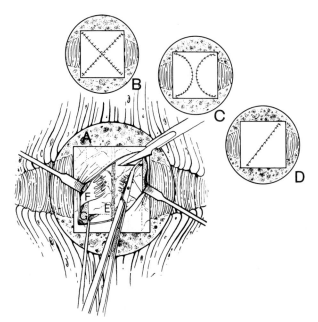

Figure 132–3 Operative approach for anterior cervical open cordotomy. *A.* Bony opening, squared up with Kerrison punch. *B.* Cruciate dural incision. *C.* Semilunar dural incisions. *D.* Oblique dural incision. The main sketch shows the dura open with the oblique dural incision to expose the anterior spinal artery, E, in the midline and the anterior roots, F. The pia is incised next to the anterior spinal artery and opened to the exact level of the dentate ligament, G, with microscissors. The upcutting cordotomy knife is then inserted at the level of the unrotated dentate ligament to a depth of 5 mm and brought upward to emerge at the line of the anterior roots. Following this the incision may be extended laterally from the border of the anterior spinal artery to the previous incision.

is chosen; otherwise, C4–C5 or C5–C6 is used. Following evacuation of the disc space, a 16-mm drill opening is made in the usual fashion centered exactly in the midline. The operating microscope is introduced. The posterior longitudinal ligament is incised with the No. 15 knife and removed with a micro-Kerrison punch. Following this it is helpful to square up the posterior aspect of the bony opening with a small Kerrison punch (Fig. 132–3). Epidural venous bleeding will respond readily to gentle packing with small Gelfoam strips; it has not been necessary to suture up the dura.

Originally it was found that a cruciate incision was difficult to close in a watertight fashion, particularly where the tips met. The dura in this region is very thin and is easily torn, and in the initial cases difficulty was experienced in obtaining a watertight closure. The author was not successful in the use of silver clips. He therefore used a semilunar incision, which permitted satisfactory watertight closure. More recently, in performing a bilateral procedure, it has been learned that a simple diagonal incision will give very satisfactory access to both sides of the cord at two different levels and, being a linear incision, is easily closed (Fig. 132–3D).[7] (A half-round swedged needle of suitable size for 7-0 suture would be highly desirable but is not manufactured at the present time.) If the diagonal dural incision is made, a small microspatula is inserted to hold the dura laterally. This fits well on the Greenberg automatic retractor. The arachnoid is opened, and the anterior spinal artery is immediately seen in the middle of the cord on the surface. The anterior roots have their takeoff at a variable distance from the midline but may be quite close to it. A small strip of cottonoid is placed laterally down to the level of the dentate ligament for suction, spinal fluid is evacuated, and an avascular area is chosen between the roots. If present, fine surface pial vessels are coagulated with fine-tipped bipolar microforceps. With a No. 11 knife the pia is opened for a short distance at approximately the level of the anterior roots, and then the microscissors are used to continue the pial opening laterally to a point flush with the dentate ligament, as shown in Figure 132–3. The ligament is clearly seen at its junction with the cord, and of course, the cord does not have to be manipulated or

rotated. At this juncture, the surgeon should survey the cord to make sure that the dentate ligament is in its normal meridional position and not located abnormally posteriorly or anteriorly. A right-angle upcutting cordotomy knife is inserted to a depth of 5 mm flush with the dentate ligament and parallel to it and brought upward to emerge at the line of the anterior roots. Over the anterior horns, the incision should not be more than 3 mm deep to avoid respiratory fibers. Following this, the pia is incised just lateral to the anterior spinal artery by inserting the No. 11 knife with the cutting edge away from the anterior spinal artery. The incision is carried laterally from the anterior spinal artery to the previous incision at the line of the anterior roots at a depth of 3 mm. In this way, the incision can be carried to the midline if especially high levels of analgesia are desired. In the limited number of cases in which this technique has been used to date it has not been possible to determine the essentiality of the medial incision.[7] Bleeding is minimal and easily controlled with Gelfoam. The dural incision is then closed with fine interrupted 7-0 sutures. Bleeding from the bone or epidural space is readily controlled by using a topical hemostatic agent (Avitene). The bone plug is taken from the analgesic hip. The wound is closed in the usual manner for the anterior Cloward procedure.

If a bilateral procedure is to be done, the diagonal linear dural opening permits the incisions to be staggered to the maximum afforded by the bone opening and still provides an easy-to-close linear incision (see Fig. 132–3D).

Commissural Myelotomy

The history of commissural myelotomy for relief of pain has been summarized by White and Sweet, Cook and Kawakami, and King.[14,44,102] First reported by Armour in England in 1927, the procedure was performed in France by Leriche in 1928 and published in 1936; in the meantime, Putnam had reported it in the United States in 1934. Since that time a number of individuals have performed the operation by using blunt dissection, radiofrequency, ultrasound, laser, and stereotaxic methods.*

---

* See references 1, 2, 14, 38, 44, 76.

Recently King was able to find reports in the literature of 200 patients who underwent commissurotomy, and published nine of his own cases. He described the microsection of the dorsal fissure, the identification of the central canal, and the opening of the anterior commissure into the anterior fissure under direct microscopic visualization.[44]

Cook and Kawakami report commissural myelotomy accomplished by blunt dissection in 24 patients. The operations were at various levels from C4 through L1, and there were good or fair immediate results in all patients but poor results in 7 of 11 long-term survivors.[14]

The procedure has been used in the cervical, thoracic, and lumbar areas. The segment of cord that must be interrupted to relieve pain in the desired area should be ascertained, and laminectomy performed at the appropriate level, frequently at T9 to T12 for lower extremity and pelvic pain. Following opening and retraction of the dura, the arachnoid is opened and the operating microscope brought into play. The midline is identified by convergence of small vessels; it does not necessarily correspond to the dorsal vein. It is usually possible to dissect the dorsal vein free and retract it to one side and identify the medial dorsal fissure. The length of the incision is demarcated, and one begins at the cephalad end by incision of the pia with a sharp knife or microscissors. The fissure usually opens easily. Very fine-bladed retractors are inserted down to the central canal, and the dorsal columns are retracted as little as possible. The anterior commissure is then identified and is opened with a blunt instrument into the dorsal aspect of the anterior fissure (see Fig. 132–1). One should look for branches of the anterior spinal artery, but the artery itself lies on the surface of the cord and is not encountered. One may continuously open the dorsal fissure and carry the procedure caudad to its termination or one may make short segmental openings into the fissure and by sweeping the instrument forward and backward may connect the transections of the anterior commissure without completely opening the dorsal fissure throughout its length. Care is taken to avoid handling the dorsal roots to avoid postoperative radicular hyperesthesia, and the least possible retraction is used to mini-

mize dorsal changes in dorsal column function and structure. Bleeding is minimal and easily controlled with small pledgets of Gelfoam or with micro–bipolar cautery.

The operation appears to be indicated for patients with carcinoma involving the lower extremities, but Cook has sounded a note of warning regarding difficulty in obtaining complete relief in patients with midline sacral involvement. The unanswered questions regarding variation in postoperative sensory findings raised by King regarding this procedure need further investigation.[44]

RESULTS

Following cordotomy the patient will have loss of pain and temperature sensation at some level below where the cord was sectioned, usually T3 to T12 after high thoracic and C2 to C7 after high cervical section. Refined physiological testing has confirmed that there is a thorough mixing of temperature and pain fibers as well as tactile fibers carried in the tract. The detailed sensory studies of White and associates showed that after anterolateral cordotomy there is abolition of perception of pain, temperature, and itching, and reduction in deep pressure and two-point discrimination. Touch, vibration, and position senses are preserved. In addition, the pain of electric current; testicular, tendon, or bone pressure; and other sensations may be preserved in reduced form. Perception of pain from unilaterally innervated visceral organs is lost.[103] After thoracic cordotomy performed for 271 cases of pain due to malignant disease, White and Sweet reported immediate relief in 70 per cent of patients with unilateral and in 40 per cent of those with bilateral procedures. Early failures were due to postoperative pain (15 per cent), inadequate denervation (6 per cent), and immediate spread of pain to the opposite side (9 per cent). Late failures occurred in 9 per cent owing to spread of the disease and in 4 per cent owing to loss of analgesia. In 70 cases in which cordotomy was performed for neuralgias and survival was prolonged, analgesia was achieved postoperatively in 86 per cent and permanently in 56 per cent, with 14 per cent showing early failure and 20 per cent late recurrence.[102] A number of authors have reported immediate relief in

50 to 75 per cent of cases, partial relief in 20 per cent, and failure in 3 to 32 per cent.* Schwartz, advocating high cervical cordotomy to take advantage of the dorsolateral shift of the pain-conducting fibers and more complete decussation, reported pain relief in 69 per cent after unilateral and 78 per cent after bilateral cordotomy for short-term follow-ups.[84] Chou and associates reported that 92 per cent of their patients with high cervical cordotomies had a C4 level of analgesia after operation, and at 12 months, 86 per cent continued to have a satisfactory level of analgesia. There was satisfactory relief of pain in 96 per cent.[10] French reported analgesia to C4 in 93 per cent of patients, with persistent C4 levels in 84 per cent of those who could be examined in 12 months.[27,28] Some of these patients were included in both series.

Tasker compared 141 percutaneous cervical cordotomies with 113 randomly selected open cordotomies performed at various sites over a 15-year period. Percutaneous cordotomy showed better results than open cordotomy (96 per cent versus 84 per cent unilateral and 83 per cent versus 53 per cent bilateral pain relief) and markedly decreased incidence of significant paresis (0 versus 15 per cent unilateral and 0 versus 39 percent bilateral), while the incidence of bowel, bladder, and sexual impairment was about the same for the two procedures (6 per cent versus 2 per cent unilateral and 21 per cent versus 25 per cent bilateral).[95]

Rosomoff, in reviewing 1279 percutaneous high cervical cordotomies, found that in only 13 per cent were analgesia levels inadequate, and that in 9 per cent analgesia disappeared, to be restored by repeat cordotomy. At follow-up, 66 per cent of patients had died or were lost to follow-up at three months and 75 per cent at one year. Hemiparesis occurred transiently in 5 per cent and permanently in 3 per cent; the latter died early. Ataxia occurred in 20 per cent and was permanent in 3 per cent. Catheterization was required temporarily in 10 per cent, permanently in 2 per cent. In 4 per cent there was a decrease in sexual sensation. Dysesthesias were seen in less than 1 per cent. Pain relief was obtained in 90 per cent postoperatively, the success rate fall-

ing to 84 per cent in three months, 60 per cent at one year, and 40 per cent at two years. Many other patients had partial relief.[79]

No long-term results have been reported for anterior cervical cordotomy. Cloward, reporting his original 10 cases followed for 18 months, found that most of the cancer patients were dead in six months and that about half had had pain relief. Of four patients operated on for pain of nonmalignant origin, one had relief for eight months, the others for less.[11] Hardy performed 13 cordotomies in 10 patients at the C4–C5 level. Levels of analgesia varied from C5 to T9; nine of ten patients were relieved of pain at discharge, and there was short-term relief of pain until death in six cases and long-term relief in one case. There was one case of transient leg paresis and one cerebrospinal fluid leak.[36]

The author has performed anterior cervical cordotomy in twelve cases. One was a bilateral procedure. Two operations were done at C2 and C3, producing analgesia at C2. The remainder were done at C5 to C7, with levels of analgesia from C5 to T4. Eleven patients had immediate complete relief of pain; one had no relief. In one case there was severe postoperative leg weakness, and in two, mild leg paresis that cleared. About half the patients complained of a very transient feeling of awkwardness or weakness in the hand on the side operated on. There were two examples of increased bladder weakness, one of bowel incontinence, and one of cerebrospinal fluid leak in an early case. Long-term follow-up is not available as yet, but there have been two instances of analgesia below T3 with dermatomic preservation of pain sensation over S1 in one and S1 to S5 in the other, with recurrence of pain in those dermatomes.[7] It is the author's impression, based on this preliminary experience, that the procedure gives excellent visualization, is very well tolerated by the patients, and is probably subject to the same deficiencies of long-term recurrence and complications as other methods of cordotomy.

For the procedure of myelotomy, King reported that short-term relief was achieved in seven of the nine patients. Two patients suffered a mild monoparesis. The sensory loss after the procedure was varied, and transient posterior column findings

---

* See references 47, 67, 72, 75, 95, 101–103.

were present, particularly in a bandlike level at the top of the incision. The pain recurred at 5, 10, and 12 months in the surviving patients.[44] Cook and Kawakami also reported good or fair immediate results in 24 patients, but poor results in 7 of 11 long-term survivors.[14]

Long-term results were particularly disappointing in eight cases of chronic adhesive arachnoiditis. Half the patients operated on had immediate postoperative hyperalgesia and dysesthesia not relieved by analgesic drugs. These sensations were temporary. Proprioception was also disturbed temporarily in half the patients, and with incisions in the thoracolumbar area there was a band of sensory disturbance about the trunk that appears to be characteristic of this procedure. The advantages of the procedure, stressed by both King and Cook and Kawakami are: the absence of deaths, the effectiveness in relieving bilateral pain, and the lack of permanent disturbance of sphincteric or motor function. The disadvantages are those of an open operation, transient sensory or motor disturbances, inconstant areas of analgesia despite pain relief, and lack of pain relief for pelvic metastases.[14,44] In addition, it is important to point out that this procedure has failed for chronic pain conditions and is, therefore, recommended only for pain due to cancer and other conditions in which survival is not likely to be long. In this it resembles all other cordotomy procedures.

White and Sweet state that in their experience the waning of anesthesia and the appearance of islands of nonanalgesia are the same for both cervical and thoracic cordotomy.[102] A similar appearance of islands of preserved sensation and loss of analgesia has been found in a small number of cases in which the anterior cervical approach was used.[7] White and Sweet in their detailed study of cordotomy have shown in their Figure 103 the late results of anterolateral cordotomy, indicating the reduction of satisfactory results from 90 per cent postoperatively to 50 per cent at one year, with poor results following secondary and tertiary cordotomies.[102] Upper cervical posterior cordotomy can be extended by appropriate ipsilateral root section from C2 through C4 for improved relief of arm pain, but prospects of prolonged arm analgesia are poor.

It is a well-known phenomenon that, as time passes, islands of return of sensation begin to appear and the level of the analgesia may decrease either immediately or after long periods of time up to a year or more. The reasons for early inadequate level of analgesia is undoubtedly an improperly performed procedure or serious anatomical variation of sensory or motor tracts. If analgesia is not absolutely complete as determined by detailed tests immediately postoperatively, recurrence of pain may be expected. Variation in sensory level may be due to variation in level of decussation, according to White and co-workers.[103] Diminution of levels of analgesia in the immediate postoperative period probably is due to pushing aside or contusion of fibers, particularly by tentative cuts rather than single incisive cordotomy incisions. This can be avoided by opening the pia and outer layers of the cord generously with the microscissors prior to doing the cordotomy, thus reducing distortion and the amount of tissue that needs to be cut by the cordotomy knife. Another important reason undoubtedly is the variability of the position of the pain fibers in terms of both their dorsal-ventral and medial-lateral disposition, and it is likely that fibers, particularly medial and dorsomedial, may be missed or only contused, only to have their function return at a later date. The most difficult result to explain is the cordotomy that produces dense analgesia and relief of pain for 1 to 15 years only to have pain return following some incident such as an accident, with examination showing that sensation of pinprick and temperature has returned. Analgesia and pain relief may follow repeat cordotomy. Although such hypotheses as regeneration of fibers, incomplete section, and others have been offered, the mechanism for return of sensation is not known at the present time. A further speculation is the possibility of other pathways having or assuming the function of pain transmission. No convincing evidence for this has been presented to date, however. Nevertheless, the case reported by Noordenbos and Wall in which the entire cord was sectioned with sparing of one ventrolateral quadrant is important. Pinprick and temperature sensation were retained contralateral to the intact ventral quadrant, but touch, pressure, and position sense and pain could be evoked by stimulation on both sides.[71] This and findings of Giesler and Willis and their co-workers suggest more diffuse sensory transport than formerly accepted.[30,71,105]

The most common cause of cordotomy failure is performance of cordotomy for the wrong reason. The marked interest in the problem of chronic pain in recent years and the expansion of knowledge through the development of pain clinics as well as new information regarding the anatomy and physiology of the pain pathways, the opiate receptor system, and the like, have made it perfectly clear that in many cases pain is the minor portion of a suffering syndrome and that very important psychological, social, and environmental factors are being expressed as chronic pain. This situation, leading to many unwarranted operations of all types, may well engender attempts to relieve pain by ill-advised cordotomies. It is generally accepted at present that cordotomy should be reserved for patients with pain due to malignant disease and short life expectancy, and is not indicated for painful conditions in which prolonged survival is expected, except under special circumstances. Hitchcock found cordotomy of any type indicated in only 5 per cent of the patients he treated for pain[38]

COMPLICATIONS OF CORDOTOMY

The complications of cordotomy vary with the condition of the patient and the level of the cordotomy. The mortality risk of open cordotomy performed in the thoracic area is approximately 10 per cent in malignant disease (usually associated with poor-risk factors associated with the carcinoma), while cordotomies performed in benign conditions are essentially free of mortality risk. Cervical cordotomies carry a higher risk due to the associated respiratory failure, particularly in patients with thoracic carcinoma who already have respiratory embarrassment.

Figure 132–1 shows in diagrammatic form the approximate location of the tracts and location of fibers serving respiratory and sphincteric functions.

Schwartz reported mortality rates of 3 per cent for unilateral and 20 per cent for bilateral procedures for high cervical section. Bladder involvement occurs in approximately 2 to 10 per cent of unilateral and 10 to 30 per cent of bilateral thoracic cordotomies, whether done in one or two stages.[84] Chou and co-workers found transient (14 per cent) and permanent (5 per cent) urinary difficulties after unilateral high cervical cordotomy, and temporary (100 per cent and permanent (92 per cent) urinary problems after bilateral high cervical cordotomy.[10] Schwartz found temporary (11 per cent) and permanent (5 per cent) bladder weakness after unilateral cervical cordotomy, and transient (42 per cent) and permanent (20 per cent) bladder problems after bilateral high cervical cordotomy.[85]

After unilateral cordotomy, difficulty with urination when present is usually temporary. Rectal complications are more difficult to analyze and are present in approximately 8 per cent of patients. In addition, unilateral cordotomy interferes with sexual function, and impotence is certain to follow bilateral procedures.[102]

Hyponatremia probably associated with vasoparalysis has been reported after bilateral cervical cordotomy.[51]

Weakness of the extremities may occur, particularly in those patients with preexisting involvement by disease and is usually found upon awakening from the operation. The incidence of serious paresis declines markedly with time, and recovery of function is the rule. White and Sweet reported a 10 per cent incidence of paresis after unilateral cervical, 5 per cent after unilateral thoracic, and 20 per cent after bilateral thoracic cordotomy.[102] Nathan and Smith reported no or slight paresis in 90 per cent after unilateral and in 76 per cent after bilateral procedures, or conversely, severe weakness after 10 per cent and 24 per cent of the unilateral and bilateral procedures respectively.[69] Tasker reported significant paresis in 15 per cent after unilateral and in 39 per cent after bilateral open cordotomy.[95] Chou and co-workers and French found 12 per cent of patients had transient and 5 per cent had permanent weakness after unilateral high cervical cordotomy, and 20 per cent had transient and 12 per cent had permanent weakness after bilateral high cervical cordotomy.[10,28] Schwartz found weakness to be present transiently in 13 per cent and permanently in 2 per cent after both unilateral and bilateral high cervical cordotomy.[85]

Respiratory complications may follow high cervical cordotomy and constitute a risk to life after bilateral procedures. Nathan, in a careful postmortem study of cords from cordotomy patients, localized the descending pathway in the reticulospinal fibers lying on the surface of the ventral horn medial to the spinothalamic tract.[68] Later studies by Hitchcock and Luce and by Fox suggest that descending fibers to the phrenic cells of origin lie medially and those to the anterior horn cells of the intercostals are more dorsolateral, corresponding to the layering of the spinothalamic tract.[24,39] Belmusto and associates reported respiratory and vascular changes after 4-mm cervical incisions in 20 patients and found a correlation of pain relief with respiratory changes, implying close correlation or intermixing of descending respiratory fibers with ascending pain fibers. These results were extended in experimental studies.[5,6]

Rosomoff and his associates, in a series of studies of respiratory function in patients undergoing percutaneous cervical cordotomy, concluded that interruption of ascending spinoreticular fibers produces sleep apnea, which was seen in 3 per cent of patients following high cervical cordotomy.[45,46,48,49,80] Others have also noted respiratory complications.[37,63,92,95,102]

French found a 22 per cent incidence of hypotension after cervical cordotomy, 5 per cent of which was permanent; and hypotension also may follow high thoracic procedures.[28,102] A common complaint formerly following cordotomy by complete laminectomy of several segments was radicular pain at the area of the cordotomy incision, but this has largely been eliminated by the more limited approaches, both posterior and anterior. A disabling complication of cordotomy is postoperative paresthesias, reported by White and Sweet to occur in 11 per cent of cases, and it is now believed that these may well be sensory disconnection paresthesias.[102]

SUMMARY

It is apparent that a number of substantial problems remain at present that make cordotomy by either open or percutaneous method less than satisfactory. Both methods can achieve a high rate of initial analgesia when performed by experienced operators. Each procedure, however, carries definite risks of failure to obtain pain relief with adequate sensory level. In addition, there are definite risks of difficulty with bowel, bladder, and sexual function, particularly with bilateral procedures; the risk of paresis; and in high cervical procedures, the risk of respiratory paralysis and sleep apnea. The risk of paresis is less with the percutaneous procedure, but the risk of sphincteric, autonomic, and respiratory complications is probably similar in the two procedures, depending on the extent of the cordotomy. It is likely that physiological testing in the awake patient during the open and the percutaneous procedures will decrease the risk of complication and increase the possibility of better levels of analgesia.

A second major practical problem with both the open and closed methods is the declining rate of satisfactory analgesia and the appearance of islands of spared sensation as time passes, so that by one year approximately 50 per cent of patients no longer have satisfactory analgesia or pain relief. In a substantial number of cases, however, such as those documented by White and Sweet, very long-term complete relief of pain can be obtained.[102] While the loss of analgesia and recurrence of pain in 50 per cent of the patients at one year can be viewed as a distinct disadvantage, nevertheless, the satisfactory relief of the other 50 per cent, many of whom are in desperate situations, can be viewed as a very worthwhile result.

A third problem, fortunately not common, is postcordotomy dysesthesia that can be disabling.

These and other problems result from the fact that at present the topographical anatomy of the pain-conducting fibers is not only not precisely established but is probably subject to considerable anatomical variation. Further, it is now well recognized that, following a generous section of the anterior lateral column, a number of modalities of pain remain.[43,102] The mechanism and pathways by which this pain sensation ascends to consciousness is not well understood.

Unless new discoveries as to physical modalities of energy application to the cord that would result in selective analgesia with sparing of other function can be made, it is unlikely that further development in the technique of cordotomy can decisively ameliorate the drawbacks to the procedure. With the development of new information regarding the pain pathways and pharmacological systems governing transmission of pain, it seems to the writer that future developments are much more likely to flow from pharmacological than from surgical methods, and it may well be that such developments will render the operation of cordotomy unnecessary in the not too distant future. In the meantime, despite the advances derived from pain clinics, psychological counseling, nerve block procedures, and the like, there remain a substantial number of patients whose pain is not controlled by nonoperative means. In these patients, particularly those with pain due to malignant disease, cordotomy remains an important modality of therapy.

REFERENCES

1. Armour, D.: Surgery of the spinal cord and its membranes. Lancet, *1*:423–430, 533–537, 691–698, 1927.
2. Ascher, P. W.: Longitudinal medial myelotomy with the laser. *In* Proceedings of Sixth International Congress of Neurological Surgery, São Paulo, Brazil, 1977. Amsterdam-Oxford, Excerpta Medica, 1978, pp. 267–270.
3. Basbaum, A. I.: Conduction of the effects of noxious stimulation by short-fiber multisynaptic systems. Exp. Neurol., *40*:699–716, 1973.
4. Beer, E.: The relief of intractable and persistent pain due to metastases pressing on nerve plexuses. J.A.M.A., *58*:1490—1493, 1912.
5. Belmusto, L., Brown, E., and Owens, G.: Clinical observations on respiratory and vasomotor disturbances as related to cervical cordotomies. J. Neurosurg., *20*:225–232, 1963.
6. Belmusto, L., Brown, E., and Owens, G.: Localization and patterns of potentials of the respiratory pathway in the cervical spinal cord of the dog. J. Neurosurg., *22*:277–283, 1965.
7. Brackett, C. E.: Unpublished data.
8. Brown-Séquard, M.: Mémoire sur la transmission des impressions sensitives dans la moelle épinière. C. R. Acad. Sci. (Paris), *31*:700–701, 1850.
9. Cadwalader, W. B., and Sweet, J. E.: Experimental work on the function of the anterolateral column of the spinal cord. J.A.M.A., *58*:1490–1493, 1912.
10. Chou, S. N., French, L. A., and Story, J. L.: The relief of pain of cancer by cordotomy. Progr. Clin. Cancer, *2*:135–142, 1966.
11. Cloward, R. B.: Cervical cordotomy by the anterior approach: Technique and advantages. J. Neurosurg., *21*:19–25, 1964.
12. Cloward, R. B.: Personal communication.
13. Collis, J. S.: Anterolateral cordotomy by an anterior approach: Report of a case. J. Neurosurg., *20*:445–446, 1963.
14. Cook, A. W., and Kawakami, Y.: Commissural myelotomy. J. Neurosurg., *47*:1–6, 1977.
15. Coulter, J. D., Foreman, R. D., Beall, J. L., and Willis, W. D.: Cerebral cortical modulation of primate spinothalamic neurons. Advances Pain Res. Ther., *1*:271–277, 1976.
16. Crue, B. L.: Pain, Research and Treatment. Academic Press, New York, 1975, pp. 417.
17. Crue, B. L., Keaton, B., and Carregal, E. J. A.: Neurophysiology of pain. Bull. Los Angeles Neurol. Soc., *41*:13–42, 1976.
18. Crue, B. L., Todd, E. M., and Carregal, E. J. A.: Posterior approach for high cervical percutaneous radiofrequency cordotomy. Confin. Neurol., *30*:41–52, 1968.
19. Edinger, L.: Vergleichend-entwicklungsgeschichtliche und anatomische Studien im Bereiche des Centralnervensystems. II. Über die Fortsetzung der hinteren Rückenmarkswurzeln zum Gehirn. Anat. Anz., *4*:121–128, 1889.
20. Edinger, L.: Vorlesunger über den Bau der nervösen Centralorgane. Liepzig, 1904.
21. Foerster, O., and Gagel, O.: Die Vorderseitenstrangdurchschneidung beim Menschen. Z. Ges. Neurol. Psychiat., *138*:1–92, 1932.
22. Foerster, O.: Vorderseitenstrangdurhschneidung in Ruckenmark zur Beseitigung von Schmerzen. Berlin. Klin. Wschr., *50*:1499–1500, 1913.
23. Fox, J. L.: Percutaneous stereotaxic cordotomy. II. A guidance technique for the anterior approach. Acta Neurochir., *18*:318–326, 1968.
24. Fox, J. L.: Localization of the respiratory motor pathway in the upper cervical spinal cord following percutaneous cordotomy. Neurology (Minneap.), *19*:1115–1118, 1969.
25. Fox, J. L.: Experimental relationship of radiofrequency electrical current and lesion size for application to percutaneous cordotomy. J. Neurosurg., *33*:415–421, 1970.
26. Frazier, C. H.: Section of the anterolateral columns of the spinal cord for the relief of pain. Arch. Neurol. Psychiat., *4*:137–147, 1920.
27. French, L. A.: Cordotomy in the high cervical region for intractable pain. Lancet, *73*:283–287, 1957.
28. French, L. A.: High cervical tractotomy: Technique and results. Clin. Neurosurg., *21*:239–245, 1973.
29. French, L. A., and Peyton, W. T.: Ipsilateral sensory loss following cordotomy. J. Neurosurg., *5*:403–404, 1948.
30. Giesler, G. L., Cannon, T. J., Urca, G., and Liebskind, J. C.: Long ascending projections from substantia gelatinosa rolandi and the subjacent dorsal horn in the rat. Science, *202*:984–986, 1978.
31. Gildenberg, P. L.: Stereotaxic lower cervical cordotomy for the treatment of intractable pain. Confin. Neurol., *34*:275–278, 1972.
32. Gildenberg, P. L.: Percutaneous cervical cordotomy. Clin. Neurosurg., *21*:246–256, 1973.
33. Gowers, W. R.: A case of unilateral gunshot injury to the spinal cord. Trans. Clin. Soc. London, *11*:24–26, 1878.
34. Graf, C. J.: Consideration in loss of sensory level after bilateral cervical cordotomy. Arch. Neurol. (Chicago), *3*:410–415, 1960.
35. Hamby, W. B.: A modified technique for spino-

thalamic cordotomy. J. Neurosurg., *11*:378–385, 1954.

36. Hardy, J., LeClerq, T. A., and Mercky, F.: Microsurgical cordotomy by the anterior approach. Technical note. J. Neurosurg., *41*:640–643, 1974.

37. Hill, G. E., and Polk, S. L.: Hypoventilation after high unilateral cervical chordotomy in a patient with preexisting injury of the phrenic nerve. Southern Med. J., *69*:718–746, 1976.

38. Hitchcock, E.: Stereotaxic spinal surgery. *In* Proceedings of Sixth International Congress of Neurological Surgery, São Paulo, Brazil, 1977. Amsterdam-Oxford, Excerpta Medica, 1978, pp. 271–281.

39. Hitchcock, E., and Luce, B.: Somatotopic representation of the respiratory pathways in the cervical cord of man. J. Neurosurg., *27*:320–329, 1967.

40. Hyndman, O., and Van Epps, C.: Possibility of differential section of the spinothalamic tract. Arch. Surg. (Chicago), *38*:1038–1053, 1939.

41. Kahn, E. A., and Rand, R. W.: On the anatomy of anterolateral cordotomy. J. Neurosurg., *9*:611–619, 1952.

42. Kerr, F. W. L.: Segmental circuitry and spinal cord proprioceptive mechanisms. Advances Pain Res. Ther., *1*:75–89, 1976.

43. King, R. B.: Post cordotomy studies of pain threshold. J. Neurol., *7*:610–614, 1957.

44. King, R. B.: Anterior commissurotomy for intractable pain. J. Neurosurg., *47*:7–11, 1977.

45. Krieger, A. J., and Rosomoff, H. L.: Sleep induced apnea. Part I. A respiratory and autonomic dysfunction syndrome following bilateral percutaneous cervical cordotomy. J. Neurosurg., *39*:168–180, 1974.

46. Krieger, A. J., and Rosomoff, H. L.: Sleep induced apnea. Part II. Respiratory failure after anterior spinal surgery. J. Neurosurg., *39*:181–185, 1974.

47. Kunicki, A.: Anterolateral cordotomy. *In* Proceedings of Sixth International Congress of Neurological Surgery, São Paulo, Brazil, 1977. Amsterdam-Oxford, Excerpta Medica, 1978, pp. 264–266.

48. Kuperman, A. S., Krieger, A. J., and Rosomoff, H. L.: Respiratory function after cervical cordotomy. Chest, *59*:128–132, 1971.

49. Kuperman, A. S., Rogelio, B., Fernandez, A., and Rosomoff, H. L.: The potential hazard of oxygen after bilateral cordotomy. Chest, *59*:232–235, 1971.

50. Lin, P. M., Gildenberg, P. L., and Polakoff, P. O.: An anterior approach to percutaneous lower cervical cordotomy. J. Neurosurg., *25*:553–560, 1966.

51. Long, D. M., and Story, J. L.: Hyponatremia following bilateral cervical cordotomy. J. Neurosurg., *25*:623–627, 1966.

52. Mansuy, L., and Sindou, M.: Physiology of pain at the spinal cord level: Neurosurgical aspects. *In* Proceedings of Sixth International Congress of Neurological Surgery, São Paulo, Brazil, 1977. Amsterdam-Oxford, Excerpta Medica, 1978, pp. 257–263.

53. Mansuy, L., Sindou, M., Fischer, G., and Brenon, J.: La cordotomie spinothalamique dans les douleurs cancereuses. Neurochirurgie, *22*:437–444, 1976.

54. Marx, J. L.: Analgesia: How the body inhibits pain perception. Science, *195*:471–473, 1977.

55. Mayer, D. J., Price, D. D., and Becker, D. P.: Neurophysiological characterization of the anterolateral cord neurons contributing to pain perception in man. Pain, *1*:51–58, 1975.

56. Mayer, D. J., Price, D. D., Becker, D. P., and Young, H. F.: Threshold for pain from anterolateral quadrant stimulation as a predictor of success of percutaneous cordotomy for relief of pain. J. Neurosurg., *43*:445–447, 1975.

57. Mehler, W. R.: Central pain and the spinothalamic tract. Advances Neurol., *4*:127–146, 1974.

58. Mehler, W. R., Feferman, M. E., and Nauta, W. J. H.: Ascending axon degeneration following anterolateral cordotomy in man. Brain, *83*:718–750, 1960.

59. Moosy, J., Sagone, A., and Rosomoff, H. L.: Percutaneous radiofrequency cervical cordotomy. J. Neuropath. Exp. Neurol., *26*:118, 1967.

60. Morin, F., Schwartz, H. G., and O'Leary, J. L.: Experimental study of the spinothalamic and related tracts. Acta Psychiat. Scand., *26*:371–396, 1951.

61. Morley, T.: Congenital rotation of the spinal cord. J. Neurosurg., *10*:690–692, 1953.

62. Müller, W.: Beiträge zur pathologischen Anatomie und Physiologie des menschlichen Rückenmarks. Leipzig, 1871.

63. Mullan, S., and Hosobuchi, T.: Respiratory hazards of high cervical percutaneous cordotomy. J. Neurosurg., *28*:291–299, 1968.

64. Mullan, S., Hekmatpanah, J., Dobben, G., and Beckman, F.: Percutaneous intramedullary cordotomy utilizing the unipolar anodal electrolytic lesion. J. Neurosurg., *22*:548–553, 1965.

65. Mullan, S., Harper, P. V., Hekmatpanah, J., Torres, H., and Dobben, G.: Percutaneous interruption of spinal pain tract by means of a strontium needle. J. Neurosurg., *20*:931–939, 1963.

66. Nashold, B., and Urban, B.: Percutaneous epidural stimulation of the spinal cord for relief of pain: Description of technique and pulmonary results. *In* Proceedings of Sixth International Congress of Neurological Surgery, São Paulo, Brazil, 1977. Ansterdam-Oxford, Excerpta Medica, 1978, pp. 285–287.

67. Nathan, P. W.: Results of anterolateral cordotomy for pain in cancer. J. Neurol. Neurosurg. Psychiat., *26*:353–362, 1973.

68. Nathan, P. W.: The descending respiratory pathway in man. J. Neurol. Neurosurg. Psychiat., *26*:487–499, 1963.

69. Nathan, P. W., and Smith, M. C.: Effect of two unilateral cordotomies on the motility of the lower limbs. Brain, *96*:471–494, 1973.

70. Noordenbos, W.: Pain: Problems Pertaining to the Transmission of Nerve Impulses Which Give Rise to Pain. Preliminary Statement. Amsterdam, Elsevier Publishing Co., 1959.

71. Noordenbos, W., and Wall, P. O.: Diverse sensory functions with an almost totally divided spinal cord. A case of spinal cord transection with preservation of part of one anterolateral quadrant. Pain, *2*:185–195, 1976.

72. O'Connell, J. E. O.: Anterolateral chordotomy

for intractable pain in carcinoma of the rectum. Proc. Roy. Soc. Med., *62*:1223–1225, 1969.

73. Onofrio, B. M.: Cervical spinal cord and dentate delineation in percutaneous radiofrequency cordotomy on the level of the first to second cervical vertebrae. Surg., Gynec. Obstet., *133*:30–34, 1971.

74. Petrén, K.: Ein Beitrag sur Frage vom Verlaufe der Bahnen der Hautsinne im Rückenmarke. Scand. Arch. Physiol., *13*:9–13, 1902.

75. Porter, R. W., Hohmann, G.W., Borse, E., and French, J. D.: Cordotomy for pain following cauda equina injury. Arch. Surg. (Chicago), *92*:765–770, 1966.

76. Putnam, T.: Myelotomy of the commissure. A new method of treatment for pain in the upper extremities. Arch. Neurol. Psychiat., *32*:1189–1192, 1934.

77. Raskind, R.: Analytical review of open cordotomy. Int. Surg., *51*:226–231, 1969.

78. Rosomoff, H. L.: Bilateral percutaneous cervical radiofrequency cordotomy. J. Neurosurg., *31*:41–46, 1969.

79. Rosomoff, H. L.: Management of pain with percutaneous radiofrequency cervical cordotomy. *In* Proceedings of Sixth International Congress Neurological Surgery, São Paulo, Brazil, 1977. Amsterdam-Oxford, Excerpta Medica, 1978, pp. 281–284.

80. Rosomoff, H. L., Krieger, A. J., and Kuperman, A. S.: Effect of percutaneous cervical cordotomy on pulmonary function. J. Neurosurg., *31*:620–627, 1969.

81. Rosomoff, H. L., Carroll, F., Brown, J., and Sheptak, T.: Percutaneous radiofrequency cervical cordotomy. Technique. J. Neurosurg., *23*:639–644, 1965.

82. Schneider, R. J., and Paul, R. L.: Body representation in the anterolateral funiculi as reconstructed by percutaneous cordotomies in benign intractable pain. Advances Pain Res. Ther., *1*:267–270, 1976.

83. Schüller, A.: Über operative Durchtrennung der Rückenmarksstränge (Chordotomie). Wien. Med. Wschr., *60*:2292–2295, 1910.

84. Schwartz, H. G.: High cervical cordotomy—technique and results. Clin. Neurosurg., *8*:282–293, 1962.

85. Schwartz, H. G.: High cervical cordotomy. J. Neurosurg., *26*:452–455, 1967.

86. Smith, M. C.: Retrograde cell changes in human spinal cord after anterolateral cordotomies. Location and identification after different periods of survival. Advances Pain Res. Ther., *1*:91–98, 1976.

87. Spiller, W. G.: The location within the spinal cord of the fibers for temperature and pain sensation. J. Nerv. Ment. Dis., *32*:318, 1905.

88. Spiller, W. G., and Martin, E.: The treatment of persistent pain of organic origin in the lower part of the body by division of the anterolateral column of the spinal cord. J.A.M.A., *58*:1489, 1912.

89. Stookey, B.: Chordotomy of the second cervical segment for relief from pain due to recurrent carcinoma of the breast. Arch. Neurol. Psychiat., *26*:443, 1931.

90. Stookey, B.: The management of intractable pain by chordotomy. Res. Publ. Ass. Res. Nerv. Ment. Dis., *23*:416–433, 1943.

91. Sweet, W. H.: Craniospinal Surgery for Pain. Avens, 1973.

92. Sweet, W. H.: Recent observations pertinent to improving anterolateral cordotomy. Clin. Neurosurg., *23*:80–95, 1976.

93. Taren, J. A.: Physiologic corroboration in stereotaxic high cervical cordotomy. Confin. Neurol., *33*:285–290, 1970.

94. Tasker, R. R.: Percutaneous cordotomy. Physiological identification of site. Confin. Neurol., *35*:110–117, 1973.

95. Tasker, R. R.: Open cordotomy. Progr. Neurol. Surg., *8*:1–14, 1977.

96. Tasker, R. R., Organ, L. W., Rowe, I. J., and Hawsylyshyn, P.: Human spinothalamic tract —stimulation mapping in the spinal cord and brainstem. Advances Pain Res. Ther., *1*:251–257, 1976.

97. Todd, E. M., Crue, B. L., and Carregal, E. J. A.: Posterior percutaneous tractotomy and cordotomy. Confin. Neurol., *31*:106–115, 1969.

98. Walker, A. W.: The spinothalamic tract in man. Arch. Neurol. Psych., *43*:284–298, 1940.

99. Wall, P. D., and Dubner, R.: Somatosensory pathways. Ann. Rev. Physiol., *34*:315–336, 1972.

100. Weaver, T. A., and Walker, A. E.: Topical arrangement within the spinothalamic tract in the monkey. Arch. Neurol. Psych., *46*:877–883, 1941.

101. White, J. C.: Cordotomy: Assessment of its effectiveness and suggestions for its improvement. Clin. Neurosurg., *13*:1–19, 1966.

102. White, J. C., and Sweet, W. H.: Pain and the Neurosurgeon. A Forty Year Experience. Springfield, Ill., Charles C Thomas, 1969.

103. White, J. C., Sweet, W. H., Hawkins, R., and Nilges, R. G.: Anterolateral cordotomy: Results, complications, and causes of failure. Brain, *73*:346–367, 1950.

104. Willis, W. D.: Spinothalamic system: Physiological aspects. Advances Pain Res. Ther., *1*:215–223, 1976.

105. Willis, W. D., Leonard, R. B., and Kenshalo, D. R.: Spinothalamic tract neurons in the substantia gelatinosa. Science, *202*:986–988, 1978.

133

STEREOTAXIC MESENCEPHALOTOMY AND TRIGEMINAL TRACTOTOMY

STEREOTAXIC MESENCEPHALOTOMY

Historical Background

During the last decade the importance of the mesencephalon in the genesis of pain and emotion has taken on greater significance. The midbrain has been found to contain polypeptides (enkephalins) that mimic the pharmacological action of opiates. Also it has been discovered that chronic pain can be relieved by electrical stimulation or a destructive lesion in mesencephalic structures.

The first report of stereotaxic mesencephalotomy and mesencephalothalamotomy for relief of pain was published by Spiegel and Wycis in 1948.[44] With the development of the stereotaxic technique for treatment of human neurological diseases the year before, it was natural that the mesencephalon would become a site for stereotaxic neurosurgical intervention. Through the pioneering efforts of Dogliotti, of Walker, and of White and Sweet, open craniotomy for mesencephalic tractotomy had already been used for relief of pain; the open operation fell into disuse, however, because of the great risk of death and morbidity and the high incidence of postoperative dysesthesia that often was more serious than the patient's original pain.[17,55,59]

It was logical to attack the pain pathways in the mesencephalon, since it was possible to interrupt not only the ascending spino- and quintothalamic systems but also the spinoreticulothalamic pathways. In 1954, Spiegel and co-workers demonstrated that spinal pain conduction could be mediated via short chains of neurons, and therefore, mesencephalotomy was performed to interrupt not only the spinothalamic tract but also portions of the ascending reticular formation in the dorsal tegmentum.[46] Spiegel and Wycis were concerned about the possible serious consequences of producing a lesion that destroyed a major part of the reticular formation, but they also believed it was important to destroy a portion of this system, particularly in patients whose pain evoked strong emotional reactions.[44] They showed that a therapeutic lesion of the dorsal medial thalamic nucleus interrupting the thalamofrontal connections greatly reduced the patient's emotional response to his pain and that such a lesion might also interrupt portions of the interlaminar nuclei and the rostral endings of the spinoreticulothalamic system.

It is of interest that their first patient with a postoperative trigeminal dysesthesia, operated on in 1947, was relieved for 18 years. The lesion involved the dorsomedial thalamus and the mesencephalon. A second patient was relieved for eight years. Of the 42 patients with pain from nonneoplastic states, however, only 31 per cent received complete or partial relief. With the increasing use of stereotaxic neurosurgical mesencephalotomy, other reports appeared from the neurosurgical clinics of Leksell, Ta-

---

B. S. NASHOLD, JR., AND B. L. CRUE, JR.

lairach, Mazars and asssociates, Riechert, Orthner and Roeder, and others.* As the neurosurgical technique evolved, slight variations in the location of the therapeutic lesion also were reported. Leksell's lesion included the spinothalamic tract as well as the medial lemniscus, while Hassler and Riechert found that the addition of a dorsomedial thalamic lesion including the nucleus ventralis posterior improved the overall therapeutic results.[21,22,26,38] Mark and co-workers noticed that the combination of thalamic midbrain lesions and midbrain reticular formation lesions was useful in the relief of pain.[28] Later, Roeder and Orthner pointed out the importance of selectively destroying most of the spinoreticular formation medial to the spinothalamic tract and adjacent to the central gray of the mesencephalon.[39] Still later, Nashold and co-workers, using chronically implanted midbrain electrodes, delineated a variety of physiological responses due to electrical stimulation of the direct and diffuse ascending pain pathways in the mesencephalon and advocated the routine use of prelesion electrical stimulation to improve the precision of the stereotaxic lesion.[33]

Anatomy

The mesencephalon, although the smallest portion of the brain, measuring 15 to 20 mm in length, contains one of the most complex neuroanatomical and physiological regions to be found within the central nervous system. The midbrain is a primordial organ for the correlation of sensory impulses, and these impulses are received by the midbrain from the eyes, ears, skin, muscles, joints, and bones, and are there correlated in the interest of producing the most effectual motor responses. The organization of certain "instinctual" reflexes for fear, flight, food, and sexual response is mediated through circuits in the mesencephalon, and the state of sentient consciousness is uniquely dependent upon its integrity. The pain pathways of interest to the neurosurgeon are located in the more dorsal aspects of the midbrain in the region of the tectum and dorsal tegmentum. The full length of the mesencephalon is tra-

versed by the sylvian aqueduct connecting the cerebral ventricles with those of the posterior fossa, and surrounding it is the central gray matter, a core of neural tissue that appears to be related to complex affective and emotional activities of the organism.

The ascending pain and temperature tracts traverse the dorsal part of the mesencephalon along with the lateral spinothalamic and the trigeminothalamic pathways and represent the primary direct paths. The lateral spinothalamic pathway conveys pain and temperature sensations from the entire contralateral surface of the body, excluding the face, and it lies in the dorsolateral angles of the dorsal tegmentum. Within it is represented a specific somatotopic scheme of the body, the lower portions of which lie lateral to the more cephalad portions. The cross-sectional area of the lateral spinothalamic tract at the superior colliculus is extremely small, 0.65 sq mm in area; and approximately 1500 fibers make up the tract at this level, although at the cervical segments it contains approximately 15,000 fibers, indicating that between the cervical and upper midbrain regions a large number of fibers leave the main tract, making connections below the level of the rostral midbrain. The trigeminothalamic pathway conveying pain and temperature sensations from the facio-oral region lies medial to the lateral spinothalamic tract and at the lateral edge of the central gray adjacent to the aqueduct. The exact organization of this pathway in man is still not completely known. The mandibular division appears to be situated more laterally than the ophthalmic division, and there is an intermingling of these facial fibers at this level with those from the seventh, ninth, and tenth cranial nerves. In other words, two body schemes related to pain perception are represented at this level of the midbrain. The surface and appendicular parts of the body are represented in the lateral spinothalamic tract, while the facial, oral, and internal body cavities are represented more medially. This has been well demonstrated by direct stimulation of the mesencephalon in awake man. In addition to these direct pathways, there are diffuse multisynaptic pathways related to the reticular formation, and these include the spinotectal and the spinocollicular tracts, which also convey noxious sensations and are old phylogenetically. The

---

* See references 26, 29, 38, 39, 48, 61.

ascending reticular fibers nearby the peri-aqueductal region are responsible for the origin of affective reaction to painful stimuli. There is also additional anatomical evidence that the pathways conveying painful sensations from the facial areas may be ipsilateral as well as contralateral, and there appears to be a large concentration of the ipsilateral trigeminothalamic fibers in the region of the central tegmental tract.

Indications for Mesencephalotomy

Wycis and Spiegel advised that stereotaxic mesencephalotomy was justifiable only after failure of all other conservative methods of treatment.[60] They pointed out that it should be given serious consideration when there was danger of drug addiction or suicide and when the patient was "desiring the relief from pain so desperately that he is willing to accept the risk of operation of which he should be properly informed." Of their original 54 patients, 31 had been treated by various other neurosurgical procedures such as nerve blocks, sympathectomy, rhizotomy, cordotomy, gyrectomy of the sensory cortex, and frontal lobotomy, or a combination of these operations. At the present time, central dysesthesias such as the thalamic syndrome, the lateral medullary plate syndrome, trigeminal dysesthesia, and under some circumstances, phantom limb pain respond satisfactorily to mesencephalotomy. The operation is strongly recommended for intractable unilateral or bilateral pain caused by carcinoma of the head, neck, and brachial region.[32]

Stereotaxic Neurosurgical Technique

Stereotaxic techniques for mesencephalotomy, target coordinates, and lesion parameters are summarized in Table 133–1.

The technique employed by Spiegel and Wycis for the introduction of a lesion electrode into the mesencephalon involved cortical puncture through a parieto-occipital burr hole, producing a tract parallel to the median plane in a plane 34 degrees behind the intraoral plane and passing through the posterior commissure (Fig. 133–1).[45,47] According to Spiegel, with this posterior oblique approach, the electrode intersects the spinothalamic system at a larger angle than with the intraoral plane, thus increasing the chance of complete interruption. Initially, they made several punctures, but later they advised that introduction of the electrode once was preferable and stressed the posterior approach in order to avoid injury to the cortical leg area, which might produce weakness of the contralateral lower limb.

At present, stereotaxic localization of mesencephalic structures is best made by using the AC–PC line designation as introduced by Talairach and co-workers.[49]

The following technique is suitable for the introduction of depth electrodes into the mesencephalon for stimulation or a therapeutic lesion. The procedure is care-

TABLE 133–1   STEREOTAXIC TECHNIQUE FOR MESENCEPHALOTOMY

	SPIEGEL AND WYCIS	LEKSELL	NASHOLD	ORTHNER	AMANO
Target coordinates					
Posterior to posterior commissure (mm)	2–3	3–3.5	5	0	14 mm posterior to coronal plane
Below posterior commissure (mm)	0–3.5	2–2.5 below midpoint of aqueduct	5	0	5–8
Distance from midsagittal plane (mm)	5.5–9.5	5–7	5–10	7.5	5–8
Lesion parameters					
Lesion	anodal direct current 10 ma	65°C	70–72° C	30 mA, 30 sec	High frequency, parameters not given
Time (sec)	60	20–30	30	30	High frequency
Type probe	3-mm stylet-string	High-frequency thermistor	thermistor, Hz 500K (high frequency)	stylet-string, Hz 500K (high frequency)	

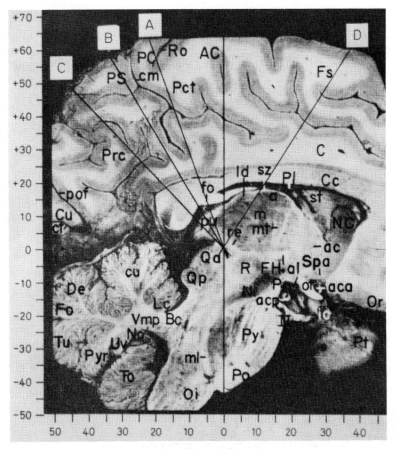

Figure 133–1   Sagittal section of brain at 5 mm lateral to midsagittal plane. The lines A, B, and C represent the direction of electrode tracts entering the mesencephalon as designated by Spiegel and Wycis. The anterior approach described by Nashold is represented by line D. (Adapted from Spiegel, E. A., and Wycis, H. T.: Stereoencephalotomy: Thalamotomy and Related Procedures, Vol. I. New York, Grune & Stratton, 1952.)

fully explained to the patient, with emphasis on the importance of patient cooperation during the stimulation session. No preoperative medication is given until the patient arrives in the operating room, where 1 to 2 ml of Innovar may be administered intravenously in the early part of the operation, usually during the placement of the burr hole and ventriculogram.

The anterior approach to the mesencephalon is the preferred route, especially if electrodes are to be implanted. The burr hole is located either on or 1 cm anterior to the coronal suture contralateral to the pain and 1.5 cm from the midsagittal plane. Using this anterior approach, the neurosurgeon can use the brain maps of the mesencephalon constructed by Nashold and coworkers.[33]

Clear identification of the third ventricle and sylvian aqueduct are essential for the accurate introduction of electrodes into the mesencephalon. A mixture of meglumine iothalamate (Conray 60 per cent) and cerebrospinal fluid injected into the ventricular system gives excellent visualization. The technique is as follows: 3 ml of 60 per cent Conray plus 3 ml of cerebrospinal fluid is shaken together in a large syringe to produce emulsification. The mixture is then injected directly into the lateral ventricles with care that it is not allowed to leak either into the substance of the brain tissue or over the cerebral cortex. Epileptic seizures have resulted from Conray spilling over the cerebral cortex; however, if proper precautions are taken, no complications occur. The roentgenograms are taken in rapid sequence with the lateral projection first followed by the anteroposterior projection (Fig. 133–2). Visualization of the posterior commissure and rostral end of the sylvian aqueduct is of prime importance in the final localization, and the electrode crosses the

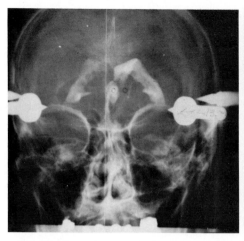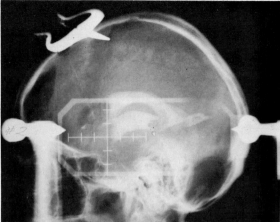

Figure 133–2   Anteroposterior and lateral roentgenograms of skull after intraventricular injection of Conray. Todd-Wells stereotaxic instrument.

AC–PC line at an approximate angle of 65 to 70 degrees, entering the dorsolateral portion of the midbrain at the level of the posterior commissure and superior colliculus. The lateromedial angulation of the electrode is between 2 and 4 degrees off the midsagittal plane. With this technique, the electrodes come to lie almost parallel to the long axis of the brain stem and pass in a rostrocaudal direction through the core of the dorsolateral ventral tegmentum as far caudally as the inferior colliculus. When an electrode with a protruding stylus is used, the localization is approximately 5 mm from the midsagittal plane. The electrode then may be rotated in a 360-degree arc and stimulation may be in any plane, but final placement of the lesion is determined by the physiological response of the awake patient. Although long-term implantation of depth electrodes has been extremely useful in localizing structures in the mesencephalon, it is not entirely necessary if careful short-term stimulation is carried out. It may, however, be noted that depth electrodes have remained in situ from weeks to months without adverse effects.

Effects of Electrical Stimulation of the Mesencephalon

Physiological responses are best produced by bipolar stimulation for which a square wave generator of the neurophysiological laboratory type and a variety of pulse widths and frequencies are used. The subjective responses produced as a result of mesencephalic stimulation were first described by Spiegel, who used short-term stimulation in the mesencephalon prior to the production of the therapeutic lesion. He noted a definite topographic pattern of referred pain that was related to the various sites of brain stimulation and reported on both ocular and auditory phenomena. Later, Nashold and associates reported the use of electrodes implanted in the mesencephalon for periods of several weeks.[33] The response of the patient to electrical stimulation of the midbrain is related to the location of the electrode in the midbrain as well as to the parameters of stimulation employed. The orientation of body pattern within the spinothalamic path, with the leg area more lateral and the facial areas medial, has already been described. Although the ascending spinothalamic and quintothalamic pathways are considered to be compact bundles of fibers, stimulation results suggest that there is a wider distribution of these fibers that mediate pain from the periphery than one can determine by their major neuroanatomical components. One of the most interesting and important observations of long-term stimulation of the medial mesencephalon was the finding that the central portion of the body seemed to be represented adjacent to the central gray. Electrical stimulation in this area resulted in the reference of unpleasant sensations through the central parts of the body, namely the cranial, oral, nuchal, thoracic, and abdominal cavities. These noxious sensations were accompanied by marked emo-

TABLE 133–2 RESPONSES TO ELECTRICAL STIMULATION OF THE DORSAL TEGMENTUM AND CENTRAL GRAY OF MESENCEPHALON IN HUMANS

FROM MIDLINE (MM)	SUBJECTIVE SENSATION	LOCUS OF SENSATION	MOTOR	AUTONOMIC	EMOTIONAL	OTHER
Posterior commissure						
0–5	Vibration	Center of face, head, chest	Eyelid closure, facial grimace, ocular movement, head movement		Terrible feeling, scared, strong response	Deep breaths, hyperventilation
5–10	Pain, burning heat, numbness	Contralateral face, arm, chest	Partial eyelid closure	Contralateral piloerection, contralateral sweating	Fright	Nausea
Superior colliculus						
0–5	Burning, cold, hurt, numbness	Head: nose, eyes, mouth Chest: contralateral head, chest, arm	Ocular movement, wide palpebral fissure, facial grimace	Pulse, respiration inhibited	Fright, "scared to death," strong response	Vocalization, speech arrest
5–10	Pain, burning, cold, chill	Contralateral face, arm, chest, trunk	Eyelid closure		Very painful	
Inferior colliculus						
0–5	Pain, hot funny feeling (severe)	Head, face, oral cavity, leg	Wide palpebral fissure, ipsilateral facial contraction, convergence, eye oscillation	Blush (face), blush (face, neck, piloerection contralateral arm, trunk)	Fright	Central pain, respiration, sighing
5–10	Pain, burning	Contralateral arm, face, shoulder	Eye movement		Cries out	EEG after discharge with pain

tional responses exhibited by the patient (Table 133–2).

Somatosensory evoked potentials were routinely recorded by Lieberson and fellow workers during mesencephalotomy.[27] When the tip of the electrode was located 5 mm below, 10 mm lateral to, and 5 mm posterior to the posterior commissure, evoked spikes were recorded during peripheral nerve stimulation (Fig. 133–3). The spike latency was 10 to 15 msec, suggesting transmission via multisynaptic relays. A lesion in the same area produced complete relief with minimal hypesthesia in five of six patients. Stimulation of the inferior maxillary or the tibial nerve also results in evoked responses from the area but with different latencies. These workers point out that the recording of evoked spikes did not necessarily correspond to transmission of pain perception and admit that the functional significance of these observations is still unknown, although they believe that the therapeutic lesion is located between the lateral and medial lemnisci in the nucleus lateralis mesencephali.

At the level of the midbrain there is a divergence of the reticular formation in two different nociceptive pathways, discriminative pain via a thalamic route (CM–PF) and motivational pain terminating in the limbic "emotional" brain. Microelectrode recordings in man during mesencephalotomy have demonstrated neurons in the midbrain formation near the central gray that respond specifically to peripheral pinprick stimulation.[1] The following phenomena have been observed on spontaneous single neuron firing from the human central gray: (1) abrupt change of background noise on entering the reticular formation, (2) firing of neurons mostly composed of small cells, (3) predominant activity of fiber components rather than firing of cell components, (4) scanty neural firing with inconstant interspike intervals, and (5) small number of large neurons not responding to peripheral pinprick stimulation (Fig. 133–4).

Clinical Observations

Mesencephalotomy is the treatment of choice for intractable unilateral or bilateral pain caused by extensive carcinoma involving the head, neck, and arm.[32] Significant

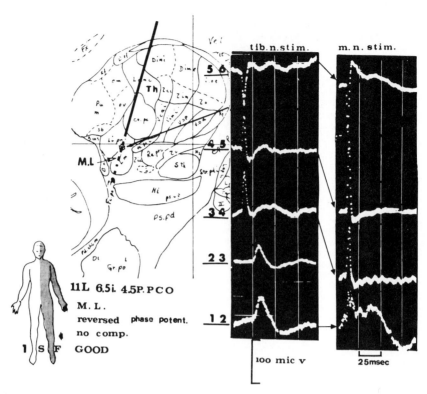

Figure 133-3   Recording of evoked sensory response from right mesencephalon in patient with intractable back and left leg pain. Stimulation of the left tibial nerve in the popliteal fossa elicited a sharp spike allegedly 4.5 mm below the intercommissural line with a phase reversal 1 mm below this line. Stimulation of the left median nerve at the wrist elicited a sharp spike (duration, about 10 msec) about 4 mm below this line with the phase reversal at the same level as in the case of the tibial nerve. The latency time of the onset of this spike is 13 msec for the tibial nerve and 11 msec for the median nerve. There was another spike of longer duration (about 25 msec) with a latency time of 25 msec recorded for the tibial nerve only. (From Lieberson, W. T., Voris, H. C., and Vernatsu, S.: Recording of somatosensory evoked potentials during mesencephalotomy for intractable pain. Confin. Neurol., *32*:185, 1970. Reprinted by permission.)

relief of pain can be expected for the life of these patients. Roeder and Orthner pointed out that facial pain was reduced if the stereotaxic lesion involved the diffuse ascending spinoreticular pathways in the medial midbrain.[39] The syndrome of pain plus

mental suffering can also be relieved by lesions interrupting the neural input of the limbic system in the dorsal mesencephalon. Patients with extensive carcinoma involving the tongue and the pharyngeal, tonsillar, or maxillary regions often experience

unit 9

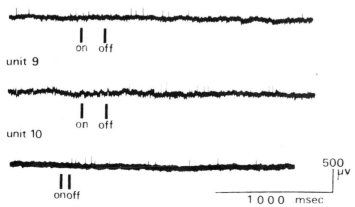

Figure 133-4   Single neuron recording from midbrain reticular formation in a 62-year-old man, nociceptive neurons responding to peripheral pinprick stimulation. (From Amano, K., Kitamura, K., Sano, K., and Sekino, H.: Relief of intractable pain from neurosurgical point of view with reference to present limits and clinical indications. A review of 100 consecutive cases. Neurol. Med. Chir. *16*:141, 1976. Reprinted by permission.)

severe pain when they cough, swallow, or chew. This pain is triggered reflexly via circuits in the dorsal mesencephalon responsible for the integration of interoceptive impulses ascending from the seventh (intermedius), ninth, and tenth cranial nerves. If the pain is strictly unilateral, the stereotaxic lesion should be placed contralaterally in the mesencephalon; in bilateral pain, a unilateral lesion usually opposite to the side of greatest involvement will result in sufficient bilateral relief. This relief of bilateral pain is in all probability due to the net effect of interrupting both the contralateral and ipsilateral pain pathways in the dorsomedial midbrain and also modifies the emotional and affective responses of the patient to his pain, often allowing for cessation of narcotics with minimal withdrawal effects. The clinical effects of these midbrain lesions closely resemble those noted after cingulumotomy. The degree of analgesia that follows midbrain lesions is often difficult to delineate clinically and is not directly related to the degree of pain relief. Walker noted that the analgesia after open mesencephalic tractotomy may extend to the midfacial regions, but he was not certain as to the degree of analgesia within the oral cavity.[55] The authors believe that the degree of relief of pain following medial mesencephalotomy is not dependent on the production of analgesia in the oral cavity.[32] Combination thalamic and midbrain lesions hold no better prognosis for relief of pain than mesencephalotomy alone. Turnbull has, in contrast, reported that combined cingulumotomy and mesencephalotomy lesions may give satisfactory relief of pain due to malignant disease; however, Voris and Whisler were not enthusiastic about combination lesions of either the cingulum, thalamus, or mesencephalon, since in their experience, mesencephalotomy alone was satisfactory.[52,54]

Central pain, such as that of the thalamic syndrome, the lateral medullary plate syndrome, postcordotomy dysesthesia, avulsion of the brachial plexus with phantom limb pain, and postherpetic pain has been successfully relieved by mesencephalotomy about 50 per cent of the time. With the passage of time, however—within a three- to five-year period—the effect wears off. Spiegel and Wycis reported a patient with postoperative trigeminal dysesthesia that was still relieved 18 years later, and

Nashold and co-workers have a group of 15 patients with central dysesthesia of whom 50 per cent continued to be relieved after five years.[43,60] The best results were obtained with phantom limb pain caused by traumatic brachial plexus avulsion. At the present time, central pain, as just described, is best treated first by the use of electrical stimulation, then by mesencephalotomy. Bilateral mesencephalotomies in a few patients have been reported, the first by Wycis and Spiegel, in which they noted bilateral perceptive deafness.[43,60] This phenomenon could not be confirmed, however, in the bilateral operation reported by Voris and Whisler.[54] The use of bilateral operations for relief of pain has little to recommend it.

The mortality rate following stereotaxic mesencephalotomy averages 3 to 5 per cent. The complication rate of 37 per cent, however, is higher than that for cingulumotomy (16 per cent) or thalamotomy (4 per cent). The complications of mesencephalotomy are due to the interruption of neural systems other than the pain pathways that are located in the small confines of the dorsal part of the mesencephalon. Changes in ocular motility occur in almost every patient, the main one being loss of upward gaze, which is usually permanent but not disabling, since most patients are unaware of the defect.[31] Transient ocular defects, such as forced ipsilateral deviations of the eyes, nystagmus retractorius, convergence nystagmus, and pupillary asymmetry can occur, but usually clear within several weeks. Diplopia, when it occurs (1 to 5 per cent), is the most disabling ocular symptom, but as a rule it will also resolve in time and can often be prevented by careful physiological testing prior to making the lesion. The midbrain lesion proposed by Amano does not interfere with conjugate eye movements but may cause transient diplopia due to skew deviation and lack of convergence (see Table 133–1).

Contralateral motor weakness, mild to moderate reductions of muscle tone and tendon reflexes have been noted following mesencephalotomy. Spiegel and Wycis reported on a patient with postoperative weakness and spasticity in the contralateral leg and thought it due to an injury of the cerebral cortical leg area following the introduction of the stereotaxic probe.[45] Torvik, however, performed postmortem examinations on two patients who died after stereotaxic mesencephalotomy; one with a lower extremity weakness had sparing of the pyramidal tract, but partial destruction of the ventral tegmentum.[51] Torvik suggested that the altered motor function was not caused by a cortical lesion but by an injury to the efferent fibers of the extrapyramidal motor system in the ventral tegmentum.

Postoperative mesencephalic dysesthesia has been considered by many neurosurgeons to be the most serious deterrent to midbrain tractotomy. Following open operation, the incidence was as high as 70 per cent according to one report; however, after the stereotaxic operation, serious postoperative dysesthesias occur in less than 15 per cent of the patients.[32,43] This complication is not considered an important deterrent in patients who will live less than two years; however, with the passage of time the chance of postoperative dysesthesia increases. The reduced incidence of central dysesthesia in recent stereotaxic mesencephalotomies may be due to the greater degree of interruption of the spinoreticular thalamic system.

Conclusions

Stereotaxic mesencephalotomy is the treatment of choice for intractable pain due to carcinoma of the head and neck regions and severe central pain syndromes. Mesencephalotomy relieves pain and suffering, particularly if the lesion involves the mediodorsal region adjacent to the central gray matter. Careful stereotaxic localization of the probe in the mesencephalon depends upon clear radiographic delineation of the ventricular system plus physiological localization by means of either direct electrical stimulation or the recording of electroencephalographic responses evoked from peripheral nerve stimulation. Although the mortality rate in mesencephalotomy is low, the morbidity rate is high, oculomotor defects and postoperative dysesthesia being the most serious complications; however, the changes in ocular motility (loss of upward gaze) per se do not constitute a serious disability. The dorsal mesencephalon represents a complex neural region of the brain where multiple afferent and efferent systems converge along with the direct and diffuse pain systems. Its role in the genesis of complex pain syndromes is important, and further studies in man are needed in order to understand the puzzle of pain.

TRIGEMINAL TRACTOTOMY

The destruction of descending fibers in the trigeminal tract in the medulla can produce ipsilateral analgesia and thus afford pain relief in patients with invasive malignant neoplasms of the face, head, and neck as well as in patients with primary trigeminal neuralgia (tic douloureux). This procedure can now be performed percutaneously and stereotaxically.

Historical Background

Operative attempts to relieve human pain and suffering have a long and interesting history.[25] Over the last decade, much has been learned concerning the control of input of information into the central nervous system, raising hope of improved methods of therapy in spite of the incredibly complex neuroanatomical, neurochemical, and neurophysiological mechanisms underlying nociception.[6] While most of the neurosurgical operative procedures that relieve pain are reserved for patients suffering from incurable malignant disease, there are a few pain syndromes of a nonneoplastic nature that may require operative intervention. Primary trigeminal neuralgia (tic douloureux) is one of these pain syndromes. In spite of a high success rate achieved by treating trigeminal neuralgia with anticonvulsants, there still remain cases that require operative intervention. While simpler, more peripheral operative techniques exist, there are also occasional cases of tic douloureux (usually after repeated failures of more conservative operative techniques), in which an operative approach to the central nervous system itself is warranted.

Walker credits Serra and Neri with attempting the destruction of the trigeminal nucleus in the pons in 1935.[41,56] It was Sjoquist, however, who made a thorough study of pain conduction in the trigeminal nerve, and tractotomy of the descending fibers of the trigeminal tract in the medulla is still referred to as the ''Sjoquist procedure.''[42]

In recent years, others such as Raney and co-workers have continued to perform a similar tractotomy.[37] Walker and others have continued to use the suboccipital approach for the Dandy procedure of partial rhizotomy of the posterior trigeminal root via the posterior fossa.[15,57] Most neurosurgeons believed, however, that the higher risk of morbidity and death inherent in a posterior fossa exploration and direct tractotomy in the medulla was unacceptable in most instances; and as more peripheral techniques were perfected, medullary trigeminal tractotomy was used less frequently.[9]

The situation changed when Mullan and Rosomoff and their co-workers demonstrated that destructive lesions could be made in the upper cervical cord at the C1–C2 level by way of a percutaneous approach.[30,40] Next, Crue and Todd and their associates performed percutaneous high cervical cordotomy from a posterior approach, using a stereotaxic procedure, with the patient prone.[7,50] In 1966 Crue's group demonstrated that, by using a similar percutaneous technique, the electrodes could be inserted above the arch of C1 and a trigeminal tractotomy could be performed stereotaxically.[14] Others, among them Hitchcock and Fox, also performed percutaneous trigeminal tractotomies but used slightly different techniques.[18–20,23,24]

Technique of Percutaneous Stereotaxic Radiofrequency Trigeminal Tractotomy from Posterior Approach

The patient is placed prone on the operating table, under local anesthesia, with the head held firmly in the Todd-Wells stereotaxic headpiece (Fig. 133–5). Instead of using the vertical electrode approach between the arches of C1 and C2 (as in anterior quadrant cordotomy in which the electrode is inserted through the spinal cord), a 30-degree cephalad angle is utilized to insert the electrode above the arch of C1 and beneath the posterior rim of the foramen magnum (Fig. 133–6). By means of x-ray localization, the midline is centered on the

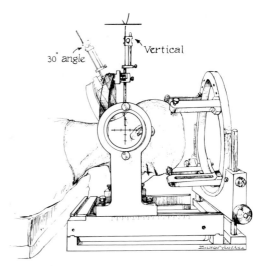

Figure 133–5 Patient placed prone in Todd-Wells stereotaxic frame for posterior approach.

odontoid process, and the electrode is aimed 6.5 mm ipsilateral to the painful side (Fig. 133–7). Contact with the dorsum of the brain stem (usually a few millimeters caudad to the obex of the fourth ventricle) can be determined by impedance monitoring. The electrode is then inserted approximately 2 to 3 mm beneath the surface. In recent years, the precise electrode placement has been verified (both for physiological recordings and prior to making a radiofrequency lesion) by the use of recorded evoked potentials.[4,5,10] The stimulating electrode is an electromyographic needle inserted percutaneously into the region of the infraorbital nerve in the infraorbital foramen (see Fig. 133–7A).

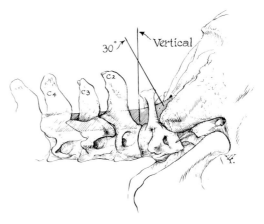

Figure 133–6 Electrode placement: vertical for cordotomy and 30-degree angle for percutaneous trigeminal radiofrequency cordotomy.

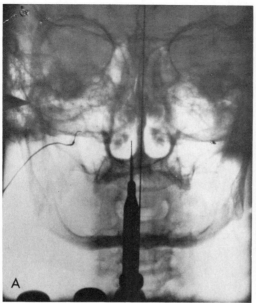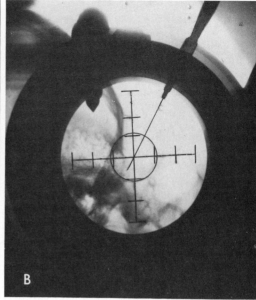

Figure 133–7   X-ray views showing electrode placement and ipsilateral infraorbital nerve stimulating needle for evoked response. *A*. Posteroanterior view. *B*. Lateral view. (From Crue, B. L., Carregal, E. J. A., and Felsoory, A.: Percutaneous stereotactic radiofrequency trigeminal tractotomy with neurophysiological recordings. Confin. Neurol., *34*:389, 1972. Reprinted by permission.)

Results

Since 1966 Crue and his associates have performed 15 such percutaneous stereotaxic radiofrequency trigeminal tractotomies. Eleven were for ipsilateral head and neck pain from a variety of uncontrolled malignant neoplasms, and four were for trigeminal neuralgia.[53] The results in the 11 cases of terminal malignant disease were rewarding, with no failure of significant pain relief and no morbidity and no deaths, but with two patients having prompt recurrence of pain. Of the four patients with trigeminal neuralgia, only two obtained significant pain relief; and there were two cases of postoperative contralateral trunk and extremity hypalgesia, and one case of transient ataxia in one hand.

The results have been sufficiently satisfying to encourage Crue and his group to experiment further with percutaneous trigeminal tractotomy in an attempt to refine it further. While percutaneous high cervical cordotomy seems to have obviated the need for medullary tractotomy for contralateral neck and shoulder pain, the necessity for trigeminal tractotomy for ipsilateral head, face, and neck pain is still occasionally encountered.[3,8,16,58]

Recent Experimental Refinement

In an attempt to utilize the stereotaxic percutaneous trigeminal tractotomy approach and improve the technique further, Crue and co-workers have recently mounted a fiberoptic endoscope on the Talairach bar of the Todd-Wells stereotaxic instrument. Through a second needle inserted percutaneously into the cisterna magna through the foramen magnum, as shown in Figure 133–8, the region of the dorsum of the upper cervical cord and lower medulla can then be readily visualized.[12] This has been done without incident, and the electrode placement (prior to both recording and lesion making) has been visualized (Fig. 133–9). Figure 133–10 shows the postmortem specimen with the radiofrequency lesion depicted in Figure 133–9.

In recent years, attempts at noninvasive *trans*cutaneous electrical stimulating techniques have become commonplace. Crue and his group have utilized cervical skin electrodes in an attempt at a "transcutaneous electrical cordotomy."[2,11] Results, however, suggested that the pain relief encountered was probably based on a "placebo" effect, and no way could be found to perform a satisfactory double-blind study.

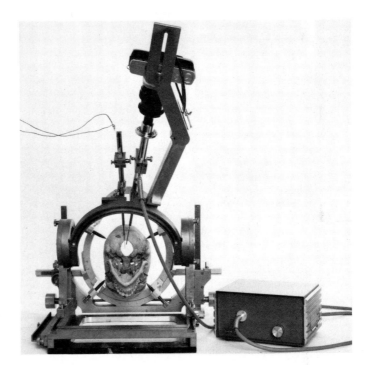

Figure 133–8 Addition of fiberoptic endoscope and camera attachment to Todd-Wells sterotaxic instrument.

Also, definitely still on an experimental basis, attempts have been made to stimulate the periaqueductal gray matter in the human mesencephalon elecrically by percutaneous insertion of an electrode. In 1974 Oliveras and co-workers had reported that in the cat analgesia could be obtained by stimulating in the midbrain, and reported the unusual finding that the tips of 17 electrodes had been found to lie within the aqueduct itself, and yet stimulation via 9 of these provided analgesia, although the neural structures that had been stimulated were unknown.[35] While mesencephalic tractotomy is an excellent operative technique in many cases, Crue and associates thought it might be better to perform an electrical stimulating mesencephalic procedure without having to resort to an operative burr hole and insertion of the electrode through neural tissues.[13] Consequently, using the fiberoptic scope as shown in Figure 133–8, and with the view as seen in Figure 133–9, in three percutaneous trigeminal tractoto-

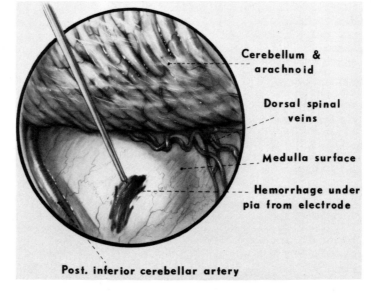

Figure 133–9 Drawing of view through endoscope as concentric bipolar recording and radiofrequency lesion making electrode is inserted in region of trigeminal tract.

Cerebellum & arachnoid

Dorsal spinal veins

Medulla surface

Hemorrhage under pia from electrode

Post. inferior cerebellar artery

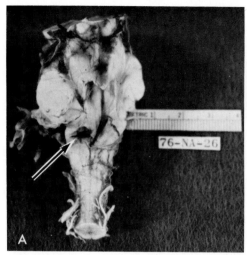
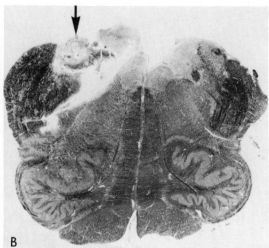

Figure 133–10 *A.* Gross postmortem specimen with lesion shown in Figure 133–9. *B.* Cross section of brain stem at level of maximum lesion (*arrow*).

mies, an attempt was made to thread a percutaneous stimulating electrode through the roof of the fourth ventricle and up the aqueduct prior to inserting the radiofrequency electrode into the trigeminal tract itself. While the results are still tentative, and the patient with pain from terminal cancer and under sedation for this operative procedure is far from an ideal test subject, it does appear possible to obtain clinical analgesia by this mesencephalic stimulating method. Further investigation and refinement of the technique are necessary before it can be considered anything but experimental.

REFERENCES

1. Amano, K., Kitamura, K., Sano, K., and Sekino, H.: Relief of intractable pain from neurosurgical point of view with reference to present limits and clinical indications. A review of 100 consecutive cases. Neurol. Medicochir. *16*:141, 1976.
2. Crue, B. L., and Felsoory, A.: Transcutaneous high cervical "electrical cordotomy." Minn. Med., *57*:204, 1974.
3. Crue, B. L., and Todd, E. M.: Vagal neuralgia. *In* Vinken, P. J., and Bruyn, G. W. eds.: Handbook of Clinical Neurology. Vol. V. Amsterdam, North Holland Publishing Co., 1968.
4. Crue, B. L., Carregal, E. J. A., and Felsoory, A.: Percutaneous stereotactic radiofrequency trigeminal tractotomy with neurophysiological recordings. Confin. Neurol., *34*:389, 1972.
5. Crue, B. L., Carregal, E. J. A., and Felsoory, A.: Percutaneous stereotactic radiofrequency trigeminal tractotomy. *In* Crue, B. L., ed.: Pain—Research and Treatment. New York, Academic Press, 1975.
6. Crue, B. L., Kenton, B., and Carregal, E. J. A.: Neurophysiology of pain—peripheral aspects. Bull. Los Angeles Neurol. Soc., *41*:13, 1976.
7. Crue, B. L., Todd, E. M., and Carregal, E. J. A.: Posterior approach for percutaneous cervical cordotomy. Confin. Neurol., *30*:41, 1968.
8. Crue, B. L., Todd, E. M., and Carregal, E. J. A.: Cranial Neuralgia. *In* Vinken, P. J., and Bruyn, G. W. Handbook of Clinical Neurolgy. Vol. V. Amsterdam, North Holland Publishing Co., 1968.
9. Crue, B. L., Todd, E. M., and Carregal, E. J. A.: Observations in the present status of the compression procedure in trigeminal neuralgia. *In* Crue, B. L., ed.: Pain and Suffering—Selected Aspects. Springfield, Ill., Charles C Thomas, 1970.
10. Crue, B. L., Todd, E. M., and Carregal, E. J. A.: Percutaneous radiofrequency stereotactic trigeminal tractotomy. *In* Crue, B. L., ed.: Pain and Suffering—Selected Aspects. Springfield, Ill., Charles C Thomas, 1970.
11. Crue, B. L., Carregal, E. J. A., Felsoory, A., and Amromin, G. D.: Preliminary report on cervical transcutaneous "electrical cordotomy." In Crue, B. L., ed.: Pain—Research and Treatment. New York, Academic Press, 1975.
12. Crue, B. L., Lasby, V., Kenton, B., and Felsoory, A.: Needle scope attached to stereotactic frame for inspection of cisterna magna during percutaneous radiofrequency trigeminal tractotomy. Appl. Neurophysiol., *39*:58, 1976–1977.
13. Crue, B. L., Lasby, V., Kenton, B., and Felsoory, A.: Needle scope attached to stereotaxic frame for percutaneous radiofrequency trigeminal tractotomy and percutaneous mesencephalic electrical stimulation. *In* Crue, B. L., ed.: Chronic Pain. New York, Spectrum Press, 1979.
14. Crue, B. L., Todd, E. M., Carregal, E. J. A., and Kilham, O.: Percutaneous trigeminal tractotomy. Case report. Bull. Los Angeles Neurol. Soc., *32*:87, 1967.
15. Dandy, W. E.: Surgery of the brain. *In* Lewis, D.

ed.: Practice of Surgery. Hagerstown, Md., W. F. Prior Co., 1945.

16. D'Errico, A.: Mesencephalic and medullary tractotomies. *In* Youmans, J. R., ed.: Neurological Surgery. Philadelphia, W. B. Saunders Co., 1973.

17. Dogliotti, M.: First surgical section in man of the lemniscus lateralis. Curr. Res. Anesth. Analg., *17*:143, 1938.

18. Fox, J. L.: Intractable facial pain relieved by percutaneous trigeminal tractotomy. J.A.M.A., *218*:1940, 1971.

19. Fox, J. L.: Delineation of the obex by contrast radiography during percutaneous trigeminal tractotomy. Technical note. J. Neruosurg., *36*:107, 1972.

20. Fox, J. L. Percutaneous trigeminal tractotomy. Variations in delineation of the obex using emulsified Pantopaque. Confin. Neurol., *36*:97, 1974.

21. Halfant, M. H., Leksell, L., and Strang, R. R.: Experiences with intractable pain treated by stereotaxic mesencephalotomy. Acta Chir. Scand., *129*:573, 1965.

22. Hassler, R., and Riechert, T.: Indikationen und Lokalisationsmethode der gezielten Hirnoperationen. Nervenarzt, *25*:441, 1954.

23. Hitchcock, E.: Stereotaxic spinal surgery. A preliminary report. J. Neurosurg., *31*:386, 1969.

24. Hitchcock, E.: Stereotactic trigeminal tractotomy. Ann. Clin. Res., *2*:131, 1970.

25. Keele, K. D.: Anatomies of Pain. Oxford, Blackwell Press, 1957.

26. Leksell, L.: Gezielte Hirnoperationen. *In* Olivecrona, H., und Tonnis, W., eds.: Handbuch der Neurochirurgie. Vol. 6. Berlin, Springer-Verlag, 1957, p. 178.

27. Lieberson, W. T., Voris, H. C., and Vernatsu, S.: Recording of somato-sensory evoked potentials during mesencephalotomy for intractable pain. Confin. Neurol., *32*:185, 1970.

28. Mark, V. H., Ervin, F. W., and Hackett, T. P.: Clinical aspects of stereotactic thalamotomy in the human. I. The treatment of chronic pain. Arch. Neurol. (Chicago), *3*:351, 1960.

29. Mazars, G, Pansini, A., and Chiarelli, J.: Coagulation du faisceau spinothalamique et du faisceau quintothalamique par stereotaxie. Rev. Neurol. (Paris), *100*:516, 1959.

30. Mullan, S., Harper, P. V., Hekmatpanah, J., Torres, H., and Dobbin, G.: Percutaneous interruption of spinal pain track by means of a strontium 90 needle. J. Neurosurg., *20*:931, 1963.

31. Nashold, B. S., Jr.: Defects of ocular motility after stereotactic midbrain lesions in man. Arch. Ophthal. (Chicago), *88*:245, 1972.

32. Nashold, B. S., Jr.: Extensive cephalic and oral pain relieved by midbrain tractotomy. Confin. Neurol., *34*:382, 1972.

33. Nashold, B. S., Jr., Wilson, W. P., and Slaughter, D. G.: Sensations evoked by stimulation in the midbrain of man. J. Neurosurg., *30*:14, 1969.

34. Nashold, B. S., Jr., Wilson, W. P., and Slaughter, D. G.: Stereotactic midbrain lesions for central dysesthesia and phantom pain. J. Neurosurg., *30*:116, 1969.

35. Oliveras, J. L., Besson, J. M., Guilbaud, G., and Liebeskud, J. C.: Behavioral and electrophysiological evidence of pain inhibition from midbrain stimulation in the cat. Exp. Brain Res., *20*:32, 1974.

36. Orthner, H., and Roeder, F.: Further clinical and anatomical experiences with stereotactic operations for relief of pain. Confin. Neurol., *27*:418, 1966.

37. Raney, R., Raney, A. A., and Hunter, C. R.: Treatment of major trigeminal neuralgia through section of the trigeminal tract in the medulla. Amer. J. Surg., *80*:11, 1950.

38. Riechert, T.: Die chirurgische Behandlung des zentralen Schmerzzustandes einschliesslich der stereotaktischen Operationen im Thalamus und Mesencephalon. Acta Neurochir. (Wien), *8*:136, 1960.

39. Roeder, F., and Orthner, H.: Erfahrungen mit stereotaktischen Eingriffen, III. Mitteilung. Uber zerebrale Schmerzoperationen, insbesondere mediale Mesencephalotomie bei thalamischer Hyperpathie und bei Anaesthesia dolorosa. Confin. Neurol., *21*:51–97, 1961.

40. Rosomoff, H. L., Carrol, F., Brown, J., and Sheptok, P.: Percutaneous radiofrequency cervical cordotomy: Technique. J. Neurosurg., *23*:639, 1965.

41. Serra, A., and Neri, V.: Die elektro-chirurgische Unterbrechung der Zentralbahnen des V. Paares am lateralen ventralen Rand des Pons Varoli als erster Behandlungsversuch von hartnäckigen Neuralgien des Trigeminus, durch Tumoren der Schädelbasis. Zbl. Chir., *63*:2248–2551, 1936.

42. Sjoquist, O.: Studies on pain conduction in the trigeminal nerve. Acta Psychiat. Scand., suppl. 17, 1938.

43. Spiegel, E. A.: Mesencephalotomy in treatment of intractable facial pain. Arch. Neurol. Psychiat., *69*:1, 1953.

44. Spiegel, E. A., and Wycis, H. T.: Mesencephalotomy for relief of pain. *In* anniversary volume for O. Poetzl, Vienna, 1948, p. 438.

45. Spiegel, E. A., and Wycis, H. T.: *In* Spiegel, E. A., ed.: Stereoencephalotomy. Vol. II. Clinical and Physiological Applications. New York, Grune & Stratton, 1962, p. 504.

46. Spiegel, E. A., Kleizkin, M., Szekely, E. G., and Wycis, H. T.: Role of hypothalamic mechanisms in thalamic pain. Neurology (Minneap.) *4*:739, 1954.

47. Spiegel, E. A., Wycis, H. T., Marks, M., and Lee, A. J.: Stereotaxic apparatus for operations on human brain. Science, *106*:349, 1947.

48. Talairch, J.: Chirurgie stereotaxique du thalamus. VI. Congr. Latinoamer, Neurochir., Montevideo 1955, p. 865.

49. Talairach. J., Hecaen, H., David, H., Monnier, M., and Ajuriaguerra, J.: Recherches sur la coagulation thérapeutique des structures sous-corticales chez l'homme. Rev. Neurol., (Paris) *81*:4–24, 1949.

50. Todd, E. M., Crue, B. L., and Carregal, E. J. A.: Posterior approach for high cervical cordotomy and trigeminal tractotomy. Confin. Neurol., *31*:106, 1970.

51. Torvik, A.: Sensory, motor and reflex changes in two cases of intractable pain after stereotactic mesencephalic tractotomy. J. Neurol. Neurosurg. Psychiat., *22*:299, 1959.

52. Turnbull, I. M.: Bilateral cingulumotomy combined with thalamotomy or mesencephalic tractotomy for pain. Surg. Gynec. Obstet., *134*:958, 1972.

53. Tytus, J. S.: Trigeminal neuralgia. *In* Youmans, J. R., ed.: Neurological Surgery. Vol. 3. Philadelphia, W. B. Saunders Co., 1973.

54. Voris, H. C., and Whisler, W. W.: Results of stereotaxic surgery for intractable pain. In press.

55. Walker, A. E.: Relief of pain by mesencephalic tractotomy. Arch. Neurol. Psychiat., *48*:865, 1942.

56. Walker, A. E.: A History of Neurological Surgery. Baltimore, Williams & Wilkins Co., 1951.

57. Walker, E., Miles, F. C., and Simpson, J. R.: Partial trigeminal rhizotomy using suboccipital approach. Arch. Neurol. Psychiat., *75*:514, 1956.

58. White, J. C.: Spinothalamic tractotomy in the medulla oblongata. Arch. Surg. (Chicago), *43*:113, 1941.

59. White, J. C., and Sweet, W.H.: Pain and the Neurosurgeon. Springfield, Ill., Charles C Thomas, 1969.

60. Wycis, H. T., and Spiegel, E. A.: Long range results in the treatment of intractable pain by stereotaxic midbrain surgery. J. Neurosurg., *9*:101, 1962.

61. Zapletal, B.: Open mesencephalotomy and thalamotomy for intractable pain. Acta Neurochir., suppl., *18*:118, 1969.

134

SYMPATHECTOMY

Interest in the sympathetic nervous system as an object of anatomical and physiological study as well as a site of operative intervention progressively increased throughout the first half of this century. Academic interest continues to expand with the development of a number of medications that can be used to modify sympathetic activity and even the structure of the system. Investigations have demonstrated numerous and varied physiological responses to modification of autonomic activity.

Indications for an operative approach to the sympathetic nervous system have become more limited if not more clearly defined by the advent of the medications that modify sympathetic activity, the refinement of direct operations on blood vessels, and better definition of some of the physiological consequences of sympathetic denervation. There are still areas in which the type of operative procedure indicated and even the desirability of sympathectomy are disputed. In this report, a review of some anatomical and physiological considerations is followed by a summary of the indications for sympathectomy and a review of some of the more commonly used techniques for resecting portions of the sympathetic chain. Subsequently, three of the more commonly encountered side effects of sympathectomy and possible forms of therapy are discussed. Also included are comments regarding sympathectomy by means of nonoperative techniques.

ANATOMICAL AND PHYSIOLOGICAL CONSIDERATIONS

The preganglionic fibers of the sympathetic nervous system are the axons of cells located in the lateral columns of the lower cervical, thoracic, and lumbar segments of the spinal cord. These axons pass out of the spinal cord into the lower one or two cervical, the thoracic, and the first two or three lumbar anterior spinal nerve roots. Most preganglionic fibers leave the anterior roots through the white rami communicantes to reach the paravertebral ganglia, which extend as a chain from the base of the skull to the coccyx. From this chain, postganglionic fibers pass back into the spinal nerves or through separate nerves or nerve plexuses to the organs innervated (Fig. 134–1).

Cervical Outflow

The question of the extent of cervical outflow to the sympathetic chain has been raised repeatedly. Palumbo reported that the upper thoracic sympathetic trunk, including the lower third of the stellate ganglion, could be removed without producing a disfiguring Horner's syndrome as long as the connections between the eighth cervical nerve and the cervical portion of the stellate ganglion were preserved.[50,51] These experiences, confirmed by many others, indicate the presence of cervical sympathetic efferent fibers that include, at least, pupillodilator fibers and some fibers to the nonstriated muscles in the upper eyelids. It is interesting that, although the pupillary changes and drooping eyelids are avoided by preserving the upper two thirds of the stellate ganglion, other sympathetic innervation to the head is still interrupted when the lower third of the ganglion and the upper portion of the thoracic sympathetic trunk are removed.[50] A more recent laboratory investigation has demonstrated that sympathetic innervation to the middle cere-

M. B. ALLEN, JR., AND W. H. MORETZ

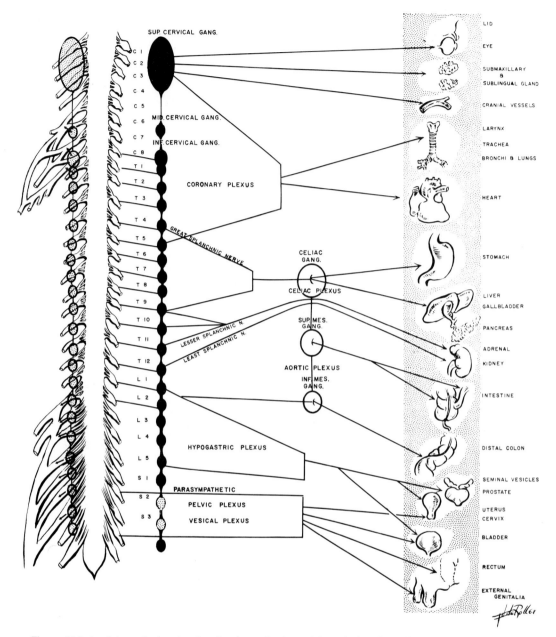

Figure 134–1 Schematic drawing showing the projections of the spinal outflow of the autonomic nervous system.

bral artery is interrupted by excision of the superior cervical ganglion, but the site in the central nervous system where the preganglionic cells are located was not identified in this study.[16]

Outflow to Upper and Lower Extremities

Preganglionic fibers leading to cells that send sympathetic impulses into the upper extremity are found in the first or second through the seventh to tenth thoracic anterior spinal roots.[56] Most of the ganglion cells are located in the upper thoracic sympathetic chain with the postganglionic fibers passing into the brachial plexus. Interruption of the sympathetic trunk between the third and fourth thoracic ganglia and decentralization of the lower third of the stellate ganglion and the second and third thoracic ganglia or excision of these elements will eliminate central influence on all of those sympathetic fibers that pass through the thoracic chain to the upper extremity.

Sympathetic innervation to the lower extremity passes out of the cord through the twelfth, and possibly the eleventh, thoracic and the upper two or three lumbar roots.[57,70] Most of the ganglionic connections are made in the lower two lumbar and the upper sacral levels with the gray rami passing to adjacent components of the lumbosacral plexus. Excision of the second and third lumbar ganglia disconnects those sympathetic fibers that pass through the sympathetic chain to the leg. Some preganglionic fibers that have influence in the thigh, however, may leave the spinal cord through anterior nerve roots of the last thoracic and first lumbar segments.

Ganglion Cells in Anterior Spinal Nerve Roots

Evaluation of patients who have had ganglionectomies in either the upper thoracic or lumbar regions has demonstrated evidence of residual sympathetic innervation, even though the ganglionectomies were known to be complete. Sweating and superficial vasoconstriction recurred over the anteromedial part of the thigh following thoracolumbar sympathectomy. Ray and Console postulated that some aberrant sympathetic fibers must bypass the sympathetic trunks.[55] Later, ganglion cells were demonstrated in the anterior roots of the first two thoracic and first two lumbar spinal roots as well as in the white and gray rami.[2] In many instances, neither the preganglionic nor postganglionic fibers passed through the sympathetic trunks. The frequency with which sympathetic ganglion cells remain within the nerve roots and proximal peripheral nerves is not known, but cases have been reported in which failures of initial ganglionectomy were converted into successes by subsequent anterior nerve root sections.

Sensitization of Smooth Muscle

Some reports have indicated that sensitization of smooth muscle fibers to circulating epinephrine occurs when sympathetic pathways are interrupted peripheral

to the ganglionic synapse.[73] Goetz and others have reported, however, that this increase in sensitivity to epinephrine is not of clinical significance.[23] Since many surgeons believe that nerve regeneration is much less likely to occur after ganglionectomy than after sectioning of preganglionic pathways for routine sympathectomy, most now use ganglionectomy for sympathetic denervation of the upper as well as the lower extremities, although some still prefer preganglionic ramisectomy as described by Smithwick.[64] One may add anterior rhizotomy at those levels indicated when there is evidence that failure of sympathectomy is due to incomplete autonomic denervation.

Sudomotor Innervation

Fairly discrete patterns of sudomotor innervation to the lower extremity have been demonstrated following ganglionectomy, the patterns following closely those of sensory innervation.[57] Sympathetic innervation in the upper extremities follows the course of sensory fibers, but denervation patterns following ganglionectomy appear to be somewhat less specific than in the lower extremities.

Afferent Fibers in Sympathetic System

The question of whether fibers carrying afferent impulses from vessels in the extremities pass through the sympathetic chains has been raised by numerous authors. There is no doubt that pain-conducting fibers accompany those sympathetic elements innervating thoracic and abdominal viscera. Since nerve fibers and plexuses to the body viscera must pass in the region of the sympathetic ganglia, it is likely that interruption of associated pain-conducting fibers accounts, at least in part, for the success of sympathectomy in relieving some pain syndromes involving body organs, i.e., angina pectoris, pancreatitis, and carcinoma of the head of the pancreas.*

The anatomy of the nerves supplying the extremities is not so simple. Pain is pro-

---

* See references 11, 24, 27, 32, 59, 60.

duced by stimulating peripheral vessels. Resulting sensations are conducted by afferent nerve fibers that pass from the blood vessels to the peripheral nerves, a course similar to that of the efferent sympathetic fibers in their peripheral segments. There is, however, no need for the sensory fibers to pass through the rami communicantes to the sympathetic ganglia, and experimental data have been conflicting on this point. It is generally conceded that the pain of causalgia is certainly moderated if not relieved by sympathectomy, but this does not necessarily imply that afferent conduction of the pain passes through the sympathetic nervous system.

INDICATIONS FOR SYMPATHECTOMY

Former Indications

Segments of the sympathetic nervous system have been resected as a form of therapy for epilepsy, exophthalmic goiter, retinitis pigmentosa, migraine headaches, cerebrovascular disease, tic douloureux, Hirschsprung's disease, atypical trigeminal neuralgia, tabes dorsalis, urinary tract disorders, and spastic paraplegia. Scrutiny of the operative results of cases falling into these categories has resulted in the elimination of these conditions as indications for sympathectomy. Though many sympathectomies have been performed for hypertension, and usually with effective lowering of blood pressure, modern drug therapy has practically eliminated this indication.

Present Indications

Most sympathectomies are performed for specific pain syndromes and selected vascular lesions of the extremities. Two recent experimental reports substantiate the advantageous effects of sympathectomy in treating frostbite.[28,29] Hyperhidrosis, when very severe, is also an indication for sympathectomy.* In addition, unilateral ptosis might be considered a cosmetic indication for a contralateral stellate ganglionectomy

---

* See references 5, 9, 17, 30, 31, 37, 62.

in selected cases. Permanent ptosis produced by stellate ganglionectomy may protect the corneas of patients with "malignant exophthalmos" that is not controlled by hypophysectomy or by orbital decompression. The same procedure has been recommended as therapy for corneal ulceration associated with cranial nerve deficits resistant to other forms of therapy. Also, a chemical sympathectomy may be combined with topical application of norepinephrine as a treatment for open-angle glaucoma.[40] Sympathectomies have also been recommended for tachycardias and arrythmias that are resistant to medical therapy, for angina pectoris, and for treatment of pain originating in other visceral organs.[24,27,32,59,60]

Post-Traumatic Extremity Pain

Pain syndromes in the extremities that are most likely to be favorably influenced by sympathectomy are causalgia or "causalgia-like" states (minor causalgia of Homans, post-traumatic sympathetic dystrophy, and post-traumatic osteoporosis). While some patients with clearly defined causalgia and many with "causalgia-like" symptoms have spontaneous remissions, sympathectomy is helpful in relieving persistent pain. Although preliminary nerve exploration has been recommended in the past as the initial therapy in causalgia, it should precede sympathectomy only if it is indicated by the type of nerve lesions involved. Phantom limb pain is no longer considered as indication for sympathetic denervation.

Sympathetic Blocks

Preliminary sympathetic blocks at the appropriate levels are often helpful in predicting the response to sympathectomy and sometimes are followed by permanent relief, rendering operative sympathetic denervation unnecessary. Complete but temporary relief of pain at the time of the first block indicates a good prognosis. Repeated blocks may be therapeutic in those patients who have a greater degree of relief or more prolonged remissions following a second or third injection. Patients with psychiatric problems frequently respond well to the first sympathetic block, but responses to repeat injections may be less favorable. Some patients with serious pain problems may be improved by sympathectomy despite failure of sympathetic blocks. In rare situations one may resort to the procedure without first obtaining complete relief by preliminary sympathetic blocks. In questionable cases, psychiatric evaluation may be helpful in identifying patients with depressive reactions who may receive little benefit from sympathectomy.

Vascular Lesions

Sympathectomy is frequently employed in the treatment of vascular lesions of the extremities; however, discrete occlusive lesions located proximally in the major arteries supplying limbs are best treated by a more direct attack on the arteries themselves; i.e., endarterectomy, resection, or bypassing procedures. It has been recommended that sympathectomy be performed in conjunction with the reconstructive procedure, since sympathectomy results in enhanced flow in the major vessels supplying an extremity, which might be associated with a significant reduction in the incidence of occlusion at the site of reconstruction.*

The value of sympathectomy in the treatment of intermittent claudication has been questioned since it has been demonstrated that the incidence of clinical improvement following the sympathectomy is very little different from the frequency of spontaneous improvement.[21,22,53] In addition, there is no significant improvement in the rate of blood flow through muscles either at rest or during or following exercise.[33,49,58,67]

There is usually an augmentation of the blood flow to the skin of the distal segments of a recently denervated extremity, evidenced by increased skin temperatures and digital plethysmography.[65] Clinical observations have demonstrated both subjective and objective improvement, at least temporarily, in patients suffering from Raynaud's phenomenon.‡ Failures have, however, frequently been recognized when sympathectomy has been applied to the treatment of large ischemic ulcers.[21,36] Recent studies have demonstrated that, while the overall flow of blood to the skin following sympathectomy is increased, most of the increase in flow is passed through arteriovenous anastomoses rather than through the capillary network that provides nourishment to the tissues.[12,14,42] It appears that sympathectomy is indicated in patients who exhibit vasospastic phenomena of the distal segments of an extremity that are initiated by exposure to cold or emotional upset, but in whom no other evidence of associated collagen or other systemic disease can be demonstrated. However, sympathectomy has limited value in the patient with an advanced collagen disease or thromboangiitis obliterans. Alteration in patterns and levels of blood flow in the presence of reactive hyperemia or during artificial warming may give a better indication of the anticipated long-term effect of sympathectomy on vascular lesions than the response to the more classic sympathetic block or heavy sedation.[48]

Angina Pectoris

The mechanism by which sympathectomy has relieved the symptoms of angina pectoris is still disputed. Undoubtedly, many afferent fibers from the heart, as well as vasomotor fibers to coronary vessels, are interrupted. Since operative denervation has been considered a major procedure for patients with serious heart disease, some surgeons have used paravertebral alcohol injection to treat patients disabled by the anginal attacks. Birkett and co-workers have reported acceptable results in moderate numbers of patients with anginal attacks who have undergone operative ablation of the upper four or five thoracic ganglia.[8]

Angina pectoris is considered to be the result of relatively insufficient blood flow to the cardiac muscle. This may be the result of occlusive lesions in the coronary vessels for which revascularization techniques are now frequently recommended. Sympathectomy has been shown to reduce the incidence of arrythmia following coronary occlusion, however, and has been recommended for patients who have anginal symptoms but whose angiograms are normal or exhibit evidence of isolated spasm.[19,27]

---

* See references 36, 52, 61, 63, 65, 71.
‡ See references 1, 4, 5, 26, 36, 65.

Dysmenorrhea

Presacral neurectomy continues to be utilized in the treatment of dysmenorrhea, although perhaps less frequently than formerly.[20] It is often performed as part of an abdominal exploration after the patient has been evaluated thoroughly for treatable pelvic disease that is resistant to medical therapy. Here, as in the treatment of other pain syndromes, psychiatric evaluation may be helpful in selecting proper candidates for the procedure.

OPERATIVE TECHNIQUES

Cervicothoracic Sympathectomy

Sympathetic denervation of the upper extremity requires resection of the lower third of the stellate ganglion and the upper two thoracic ganglia or, at least, proximal ramisectomy of the lower third of the stellate ganglion and the sympathetic ganglia at the second and third thoracic levels and sectioning of the upper thoracic sympathetic trunk below the third segment. Some surgeons prefer to resect the second to the fifth thoracic ganglia. Four basic approaches have been used to accomplish this objective: the anterior cervical, the posterior thoracic, the anterior transpleural, and the axillary. To these basic approaches must be added a variation, an endoscopic technique described recently by Kux of Vienna.[43]

Anterior Cervical Approach

Through a transverse incision above the clavicle, the inferior extremity of the sternocleidomastoid, the omohyoid, and the anterior scalene muscles are divided. One may visualize the subclavian artery with its branches and the stellate ganglion lying behind the origin of the vertebral artery. In order to resect the upper thoracic ganglia, the pleura must be separated from the bodies of the first three thoracic vertebrae and the adjacent portions of the first three ribs. The rami of the stellate ganglion, which is seen lying on the head of the first rib, are divided after the ganglion is lifted. One may then grasp the stellate ganglion and resect the second and perhaps the third thoracic ganglia. It is difficult to expose more of the sympathetic chain through this

approach. Indeed, if bleeding is encountered deep in the wound, one may have difficulty controlling it. This approach is recommended for simple stellate ganglionectomy and has been utlized when sympathectomy is performed in conjunction with division of the anterior scalene muscle or resection of a cervical rib in patients with the thoracic outlet syndrome.

A variation of the anterior approach has recently been described whereby the exposure is completed down to the third thoracic ganglion before an attempt is made to resect the sympathetic ganglia.[38] After interruption of fibers between the third and fourth ganglia, the third and second ganglia are disconnected from adjacent intercostal nerves and the lower lip of the stellate ganglion is resected. This variation has the advantage of avoiding permanent ptosis in most cases.

Posterior Approach

Through a paraspinal cervicothoracic incision, the trapezius muscle is divided and the paraspinal muscles are separated, exposing the angles of the second and third ribs. The transverse processes of the second and third thoracic vertebrae along with proximal segments of the associated ribs are resected. The pleura may then be separated from the upper thoracic vertebrae and the adjacent rib sections, exposing the upper sympathetic chain. Resection of the chain together with proximal segments of the second and third thoracic nerves may be performed. Some surgeons prefer Smithwick's method of resecting the second and third thoracic nerves with their rami communicantes, dividing the sympathetic chain between the third and fourth ganglia, swinging it posteriorly, and suturing the free end to the paraspinal muscles. This separates it from the remaining chain and reduces the possibility of regeneration.[64]

Cloward described a variation of the posterior approach that permits bilateral sympathectomy through a single midline incision.[9] With the patient prone, the skin incision extends from C7 to T4. Muscle and ligamentous attachments of the upper three thoracic spines are divided. After a bilateral costotransversectomy of T2, the sympathetic chain is identified and attachments of the second and third ganglia are divided, the third ganglion being brought out of the chest and attached to the muscle to prevent regeneration.

Anterior Transpleural Approach

This was the first transpleural approach and is accomplished with the patient in the supine position, the ipsilateral arm being abducted and the elbow flexed.[50] An incision is made through the anterior chest wall, passing through the pectoralis major muscle and the third intercostal space. The third costochondral junction is divided, the ribs separated, and the apex of the lung depressed, exposing the upper portion of the thoracic vertebrae and the sympathetic chain. When devised, this approach offered considerable improvement in exposure of those fibers passing to the heart. Alternatively, a more limited denervation of the heart may be accomplished by resecting the preaortic plexus.[27]

Axillary Approach

Recently, the axillary transpleural approach has been recommended and is becoming popular for unilateral upper thoracic sympathectomies.[35,39,44,45,68] It is a simple approach that offers direct exposure of the upper portion of the sympathetic chain. The patient is placed in the lateral decubitus position with the superior arm abducted 100 to 120 degrees, extended 30 degrees, and fixed to an overhanging bar. Through a transverse incision from the lateral edge of the pectoralis major and centered over the second intercostal space, the long thoracic and thoracobrachial nerves are identified. Any inconstant third thoracic contribution to the latter is divided. Other portions of these nerves are carefully preserved as the axillary fat pad is swept cephalad. The thorax is entered through the second interspace, and the apex of the lung is retracted. The upper portion of the sympathetic chain is in direct view of the operator, allowing discrete identification of the respective elements. After opening the parietal pleura, one may have adequate access to the thoracic sympathetic ganglia.

Lumbar Sympathectomy

Several approaches to the lumbar sympathetic trunk have been described. When resection is to be limited to these segments, the approach is usually through the flank. One popular technique is performed with the patient lying in the supine position, the side to be operated upon being slightly elevated. Through an oblique incision extending approximately 18 cm inferomesially from the lower costal margin, the external oblique muscle and fascia and the internal oblique muscle are split in the line of their fibers. After separation of the internal oblique from the transversalis muscle and fascia, retractors are inserted and the transversalis muscle and its fascial continuation are divided in the direction of their fibers, exposing the retroperitoneal fat.

The peritoneum is separated from the quadratus lumborum and iliacus muscles by finger dissection that is extended inward, upward, and medially below the twelfth rib and behind the kidney. Dissection continues until the sympathetic trunk is identified along the vertebral column at the anteromedial aspect of the iliopsoas muscle. The peritoneum, ureter, and vena cava or aorta are protected from a broad flat retractor by a gauze pad. The fascia of the medial lumbocostal arch of the diaphragm must be divided if the first lumbar ganglion is to be visualized. Care must be taken not to tear tributaries of the vena cava that may cross the sympathetic chain. The desired portions of the sympathetic trunk are excised.

An alternate approach places the patient in the lateral decubitus position. The incision is then made in the same direction but located more posteriorly.

A transperitoneal approach is sometimes utilized when this procedure is being combined with plastic procedures upon the intra-abdominal blood vessels. Some surgeons have found this approach so simple that they have recommended it as a routine technique for sympathectomizing the lower extremities.[66]

Thoracolumbar Resection

For thoracolumbar resections, formerly performed in great numbers for hypertension, the approach was usually through rib beds, the parietal pleura being separated from the chest wall. Extensive resections of the sympathetic trunk were combined with splanchnicectomy. Modifications of this procedure are now utilized, on rare occasions, for abdominal pain syndromes, e.g., pancreatitis.

Presacral Neurectomy

Presacral neurectomy is performed through a transperitoneal approach. A longitudinal incision is made in the peritoneum from the aortic bifurcation to the region of the third sacral segment. The superior hypogastric plexus is identified as two or three nerve bundles overlying the aorta when the peritoneum is retracted. Most authors advocate identification of the various segments of the plexus, but others would simply resect all nerve and connective tissue in the area. Care must be taken not to leave fibers attached to the peritoneum. Dissection is continued down to a base formed by a line drawn between the origins of the hypogastric arteries. The communicating fibers from the lower lumbar ganglia must be interrupted. The lower end of the pedicle is ligated securely before it is cut.

SIDE EFFECTS OF SYMPATHECTOMY

Undesirable responses to sympathectomy include postsympathectomy neuralgia, which characteristically appears about one week to 10 days after sympathectomy. The pain is continuous and sometimes intensely severe with exacerbations at night. Usually the pain subsides spontaneously after a period that may vary from a few weeks to a maximum of about three months. Until it subsides, it can be extremely annoying, requiring reassurance that it will subside spontaneously. Limitation of physical activity during the day and the administration of mild sedatives may help to reduce the nocturnal exacerbations. A recent report indicates that diphenylhydantoin and carbamazepine may be helpful in relieving the pain.[54]

"Paradoxical gangrene" may be due to opening of arteriovenous shunts in an extremity and consequent shunting of blood away from ischemic areas. It is most likely to occur when sympathectomy is performed in an extremity with severe obliterative vascular disease.

Return of vasomotor activity occurs routinely, but in varying degrees. It is of considerable importance in those patients in whom sympathectomy is being performed for vascular lesions but of virtually no consequence in patients being operated upon for pain.

SYMPATHECTOMY BY DRUGS OR IMMUNOLOGICAL TECHNIQUES

Several drugs are known to reduce catecholamine responses temporarily. This is the basis for many medical treatments of hypertension. During the last two decades it has been shown that the administration of guanethidine or 6-hydroxydopamine under experimental conditions will produce chemical sympathectomy.[18,41,69] Sympathectomy may also be accomplished experimentally by immunological techniques.[7,74] Immunological sympathectomy and chemical sympathectomy with guanethidine have been reported most commonly in very young animals.[18,74] The effects of systematically administered 6-hydroxydopamine appear to be widespread.[10,13,34] Although localized sympathectomy may be accomplished with 6-hydroxydopamine, studies on animals demonstrate that systemic effects still result.[3,6,15] General clinical use of this technique appears to be unlikely for some time in the future even though a few clinical cases involving chemical sympathectomy have been reported.[40]

REFERENCES

1. Aldasoro, G. E., Herrera, O. R., Enriquez, J. L. A., de Baca, G. N., de la Torre, I., and de Escobar, S. C.: Surgical treatment of livedo reticularis. Int. Surg., 60:44–45, 1975.
2. Alexander, W. F., Kuntz, A., Henderson, W. P., and Ehrlich, E.: Sympathetic conduction pathways independent of sympathetic trunks—their surgical implications. J. Int. Coll. Surg., 12:111–119, 1949.
3. Antebi, E., Berman, H. J., Giron, F., Angelakos, E. T., and Soroff, H. S.: Localized sympathectomy by single intra-arterial injection of 6-hydroxydopamine. J. Surg. Res., 15:117–121, 1973.
4. Arnulf, G.: Physiological basis of sympathetic surgery for the upper limb in Raynaud's disease. J. Cardiovasc. Surg. (Torino), 17:354–357, 1976.
5. Atkinson, L.: Upper dorsal sympathectomy. Med. J. Aust., 1:267–70, 1975.
6. Barrie, W. W., and Schenk, W. G., Jr.: Experi-

mental chemical sympathectomy. Regional and systemic effects of intraarterial injection of 6-OH dopamine. J. Surg. Res., *19*:333–340, 1975.

7. Berkowitz, B. A., Spector, S., and Tarver, J. H.: Resistance of noradrenaline in blood vessels to depletion by 6-hydroxydopamine or immunosympathectomy. Brit. J. Pharmacol., *44*:10–16, 1972.

8. Birkett, D. A., Apthorp, G. H., Chamberlain, D. A., Hayward, G. W., and Tuckwell, E. G.: Bilateral upper thoracic sympathectomy in angina pectoris: Results in 52 cases. Brit. Med. J., *2*:187–190, 1965.

9. Cloward, R. B.: Hyperhydrosis. J. Neurosurg., *30*:545–551, 1969.

10. Consolo, S., Garattini, S., Ladinsky, H., and Thoenen, H.: Effect of chemical sympathectomy on the content of acetylcholine, choline and choline acetyltransferase activity in the cat spleen and iris. J. Physiol. (London), *220*:639–646, 1972.

11. Cooper, T.: Surgical sympathectomy and adrenergic function. Pharmacol. Rev., *18*:611–618, 1966.

12. Cronenwett, J. L., and Lindenauer, S. M.: Direct measurement of arteriovenous anastomotic blood flow after lumbar sympathectomy. Surgery, *82*:82–89, 1977.

13. DeCamara, D., Moss, G. S., Das Gupta, T. K.: Alterations in pulmonary surfactant following sympathectomy. Surg. Forum, *27*:182–184, 1976.

14. Delaney, J., and Scarpino, J.: Limb arteriovenous shunting following sympathetic denervation. Surgery, *73*:202–206, 1973.

15. Eddy, C. A., and Black, D. L.: Chemical sympathectomy of the rabbit oviduct using 6-hydroxydopamine. J. Reprod. Fertil., *33*:1–9, 1973.

16. Edvinsson, L., Aubineau, P., Owman, C., Sercombe, R., and Seylaz, J.: Sympathetic innervation of cerebral arteries: Prejunctional supersensitivity to norepinephrine after sympathectomy or cocaine treatment. Stroke, *6*:525–30, 1975.

17. Ellis, H.: The surgical treatment of hyperhidrosis. Practitioner, *217*:416–419, 1976.

18. Eränkö, O., and Eränkö, L.: Histochemical evidence of chemical sympathectomy by guanethidine in newborn rats. Histochem. J., *3*:451–456, 1971.

19. Fowlis, R. A. F., Sang, C. T. M., Lundy, P. M., Ahuja, S. P., and Colhoun, H.: Experimental coronary artery ligation in conscious dogs six months after bilateral cardiac sympathectomy. Amer. Heart J., *88*:748–757, 1974.

20. Freier, A.: Pelvic neurectomy in gynecology. Obstet. Gynec., *25*:48–55, 1965.

21. Fulton, R. L., and Blakeley, W. R.: Lumbar sympathectomy: A procedure of questionable value in the treatment of arteriosclerosis obliterans of the legs. Amer. J. Surg., *116*:735–744, 1968.

22. Gillespie, J. A.: The current status of lumbar sympathectomy in the management of the ischaemic leg. Scand. J. Clin. Lab. Invest., suppl. 128, *31*:67–70, 1973.

23. Goetz, R. H.: The diagnosis and treatment of vascular diseases with special consideration of clinical plethysmography and the surgical physiol-

ogy of the autonomic nervous system. Brit. J. Surg., *37*:25–40, 1949.

24. Gorbitz, C., and Leavens, M. E.: Alcohol block of the celiac plexus for control of upper abdominal pain caused by cancer and pancreatitis. Technical note. J. Neurosurg., *34*:575–579, 1971.

25. Greenwood, B.: The origins of sympathectomy. Med. Hist., *11*:165–169, 1967.

26. Grima, M. R.: Bilateral cervical sympathectomy for acrocyanosis. Nurs. Times, *71*:1850–1852, 1975.

27. Grondin, C. M., and Limet, R.: Sympathetic denervation in association with coronary artery grafting in patients with Prinzmetal's angina. Ann. Thorac. Surg., *23*:111–117, 1977.

28. Gulati, S. M., Kapur, B. M. L., and Talwar, J. R.: Sympathectomy in the management of frostbite: An experimental study. Indian J. Med. Res., *58*:343–351, 1970.

29. Hardenbergh, E., and Miles, J. A., Jr.: The effect of sympathectomy on tissue loss after experimental frostbite of the rabbit ear. J. Surg. Res., *3*:126–134, 1972.

30. Harris, J. D., and Jepson, R. P.: Essential hyperhidrosis. Med. J. Aust., *2*:135–138, 1971.

31. Hartfall, W. G., and Jochimsen, P. R.: Hyperhidrosis of the upper extremity and its treatment. Surg. Gynec. Obstet., *135*:586–588, 1972.

32. Heisey, W. G., and Dohn, D. F.: Splanchnicectomy for the treatment of intractable abdominal pain. Cleveland Clin. Quart., *34*:9–25, 1967.

33. Hirai, M., Kawai, S., and Shionoya, S.: Effect of lumbar sympathectomy on muscle circulation in dogs and patients. Nagoya J. Med. Sci., *37*:71–77, 1975.

34. Imbach, A.: Metabolic alterations following chemical sympathectomy with 6-hydroxydopamine in the rat. Rec. Adv. Stud. Cardiac Struct. Metab., *9*:259–267, 1976.

35. Jochimsen, P. R., and Hartfall, W. G.: Per axillary upper extremity sympathectomy: Technique reviewed and clinical experience. Surgery, *71*:686–693, 1972.

36. Keates, J. S., Beemann, J., Pasternak, G., and Sawyer, P. N.: Assessment of sympathectomy in the treatment of peripheral vascular disease. Bibl. Anat., *13*:396–397, 1975.

37. Keaveny, T. V., Fitzpatrick, J., and Fitzgerald, P. A.: The surgical treatment of hyperhidrosis. J. Irish Med. Ass., *67*:544–545, 1974.

38. Khanna, S. K., Sahariah, S., and Mittal, V. K.: Supraclavicular approach for upper dorsal sympathectomy. Vasc. Surg., *9*:151–159, 1975.

39. Kirtley, J. A., Riddell, D. E., Stoney, W. S., and Wright, J. K.: Cervicothoracic sympathectomy in neurovascular abnormalities of the upper extremities: Experiences in 76 patients with 104 sympathectomies. Ann. Surg., *165*:869–879, 1967.

40. Kitazawa, Y., Nośe, H., and Horie, T.: Chemical sympathectomy with 6-hydroxydopamine in the treatment of primary open-angle glaucoma. Amer. J. Ophthal., *79*:98–103, 1975.

41. Krakoff, L. R., and Ginsburg, S. M.: Effect of chemical sympathectomy on pressor responses to norepinephrine, angiotensin and tyramine. Experientia, *29*:995–997, 1973.

42. Kreuzer, W., and Schenk, W. G., Jr.: Hemodynamic responses to lumbar sympathectomy. An

experimental study of changes in blood flow and limb oxygen consumption in the dog with acute or chronic arterial obstruction. J. Cardiovasc. Surg. (Torino), *13*:532–537, 1971.

43. Kux, M.: Thoracic endoscopic sympathectomy for treatment of upper-limb hyperhidrosis. Lancet, *1*:1320, 1977.

44. Little, J. M., and May, J.: A comparison of the supraclavicular and axillary approaches to upper thoracic sympathectomy. Austr. New Zeal. J. Surg., *45*:143–146, 1975.

45. Man, B., Kraus, L., and Motovic, A.: Axillary sympathectomy for upper extremities. Vasc. Surg., *10*:138–143, 1976.

46. Munro, P. A. G.: Sympathectomy, An Anatomical and Physiological Study with Clinical Applications. London, New York, Toronto, Oxford University Press, 1959.

47. Myers, K. A., and Irvine, W. T.: An objective study of lumbar sympathectomy. I. Intermittent claudication. Brit. Med. J., *1*:879–883, 1966.

48. Myers, K. A., and Irvine, W. T.: An objective study of lumbar sympathectomy. II. Skin ischemia. Brit. Med. J., *1*:943–947, 1966.

49. Nakata, Y., Suzuki, S., Kawai, S., Hirai, M., Shinjo, K., Matsubara, J., Ban, I., and Shionoya, S.: Effects of lumbar sympathectomy on thromboangiitis obliterans. J. Cardiovasc. Surg. (Torino), *16*:415–425, 1975.

50. Palumbo, L. T.: Anterior transthoracic approach for upper thoracic sympathectomy. Arch. Surg. (Chicago), *72*:659–666, 1956.

51. Palumbo, L. T.: A new concept of the sympathetic pathways to the eye, a new technique to avoid a Horner's syndrome. Surgery, *42*:740–748, 1957.

52. Perrin, M.: Is lumbar sympathectomy liable to influence the results of reconstructive arterial surgery? J. Cardiovasc. Surg. (Torino), *16*:381–383, 1975.

53. Postlethwaite, J. C.: Lumbar sympathectomy. A retrospective study of 142 operations on 100 patients. Brit. J. Surg., *60*:878–879, 1973.

54. Raskin, N. H., Levinson, S. A., Hoffman, P. M., Pickett, J. B. E., III, and Fields, H. L.: Postsympathectomy neuralgia. Amelioration with diphenylhydantoin and carbamazepine. Amer. J. Surg., *128*:75–78, 1974.

55. Ray, B. S., and Console, A. D.: Residual sympathetic pathways after paravertebral sympathectomy. J. Neurosurg., *5*:23–50, 1948.

56. Ray, B. S., Hinsey, J. C., and Geohegan, W. A.: Observations on the distribution of sympathetic nerves to pupil and upper extremity as determined by stimulation of anterior roots in man. Ann. Surg., *118*:647–655, 1943.

57. Richter, C. P., and Woodruff, B. G.: Lumbar sympathetic dermatomes in man determined by the electrical skin resistance method. J. Neurophysiol., *8*:323–338, 1945.

58. Rogers, W., Reller, C. R., Jr., Sheridan, J. D. and Aust, J. B.: Tissue blood flow in the canine lower limb following lumbar sympathectomy. Vasc. Surg., *6*:227–238, 1973.

59. Sadar, E. S., and Cooperman, A. M.: Bilateral thoracic sympathectomy-splanchnicectomy in the treatment of intractable pain due to pancreatic carcinoma. Cleveland Clin. Quart., *41*:185–188, 1974.

60. Schoonmaker, F. W., Carey, T., and Grow, J. B., Sr.: Treatment of tachyarrhythmias and bradyarrhythmias by cardiac sympathectomy and permanent ventricular pacing. Ann. Thorac. Surg., *19*:80–87, 1975.

61. Shanik, G. D., Ford, J., Hayes, A. C., Baker, W. H., and Barnes, R. W.: Pedal vasomotor tone following aortofemoral reconstructions: A randomized study of concomitant lumbar sympathectomy. Ann. Surg., *183*:136–138, 1976.

62. Shoenfeld, Y., Shapiro, Y., Machtiger, A., and Magazanik, A.: Sweat studies in hyperhidrosis palmaris and plantaris. A survey of 60 patients before and after cervical sympathectomy. Dermatologica (Basel), *152*:257–262, 1976.

63. Skilton, J. S., Ashton, F., and Slaney, G.: Lumbar sympathectomy in the salvage of ischaemic limbs. Brit. J. Clin. Pract., *28*:339–342, 1974.

64. Smithwick, R. H.: Rationale and technic of sympathectomy for relief of vascular spasm of extremities. New Eng. J. Med., *222*:699–703, 1940.

65. Smithwick, R. H.: Sympathectomy, splanchnicectomy and vagotomy. Rev. Surg. (Phila.), *30*: 153–173, 1973.

66. Sproul, G., and Pinto, J.: Transabdominal sympathectomy. Vasc. Surg., *6*:55–58, 1972.

67. Stein, I. D., Harpuder, K., and Byer, J.: Effect of sympathectomy on blood flow in the human limb. Amer. J. Physiol., *152*:499–504, 1948.

68. Sundaresan, N., Rajakulasingam, K., Lawrence, E. P., and Wetzel, N.: Transaxillary transthoracic sympathectomy. Surg. Neurol., *7*:149–152, 1977.

69. Thureson-Klein, A., Lagercrantz, H., and Barnard, T.: Chemical sympathectomy of interscapular brown adipose tissue. Acta Physiol. Scand., *98*:8–18, 1976.

70. Ulmer, J. L., and Mayfield, F. H., Causalgia; study of 75 cases. Surg. Gynec. Obstet., *83*: 789–796, 1946.

71. Van der Stricht, J.: The influence of lumbar sympathectomy on the permeability of reconstructions. J. Cardiovasc. Surg. (Torino), *16*:552–553, 1975.

72. White, J. C., and Smithwick, R. H.: The Anatomic Nervous System. New York, Macmillan Publishing Co., 1941.

73. White, J. C., Okelberry, A. M., and Whitelaw, G. P.: Vasomotor tonus of denervated artery: control of sympathectomized blood vessels by sympathomimetic hormones and its relation to the surgical treatment of patients with Raynaud's disease. Arch. Neurol. Psychiat., *36*: 1251–1276, 1936.

74. Zaimis, E.: Immunological sympathectomy. Sci. Basis Med. Ann. Rev., pp. 59–73, 1967.

135

AFFECTIVE
DISORDERS
INVOLVING PAIN

The complaint of pain continues to challenge our best therapeutic efforts, particularly when it involves the behavioral disability associated with a painful, healed, and nonprogessive lesion. In this situation the problem arises from the patient's reaction to and concern about the static input of pain, as contrasted with the positive reaction associated with the dynamic input of pain from a destructive lesion such as cancer. In both patients, however, the emotional impact of the physical future is a major factor in the continuing "pain" and disability. In the non-cancer patient, the uncertainty for the future, the fear of possible death from his nonprogressive lesion, the reliance on a complaint of "pain" because of the psychological need for dependence on someone, and even the subconscious reliance on "pain" for financial gain may be the truly basic causes of disability. In the cancer patient, some of these same mechanisms play a role in the disability from pain as well as in the fundamental reaction of dependence when he fully realizes death from his cancer is inevitable and not too distant. This multifaceted reaction may be termed "suffering" in all such patients. This secondary or reactive manifestation of the disease may be overwhelming and more disabling than the primary organic disease itself.

PSYCHOPATHOPHYSIOLOGY UNDERLYING "PAIN"

The basis of the psychological aspects of suffering and its role in the total pain response of a patient is discussed in Chapter 116. The various ablative techniques directed at the pain pathways and their importance in controlling pain of a progressive nature, particularly in carcinoma and other destructive lesions, are summarized in other chapters of this book.

The nonprogressive, nondestructive, healed lesion that hurts is the subject of this chapter, the sort of case for which White and Sweet give the following sage advice:

Here eventual failure is most common and we are generally reluctant to intervene until the emotional background has been investigated and it is evident that the subject can no longer live with his discomfort without recourse to habit-forming drugs.[52]

Additional experience with the long-term follow-up of over 1000 such cases strongly supports this advice.[3,10] In these cases, careful evaluation reveals the input of pain from the healed and stable lesion to remain quite constant, but the suffering and behavioral reaction to vary with the life situations faced by the patient. Simply to modify the character of the input does little to decrease the labile suffering of the patient. This fact can explain many of the failures of pain pathway operations.

The term commonly used at the end stage of therapeutic trials for pain control is "psychogenic pain," which to the patient means he is "imagining" it, whereas to the physician it means he admits defeat. Few painful states are spontaneously generated. Most of them have an organic basis at least in their origin. The problem is one of psychic magnification in which the pain be-

---

E. L. FOLTZ AND L. E. WHITE, JR.

comes a disease in its own right, creating a social disability in the otherwise healthy and sound individual. As such the pain is intractable to the usual forms of disease-oriented therapeutic management and broadcasts itself to the physician and society through affective emotional behavior. Therefore, truly intractable pain can be looked upon as an affective disorder.

The mechanistic tendency to look upon pain as strictly stimulus oriented, and therefore reversible by removing the stimulus, overlooks the capability of the conscious individual to perceive bodily differences, to remember and dwell upon the consequences of a painful disease or injury after it has healed. These observations led Cobb to state dogmatically,

I do not believe in "imaginary pain" . . . it is not a case of "real" pain or "imaginary" pain but a matter of how much pain and how the patient reacts to it.[15]

Furthermore, the importance of the protective concept of pain to the productive survival of the organism from which is derived Sternbach's definition:

Pain is an abstract concept which refers to (1) a personal, private sensation of hurt, (2) a harmful stimulus which signals current or impending tissue damage, (3) a pattern of responses which operate to protect the organism from (psychic or physical) harm.[46]

Therefore, the classic pain response of the patient, withdrawal and protection, is modulated by the more versatile associative aspects of intellectual brain function adding the dimension of suffering by which the patient communicates his interpretation of the consequences of the pain stimulus.

The medical evaluation of pain is difficult, and particularly so in the patient with intractable pain. Stead has emphasized this by describing the first step in evaluation of any complaint—"is the patient ill or well?"[45] The importance of making this first judgment is little emphasized, but to treat a basically well person as though he were ill tends to reinforce the assumption that directed him in search of aid in the first place.

In the evaluation and management of patients with pain, the importance of the individual basic conception of pain cannot be overemphasized. When disease and illness are involved, pain is only a symptom and

can be removed simply by removing the stimulus or blocking its normal transmission to the level of consciousness. When the patient is healthy and without disease, or healed and only structurally changed from the disease that is now "cured," and pain persists, it becomes an illness in its own right, intractable pain. As an affective disorder it must be managed as such. The patient is biologically healthy but sick with the intellectual phenomenon of pain.

Accepting these truisms, the majority of patients will do well with a careful evaluation and an anatomical diagnosis of the source of the discomfort. They will readily accept, if it is suitably documented and explained, the fact that their bodies are sound and healthy and the discomfort they feel is not evidence of disease but the persistent disability of a healed disease. The general tendency of physicians is to avoid this approach and to rely on the scientific method. The latter approach makes is easy to explain to an amputee with true phantom limb pain that he cannot grow a new leg, but it is difficult to convince him that the feeling of painful absence of the leg will never be totally relieved and can be modified only to a level that is tolerable by a combination of therapeutic efforts.

The conservative management of an affective disorder must be based on as accurate a diagnosis as possible and the patient's complete understanding of the problem. Confidence in the physician or physicians managing the problem and consistency of approach between physicians cannot be overemphasized. Success depends upon the reorientation of the patient's expectations as to recovery and his motivation to rehabilitate himself.

The crash approach to this form of management is hypnosis. Through such concentration the patient consciously blocks the behavioral pattern associated with the pain, therefore no longer communicating it to others. Barber has reviewed the effects of hypnosis on pain and has shown that the physiological components of the destructive stimulus are usually not blocked by hypnotic trance, but the patient's conscious perception of them and desire to communicate this meaningfully to others is blocked.[4] Similar observations have been made by Beecher in patients receiving placebos or being injured in athletics or war. In these latter situations, the consequences of the destructive stimulus are volitionally modified owing to the context in which the perception of pain is reaching consciousness.[8,9]

Similarly, a more profound approach can be taken through the psychological approach of conditioning. Fordyce and co-workers have shown that with adequate therapeutic tests, patients can be conditioned positively to rehabilitate themselves.[25] Skinner and others have described this behavior as operating in a realistic sense with the environment, the result termed "operant conditioning."[43] Therefore, these patients learn to live with their chronic stable pain. A surprisingly large number of them learn to ignore their discomfort completely. Similar results have been accomplished by a team of specialists working through a referring or coordinating physician.[3,10] The function of the specialists is to confirm the diagnosis and recommend forms of management through the referring physician. Through the comparison of various specialty opinions the problem is established as an intractable and healed one involving the disability of persistent suffering. The managing physician uses the collective opinions of the specialists to approach the patient in a "positive" fashion, supporting the patient's own desire to recover. The initial results of this conservative clinical approach have shown better than 50 per cent good results in rehabilitating patients with intractable pain.[53]

The patient with intractable pain who does not respond to supportive care and shows the physiological and psychic deterioration that accompany persistent suffering creates a challenge to the surgeon. The physiological changes result from unconscious protective reflexes and the habitual use of pain-relieving medication. The classic trophic changes of the skin ensue—the loss of hair, edema, smoothness, and poverty of motion first emphasized by Weir Mitchell. Certain autonomic phenomena can be learned or acquired under experimental conditions, as has been shown by Miller.[39] To this is added cachexia associated with weight loss and shift to the ratio of albumin to globulin. Early renal and liver failure is usually superimposed because of prolonged use of many drugs. The usual psychic picture is one of withdrawal, brooding, and severe depression associated with the acute anxiety and tension of the chronic sufferer.

White and Sweet have emphasized that this form of chronic pain is refractory to the usual pain operation.[52] Operation fails because it is aimed at modifying the perceived pain stimulus. As outlined, existing evidence supports the premise that the problem is an affective one involving suffering and that it signals the unconscious disruption of the normal homeostatic mechanisms of the body. Obviously, when such intractable pain is diagnosed, the physiological approach toward therapy should not be directed toward removal of the pain stimulus but toward the relief of the basic psychological chronic suffering.

NEUROPHYSIOLOGICAL HOMEOSTASIS AND SUFFERING

Several early investigators observed the relationship of the medial aspect of the hemisphere to the more primitive aspects of emotional behavior. Darwin documented the evolutional characteristics of emotion, and Herrick suggested that the limbic lobe may serve as a nonspecific activator of all cortical activities, influencing "the internal apparatus of general bodily attitude, disposition and affective tone."[17,30] Subsequently, Papez made his historic postulate of an emotional mechanism involving the limbic lobe, anterior thalamus, and hypothalamus.[42] These observations do not preclude the function of the neocortex, but they indicated to Cobb that the meso-allo-cortex of the limbic lobe ". . . set the emotional background on which man functions intellectually."[14]

The importance of the limbic lobe of the brain to the basic development of the cerebral hemispheres and its possible relationship to homeostatic function can be documented both by phylogenetic and by ontogenetic data.[54] The absence of a specific phylogenetic promammalian representative is not surprising, but its importance cannot be overemphasized. The basic need for relative homeostatic control is necessary for simple survival. Therefore, it is consistent to assume that the area of the cerebral cortex related to this function differentiated first. Elliot Smith diagrammed the hypothetical extinct promammalian brain in 1910 and documented its primary position in setting the stage for the subsequent differentiation of the remainder of the neocortical elements of the telencephalon (Fig. 135–1).[18] At this transition stage almost the entire cerebral hemisphere is made up of limbic lobe structures. Ontogenetic observations led Hines to state that the hippocampus is the earliest of cerebral structures to differentiate in man.[31] Furthermore, neuropathological observations of arrhinencephalic monsters, as experiments of nature, emphasize the massive primary distortion of limbic structures when teratogenic agents strike early in the process of telencephalic differentiation.[55]

Physiological observations directed at this primitive and basic cortex of the telencephalon further confirm its pre-eminence in basic homeostatic behavioral mechanisms. First, it has been noted by Brobeck and co-workers that basic satiation is controlled in the hypothalamus but that lesions in these same areas evoke rage or "sham rage" in animals.[1,5,12] Second, removal of the neocortex does not produce a hyperirritable animal, but rage occurs if subsequent lesions are placed in the limbic cortex, as shown by Bard and co-workers.[6,7] Third, lesions of the medial temporal cortex

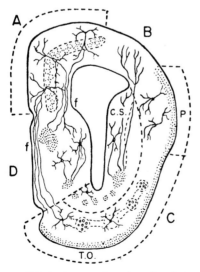

Figure 135–1 A coronal section of half of the telencephalon of a possible promammalian brain. A, archipallium; B, neopallium; C, paleopallium; D, telencephalon medium; C.S., corpus striatum; f, fornix; p, piriform cortex; T.O., olfactory tubercle. (Modified from Elliot Smith, G.: Some problems relating to the evolution of the brain. Lancet, *1*:147, 1910.)

involving entorhinal cortex and amygdala produce animals with no apparent fear, anomalous sexual behavior, and peculiar oral tendencies, as originally described by Kluver and Bucy.[35] Fourth, lesions of the anterior cingulate gyrus and cingulum fasciculus produce animals that behaviorally seem to have lost their social conscience, a modification that cannot be qualitatively increased by additional ablation of the frontal lobe cortex.[21,48] The variability and pluripotentiality of behavioral responses from these rudimentary limbic areas have been demonstrated by numerous experiments in awake, freely functioning animals.[11,34] Following limbic lobe lesions, addicted animals are protected from death when exposed to the threat of nalorphine-precipitated withdrawal.[21]

Present anatomical and physiological knowledge emphasizes the importance of limbic structures in what Cobb referred to as setting the "emotional background" for subsequent behavioral function, in more functional terms the areas responsible for maintenance of homeostasis.[15]

The preceding analysis of the affective disability of intractable pain suggests a behavioral disability of self-protection or an overactivity of the normal homeostatic mechanisms. Such being the case, it is not surprising that lesions primarily involving the limbic lobe are useful in relieving the suffering patient. Likewise, even with alleviation of suffering, the fact that pain perception is not altered is readily confirmed and consistent—for the limbic cortex has little to do with the perception of pain but rather is concerned with the organism's reaction to the anticipated consequences of the pain perception.

These observations have led to a clinical concept of the limbic lobe that can be applied in the operative management of the affective disorders of suffering in the intractable pain syndrome.[13,23,54] This concept represents a hypothetical distillate of clinical and experimental observations. On the basis of phylogenetic, ontogenetic, and historical material, the limbic lobe can be readily divided into two almost concentric anatomical rings, the "inner limbic ring" and the "outer limbic ring" (Fig. 135–2). This anatomical relationship is consistent with physiological data about this system wherein reverberating circuits and positive feedbacks are prominent. Interaction is free

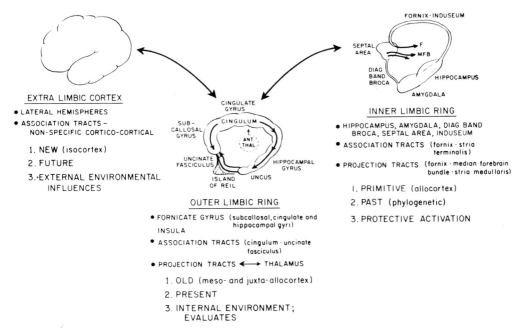

Figure 135–2 Limbic system: schematic comparison and correlation of anatomy and function of "inner limbic ring," "outer limbic ring," and "extralimbic cortex." (From Foltz, E. L., and White, L. E., Jr.: Rostral cingulumotomy and pain "relief." *In* Knighton, R. S., and Dumke, P. R., eds.: Pain. Boston, Little, Brown & Co., 1966. Reprinted by permission.)

between these two cortex-fiber systems. The "inner limbic ring" consists of the hippocampus, fornix, septal area, diagonal band of Broca, medial amygdala, and stria terminalis. Its interrelationships with the brain stem allow direct autonomic effector action via the projection system consisting of the fornix, medial forebrain bundle, and stria medularis. The cortical structure is allocortex oriented to the phylogenetic past, and the basic function is probably to produce or allow "protective activation" of the organism.

The "outer limbic ring" is made up of the fornicate gyrus (subcallosal, cingulate, and hippocampal gyri) plus the uncus and the insula (island of Reil) with association tracts in the cingulum and uncinate fasciculus, and projection pathways with the anterior thalamus. This cortex is intermediate in type and is made up of mesocortex and juxta-allocortex. Its function presumably relates primarily to the immediate present, especially the consequences of environmental change on the internal environment of the organism. It has functional interplay via afferent and efferent pathways with the inner limbic ring and with the extralimbic cortex, thereby possibly evaluating internal and external factors in light of

the past as well as the present. It may relate to future elements on the basis of its interrelationships with the "extralimbic cortex."

The "extralimbic cortex," physically massive by comparison, consists of the large lateral hemispheres in which the cortex is fully differentiated isocortex and is related to receptive and associative function. This cortex is highly structured with numerous association tracts and projects through the internal capsule system onto the brain stem and spinal cord. Its primary function presumably is related to external environmental features and their significance.

Through the outer limbic ring, the limbic lobe is in a position to interact with both the extralimbic cortex with its future-related external environmental influences and the inner limbic ring with its basically protective autonomic influences. The resulting "evaluation" via its own interaction with the thalamus and the other centers thereby modulates the motivated responses in terms of both somatic and autonomic tone. Therefore, through the interaction of these three basic cerebral parts, the limbic lobe functions to maintain homeostasis and control emotional tone.

This predominantly morphological and

empirical clinical model of homeostasis has begun to reveal its physiological secrets. The use of fluorescence microscopy revealed the presence of biogenically active amines within the central nervous system.[28] These putative transmitters are intimately associated with the medial aspects of the brain stem and the limbic structures. Although these substances can be found in varying concentrations throughout the central nervous system, they are largely distributed through the medium of the medial forebrain bundle and the association fasciculi of the limbic lobe (cingulum, uncinate fasciculus, and fornix systems). The major mechanism of distribution is through the active process of orthodromic axoplasmic flow. The biogenically active amines are metabolically generated within certain areas of the central brain stem extending from the lower medulla (A1) to the midline region of the thalmus (A14) for the catecholamines (dopamine and norepinephrine) and areas (V1–B9) for the indolamines (serotonin). It is through the modulation of these systems that the major and minor tranquilizers seem to bring about their therapeutic responses.

Similarly, it has been recently discovered that specific opiate receptors can be found within the same general areas of the brain stem and the substantia gelatinosa of the spinal cord.[44] These opiate receptors are normally responsive to enkephalin, a newly defined and naturally occurring polypeptide. Both the naturally occurring enkephalin polypeptides and morphine-like drugs are inhibited by morphine antagonists. These receptor sites are prominent in the periaqueductal gray matter and seem to project into the region of the caudally located serotonergic raphe nuclei (raphe magnus). This region in turn projects into the dorsal horn gray matter through an ill-defined projection system within the dorsolateral funiculus of the spinal cord.[19] The importance of this newly defined relationship is emphasized by the recent observations that long-term stimulation of the periaqueductal gray matter is followed by prolonged analgesia lasting from several minutes to hours in animals and in humans, a response that is inhibited by morphine antagonists. It is not fortuitous that these same midline zones were found by behavioral researchers to house the so-called "pleasure centers."

Although not applying the present concept, the startling taming effect following frontal lobe amputation in the chimpanzee "Becky" led to the development of frontal lobotomy, which also helped the patient suffering from intractable pain problems.[50] Anatomical evaluation of the various procedures—frontal lobotomy, supraorbital topectomy, anterior cingulate gyrus topectomy, cingulumotomy, and anterior thalamotomy—effective in relieving suffering reveals a common involvement of the major association tracts or cortex of the outer limbic ring or its major projection system with the anterior thalamus.[52]

The close interrelationship of the anterior thalamus to the limbic cortex has been submitted to careful study by Yakovlev and his colleagues.[57] These studies indicate an anterior thalamic interplay upon the entire mesocortical rim of the limbic lobe. Similar findings have been confirmed in animals following electrical stimulation.[56] It is important to note that the major portion of the anterior thalamic fibers to the cingulate gyrus course laterally in the internal capsule to join the cingulum bundle in the coronal plane of the anterior commissure.[37] Therefore, lesions anterior to this plane and deep to the cingulate cortex are confined largely to the major association tract of the outer limbic ring—the cingulum. Lesions anterior to the corpus callosum in the depths of the frontal lobe also sever the collecting fibers of the cingulum as well as thalamic projections to the orbital limbic cortex. It has been suggested that the "laconic" post-lobotomy state in man may be due to the separation of the frontal lobe cortex from its normal reticular activating mechanisms via the thalamus.[26]

Watts and Freeman, and Koskoff and co-workers described the initial effects of lobotomy on pain syndromes and made a distinction between pain and suffering.[36,51] They emphasized that frontal lobotomy was an operation for the relief of suffering and had no effect on pain threshold. Furthermore, Koskoff and associates emphasized that the effects of frontal lobotomy were due to ". . . interruption of association pathways forming part of a vicious circle."[36]

The results of the various operations to modify suffering are clouded by the patient who responds adversely with apathy and deterioration of personality.[38] On the basis of the foregoing data, however, the smallest lesion productive of relief of suffering is ideal. Furthermore, the overall results reported by White and Sweet encourage making as specific a lesion as possible, graded in extent by the use of indwelling electrodes.[52]

The technique of electrolytic frontal lobotomy minimized the size of the lesion and confined it to the primary frontal collection system of the cingulum bundle and the orbital projections of the thalamus.[29] Development of this procedure by Grantham and the observation of Ward following anterior cingulate gyrus resection in man and animals led to the logical placement of electrolytic lesions in the cingulum bundle deep to the anterior cingulate gyrus specifically for the management of intractable pain.[22,23,49] These limited procedures seem to minimize the psychic deterioration of the patient and maximize pain ''relief'' by modifying ''suffering'' reactions.

The striking effect on suffering of the limited cingulum lesion as well as the subsequent behavioral reorientation of the patient leads to an attractive notion. Could these responses be due to the imparted discontinuity of the catecholamine distribution system of the cingulum bundle in much the same way that the responses of parkinsonian patients to thalamotomy were due to dopamine depletion within the striatum? This development could lead to an adjustment of the enkephalin response, currently identified as a biological response by opiate receptor areas that inhibits interpretation of pain stimuli as pain experience. This response may be less inhibited after the cingulum lesions. Effectively, the operation produces augmentation of the enkephalin response. Studies of this hypothesis are still needed.

ROSTRAL CINGULUMOTOMY

The technique of electrolytic cingulumotomy has two outstanding features. First, the operative approach is simple yet precise. It uses local anesthesia throughout, thus allowing observation on the effects of brain stimulation or destruction on behavior or autonomic systems. Second, the stereotaxis involved can be simple hand-directed placement of electrodes into the rostral cingulum bilaterally under x-ray control using biplane frontal horn ventriculography.

Morphological Intent of Cingulumotomy

The morphological intent of the cingulum lesions is demonstrated in Figure 135–3. This figure depicts diagrammatically the median sagittal section of the human brain wherein the cingulum bundle is shown above the corpus callosum with the target area for destruction outlined by the dotted line. The lesion is placed to interrupt the cingulum bundle deep to the cingulate gyrus.

Figure 135–4 shows the uncinate fasciculus and the cingulum fasciculus in a coronal section simply for morphological orientation. This stereotaxic approach is reasonably safe and has few complications.

Figure 135–5 diagrams the microscopic complexity of the primary cingulum fasciculus, showing that this fasciculus is made up of fibers coming from neurons in the cingulate gyrus as well as from the supralimbic cortex. The cingulum is a complex fasciculus made up of fibers both short and long, some traversing the entire extent of the bundle. In the anterior portion they go more anteriorly. In the posterior portion, the fibers are largely directed toward the hippocampal formation as shown at site 7 in Figure 135–5. There are projections coming from this axial bundle that leave the

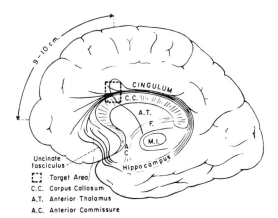

Figure 135–3 Median sagittal diagram to illustrate target site of rostral cingulumotomy. (From Foltz, E. L., and White, L. E., Jr.: Rostral cingulumotomy and pain ''relief.'' *In* Knighton, R. S., and Dumke, P. R., eds.: Pain. Boston, Little, Brown & Co., 1966. Reprinted by permission.)

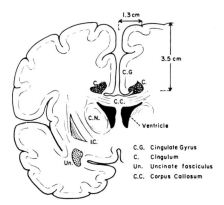

Figure 135–4 Coronal section diagram of rostal cingulum, its fiber pathway projections, and target site of rostral cingulumotomy. (From Foltz, E. L., and White, L. E., Jr.: Rostral cingulumotomy and pain "relief," *In* Knighton, R. S., and Dumke, P. R., eds.: Pain. Boston, Little, Brown & Co., 1966. Reprinted by permission.)

bundle, cross the corpus callosum to the opposite side, cross part of the corpus callosum to go to the septal area, or may stay on the homolateral side projecting to the anterior thalamus and striatum.

Method of Cingulumotomy

Cingulum destruction involves the insertion of electrodes into the cingulum fasciculus as shown in Figure 135–6, under x-ray control and with air placed in the ventricles so that the proper positioning of the electrodes in the cingulum bundle can be assured. The measurements shown in Figures 135–3 and 135–4 are applied to the x-ray done at the time the cingulum de-

struction is to be accomplished by radiofrequency current. Figure 135–7 shows the lateral skull x-ray of the same patient. The electrodes shown in these figures were slightly deeper than they should be and were withdrawn to point Y, at which place the lesions were made.

The anterior-posterior position of the lesions is important. It should be emphasized that in a stage I cingulumotomy the lesion is anterior to the coronal suture line. If the clinical result is inadequate, a second stage can be done as shown in Figure 135–8. The small air-containing space appearing as an outpocketing of the ventricle is the site of the cingulum bundle lesions made two years prior to the stage II cingulumotomy. The patient had recurrent symptoms of augmented emotional response to the pain problem, and a second stage procedure was performed in this manner. If proper positioning of the electrodes is achieved, a cingulumotomy is a relatively safe procedure. Adequate patient selection for cingulumotomy, of course, is still the single most important criterion for a successful result.

Figure 135–9 is a photomicrograph that shows a cross section of the cingulum fasciculus within the cingulate gyrus located above the corpus callosum and demonstrates the degree of destruction from a typical cingulumotomy.

Results

Existing evidence strongly supports the use of bilateral small lesions for lasting results rather than unilateral lesions.[2,23] This

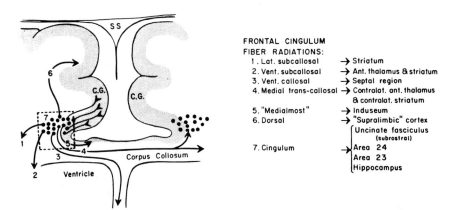

Figure 135–5 Coronal diagram to show rostral cingulum fiber radiations. (From Foltz, E. L., and White, L. E., Jr.: Rostral cingulumotomy and pain "relief." *In* Knighton, R. S., and Dumke, P. R., eds.: Pain. Boston, Little, Brown & Co., 1966. Reprinted by permission.)

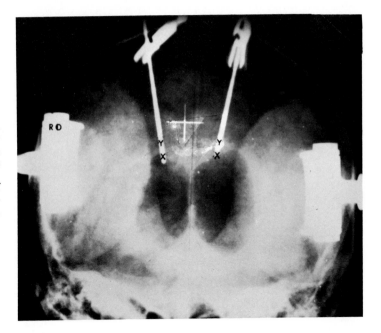

Figure 135–6 X-ray, antero-posterior view, shows cingulumotomy electrodes in place, x-ray control by air in ventricles. Lesion was made at "Y" after electrode tips were slightly withdrawn. (From Foltz, E. L.: The role of the limbic system in pain interpretation. Ariz. Med., 26:1033–1040, 1969. Reprinted by permission.)

is particularly true in the intractable pain problems unrelated to malignant disease in which the affective syndrome of suffering is paramount. Similarly, comparative observations suggest that bilateral severance of the cingulum bundle deep to the anterior cingulate gyrus results in less persistence of apathy and more lasting relief of suffering. It is tempting to suggest that the less persistence of apathy is due to minimal involvement of the thalamic projections and the more lasting relief of suffering is due to

maximal involvement of one of the major association tracts of the outer limbic ring.

The latter point is important in managing the affective aspects of suffering in the intractable pain problem that is not related to malignant disease. Similar observations would suggest that in terminal cancer pain the attendant apathy of frontal lobotomy is of added value because the fear of death and progression of the disease is a prominent factor.

Complications of the procedure other

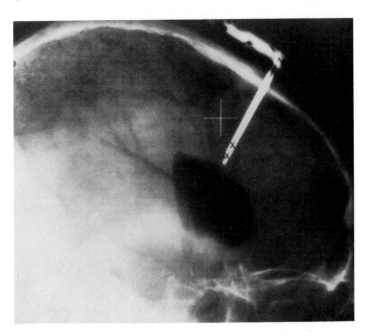

Figure 135–7 X-ray, lateral view, of same patient as in Figure 135–6. (From Foltz, E. L.: The role of the limbic system in pain interpretation. Ariz. Med., 26: 1033–1040, 1969. Reprinted by permission.)

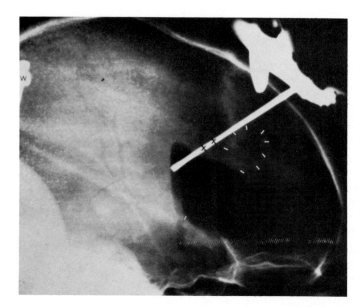

Figure 135–8 Stage II cingulumotomy, lateral skull x-ray; lesion made posterior to position shown in Figure 101–6; note porencephaly (*arrows around air pocket*) where previous lesions were made anterior to present electrode position. (From Foltz, E. L.: The role of the limbic system in pain interpretation. Ariz. Med., *26*:1033–1040, 1969. Reprinted by permission.)

than those due to operative manipulation are encountered if the lesion is placed too far back in the cingulum bundle.[2,23] In those cases a syndrome described by Meyer as marasmus is encountered.[38] It consists of a severe unresponsiveness associated with akinesia, mutism, and lack of spontaneity. These changes may be due to involvement of the anterior thalamic projections and are avoided if the lesion is anterior to the plane of the anterior commissure.

Patients with primary complaints of intolerable pain may respond well to rostral cingulumotomy. Included in this catagory are patients with "psychogenic pain," paroxysmal pain from obviously nonneoplastic organic lesions that nevertheless have an emotional relationship, and patients with neoplastic disease compounded by emotional factors. Long-term follow-ups of these patients show that the results must be measured in behavior patterns and not in

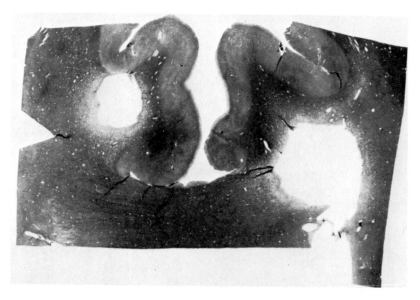

Figure 135–9 Photomicrograph of bilateral cingulum lesions (From Foltz, E. L., and White, L. E., Jr.: Rostral cingulumotomy and pain "relief." *In* Knighton, R. S., and Dumke, P. R., eds.: Pain. Boston, Little, Boston & Co., 1966. Reprinted by permission.)

verbal complaints. Cingulumotomy is only a step in the long-term supportive care of such patients.

CONCLUSION

Review of the structure of the pain pathways, the physiological and behavioral data that relate this system with the limbic lobe, and recent data on the pharmacology of the putative transmitters of the cerebral nervous systems establishes a clear relationship between these areas and the clinical notions of pain and suffering. Empirical clinical data clearly indicate that disruption of the classic pain pathways is effective in controlling pain generated by a destructive process such as cancer or inflammation.[52] Similar lesions produced to control the pain of a nondestructive, apparently healed process, however, is singularly unrewarding. Therapeutically, the neurological surgeon must consider this distinction when evaluating the patient with severe pain.

Both empirical clinical data and mounting laboratory information suggest that there are two origins of the complaint of pain. First, a "dynamic" situation exists in which tissue destruction is taking place. In this situation, anatomically adequate operations on the primary pain pathway have almost uniformly good results. Second, there is a "static" situation in which a nondestructive healed lesion exists but is perceived as pain by the individual. It is in this situation that destructive operations on the primary pain pathway usually fail. Anxiety and depression are commonly associated with the latter and, when resistant to the usual therapeutic forms of management, may be helped by operative interruption of transmission pathways within the limbic lobe.

Since the enkephalin response by opiate receptor areas of the brain produces considerable mitigation of the pain response, similar in nature to the effect of morphine itself, it is reasonable to postulate that new techniques will be developed that are designed to activate that chemical system. Possibly cingulumotomy already acts in this manner by reduction or partial destruction of an inhibitory control system to the enkephalin response.

Cingulumotomy for intractable pain as an affective disorder is not an end-stage procedure. The procedure does nothing to alter the perception of pain. Rather, operative damage to the limbic structures allows the individual to restore homeostatic balance and live with his pain. Those responsible for the aftercare of these individuals must continue supportive measures to maintain homeostatic balance. These patients must have proper long-term care. Otherwise many of them will simply revert to their preoperative status and be considered failures. This reversion appears to be due to the fact that the ability to suffer is as basic as life itself.

REFERENCES

1. Anand, B. K., and Brobeck, J. R.: Localization of a "feeding center" in the hypothalamus of the rat. Proc. Soc. Exp. Biol. Med., 77:323, 1951.
2. Atkinson, J. R.: Personal communication, 1968.
3. Atkinson, J. R.: Pain Clinic. Phoenix, Ariz., Barrow Neurologic Institute, 1968.
4. Barber, T. X.: The effects of "hypnosis" on pain. Psychosom. Med., 25:303, 1963.
5. Bard, P.: Central nervous mechanisms for the expression of anger in animals. In Reymert, M. L., ed.: Feelings and Emotions. New York, McGraw Hill Book Co., 1950, p. 211.
6. Bard, P., and Mountcastle, V. B.: Some forebrain mechanisms involved in expression of rage with special reference to suppression of angry behavior. Ass. Res. Nerv. Ment. Dis., 27:362, 1948.
7. Bard, P., and Rioch, P. M.: A study of four cats deprived of neocortex and additional portions of the forebrain. Bull. Johns Hopk. Hosp., 60:73, 1937.
8. Beecher, H. K.: Pain in men wounded in battle. Ann. Surg., 123:96, 1946.
9. Beecher, H. K.: Relationship of significance of wound to pain experienced. J.A.M.A., 161:1609, 1956.
10. Bonica, J., and White, L. E., Jr.: Pain Clinic, University of Washington School of Medicine, Seattle Wash., 1965.
11. Brady, J. V.: Emotional behavior. In Magoun, H. W., ed.: Handbook of Physiology. Sec. I, Neurophysiology. Vol. III. Baltimore, Williams & Wilkens Co., 1960, 1529.
12. Brobeck, J. R.: Regulation of feeding and drinking. In Magoun, H. W., ed.: Handbook of Physiology. Sec. I, Neurophysiology. Vol. II. Baltimore, Williams & Wilkins Co., 1960.
13. Chronister, R. B., and White, L. E., Jr.: Fiberarchitecture of the hippocampal formation: Anatomy, projections, and structural significance. In Isaacson, R. L., and Pribram, K. H., eds.: The Hippocampus. Vol. I. New York, Plenum Press, 1975, p. 9.
14. Cobb, S.: Emotions and Clinical Medicine. New York, W. W. Norton & Co., 1950.
15. Cobb, S.: A pain in the neck. Harvard Med. Alumni Bull. p. 9, Feb. 1960.
16. Crawford, M. P., Fulton, J. F., Jacobsen, C. F.,

and Wolfe, J. B.: Frontal lobe ablation in chimpanzee: A resume of "Becky" and "Lucy." Ass. Res. Nerv. Ment. Dis., 27:3, 1948.

17. Darwin, C. R.: The Expression of the Emotions in Man and Animals. New York, D. Appleton & Co., 1873.

18. Elliot Smith, G.: Some problems relating to the evolution of the brain. Lancet, 1:1, 147, 221, 1910.

19. Fields, H. L., Clanton, C. H., Basbaum, A. I., and Anderson, S. D.: Medullary control of spinal dorsal horn neurons. Neurosci. Abstr., 2:934, 1976.

20. Foltz, E. L.: The role of the limbic system in pain interpretation. Ariz. Med., 26:1033, 1969.

21. Foltz, E. L., and White, L. E., Jr.: Experimental cingulumotomy and modification of morphine withdrawal. J. Neurosurg., 14:655, 1957.

22. Foltz, E. L., and White, L. E., Jr.: Pain "relief" by frontal cingulumotomy. J. Neurosurg., 19:89, 1962.

23. Foltz, E. L., and White, L. E., Jr.: Rostral cingulumotomy and pain "relief." In Knighton, R. S., and Dumke, P. R., eds.: Pain. Boston, Little, Brown & Co., 1966.

24. Foltz, E. L., and White, L. E., Jr.: The role of rostral cingulumotomy in "pain" relief. Int. J. Neurol., 6:353, 1968.

25. Fordyce, W. F., Fowler, R. S., and Lehman, J. F.: Some implications of learning in problems of chronic pain. J. Chron. Dis., 21:179, 1968.

26. French, J. D., von Amerongen, F. K., and Magoun, H. W.: An activating system in brain stem of monkey. Arch. Neurol. Psychiat., 68:577, 1952.

27. Fulton, J. F. Frontal Lobotomy and Affective Behavior. New York, W. W. Norton & Co., 1951.

28. Fuxe, K., Hökfelt, T., and Ungerstedt, U.: Morphological and functional aspects of central monoamine neurons. Int. Rev. Neurobiol., 13:93, 1970.

29. Grantham, E. G.: Prefrontal lobotomy for relief of pain. J. Neurosurg., 8:405, 1951.

30. Herrick, C. J.: The functions of the olfactory parts of the cerebral cortex. Proc. Nat. Acad. Sci., 19:7, 1933.

31. Hines, M.: Studies in the growth and differentiation of the telencephalon in man. J. Comp. Neurol., 34:73, 1922.

32. Hosobuchi, Y., Adams, J. E., and Linchitz, R.: Pain relief by electrical stimulation of the central gray matter in humans. Neurosci. Abstr., 2:940, 1976.

33. Jacobson, C. F.: Functions of frontal association areas in primates. Arch. Neurol. Psychiat., 33:558, 1935.

34. Kaada, B. R.: Cingulate, posterior orbital, anterior insular and temporal pole cortex. In Handbook of Physiology. Sec. I, Neurophysiology. Vol. II. Baltimore, Williams & Wilkins Co., 1960.

35. Kluver, H., and Bucy, P. C.: An analysis of certain effects of bilateral temporal lobectomy in the rhesus monkey, with special reference to "psychic blindness." J. Psychol. 5:33, 1938.

36. Koskoff, Y. D., Dennis, W., Lazovik, D., and Wheeler, E. T.: The psychological effects of frontal lobotomy performed for the alleviation of pain. Ass. Res. Nerv. Ment. Dis., 27:723, 1948.

37. Krieg, W. J. S.: Connections of the frontal cortex of the monkey. Springfield, Ill., Charles C Thomas, 1954.

38. Meyer, A., and Beck, E.: Prefrontal leucotomy and related operations. Edinburgh, Oliver & Byrd Ltd., 1954.

39. Miller, N. E.: Learning of visceral and glandular responses. Science, 163:434, 1969.

40. Moniz, E.: Tentative Operations dans le Traitement de Certaines Psychoses. Paris, Masson & Cie, 1936.

41. Oliveras, J. L., Hosobuchi, Y., Redjemi, F., Guilbaud, G., and Bessen, J. M.: Opiate antagonist, naloxone, strongly reduces analgesia induced by stimulation of a raphe nucleus (centralis inferior). Brain Res., 120:221–229, 1977.

42. Papez, J. W.: A proposed mechanism of emotion. Arch. Neurol. Psychiat., 38:728, 1937.

43. Skinner, B. F.: The Behavior of Organisms: An Experimental Analysis. New York, Appleton-Century Co., 1938.

44. Snyder, S. H., and Simanton, R.: The opiate receptors and opiod peptides. J. Neurochem., 28:13–20, 1977.

45. Stead, E. A., Jr.: Why doctoring is difficult. Res. Staff Physician, p. 37, Nov. 1969.

46. Sternbach, R. A.: Pain: A Psychophysiological Analysis. New York, London, Academic Press, 1968.

47. Walker, A. E.: Afferent connections. In Bucy, P. C., ed.: The Precentral Motor Cortex. Urbana, Ill., University of Illinois Press, 1944.

48. Ward, A. A., Jr.: The cingular gyrus. Area 24. J. Neurophysiol., 11:15, 1948.

49. Ward, A. A., Jr.: The anterior cingulate gyrus and personality. Ass. Res. Nerv. Ment. Dis. Proc., 27:438, 1947.

50. Watts, J. W.: and Freeman, W.: Psychosurgery in the relief of unbearable pain. J. Int. Coll. Surg., 9:679, 1946.

51. Watts, J. W., and Freeman, W.: Frontal lobotomy in the treatment of unbearable pain. Ass. Res. Nerv. Ment. Dis. Proc., 27:715–722, 1948.

52. White, J. C., and Sweet, W. H.: Pain and the Neurosurgeon. Springfield, Ill., Charles C Thomas, 1969.

53. White, L. E., Jr.: Pain Clinic Concept. Pain Clinic; University of Washington, College of Medicine, unpublished observations, 1970.

54. White, L. E., Jr.: A morphologic concept of the limbic lobe. Int. Rev. Neurobiol., 8:1, 1965.

55. White, L. E., Jr., and Alvord, E. C., Jr.: Embryologic significance of variations in arrhinencephalic anomalies. Anat. Rec., 145:356, 1964.

56. White, L. E., Jr., Nelson, W. M., and Foltz, E. L.: Cingulum fasciculus study by evoked potentials. Exp. Neurol., 2:406, 1960.

57. Yakovlev, P.: In White, J. C., and Sweet, W. H., eds.: Pain and the Neurosurgeon. Springfield, Ill., Charles C Thomas, 1969, p. 773.

136

INTRACEREBRAL ELECTRICAL STIMULATION FOR THE RELIEF OF CHRONIC PAIN

Relief of chronic pain by stimulation of electrodes implanted in the human brain was first reported by Heath in 1954 and by Pool and associates in 1956.[10,31] To targets in the septal area just anterior and lateral to the anterior columns of the fornix they delivered currents of about 4 ma. They made the observation, often confirmed at many cerebral and other neural sites since, that when relief of pain occurred it might long outlast the stimulus. In some cancer patients relief persisted as long as two to three weeks following a single session of stimulation, and these results were repeatable. In 1960 Heath and Mickle reported that septal stimulation relieved intractable pain in six nonpsychiatric patients—two with rheumatoid arthritis and four with advanced cancer. Not only was relief immediate upon starting stimulation, but the patients "appeared alerted" and "spoke more rapidly" as well. Almost daily stimulation was necessary, but it yielded repeatable relief.[11] In Gol's series of six patients who received septal stimulation, however, satisfactory relief of pain occurred in only one of them.[9] A minor complication in one of Pool's patients, whose electrodes apparently were over the supraoptic nuclei, was diabetes insipidus for three days after a session of stimulation at 3 ma. Initially, stimulation in this area evoked smiles, pleasant feelings, and a cessation of pain. Not quite so minor were temporary rage reactions, which in two other cancer patients followed stimulation near the anterior commissure.[21]

At an electrode in the caudate nucleus, the target chosen by Ervin, Brown, and Mark, stimulation yielded not only pain relief but also some cheerfulness in a previously most unhappy man with an advanced cancer that was invading the pharynx and cranial base. Like stimulation in the septal area, stimulation in the caudate nucleus was effective in relieving pain but caused no sensation anywhere in the body and no objective neurological changes. This finding permitted the Ervin group to make double-blind studies that confirmed that both the patient and an observer could note the favorable effects on pain and mood that were coincident only with actual stimulation.[6] Gol, however, was unable to achieve any fruitful response from a wide range of stimuli delivered to 6 to 12 electrodes in the caudate nucleus in each of four patients.[9] The only recent use of targets in septal or caudate nuclei or both has been by Martin-Rodriguez and colleagues in five patients; a long-term follow-up has not been reported.[23]

AREAS OF STIMULATION

The thalamic nucleus ventralis posteromedialis or posterolateralis, the posterior limb of the internal capsule lateral to these nuclei, and the periventricular gray matter

---

W. H. SWEET

lying in the inferoposteromedial thalamus adjoining the wall of the third ventricle near the posterior commissure are now the three most extensively used sites.

Nuclei Ventralis Posterior Medialis and Ventralis Posterior Lateralis

Target coordinates, as given by Mazars; are 5 to 10 mm in front of and at a horizontal level 0 to 1 mm above the line from posterior commissure to foramen of Munro; distance from midline for lower limb 14 to 18 mm; for upper limb 9 to 14 mm; for face 7 to 9 mm.[27] The position of the electrode is checked by noting a sharply local reference of stimulus-evoked sensation and evoked action potential typical of the response from the nucleus ventralis posterior medialis or ventralis posterior lateralis.

The first implantations into this area were done by Mazars. His successes have led to his building up the largest series of intracerebral electrode placements in the world, and to the adoption of this site of placement by many other neurological surgeons. Beginning in 1961, he left electrodes in some portion of the thalamic nucleus ventralis posterior for periods of days up to as long as two months. Such a temporary placement was performed in 17 patients during circa 10 years until 1972, often yielding months to years of relief.[26]

In 1966 Adams was treating a patient with pain due to a peripheral nerve injury in the arm. Upon stimulation to locate the nucleus ventralis posterior lateralis before making a lesion therein, he found that evocation of sensory paresthesias immediately suppressed the patient's pain.[3] Adams and his associates began implantation of electrodes in the thalamus in 1971.[15]

Mazars soon discovered that none of his patients with cancer pain secured relief from such stimulation, and he proceeded cautiously to expand his observations on patients whose chronic pain was from nonlethal causes until he had excluded the possibility that the relief was based on a psychotherapeutic or placebo effect. From 1972 until 1975 he implanted electrodes in the thalamic nucleus ventralis posterior in 27 more patients, having established that some individuals secured relief from low intensities of stimulation that caused no subjective sensation. The leads were con-

nected to a battery placed in an infraclavicular subcutaneous pocket.[27]

Current Methods

The implanted battery has been replaced by an implanted subcutaneous radiofrequency receiver activated by an external power source via leads to a circular antenna that is applied to the skin over the receiver. In general, wherever the intracerebral electrodes are placed, a preliminary testing as developed both by Mazars and by Hosobuchi, Adams, and Rutkin is used.[15,27]

One or several electrodes can be inserted into one or more intracerebral targets; their leads are passed through the scalp and then attached to an external battery-supplied source of current. The degree of pain relief following stimulation at each of the target sites is then assessed for one to many weeks. If worthwhile relief is obtained, the leads are placed internally and connected to the subcutaneously implanted receiver for long-term use. A criterion for correct electrode placement in the thalamic specific-sensory relay nuclei—ventralis posterior medialis for the face, ventralis posterior lateralis for the other parts of the body—and in the posterior limb of the internal capsule as well, is the occurrence on stimulation of sensations referred to the contralateral clinically painful area. The thresholds for these stimulus-induced paresthesias vary greatly within the same structure—e.g., from lows of 0.15 to 0.30 ma up to 5 to 7 ma as recorded by Boëthius and co-workers. Pulse duration can also be critical; in one case increase from 100 to 300 μ-sec caused the paresthesias to spread from the hand and face to the entire half of the body.[5] Bipolar stimulation here and at the other sites to be discussed has come to be preferred to monopolar stimulation. The electrode itself is usually a cylinder about 1 mm in diameter by 1 to 2 mm in height. Stainless steel electrodes, used originally by Hosobuchi and associates for a temporary implant, tend to develop increased resistance around them —from 2000 to 5000 ohms in nine months in one patient.[15] Platinum electrodes are much less likely to develop this problem. A systematic exploration of the parameters of pulse duration and of frequency and amplitude of stimulus is advisable in each patient.

The first patient of Hosobuchi and co-workers found that the facial pain of his trigeminal anesthesia dolorosa was relieved within a few seconds of the beginning of stimulation. The pain recurred, however, in 60 to 90 seconds. If the current was turned off the pain disappeared within another few seconds, only to recur in another one to one and a half minutes. Continuing relief was achieved by designing a generator to produce a "ramp-type" signal that increased linearly from 0.5 to 4.5 v for about 30 seconds, then shut off and repeated.[15]

Therapeutic stimulation must be used sparingly—at most a few hours a day—in order to avoid the development of tolerance, the electrical analog of tachyphylaxis to drugs. If adaptation with decreasing efficacy appears, useful relief can sometimes be regained if all stimulation is stopped for days or weeks. In this respect the behavior is similar to that often seen after stimulation of posterior columns of the cord or peripheral nerves. In the most favorable cases, however, including some of the earliest of Mazars, long-term relief (i.e., for years) ensues after a few interrupted minutes or hours of stimulation. One of Mazar's first patients required only a few few-minute bursts of stimulation over a three-day period to achieve a suppression of his pain that continues 13 years later; the chronic pain had been persisting in the chest following avulsion of intercostal nerves.[27]

Electrode Placements

By 1978 Mazars had 121 patients with electrodes in the nucleus ventralis posterior medialis or ventralis posterior lateralis. His best success rate was in patients with "deafferentation pain." This expression has come to be applied to the chronically painful disorders listed in Tables 136–1 and 136–2. Mazar's ranking of his results is given in Table 136–1. All his patients with good results had some objective sensory deficit due to the lesion causing the pain, although many of the failures also showed such deficits. One patient had burning pain in one side of the face and the corresponding upper limb following pontomesencephalic infarction. This pain was relieved by the thalamic stimulation that did not help later pain due to newly developing gouty tophi in the thumb on the same painful side. Colchicin did stop the latter pain. The failure to relieve the pain of gout is evidence

TABLE 136–1   RESULTS OF STIMULATION AT NUCLEI VENTRALIS POSTEROMEDIALIS AND POSTEROLATERALIS*

TYPE OF PAIN	SUCCESS	FAILURE
Deafferentation pain		
Anesthesia dolorosa	8	1
Brachial plexus lesion	11	2
Brain stem infarct	5	1
Cord injury	2	0
Hand operation	18	0
Phantom limb	22	1
Postherpetic	5	6
Postradiation arm pain		
with edema	3	0
Post-traumatic hyperpathia	2	0
Thalamic	0	6
Miscellaneous	10	0
Total	84	17
Other Pain		
Cancer	0	17
Rhizopathy	0	4
Tic douloureux	0	1
Total	0	22

* Data from Mazars, G.: État actuel de la chirurgie de la douleur. Neurochirurgie (suppl.), 22:1–164, 1976, and as cited by Meyerson, B. A.: "European" Study on Deep Brain Stimulation. Resumé of the 3rd European Workshop on Electrical Neurostimulation, Megeve, March 30–31, 1979.

that a procedure that helps centrally induced pain may not affect a peripherally caused chronic pain. Mazars regards the case of the patient with gout and his results as a whole as being explained by the fact that those pains accompanied by sensory deficits may be relieved by stimulation of the portion of the thalamus that subserves the area with the deficit. On the other hand, those patients without a sensory deficit in whom there is in his phrase "an excess of nociception" do not secure relief from such stimulation. In addition to Mazar's uninterrupted series of failures in his "other" group, his patients without sensory deficit, he found central pains of "thalamic" type to be in the same category. Postherpetic neuralgia also was helped in less than 50 per cent of the patients. He does not describe any correlation between degree of objective sensory loss and degree of pain relief in any of these groups.[26,27]

Thresholds to pain evoked by pinprick or other pain-provoking tests are not raised by stimulation at the low therapeutic intensities. At higher current intensities, however, and at frequencies from 50 to 100 per second that evoke intense paresthesias, there is a higher threshold not only to various tests for pain but also to tests of sensory discrimination.

TABLE 136-2   RESULTS OF PERMANENT ELECTRODE IMPLANTATION OR PERCUTANEOUS TEST STIMULATION*

	ELECTRODE SITE							
	Periventricular Gray				Nuclei Ventralis Posterolateralis and Posteromedialis		Posterior Limb of Internal Capsule	
	Richardson		Cooperative Study					
	Patients Relieved†		Patients Relieved†		Patients Relieved†		Patients Relieved†	
TYPE OF PAIN	>50%	<50%	>50%	<50%	>50%	<50%	>50%	<50%
Deafferentation pain								
Anesthesia dolorosa		—	3(1)	12	7(2)	14	(1)	1
Brachial plexus lesion	1	0	9	7	1	2	0	2
Cord injury	2	3	2	4	1	2	1	5
Phantom limb	0	1	3	8	2(1)	3	1	0
Postcordotomy	—		—		1	0	3	1
Postherpetic	0	1	0	3	1	3	—	
Thalamic	1	1	2	6	1	11	4	12
Non-specified	—		0	17	—		—	
Total	4	6	19(1)	57	14(3)	35	9(1)	21
"Neurogenic" pain								
Low back syndrome	7	5	20(2)	4	(1)	0	—	
Cervical rhizopathy	—		1	0	—		—	
Peripheral nerve lesion	—		3	2	—		—	
Scoliosis and arthritis	3	0	—		—		—	
Other	1	0	(1)	1	—		—	
Total	11	5	24(3)	7	(1)	0		
Cancer pain								
Visceral	—		3(3)	1	—		—	
Metastatic	—		11	15	—		—	
Non specified	3	1	3(1)	3	—		—	
Total	3	1	17(4)	19	—		—	
Grand total	18	12	60(8)	83	14(6)	35	9(1)	21

* Data from reports of international cooperative study (Meyerson, B. A.: "European" Study on Deep Brain Stimulation Resumé of the 3rd European Workshop on Electrical Neurostimulation, Megeve, March 30–31, 1979) and of Richardson and Akil (Pain reduction by electrical brain stimulation in man. Part 1. Acute administration in periaqueductal and periventricular sites. J. Neurosurg., 47:178–183, 1977; Pain reduction by electrical brain stimulation. Part 2. Chronic self-administration in the periventricular gray matter. J. Neurosurg., 47:184–194, 1977; Long term results of periventricular gray self-stimulation. Neurosurgery, 1:199–202, 1977).

† Numbers in parentheses indicate cases with decreasing effect during follow-up.

By 1977 Adams and colleagues had implanted electrodes in the specific-sensory nuclei in only 11 of their 39 patients who had permanent intracerebral placements. (There were also 27 patients who did not obtain relief upon temporary implantation whose electrodes were withdrawn.) Facial pain associated with anesthesia or analgesia or both was the problem in 7 of these 11; in all 7 the nucleus ventralis posterior medialis was the target. These investigators record the resulting relief as "+" if the pain no longer requires medication, as "±" if continuing stimulation enables the patient to reduce his intake of medication, and as "0" if there is no relief. In the group with facial pain three patients were in the "+" category, three were in the "±" category, and one moved into the "0" group after 15 months in the "±" group.

A cooperative study involving 13 groups of neurosurgeons from three continents has been undertaken, and the preliminary results in 203 cases have been assembled by Meyerson.[29] The two large series of Richardson and of Mazars are not included. The 56 cases from the Adams-Hosobuchi group form the largest single component of the cooperative study.

Table 136–2 records the combined results of this group both for the patients with temporary electrodes and for the individuals who later had the electrodes permanently implanted. The patients were classified as having either more than 50 per cent or less than 50 per cent relief of pain. Those indicated by the numbers enclosed in parentheses began with relief that was more than 50 per cent but decreased during follow-up. The results of Richardson and Akil, indicated separately, are classified in the same fashion.[36]

Of the 52 patients in the "deafferentation" group with electrodes in the nucleus ventralis posterior medialis or ventralis posterior lateralis, nearly half had anesthesia dolorosa. Only 7 of the 23 were maintaining 50 per cent relief, a degree of alleviation that was probably not satisfactory for some of them. In agreement with Mazars' findings, the group had their worst results with thalamic pain.

Turnbull and colleagues describe complete relief obtained with ventralis posterior medialis or ventralis posterior lateralis implants in 7 of 11 patients, 8 with lumbar arachnoiditis and 3 with post-traumatic neuropathy. Relief was probably greater than 50 per cent in two more of these. Although the authors classify them all as having a "neuropathic pain" of deafferentation, most neurological surgeons do not include such patients in the deafferentation category and have not treated them by using electrodes in the nucleus ventralis posterior medialis or ventralis posterior lateralis. The Turnbull group has achieved successes in three patients in the orthodox deafferentation category—complete relief of pain after a midbrain injury and probably more than 50 per cent relief in one patient with avulsion of the brachial plexus and another with a painful amputation stump.[38]

Posterior Limb of Internal Capsule

Coordinates for the target site in the posterior limb of the internal capsule lateral to thalamic specific-sensory relay nuclei, as given by Adams and co-workers, are: Horizontal plane: from 8 mm behind the midpoint of the line between anterior and posterior commissures to the posterior commissure point; Coronal plane: 1 mm below to 4 mm above the midpoint of the anterior commissure to posterior commissure line; Parasagittal plane: 20 to 24 mm lateral to the midline.[1]

An unplanned lateral shift of the implanted electrode into the posterior limb of the internal capsule in one of Adams's cases led to the adventitious but astute observation that this could be a rewarding site of stimulation for suppression of pain. The first patient in whom Adams deliberately implanted electrodes in the posterior limb

of the internal capsule had excruciating spontaneous pain and hyperpathia in the distal halves of both left limbs following a major right temporoparietal injury. Acting on the assumption that the injury had destroyed some of the normal cortical suppressor mechanisms for pain, Fields and Adams sought to reinforce the remaining suppressor mechanism by stimulating the pathways to or from the right cerebral cortex. Stimulation here may well involve a higher-order neuron than does stimulation of the nucleus ventralis posterior lateralis or ventralis posterior medialis. In any event, their success was spectacular with this patient. In this patient and in others, correct electrode placement in the posterior limb of the internal capsule is demonstrated by paresthesias such as light tingling and vibration referred to the affected areas. Slight increases in the amplitude or frequency of the stimulus increase the intensity of the sensation, and further increases may induce muscle contraction. Days of complete relief may follow minutes of low-intensity stimulation. At times pain relief ensues from electrical input so small that there are no stimulation-induced paresthesias, but most patients usually are aware of some sensation when effective stimulation is being delivered. In the first patient of Fields and Adams the inhibiting effect was remarkably specific in stopping the spontaneous pain and the hyperpathia such as the spreading electrical sensations evoked by repeated pinprick. Yet, interestingly enough, stimulation, if anything, "enhanced the sharpness and hurting quality of the local sensation to pinprick *to the same area*." There was no improvement in the impaired two-point discrimination or stereognosis during or following stimulation.[7] Boëthius and associates have confirmed that stimulation both in the posterior limb of the internal capsule and in the nuclei ventralis posterior medialis and ventralis posterior lateralis does not change the thresholds for tactile, vibratory, thermal, or mechanical painful stimuli either inside or outside the area of clinical pain. Moreover, these thresholds remain the same whether the stimulation does or does not relieve the clinical pain.[5]

Lesions of the cerebral hemispheres that provoke chronic pain are rare. The results of stimulation in the posterior limb of the internal capsule for pain of other causes have become poorer as the patients have been viewed more critically and the follow-ups have lengthened. Thus Adams and his colleagues reported 50 per cent or better relief in their first 3 patients with the thalamic syndrome, and Hosobuchi reported that 8 of 10 patients with the thalamic syndrome responded well to long-term stimulation of the posterior limb of the internal capsule.[1,13] In another report of results from the same group, however, none of these 10 patients was placed in their plus column.[3] In the "deafferentation pain" categories as reported by the cooperative study, only that for postcordotomy dysesthesias shows a majority of patients with more than 50 per cent pain relief. In the cooperative study about one third of the patients sustained relief greater than 50 per cent; a bit better than the results of stimulation for deafferentation pain at the other sites.[29]

Periventricular Gray Matter of Inferoposteromedial Thalamus

Target coordinates for the site in the periventricular gray matter of the inferoposteromedial thalamus adjoining the wall of the third ventricle near the posterior commissure, as given by Richardson and Akil (from the Schaltenbrand-Bailey Atlas), are Horizontal plane 0; Coronal plane posterior 10; Parasagittal plane 3 to 7 mm, depending on width of third ventricle.[35]

Animal experimentation, as reported first by Reynolds in rats, has revealed that unilateral electrical stimulation at the perimeter of the mesencephalic central gray matter lateral to the aqueduct produces such an effective generalized analgesia to acute painful stimuli that paws and tail can be pinched with a hemostat and a laparotomy can be performed with no aversive movements. Yet the animals struggle in response to quick movements in their visual fields or to loud noises.[32] Other work has shown that in most rats the peripheral field of analgesia is usually restricted to half of one quadrant of the body. Studies from other laboratories have confirmed this basic observation, extended it to other species, and presented evidence that the potent suppressor effect specifically on acute noxious stimuli is mediated both by descending pathways to cells in the cord's posterior horns and by ascending pathways.[25]

The state of analgesia to acute noxa outlasted by only a few minutes the termination of stimulation. The animals were otherwise behaviorally normal even after several months of long-term stimulation. Electrolytic lesions in this central gray area did not produce analgesia, further evidence that an active inhibitory mechanism for pain was operative.[20]

Richardson and Akil were the first to assay the effectiveness of stimulation of these areas in man. Working first with four patients with chronic pain who were scheduled for thalamic lesions, they explored the medial thalamus and the length of the periaqueductal mesencephalic gray matter with a stimulating electrode. They quickly established that stimulation at tegmental and periaqueductal mesencephalic sites was likely to cause unacceptable dizziness, dyspnea, nystagmus, and other oculomotor or visual disturbances. Hence the sites that were most effective in animals were not feasible in man. In three of the four patients, however, stimulation in the posterior medial thalamus, especially at the nucleus parafascicularis, relieved the chronic pain. The fourth patient, with cancer pain, was not relieved. Neither he nor two of the patients who were relieved had any reduction of pinprick sensation, but the third patient who was relieved—of intense pain in an arm and leg associated with the thalamic syndrome—had "complete bilateral analgesia to pinprick that outlasted the stimulation by three to five minutes."[34] In general, they found that unilateral electrode stimulation might relieve bilateral pain, but with greater relief contralaterally. Of the first five patients with implants, all had some reduction in pinprick sensation bilaterally during stimulation—but by no means the unresponsiveness described as analgesia to crushing pinch that was seen in animals. The patients also had a modest elevation of their pain thresholds both to graded radiant heat and to controlled ischemia. These increases were correlated with good clinical results. In another patient with poor pain relief, the thresholds to pain of pinprick and radiant heat were unaltered.[35] Boëthius and co-workers also found that in man such stimulation might raise pain thresholds to pinprick, heat, and cold in all four limbs, whereas thresholds for vibratory stimuli were unchanged.[5] The initial good results of Richardson and Akil led them to place temporary implants in the periventricular gray matter in 30 patients and to make these permanent in 27 of them within 1 to 13 weeks. Any paresthesias evoked during low-intensity stimulation were *usually not related to the sites of chronic pain*—a marked difference between this response and that evoked from the other two sites. A sensation of heat or cold either fairly focal or involving the whole trunk, however, usually indicated a good electrode placement for pain control. This response was seen in 16 patients; tingling and other paresthesias occurred in 11; visual symptoms, mainly blurred vision with nystagmus noted in 8, and startle or nervousness in 4 patients completed the principal subjective responses to stimulation. By careful selection of the minimal parameters giving pain relief, disagreeable responses could usually be avoided. Typically patients were able to reduce their stimulation gradually so that 30-minute periods two or three times per day sufficed. In their fourth patient, in whom the stimulation was becoming ineffective, the good result was recouped by adding 150 mg amitriptyline and 3 mg fluphenazine per day to the regimen. These drugs alone were ineffective, but they did increase the effectiveness of the brain stimulation and enabled the patient to resume full-time work. This finding led Richardson and Akil to prescribe amitriptyline routinely, 100 mg daily at bedtime, for all patients. The electrode has been placed on one side only; for bilateral pain the side opposite the more intense pain is chosen. If the pain is equal on the two sides, implantation is in the nondominant hemisphere.[35,36] Although Hosobuchi and Adams have used two electrode arrays, they too usually place them on one side only.[2,13]

Results in Periventricular Gray Matter

Richardson and Akil have confined their electrode placements to the periventricular gray area, and the results they report have been tabulated separately in Table 136–2. Two thirds of their patients, 18 of 30, had greater than 50 per cent relief of pain. In a particularly vexing group of patients, those who had had multiple operations on the lower part of the back, they not only achieved this degree of relief in 7 of 12 but they returned all 7 either to work or to ac-

tivity levels consistent with their physical defects.[36] Hosobuchi and Plotkin both describe even better results with scores, respectively, of 8 (1) and 3 and 12(1) and 1, (lumped together in Table 136–2 as 20(2) and 4.[14,30] These were the only two surgeons in the cooperative study who did this operation for the "low back syndrome."

The generalization ventured by Mazars is that pains due to "an excess of nociception" are unaffected by stimulation to the specific-sensory thalamic nuclei, and those accompanied by sensory deficit are almost certain to be helped. His two exceptions to the latter half of the rule are the thalamic syndrome and postherpetic neuralgia.[27] The results of other surgeons do not accord quite so well. Thus for deafferentation pain the cooperative group reports only 27 per cent good results from stimulating the ventralis posterior lateralis–ventralis posterior medialis nuclei, actually worse than their 33 per cent good results from periventricular gray. Richardson records 40 per cent good results from periventricular gray in these patients.

The results in cancer pain are difficult to evaluate because, as Meyersen points out, these patients become less motivated to continue stimulation as their condition deteriorates and often prefer to resume taking medication.[29] If the electrode leads are conducted through a long subgaleal course and then out through the scalp, it is likely that they can be left in position for many months until the patient dies. Thus, the extra expense of internalizing the system can be eliminated. If cancer pain is to be treated by stimulation, the patient should have a life expectancy of at least four to six months.

Complications

Mazars, Adams and co-workers, and Richardson and Akil have all described their problems as being principally of a technical character with relatively few infections and operatively induced neurological deficits.[3,26,36] A detailed breakdown of the complications in the patients of Richardson and Akil was: broken wiring in three, migration of electrode in two, electronic failure of device in one, meningitis in three, infected device in one, hemiparesis in one, and transient hemiparesis in two.[36]

MECHANISMS OF RELIEF

Opiate receptors—structures that stereo-specifically bind morphine and its analogs —have been identified in high concentration in certain parts of the brain, of which one of the areas with the highest concentration is the midbrain periaqueductal gray matter.[19] The opiate receptors have apparently developed to bind endogenous substances, "the brain's own morphine." Hughes and colleagues have established the precise composition of two pentapeptides in the brain, named by them met- and leu-enkephalin. These mimic morphine by binding to the same "opiate receptor" sites, including the periaqueductal gray area.[18] This area contains dense concentrations of both enkephalin terminals and enkephalin cell bodies, as shown by Hökfelt and associates, and microinjections of met-enkephalin into this area produce analgesia.[8,12] This analgesia like that of morphine is effectively antagonized by the drug naloxone.[21] There is a cross-tolerance between morphine and stimulation in the periventricular gray, a fact that also points to involvement of the same neural system for both of them.[24]

These animal studies concerning pain were placed on a firmer basis by observations in patients, about the occurrence of whose pain one can be more positive. Adams has reported a patient whose chronic pain was completely relieved by stimulation in periventricular gray matter. Naloxone in a total dose of 0.6 mg intravenously completely counteracted this pain relief, which, however, reappeared about one hour after the final increment of naloxone.[2] The Adams group later reported this same naloxone reversal of pain relief in five of six patients.[16] Akil and colleagues, testing several patients whose pain was relieved by stimulation in the periventricular gray area, also found the relief to be partially reversible by naloxone in 80 per cent of those tested. In their eight patients they measured the concentration of "enkephalinlike material" in the third ventricle before and during stimulation. A 50 to 80 per cent increase over the baseline level was seen in seven of the eight patients.[4] Hosobuchi and colleagues have also found an increase from 60 to 700 per cent above baseline values for "immunoreactive β-endorphin" in ventricular fluid collected at the foramen of Munro in three patients during pain relief while the periventricular gray was being stimulated and again 30 minutes after stimulation stopped. In three other patients with "deafferentation" pain, however, relief from stimulation in the nucleus ventralis posterior lateralis was accompanied by no change in β-endorphin levels in cerebrospinal fluid collected at the same site.[14] (β-Endorphin is the naturally occurring peptide found in the hypothalamus and diencephalon but principally in the pituitary gland as residues 61–91 in the larger pituitary peptide β-lipotropin.) The suggestion is that endogenous enkephalin and endorphin are involved in pain relief related to stimulation of the periventricular gray but not to that of the ventralis posterior lateralis–ventralis posterior medialis nuclei.

GENERAL APPRAISAL OF THE METHOD

There is a striking discrepancy between the results reported by the original proponents of the three sites of stimulation and those of their successors in these efforts. Thus Mazars reports 82 per cent success in treating deafferentation pain via electrodes in ventralis posterior lateralis and ventralis posterior medialis nuclei (cf. Table 136–1).[27,28] This contrasts sharply with the 27 per cent success rate in the cooperative study in such patients recorded in Table 136–2. Likewise the 40 per cent success rate of Richardson and Akil for electrodes in periventricular gray in deafferentation pain contrasts with the success rate of 25 per cent in the cooperative study. In 1977 Adams and co-workers reported only two cases in the category of low back pain— one as a failure and the other in their ± group.[3] Yet in 1980 Hosobuchi describes an additional 12 apparently consecutive successful cases in this category.[14] The result is a dilemma of trying to decide whether the original advocates are too enthusiastic or whether they have acquired skills not yet possessed by the later comers in the field.

The latter conclusion is suggested by Richardson, who informs the author that his rate of achievement of greater than 50 per cent relief is now approaching 90 per cent. He attributes the improvement to more critical selection of patients by means of initially thorough diagnosis and intensive medically and psychiatrically oriented therapy, an approach that has led to fewer but more successful operations.[33]

It is worth noting that a destructive thalamotomy, in which virtually this same area was the target site for the lesion, was an operation initiated by Mark and colleagues in 1960 and 1963.[22] For over a decade this operation was the most frequently performed stereotaxic brain operation for relief of pain from cancer of the head and neck. A summary of the results from 17 centers was provided recently.[37] It should not be a surprise that stimulation of a zone will not invariably stop pain when destruction of that area has such a result in a gratifyingly high percentage of cases. It is known that not only every cluster of neurons but every neuron in that cluster has playing on it both excitatory and inhibitory impulses. Electrical stimulation indiscriminately activates both types of fibers. With luck, the effect that is sought predominates. When it is possible stereotaxically, intradural introduction of chemicals that will perturb the system in only the desired direction is perhaps likely to achieve more consistent results. Stimulation via intracerebral electrodes for relief of pain is probably only a temporary way station in the quest for understanding of mechanisms of pain and how to control them. If others can, like Turnbull and colleagues, achieve the good results of the original proponents, it will be an attractive way station.[38]

Acknowledgment. The author is grateful for the financial assistance from the Neuro-Research Foundation during the preparation of this manuscript.

REFERENCES

1. Adams, J. E., Hosobuchi, Y., and Fields, H. L.: Stimulation of internal capsule for relief of chronic pain. J. Neurosurg., *41*:740–744, 1974.
2. Adams, J. E.: Naloxone reversal of analgesia produced by brain stimulation in the human. Pain, *2*:161–166, 1976.
3. Adams, J. E., Hosobuchi, Y., and Linchitz, R.: The present status of implantable intracranial stimulators for pain. Clin. Neurosurg., *24*:347–361, 1977.
4. Akil, H., Richardson, D. E., Hughes, J., and Barchas, J. D.: Enkephalin-like material elevated in ventricular cerebrospinal fluid of pain patients after analgetic focal stimulation. Science, *201*:463–465, 1978.
5. Boëthius, J., Lindblom, U., Meyerson, B. A., and Widén, L.: Effects of multifocal brain stimulation on pain and somatosensory functions. *In* Zotterman, Y., ed: Sensory Functions of the Skin. Oxford and New York, Pergamon Press, 1976, pp. 531–548.
6. Ervin, F. R., Brown, C. E., and Mark, V. H.: Striatal influence on facial pain. Confin. Neurol., *27*:75–86, 1966.
7. Fields, H. L., and Adams, J. E.: Pain after cortical injury relieved by electrical stimulation of the internal capsule. Brain, *97*:169–178, 1974.
8. Frenk, H., McCarty, B. C., and Liebeskind, J. C.: Different brain areas mediate the analgesic and epileptic properties of enkephalin. Science, *200*:335–337, 1978.
9. Gol, A.: Relief of pain by electrical stimulation of the septal area. J. Neurol. Sci., *5*:115–120, 1967.
10. Heath, R. G.: Studies in Schizophrenia. Cambridge, Mass., Harvard University Press, 1954.
11. Heath, R. G., and Mickel, W. A.: Evaluation of seven year's experience with depth electrode studies in human patients. *In* Ramey, E. R., and O'Doherty, D. S., eds: Electrical Studies in the Anesthetized Brain. New York, Hoeber Medical Division, Harper & Row, 1960, pp. 214–247.
12. Hökfelt, T., Ljungdahl, Å., Terenius, L., Elde, R., and Nilsson, G.: Immunohistochemical analysis of peptide pathways possibly related to pain and analgesia: Enkephalin and substance P. Proc. Nat. Acad. Sci. U.S.A., *74*:3081–3085, 1977.
13. Hosobuchi, Y.: Chronic brain stimulation for the treatment of intractable pain. Res. Clin. Stud. Headache, *5*:122–126, 1978.
14. Hosobuchi, Y.: Endorphin and analgesic brain stimulation. Presented to Society of Neurological Surgeons, San Francisco, May 26, 1980.
15. Hosobuchi, Y., Adams, J. E., and Rutkin, B.: Chronic thalamic stimulation for the control of facial anesthesia dolorosa. Arch. Neurol. (Chicago), *29*:156–161, 1973.
16. Hosobuchi, Y., Adams, J. E., and Linchitz, R.: Pain relief by electrical stimulation of the central gray matter in humans and its reversal by naloxone. Science, *197*:183–186, 1977.
17. Hosobuchi, Y., Rossier, J., Bloom, F. E., and Guillemin, R.: Stimulation of human periaqueductal gray for pain relief increases immunoreactive β-endorphin in ventricular fluid. Science, *203*:279–281, 1979.
18. Hughes, J., Smith, T. W., Kosterlitz, H. W., Fothergill, L. A., Morgan, B. A., and Morris, H. R.: Identification of two related pentapeptides from the brain with potent agonist activity. Nature, *252*:734–735, 1975.
19. Kuhar, M. J., Pert, C. B., and Snyder, S. H.: Regional distribution of opiate receptor binding in monkey and human brain. Nature, *245*:447–450, 1973.
20. Liebman, J. M., Mayer, D. J., and Liebeskind, J. C.: Mesencephalic central gray lesions and fear-motivated behavior in rats. Brain Res., *23*:353–370, 1970.
21. Lord, J. A. H., Waterfield, J., Hughes, H., and Kosterlitz, H. W.: Endogenous opioid peptides: Multiple agonists and receptors. Nature, *267*:495–499, 1977.
22. Mark, V. H., Ervin, F. R., and Yakovlev, P.: Stereotactic thalamotomy. III. The verification

of anatomical lesion sites in the human thalamus. Arch. Neurol. (Chicago), *8*:528–538, 1963.

23. Martin-Rodriguez, J. G., Delgado, J. M. R., Obrador, S., Santo-Domingo, J., and Alonso, A.: Intractable pain: Dynamics of its psychoneurosurgical approach and brain stimulation. *In* Sweet, W. H., et al., eds: Neurosurgical Treatment in Psychiatry, Pain, and Epilepsy. Baltimore, University Park Press, 1977, pp. 639–649.

24. Mayer, D. H., and Hayes, R. L.: Stimulation produced analgesia: Development of tolerance and cross-tolerance to morphine. Science, *188*:941–943, 1975.

25. Mayer, D. J., Wolfle, T. L., Akil, H., Carder, B., and Liebeskind, J. C.: Analgesia from electrical stimulation in the brainstem of the rat. Science, *174*:1351–1354, 1971.

26. Mazars, G.: Intermittent stimulation of nucleus ventralis posterolateralis for intractable pain. Surg. Neurol., *4*:93–95, 1975.

27. Mazars, G.: État actuel de la chirurgie de la douleur. Neurochirurgie (suppl.), *22*:1–164, 1976.

28. Mazars, G.: cited by Meyerson, B. A., 1979.

29. Meyerson, B. A.: ''European'' Study on Deep Brain Stimulation. Resumé of the 3rd European Workshop on Electrical Neurostimulation, Megeve, March 30–31, 1979.

30. Plotkin, R.: cited by Meyerson, B. A., 1979.

31. Pool, J. L., Clark, W. D., Hudson, P., and Lombardo, M.: Hypothalamic-hypophysial interrelationships. Springfield, Ill., Charles C Thomas, 1956.

32. Reynolds, D. V.: Surgery in the rat during electrical analgesia induced by focal brain stimulation. Science, *164*:444–445, 1969.

33. Richardson, D. E.: Personal communication, 1980.

34. Richardson, D. E., and Akil, H.: Pain reduction by electrical brain stimulation in man. Part 1. Acute administration in periaqueductal and periventricular sites. J. Neurosurg., *47*:178–183, 1977.

35. Richardson, D. E., and Akil, H.: Pain reduction by electrical brain stimulation. Part 2. Chronic self-administration in the periventricular gray matter. J. Neurosurg., *47*:184–194, 1977.

36. Richardson, D. E., and Akil, H.: Long term results of periventricular gray self-stimulation. Neurosurgery, *1*:199–202, 1977.

37. Sweet, W. H.: Central mechanisms of chronic pain. *In* Bonica, J. J., ed: Pain. New York, Raven Press, 1980, pp. 287–303.

38. Turnbull, I. M., Shulman, R., and Woodhurst, W. B.: Thalamic stimulation for neuropathic pain. J. Neurosurg., *52*:486–493, 1980.

137

MANAGEMENT OF
CHRONIC PAIN
REFRACTORY TO
SPECIFIC THERAPY

Management of any patient with pain begins with an attempt to determine the etiology of the pain so that specific therapy can be directed toward the cause rather than toward the pain as a symptom. Unfortunately, this approach is not always successful. The cause may be a condition, widespread metastatic disease for example, that defies successful specific treatment. In other patients, efforts to isolate specific causes of pain may be fruitless. A third group of patients in whom the painful condition began with a specific cause that was treated appropriately may, with or without objective signs of the original condition, continue to complain of pain.

Treatment of pain secondary to metastatic disease is discussed in other chapters and is not addressed here. Of the remaining patients with pain, those whose pain has persisted for months or years without signs of spontaneous remission or response to simple palliative measures are the primary focus of this chapter.

DEFINITION OF PAIN

The subjective nature of pain perception, conceptualization, and description presents a problem that pervades the evaluation and management of patients with pain. The designations "physiological," "pathological," "psychological," "acute," and "chronic" provide a clinical vocabulary for discussing the origins, physical and emotional components, duration, and amenability to treat-ment of pain. They cannot, however, assure that "pain" means the same thing to all who experience it, describe it, evaluate it, or treat it.

Clinically, pain can be labeled physiological, pathological, or psychological. *Physiological pain* is an appropriate sensation resulting when a noxious stimulus (one with the potential for producing tissue damage) is applied to a body with an intact nervous system in which the appropriate pathways concerned with pain perception are active. An example of acute physiological pain is that resulting from a fracture; an example of chronic physiological pain is that resulting from a bony metastasis. *Pathological pain* is a sensation perceived as pain because of an abnormality or malfunction of the nervous system, which improperly processes nonnoxious incoming information. An example of pathological pain, in which a minor stimulus may be perceived as pain, is that resulting from peripheral neuritis or from a radiculopathy caused by compression from a herniated intervertebral disc in which the nerve root fires with no or minimal peripheral stimulus. Pain pathway firing may be initiated by misfiring of abnormal peripheral or central neurons. *Psychological pain* occurs without external stimulus or firing of lower pain pathways. An example is hysterical pain or pain that an individual has learned or been conditioned to perceive.

In addition, it is clinically imperative to differentiate between acute and chronic pain—a process all too often omitted. Fre-

P. L. GILDENBERG AND R. A. DeVAUL

quently *acute pain* is physiological or pathological. It lasts for a relatively short time. Management is primarily directed toward defining and treating the underlying cause rather than the pain symptom. It may be possible to suppress the pain temporarily by the use of narcotic or nonnarcotic medications. Attention is directed toward treating the patient, whose involvement is often passive and who is encouraged to decrease his activity and to rest in anticipation that the pain will abate and allow him to return to his prior activities.

Chronic pain is much different. It is common for patients with chronic pain to have any one or a combination of the three types of pain just mentioned, especially a combination of pathological and psychological pain. At the time of presentation, the pain has lasted for weeks to months, and the patient's anticipation of successful treatment or eventual relief has waned. The patient has become depressed and anxious. Ordinary analgesic drugs are of limited use in chronic pain, and their continued administration may increase the patient's depression and introduce other serious problems, such as addiction and tolerance.[39] Attention is directed toward the pain symptom itself in hopes of either alleviating it or teaching the patient to live more satisfactorily despite the pain. The patient must do much of this himself and is encouraged to increase his activity in hopes of regaining as normal a life style as possible. Realistic goals must be set, since it may not be possible for the patient to return to his previous life style or occupation.

When the patient describes his disagreeable sensation as simply "pain," he may be referring to a specific painful sensation or to something altogether different. His discomfort can be defined and measured only by his perception and conceptualization of it. Therefore the physician must make every effort to interpret that description properly. This requires looking beyond what the patient verbalizes.

PATIENT EVALUATION

All too often, when faced with a patient complaining of chronic pain, the physician responds reflexly to the word "pain" and writes a prescription for an inappropriate analgesic.[50,78] Greater attention must be paid to evaluation of the patient with pain before any steps toward treatment are taken. Among the more useful diagnostic tools are listening carefully to the patient's description of his pain, asking questions about his activities and his ideas about his pain problem, observing his actions throughout the interview and examination, talking with his accompanying spouse or caretaker, and obtaining a comprehensive clinical history. In conjunction with a thorough physical examination, these steps can offer clues for the patient's management.

The patient's description of the nature of his pain is often helpful. Disagreeable sensations may not really involve the pain pathways, even though the patient may call them pain. Unless the patient describes what is classically pain, procedures involving interruption or stimulation of the pain pathways are of little benefit. Patients may describe their pain as pulling or pressure sensations not defined clinically as pain. A patient with a malignant rectal tumor may describe his "pain" as, "It feels like I'm sitting on a rock," or "It always feels like I have to move my bowels." A dramatic description or a report of pain more intense than the patient appears to have may indicate significant psychological components of the pain. Thus, "It feels like a hundred elephants are pulling on my arm," or "This is just like the pain my wife had before she died of cancer," may be helpful leads in determining the meaning of the discomfort.

Statements of what makes the pain worse and what makes it better may reveal a significant mechanical or emotional factor and give clues for treatment. Such observations as, "The pain seems to be worse when I'm tired," or "The pain gets worse when I'm nervous," are significant. Especially revealing might be, "The pain gets worse when I try to have intercourse, so we just don't do that anymore." Knowing what makes the pain better may likewise lead to recognition of mechanical factors involved with the pain and may suggest the best therapy. If the pain is relieved by lying down, how long does it take to achieve relief?

Often the patient will not admit that narcotic medication is ineffective, but may insist that he continue medication "just to take the edge off." Closer questioning may reveal withdrawal symptoms with increased pain if the patient fails to take narcotics at the prescribed intervals. In such instances, successful discontinuation of the drug may provide significant pain relief.

The patient should be questioned closely about the distribution of his pain, since his initial description may be misleading. If he complains of back pain, is it really at the site of a prior laminectomy or has it now changed to the renal area? If the patient complains of leg pain, is it truly in a radicular distribution, or might it be hip pain? In some cases it is helpful to ask the patient to describe first the back pain and then the leg pain, whereupon it may be discovered that these two pains are separate. It is surprising how often patients who have had several unsuccessful laminectomies are actually complaining of a disabling back pain with only minor or occasional leg pain. Close examination or trigger point blocks may indicate a myofascial syndrome, which can be treated locally, rather than a recurrent disc problem, which might require a repeat laminectomy.

Information about the patient's activities may provide a better index for judging the severity of his pain than his description of the pain. A patient who describes "unbearable" pain may tell of participating in activities and hobbies that such severe pain would preclude.

It is often interesting to ask the patient what he would do if the pain were suddenly relieved. Patients whose answers show that they have not thought realistically of this possibility may have already decided that their pain will not be relieved despite any and all treatment. It is also advisable to consider early in the program what might be practical goals for treatment, what the patient's own goals are, and whether the patient has a realistic understanding of his problem.

If possible, at least part of the interview should be conducted with the spouse or caretaker present. Observing the interaction between the patient and his family member may be more revealing than the most sophisticated electronic diagnostic test. Is the spouse supportive despite the patient's disability? Is the spouse too supportive? Does the spouse's support promote the disability or encourage rehabilitation?

A detailed history should be taken in an attempt to define the cause of the pain. Beware of the urge to accept labels put on the patient by himself or by his physicians.

Consider that the patient's continued pain may be the result of misdiagnosis and inappropriate treatment. Sometimes a fresh start by a new physician allows consideration of a cause not previously considered. The tendency to forget about other possible causes once the pain has been categorized is an error that should not prejudice a reevaluation.

Physical examination begins with the same thorough examination one would provide any other new patient. It should likewise include a search for underlying causes as well as whatever procedures are necessary to verify a diagnosis. Although old histories and reports can be very helpful, they can also be very misleading. Accept the accounts of factual information, but not necessarily opinions expressed in those reports. One should examine x-ray films personally or have them repeated, particularly if much time has passed.

In addition to the detailed routine examination, several aspects of the initial interview particularly concern patients with chronic pain. Does the patient walk down the hall to the examination room in a manner that reflects his description of the pain? Is there a difference in the patient's movement when he does not recognize that he is being observed and his movement during the examination? Inappropriate responses during the examination should be noted. The patient who dramatically reports pain on deep palpation of a muscle area and then responds just as dramatically to compression of a fold of overlying skin and subcutaneous fat between the fingers may be experiencing no muscle group tenderness at all. On the other hand, deep palpation of muscles in spasm or tender nodules in the muscle may give credence to the patient's report of tenderness. One must be suspicious of the patient who exhibits extreme distress on straight leg raising to 5 or 10 degrees during the testing if the examiner can elevate the straight leg to 60 or 80 degrees while distracting the patient with some other part of the examination. The claims of a patient who is unable to bend more than 5 degrees during the examination but is able to tie his own shoe laces with no difficulty after the examination are certainly suspect.

One curious sign noted during interviews of patients with pain and other neurosurgical disorders is the "tissue clutching sign." Those patients, particularly female, who sit throughout the interview clutching paper tissues in their hands have invariably demonstrated significant functional overlay to their complaints.

Diagnostic blocks with local anesthetic can be very helpful, even during initial evaluation of the patient.[10,71] Their results must be accepted with extreme caution, however, since they may be associated with considerable placebo effect. A patient who is enthusiastically hopeful of pain relief may obtain a surprising amount of temporary benefit from an injection of any kind. Important to diagnosis is not only whether the patient has immediate relief on administration of the local anesthetic but also whether the pain returns after the local anesthetic wears off or may even be somewhat worse from the trauma of the injection. Although pain relief may outlast the duration of anesthesia in some patients with a myofascial syndrome, a patient who has too much relief from a local anesthetic block is just as worrisome as a patient who has insufficient relief. As a general rule, diagnostic blocks should be repeated at least four times before they can be used in making a decision about an invasive therapeutic procedure. At least one of those four injections should be with a small volume of saline, possibly subcutaneously, as a "mock block."

One particularly helpful maneuver in evaluating patients with chronic intractable back pain is the search for trigger points.[117,118] The patient lies prone. The examiner presses firmly about the general area of pain, searching for points that are tender or painful on deep palpation. Often pressure on such trigger points will reproduce the patient's pain or may even cause pain that travels down the leg in a seemingly radicular distribution. The most common sites in the low back for such trigger points are the posterior iliac spine, the crest of the sacrum, the upper end of the sacroiliac joint (where the long muscles of the back attach to the upper margin of the sacrum and adjacent ilium), just lateral to a laminectomy or fusion incision, at the iliac crest, over the sacral foramina, or over the donor site after a fusion operation. Injection of these trigger points with local anesthetic may cause dramatic alleviation of the patient's pain. The trigger points are marked on palpation of the back, the needle

is inserted at a mark and is advanced until the patient's report of pain indicates that the tip of the needle has entered the trigger area. This area is most often just at the depth of the bone or the muscular attachment to bone. Two to five milliliters of local anesthetic may be injected at each area. Significant alleviation of the patient's pain is some evidence that the pain originates in the muscle and fascia of the lower back rather than at the nerve root itself.

The story of a patient with the onset of severe low back pain on lifting, bending, or jolting the back is common, as is the problem of posterior cervical pain after a rear-end automobile collision. Such pain, when due to tearing of muscle or fascia, may persist for many weeks and be accompanied by local muscle spasms. It is not uncommon for such patients to report for evaluation with unimproved or worse back pain after one or two unsuccessful laminectomies, often based on equivocal myelograms.

If a thorough initial evaluation and appropriate diagnostic procedures fail to reveal additional information about the cause of the pain, the patient and the physician can be reassured that it is fitting to embark on a program to control chronic pain rather than a program to treat acute pain.

Psychological Factors in Chronic Pain

Consideration of psychological factors is an important part of the evaluation of any patient with chronic pain or illness. Professional distinction between a neurosurgeon or anesthesiologist and a psychiatrist is an artificial one, and *any* physician who takes on the responsibility of treating patients with pain must likewise assume the responsibility of considering psychological factors. If the patient's psychological problems exceed the capabilities of the primary physician, professional psychiatric opinion should be sought. One must bear in mind, however, that many psychiatrists have little or no experience with patients with chronic illness or chronic pain, so that excellent communication must be maintained between the primary physician and a practical empathetic psychiatrist. Primary physician or psychiatrist must determine two things —the effect of the chronic pain on the patient's psychological adjustment and the extent to which the patient's complaint of pain is secondary to psychological maladjustment.

Patients may regard the suggestion that they receive psychiatric evaluation as an accusation that "the pain is all in your head." Frequently those who would profit most from this assessment object most strenuously to the suggestion. These patients might be told that a person with chronic pain from any cause is under considerable chronic stress, and that it is normal for such chronic stress to produce anxiety, tension, and depression. When these occur, they often reduce the patient's ability to tolerate pain and, hence, increase his perception of pain. As his perception of pain sharpens, the depression, anxiety, and tension grow worse, further reducing his ability to tolerate the pain. Ideally this cycle should be broken in as many places as possible with physical management of the pain as well as treatment of contributing psychological factors. The appropriate physical treatment may fail if the patient is too depressed to participate effectively in the treatment program or if he is not prepared for the social readjustment that accompanies relief from disability.

Patients with chronic pain generally present a typical pattern of features. Most resist the idea of psychiatric consultation at first, but soon respond enthusiastically to the forum for their complaints that the psychiatrist provides. They relate their histories expansively, professing disappointment at therapeutic failures. Such disappointment has not prejudiced them, however, against further treatment of whatever kind to effect relief from their incapacitating pain. They insist that their pain is an isolated, undiagnosed, physical condition. Although information from other family members usually identifies personal, social, financial, or work-related problems, the patient denies either that his pain is related to such situations or that such problems even exist.

The psychiatric interview often indicates that the pain is serving the patient in some way, perhaps providing special status, granting desired attention, or relieving him of unwanted responsibilities. Patients with such emotional components to their pain behavior commonly display (1) evidence of psychological regression, (2) a need to be identified as acutely ill, (3) nonresponse to drug treatment, and (4) conditioned pain behavior.

Psychological regression (return to a more childlike state) is a common reaction to both chronic and acute illness.[37,81,93] Regression manifests itself as a marked increase in egocentricity, a preoccupation with bodily perceptions, a significantly reduced scope of interests, and a noticeable increase in dependency, frequently accompanied by a demanding and manipulative insistence on attention. By these criteria, most patients with chronic pain are moderately regressed. The degree of regression varies widely from patient to patient and is related to the nature and length of illness, personality, and cultural and situational factors.[81] It is of particular note that the expectations inherent in the acute medical sick role and the hospital or clinic environment foster regression through enforced passivity, anxiety caused by medical diagnostic procedures or intervention, and the implied promise that if a patient is good his primary needs will be met.[80,81]

The ability to convey a *sense of urgency* about their difficulty to the evaluating physician is a prominent feature of this patient group. They frequently regard their condition as acute, and their presentation would be understandable if they were acutely ill. In essence, they define their pain as an illness, contending that there is nothing wrong with them except the pain, and that everything would be fine if the doctor would do his job and treat the pain problem. These expectations are unsuited to successful management of chronic illness in which the patient's participation is important.

A third and striking feature in patients with chronic pain is a lack of response or a report of worse pain following repeated attempts at short-term medical or operative treatment. Patients may sometimes report temporary relief, but generally the pattern is one of an unchanging or steadily deteriorating condition despite the treating physician's increasingly heroic attempts to relieve pain. Specifically, most patients take multiple medications, including narcotics, if their physicians prescribe them. Most patients will volunteer or admit upon inquiry that they receive no significant relief from any of the analgesics or narcotics. *Nonresponse to narcotics* appears to be a characteristic identifying feature of the chronic pain syndrome with a major emotional basis.[16]

A final feature of emotional involvement in the chronic pain syndrome is *conditioned pain behavior*.[27,29] If one were to design an experimental protocol to condition an animal to exhibit a particular type of behavior, he would confine the animal, reward it for exhibiting the desired behavior, and punish it for exhibiting contrary behavior. With classic conditioning techniques, it is quite simple to modify behavior so that the animal acts in a manner that may not be normal and may even be contrary to that of an unconditioned animal of his species. Such conditioning techniques are well recognized and accepted.[102]

What is not so well recognized is that society, family, and well-meaning physicians often construct an environment that conditions certain patients to exhibit pain behavior. Either because pain behavior is rewarded and pain-free behavior is not reinforced, or because of a psychological need to have overt behavior agree with their feelings and affect, such patients can be conditioned to have pain that is as real to them as any other pain.

A sample scenario might be as follows: A miner has been working at the same underground job for 12 years. He has no chance for advancement or of finding a less disagreeable occupation. He has come to fear his job, having seen many fellow miners injured or killed. He detests his foreman, who dislikes him also. His wife has always been too busy taking care of their children to pay much attention to him, and the romance disappeared from their relationship many years ago. Now that the children are in their late teens, his wife feels useless and depressed, which drives them farther apart. He spends most evenings killing time at the local tavern and has neither the intellectual capacity nor the background to develop rewarding interests.

One day while lifting a railroad tie, he feels a sudden tearing sensation in his back and is unable to stand erect. The company doctor releases him from work to spend three weeks resting at home at full pay. During those three weeks he remains essentially sedentary, in marked contrast to the physically active day he formerly spent on the job. His wife is suddenly attentive and finds that taking care of him gives her, at last, some pride and purpose. When he moans, she is quick to respond with loving sympathy. She rubs his back, serves him his favorite foods, and assumes a role of subservience compatible with both their personalities. Despite his sore back, the new relationship he has with his wife revitalizes their interest and enjoyment in sex. The time he spends out of bed is spent in an easy chair in front of the television set with beer and pretzels. As additional reinforcement, if he complains sufficiently, every three or four hours he receives a pill prescribed by the doctor, which makes him feel pleasantly high.

By the end of three weeks, the conditioning process is well under way. He is able to perpetuate his idyllic state by insisting that he still has too much pain to return to work, since company policy does not allow for return to any lighter duty than he had before. He is given a six-week extension of his sick leave, during which time he is examined by another physician who takes his complaint of pain at face value. Despite a physical examination that objectively discloses only mild muscle spasm in the low back area, the patient's display of pain and accompanying subjective evidence of an abnormal condition prompt the physician to admit the patient to the hospital, where some minor asymmetry on a myelogram leads to a diagnosis of herniated lumbar disc, and a laminectomy is performed. The operation provides the patient with an additional three months' immersion in the conditioning process. As long as he has pain (i.e., exhibits pain behavior), he obtains the positive reinforcement of spending his time at leisure, receiving the pleasant side effects of narcotics, perpetuating his new romantic relationship with his wife, and getting sympathy from friends for having suffered such a severe injury. Although he is no longer on full pay, his disability and union benefits provide him with 80 per cent of his former income, and with the tax benefits extended to disabled persons, he finds that his income has not diminished significantly. His expenses, however, have decreased, since he does his drinking at home instead of at the local tavern.

In addition to this positive reinforcement, the patient also avoids returning to what was an intolerable work situation as long as he still has pain. Indeed, he avoids all responsibility and has become passive and dependent, as was always his natural inclination. By the time his case is reviewed by the disability commission six months after his injury, he has undergone an extensive conditioning procedure that has taught him to have pain. Were his pain to cease, his situation would be worse than it was before his injury, since six months of complete physical rest have made him incapable of performing the only occupation for which he was qualified. It can readily be seen from this overall picture that no cordotomy or nerve block will enable this patient to return to his previous life style.

Psychological Testing

Unfortunately no psychological tests exist that perform the essential function of aiding in the differential diagnosis of psychogenic and organic pain. The most widely used test, frequently misused for this purpose, is the Minnesota Multiphasic Personality Inventory (MMPI). On the basis of a literature review and his own work, Sternback concludes that neurotic MMPI patterns are seen in both patients with psychogenic pain and those with chronic organic pain syndromes without significant differences.[108] The importance of Sternback's findings cannot be stressed too much, since considerable weight may erroneously be given to MMPI results in choosing elective invasive procedures. The real value of this test and other psychological tests lies in the documentation of psychological problems that require attention for effective management and the delineation of profiles that may dictate specific psychological intervention.

Differentiation of Chronic Pain Syndrome from Primary Psychogenic Pain

Chronic pain syndromes with physiological or pathological causes are invariably accompanied by emotional factors that affect successful management. Conversely, psychogenic pain is often attended by physiological symptoms that mask its *primary* emotional origin. The patient with psychogenic pain may experience paresthesia, motor weakness, or other motor dysfunctions.[121] Because of this evidence, unnecessary diagnostic or therapeutic procedures are sometimes recommended. In the absence of definitive diagnostic tools, the physician must rely upon medical histories and direct observation of the patient. From these two sources a behavior pattern characteristic of psychogenic pain behavior may emerge. Such behavior can be rather accurately classified according to the specific emotional condition from which it arises, or the specific emotional need that it serves.

Pain as a Symptom of Depression

It is understandable that persons with chronic pain may suffer some depression. Unrelieved pain results in the feelings normally associated with a depressed emotional state. In a particular type of psychogenic pain the cause and effect relationship is reversed so that the patient's depression is the source of his pain experience.[107] In this latter instance, the symptoms of depression precede the onset of pain. The patient may be unaware that he is depressed, in which case his family should be questioned about such objective indicators of depression as loss of appetite and weight, insomnia, unprovoked crying, withdrawal from personal contact, lack of interest in sex, constipation, and talk of suicide.

Delusional Pain

Delusional pain may accompany any illness in which the patient's perception of reality is impaired, either as a result of emotional disorders like schizophrenia and hysteria or as a result of organic brain syndromes such as toxic and withdrawal delirium.[18,20,21] Frequently the patient "knows" the cause of his pain and will describe a mechanical process of a nonmedical or even unnatural kind ("ants eating my shoulder joint"), while his demeanor suggests that this bizarre explanation is credible to him. Medical assurance that what he describes is not taking place has no effect on his pain, which has become a fixed entity. Patients with less severe delusionary pain disturbances may be more difficult to recognize, but some evidence of the impairment of their perception of reality usually emerges during extensive interviewing and oblique questioning. Such patients should be referred for psychiatric treatment.

Pain as a Conversion Symptom

Pain as a conversion symptom is a neurotic solution to a personal conflict, its characteristics often including (1) a description of pain that touches upon the underlying personal conflict, (2) inappropriate indifference to the pain despite its continued presence, (3) the sudden onset of pain coincidental with an emotionally charged situation, (4) the description of a pain that defies neuroanatomical boundaries, and (5) gratification of dependency and release from responsibilities that the patient would find unacceptable in good health.[19]

In such patients an intense neurotic need to avoid some situation or obtain some goal has resulted in the onset of pain. Ends toward which the behavior is directed might be resolution of a personal conflict, explanation for an inability to perform, or perpetuation of a disabled condition.

Pain as a Symptom of Unresolved Grief

It is not uncommon for those who have just lost a close friend or relative to experience symptoms similar to those suffered by the deceased.[15,56,79,127] During the normal grieving process these symptoms abate. In cases of unresolved grief reaction, the patient has for some reason been unable to grieve properly, and his identification symptoms persist. As in the preceding kinds of psychogenic pain disorders, the chief diagnostic clue is provided by the patient's description of his pain. In this instance, he frequently explains his discomfort in the pain vocabulary used to describe symptoms associated with the illness of the deceased.

Pain as a Symptom of a Need to Suffer

The patient's history is of greater help in identifying this source of pain than the description of the presenting symptom. There is a pattern, usually from childhood onward, in which pain and illness provide respite from work and accord the sufferer special attention. Possibly there is another family member with chronic problems of some sort from whom the patient learned the value of pain behavior. What appear at first to be many misfortunes in the history may actually be situations over which the patient could have exercised some control. The need to suffer so determines the behavior of this person that often in times of true stress from external sources his pain ceases, only to return in the absence of the stressful situation. This patient, since he is seeking help for the present pain, is likely to say, "Things would be fine right now if it weren't for this pain.[11,18,20,68,120]

The Manipulative Patient

The manipulative patient with chronic pain feels the need to define himself as an acutely ill person with legitimate demands for excessive medical attention. If this misrepresentation is not appreciated during evaluation, all forms of pain management may fail, causing patient and physician alike to become discouraged. The most dangerous aspect of the manipulative patient, both for the patient and for the physician, is that frequently the physician fails to recognize the extent to which he is being manipulated. After many months in "the pain game" and with the psychological need to perpetuate pain behavior, the patient may become more sophisticated than the physician. The initial step in dealing with such patients is to recognize that they are manipulative. Recognition of a skillfully manipulative patient may not be as easy as one would think.

Usually the manipulation consists of attempts to convert the chronic pain situation into an acute event that the physician feels required to treat. A decision to perform an operation may be made by the patient rather than the physician, who may later be called upon to defend the decision, especially if the patient becomes worse after the operation.

It is important for the physician to indicate at the initial encounter that, "Under no circumstances will I prescribe narcotics for you." The physician can expect that his resolve will be tested, and once the manipulative patient senses even the slightest vacillation, efforts at manipulation will be intensified.

To deal successfully with the manipulative patient, the physician must assert control over medical and operative procedures and drug dispensing. It is perfectly justifiable for the physician to state that there is no treatment for the patient's pain, an option that is unfortunately not often enough exercised. Treatment should then be directed toward helping the patient function better despite his chronic pain state. The patient may reject the physician's terms for management, but he must not be allowed to assume the role of physician.

As with patients with chronic pain in general, it is helpful to have a single physician make all decisions concerning the patient, even though he may consult with other members of a multidisciplinary team. This approach reduces the patient's opportunity to manipulate by playing one physician against the other.

It is often wise for patient and physician to draw up a written contract at the beginning of the program. This document should state the specific goals of the regimen and the parts to be played by patient and physician in their achievement. It might be stipulated that no operative intervention will be considered before the resources of the conservative management plan have been exhausted. So that this last part of the agreement does not encourage the patient to fail in his attempt at pain control in order to qualify for an operation, he should be told that he will not be evaluated for any procedure until after he has conscientiously completed the comprehensive program.

The cardinal rule in dealing with the manipulative patient is not to vacillate or appear indecisive but to be guided by what is in the patient's best long-term interest, even though he may object to it. The patient, in part because of the regression associated with chronic illness, is not unlike a child who, although he tries to manipulate his parent, feels more secure when he fails and the parent acts in the child's best interest.

In summary, the psychological evaluation should define the meaning the pain has for the patient, differentiate psychogenic pain if it exists, furnish information about the patient's personality, and make recommendations for successful management of the chronic problem.[17,113] Kahana and Bebring offer an excellent discussion of management strategies for patients with various types of personality.[48]

MANAGEMENT AND TREATMENT OF THE CHRONIC PAIN SYNDROME

Redefinition of the Problem

Redefinition of the problem precedes all treatment in the management of the diagnosed chronic pain syndrome. The patient has assumed the attributes of an acutely ill person—passivity, suffering, regression, abdication of responsibility—all of which militate against successful management of a chronic problem.[17,37,80,81,93] He must be made to understand that his problem is not similar to that of an acutely ill person. Though medical, surgical, psychological, and social resources will be tapped when necessary, he will be expected to take an active role in the control of his own pain. Control of the patient's perception of pain will replace cure of an acute disorder as goal for patient and physician. Energy the patient has directed toward maximizing his special status as a sufferer must be channeled toward returning to a normal life despite possible residual disability.

Medical Intervention

As noted previously, most patients with chronic pain experience some symptoms of depression secondary to their continued pain and disablement. Analgesics, tranquilizers, and narcotics prescribed for pain can also produce depression. These drugs are not only ineffective treatments for the chronic pain syndrome but also introduce the risks of addiction and tolerance. Depression from whatever source lowers the patient's tolerance of pain, inducing him to take more medication. This depression-pain-medication cycle can usually be broken by withdrawal of simple tranquilizers and narcotic and analgesic substances, and substitution of tricyclic antidepressants. The latter have been used successfully to remedy secondary depression and reduced pain tolerance.

Usually, it is advisable to discontinue all addicting drugs prior to or simultaneously with embarking on the treatment program. Otherwise the patient's need to have his pain may continue in order to justify taking the medication to which he is addicted.

Also, the patient may experience pain or an exacerbation of the pain he complains of as part of the withdrawal syndrome, reinforcing his notion that he needs the drug. Since most patients complain that narcotics do not adequately relieve their pain, they should be made to understand that, conversely, withdrawing the medication will not aggravate their condition and may improve it significantly.

As a rule, narcotics should be withdrawn abruptly, unless the patient experiences extreme withdrawal effects. Barbiturates or diazepam should be withdrawn gradually if the patient has been taking large doses continually and over a protracted period. Other medications can begin when narcotics, tranquilizers, and inappropriate analgesics are discontinued. The tricyclic antidepressants, because of their delayed effectiveness, may be started several weeks before withdrawal of other medications.

A standard withdrawal regimen that prevents serious or unpleasant withdrawal symptoms regardless of the drug class is as follows: (1) An estimation of the daily drug intake is made. (2) The patient's condition is stabilized at the calculated dosage, and he is observed for several days to insure that no withdrawal symptoms appear. (3) The dosage is then decreased by 10 per cent daily for 10 successive days. A drug similar to the addictive drug and in its same class may be substituted during the withdrawal process. For instance, if the patient is addicted to short-acting barbiturates, a smoother withdrawal is effected by using equivalent doses of longer-acting phenobarbital.

If tricyclic antidepressants are to be substituted, a dosage of at least 150 mg of amitriptyline hydrochloride (Elavil) or its equivalent should be used. A workable outpatient dosage regimen begins with 25 mg of amitriptyline at night increased by 25 mg every other night until 150 mg is reached. Tricyclic antidepressants are not benign medications, and the prescribing physician should be aware of drug side effects and potential hazards. One such hazard is possible cardiac intoxication, particularly in patients over 40 years of age or those in whom there is evidence or history of heart disease. This hazard is not a contraindication but requires careful medical supervision. A pretreatment electrocardiogram is recommended. Doxepin produces fewer cardiac toxic effects, but in clinical experience has not been as successful as amitriptyline hydrochloride in treatment of depression or modification of tolerance.

One technique for safe and efficient withdrawal of undesired medications that can be employed in an inpatient unit, such as a chronic pain treatment center, combines the drug withdrawal regimen with a behavior modification program, since it takes away the reward aspect of drug administration.[39] The program entails administering all the patient's medication on a schedule rather than on demand. No longer is the patient rewarded for complaints of pain or for pain behavior by having a nurse appear with a pill or shot. Medications are given in a solution of quinine water, the bitter taste of which serves both to mask the taste of the drugs and as negative reinforcement. Initially, the solution can be given every four hours around the clock, the patient being awakened for his medication at night until he himself requests that this no longer be done. All medications are given orally. If the patient was taking intramuscular narcotics, an equivalent dosage of methadone is substituted for the usual narcotic—approximately 1 mg per 1 mg compared with morphine. The initial dose of medication over 24 hours should be as great as, or greater than, the dose the patient was taking himself, and he should be thus informed. Without informing the patient of the specific dosage, however, all medication can be decreased by approximately 10 to 15 per cent daily, so that at the end of the week the patient is receiving the quinine water alone, perhaps with the daily dose of amitriptyline hydrochloride added to the evening administration. It is interesting that even after patients are told that the quinine water no longer contains medication, some still request that they be allowed to take it, since it gives them a feeling of control over their pain.

Psychological Intervention

The thorough psychiatric evaluation outlined earlier and encouraged as part of comprehensive diagnosis for the pain patient helps to isolate treatable psychological factors that might relate to pain perception. If the psychiatric report discloses ways in which pain is emotionally beneficial to the patient or problems the patient is using his pain to avoid or solve, the physician can recommend psychological treatment in conjunction with any medical or operative intervention that is indicated. Psychological management is likely to include one or more of the following: behavior modification, relaxation techniques, control of autonomic processes through use of biofeedback aids, hypnosis, and psychotherapy.

Behavior modification techniques derive from learning theory. One theory, described in some detail earlier in this chapter, assumes that behavior is learned and controlled to a large degree by consequences in the environment. One can change behavior, the theory holds, by changing its consequences rather than its cause. This model can be used to modify types of pain behavior that appear to be maladaptive to recovery.[28,29] If learned and reinforced, maladaptive pain behavior may continue in the absence of significant pain. For example, a patient's pain behavior often is encouraged (reinforced) by attention, sympathy, relief from adult responsibility, rest, absence of stress, medication, or compensation. Specific recommendations for nonreinforcement of illness behavior include the discontinuation of pain medication on demand, the substitution of a medication time schedule, and the introduction of physical exercise.

Remobilization is a key component in any program for rehabilitation of patients with chronic pain, who are often completely sedentary for months. One can readily imagine that a healthy individual put to bed for several months would have pain on resumption of activity. Many patients use this phenomenon to demonstrate to physicians, spouses, and disability officers that their pain is real. It is not uncommon for patients to complain that any physical activity at all makes their pain worse, then to attempt vigorous work (such as mowing a lawn) on their first day out, and to complain that it made their pain worse.

Two keys to successful mobilization of the patient are encouragement (or coercion) and a program that allows gradual increase of activity with no large increments in level of activity from day to day. Exercise should not be prescribed to tolerance but to a predetermined level short of the precipitation of severe pain. Exercise within limits allows rest and encouragement as rewards for behavior that is non pain producing. Mobilization should begin under supervision and increase over many weeks. If suitable facilities for such instruction are not available, a simple progressive exercise program such as that set forth in the *Royal Canadian Air Force Exercise Plans for Physical Fitness* manual may be helpful.[90]

The encouragement, direction, and understanding that a good physical therapist can supply is a desirable adjunct to the program of behavior modification and mobilization. Physical therapy is of particular rehabilitative value in cases in which tight joints and shortened muscles must be overcome. Joints with limited range of motion from prolonged disuse, muscles atrophied or shortened from prolonged disuse, and tight or spastic muscles might profit from local physical therapy. Incorporation of physical therapy into the program reassures the patient, who is perhaps concerned about the attention to psychiatric considerations, that the physician does not think the pain is all in his head.

Patients whose disability will involve permanent restriction of motion or activities can benefit considerably from an activities-of-daily-living program, which concentrates on teaching them to utilize the physical resources they still have to compensate for those that have been lost. A patient with weakness of one or more extremities may learn to dress himself, feed himself, and provide himself with maximal care, thereby reducing the dependency that can accompany the chronic pain state.

Relaxation techniques are simple and useful tools for modifying pain perception and in particular for assisting patients whose pain problems have a muscle tension component.[24] Their major advantages appear to be their use as substitutes for minor tranquilizers and, more importantly, their success in proving to the patient that he can take active control in altering his perception of pain without resort to drugs.

Biofeedback is a technique of training one to become better able to control physiological processes. Its effectiveness in management of pain is still undetermined, but evidence indicates that it can be particularly useful for relief of tension headaches and other muscular tension–based problems.[9,86] The biofeedback monitor produces a signal, either auditory or visual, generated by the electrical activity in some part

of the patient's body. The patient attempts
to reduce the activity of the monitored area
consciously, and is rewarded and encouraged by diminution of the reported signal. The technique enhances relaxation and
hence reduces pain. In the more usual
form, muscle activity in the area where tension or spasms are suspected is monitored.
This form is particularly helpful when the
low back or posterior cervical muscles are
involved. In another form of the technique,
the occipital electroencephalogram is used
as the biofeedback signal. Since the presence of alpha waves may dominate periods
of relaxation, the patient is presented with a
signal that represents alpha wave activity
and is asked to reproduce the signal voluntarily under the presumption that such an
effort will result in relaxation.

Hypnosis is a learned state of selective
concentration and is of documented use in
altering pain perception. The operative
mechanisms are unknown, and paradoxi-
cally it is much more effective in pain of primary organic origin (especially that related
to terminal cancer) than in pain that has significant emotional content or pain that is
used primarily for personal gain. Its usefulness in management of the chronic pain
syndrome is limited, since those conditions
in which hypnosis is most effective are
those with an organic cause that respond to
other anesthetic techniques also. Hypnosis
can, however, be incorporated into a comprehensive program for controlling chronic
pain, particularly as an agent for reducing
medication requirements.[76]

Social Intervention

The likelihood that a patient with chronic
pain will display regressive behavior has already been discussed. Efforts to reverse
this behavior pattern must include the people around the patient who foster or tolerate such behavior, primarily parents or
spouse. These relatives must have the
chronic pain problem redefined for them as
it was for the patient so that their relationship as caretakers can be altered. Hence-
forth they will be expected to encourage
well behavior and independence rather than
pain reporting and dependency. They will
be as important a part of the behavior modification program as the patient and physi-

cian. The social aspect of management of
chronic pain can be decisive, for without
substituting and reinforcing a repertoire of
types of well behavior, it is almost impossible to reverse maladaptive behavior.

Physical and Neurosurgical Intervention

Only a minority of the patients referred
to a neurosurgeon qualify for operative intervention. An informal survey revealed
that only 3 to 10 per cent of the patients referred to several pain clinics for pain other
than that of malignant disease were treated
by invasive types of intervention, and of
those only 50 to 60 per cent obtained satisfactory relief for a reasonable period of follow-up.[33] All had undergone extensive evaluation prior to the procedure, and many
were found to have psychological or physical factors contraindicating such types of
intervention. In contrast, 90 per cent of patients with pain secondary to malignant disease qualified for some sort of procedure.
There is no reason to suspect that the distribution of patients referred to the average
neurosurgeon for treatment of pain is any
different. Consequently, any neurosurgeon
who assumes the responsibility for employing operative intervention to alleviate intractable pain likewise assumes the responsibility for undertaking the type of
extensive patient evaluation described earlier. The majority of patients referred to
neurosurgeons for pain-relieving procedures should be declined and possibly referred to the primary physician, a psychiatrist, or a multidisciplinary group for a
comprehensive nonoperative treatment
program. With the few who do qualify for
procedural intervention, it is better to initiate the behavior-modifying part of the
program and have the patient's drug intake
within acceptable limits prior to embarking
on any invasive neurosurgical treatment.

Nonspecific pain-relieving procedures
can be divided into two groups—stimulation procedures (which depend upon blocking of pain pathways or stimulation of inhibitory pathways, do not ordinarily result
in the destruction of tissue, and are therefore reversible), and destructive lesions or
ablative procedures (which interrupt the
pain pathways somewhere along their

course and deprive the patient of pain and possibly of other sensation, perception, or emotional response).

As with any operative procedure, the decision involves assessment of the risk-to-benefit ratio. Nonoperative techniques carry the least risk, frequently are of significant benefit, and should be considered first. Stimulation techniques ordinarily do not result in permanent alteration of neurological function and, where indicated, might be considered next. Ablative procedures should be reserved for those patients in whom, because of the etiology of the pain, there is significant chance of success, since the risk is greatest in such procedures.

Although stimulation procedures do not in themselves necessarily result in permanent neurological dysfunction, greater risk is associated with some than others, and selection of patients for intervention should reflect awareness of this scale of risk. For example, most patients may be candidates for a trial of transcutaneous stimulation somewhere in their treatment process, but few will qualify for trial stereotaxic stimulation of deep brain structures. Potential risk and long-term benefit must be considered, since many procedures are known to result in only temporary improvement of the conditions.

Candidates for ablation procedures must be screened and chosen with very great care, since the desired therapeutic effect implies irreversible neurological deficit. There are some chronic pain conditions for which destructive techniques may be indicated, but few of these (less than 5 per cent) involve chronic pain of benign origin. They are most often conditions resulting from specific trauma to peripheral nerves or to the nervous system, with well-defined, discretely localized causes. Generally, the higher in the nervous system a lesion is made, the less likelihood there is for permanent pain relief. This phenomenon may be a function of the increasing complexity and redundancy of pain-perceiving systems as the central nervous system ascends toward the brain. Taking this situation into consideration, a peripheral neurectomy to treat chronic pain of a discrete neuroma would be sanctioned much more readily than a thalamotomy for a diffuse pain of indefinite etiology.

It cannot be stressed too emphatically that (1) destructive procedures do not frequently have a place in the management of chronic pain of nonmalignant origin, (2) the potential benefit from such procedures is not as great as might be expected from a comparable procedure performed to relieve pain of malignant disease, (3) they are to be considered only when a specific organic pathological condition indicates the painful nature of the condition, and (4) they should be selected for use in order of increasing risk so that the most peripheral procedures are considered first.

Stimulation Procedures

Transcutaneous stimulation, in which a controlled electrical stimulus is applied via electrodes taped to the skin, has been helpful in up to 50 per cent of patients with chronic pain. Transcutaneous stimulation for the treatment of pain was discovered empirically many years ago, and at one time a number of battery-operated stimulators were freely available commercially.[99] The application of a stimulating current at a nonpainful level results in relief not unlike that obtained from rubbing a part of the body that is acutely injured.

With the introduction of the Melzack and Wall gate theory, a more scientific basis for such pain relief has been found.[67] According to the gate theory, firing of small neurons transmitting pain competes with firing of large fibers stimulated by nonnoxious stimuli to open or close a "gate" or pathway for transmitting sensory information toward the brain. When small-fiber activity predominates, the gate is opened, and second-order neurons are allowed to fire, sending their pain information toward the brain. When large-fiber activity is increased by adding a nonpainful stimulus, however, the gate may close and the pain sensation may decrease or cease.

Electrodes are taped to the skin over the area of the pain or adjacent to it. Contact jelly is used to assure reliable electrical transmission. The patient adjusts the voltage of the battery-operated stimulator himself so that a nonpainful stimulus is applied. Regardless of the cause of the pain, a significant number of patients obtain appreciable relief with this technique.[6,58,99] For treatment of widespread pain, transcutaneous stimulators are available with two channels of two electrodes each.

Dorsal column stimulation applies a train of electrical stimuli to the dorsal aspect of the spinal cord by means of an apparatus that can also be controlled by the patient.[59,100,101,111] A further outgrowth of the Melzack-Wall pain theory, this procedure attempts to stimulate the collaterals of the large sensory fibers as they ascend in the dorsal columns of the spinal cord. Fortuitous anatomical circumstance affords collateral access to a pure population of virtually all the large fibers below the stimulated spinal level. The impulse flows retrograde down the axon in the dorsal column to increase the large-fiber input to the substantia gelatinosa, theoretically closing the gate and inhibiting perception of pain from caudal areas.

The original technique for implanting a dorsal column stimulator called for laminectomy and placement of the electrode in the subarachnoid or subdural space, in a pocket within the dura, or epidurally.[60] The implanted electrode is connected by subcutaneous leads to a radio receiver implanted in a subcutaneous pocket at some convenient location, usually the chest just below the clavicle or the upper abdomen. The radio receiver is passive, that is, does not contain a power supply. It depends on a radiofrequency signal transmitted through the skin for both control and power, and converts the signal into stimulus impulses delivered to the electrode at the spinal cord. The patient controls the stimulus by adjusting a battery-operated radio transmitter he can carry with him.

Percutaneous insertion of stimulating electrodes now allows a nonoperative trial to see if pain is successfully alleviated by dorsal column stimulation, so that only patients who obtain relief over a period of several days are considered for implantation of a stimulator.[21,75] Present techniques allow incorporation of percutaneously inserted electrodes into a permanent system by connecting them to an implanted radio receiver under local anesthesia, making the laminectomy unnecessary in some cases.[74]

Patients whose pain affects the lower part of the body, certainly below the shoulder or neck area, might be candidates for dorsal column stimulation. The patients should be emotionally stable and be willing to undertake a comprehensive pain program. Ideally they should have a definite known physical cause for their pain. There

should be no adverse compensation incentive or impending litigation that might unfavorably bias the patient's response. Ideally, trial percutaneous subarachnoid or epidural stimulation should be performed to assure that the patient is reasonably likely to obtain pain relief from a permanent stimulator, as well as to assure that the patient is intellectually and psychologically capable of maintaining and tolerating his stimulation device.

Patients with neuropathic pain originating in an individual peripheral nerve sometimes respond to stimulation of the peripheral nerve. Again, according to the Melzack-Wall gate theory, if the peripheral nerve receives a stimulus of intensity sufficient to activate the low-threshold large fibers but not great enough to include the high-threshold small pain fibers, the resultant large-fiber stimulation might close the gate and afford pain relief. On the basis of this consideration, Sweet first inserted an electronic device similar to that just described for dorsal column stimulation, except that the electrode was wrapped around a peripheral nerve.[110] Indications for peripheral nerve stimulation are essentially the same as for dorsal column stimulation, except that the pain arises from neuropathy of a single peripheral nerve that has a normal proximal segment available to which to apply the stimulation.

An outgrowth of the development of hardware for dorsal column and peripheral nerve stimulation, deep brain stimulation is still an experimental procedure at the time of this writing. A radio receiver attached to a multicontact electrode is inserted stereotaxically into a target deep within the brain. At present, three such targets are considered. The internal capsule and ventral posterior nuclear complex have been found to be useful implantation sites for patients with denervation pain, that is, patients whose pain is secondary to spinal cord lesions, thalamic syndrome, or phantom limb pain.[2,3,45] A third target is predicated on experimental findings by Reynolds in 1969 and later by Liebeskind, Mayer, and Akil, who demonstrated that stimulation of the periventricular or periaqueductal gray matter results in analgesia over wide areas of the body in experimental animals.* Al-

---

* See references 4, 36, 51–54, 62, 64, 65, 82, 91.

though stimulation of these same areas in man may not result in overt analgesia, there may be significant alleviation of chronic intractable pain.* The response appears to be related to narcotic or endorphone analgesia, since it can be blocked by naloxone and has a partial cross-tolerance to morphine.[1,63] These observations, especially in man, have opened the door to new insights in pain perception and control.

Ablative Procedures

Although treatment of pain by regional anesthetic and peripheral blocks is discussed in other chapters, several techniques are of sufficient interest in the management of chronic pain to be mentioned here, especially since much chronic pain is secondary to low back or intraspinal problems.

The simplest block procedure most often employed in treatment of the chronic pain syndrome is the trigger point block. The technique for identifying trigger points is discussed earlier. Once it has been ascertained that the patient's pain can be significantly but temporarily alleviated by local anesthetic blocks at trigger points, a program to obtain prolonged relief can begin. Patients are seen at weekly intervals. For the first three weeks a local anesthetic such as lidocaine is used. Occasionally relief may outlast duration of the local anesthetic by longer and longer periods, in which case local anesthetic alone may be sufficient. If after three series of trigger point injections the patient's pain continues to return as the local anesthetic wears off, a steroid preparation such as triamcinolone or hydrocortisone might be mixed with the local anesthetic. Patients who still fail to obtain long-lasting benefit might then proceed to the next level of treatment. Local anesthetic is injected into each trigger point as previously. A maximum of 2 ml of lidocaine is used. The needle is left in place, but the syringe is replaced with one containing a solution of phenol crystals dissolved in saline (100 mg per milliliter). One or two milliliters of the phenol solution is injected into the anesthetized trigger point. As many as 8 or 10 trigger points can be thus treated on a weekly basis. Often, with the addition

of the phenol to the program, the relief begins to outlast the duration of the local anesthetic.

Many patients with chronic pain of radicular origin or arachnoiditis may not have a demonstrably treatable anatomical lesion. Once a nerve has been traumatized, it may not return to its normal state even after it has been decompressed, and radicular pain may persist or adhesive arachnoiditis may occur. Relief either from the chronic pain of this condition or from its intermittent acute exacerbations can frequently be obtained with intrathecal methylprednisolone (Depo-Medrol, Upjohn).[97] A lumbar puncture is performed and methylprednisolone, 40 mg, is instilled at weekly intervals for a maximum of three injections. Since the methylprednisolone eventually is absorbed, one must be concerned about prolonged systemic administration of steroids by this route. In reported experience, as many as half of the patients with acute radiculopathy and as many as one third of those with chronic radicular pain have responded to such a series of injections.

In some cases of persistent radicular pain, it may be possible to obtain relief by the intrathecal injection of an agent toxic to the nerve roots. Unfortunately, patients with pain secondary to failure of operations on the intervertebral disc usually obtain no long-term benefit from this procedure, perhaps because the pathological change has affected more proximal structures or because of the complex psychological and compensation milieu often surrounding these patients. The classic substance employed has been alcohol, but it has the disadvantage of being difficult to control, and it may spread to adjacent roots where destruction of nerve fibers is undesired. For selective lumbar chemical rhizotomy of multiple roots, phenol is more reliable and less dangerous. Phenol crystals are dissolved in Pantopaque at a concentration of 100 to 200 mg per milliliter, depending on how dense an analgesia is required. The patient is placed in a lateral position on the myelogram table. A lumbar puncture is performed and 1 ml of plain Pantopaque is introduced. The table is tilted so that the Pantopaque lies right in the center of those roots to be treated. Then 3 to 6 ml of the Pantopaque-phenol mixture is introduced under fluoroscopic guidance, and the table tilted so that the pool of Pantopaque sur-

---

* See references 2, 38, 45, 70, 83–85.

rounds only the desired roots and no other. The patient remains in this position for 10 minutes, after which the Pantopaque may be removed if so desired. The patient must of course be warned that such a procedure may influence the motor fibers as well and weakness may result. By beginning with lower concentrations of phenol and fractionating the treatment, it is usually possible to affect the smaller fibers first and obtain a significant decrease in pain sensation without weakness. It may be necessary to repeat the block two or three times to obtain permanent relief. In adhesive arachnoiditis, the phenol solution cannot get to the involved nerve roots.

A related procedure can be employed with patients who are suffering severe perineal pain from malignant disease and who have already lost bowel and bladder function.[112] Four hundred milligrams of phenol crystals is dissolved in two milliliters of Pantopaque, which in this instance is used because it is hyperbaric. A lumbar puncture is made with the patient in a sitting position, and the phenol-Pantopaque mixture is instilled. It will run to the lower end of the arachnoidal sac and affect preferentially the lower sacral nerve roots. The patient remains sitting for 10 minutes, following which the Pantopaque may or may not be removed as desired. This procedure is extremely simple, readily tolerated, and in well-selected patients can be quite effective.

Although the classic theory of a three-neuron chain involving small fibers of peripheral nerves, spinothalamic tract, and thalamocortical radiations has been found deficient in many respects, it still constitutes the basis for ablative techniques for the treatment of pain.[67] These procedures are designed to obliterate the perception of pain (and sometimes other sensations) from certain areas of the body or to obliterate the appreciation of the suffering involved with chronic pain. They are described in detail in other chapters and are mentioned here only briefly.

Peripheral neurectomy may be useful in treating pain of neuroma or trauma to the individual nerves. If there is a reflex sympathetic component to the pain, however, this must be identified and treated separately by sympathetic blocks or sympathectomy. The neurectomy limits loss of sensation to the distribution of only a single nerve, but

the activity of that nerve is completely abolished, so all sensations and motor function are likewise interrupted.

Intercostal neurectomy is sometimes helpful in patients who have pain secondary to a neuroma of a traumatized intercostal nerve, whether it be from rib fracture or thoracic operations. It has been found to be of little help in postherpetic neuralgia pain or diffuse pain over the thorax or abdomen. Since innervation is by overlapping segments, it is necessary to interrupt a minimum of three intercostal nerves or dorsal roots to effect loss of sensation in any one dermal segment.

Dorsal rhizotomy can be used to interfere with pain in various areas of the body. A laminectomy is performed so that the rhizotomy can be done under direct vision. To obtain complete obliteration of sensation it is necessary to interrupt multiple dorsal roots in any area. The procedure is recognized to have less and less use in the treatment of chronic pain, and long-term results of rhizotomy for lumbar radiculopathy have been particularly poor.[122]

There have been reports of some success with radiofrequency denervation of lumbar nerve roots for treatment of so-called postlaminectomy pain or laminectomy failure.[11,49,66,95,98] This is likewise described in another chapter.

Cordotomy has been the classic procedure for alleviating pain by interrupting the lateral spinothalamic tract. It is still extremely useful in patients with cancer pain, and in a few very carefully selected patients with benign pain. As classically performed, a laminectomy is done and the anterolateral quadrant of the spinal cord is severed under direct vision.[47,125] Techniques have, however, been available since 1963 for interrupting the lateral spinothalamic tract with a radiofrequency current applied through a needle electrode inserted percutaneously under x-ray guidance at either the C2 level or lower.*

Closely related procedures involve stereotaxic insertion of an electrode into the descending trigeminal nucleus for treatment of head and face pain.[43,44,94,96] Hitchcock and Schvarcz devised a procedure whereby the electrode is stereotaxically inserted in the midline at the cervicomedul-

---

* See references 12, 13, 31, 32, 34, 35, 55, 72, 88, 89, 115, 116.

lary junction to produce a central myelotomy for the treatment of body pain.[42,95]

Mesencephalotomy might be considered in cases of central neurogenic pain, and there are case reports of successful treatment of thalamic syndrome pain by this stereotaxic procedure.[70,73,87,104,126] Newer stimulation techniques may, however, have completely supplanted it for this indication. Mesencephalotomy is still valuable for treatment of cancer pain of the head and face.[103,104,119] The lesion can be directed either to the spinothalamic pathway as it ascends through the mesencephalon along the base of the thalamus, or it can be extended toward the central gray to interrupt the multisynaptic paleospinothalamic pathway. As an alternative, a stereotaxic lesion can be made slightly higher at the base of the thalamus to interrupt these two pathways.* The higher lesion is farther from the oculomotor fibers and can be extended into the interlaminar area of the thalamus to interrupt the diffuse pain pathways.

Alternatively, the lesion can be directed to interrupt the limbic system in the cingulum or centrum medianum, although these procedures are generally reserved for patients with cancer.†

In summary, ablative procedures are being used less and less frequently for the treatment of pain of benign origin. It is to be hoped that fewer inappropriate procedures are performed, since they so often involve the doctor in more and more procedures while the patient's problem becomes worse and worse.

REFERENCES

1. Adams, J. E.: Naloxone reversal of analgesia produced by brain stimulation in the human. Pain, 2:161–166, 1976.
2. Adams, J. E.: Technique and technical problems associated with implantation of neuroaugmentative devices. Appl. Neurophysiol., 40:111–123, 1977–1978.
3. Adams, J. E., Hosobuchi, Y., and Fields, H. L.: Stimulation of internal capsule for relief of chronic pain. J. Neurosurg., 41:740–744, 1974.
4. Akil, H., Mayer, D. J., and Liebeskind, J. C.: Psychophysiologie - comparison chez le rat entre l'analgésie induite par stimulation de la substance grise péri-aquéducale et l'analgésie morphinque. C.R. Acad. Sci., Paris, 274:3603–3605, 1972.
5. Albe-Fessard, D., Dondey, M., Nicolaidis, S., and LeBeau, J.: Remarks concerning the effect of diencephalic lesions on pain and sensitivity with special references to lemniscally mediated control of noxious afferences. Confin. Neurol., 32:174–184, 1970.
6. Appenzeller, O., and Atkinson, R.: Transkutane nervenbeizung zur Behandlung der Migrane und anderer Kopfschmerzen. Munchen. Med. Wschr., 117:1953–1954, 1975.
7. Ballantine, H. T., Jr., Cassidy, W. L., Flanagan, N. D., and Marino, R., Jr.: Stereotaxic anterior cingulotomy for neuropsychiatric illness and intractable pain. J. Neurosurg., 26:488–495, 1967.
8. Bettag, W., and Yoshida, T.: Über stereotaktische Schmerzoperationen. Acta Neurochir., Wein, 8:299–317, 1960.
9. Blanchard, E. B., and Young, L. D.: Clinical application of biofeedback training: A review of evidence. Arch. Gen. Psychiat. 30:573–589, 1974.
10. Bonica, J. J.: Clinical Applications of Diagnostic and Therapeutic Nerve Blocks. Springfield, Ill., Charles C Thomas, 1959.
11. Burton, C.: Percutaneous radiofrequency lumbar rhizolysis (rhizotomy). Appl. Neurophysiol., 39:87–96, 1976–1977.
12. Crue, B. L., Todd, E. M., and Carregal, E. J.: Posterior approach for high cervical percutaneous radiofrequency cordotomy. Confin. Neurol., 30:41–52, 1968.
13. Crue, B. L., Todd, E. M., and Carregal, E. J.: Percutaneous radiofrequency stereotactic tractotomy. In Crue, B. L., ed.: Pain and Suffering. Springfield, Ill., Charles C Thomas, 1970, pp. 69–79.
14. Davis, R. A., and Stokes, J. W.: Neurosurgical attempts to relieve thalamic pain. Surg. Gynec. Obstet., 123:371–384, 1966.
15. DeVaul, R. A., and Zisook, S.: Unresolved grief, clinical considerations. Postgrad. Med., 5:267–271, 1976.
16. DeVaul, R. A., Hall, R. C. W., and Faillace, L. A.: Drug use by the polysurgical patient. Amer. J. Psychiat., 135:682–685, 1978.
17. DeVaul, R. A., Zisook, S., and Lorimor, R.: Patients with chronic pain. Med. J. St. Joseph Hosp. Houston, 12:59–63, 1977.
18. DeVaul, R. A., Zisook, S., and Stuart, J. H.: Patients with psychogenic pain. J. Fam. Prac., 4:53–55, 1977.
19. Diagnostic and Statistical Manual of Mental Disorders. Washington, D. C., American Psychiatric Association, 1968.
20. Engel, G. L.: Psychogenic pain and the pain-prone patient. Amer. J. Med., 26:899–918, 1959.
21. Erickson, D. L.: Percutaneous trial of stimulation for patient selection for implantable stimulating devices. J. Neurosurg., 43:440–444, 1975.
22. Faillace, L. A., Allen, R. P., McQueen, J. D., and Northrup, B.: Cognitive deficits from bilateral cingulotomy for intractable pain in man. Dis. Nerv. Syst., 32:171–175, 1971.
23. Fairman, D.: Stereotactic treatment for the alle-

---

* See references 5, 8, 14, 23, 40, 57, 61, 92, 104, 105, 106, 114, 123, 124.

† See references 7, 22, 25, 26, 41, 77, 95.

viation of intractable pain: Reassessments and limitations. Confin. Neurol., *32*:341–344, 1970.

24. Ferguson, J. M., Marquis, J. N., and Taylor, C. B.: A script for deep muscle relaxation. Dis. Nerv. Syst., *38*:703–708, 1977.

25. Foltz, E. L., and White, L. E., Jr.: Pain ''relief'' by frontal cingulumotomy. J. Neurosurg., *19*:89–100, 1962.

26. Foltz, E. L., and White, L. E.: The role of rostral cingulumotomy in ''pain'' relief. Int. J. Neurol., *6*:353–373, 1968.

27. Fordyce, W. E.: Pain viewed as learned behavior. Advances Neurol., *4*:415–422, 1974.

28. Fordyce, W. E.: Treating chronic pain by contingency management. Advances Neurol., *4*:583–589, 1974.

29. Fordyce, W. E., Fowler, R. S., Jr., Lehmann, J. F., DeLateur, B. J., Sand, P. L., and Trieschmann, R. B.: Operant conditioning in the treatment of chronic pain. Arch. Phys. Med., *54*:399–408, 1973.

30. Fox, J. L.: Percutaneous trigeminal tractotomy for facial pain. Acta Neurochir., *29*:83–88, 1973.

31. Gildenberg, P. L.: Angle-meter to indicate the proper angle of insertion in anterior percutaneous cervical cordotomy. Technical note. J. Neurosurg., *34*:244–247, 1971.

32. Gildenberg, P. L.: Percutaneous cervical cordotomy. Clin. Neurosurg., *21*:246–255, 1974.

33. Gildenberg, P. L.: VA symposium on Chronic Pain. Washington, D. C., 1977.

34. Gildenberg, P. L., Lin, P. M., Polakoff, P. P., II, and Flitter, M. A.: Anterior percutaneous cervical cordotomy: Determination of target point and calculation of angle of insertion. Technical note. J. Neurosurg., *28*:173–177, 1968.

35. Gildenberg, P. L., Zanes, C., Flitter, M., Lin, P. M., Lautsch, F. V., and Truex, R. C.: Impedance measuring device for detection of penetration of the spinal cord in anterior percutaneous cervical cordotomy. Technical note. J. Neurosurg., *30*:87–92, 1969.

36. Goodman, S. J., and Holcombe, V.: Selective and prolonged analgesia in monkey resulting from brain stimulation. *In* First World Congress on Pain. Seattle, Wash., Int'l Assoc. for the Study of Pain, 1975, p. 264.

37. Gunther, M. S.: Psychiatric consultation in rehabilitation hospital: A regression hypothesis. Compr. Psychiat., *12*:572–585, 1971.

38. Gybels, J., van Hees, J., and Peluso, F.: Modulation of experimentally produced pain in man by electrical stimulation of some cortical, thalamic and basal ganglia structures. *In* Zotterman, Y., ed.: Sensory Functions of the Skin in Primates, with Special Reference to Man. Wenner-Gren Center International Symposium Series. Oxford, Pergamon Press, 1976.

39. Halpern, L. M.: Treating pain with drugs. Minn. Med., *57*:176–184, 1974.

40. Hassler, R., and Reichert, T.: Kliniche und anatomische Befunde bei stereotacktichen Schmerzoperationen in Thalamus. Arch. Psychiat., *200*:92–122, 1959.

41. Hecaen, H., Talairach, J., David, M., and Dell, M. B.: Coagulations limitées du thalamus dans les algies du syndrome thalomique. Résultats thérapeutiques et physiologiques. Rev. Neurol., (Paris), *81*:917–931, 1949.

42. Hitchcock, E. R.: Stereotactic cervical myelotomy. J. Neurol. Neurosurg. Psychiat., *33*:224–230, 1970.

43. Hitchcock, E. R.: Stereotactic trigeminal tractotomy. Ann. Clin. Res., *2*:131–135, 1970.

44. Hitchcock, E. R., and Schvarcz, J. R.: Stereotactic trigeminal tractotomy for postherpetic facial pain. J. Neurosurg., *37*:412–417, 1972.

45. Hosobuchi, Y., Adams, J. E., and Rutkin, B.: Chronic thalamic stimulation for the control of facial anesthesia dolorosa. Arch. Neurol. (Chicago), *29*:158–161, 1973.

46. Hosobuchi, Y., Adams, J. E., and Weinstein, P. R.: Preliminary percutaneous dorsal column stimulation prior to permanent implantation. Technical note. J. Neurosurg., *37*:242–245, 1972.

47. Joyner, J., Merley, J., Jr., and Freeman, L. W.: Cordotomy for intractable pain of nonmalignant origin. Review of twenty cases. Arch. Surg. (Chicago), *93*:480–486, 1966.

48. Kahana, R. J., and Bebring, G. L.: Personality types in medical management. *In* Zinberg, N. E., ed.: Psychiatry and Medical Practice in a General Hospital. New York, International University Press, 1964, pp. 108–123.

49. Leksell, L., Meyerson, B. A., and Forster, D. M. C.: Radiosurgical thalamotomy for intractable pain. Confin. Neurol., *34*:264, 1972.

50. Lewis, J. R.: Misprescribing analgesics. J.A.M.A., *9*:1155–1156, 1974.

51. Liebeskind, J. C.: Behavioral and electrophysiological evidence of pain inhibition from midbrain stimulation in the cat. Exp. Brain Res., *20*:32–44, 1974.

52. Liebeskind, J. C.: Pain modulation by central nervous system stimulation. *In* Bonica, J. J., and Albe-Fessard, D., eds.: Advances in Pain Research and Therapy. Vol. 1. New York, Raven Press, 1976, pp. 445–453.

53. Liebeskind, J. C., Mayer, D. J., and Akil, H.: Central mechanisms of pain inhibition: Studies of analgesia from focal brain stimulation. Advances Neurol., *4*:261–268, 1974.

54. Liebeskind, J. C., Guilbaud, G., Besson, J. M., and Oliveras, J. L.: Analgesia from electrical stimulation of the periaqueductal gray matter in the cat: Behavioral observations and inhibitory effects on spinal cord interneurons. Brain Res., *50*:441–446, 1973.

55. Lin, P. M., Gildenberg, P. L., and Polakoff, P. P.: An anterior approach to percutaneous lower cervical cordotomy. J. Neurosurg., *25*:553–560, 1966.

56. Lindemann, E.: Symptomatology and management of acute grief. Amer. J. Psychiat., *101*:141–148, 1944.

57. Logue, V., and Watkins, E. S.: The treatment of intractable pain by stereotaxic thalamotomy. Report to Medical Research Council, Great Britain, London, 1962.

58. Long, D. M.: Cutaneous afferent stimulation for relief of chronic pain. Clin. Neurosurg., *21*:257–268, 1974.

59. Long, D. M., and Erickson, D. E.: Stimulation of the posterior columns of the spinal cord for relief of intractable pain. Surg. Neurol., *4*:134–141, 1975.

60. Long, D. M., and Hagfors, N.: Electrical stimulation of the nervous system. The current sta-

tus of electrical stimulation of the nervous system for relief of pain. Pain, *1*:109–123, 1975.

61. Mark, V. H., and Ervin, F. R.: Stereotactic surgery for relief of pain. *In* White, J. C., and Sweet, W. H.: Pain and the Neurosurgeon. Springfield, Ill., Charles C Thomas, 1969, pp. 843–887.

62. Mayer, D. J.: Pain inhibition by electrical brain stimulation: Comparison to morphine. Neurosci. Res. Program Bull., *13*:94–99, 1975.

63. Mayer, D. J., and Hayes, R. L.: Stimulation produced analgesia: Development of tolerance and cross-tolerance to morphine. Science, *188*:941–943, 1975.

64. Mayer, D. J., and Liebeskind, J. C.: Pain reduction by focal electrical stimulation of the brain: An anatomical and behavioral analysis. Brain Res., *68*:73–93, 1974.

65. Mayer, D. J., Wolfle, T. L., Akil, H., Carder, B., and Liebeskind, J. C.: Analgesia from electrical stimulation in the brain stem of the rat. Science, *174*:1351–1354, 1971.

66. McCulloch, J. A.: Percutaneous radiofrequency lumbar rhizolysis (rhizotomy). Appl. Neurophysiol., *39*:87–96, 1976–1977.

67. Melzack, R., and Wall, P.D.: Pain mechanisms: A new theory. Science, *150*:971–979, 1965.

68. Menninger, K. A.: Polysurgery and polysurgical addiction. Psychoanal. Quart., *3*:173–199, 1934.

69. Menzel, J., Piotrouski, W., and Penzholz, H.: Long-term results of Gasserian ganglion electrocoagulation. J. Neurosurg., *42*:140–143, 1975.

70. Meyerson, B. A., Boëthius, J., and Carlsson, A. M.: Percutaneous central gray stimulation for cancer pain. Appl. Neurophysiol., *41*:57–65, 1978.

71. Moore, D. C.: Regional Block. Springfield, Ill., Charles C Thomas, 1965.

72. Mullan, S., Hekmatpanah, J., Dobbin, G., and Beckman, F.: Percutaneous intramedullary cordotomy utilizing the unipolar anodal electrolytic lesion. J. Neurosurg., *22*:548–553, 1965.

73. Nashold, B. S., Jr., Wilson, W. P., and Slaughter, D. E.: Stereotactic midbrain lesions for central dysesthesia and phantom pain. J. Neurosurg., *30*:116–126, 1969.

74. North, R. B., Fischell, T. A., and Long, D. M.: Chronic dorsal column stimulation via percutaneously inserted epidural electrodes: Preliminary results in 31 patients. Appl. Neurophysiol., *40*:184–191, 1977–1978.

75. Onofrio, B. M.: Radiofrequency percutaneous Gasserian ganglion lesions; results in 140 patients with trigeminal pain. J. Neurosurg., *42*:132–139, 1975.

76. Orne, M. T.: Pain suppression by hypnosis and related phenomena. Advances Neurol., *4*:563–572, 1974.

77. Orthner, H.: Weitere Klinische und anatomische Erfahrungen mit zerebralen Schmerzoperationen. Confin. Neurol., *27*:71–74, 1966.

78. Owen, W. H. P.: Pills for personal problems. British Med. J., *27*:749–751, 1975.

79. Parkes, C. M.: Bereavement: Studies of Grief in Adult Life. New York, International University Press, Inc., 1972.

80. Parsons, T.: The Social System. New York, Free Press, 1951, pp. 428–479.

81. Peterson, B. H.: Psychological reactions to acute physical illness in adults. Med. J. Aust., *1*: 311–316, 1974.

82. Reynolds, D. V.: Surgery in the rat during electrical analgesia induced by focal brain stimulation. Science, *164*:444–445, 1969.

83. Richardson, D. E., and Akil, H.: Pain reduction by electrical brain stimulation in man. Part 1: Acute administration in periaqueductal and periventricular sites. J. Neurosurg., *47*:178–183, 1977.

84. Richardson, D. E., and Akil, H.: Pain reduction by electrical brain stimulation in man. Part 2: Chronic self-administration in the periventricular gray matter. J. Neurosurg., *4*:184–194, 1977.

85. Richardson, D. E., and Akil, H.: Pain reduction by electrical stimulation in man: Long-term results of periventricular gray self-stimulation. Pain, in press.

86. Roberts, A. H.: Biofeedback techniques: Their potential for the control of pain. Minn. Med., *57*:167–171, 1974.

87. Roeder, F., Orthner, H., and Müller, D.: Studies with stereotactic surgery in the Gasserian ganglion and mesencephalon, in combination with other methods (additional thalamotomy). *In* Janzen, R., Keidel, W. D., Herz, A., and Steichele, C., eds.: Pain. Baltimore, Williams & Wilkins Co., 1972, pp. 200–202.

88. Rosomoff, H. L.: Bilateral percutaneous cervical radiofrequency cordotomy. J. Neurosurg., *31*:41–46, 1969.

89. Rosomoff, H. L., Brown, C. J., and Sheptak, P.: Percutaneous radiofrequency cervical cordotomy: Technique. J. Neurosurg., *23*:639–644, 1965.

90. Royal Canadian Air Force Exercise Plans for Physical Fitness. New York, Simon and Schuster, 1962.

91. Ruda, M., Hayes, R. L., Dubner, R. and Price, D. D.: Analgesic and electrophysiological effects of stimulation of medial mesencephalic and diencephalic structures in the primate by electrical current or narcotic microinjection. Soc. Neurosci. Abstracts, Vol. 2. Bethesda, Society for Neuroscience, 1976.

92. Sano, K., Yoshioka, M., Ogashiwa, M., Ishijima, B., and Ohye, C.: Thalamolaminotomy. A new operation for the relief of intractable pain. Confin. Neurol., *27*:63–66, 1966.

93. Sargent, D. A.: Confinement and ego regression: Some consequences of enforced passivity. Int. J. Psychiat. Med., *5*:143–151, 1974.

94. Schvarcz, J. R.: Stereotactic trigeminal tractotomy. Confin. Neurol., *37*:73–77, 1975.

95. Schvarcz, J. R.: Spinal cord stereotactic techniques re trigeminal nucleotomy and extralemniscal myelotomy. Appl. Neurophysiol. *41*:99–112, 1978.

96. Schvarcz, J. R.: Stereotactic trigeminal nucleotomy: Evaluation of 100 cases. In preparation.

97. Seghal, A. D., Gardner, W. J., and Dohn, D. F.: Pantopaque "arachnoiditis." Treatment with subarachnoid injections of corticosteroids. Cleveland Clin. Quart., *29*:177–188, 1962.

98. Shealy, C. N.: Facets in back and sciatic pain. A new approach to a major pain syndrome. Minn. Med., *57*:199–203, 1974.

99. Shealy, C. N.: Transcutaneous electrical stimulation for control of pain. Clin. Neurosurg., *21*:269–277, 1974.

100. Shealy, C. N., Mortimer, J. T., and Hagfors, N. R.: Dorsal column electroanalgesia. J. Neurosurg., *32*:560–564, 1970.

101. Shealy, C. N., Mortimer, J. T., and Reswick, J. B.: Electrical inhibition of pain by dorsal column stimulation: Preliminary clinical report. Anesth. Analg. (Cleveland), *46*:489–491, 1967.

102. Skinner, B. F.: Beyond Freedom and Dignity. New York, Knopf, 1971.

103. Spiegel, E. A., and Wycis, H. T.: Mesencephalotomy in treatment of "intractable" facial pain. Arch. Neurol. Psychiat., *69*:1–12, 1953.

104. Spiegel, E. A., and Wycis, H. T.: Stereoencephalotomy. Part II: Clinical and Physiological Applications. New York, Grune & Stratton, 1962.

105. Spiegel, E. A., Wycis, H. T., Szekely, E. G., and Gildenberg, P. L.: Medial and basal thalamotomy in so-called intractable pain. *In* Knighton, R. S., and Dumke, P. R., eds.: Pain. Boston, Little, Brown & Co., 1966, pp. 503–517.

106. Spiegel, E. A., Wycis, H. T., Szekely, E. G., Gildenberg, P. L., and Zanes, C.: Combined dorsomedial intralaminar and basal thalamotomy for the relief of so-called intractable pain. J. Int. Coll. Surg., *42*:160–168, 1964.

107. Sternbach, R. A.: Pain and depression. *In* Kiev, A., ed.: Somatic Manifestations of Depressive Disorders. Excerpta Medica, New York, American Elsevier Publishing Co., 1974.

108. Sternbach, R. A.: Pain Patients, Traits and Treatment. New York, Academic Press, 1974.

109. Sugita, K., Mutsuga, N., Takaoka, Y., and Doi, T.: Results of stereotaxic thalamotomy for pain. Confin. Neurol., *34*:265–274, 1972.

110. Sweet, W. H.: Control of pain by direct electrical stimulation of peripheral nerves. Clin. Neurosurg., *23*:103–111, 1976.

111. Sweet, W. H., and Wepsic, J. C.: Stimulation of the posterior columns of the spinal cord for pain control: Indications, techniques and results. Clin. Neurosurg., *21*:278–310, 1974.

112. Swerdlow, M.: Intrathecal and extradural block in pain relief. *In* Swerdlow, M., ed.: Relief of Intractable Pain. Excerpta Medica, New York, American Elsevier Publishing Co., 1974, pp. 148–175.

113. Szasz, T., and Hollender, M.: A contribution to the philosophy of medicine: The basic models of the doctor-patient relationship. Arch. Intern. Med. (Chicago), *97*:585–592, 1956.

114. Tasker, R. R.: Thalamotomy for pain-lesion localization by detailed thalamic mapping. Canad. J. Surg., *12*:62–74, 1969.

115. Tasker, R. R., and Organ, L. W.: Percutaneous cordotomy: Physiological identification of target site. Confin. Neurol., *35*:110–117, 1973.

116. Todd, E. M., Crue, B. L., and Carregal, E. J. A.: Posterior percutaneous tractotomy and cordotomy. Confin. Neurol., *31*:106–115, 1969.

117. Travell, J.: Myofascial trigger points: Clinical view. *In* Bonica, J. J., and Albe-Fessard, D., eds.: Advances in Pain Research and Therapy Vol. 1. New York, Raven Press, 1976, pp. 919–926.

118. Travell, J., and Rinzler, S. H.: The myofascial genesis of pain. Postgrad. Med., *11*:425–434, 1952.

119. Voris, H. C., and Whisler, W. W.: Results of stereotaxic surgery for intractable pain. Confin. Neurol., *37*:86–96, 1975.

120. Wahl, C. W., and Golden, J. S.: The psychodynamics of the polysurgical patient: Report of sixteen patients. Psychosomatics, *7*:65–72, 1966.

121. Walters, A.: Psychogenic regional pain alias hysterical pain. Brain, *84*:1–18, 1961.

122. Watkins, E. S.: The place of neurosurgery in the relief of intractable pain. *In* Swerdlow, M., ed.: Relief of Intractable Pain. Excerpta Medica, New York, American Elsevier Publishing Co., 1974, pp. 21–58.

123. Watkins, E. S.: Stereotactic thalamotomy for intractable pain. Presented at the meeting of the Harvey Cushing Society, St. Louis, 1966.

124. Wepsic, J. G.: Complications of percutaneous surgery for pain. Clin. Neurosurg., *23*:454–464, 1976.

125. White, J. C., and Sweet, W. H.: Pain and the Neurosurgeon: A 40 Year Experience. Springfield, Ill., Charles C Thomas, 1969.

126. Wycis, H. T., and Spiegel, E. A.: Long-range results in the treatment of intractable pain by stereotaxic midbrain surgery. J. Neurosurg., *19*:101–107, 1962.

127. Zisook, S., and DeVaul, R. A.: Grief-related facsimile illness. Int. J. Psychiat. Med., *7*:329–336, 1977.

XIII

NEURO-PHYSIOLOGICAL AND ABLATIVE PROCEDURES

138

CRANIAL RHIZOPATHIES

Several "idiopathic" disorders of the cranial nerves have defied attempts at categorization, clarification of etiology, elaboration of mechanism, and definitive treatment despite study by investigators in several disciplines.[29] Theories about the cause of such apparently diverse "diseases" as trigeminal neuralgia, hemifacial spasm, Meniere's syndrome and its variants, paroxysmal vertigo, and glossopharyngeal neuralgia have been proposed but not verified.[17,28,58] These problems constitute the hyperactive dysfunction syndromes, each with a similar etiology. Another category exists, the hypoactive dysfunction syndromes, which include trigeminal neuropathy, Bell's palsy, vestibular neuritis and neuronitis, and probably some cases of idiopathic sensorineural hearing loss. Disorders in this category again appear to have a common etiological factor. In 1966, during an attempt at selective section of the trigeminal nerve at the brain stem for trigeminal neuralgia, it was noted that the trigeminal nerve root was cross-compressed and distorted by a small artery at its entry zone into the pons.[34] Later in 1966, a 41-year-old man was relieved (and has remained so to the present) of hemifacial spasm by coagulation and division of a small pontomedullary vein that was compressing and distorting the facial nerve exit zone at the brain stem.

The operation to relieve vascular compression of the cranial nerves was planned and performed as an extrapolation of the observations from the three original trigeminal neuralgia cases. It was based on the thesis that the compression caused a hyperactive dysfunction in a sensory nerve, the trigeminal, causing pain, and should also be true in the facial, causing twitching, or hemifacial spasm. A compressing vessel was noted in the former problem and should therefore be a distinct possibility in the latter. This premise proved to be valid. The natural extension to glossopharyngeal neuralgia and tinnitus and vertigo is obvious.

From 1966 to 1977, the author has explored and performed vascular decompression of the appropriate cranial nerve in 274 patients with trigeminal neuralgia, 85 with hemifacial spasm, 20 with acoustic nerve dysfunction, and 6 with glossopharyngeal neuralgia.* In the hyperactive dysfunction syndromes considered here, an abnormality of the root entry zone of the affected cranial nerve has been noted in almost every patient and has been treated by relocation and removal of the abnormality, eliminating the hyperactive neural function and lessening the neural hypofunction.[31]

In 1972, a 51-year-old woman was operated upon for an intractable lower cranial nerve problem unrelated to the subject of this discussion. Her history revealed that seven years earlier, she had suffered from Bell's palsy on the ipsilateral side and had recovered completely. At operation, the facial nerve was found to be stretched by an arterial loop a short distance from the brain stem. The relationships were left undisturbed. It was thought that the vascular compression of the facial nerve had caused the hypofunction of the nerve, i.e., Bell's palsy. As a result of this observation, this approach has been used in a small series of patients with hypoactive dysfunction symptoms.[32] They include 3 patients with trigeminal neuralgia, 12 with Bell's palsy, 4 with vestibular neuronitis, and 1 with hypoglos-

---

* See references 25–28, 30, 35, 38, 49.

P. J. JANNETTA

sal neuropathy. In the discussion of this group, Bell's palsy is used as the example.

VASCULAR DECOMPRESSION IN CRANIAL NERVE SYNDROMES

The hyperactive types of cranial nerve dysfunction are caused by vascular cross-compression at the root entry zone of the nerve. More peripheral vascular compression does not cause these problems. Because the root entry zone of the trigeminal nerve extends distally for quite some distance on the lateral side, a more peripheral vessel on the lateral side of the nerve can cause tic douloureux, usually in the distribution of the second division of the fifth nerve. In contrast, in the hypoactive dysfunction syndromes, the nerve is stretched by an arterial loop that apparently has shifted, and the site of the abnormality is not necessarily at the root entry zone.

Operative Technique and Assessment

In all patients the operation has consisted of a small (5.0 cm or less in diameter) retromastoid craniectomy with micro-operative exploration of the cerebellopontine angle performed in a modified sitting or lateral position. A superolateral cerebellar exposure has been used for the trigeminal nerve and an inferolateral cerebellar exposure for the lower cranial nerves. The most frequently noted abnormality has been vascular cross-compression of the nerve root at the brain stem by an arterial loop. Intrinsic or bridging veins also can cause the syndrome. The offending artery, although usually an elongated loop, has appeared to be normal except in elderly patients in whom arteriosclerotic plaques have been found. A small piece of muscle from the neck incision, silicone sponge, Teflon felt, or plastic sponge carved to fit the region has been used to hold the vessel away from the cranial nerve root entry zone by changing the axis of the loop after the vessel has been mobilized. Veins found to be compressing the root entry zone have been treated similarly or have been coagulated and divided. Tumors (often unrecognized before operation) were the cause of the symptoms in 21 patients and were resected. These tumors are extra-axial and benign, and appear to cause the symptoms by causing associated vascular compression of the nerve. Selective section of the sensory portio major of the trigeminal nerve has been performed in trigeminal neuralgia that was due to multiple sclerosis (seven cases) and when the vessel could not be mobilized safely (four cases).

In the present series, each patient was evaluated independently, before and after operation, by another neurosurgeon or a neurologist, and those with eighth nerve dysfunction were examined similarly by an otolaryngologist. Computed tomography, usually with enhancement, has been performed in all patients since 1975. Vertebral angiography was performed in selected patients. Operative findings were documented by 16-mm color motion picture films, videotapes, or 35-mm color slides. In addition, patients were assessed by preoperative and postoperative movies and special testing such as electromyography of the facial or temporalis and masseter muscles and otovestibular testing when indicated.

Case Material

From February 1966 to June 1977, observations were made on 399 patients. More than 600 patients have been operated upon subsequently, but are not included in this report. All patients had severe and disabling symptoms that were refractory to medical treatment or had recurred after a prior operation.

HYPERACTIVE DYSFUNCTION SYNDROMES

Trigeminal Neuralgia

This group was composed of 274 patients (119 men and 155 women, ages 31 to over 75 years). Of these, 158 had right-sided, 111 had left-sided, and 5 had bilateral tic douloureux. The majority of patients had developed recurrence of pain or carbamazepine intoxication. Lower facial tic (second or third division of the fifth nerve, or both) was usually correlated with nerve root compression from the anterocephalad direction (Fig. 138–1). Upper facial tic (first or first and second divisions) was associated with compression from the caudolat-

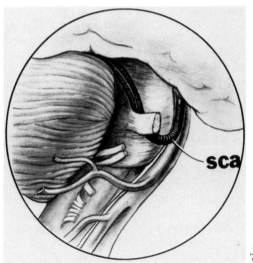

Figure 138–1 Lower facial trigeminal neuralgia (second division, third division, or both) caused by cross-compression of the trigeminal nerve root entry zone by the superior cerebellar artery (sca).

eral direction (Fig. 138–2). The most frequent cause of trigeminal nerve root compression was a looping superior cerebellar artery, found in over 80 per cent of patients, while the anterior inferior cerebellar artery was the cause in four. A vein was incriminated in 10 per cent of the patients. Tumors were found in and removed from 20 patients. Of the first 14 tumors, which occurred in the first 174 patients, the diagnosis of tumor was made preoperatively in only 3 patients.

The longest follow-up period after de-

compression as the sole treatment is now over 13 years. It is of interest that some patients, those in whom the trigeminal nerve was not touched at operation, had mild trigeminal neuralgia postoperatively. This gradually decreased and then disappeared. Recurrence of severe pain with headache occurred in four patients in the early postoperative period. Re-exploration showed that the implant had slipped and that the artery was once again compressing the nerve. Reinsertion of the implant was successful in stopping pain in three of the four. Additional discussion of trigeminal neuralgia is given in Chapters 119 through 123.

Hemifacial Spasm

Observations were made of 85 patients with classic hemifacial spasm (30 men and 55 women, ages 20 to 75 years). The mean was 51.1 years. Twenty-four patients had right-sided and 61 had left-sided symptoms. Eighty-two patients had vascular cross-compression or distortion of the facial nerve at the brain stem, usually by the vertebral artery, the posterior inferior cerebellar artery complex, or the anterior inferior cerebellar artery (Fig. 138–3). Of the remaining three patients, one, who had undergone two prior unsuccessful peripheral facial rhizotomies, had an epidermoid tumor 2.5 cm in diameter that compressed the facial nerve at its exit zone from the

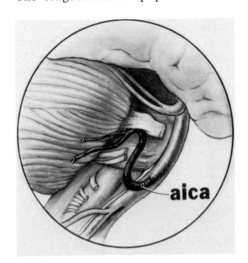

Figure 138–2 Upper facial trigeminal neuralgia (first division or first and second divisions) caused by compression of the trigeminal nerve root entry zone by the anterior inferior cerebellar artery (aica).

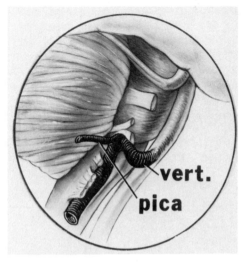

Figure 138–3 Hemifacial spasm caused by cross-compression of the facial nerve root exit zone by the vertebral artery (vert.)–posterior inferior cerebellar artery (pica) complex.

brain stem. Its removal relieved the symptoms. The second patient had a small arteriovenous malformation as the cause of the compression. The compression could not be eliminated adequately, and the symptoms persisted. The third patient had an aneurysm of the posterior inferior cerebellar artery causing the vascular compression. This woman had a history compatible with subarachnoid hemorrhage, and the diagnosis of aneurysm was established preoperatively. Eight patients had undergone prior unsuccessful peripheral or other nondefinitive procedures, one having had two suboccipital craniectomies without obtaining relief. The facial nerve was successfully decompressed and the aneurysm was clipped.

Pathological findings are listed in Table 138–1. In one elderly woman, operated upon in the lateral position, the vertebral artery was mobilized from the nerve without achieving relief. At re-operation in the modified sitting position it was found that the posterior inferior cerebellar artery was medial to the vertebral artery loop and was cross-compressing the facial nerve at the brain stem. It had been missed at the prior procedure. Mobilization of this vessel relieved the symptoms.

The vascular compression was relieved successfully in all patients in whom "normal" looping vessels were causing the trouble, but only temporarily in the one patient who had a small arteriovenous malformation in this area. Early replacement of the small plastic sponge implants, which had slipped out of position, was necessary in three patients. Re-exploration in a fourth patient whose hemifacial spasm had not improved 10 days postoperatively showed that the implant was in the proper place. Nothing further was done, and the spasm gradually disappeared.

An initially poor result, but one that provided important information, was noted in 1972 in a woman who developed ipsilateral peripheral facial palsy with hearing loss starting three days after the verbetral artery had been moved laterally away from the brain stem exit zone of the facial nerve. At re-exploration on the ninth postoperative day, a loop of the anterior inferior cerebellar artery, which had been horizontal, was found to be vertical, apparently mobilized by the lateral displacement of the vertebral artery or pia-arachnoid dissection. It was compressing the cochlear and facial nerves between the brain stem and porus acusticus. Postoperatively, facial weakness and hemifacial spasm persisted with some decrease in hearing on the same side. A second re-exploration was undertaken because of continuing mild spasm and facial weakness, and after placement of a new implant, her symptoms abated. Hearing was not improved. She is Case III in the Bell's palsy series.

Six patients had ipsilateral postoperative deafness (Table 138–2). This complication was due to technical error in one, was unavoidable in a second one because of severe scarring in the region from a prior course of radiation for pituitary adenoma, and although inexplicable in the remainder, was probably due to compression by the relatively hard plastic sponge inplant that was being used at the time or to operative trauma. The postoperative results are given in Table 138–3. Note that improvement of both strength and spasm is gradual after microvascular decompression.

Spasm, if present postoperatively, usually will be gone in 7 to 30 days. It persisted for nine months in one patient and for four and one half months in another. Return

TABLE 138–1 CAUSE OF HEMIFACIAL SPASM

CAUSE	NUMBER OF PATIENTS	
Vessel		83
Artery (single)	66	
Artery (multiple)	13	
Vein	2	
Artery and vein	2	
Tumor (cholesteatoma)		1
Arteriovenous malformation		1
Total		85

TABLE 138–2 COMPLICATIONS IN HEMIFACIAL SPASM PATIENTS

COMPLICATIONS	NUMBER OF PATIENTS
Temporary	
Air embolism	12
Herpes perioralis	7
Facial weakness	43 (present preoperatively in all but six)
Decreased hearing	15
Decreased IX, X nerve function—at least	5
Permanent	
Stance and gain ataxia, mild	1
Significant hearing loss	6
Persistent facial weakness	3

TABLE 138-3 RESULTS IN HEMIFACIAL SPASM (85 PATIENTS)

RESULT	EARLY	LATE
Excellent	45	74
Good	27	2
Fair	7	4
Poor	6	5
Recurrence (permanent after discharge)		1

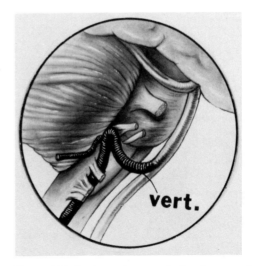

Figure 138-4 Acoustic nerve dysfunction caused by compression of the acoustic nerve root entry zone by the vertebral artery (vert.).

of normal strength of the muscles of facial expression is slower, although the face is usually stronger immediately postoperatively than it was preoperatively. This is especially true in those patients who have had a prior nerve section or crush.

Two other patients with atypical hemifacial spasm had cross-compression of the facial nerve root by the cochlear artery between the facial and acoustic nerves. Adequate decompression was not technically possible in either patient, and they are among those with poor results. More recently, the author has been able to decompress the nerve in patients with atypical hemifacial spasm in a series that is not included in the patient population reviewed for this chapter.

Acoustic Nerve Dysfunction

This group was composed of 20 patients with tinnitus and hearing loss, paroxysmal vertigo, or all three. The last-mentioned patients often meet the criteria for Meniere's disease.[1] Vascular cross-compression of the appropriate part of the acoustic nerve (cochlear, vestibular, or both) was noted in all patients. In this small group of patients, those with pure vestibular or combined cochlear-vestibular hyperactive dysfunction, and two with pure cochlear symptoms had vascular cross-compression at the root entry zone of the appropriate part of the acoustic nerve (Fig. 138-4). Three patients with pure cochlear involvement had a more peripheral compression of the cochlear nerve: in this group results were poor in one and fair in two. The failures were in this latter group and appear to be related to the technical difficulties of attempting to interpose a small prosthesis between the distal cochlear nerve medial to the porus acusticus and an underlying artery when "brain-sag" had drawn the eighth nerve down to the floor of the posterior fossa. Improvement in hearing on formal testing was not as striking as useful return of hearing due to a decrease in tinnitus in the patients with cochlear nerve dysfunction.

Those patients with vertigo and intercurrent unsteadiness have done well after microvascular decompression. Of 15 such patients, 11 are well clinically. Two have had late recurrence of symptoms; one was relieved by endolymphatic shunt. One older woman developed an internuclear ophthalmoplegia on her second postoperative day, which has persisted. She complains of more severe vertigo now than she had preoperatively. One is improved to a significant degree but is not asymptomatic. Improvement in tinnitus is variable. Some patients have had improvement in tinnitus, some are unchanged, none are worse. The author believes that microvascular decompression should be performed for tinnitus alone if it is disabling.

Glossopharyngeal Neuralgia

Observations were made of six patients with glossopharyngeal neuralgia, all of whom had cross-compression of the glossopharyngeal and vagus nerve fascicles at the brain stem root entry zone (Fig. 138-5). The vessel involved was the vertebral artery or posterior inferior cerebellar artery. Decompression in one of these patients was followed by a hypertensive crisis in the re-

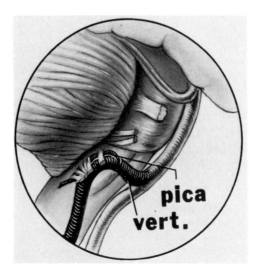

Figure 138–5 Glossopharyngeal neuralgia caused by compression of the glossopharyngeal and vagal nerve root entry zones by the vertebral artery (vert.)–posterior inferior cerebellar artery (pica) complex.

covery room and a large hemispheric intracerebral hemorrhage that resulted in the patient's death. This course of events occurred despite the absence of any history of hypertension. A second patient had hypertension for one week. This worrisome sequence has intriguing implications regarding medullary compression.[20,33,54] The left side of the heart is innervated by the left vagus nerve, and early experience with "essential" hypertension in both the clinical and laboratory setting suggests that arterial loops causing pulsatile compression of the left vagus nerve and anterior lateral medulla oblongata are a common factor in this clinical problem. Because of the risk of cardiovascular complications and the minimal morbidity of nerve section, the author is unsure about the place of microvascular decompression for glossopharyngeal neuralgia on the left. It appears to be safe on the right side. Medullary compression or stretching of the nerve must be avoided.

Discussion

A number of cranial nerve dysfunction syndromes occur that have several characteristics in common:

1. The nerves (V, VII, VIII, IX, X) are located in the posterior fossa and specifically in the cerebellopontine angle, where they are surrounded by normal arteries and veins.

2. The onset of symptoms of disordered hyperactivity in the involved nerve is gradual, and they become more severe, more frequent, and more prolonged.

3. The symptoms usually begin in midlife or later, when the arteries of the body may become tortuous and elongated owing to arteriosclerosis, and the brain may "sag."

4. In time, the symptoms of hyperactivity are superseded by progressive, although usually mild, decrease of hyperactivity and then progressive loss of function. This may progress to loss of the initial hyperactivity and total loss of function.

5. Standard operative treatment has usually consisted of a procedure involving the peripheral portion of the nerve, causing loss or decrease of function in the area of representation of the nerve.

6. These disorders appear, however, to be due to mechanical compression, usually vascular, of the nerve at the root entry or exit zone. Furthermore, symptoms of hyperfunction are relieved and those of hypofunction reversed by decompression.

7. These syndromes include trigeminal neuralgia, hemifacial spasm, tinnitus and vertigo, and glossopharyngeal neuralgia.

In all of these syndromes loss of function may gradually supervene in the prolonged course of the illness so that the early hyperfunction is accompanied by progressive loss of function in the pertinent cranial nerve. This is certainly true of trigeminal neuralgia in which, on careful examination, mild sensory abnormality is found in many patients (such was the case in 15 of 46 consecutive patients in this series who had not previously had any operation), in which constant burning facial pain is frequently observed after many years of illness, and in which electromyographic abnormalities consistent with denervation of the temporalis and masseter muscles may be found (40 per cent of patients tested in this series). This phenomenon was first noted by Saunders and co-workers.[52] In the author's patients, these abnormalities have returned to or toward normal after vascular decompression. For example, postoperative electromyography, performed in a small number of patients who had shown preoperative denervation, was normal. The sensory abnormality rapidly returned to normal in the patients with preoperative deficit.

Mild peripheral facial weakness gradually develops in patients with prolonged hemifacial spasm. Preoperative electromyographic data in the author's patients almost always showed evidence of denervation as well as changes due to overactivity. The electromyogram gradually returned to normal postoperatively in all 30 patients tested.

The correlation between elongation of intracranial arteries with arteriosclerotic cerebrovascular disease and the development of symptoms in most patients with these cranial nerve dysfunction syndromes is quite appropriate. Lewy and Grant, in 1938, discussed the role of arteriosclerosis in the etiology of tic douloureux, but then placed the theoretical arteriosclerotic abnormality within the brain.[40] Abnormalities of the cranial nerves in some cases of trigeminal neuralgia and hemifacial spasm were noted by several early investigators.[11–14,18–22] None of them had access to the operating microscope, and only one of them, Dandy, inspected the brain stem entry-exit zone of the trigeminal nerve in a large number of patients. Although handicapped by looking without magnification from a caudolateral direction, he still noted abnormalities in an increasingly large percentage of his patients. He noted similar abnormalities in a small percentage of his patients with Meniere's disease, but he did not inspect the nerve at the brain stem.[12–14] In reported series, unless the vascular abnormalities were gross, they generally were not seen, and in those patients who had obvious aneurysms or tumors, the diagnosis was usually changed from "trigeminal neuralgia" to "symptomatic trigeminal neuralgia," the primary diagnosis being aneurysm or tumor. In summary, up to the present era, when the micro-operative techniques have come into use, only Dandy had systematically looked at the lower cranial nerves at operation in cases of cranial nerve dysfunction syndromes, with or without magnification.

Observations in three types of control subjects have been utilized to compare the findings of the present study with the normal population: (1) careful inspection via the microscope of cranial nerve root entry or exit zones in patients operated upon for other problems (over 70 in number); (2) studies of cadavers who did not have trigeminal neuralgia in life (over 250 in number); and (3) two postmortem dissections of patients who did have trigeminal neuralgia in life.[23] Although the cranial nerves are normally surrounded by many vessels, as Sunderland has noted, specific cross-compression at the brain stem was rarely seen and was not remarkable when present in any of the asymptomatic subjects in the first two categories.[57] In the brains of the two who had trigeminal neuralgia in life, however, definite cross-compression and distortion of the ipsilateral (but not the contralateral) trigeminal nerve root at the entry-exit zone was found.

Neurovascular compression and distortion of cranial nerves has now been observed and relieved safely by a number of neurological surgeons.* In the present series, the compression and distortion had a vascular cause in all patients except 20 with trigeminal neuralgia and 1 with hemifacial spasm, who had a cholesteatoma. It was located precisely at the nerve root entry or exit zone in all patients in the series save five who had purely cochlear nerve dysfunction. It is of interest that central nervous system (oligondendroglial) myelin is present in the region of the porus acusticus in the cochlear nerve, in contrast to the other nerves discussed, in which the junction of central and peripheral myelin is at the nerve root entry or exit zone.

Abnormalities of myelin that have been noted in the trigeminal nerve in trigeminal neuralgia and in the facial nerve in hemifacial spasm may be due to compression; if so, decompression might result in remyelination.[7,8,49] There is some unpublished evidence, however, that some of these changes may be nonspecific and due to aging.[7,8,29] When the involved nerve was not touched, stroked, or manipulated at operation, the symptoms or signs (or both) of hyperactivity persisted postoperatively, although to a lesser degree than preoperatively. They gradually regressed in severity and frequency until they disappeared entirely with return of normal function of the involved nerve. Symptoms and signs of hypofunction gradually or rapidly disappeared in the postoperative period. This sequence clearly belies operative trauma as the cause of improvement.

It must be emphasized that etiology as discussed here must not be confused with

---

* See references 6, 9, 24–32, 34, 35, 38–41, 45, 46.

mechanism. Much discussion has been focused upon "central" versus "peripheral" mechanism in these symptom complexes, and discussants have frequently confused questions of mechanism with those of etiology. All pain certainly must have a central mechanism to be perceived, and the hyperactive motor abnormalities such as are found in hemifacial spasm may also denote central action, but central mechanism does not imply a central cause.

It must be further emphasized that the available evidence regarding acoustic nerve dysfunction and glossopharyngeal neuralgia is sufficient only for a preliminary statement regarding a vascular compressive etiology, in contrast to the more extensive and convincing evidence in trigeminal neuralgia and hemifacial spasm. Normal vessels have been found to distort cranial nerves peripherally in a high percentage of routine autopsy cases. They are not thought to cause symptoms.[57] This may or may not be true, but further observations with careful clinical correlation are necessary before this point can be clarified.

HYPOACTIVE DYSFUNCTION SYNDROMES

Bell's Palsy

Bell's palsy is one of a number of hypoactive cranial nerve dysfunction syndromes. It consists of rapid or sudden loss of function of the nerve, with a high incidence of rapid or slow, complete or partial recovery. Other syndromes include idiopathic loss of trigeminal function, the Ramsay-Hunt syndrome, vestibular neuronitis, and sudden sensorineural hearing loss. In the course of the foregoing experience with procedures for hyperactive dysfunction cranial nerve disorders, the author noted stretch of the facial nerve by an arterial loop in the cerebellopontine angle in a patient who had had Bell's palsy that had resolved (Case 1). Upon this first observation the present discussion is based.[25] The series now includes 12 patients with Bell's palsy, 3 with trigeminal neuropathy, 4 with vestibular neuronitis, and 1 with hypoglossal neuropathy. For discussion, Bell's palsy is used as the example of the loss of function syndromes.

Case 1

A 57-year-old housewife underwent right nervus intermedius section through a retromastoid craniectomy for intractable nervus intermedius neuralgia. She had a history of Bell's palsy on the right seven years before admission. There had been complete resolution of the facial weakness. At operation, the facial nerve was noted to be stretched by an arterial loop about 1 cm from the brain stem. The artery was left undisturbed.

Case 2

A 29-year-old telephone operator had Bell's palsy on the left six years before admission, with nearly complete recovery. One year before admission she developed rapidly progressive left facial weakness estimated at 60 to 75 per cent loss of function with abnormal motor movements of the ipsilateral muscles of facial expression (synkinesis). In July 1973, micro-operative exploration through a retromastoid craniectomy showed that an arterial loop, the anterior inferior cerebellar artery, was cross-compressing and stretching the facial nerve about 1 cm from the brain stem (Fig. 138–6). The arterial loop was mobilized away from the nerve. Postoperatively, the abnormal movements rapidly decreased to a low level with occasional residual mild spasm of the corner of the mouth. Facial muscle strength improved slowly to an estimated 80 to 90 per cent recovery.

Case 3

A 59-year-old housewife underwent left retromastoid micro-operative craniectomy in September 1972 for hemifacial spasm of three years' duration. The left vertebral artery was

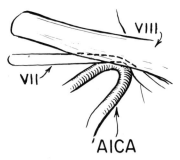

Figure 138–6 The relationship of facial nerve and artery in Bell's palsy. An arterial loop, the anterior inferior cerebellar artery (AICA), was cross-compressing and stretching the facial nerve (VII) about 1 cm from the brain stem. (Drawings for Figures 138–6 through 138–10 were made from slides or movies of view through operating microscope. Exposure is via retromastoid craniectomy, and the cerebellopontine angle is seen from behind.)

Figure 138–7 The relationship of facial nerve and artery in Bell's palsy. *a*. The left vertebral artery was found to be cross-compressing the facial nerve (VII) at the root entry zone and was mobilized from the nerve, with immediate improvement in spasm. Postoperatively the patient developed facial weakness and hearing loss. *b*. At exploration 10 days later the facial and cochlear nerves were found to be cross-compressed and stretched halfway between the brain stem and internal auditory meatus by a vertical loop of the anterior inferior cerebellar artery. (Drawings for Figures 138–6 through 138–10 were made from slides or movies of view through operating microscope. Exposure is via retromastoid craniectomy, and the cerebellopontine angle is seen from behind.)

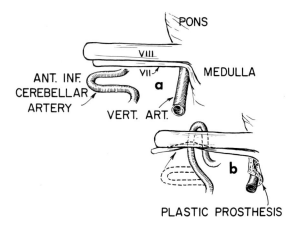

found to be cross-compressing the facial nerve at the root entry zone (Fig. 138–7*a*). The looping artery was mobilized from the nerve by interposition of a small piece of plastic sponge between the artery and adjacent brain stem, with immediate and progressive improvement in the spasm. But beginning at about 48 hours postoperatively, the patient developed progressive ipsilateral facial weakness and hearing loss. At exploration 10 days later the facial and cochlear nerves were found to be cross-compressed and stretched halfway between the brain stem and the internal auditory meatus by a vertical loop of the anterior inferior cerebellar artery (Fig. 138–7*b*). This loop had been horizontal at the first operation. A pledget of gelatin sponge was placed between the artery and the nerves, and moderate return of facial strength and hearing ensued. All symptoms, including the spasm, gradually recurred. At re-exploration in April 1974, it was noted that the vertebral artery was again cross-compressing the facial nerve at the brain stem, the plastic prosthesis having slipped, and the smaller artery was again stretching the facial and cochlear nerves in the midportion. Placement of a new plastic prosthesis was only partially successful in relieving hearing loss and facial weakness, and more successful in relieving the spasm.

Case 4

A 48-year-old interior designer underwent left retromastoid craniectomy with micro-operative exploration of the facial nerve for intractable Bell's palsy of 41 days' duration. He had some mild vertigo early in the course and severe ipsilateral occipital headache and tenderness. He had no motor or sensory facial nerve function preoperatively. At operation in March 1974, the facial-acoustic nerve bundle was found to be stretched and compressed from the anterior aspect of the facial nerve by a laterally-coursing loop of anterior inferior

cerebellar artery midway between brain stem and internal auditory meatus (Fig. 138–8*a*). When the arterial loop was mobilized forward, a taut bowstring of apparently arachnoidal tissue coursing from the apex of the loop to the dura of the petrous bone immediately filled with arterial blood. It was indeed an arteriole (Fig. 138–8*b*). The artery was mobilized from the facial nerve with a piece of plastic sponge. Buccinator muscle function began to return in the postanesthesia recovery room. Functional return continued slowly. Six months later the patient demonstrated 90 per cent recovery of facial function with a trace of residual synkinesis on severe forced motion of the muscles of facial expression.

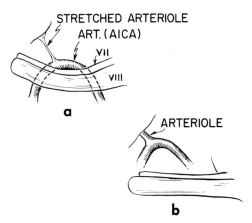

Figure 138–8 The relationship of facial nerve and artery in Bell's palsy. *a*. The facial (VII) and acoustic (VIII) nerve bundle was stretched and compressed by a laterally coursing loop of anterior inferior cerebellar artery midway between brain stem and internal auditory meatus. *b*. A bowstring of apparently arachnoidal tissue from the apex of the loop to the dura of the petrous bone was, in fact, an arteriole. (Drawings for Figures 138–6 through 138–10 were made from slides or movies of view through operating microscope. Exposure is via retromastoid craniectomy, and the cerebellopontine angle is seen from behind.)

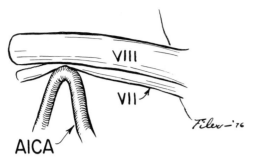

Figure 138–9 The relationship of facial nerve and artery in Bell's palsy. The facial nerve (VII) was stretched and cross-compressed by an arterial loop from the under side. (Drawings for Figures 138–6 through 138–10 were made from slides or movies of view through operating microscope. Exposure is via retromastoid craniectomy, and the cerebellopontine angle is seen from behind.)

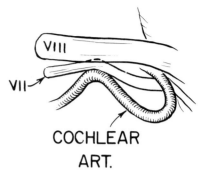

Figure 138–10 The relationship of facial nerve and artery in Bell's palsy. The facial nerve (VII) was doubly crossed, stretched, and compressed in the midportion and at the root entry zone by a long redundant loop of the cochlear artery. (Drawings for Figures 138–6 through 138–10 were made from slides or movies of view through operating microscope. Exposure is via retromastoid craniectomy, and the cerebellopontine angle is seen from behind.)

Case 5

A 73-year-old housewife developed synkinesis on the left following Bell's palsy in 1964. Peripheral facial nerve selective sections were performed elsewhere in 1967 and 1968 without relief. In May 1975, left retromastoid craniectomy with micro-operative exploration of the cerebellopontine angle was performed. The anterior inferior cerebellar artery gave off a cluster of small arteries under the facial nerve 4 mm medial to the internal auditory meatus. The facial nerve was yellowed, stretched, and cross-compressed from the under side by one of the arterial loops (Fig. 138–9). A small piece of plastic sponge was inserted between the artery and facial nerve, bringing temporary relief of symptoms, but on the third day spasms recurred. It is presumed that the prosthesis became dislocated.

Case 6

A 43-year-old attorney had left-sided Bell's palsy in 1971 with residual weakness, estimated at 30 to 40 per cent, and abnormal facial movements, felt to be compatible with post–Bell's palsy synkinesis. The movements were exacerbated severely when the patient talked, resulting in prolonged contraction that closed the eye and caused sustained hemifacial grimacing. Left retromastoid craniectomy with micro-operative exploration of the cerebellopontine angle was performed in November 1975. The facial nerve was doubly crossed, stretched, and compressed in the midportion and at the root entry zone by a long redundant loop of the cochlear artery (Fig. 138–10). This vessel was mobilized and held away from the nerve with a small prosthesis of plastic sponge, carved to fit the region. Postoperatively, the patient's facial strength improved

and there was concomitant decrease in the abnormal facial movements. He has continued to improve slowly since discharge, but some weakness and abnormal associated movement persists.

Discussion

Three major theories prevail regarding the etiology of Bell's palsy; namely, vascular ischemia, viral infection, and heredity. The vascular ischemia theory postulates that dysfunction of the autonomic nervous system leads to arteriolar spasm and thrombosis of the vessels supplying the nerve.[10] Experimental models have been designed to support the theory. Anatomical investigations reviewing the degree of anastomosis and overlapping of blood vessels that provide a highly adequate blood supply to the facial nerve seem to contradict this theory. Also, stripping of the peripheral nerve for 15 cm has produced no loss of function.

A second theory, postulating a viral cause for Bell's palsy, is currently popular. This theory is attractive because Bell's palsy closely resembles viral neuropathy in other peripheral nerves. It has been noted in association with polio, mumps, rubella, rubeola, and infectious mononucleosis. Herpes simplex virus is the organism most frequently cited as the insulting agent. It purportedly takes up residence within the peripheral nerve cell axon or sensory ganglion, where it is protected from neutralizing antibody and sensitized mononuclear immunocytes.[3,43] A number of authors have utilized complement-fixing antibody titers, serological testing, examination of serum and cerebrospinal fluid immunoglobulins, and isolation of the virus to support this etiological theory.[15,37,50] In contradiction are reports indicating that a large percentage (85 per cent) of control patients harbor antibodies to the herpes simplex virus as did the patients with Bell's palsy.[2,32,50] In addition, pathological examination such as that performed by Sadé revealed no evidence of edema, inflammatory changes, or blood vessel abnormalities in biopsy specimens of the nerve sheath epineurium.[2,50]

It has been suggested that Bell's palsy may represent a polyneuritis similar to herpes zoster oticus, as evidenced by the vestibular disturbances in the Ramsay-Hunt syndrome. Unequivocal pathological changes in the geniculate ganglion consistent with previous herpetic inflammation have been reported, the conclusion being that the eponym "Ramsay-Hunt syndrome" should be used only for cases of herpes zoster oticus with facial paralysis.[3,5] In addition, hypoesthesia may occur in the distribution of the fifth cranial nerve during the early stages of Bell's palsy, perhaps lending support to the suggestion that Bell's palsy is a polyneuritis. However, specific antibody studies for herpes zoster virus have not confirmed this hypothesis.[5] McGovern, to the contrary, considers the combination of the fifth and seventh nerve paralysis to be best explained by the vascular theory.[44] Brackmann has noted a number of studies that indicate that there is little concrete evidence to support the viral theory. Included in this monograph are references to the pathological studies of Sadé and associates, and to a prospective viral study of 27 patients with Bell's palsy and 14 matched control subjects, conducted by Brackmann, which revealed an abnormally increased protein level in only one patient who was subsequently found to have a herniated lumbar disc.[10,51] In addition, viruses could not be isolated from the gastrointestinal tract, nor could an increasing titer of any of the agents tested be observed.[10]

Hereditary factors resulting in Bell's palsy have been reported by Edgerton and co-workers, Willbrand and co-workers, and Singh and Singh.[16,55,59] Dispute persists with regard to this theory as well.

The clinical characteristics of the syndrome of rapid or sudden unilateral loss of facial nerve function have some intriguing aspects that have defied clinicopathological correlation to date. It is of interest that the loss of facial motor function may be almost instantaneous or slowly progressive, and partial or complete. Sensory facial nerve (nervus intermedius) dysfunction may occur, and appears more likely to occur in the patients with more severe facial motor loss. The syndrome at onset, and for a variable time thereafter, is accompanied by ipsilateral occipital headaches and frequently by tenderness over the ipsilateral occipital bone. The patient may develop ipsilateral tinnitus, vertigo, and hearing loss, which appears more likely to occur in the severely afflicted.

Synthesis of the foregoing clinical data with the operative findings in this small series demonstrates the following hypothetical explanation for the sequence:

It is well known that the arteries of the body elongate and become tortuous with age and may do so even in the relatively young, i.e., third decade of life. The brain stem and lower cranial nerves are surrounded by many arteries, which frequently impinge upon these nerves and are said to cause no harm. This condition has been described at postmortem examination, but without clinical correlation.[33,57] Nervous tissue is most tolerant to slow distortion or stretch, but quite intolerant to rapid distortion or stretch. Mild stretch of peripheral nerves is followed by recovery of function in most cases.

The sequence of clinical events just noted may thus correlate with the sudden shift of an arterial loop in the cerebellopontine angle, stretching the facial-acoustic nerve bundle between the brain stem and the internal auditory meatus from the anterior aspect (facial nerve side) for the following reasons:

The patient with Bell's palsy, on questioning, may observe that he "felt something" or that "something happened" in his ipsilateral suboccipital region at the onset of facial weakness. It is conceivable that this event may be the actual shift of the arterial loop. Ipsilateral occipital headache is common. The pain is conceivably due to the stretch or distortion of arachnoidal septa, dura mater, or arterioles (Case 3), or to nervus intermedius dysfunction.

The facial nerve may lose motor function partly or completely, and there may also be loss of sensory (nervus intermedius) function, especially in those patients who have severe loss of motor function. The arteries in the cerebellopontine angle are small, and the largest in the region capable of shifting to cause facial palsy should be the vertebral, basilar, anterior inferior cerebellar, and posterior inferior cerebellar. Smaller branches of these arteries may be responsible, or the shift of an arterial loop may be moderate, causing only partial loss with excellent recovery. There may be a more severe stretch of the adjacent nervus intermedius fascicles. This, rather than a medial-lateral problem, would seem a reasonable explanation of loss of sensory function in the facial nerve.

Loss of motor facial nerve function may also be accompanied by acoustic nerve dysfunction. This consists of tinnitus, vertigo, and hearing loss, and appears to be more frequent in those patients with more severe loss of facial function. This sequence may imply a more severe stretch of the facial-acoustic bundle by the shifting arterial loop.

Herpes simplex virus has now been cultured from most sensory ganglia both in patients and cadavers who did have and in those who never had dysfunction of the associated nerves. It is clear that resident viruses are stimulated by trauma such as section of a nerve. If Bell's palsy is the result of an injury to the facial nerve, the trauma may stimulate viruses residing in the geniculate ganglion to cause clinical cutaneous vesicles in some cases.

The facial-acoustic nerve bundle recovers variably from the hypofunctional state. This may depend on the size of the artery, the degree of stretch and compression, and the subsequent capacity of the specific neural tissue to recover.

Trigeminal neuropathy appears to be the sensory counterpart of Bell's palsy in the trigeminal nerve. Electrographic evidence of denervation in the temporalis and masseter muscles on the involved side is a frequent concomitant of this syndrome of ipsilateral facial numbness of sudden or rapid onset. Pain, mild to severe, constant in duration, and aching in character is also common. All but one of the author's patients had superior cerebellar arterial loops severely stretching the trigeminal nerve in the cerebellopontine angle. The motor proprioceptive fascicles, located on the anterocephalad side of the nerve as it approaches the pons, were seriously compromised by the apparently shifted, elongated arterial loop in all patients. Relief of numbness and pain is rapid; relief of motor weakness and denervation, slower after microvascular decompression.

Our patients with vestibular neuronitis all had sudden onset of vertigo and decreased vestibular function that persisted and was intractable. The vestibular nerves were stretched and compressed in the angle in all cases by arterial loops. Vestibular function improved slowly, with both vertigo and unsteadiness improving more rapidly, postoperatively.

One isolated case of hypoglossal neuropathy occurred in a 29-year-old man who was operated upon primarily for atypical trigeminal neuralgia. The left side of the tongue had been noted to be atrophic preoperatively. Special roentgenographic studies were normal. At operation, after microvascular decompression of the fifth nerve, a small medullary arterial loop was found to be abrading the stretched, thinned hypoglossal nerve against the basal dura. This was decompressed by using two small implants of soft plastic sponge. The patient remains free of pain, and his tongue gradually increased in strength, mobility, and muscle bulk.

The author's group is currently making observations on a number of other problems that appear similar to the aforementioned syndromes, all common concomitants of the aging process. These include a number of syndromes affecting the same cranial nerves, which may be due to peripheral cross-compression, to gradual stretch of the nerve in the cerebellopontine angle by elongating arterial loops and by veins, or to both. As Apfelbaum has stated, these procedures are "unforgiving," and thorough knowledge of cerebellopontine angle anatomy, extensive experience in procedures on the hindbrain, and expertise with the microscope are necessary if one is to make valid observations and operate safely.[6]

REFERENCES

1. Adour, K. K., and Wingerd, J.: Nonepidemic incidence of idiopathic facial paralysis. J.A.M.A., 227:653–654, 1974.

2. Adour, K. K., Bell, D. N., and Hilsinger, R. L.: Herpes simplex virus in idiopathic facial paralysis (Bell's palsy). J.A.M.A., *233*:527–530, 1975.

3. Aleksic, S. N., Budzilovich, G. N., and Lieberman, A. N.: Herpes zoster oticus and facial paralysis (Ramsay-Hunt syndrome). J. Neurol. Sci., *20*:149–159, 1973.

4. Alford, B. R.: Meniere's disease: Criteria for diagnosis and evaluation of therapy for reporting. Trans. Amer. Acad. Ophthal. Otolaryng., *76*: 1462–1464, 1972.

5. Antoli-Candela, F., and Stewart, T.; The pathophysiology of otologic facial paralysis. Otolaryng. Clin. N. Amer., *7*:309–330, 1974.

6. Apfelbaum, R. I.: A comparison of percutaneous radiofrequency trigeminal neurolysis and microvascular decompression of the trigeminal nerve for the treatment of tic douloureux. Neurosurgery, *1*:16–21, 1977.

7. Beaver, D. L., Moses, H. L., and Ganote, C. E.: Electron microscopy of the trigeminal ganglion II. Autopsy study of human ganglia. Arch. Path. (Chicago), *79*:557–570, 1965.

8. Beaver, D. L., Moses, H. L., and Ganote, C. E.: Electron microscopy of the trigeminal ganglion III. Trigeminal neuralgia. Arch. Path. (Chicago), *79*:571–582, 1965.

9. Becker, D. P.: What's new in neurologic surgery. Amer. Coll. Surg., Bull., pp. 23–27, January, 1978.

10. Brackmann, D. E.: Bell's palsy: Incidence, etiology and results of medical treatment. Otolaryng. Clin. N. Amer., *7*:357–368, 1974.

11. Campbell, E., and Keedy, D.: Hemifacial spasm: A note of the etiology in two cases. J. Neurosurg., *4*:342–347, 1944.

12. Dandy, W. E.: The treatment of trigeminal neuralgia by the cerebellar route. Ann. Surg., *96*:787–795, 1932.

13. Dandy, W. E.: Concerning the cause of trigeminal neuralgia. Amer. J. Surg., *24*:447–455, 1934.

14. Dandy, W. E.: Trigeminal neuralgia and trigeminal tic douloureux. *In* Lewis' Practice of Surgery. Hagerstown, Md., W. F. Prior Co., 1963, pp. 167–187.

15. Djupesland, G., Berdal, P., Johannessen, T. A., et al.: The role of viral infection in acute peripheral facial palsy. Acta Otolaryng. (Stockholm), *79*:221–227, 1975.

16. Edgerton, M. T., Tuerk, D. B., and Fisher, J. C.: Surgical treatment of Moebius syndrome by platysma and temporalis muscle transfers. Plast. Reconstr. Surg., *55*:305–311, 1975.

17. Friedmann, I. Pathology of the Ear. Oxford, Blackwell Scientific Publications, 1974, pp. 476–489.

18. Gardner, W. J.: The mechanism of tic douloureux. Trans. Amer. Neurol. Ass., *78*:168–173, 1953.

19. Gardner, W. J.: Concerning the mechanism of trigeminal neuralgia and hemifacial spasm. J. Neurosurg., *19*:947–957, 1962.

20. Gardner, W. J., and Dohn, D. F.: Trigeminal neuralgia—hemifacial spasm—Paget's disease—significance of this association. Brain, *89*: 555–562, 1966.

21. Gardner, W. J., and Miklos, M. V.: Response of trigeminal neuralgia to "decompression" of sensory root: Discussion of cause of trigeminal neuralgia. J.A.M.A., *170*:1773–1776, 1959.

22. Gardner, W. J., Todd, E. M., and Pinto, J. P.: Roentgenographic findings in trigeminal neuralgia. Amer. J. Roentgen., *76*:346–350, 1956.

23. Haines, S. J., Martinez, A. J., and Jannetta, P. J.: Arterial cross compression of the trigeminal nerve at the pons in trigeminal neuralgia. Case report with autopsy findings. J. Neurosurg., *50*:257–259, 1979.

24. Hankinso, H. L., and Wilson, C. B.: Microsurgical treatment of hemifacial spasm. Western J. Med., *124*:191–193, 1976.

25. Jannetta, P. J.: Arterial compression of the trigeminal nerve in patients with trigeminal neuralgia. J. Neurosurg., *26*:suppl.:159–162, 1967.

26. Jannetta, P. J.: Microsurgical exploration and decompression of the facial nerve in hemifacial spasm. Curr. Top. Surg. Res., *2*:217–220, 1970.

27. Jannetta, P. J.: Neurovascular compression of the facial nerve in hemifacial spasm: Relief by microsurgical technique. *In* Merei, F. T., ed.: Reconstructive Surgery of Brain Arteries. Budapest, Publishing House of the Hungarian Academy of Science, 1974, pp. 193–199.

28. Jannetta, P. J.: Neurovascular cross-compression in patients with hyperactive dysfunction symptoms of the eighth cranial nerve. Surg. Forum, *26*:467–468, 1975.

29. Jannetta, P. J.: Microsurgical approach to the trigeminal nerve for tic douloureux. Progr. Neurol. Surg., *7*:180–200, 1976.

30. Jannetta, P. J.: Treatment of trigeminal neuralgia suboccipital and transtentorial cranial operations. Clin. Neurosurg., *24*:538–549, 1977.

31. Jannetta, P. J.: Observations on the etiology of trigeminal neuralgia, hemifacial spasm, acoustic nerve dysfunction and glossopharyngeal neuralgia. Definitive microsurgical treatment and results in 117 patients. Neurochirurgia, *20*:145–154, 1977.

32. Jannetta, P. J., and Bissonette, D. J.: Bell's palsy: A theory as to etiology. Observations in six patients. Laryngoscope, *88*:849–854, 1978.

33. Jannetta, P. J., and Gendell, H.: Observations on the etiology of "essential" hypertension. Surg. Forum, *30*:431–432, 1979.

34. Jannetta, P. J., and Rand, R. W.: Transtentorial subtemporal retrogasserian neurectomy in trigeminal neuralgia by microsurgical technique. Bull. Los Angeles Neurol. Soc., *31*:93–99, 1966.

35. Jannetta, P. J., Abbasy, M., Maroon, J. C., Morales Ramos, F., and Albin, M. S.: Hemifacial spasm: Etiology and definitive microsurgical treatment. Operative techniques and results in forty-seven patients. J. Neurosurg., *47*:321–328, 1977.

36. Knight, G.: Herpes simplex and trigeminal neuralgia. Proc. Roy. Soc. Med., *47*:788–790, 1954.

37. Korczyn, A. D., Swirski, R., and Henig, E.: Bell's palsy and viral infections, Eur. Neurol., *10*:191–196, 1973.

38. Laha, R. K., and Jannetta, P. J.: Glossopharyngeal neuralgia. J. Neurosurg., *47*:316–320, 1977.

39. Lazar, M. L.: Trigeminal neuralgia: Recent advances in management. Texas Med., *74*:45–48, 1978.

40. Lewy, F. H., and Grant, F. C.: Physiopathologic and pathoanatomic aspects of major trigeminal neuralgia. Arch. Neurol. Psychiat., *40*:1126–1134, 1938.

41. Loeser, J. D.: What to do about tic douloureux. J.A.M.A., *239*:1153–1155, 1978.
42. Malis, L. I.: Petrous ridge compression and its surgical correction. J. Neurosurg., *26*:163–167, 1967.
43. McCormic, D. P.: Herpes simplex virus as a cause of Bell's palsy. Lancet, *1*:937–939, 1972.
44. McGovern, F. H.: Trigeminal sensory neuropathy and Bell's palsy. Arch. Otolaryng. (Chicago), *94*:466–470, 1971.
45. Petty, P. G.: Arterial compression of the trigeminal nerve at the pons as a cause of trigeminal neuralgia. Inst. Neurol. Madras, Proc., *6*:93–95, 1976.
46. Petty, P. G., and Southby, R.: Vascular compression of lower cranial nerves: Observations using microsurgery, with particular reference to trigeminal neuralgia. Aust. New Zeal. J. Surg., *47*:317–320, 1977.
47. Reis, D. J., and Doba, N.: Fulminating hypertension from restricted lesions of brainstem. Trans. Amer. Neurol. Ass., *98*:219–221, 1973.
48. Rhoton, A., Jr.: Microsurgery of the internal acoustic meatus. Surg. Neurol., *2*:311–318, 1974.
49. Ruby, J. R., and Jannetta, P. J.: Ultrastructural changes in the facial nerve induced by neurovascular compression. Surg. Neurol., *4*:369–370, 1975.
50. Sadé, J.: Pathology of Bell's palsy. Arch. Otolaryng. (Chicago), *95*:406–414, 1972.
51. Sadé, J., Levy, E., and Chaco, J.: Surgery and pathology of Bell's palsy. Arch. Otolaryng. (Chicago), *82*:594–602, 1965.
52. Saunders, R. L., Krout, R., and Sachs, E., Jr.: Masticator electromyography in trigeminal neuralgia. Neurology (Minneap.), *21*:1221–1225, 1971.
53. Scoville, W. B.: Hearing loss following exploration of cerebellopontine angle in hemifacial spasm. J. Neurosurg., *31*:47–49, 1969.
54. Segal, R., Gendell, H., Canfield, R., Dujovny, M., and Jannetta, P.: Cardiovascular response to pulsatile pressure. Surg. Forum, *30*:433–435, 1979.
55. Singh, H., and Singh, J.: An unusual presentation of peripheral facial paralysis in a family. J. Ass. Physicians India, *21*:905–907, 1973.
56. Snyder, R. D.: Bell's palsy and infectious mononucleosis. Lancet, *2*:917–918, 1973.
57. Sunderland, S.: The arterial relations of the internal auditory meatus. Brain, *68*:23–27, 1945.
58. Wartenberg, R.: Hemifacial Spasm. A Clinical and Pathophysiological Study. New York, Oxford University Press, 1952.
59. Willbrand, J. W., Blumhagen, J. D., and May, M.: Inherited Bell's palsy. Ann. Otol., *83*:343–346, 1974.

139

PRINCIPLES OF STEREOTAXIC SURGERY

This chapter does not present an exhaustive review of stereotaxic minutiae. For the surgeon considering the use of stereotaxic procedures it does provide some general principles upon which to base selection of a method or to devise apparatus of his own. For the more experienced stereotaxic surgeon it provides a review of the ideas of others and some references with which to further study the problems.

X-RAY LOCALIZATION

Reduced to its essentials, a stereotaxic operation consists simply of locating the target zone; inserting the electrode, probe, or other instrument after appropriate adjustments of the stereotaxic instrument; and verifying by x-ray and other means that the target zone has indeed been entered. Of the three steps, the localization of the target zone is the most difficult, since it is subject to errors in the x-ray localization of anatomical landmarks and individual variations in the relationship of these landmarks and the target zone. There is considerable literature regarding the varying relationships of x-ray landmarks and diencephalic targets in the "normal" brain and cranium, but practically nothing is known about possible variables introduced by disease.

Selection of Stereotaxic Landmarks

Perhaps the cardinal feature in selection of an x-ray landmark is that it should be as close as possible to the selected target. Thus it would be poor judgment to use landmarks in the third ventricle to place lesions in the amygdala when the posterior border of this nucleus may be directly visualized with a contrast medium in the tip of the temporal horn.[223]

The choice of a landmark becomes less obvious when the target cannot be directly visualized. Stereotaxic work in lower animals led to the hope that graphic reconstructions from the bony cranium might prove sufficient for stereotaxic localizations in man. Several investigators attempted to do this, but further study has shown the futility of these efforts.[82,117,187,200,213] It is generally accepted that the most reliable landmarks are intracerebral.[202,211]* The most commonly used points in the diencephalon are the foramen of Monro or the anterior commissure, the posterior commissure, and the midline of the third ventricle, since they may be readily demonstrated with standard x-ray techniques. It should be noted that changes in ventricular dimensions occur after lumber or ventricular air injection. The third ventricle (and the anterior and posterior commissures) seems less affected, but changes in the position of the commissures in relation to skull structures may range up to ±2 to 4 mm three to six hours after ventricular filling.[51,155,200]

To locate any site in space, three reference points are required corresponding to the x, y, and z axes in three-dimensional graphic plotting. Although this concept seems elementary, apparently much stereo-

---

* Mundinger's group has reopened the question by using several bony landmarks correlated with a computer to localize the target.[108] It is not clear, however, that this method can match the accuracy with which target sites can be derived from ventricular landmarks.

J. M. VAN BUREN AND R. A. RATCHESON

taxic surgery has been done with visualization of only two (e.g., the foramen of Monro on the lateral view and the third ventricular outline on the sagittal view). Good results have been reported from these procedures, but they would seem more a tribute to the intuitive skill of the surgeon than to the method. Since radiographic techniques are now available for the reliable demonstration of the required three reference points, there seems little reason to rely on partial evidence.

Contrast Demonstration of Stereotaxic Landmarks

Pneumoencephalography

Fractional pneumography following Lindgren's technique has made possible the routine demonstration of many intracerebral details, including those important for stereotaxic localization.[68,137-139] The technique, however, requires care and patience and cannot be profitably left to untrained assistants. A further difficulty lies in the necessity for careful positioning of the patient. Although this is possible in the operative situation described by Talairach and co-workers, it may not be possible in other theaters.[213] Furthermore, it is usually not possible to demonstrate both commissures on the same film. This necessitates combining films that show each of the commissures so that the anterior commissure–posterior commissure (AC–PC) line can be constructed. The technique is outlined here, as it is occasionally useful, but under most circumstances, a ventriculographic technique is more accurate.

At the start of the pneumoencephalogram, after the patient has been properly positioned in the sitting position with the head sharply flexed forward, introduction of 15 to 25 cc of air (without removal of spinal fluid) will show the aqueduct of Sylvius, the posterior commissure, and the posterior portion of the third ventricle. The exposure should be made within a few seconds of the end of the air injection to avoid loss into the ventricles above. An anteroposterior view to show the midline of the body of the third ventricle can be made at this time after slightly extending the head. More air may then be introduced and the remainder of the routine pneumoencephalogram completed.

It should be remembered, however, that collections of air over the insula often interfere with visualization of the anterior commissure on the lateral views. As a final step the patient is placed in the supine position, and the head is allowed to fall back over the end of the table to allow air from the lateral ventricles to re-enter the third ventricle. With this manipulation, the anterior commissure can be reliably visualized on the lateral view and the anteroposterior exposure will demonstrate the transverse position of the anterior part of the third ventricle. These exposures are left to last, since loss of ventricular air back down the aqueduct may occur.

Reconstruction of Landmarks from the Calvarium

Establishing the AC–PC line on a single lateral x-ray of the head when the commissures are separately demonstrated by pneumoencephalography necessitates the reconstruction of one of the commissures. Commissural reconstruction is also useful to localize implanted electrodes or other radiopaque objects once the contrast medium has left the ventricular system. The method, originally described by Mundinger and Riechert, was later investigated by Flamm and Van Buren using the stereotaxic pneumoencephalograms of patients in whom two had been done and reconstructing the AC–PC line from the first study onto the second.[82,157] Statistical study of the error between the actual and the reconstructed commissural positions showed a standard deviation of 1 to 2 mm for the sagittal and vertical differences of both commissures. Thus for localizations within the thalamus and upper brain stem the error appeared acceptable. Owing, however, to the possibility that the AC–PC line could be tilted by additive errors in the commissural positions (i.e., one up and the other down), caution should be exercised in interpreting localizations farther from the AC–PC line (Fig. 139–1). In the transverse plane the standard deviation of the error in reconstructing the midline of the third ventricle from the external tables of the temporal fossae was 0.8 mm.

The graphic method for reconstructing the ventricular landmarks is as follows (Fig. 139–2): On the base of the skull two points are selected; one, a well-defined bony irreg-

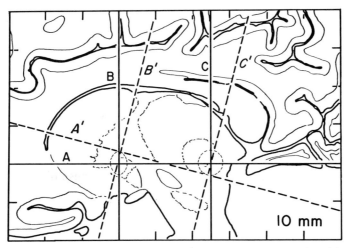

Figure 139–1 An evaluation of summed errors introduced by graphic reconstruction of the commissures from basal bony landmarks. On this section, 10 mm from the midline, the lateral projections of the anterior and posterior commissures are indicated by the intersections of line A with B and C, respectively. The areas around the commissures enclosed by broken lines have major diameters equal to 4 standard deviations of the mean difference between the actual and reconstructed commissures. Broken lines A', B', and C' indicate the maximum displacement of the AC–PC axis, assuming all errors are additive. The margins of the drawing are marked at 1-cm intervals. Outlines of the main thalamic mass, centrum medianum, subthalamic nucleus, substantia nigra, pallidum (medial and lateral parts), caudate nucleus, and optic tract are indicated on the drawing. (From Flamm, E. S., and Van Buren, J. J.: The reliability of reconstructed ventricular landmarks for localization of depth electrodes in man. J. Neurosurg., 25:67–72, 1966. Reprinted by permission.)

ularity in the vicinity of the base of the dorsum sellae, and the other on the planum sphenoidale at a point halfway between the outlines of the temporal fossae. These points define a line forming the base of two triangles having the anterior commissure and the posterior commissure as their respective apices. Differences in magnification between the original and later films can be judged either by external scales or by distances between distinctive landmarks in the skull itself. A draftsman's proportional dividers are adjusted to compensate for any difference in magnification on the two films, the bony landmarks are marked on the new film, and the commissures are reconstructed with the dividers. In the anteroposterior x-rays, the midline of the third ventricle is related to the external surface of the temporal squamae along a line parallel to the orbital roofs, which is arbitrarily accepted as parallel to the horizontal plane of the brain.

Because the commissures are centrally located and the reference points on the skull base are near the center of rotation of the head, they are relatively little influenced by change in skull position (Fig. 139–3). Although this should not permit one to be careless in positioning the head for x-ray films, it affords some reassurance

that minor differences in projection are not of great significance to the localization.

Ventriculography

Ventriculography, since it demonstrates the ventricular landmarks at the time of electrode insertion, is probably the most accurate method. Provided that visualization is adequate, one is spared the inaccuracies attending transfer of landmarks from the preoperative pneumogram to the film taken in the operating theater. Care must be taken to fix the head and x-ray tube positions for sequential films, and if films are to be taken in the supine position, x-ray equipment that is installed in the ceiling is desirable. As always, there is no substitute for care and patience in positioning the patient and aligning the x-ray tube as precisely as possible.

Positive Contrast Media

Unfortunately, at the present time there is no ideal positive contrast medium for intracranial examinations. Iophendylate (Pantopaque) is so widely used for myelography that its use is accepted rather casually. This has been fostered by the practice at the National Hospital, Queen

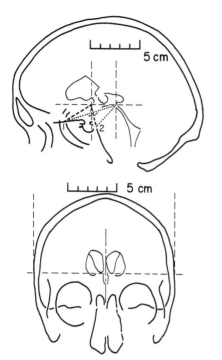

Figure 139–2 Method of relating the anterior and posterior commissures to basal bony landmarks for reconstructing these reference points on later films without contrast medium in the ventricular system. On the lateral view, point 1 lies on the planum sphenoidale between the outlines of the temporal fossae. Point 2 is a well-defined bony irregularity near the dorsum sellae. These form the base from which triangles may be erected to the commissures (dashed and dotted lines). On the sagittal view the midline of the third ventricle is related to its distance from the lateral aspects of the temporal fossae. (From Flamm, E. S., and Van Buren, J. M.: The reliability of reconstructed ventricular landmarks for localization of depth electrodes in man. J. Neurosurg., 25:67–72, 1966. Reprinted by permission.)

Square, London, of leaving all contrast medium in situ after myelography. Follow-up study of their patients by Davies showed that of 115 patients, 76 had varying subsequent symptoms; of 5 patients on whom exploratory operations were later performed, 4 had evidence of arachnoiditis of the cauda equina.[64] Finally, three cases coming to postmortem examination had thickening of the basilar meninges of the brain. Experimental studies have consistently demonstrated evidence of a chemical meningitis, often with a granulomatous response, after administration of Pantopaque, and this is apparently aggravated by the presence of blood in the cerebrospinal fluid.[81,112,114] There seems little reason to doubt that there is a definite untoward reaction to Pantopaque in the cerebrospinal fluid path-

ways. Fortunately, this usually remains subclinical, particularly when care is taken to remove as much of the iodized oil as possible after myelography. Serious clinical reactions and even death have been ascribed to its use, however, and the material should be avoided if other means are available.[73,146,184,214,216] The objection to its use in ventriculography is stronger than in myelography, since the possibility of removing a significant amount of the oil after ventriculography is much less. Nevertheless, the convenience of the method has prompted its continued use by various workers.[77,241] Wycis and Gildenberg have reported the use of impedance methods to localize the ventricle accurately and reduce the instillation of oil in areas where it is not wanted.[241]

Owing to these difficulties, attention has turned in recent years to the substitution of water-soluble contrast materials. The one most extensively investigated has been monoiodomethane sulfonate (methiodal sodium, Abrodil, Skiodan, Kontrast U). In animals it has proved to be highly irritating, causing muscle spasms, blood pressure changes, and breakdown of the blood-brain barrier in the spinal cord as judged by trypan blue injections.[89] Varying degrees of cord damage and inflammatory reaction were also found.[90,100] Clinical use of the medium for myelography requires spinal anesthesia to control muscle spasm and pain, and a few cases of paralysis of the legs or sphincters or both have resulted.[136,195] Diatrizoate sodium (Hypaque) has also been found to be highly irritating.[221]

Trials of meglumine iothalamate (Conray) have shown it to be irritating, though possibly less so than the other materials mentioned.[65] A convulsion has been reported as one of the complications in a patient; and in dogs and monkeys, epileptiform activity has resulted from its application to the cerebral cortex.[46,65,71]

Kandel and Chebotarynova found that 3.7 per cent of 320 Conray ventriculograms were followed by seizures, and one patient died.[119] Heimburger and co-workers reported 102 Conray ventriculograms with two deaths.[106] Dimer-X has been successfully employed for ventriculography.[108] Although this agent appears to be less irritating than Conray 60, about 2 per cent of the ventriculograms are attended by seizures.[2]

Hyperbaric positive contrast media offer

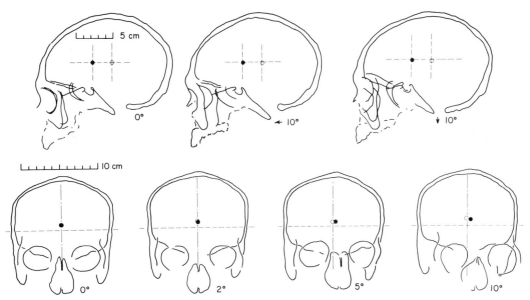

Figure 139–3   Effects of skull rotation upon the relation of the anterior (·) and posterior (○) commissures to the commissures reconstructed from a true lateral and anteroposterior view by the method given in Figure 139–2 and the text. The reconstructed commissures situated at the intersection of the perpendiculars and the AC–PC line are shown by broken lines. The arrow indicates the direction of movement of the side of the skull toward the x-ray tube. On the anteroposterior view the midskull is shown by the center line reconstructed in relation to the lateral aspects of the temporal fossae. The horizontal broken line parallel to the orbital roofs is assumed to be parallel to the horizontal axis of the brain. The degrees of skull rotation are approximate. (From Flamm, E. S., and Van Buren, J. M.: The reliability of reconstructed ventricular landmarks for localization of depth electrodes in man. J. Neurosurg., 25:67–72, 1966. Reprinted by permission.)

two advantages in stereotaxic operations. In the sitting position, if care is taken to prevent undue loss through the aqueduct, a few milliliters will fill the third ventricle and thus provide the commissural and ventricular landmarks. Perhaps more important for the surgeon, who needs the information urgently, is the density to x-rays that permits exposures on rapidly processed film (Polaroid) although it offers relatively poor contrast.

Positive-Pressure Air Ventriculography

For stereotaxic purposes, ordinary ventriculography performed with the vertex up and air exchanged for ventricular fluid has two disadvantages. Because there is relatively little difference in density to x-rays between air and brain substance, conventional films must be used, preferably with special fine line grids for maximum definition. This entails time-consuming wet processing, but automatic processing equipment now available reduces this to about five minutes. The second drawback, which also applies to pneumoencephalography, is

the difficulty in simultaneously visualizing both commissures in the third ventricle. This is overcome by injecting air into the ventricles with sufficient pressure to fill the third ventricle and displace the fluid down the aqueduct with the patient in the brow-up position. Visualization has been reliable and without serious complications apart from some headache, which, in general, is less severe than after pneumoencephalography.[25,40]

Positive-pressure air ventriculography is the most generally satisfactory and least hazardous method known to the authors for demonstrating stereotaxic landmarks. The possibility that the brain is significantly "blown up" or distorted by the procedure appears unlikely. Superimposed tracings of ventricular outlines following the initial injection with sufficient pressure to force air down the aqueduct and after release of this pressure show no striking differences (Fig. 139–4). This comparison cannot be said to be absolutely conclusive, since the degree of visualization differs on the two sets of films. Still, the outlines of the lateral ventricles are roughly the same, and these would seem to be most susceptible to change.[134]

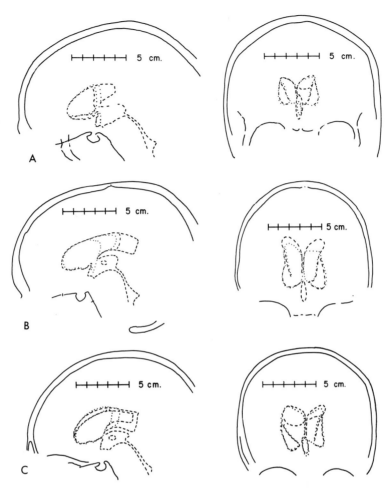

Figure 139–4   Examples of the effects of pressure air ventriculography on the size of the ventricles of a case with mild symmetrical dilatation (*B*) and asymmetrical dilatation (*C*) evaluated by superimposing the outlines before (dashed lines) and after (dotted lines) the release of ventricular pressure. Observations of this type have convinced the authors that distortion of the ventricular outline by pressure air ventriculography is negligible.

X-Ray Technique

The vast majority of the difficulties experienced in stereotaxic surgery are the result of inadequate ventricular filling with contrast medium, improper positioning of the patient, and incorrect x-ray exposure.

A number of the current stereotaxic instruments provide for rigidly fixing the head by pins directly inserted in the outer table of the skull. Fixation of this type is comfortable for the patient, but should incorporate a breakaway device so that the patient's head can be freed quickly in case of vomiting or some other threat to his airway. Its most important function is to hold the head securely once it has been aligned with the midsagittal plane of the brain parallel with the x-ray cassette and perpendicular to the central beam of the x-ray. Alignment of the central beam is not an easy matter but is much aided by centering a projected visible light source that coincides with the central beam. Checking that the central beam and the projected light beam actually coincide should not be neglected, and a technique is given by Talairach and associates.[213]

Although the work can be done with a portable x-ray unit, this is at best a makeshift for stereotaxic work, and permanent units installed in the ceiling and wall of the operating theater immensely increase both speed and precision. In some techniques the x-ray tube and stereotaxic instrument are locked together by an intervening frame. This permits consistent relationships of the tube head and cassette, but it precludes the use of the longer projection distances that offer certain advantages. Sometimes cranial asymmetry makes it difficult to position the patient accurately. Fortunately, as shown in Figure 139–3, minor degrees of malposition do not introduce large errors for targets in the vicinity of the third ventricle.

The notion that x-ray magnification increases with the distance from the central beam reappears from time to time in the literature despite the proof to the contrary supplied by Spiegel and Wycis.[186,197] The matter may be easily settled in a practical way by making an x-ray exposure of uniform wire netting placed at a distance from, but parallel to, the cassette and exposed with the central beam perpendicular to the cassette. Although the netting will be magnified, the size of the interstices will be found to be uniform throughout the film without regard to the position of the central x-ray beam.

In most stereotaxic techniques it is important to know the degree of magnification on the x-ray film. When the target and instrument reference sites lie on different planes in the x-ray projection, correction must also be made for parallax. Since the means of correcting for these sources of error differs with each group of instruments, the matter is discussed in the section concerning stereotaxic instruments.

CEREBRAL VARIATION AND X-RAY LANDMARKS

Opinion regarding the importance of individual diencephalic variation in stereotaxic surgery has varied from those who are quite content to use coordinates from a "model" brain for all applications to those who place little reliance on the localization found on x-ray examination and try physiological methods to control the lesion site. As in most other problems, the solution probably lies somewhere between the extremes. It is obvious that no physical method can ever be mathematically accurate, and certainly not when biological variation is also involved. On the other hand, safety is possible when the degree of inaccuracy is known and when provision is made to stay within the proper confines of the system.

Proportional Corrections

Proportional correction factors have been much in vogue, and the additional effort with the slide rule in applying them gives an added sense of precision to the localization.[41,66,104,211,213] All such factors, however, make the implicit assumption that large and small brains and all their contained structures are made to the same relative measurements and are simply reproduced at different scales. The cranial variation with its lack of fixed points is well known to anthropologists. A special study for fitting gas masks during World War II illustrated similar cranial incongruities. It is perhaps wishful thinking to suppose that the brain should be consistently arranged while its container is not.

In applying proportional corrections it has been hoped that the demonstration of some radiographic interval might by analogy give an indication of the extent of a structure not apparent on the film. On the anteroposterior projection one such interval is from the midline to the lateral aspect of frontal horn of the lateral ventricle. Brierley and Beck and Talairach and co-workers found this to be unreliable in predicting the thalamic width.[41,211] The latter authors also found that the interval from the midline to the lateral border of the hippocampus did not form a useful interval upon which to base a proportional correction on the transverse axis. A vertical correction factor based upon the interval from the AC–PC line to the dorsal surface of the thalamus on the lateral x-ray view with the ventricles outlined by air has been used by some surgeons. Studies by Brierley and Beck demonstrated that this was unreliable.[41] Two intervals in the sagittal axis have been proposed: specifically, the anterior commissure—posterior commissure interval and the "total thalamic length" corresponding to the length of the line drawn from the lower border of the interventricular foramen through the nearest point on the posterior commissure and ending at the posterior surface of the pulvinar.[41,211] Statistical studies of measurements in 16 specially prepared brains failed to show that localizations scaled by correction factors derived from either of these intervals were more accurate than those achieved by the use of mean values for the

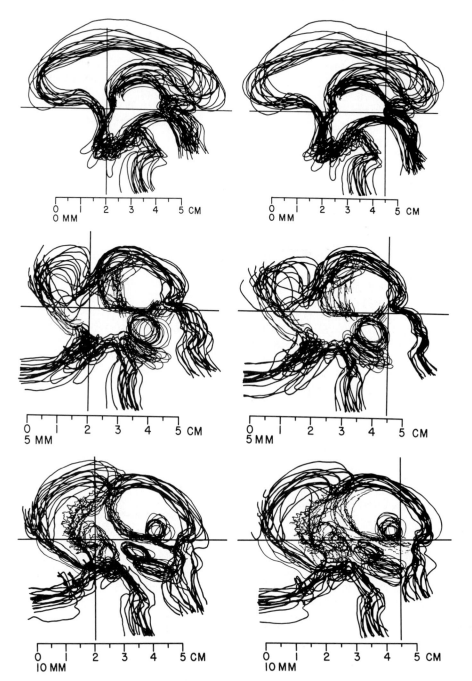

Figure 139–5 Superimposition sagittal variation diagrams at the stated distance from the midline (0 to 20 mm) prepared from 16 specimens. On the left all sections are aligned by the lateral projection of the center of the anterior commissure; on the right all sections are aligned by the lateral projection of the center of the posterior commissure. (From Van Buren, J. M., and Maccubbin, D. A.: An outline atlas of the human basal ganglia with estimation of anatomical variants. J. Neurosurg., *19*:811–839, 1962. Reprinted by permission.)

Illustration continued on opposite page

series.[228] The microelectrode studies of Bertrand and co-workers likewise throw doubt upon the value of these sagittal scaling factors under operative conditions.[28]

It is possible that more complicated interrelationships exist, however. For example, on the superimposition drawing of the diencephalon, 10 mm from the midline, the nu-

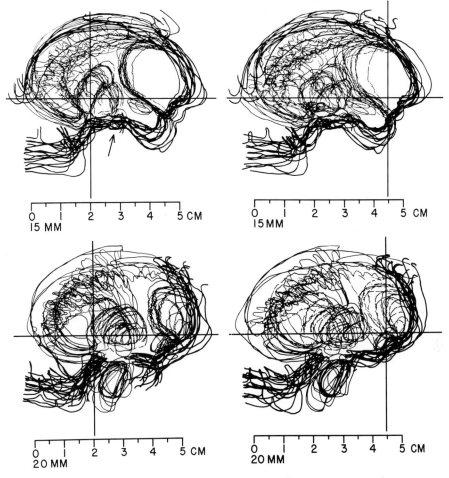

Figure 139–5 (*continued*)

cleus subthalamicus appears to show less variation when aligned by the anterior commissure and the AC–PC line than by use of this same line and the posterior commissure (Fig. 139–5). This appears not to follow the principle that variation is less with a landmark closer to the point to be localized, because the nucleus subthalamicus is about equidistant between the two commissures. It may be that stable topographical relationships between two structures are more related to their interconnections or their ontogenetic patterns than to any simple pattern applicable to all structures. Much more study is needed in this difficult field.

Since there is little justification for using scaling factors, it is necessary to develop another concept in order to place the accuracy of radiographic localizations in the human brain in proper perspective. This concept may be called the "spheroid of error" and consists of plotting the locus at the center of a sphere or ovoid in which the diameter or diameters are related to the standard deviations of the anatomical variation at the point in question. Figure 139–6 illustrates such a charting in which the variations are illustrated on a plane by "circles of error" related to a system based on the anterior commissure, the AC–PC line, and the midsagittal plane. Thus in charting a physiological response, the site of origin should be indicated as an area, not a point. Some time ago, an investigator reported localizing and recording unit activity from the nucleus reticularis thalami in man. Since the thickness of the nucleus is somewhat less than 1 mm, the value of this statement is only too apparent. More data are needed before the "spheroid of error" becomes a truly quantitative tool; this is at present under further study.[229]

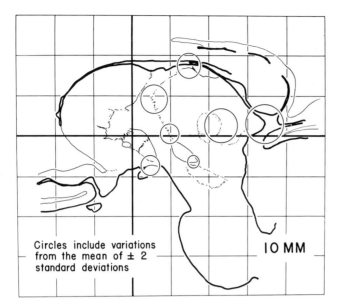

Circles include variations from the mean of ± 2 standard deviations

I0 MM

Figure 139–6 On the standard outline of the brain 10 mm from the midline (which was defined by the mean measurements of 16 brains) a number of loci have been plotted at the center of circles. The diameters of the circles are 4 standard deviations of the mean of the distance between the locus in question and the lateral projection of the center of the anterior commissure (for the sagittal axis) and the anterior commissure–posterior commissure line (for the vertical axis). (From Van Buren, J. M., and Maccubbin, D. A.: A standard method of plotting loci in human depth stimulation and electrography with an estimation of errors. Confin. Neurol., 22:259–264, 1962. Reprinted by permission.)

Normal Variations

The importance of knowledge of the variations of "normal" was apparent early to Spiegel and Wycis, and the earliest variation studies in support of human stereotaxic surgery came from their laboratory.[15,16,22,197,201] In general, studies of this kind have consisted of a series of measurements between a radiographic landmark and a point related to an operative target. Although this is useful, it is impractical to calculate the variations of all possible points. To solve this problem, the use of superimposition variation diagrams was introduced (Fig. 139–5).[228] These illustrations, although not immediately providing numerical data, allow the surgeon to make a quick estimate of the variations in the anatomical margins of a variety of target areas and permit a freedom of movement unobtainable with studies of the variations of fixed points.

Preparation of Material

It is important that the stereotaxic surgeon give thought to the origin of variation statistics. Variations introduced by the preparation methods cannot later be distinguished from true anatomical variation.

Perfusion fixation of the brain, although the method of choice in experimental animals, is probably not ideal with ordinary postmortem human material. Owing to the delay between death and autopsy, clotting in the major cerebral venous sinuses is an unavoidable, or at least a variable, factor and interferes with adequate clearing of the vascular system prior to infusion of the fixative. Marked swelling of the brain has been observed by one of the authors and by others during perfusion under these conditions.[8,191,228] In the authors' hands, immersion fixation with the dural cap in place has not led to the gross artifacts in the brain stem–cerebral relationships that have been feared by some.[197] Furthermore, the reported swelling (or shrinkage) of tissue in formalin fixation has proved, in measurements of weight and displacement, not to be a consistent or significant factor.[144,205,229]

In studies in which intervals are measured at a particular level, inquiry must be made as to how closely this approaches the true desired level. Although many studies would have us suppose that the true level was always achieved, it is certain that most macrotomes are inaccurate instruments. In their study, Amador and associates reported that section taken from various brains might vary ±4 mm around the indicated plane.[8] By using agar or Jeltrate embedding and mechanical sectioning with a rotary blade, it was possible to reduce this to ±1 mm.[228] It is possible that Slaughter and Nashold's method of using a rack of ribbon blades at set intervals (5 mm) will add further precision to the method of macrosection.[191]

Although photographic reproduction is the most accurate, many errors plague this method. These include asymmetrical prints owing to poorly centered or poorly adjusted cameras or enlargers, parallax encountered when grids or rulers are superimposed upon the specimen, and shrinkage or swelling of the print material itself. In general, statistics are only as good as the material upon which they are based.

Variations in the Sagittal Plane and a "Model" Brain

Although the sagittal plane is usually neglected in neuroanatomical textbooks, it is uniquely important to the stereotaxic surgeon, especially because usually both the sagittal and vertical coordinates are calculated from the lateral x-ray view while only the transverse factor is determined from the anteroposterior x-ray. Figure 139–5 shows the superimposed major outlines of 16 nor-

mal brains. Figure 139–7 shows sections at 5 mm, 10 mm, 15 mm, and 20 mm from the midline. This "model" brain series has an AC–PC interval of 25 mm and may prove useful in charting lesions and sites of physiological importance.[228,229]

Variations Due to Disease

Since human stereotaxic surgery is, obviously, employed only in the treatment of disease of the brain, knowledge of the variations in brain relationships introduced by disease is a basic need. Such information, however, is almost completely lacking.

There is evidence that the landmarks about the third ventricle remain relatively stable. This has been reported in hydro-

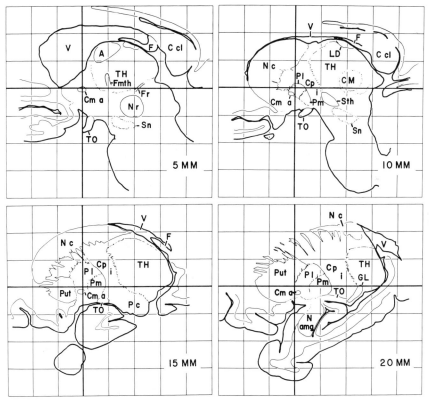

Figure 139–7 Standard sagittal brain sections labeled to show the structures illustrated in the superimposition diagrams in Figure 103–5 and the standard unlabeled sections. Squares are 1 cm. A, nucleus anterior thalami; C cl, corpus callosum; CM—nucleus centralis thalami (centrum medianum); Cm a, commissura anterior; Cpi, capsula interna; F, fornix; Fmth, fasciculus mammillothalamicus; Fr—fasciculus retroflexus; GL, corpus geniculatum laterale; LD, nucleus lateralis dorsalis thalami; N amg, nucleus amygdalae; Nc, nucleus caudatus; Nr, nucleus ruber; Pc, pedunculus cerebri; Pl, pallidum laterale; Pm, pallidum mediale; Put, putamen; Sn, substantia nigra; Sth, nucleus subthalamicus; TH, main thalamic mass; TO, tractus opticus; V, ventriculus laterale. Intervals are indicated in millimeters from the midline. The outline follows the mean values for 16 brains. The AC–PC interval is 25 mm. (From Van Buren, J. M., and Maccubbin, D. A.: An outline atlas of the human basal ganglia with estimation of anatomical variants. J. Neurosurg., *19*:811–839. Reprinted by permission.)

cephalus.[134] Talairach and co-workers studied the effect of widening of the third ventricle on the relationship of the paramedian structures to the midline.[211] Providing the true width of the third ventricle remained less than 9 mm, he found no significant displacement. This conclusion has been supported by the microelectrode studies of Bertrand and his associates at the time of therapeutic thalamotomy.[28]

Computer Aid in Stereotaxic Surgery

Atlas Display and Scaling

Programs are available to permit the display of standard brain atlas cross sections and their scaling to conform to correction factors.[32,33,217,218] As an added convenience, the electrode position may be added to the plot and the plot itself altered to conform to the electrode trajectory when this lies in a plane that does not coincide with the standard atlas planes.[33,218]

Translation of Instrument Movement into Rectilinear Coordinates

Although the use of an atlas made up of a series of plane sections invites one to think in terms of rectilinear movements, many instruments are not equipped to do this directly (exceptions include the Leksell, Talairach, and Van Buren designs). Programs devised to solve the trigonometric problems and permit an instrument employing polar coordinates (Riechert-Mundinger instrument) to move in a rectilinear fashion are available.[34,35] The complicated relationships of the Leksell instrument inherent in relating the frame landmarks and the target (all of which lie in different planes) to the central x-ray beam may now be solved by a computer program rather than by the original graphic method.[67] Other programs relating instrument coordinates to x-ray landmarks include those of Neroth and of Colloff and their associates.[53,164] The latter group has also provided a secondary program to take the probe through two specific targets, which would be of interest for investigational purposes.

The side-protruding electrode, as originally devised by Spiegel and Wycis, offers the unique convenience of permitting lesions somewhat eccentric to the puncture site.[197] Since the stylet angle to the shaft, the shaft rotation, and the shaft angulation related to the atlas planes can all be determined, the solution to the problem of the electrode position can be derived more quickly by computer.[97,172]

Hoefer and co-workers provide a program to assist in localizing the foramen of Monroe and approximate target sites from bony landmarks.[108]

Data Collection and Display

Bradley and co-workers have devised a program to study the effect of stimulation on the excitability curves of spinal reflexes. The electrode may be driven by the computer, and stimuli may be applied to two regions to study their interaction. Results are immediately available in graphic form. A subroutine was included for averaging sampled potentials.[39]

Tasker and associates describe a technique to display the corrected atlas section in which the electrode lies and the quality and localization of sensory responses entered on a figurine. Data could be stored for summary plotting on appropriate brain stem sections.[217]

PHYSIOLOGICAL ADJUNCTS TO LOCALIZATION

Radiological information concerning structural localization within the human diencephalon can be supplemented by neurophysiological methods that previously were limited to the experimental laboratory. While at present not all the methods described here have found general acceptance, their growing influence as safeguards in stereotaxic surgery merits their inclusion.

Stimulation

Observation of the conscious patient's responses to electrical stimuli applied to an electrode inserted in the brain is perhaps the most commonly used method and, superficially, a simple one. The responses, however, are influenced by the patient's degree of sedation, his emotional state, and the difficulties the surgeon may experience in observing or communicating with the patient. While readily apparent, these problems are brought into critical focus under operating conditions. The physiological response is influenced by the pulse form, duration, amplitude, and frequency of the electrical stimulus. In general, the response is a function not so much of the power employed as of the repetition rate, the rise time of the pulse, and the peak-to-peak current difference. Frequencies between 50 and 100 Hz are probably most efficient for motor and sensory responses with a square wave form or its first differential. If a square wave generator is used, the output should be biphasic (this is inherent in a differentiated unidirectional square pulse), as biphasic stimuli show less tissue damage than interrupted direct currents when equated on the basis of equivalent physiological responses.[135] Pulses over 1 msec in duration are generally inefficient and increase tissue damage.

If any importance is to be attached to the thresholds of stimulation, current- rather than voltage-controlled pulses must be used, as the electrode-brain interface presents a varying impedance producing variable stimulus intensity if the voltage is kept constant. With implanted electrodes, thresholds established at one sitting may be found changed at a later session. This is particularly so with sensory responses and may be due to a variety of factors, including damage about the stimulation site, the patient's awareness of what to expect, and presumably, fluctuations in the central excitatory state.

The current density diminishes about an electrode as the square of the distance, and it is reasonable to assume some relation between the site of stimulation and the response. However, since the current densities needed to depolarize nerve cells and fibers in a given situation in vivo remain essentially unknown, much caution is needed in evaluating the discreteness of the localization of a response. Sites that show sensory responses at from 2 to 4 ma should be coagulated cautiously in small increments, while in those that require over 4 ma the likelihood of sensory disturbance is very small. This observation suggests that effective current densities for excitations are reached at 2 to 3 mm from the electrode (the radius of the coagulum in vitro) when

about 2 ma is applied. These parameters are useful only with this specific experimental condition.

Investigators have utilized an advancing electrode to elicit motor responses and changes in stimulation threshold to identify the internal capsule.[24,181] Bertrand and co-workers, using a retractable searching electrode, found the motor fibers in the posterior limb of the internal capsule only behind a transverse plane halfway between the anterior and posterior commissures.[31] To avoid the anterior portion of the posterior limb or the genu of the internal capsule, other criteria must be used.

In interpreting the localizing significance of sensory responses to stimulation, caution must be exercised. A variety of sensations have been reported from the expected position of the thalamic sensory relay nuclei, and the conventional medial-to-lateral, face-to-leg organization has been confirmed in man.[30,74,105,133,166] A study of sensory responses to currents of 2 to 4 ma peak-to-peak amplitude (biphasic pulses of 2 msec total duration at 60 per second) intentionally applied outside the calculated position of the sensory relay nuclei showed wide distribution of effective stimulus sites in the thalamus and even in the corpus striatum.[227] The possibility of pathways transmitting sensation outside the classic thalamocortical system must be seriously considered.

The effect of stimulation on the patient's involuntary motor activity has served as a guide for the placement of stereotaxic lesions.[7,9,188,203,206] Facilitation or inhibition of tremor and dystonic movements has been reported from the pallidum,[78,79,105] the subthalamic region, Forel's field, the ventrolateral nucleus, the centrum medianum, and other areas.* Alberts and co-workers have not found a correlation between the threshold of the stimulus necessary to augment or initiate tremor and postoperative clinical improvement.[7] In the authors' experience, coagulation of sites from which tremor was blocked by stimulation proved more generally followed by favorable clinical results. Tremor may be precipitated by any startling event including the rather ubiquitous sensory responses to stimulation.

---

* See references 6, 9, 78, 79, 105, 175, 203.

Evoked Activity and Macroelectrode Recording

Attempts have been made to confirm localization by study of the cortical response to thalamic and basal ganglia stimulation. The existence of relatively long latency cortical recruitment has been reported in man from a variety of thalamic areas.* The diffuse nature of the response, unfortunately, negates its value in localization.

Better localization of an evoked response is seen with the "augmentation response" reported by Housepian and Purpura and by Yoshida and associates.[111,243] This was used in the anesthetized patient to identify placement in the ventrolateral nucleus by the appearance of a negative-positive potential complex with brief initial positivity and frequency dependence in the ipsilateral frontoparietal region. It has been considered to disappear at the lower border of the ventrolateral nucleus.[167] Stimulation of the globus pallidus and ansa lenticularis has not produced information of sufficient specificity to be useful in localization.[105,111,175] It must be realized that the conclusions regarding the localization of electrode placement have been drawn from materials subject to both x-ray errors and anatomical variations. Assuming complete accuracy in x-ray localization, variations in anatomical margins amount to ± 2 to 5 mm, rendering reports of placements in such narrow structures as the nucleus reticularis and nucleus intralaminaris outside the limits of proper evidence. Even the anatomical definition of such "well-known" structures as the nucleus ventralis lateralis rests on a rather insecure basis in man.[229]

Identification of the specific sensory relay nuclei (n. ventralis posteromedialis and n. ventralis posterolateralis [VPM, VPL]) have been successfully carried out by evoked responses from peripheral stimulation.[75,125]

Using averaged response data with which small changes in response latency can be detected, Narabayashi reported successful localization in the nucleus ventralis intermedius immediately anterior to the sensory relay nuclei.[161] As apparatus for response averaging becomes more available, this approach may assume a greater functional importance.

---

* See references 78, 105, 111, 175, 200, 234, 243.

Microelectrode Recording

The information of localizing value to be gained by microelectrode recording falls largely into the categories of the presence or absence of unit activity (presumed in the present discussion to be derived from the soma of the nerve cell); the possibility that particular patterns of resting activity may be characteristic of certain neural aggregates; the modification of resting unit activity by sensory or other stimuli (evoked activity); and the possibility that certain characteristics of unit activity may indicate the site of or participation in a pathological process.

At the outset it must be recognized that the use of electrodes with tips small enough to record activity of single cells implies a high electrical impedance. The latter characteristic makes them susceptible, even under the best circumstances, to electrical interference from a variety of sources, especially diathermy and electrosurgical apparatus. Furthermore, the apparatus needed for recordings of this type tends to be unstable in the operating room environment. Delays for servicing, while tolerable in animal experiments, cannot be permitted in operations on humans and, if they occur, will usually prevent the use of the apparatus for the particular patient. The surgeon may wish to consider using duplicate systems as a permanent part of the recording unit. Finally, it is desirable to have a means of testing the functional capacities of the electrode in situ. Ordinary measures of resistance with an applied current should not be used, but capacitance methods that do not harm the electrode and give a useful though rough index of electrode function can be utilized. It is likely that commercial sources of both stable apparatus and electrodes will soon appear; the surgeon should make their full acquaintance in the experimental laboratory before attempting to apply them and interpret the findings in man.

Presence of Unit Activity

When used in conjunction with good x-ray localization methods, the appearance of unit activity signals the entrance into a nuclear mass such as the thalamus or pallidum from the silent white matter or cerebral ventricle.[3,94] Loss of unit activity may also assist in judging the junction between the thalamus and the tegmental region or the cerebral ventricle.

Characteristic Resting Activity of Neural Aggregates

Although there have been some reports of locally specific resting activity, it is unlikely that this should be considered as a reliable means of localization. Some criteria, such as increased unit activity in the lower regions of the thalamus as opposed to the dorsal part, may be of value in specific instances.[99,215]

Evoked Activity

Although evidence of this type has probably the greatest localizing value, the area for an effective therapeutic lesion in the thalamus lies outside the sensory relay area and hence may not be subject to positive verification by this means.

Evoked responses to tactile stimulation, as reported by many investigators, have shown the expected medial-to-lateral, face-arm-leg somatotopic distribution.*

Localization of these responses to the nucleus ventralis posterior is inferred. Lying just rostral to the area of tactile responses are cells responsive to deep pressure and extremity movement but not to touch that were thought to correspond to the nucleus ventro-intermedius and nucleus ventro-oralis posterior of Hassler.[48,102,115] Farther forward, in what was considered the nucleus ventro-oralis anterior of Hassler, it has been reported that activation of unit activity or a periodic burst of slow waves at 20 to 26 cps occurred when the patient was asked to prepare to move the contralateral limb.[99,102,222] The latter is interesting as perhaps being analogous with the precentral beta blocking described by Penfield and Jasper as the patient prepares to move the extremity.[173] Others report the presence of unit activity in the nucleus ventro-oralis posterior and adjacent regions that may show either a rise or fall in firing rate with voluntary movement.[63] With the possible exception of the tactile evoked responses in the nucleus ventralis posterior, it is doubtful if the responses are consistent enough to form a localization guide upon which the surgeon can rely.

* See references 3, 20, 30, 48, 91, 99.

Pathological Patterns of Unit Activity

Rhythmic firing of groups of thalamic neurons at about the frequency of parkinsonian tremor is readily recorded. Units may fire in synchrony with recorded tremor or in the absence of tremor (whether the tremor involved a peripheral site from which no recording was made is a moot point). The crucial question whether these cells are simply responding to periodic afferent volleys from the periphery or indeed are part of the mechanism driving the tremor is difficult to decide. Jasper and Bertrand point out that posterior rhythmic units (presumed to be in the nucleus ventralis posterior) respond to touch, and that those responding to joint movement occupy an anterior position, while cells with rhythmic activity but that respond to neither are apt to be yet more rostral, perhaps in the nucleus ventro-oralis.[102,115] Recent study of units in rhythmic bursts of four to six per second by means of cross-correlation techniques showed that most were not synchronous with tremor.[63] Since parkinsonian tremor may be asynchronous in different parts of the body, it may be difficult to solve this problem.

Practical use has been made of evoked activity. Lesions placed just anterior to the tactile representation of the thumb and the corner of the mouth produced good results in the treatment of upper extremity tremors, while for the leg, good results followed lesions anterior to the site where responses were evoked in the fourth and fifth digits.[215]

Impedance Techniques

The appreciable differences in the electrical impedance of white and gray matter and the fluid in the cerebral ventricles has encouraged evaluation of impedance measurement as an aid to stereotaxic localization.[70,123,179] In practice, the current employed must be lower than that producing stimulation effects or tissue destruction, and measurements must be taken while the electrode is being advanced, as blood, fluid, or air in the withdrawal tract interferes with accurate recording.[1] A motor drive has been used with success.[179,180] Bipolar electrodes may give faulty readings because of tissue or fluid bridges that develop between the poles.

Under proper conditions it is possible in man to detect the low impedance profile of the ventricle, the maximum impedance of the myelin-rich internal capsule, and penetration of the area of lower impedance in the thalamus.[70,170,196] Laitinen and associates, while failing to obtain the accuracy of 0.01 mm in localization claimed by Robinson and Tompkins, have been able to detect in man a 15 to 45 per cent maximum difference between gray and white matter in locating the boundaries of thalamus and pallidum and as an aid to identification of the subthalamus.[124,179]

The Trial Lesion

The ideal trial lesion in any ablative procedure would be one in which the region for destruction was totally inactivated in a totally reversible fashion. To be effective, one must assume that the final lesion is the precise counterpart of the reversible one and that all the effects of the damage are present and constant from the start. Although it is doubtful if the last conditions can ever be fully met, the surgeon should seriously consider using a trial lesion in some form. The major methods are considered briefly:

Pressure

Cooper's cannula with a terminal balloon that could be inflated at the proposed site of the lesion was useful, but the use of a sclerosing fluid for lesion production, which is inherent in the method, has disadvantages that are discussed later.[60] Gildenberg quite correctly observed that, because of its large diameter (3 mm), the cannula itself caused permanent damage and was not entirely suitable for a physiological test. Bertrand was also able to produce temporary physiological effects by opening his spring wire leukotome.[24] This effect, like the others, was probably the result of a lesion too small to have permanent effect and was similar to the transient benefit that may be seen with a properly placed implanted electrode.

Chemical Agents

Narabayashi and Okuma have injected procaine into sites proposed for therapeutic lesions as a reversible test.[162] The effect lasted several to 20 hours and could be prolonged if the highly viscous mixture utilized for permanent lesion production was used. Others have employed this method to search for the most favorable therapeutic site by injecting 0.25 ml increments of procaine at 5-mm intervals and by placing their lesion at a site where injection alleviated the symptoms.[54] Difficulty in controlling the fluid and the likelihood of its migration along the cannula shaft may lead to uncertainties.

Heating with High-Frequency Current

With radiofrequency (RF) current, Brodkey and co-workers demonstrated physiological inhibition of the Edinger-Westphal nucleus in the cat by heating a thermistor monitored probe to 44 to 49° C.[42] Histological studies failed to reveal evidence of heat damage. These authors successfully placed reversible heat lesions in patients undergoing stereotaxic operations for movement disorders. Zervas, using an eccentrically insulated electrode and a focal ground point, produced directionally specific reversible radiofrequency lesions that provided information concerning the direction in which an electrode should be moved if not exactly on target.[244]

Care must be taken with the heating method, as the temperature difference between a reversible and an irreversible lesion is relatively small. The method has the advantage that lesion tests and coagulation, as well as macrorecording and stimulation, may all be carried out through the same electrode. In practice it should be recalled that although stimulation and recording can be done with a very fine wire electrode, satisfactory work with radiofrequency currents requires a somewhat larger conductor.

Cooling

Electrophysiological studies have shown that evoked activity is enhanced in neural tissue cooled to between 37° C and 27° C.[173] From 27° to 20° C no change is detectable, while from 20° to 0° C evoked activity is progressively decreased until it disappears at zero. This information has been utilized in man for testing the therapeutic efficacy of a proposed lesion. The temperature used for testing should be sufficient to depress activity yet far enough from freezing to guard safely against the production of a permanent lesion. Seven degrees centigrade has been suggested by Le Beau and co-workers.[129]

There is a sharp gradient of temperature about the cold probe.[61] When the tip is cooled to $-80°$ C, the temperature at 0.1 mm from the tip is $-33°$ C; at 1.4 mm it is $-15°$ C; and at 3 mm it is $3°$ C.

Some difficulties have been reported with the use of cold to produce trial lesions. Siegfried found in one third of his cases that a reversible cold lesion produced no clinical response even though the permanent lesion in the area resulted in the desired therapeutic effect.[189] It is possible that this is simply due to the sharp temperature gradient about the cold source and hence the small size of the trial lesion as opposed to the final volume of tissue destruction.

Ultrasonic Irradiation

Reversible physiological inhibition of neural activity utilizing ultrasonic techniques has been demonstrated by Fry and co-workers.[85] By utilizing the evoked cortical response to photic stimulation, graded ultrasonic irradiation of the lateral geniculate body in the cat was shown to inhibit this response. The response recovered completely within one to five minutes following cessation of irradiation. It has also been possible to use this physiological response in the functional mapping of the intact animal brain.[87] Meyers and associates reported successful reversible inhibition of tremor in one patient with Parkinson's disease.[149] While at present the technique of ultrasonic irradiation is not practical for general use, with anticipated technological development, the property of reversible physiological inhibition of subcortical structures may add another significant safeguard to the technique.

Incremental Coagulation

Many of the clinical failures in stereotaxic surgical treatment have at the time of initial lesion placement appeared to be successful. Often parkinsonian tremor and rigidity will disappear following lesion production or upon electrode placement, only to return a few days later. Conversely, persistent attempts to alleviate symptoms by continued coagulation in the operating room may be followed four to six hours later by hemiparesis or mental deterioration, indicating a lesion of excessive size for that particular patient.

The use of implanted electrodes permits the lesion to be made later outside the operating room when the patient has fully recovered from the effects of the operation and is more accessible to physical and mental examination by the surgeon. In practice the electrode is allowed to stay in position for four to five days following insertion and it is checked radiographically. After the effects of stimulation are evaluated, a small radiofrequency lesion is placed. The patient is then observed for two days. Often the maximum benefit is not seen immediately and may not become apparent for at least 24 hours. Lesion production in this way takes more of the surgeon's and patient's time but appears to reduce the magnitude and incidence of complications, since if untoward effects appear with a small lesion (e.g., mental confusion), the size can be limited to prevent persistent symptoms.

Since the size of the radiofrequency lesion is a function of the size and shape of the exposed coagulating tip, this must be carefully evaluated in animals or egg white. It is unlikely that consistently good clinical results can be obtained with lesions smaller than a volume equivalent to an ovoid with major and minor diameters of 9 and 6 mm respectively.[224,226]

STEREOTAXIC INSTRUMENTS

Perhaps no other aspect of neurosurgery has so intrigued the mechanically minded surgeon as has sterotaxic surgery. Since the advent of the first practical instrument for human use in 1947, new models and modifications of older models have continually appeared.[202] Many instruments are similar and may be grouped under a few general categories. If the man starting in stereotaxic surgery has a firm grasp of the nature and dimensions of the problems involved and the principles that govern the function of the instruments, he will be well on his way to choosing a current or future model sufficient for his needs.

Quite obviously there is no "best"

model. All will guide a probe to the target with adequate accuracy, provided the operator attends carefully to his technique. Since all localization is based upon relations of the target to the midsagittal plane, the importance of aligning this parallel to the x-ray cassette and the central x-ray beam perpendicular to both cannot be overemphasized. As might be expected, simplicity and relatively low cost of an instrument are generally bartered for flexibility and vice versa. Methods using dense ventricular contrast materials permit localization with rapid x-ray techniques (image intensifier fluoroscopy or Polaroid films), although one should be wary about the late effects of retained iophendylate (Pantopaque). Air contrast methods require longer film processing. Unfortunately, portable apparatus is more difficult to control and hence more error prone than apparatus fixed to the operating table with built-in or rigidly attached x-ray equipment.

In general, the two major problems to be overcome in stereotaxic localization are magnification and parallax. In evaluating new apparatus, the surgeon should gain a clear insight as to how each is solved. If adequate correction is not made, he should estimate the degree of inaccuracy introduced.

The following discussion is necessarily brief and does not supplant the operating instructions that are usually provided in great detail by the manufacturer. It seems worthwhile, however, to illustrate the major types of instruments with some specific examples and give a brief resumé of how each solves the problem of stereotaxic localization.

The Parallel X-Ray Beam Instrument

Talairach and co-workers essentially eliminated magnification and parallax at the start by using an x-ray source at 15 meters from the subject.[211,213] This permitted a very simple localizing technique consisting of a pair of metal grids with coaxial holes located on either side of the head. Localization was accomplished by lining these up by x-ray so that the holes on one side were superimposed on analogous holes in the opposite grid and the intervening ventricular landmarks.

Polar Coordinate Instruments

In this group are instruments designed by Cooper, Bleasel and associates, Ward, and Walker (Figs. 139–8 and 139–9).[36,55,59,231,236] In principle, the target site is found on the lateral and sagittal x-ray films, and a line is drawn from this through the point of electrode insertion in the calvarium. Further extracranial projection of this line will intersect radiopaque protractors to give the proper angulation needed in two planes to define the line of the electrode tract to the target. The depth of penetration required to reach the target is usually estimated by comparison of a known extracranial interval (e.g., radiopaque ruler) with the intracranial interval drawn on the film. No problem arises when the line of insertion is parallel to a major x-ray localization plane (e.g., the midsagittal plane), but when the trajectory of the electrode is oblique to both planes used for x-ray localization, the extracranial known interval, if it lies on the extracranial projection of the electrode tract, does not lie on the same plane as the intracranial trajectory and will be magnified somewhat differently. If this error is small it can be ignored; if larger, the problem can be solved by trigonometry as in the Spiegel-Wycis technique. Alternatively, it may be done by trial and error, checking the results by rapid Polaroid films.

Its proponents have cited the small size and weight of the instrument as advantages that allow it to be fixed to the cranial burr hole. Whether this is a true advantage is questionable since there is little doubt that secure bony fixation of the head is essential if carefully positioned and reproducible x-rays are to be made. These, of course, are as needed with this technique as with any other, and a head frame fixed to the table is advocated by Cooper.[55] Furthermore, two sets of preliminary films may be needed— one to set up the angle of entry and the other to determine the depth of entry.[36]

The Spiegel-Wycis stereoencephalotome may be considered as belonging with this group. It is of historical importance as the first method actually used in patients.[200,240]

Phantom Target Instruments

In general these instruments locate the intracranial target in relation to landmarks

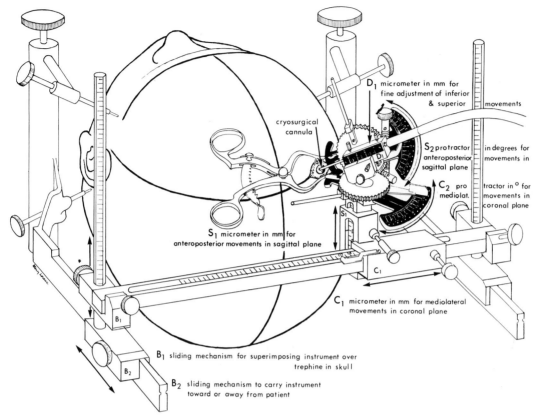

D_1 micrometer in mm for fine adjustment of inferior & superior movements

S_2 protractor anteroposterior sagittal plane in degrees for movements in

C_2 pro mediolat. tractor in° for movements in coronal plane

cryosurgical cannula

S_1 micrometer in mm for anteroposterior movements in sagittal plane

C_1 micrometer in mm for mediolateral movements in coronal plane

B_1 sliding mechanism for superimposing instrument over trephine in skull

B_2 sliding mechanism to carry instrument toward or away from patient

Figure 139–8 The Cooper instrument. (From Cooper, I. S.: Cryothalamectomy—surgical technique. *In* Rand, R. W., Rinfret, A. P., and von Leden, H., eds.: Cryosurgery. Springfield, Ill., Charles C Thomas, 1968. Reprinted by permission.)

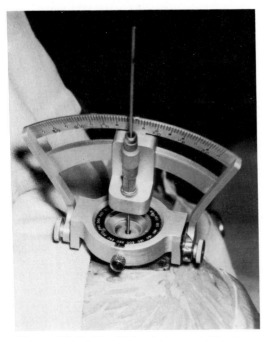

Figure 139–9 The Walker instrument. (Courtesy of Dr. Earl Walker.)

on the operative base frame of the apparatus applied to the patient's head. On a similar "phantom" base frame the target position is set up from these relationships. Next, the site of cranial puncture is chosen, then reproduced with the same relationships to the base frame on the phantom by a small ring or other guide. The electrode guide is then positioned on the phantom so that the electrode passes through the reproduced site of cranial puncture and strikes the target. When the electrode supports are moved en bloc from the phantom base frame to the operative base frame, the electrode tip position and trajectory will be reproduced.

Since the reference landmarks on the frame are a considerable distance from the target plane, particular care must be taken to guard against parallax. In the apparatus of Mundinger and Riechert this is achieved by lining up similar holes drilled in the opposite sides of the base frame, using external rings and crosshairs oriented by a visi-

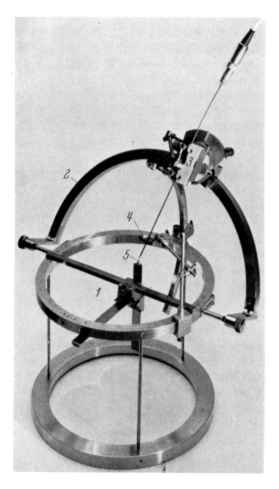

Figure 139–10 The phantom base ring of Riechert's instrument with the phantom target point erected. The electrode passes through a small ring locating the site of cranial puncture. The electrode guide is supported by two arcs supported in turn by the phantom base ring. For actual insertion these arcs are moved to the identical operative base ring mounted on the patient's head. (From Mundinger, F., and Riechert, T.: Die stereotaktischen Hirnoperationen zur Behandlung extrapyramidaler Bewegungsstörungen (Parkinsonismus und Hyperkinesen) und ihre Resultate. Fortschr. Neurol. Psychiat., *1*:1–120, 1963. Reprinted by permission.)

ble light beam parallel to the central x-ray beam (Fig. 139–10).[76,156,157]

These instruments have the advantage of secure cranial fixation so that the projection of serial x-ray exposures is identical. To be accurate much care must be used in positioning the central x-ray beam. This, however, is a technical point and is accomplished in various ways.

Instruments Aligned by the Central X-Ray Beam

In essence, instruments of this type avoid the errors of parallax by having a focal point, which is the target of the therapeutic probe and through which the central beam of the localizing x-ray apparatus also passes. In practice the intracranial target is located and brought to this focal point by graduated movements of the patient's head or of the apparatus.

The Bertrand instrument method moves the patient's head.[25,26] The apparatus consists of a frame supported by the operating table, which in turn supports the electrode guide and holds the patient's head by bony fixation. Graduated movements of the inner frame holding the head permit the target to be brought into the central x-ray beam. The positioning is checked on a small fluorescent screen.

On the instrument designed by Guiot and modified by Gillingham two rings on opposite sides of the head (which are fixed to each other by a bar across the top of the head) are moved to the target site, and then will mechanically guide an electrode to a point on the transverse line joining the centers of the rings.[96] The displacement from the midline of this sagittally oriented electrode is determined from the anteroposterior x-ray film. A modification of this instrument has been proposed recently.[220]

Because accurate centering of the central x-ray beam is necessary, the use of an image intensifier x-ray fluoroscope as suggested by Gillingham seems important as a time saver.[95] The basic instrument permits a rather limited sagittal trajectory for the therapeutic electrode, but a modification by Gillingham permits more flexibility in the operative approach.

Triplane Stereotaxic Instruments

These instruments are capable of graduated movement in three planes and, when suitably aligned, permit one to enter multiple target sites without repeating the basic biplane x-rays and computations. Leksell and Van Buren have designed instruments of this type.[130,225] The Leksell instrument permits movements at 2-mm intervals in the sagittal and vertical axes and continuous movement in the transverse axis. The Van Buren instrument permits continuous movement in all planes. Both instruments use Leksell's arcuate electrode carrier and thus do not require a set trajectory for the entry of the electrode or lesion-making instrument.

The Leksell instrument consists essentially of a square frame that is supported by bony fixation to the skull. The sagittal members (x-axis), vertical members (y-axis), and transverse members (z-axis) on either side of the head carry radiopaque graduations. The electrode carrier is a hemicircle and is fixed to the frame by supporting bars along the diameter of the hemicircle. These bars are graduated and permit movements in the transverse plane. The arcuate electrode carrier with the electrode equal in length to the radius of the arc and inserted perpendicular to its tangent introduces an important principle: the electrode may be introduced at any point on the brain surface to hit a given target point without computation to compensate for the angle of introduction. Thus the operator is free to choose which structures he wishes to pass through or to avoid on the way to the target site.

The difficulty with the apparatus is that the scales used for aligning the target lie outside the plane of the target. This circumstance requires special corrections to compensate for parallax and the differing magnifications at the target and instrument scales. Leksell has incorporated the mathematical corrections into his spiral diagram.[130] This permits the transfer of a target in a "model" brain to the magnified image of the patient's ventriculogram and from this determines the coordinates of the target on the radiopaque scales of the stereotaxic frame. On the lateral views the standard commissural reference points are used, and on the sagittal view, the midline of the third ventricle is used. A description of this procedure with computation methods is provided by Feinstein and colleagues.[80] The method is sensitive to minor rotations about the x-, y-, and z-axes, and mathematical correction procedures for the x- and z-axes are available.

A further difficulty is that when the electrode is in the target in the brain the tip is hidden on the lateral x-ray view by the supports for the arcuate electrode carrier. This prevents verification of the electrode position. This fault has been overcome by G. Bertrand, who has replaced the post supporting the electrode carrier by a ring of sufficient diameter to expose the target area and thus permit radiographic verification of the electrode in the target (Fig. 139–11).[29]

The Van Buren triplane instrument incorporates the advantages of the Leksell arcuate electrode carrier with the freedom of three-plane graduated stereotaxic movement (Fig. 139–12).[225] Gimbals at the base permit alignment of the axes of the instrument with the desired intracranial planes. Once the instrument planes are set, multiple targets may be reached simply by suitable triplane adjustments of the stereotaxic racks. Since the arcuate electrode carrier may pivot about its support radius, which is identical with the vertical axis of the instrument, it will define a portion of the surface of a sphere. Any probe equal in length to the radius of this sphere (24 cm) and inserted perpendicular to a plane tangent to the sphere will of necessity pass through the center of the sphere. In essence, it is the center of this imaginary sphere, the "impact point," that is moved by the stereotaxic apparatus.

MODES OF LESION PRODUCTION

Electrolytic Lesions

Electrolysis, first described by Sellier and Verger in 1898, is one of the oldest techniques for the production of lesions.[47] Horsley and Clarke found that, because gas

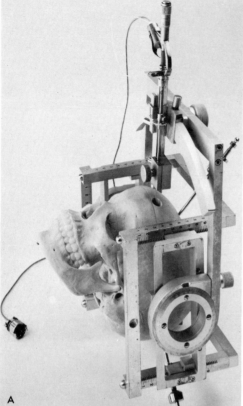

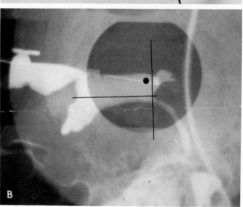

Figure 139–11 *A.* The G. Bertrand modification of the Leksell instrument permits x-ray verification of the relationship of the electrode and the target area. *B.* Pantopaque ventriculogram with recording microelectrode in place with G. Bertrand modification. (From Bertrand, G., Jasper, H., Wong, A., Mathews, G.: Microelectrode recording during stereotactic surgery. Clin. Neurosurg., *16*:328–355, 1969. Reprinted by permission.)

was produced at the cathode, a unipolar anodal lesion was smaller and better controlled.[109] It has been found that there is direct proportionality between the lesion volume and the quantity of charge (coulombs) passed even with large variations in current flow, voltage, and resistance.[141,182]

Although heating forms a relatively small part of the effect of electrolytic lesions, in vitro trials in egg white may be misleading, since the heat dissipating potential of the circulation is not in operation. Several studies have found a degree of unpredictability in the size and the shape of anodal lesions.[176,239] Carpenter and Whittier felt that use of a unipolar anodal current at 5 ma or less for less than 30 seconds resulted in a predictable lesion.[47] If the current were increased, the lesion would be more irregular in size and shape owing to increase in gas production and vascular damage. If the coagulation time were doubled from 15 to 30 seconds the lesion size would increase fourfold, while doubling the time again from 30 to 60 seconds would produce only a twofold increase. The fresh lesions were spherical; older lesions tended to be distorted by scar formation. Bipolar lesions were larger and more irregular, apparently because of cathodal gas production. Further work showed that biphasic pulses during coagulation resulted in a smaller lesion because of a decreased net change in charge flow up to a rate of about 20 cps.[183] This factor may in the future be incorporated to provide physiological safeguards or lesion reversibility, thus adding to the electrolytic method some of the advantages of other currently employed techniques.

After utilizing unipolar anodal lesions in the medulla oblongata of man, Sweet and Mark felt that because of hemorrhage and uncontrollable variability the technique was not suitable for clinical use.[208] The method, however, has been successfully employed by Spiegel and Wycis, who used a side-protruding retractable stylet electrode and were able to produce effectively shaped electrolytic lesions.[197,198,200] Mullan and associates reported that using low current (below 2 ma) applied over long intervals (e.g., 30 minutes) with a fine electrode, very discrete lesions could be made.[154] Further laboratory studies have shown the electrolytic lesion to be less variable than those produced by most other methods when made with constant current and adequate control of other variables.[83,92,209]

Surgical Lesions

Several early surgical instruments for the production of subcortical lesions were described by Clarke.[50] Bertrand's leukotome,

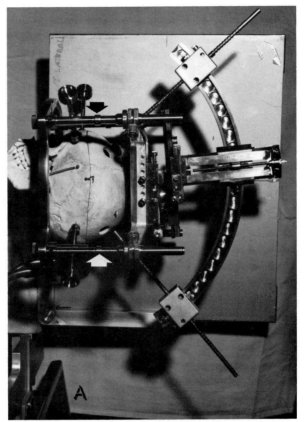

Figure 139–12   Van Buren instrument in position for lateral ventriculogram without drapes. Arrow indicates joint in instrument support. Before applying instrument, the plastic field drape is applied to the head and the frame to the left of the joint. All instruments to the right of the joint remain sterile, and the junction to the base is effected by a pointed screw in the support bar, which pierces the plastic drape. The x-ray localization bars are on the arcuate electrode carrier. Pan to hold cassette for sagittal view (A) is here folded down out of the way.

adapted from Moniz, consisted of a 16-gauge needle tubing containing a fine piano wire loop that could be protruded through a lateral slit to a distance of 6 mm from the shaft.[23] In using the instrument, care must be taken to rotate it no more than 45 degrees before closing it to prevent excessive traction and tearing of blood vessels. Five hundred consecutive cases in which this instrument was used with no deaths were reported.[27] Housepian and Pool modified their leukotome with two opening and closing blades to obtain biopsy specimens during stereotaxic procedures.[110] Aspiration biopsies with fine canulas have proved suitable for examination with the electron microscope.[98] Other mechanical devices have been described.[49,165]

Although studies by Papez and Carpenter and Whittier showed that mechanically produced lesions tended to be irregular and hemorrhagic, in practice the method has proved useful.[47,171] The lesion, however, should be made in small increments with a relatively dull cutting edge.

Lesions Produced by Injection

Corrosive and Sclerosing Fluids

The technique was first used by Beaunis, who injected a mixture of zinc chloride and aniline blue to produce a focal lesion.[21] Cooper reported successful utilization of absolute alcohol to produce basal ganglia lesions.[54] Other authors found that the lesions were too large and too irregular to be predictable.[147,199] When a radiopaque marker material was added to the injection material, migration along the needle tracts, along tissue planes, or even over the cortex and the subarachnoid space was observed. These dangers prevented the injection of low-viscosity materials from achieving great popularity.

Combined Bulk and Local Damage from Liquid

Efforts to reduce the irregularity of lesions produced when using fluids of low viscosity have centered upon the use of

Ectopalin, an 8 per cent solution of ethyl cellulose in 95 per cent ethyl alcohol that forms a coagulum upon injection, and procaine in an oil-wax colloidal mixture that forms a discrete intracerebral foreign body.[60,147,160,162,163]

Procaine mixed with vegetable oil and wax remains in a round or oval form as a permanent foreign body and exerts its therapeutic influence by mechanical destruction of the injected area. The usual dose of 0.5 to 1 ml is injected in 0.05-ml increments, and undesirable signs are checked for. It is not suitable for deep lesions via a transventricular approach because of the serious complications possible if the mixture were to enter the ventricles. Because its action is chiefly mechanical, it is not suited for destruction of thin nuclei or tracts. Occasionally the resultant lesions are not sufficient to produce the desired therapeutic effects and must be supplemented with electrocoagulation.[162]

The injection of Ectopalin into unprepared cerebral tissue, while reducing diffusibility, still produced lesions of significant variability.[199] In 1958 Cooper introduced a balloon that was connected to a cannula and inflated with Hypaque[60] at the site of a proposed lesion. The balloon formed a cavity into which, after 24 to 48 hours, Ectopalin or alcohol could be injected, theoretically, without significant danger of spread or reflux. Five to ten milliliters of the material could be injected two or three times over a seven-day period, and it was claimed that large lesions could be produced in this manner without the undesirable side effects associated with lesions of this size that were made abruptly. In attempts to further reduce any tendency for the material to diffuse, Ectopalin has been mixed with other materials such as kaolin powder.[147] Studies of the balloon technique, however, have found the unpredictable size and irregularity of the tissue cavity associated with tissue destruction and bleeding.[93] Clinical reports have indicated a higher complication rate with Ectopalin and Cooper's balloon cannula than with other widely used techniques.[233] Postmortem comparative studies indicate that the resultant lesion is caused by a combination of pressure from a foreign body and disruption of tissue.[192,194] Destruction of tissue and hemorrhage into the cavity appear to be histological features of the lesion. The lesions are from three to ten times as great in volume as those produced by unipolar diathermy.[194,233] The decline of popularity of this method may be attributed to the development of more reliable techniques.

Lesions Produced by Heat

High-Frequency Current

In 1932 Hess described the use of a high-voltage diathermy instrument for producing lesions in animals. Wyss devised a high-frequency apparatus that generated sine waves at 500 kHz, which was employed in studies relating the duration and power needed for lesion production after tissue resistance was measured.[113,242] This device was later successfully used in man. The method has gained considerable popularity, since the lesion can be well predicted on the basis of the power output of the apparatus and the size and shape of the coagulating electrode, and the same electrode may be used prior to lesion production for recording and stimulation.

Coagulation of tissue satisfactory for stereotaxic lesions occurs when the current passed is between frequencies of 0.2 MHz and 4 MNz over a wide range of current values.[5] Most commonly a frequency of 2 MHz is employed. While the dimensions of the lesion are related to the power input, specifically the temperature obtained, the current, and the duration of current, other specific characteristics such as the geometry of the electrode and the character of the tissue are also operative in determining the final result (Fig. 139–13). In general, the size of the lesion may be more reliably adjusted by changing the size of the electrode than by substituting other parameters. Within the range of frequencies just mentioned, only a minor portion of the tissue destruction is due to resistive heating of the electrode and is independent of the frequency. The major tissue destruction is the result of a frequency-dependent dielectric effect in the tissues when electrical energy is converted into heat.[12,174] The most important factors appear to be the density of current flow through the tissue and the ohmic resistance of the tissue. The influence of inductive and capacitive reactance are small in comparison.[5,159] A self-limiting factor in this type of coagulating unit is the effective

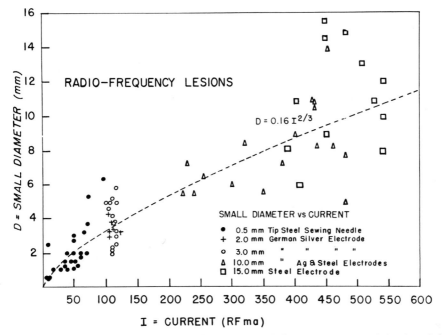

Figure 139–13 The relationship between the diameter of the lesion, the current, and the size of the source electrode. (From Aronow, S.: The use of radiofrequency power in making lesions in the brain. J. Neurosurg., *17*:431–438, 1960. Reprinted by permission.)

blockade of the current by gas evolution at the radiofrequency source. This results in a reduction in the surrounding tissue temperature despite continued application of the current.

Cerebral lesions dependent upon heat for their production are influenced by the presence of blood vessels, the spatial relationship to the cerebrospinal fluid pathways, and the tissue resistivity.[12,69] The greater vascularity of the gray matter and its greater ability to dissipate heat will require more power than is needed to produce a lesion of equal size in the white matter. The duration of current flow is exponentially related to the size of the lesion, and at 80° C an equilibrium state is obtained in which the growth of the lesion ceases after two minutes despite continued current flow.[159] Watkins has measured the heat gradient of tissue and found that with a temperature of 62° C, after 60 to 90 seconds there is an increase of 10° C 3 mm from the tip, 6° to 9° C at 4 mm, and 4° to 7° C at 6 mm.[237]

On histological examination the lesion consists of a central core produced by the electrode in which some blood is surrounded by a zone of coagulative necrosis that is enclosed by a zone of incomplete parenchymatous damage. Around this is a zone of liquefaction in which all cells and fibers are lost, bordered by a layer of demyelination.[69,103] The peripheral location of the liquefaction necrosis is said to be due to the spatial configuration of the heat radiance in which the temperature of the tissue at 2 mm from the tip is said to be greater than at the tip itself. It might be mentioned, however, that in simple observation of the coagulum forming in egg white about an electrode supplied with 2 MHz current, the coagulum starts at the electrode itself and then moves steadily peripherally.

In adapting the method to the surgical situation, the size and form of the electrode are of greatest importance, as they largely determine the size and shape of the final lesion.[69] Controllable variations may be introduced by using an electrode in which the tip exposure and direction of protrusion can be controlled or by insulating the electrode eccentrically and modifying the position of the focal ground electrode to produce alterations in the configuration of the lesion.[210,244]

Perhaps the most serious complication inherent in the method is the possibility of producing about the electrode a coagulum that is firmly attached, resulting in tissue tearing and extensive hemorrhage when the electrode is removed. In order to reduce this danger, lesion production in the vicinity of 60° C is advocated. A mechanism resulting in late hemorrhage has been discussed by Mundinger and co-workers; local heating of a vessel wall was later followed by aneurysmal dilatation and rupture.[159]

In practice it has been found that simple auscultation of the head during coagulation and interruption of the current as soon as the low popping sounds that accompany steam production appear will produce lesions safely. Further refinements have, however, been undertaken to increase the safety and control of the method. Local monitoring of temperature permits lesions to be made with a constant tip temperature over a fixed time.[4,80,237] Further safeguards can be added by using make-break feedback circuits that automatically control the tip temperature and keep it below that associated with adherence of the tissue to the electrode tip.[158,230]

In general, autopsy and experimental materials indicate that lesions made about a unipolar electrode tend to be spherical or oval in shape and more regular.[80,192–194,237] The use of bipolar electrodes tends to result in asymmetrical dumbbell-shaped, or occasionally separate, lesions about each pole of the electrode even when temperature monitoring techniques are employed.

Because of the ease with which high-frequency current can be used, the high degree of safety, and the relative simplicity of the method, a great many surgeons have made this their preferred method of lesion production in stereotaxic surgery.[158,207]

Induction Heating

When a conductive metal is placed in a time-varying magnetic field, induction heating occurs. "Eddy currents" are created in the metal, which then encounters electric resistance; this resistance causes the electric energy of the currents to be dissipated as heat. Hysteresis (lagging response of the magnetizable metal to the varying applied magnetic field) is produced by friction between microscopic magnetic polar regions of the metal and results in additional heat dissipation. This information was utilized by Carpenter and Whittier when they inserted "magnetic wires" into subcortical structures in the experimental animal to produce cerebral lesions.[47] The head was placed in an electromagnetic field generated by a high-frequency induction heating unit.

Resultant lesions were of uniform size and shape with a circular configuration and were unaccompanied by distant intracerebral injury.

Induction heating for placement of intracerebral lesions has been developed for human therapeutics by Walker and Burton.[232] Their technique of repeated exposure to radiofrequency induction seems well suited for the treatment of conditions that may commonly recur during a period of time over which it would be impractical to leave an implanted electrode. Through a hollow needle an intracerebral pocket is produced by extending a stylet past the needle tip. An 8-mm by 1.6-mm solid stainless steel cylinder is then inserted through the needle into the pocket. The patient's head is then placed in an induction coil through which radiofrequency current (greater than 200 kHz) is passed and the "Electroseed" is heated. This procedure has been repeated numerous times without the occurrence of reaction in the intervening tissues.

Migration of the implanted stainless steel cylinder has not occurred over a five-year follow-up period.[43] This can be explained by adherence of the heated cylinder to the protein coagulum. The experience of others indicates that there is danger of the unheated cylinder migrating.[94] The approximately fusiform lesion has been found to be asymmetrical owing to the influence of blood vessels and cerebrospinal fluid pathways. In some instances coagulation of blood vessels has caused infarction of tissue and an increased asymmetry. It has not been possible to predict the size and shape of the lesions accurately. When this technique is used, the application of heat is continued until the desired clinical effect is achieved. Complications of the method have been few, although a case in which unexplained death followed post-heating convulsions has been described.[232] Histopathologically, the lesion is essentially similar to that produced by the radiofrequency method.[245] For the treatment of recurrent maladies, induction heating may offer significant advantages.

Lesions Produced by Cooling

Although a number of biological factors have been pointed out as being important in the production of the hypothermic lesion, these are relatively constant features, whereas the surface area of the cooling probe, the thermal properties of the material from which it is composed, the refrigerant, its temperature and flow, and the final effective freezing rate are more important in practical application.[57,61] A number of variants in the cryoprobe have been developed to restrict the freezing area to the tip of the probe.[56-58,61,62] This has been variably accomplished by heating the body of the probe or using a vacuum insulated cannula. In one of the more recent models the temperature of the uninsulated probe tip was monitored and the flow of nitrogen controlled by a servomechanism operating to maintain the tip at a preselected temperature. This apparatus, which consisted of a 2.2-mm insulated cannula, after three minutes of cooling produced a 6-mm frozen sphere at $-40°$ C, an 8-mm sphere at $-50°$ C, and a 12-mm sphere at $-100°$ C. The expanding edge of the lesion was thought to be reversible within the first 30 seconds, which added a safety factor during the production of the lesion.

There has been some discussion as to the essential nature of the cryogenic lesion. Some have considered it to be largely an ischemic infarction with very little hemorrhage and of discrete and predictable size.[18,101,116,118,178] A number of investigators have found it difficult to predict the size and shape of the lesions and have also noted the subsequent appearance of hemorrhage within the lesion and edema surrounding it.[52,145,150,169,238] Careful control of the temperature, however, appeared to decrease the incidence of hemorrhage.[238] Hemorrhage appeared less in lesions produced at temperatures above $-50°$ C than in those produced at between $-50°$ and $-160°$ C. Proposed mechanisms of hemorrhage included the adherence of frozen tissue to the cooling probe with vascular rupture on withdrawal, and tissue damage associated with pulsation of the brain at its natural frequency (10 Hz) against the large immobile stereotaxic cooling cannula.[159] In sum, the cold probe has proved to be a useful way of producing lesions and, when temperature can be closely controlled, it possesses the safety factor of permitting study of the trial lesion before the final production of the permanent lesion. The cannula, however, is larger than the probe used

in most other methods. Statistics regarding the mortality and complication rates in this method indicate that its effectiveness and safety are equivalent to others such as the radiofrequency method of lesion production.[235]

Ultrasonic Lesions

The production of cerebral lesions by ultrasonic irradiation promises to fulfill the requirements for the ideal lesion while providing a degree of safety associated with no other technique. This method has had limited use an an investigative tool in experimental animals and man. The complexity of the technique fails to encourage wide application.[140,149] Ultrasound is the term employed for sound waves of a greater frequency than human audibility (15,000 to 20,000 Hz). The waves can be generated by a quartz crystal, which upon proper electrical excitation will vibrate in resonance. If the sound is focused by an appropriate lens or reflector, a beam can be focused to a small diameter and transmitted from the lens to tissue. Small discrete cerebral lesions can be produced in animals and in man.[19,86,88,149] Because of the difference in acoustic impedance of bone and tissue, reflection and refraction of ultrasonic irradiation would occur when the beam strikes bone. Also, the absorption of irradiation by bone would produce local heat. The acoustic impedance of air is much smaller than that of brain tissue, and acoustic energy incident upon the air-brain interface would be randomly reflected. It is necessary for the bone to be removed so that the acoustic energy can be transmitted to the brain in a gas-free fluid medium for the accurate focal delivery of ultrasound to subcortical structures. Stereotaxic aiming can be performed in a number of ways, but radiological landmarks must be demonstrated. Ventriculography, the only transdural transgressor, must be performed with a radiopaque material that has an acoustic impedance similar to brain. Following air ventriculography, sufficient time must be allowed for resorption of air before acoustic radiation. The lesion is controlled by aiming of the focused beam, alteration of intensity of the exciting voltage across the crystal, and changes in the duration of exposure. Tissue absorption is a fixed fraction of the energy at specific frequencies. As frequency is increased so is absorption; at frequencies greater than 1 MHz, intervening tissue could be affected if the target site were very deep. At 1 MHz, a 1-mm diameter lesion, which histologically forms an island-moat pattern with peripheral necrosis and a relatively spared central area, can be made in the human brain.[17] The lesions have been found to be free of hemorrhage, appearing to spare blood vessels. Edema, which is commonly found surrounding cerebral lesions, is absent.[17,19] Increasing the dose will proportionately increase the lesion size. With correct focusing of the beams and the proper dosage, no lesion is encountered in intervening tissues. White matter is affected by lower energy levels than gray, enabling the destruction of specific fiber tracts while sparing a surrounding cellular area.[19] The precise physical mechanism responsible for the lesion is not known but has been shown not to be primarily a temperature response, although the threshold for lesion production can be lowered with higher body temperature.[19,87]

Advantages of the method when employed in stereotaxic surgery are readily seen. With blood vessels spared, the danger of hemorrhage and distant effects secondary to vascular interruption would be alleviated. Multiple small lesions could be made to form a larger lesion of any desired configuration.

Meyers and co-workers successfully performed ultrasonic irradiation on a number of patients with movement and pain disorders; however, the technique has not been universally accepted.[149] The instrumentation is expensive and elaborate, requiring a great deal of time in preoperative and postoperative maintenance and calibration. It was necessary to spend a total of 12 to 14 hours in two separate periods in an operating room. A large craniotomy flap had to be made prior to the procedure so that the bone could be removed to accommodate the focused beams. Other criticism involved the lack of physiological and radiological monitoring of the lesion site. While Meyers demonstrated the applicability of ultrasonic irradiation to human stereotaxic surgery, without the development of certain technological features, wide use of the method is impractical. Efforts to achieve a system compatible with wider utilization have led to the development in the experimental animal of an acoustic system with which ventricular outline and intracerebral structures may be located without ventriculography. A physiologically acceptable, acoustically transparent, rigid window has also been designed that, when replacing bone, would allow ultrasonic visualization of cerebral structures and ultrasonic irradiation through the intact skin.[84] These advances have yet to be tested in human stereotaxic surgery.

Radiation Lesions

Implanted Sources

Radioactive energy delivered to subcortical structures by means of implanted sources is a method of lesion production that offers unique advantages along with its peculiar disadvantages. Considerable attention has been paid to the use of specific isotopes whose emission, energy, and half-life are best suited for the safe destruction of neural tissue.

Bagg and Edwards and Bagg demonstrated that sharply circumscribed subcortical lesions could be produced with an implanted radiation source.[13,72] The size of their lesion was found to be dependent upon time. Stein and Peterson, using stereotaxic techniques in monkeys, produced subcortical lesions with implanted radon.[204] Advantages claimed for their method included the production of large subcortical lesions of symmetrical shape with small entry wounds produced gradually rather than abruptly, thereby allowing neurological accommodation. In addition, the position of the implanted source can be radiologically identified both at the time of implantation and at any later date.

The biological effectiveness of a particular isotope depends upon the type and level of energy emitted. Because of their low penetration, alpha particles have no therapeutic usefulness. Most gamma rays are of limited therapeutic value because they have a large effective range in tissue and produce diffuse rather than sharp focal lesions.[14] Beta particles with maximum ranges of less than a centimeter in tissue constitute the ideal radiation for implanted sources. Lesion size is dependent upon the mean path in tissue of the particle and the duration of exposure. The mean path is determined by the energy of emission, as is the tissue effect, which is a function of the dose received. The dose is dependent upon the amount of emitted energy that is absorbed in the tissue. By selection of an isotope with suitable energy and half-life, appropriate size can be achieved. Using unfiltered beta emitters, Borison and Wang correlated dose and exposure with the lesions produced.[37] The lesions were of predictable size and shape, achieving maximum extent in 9 to 10 days. Edema, which was evident on the third day, subsided by the fortieth day. The artificial isotopes palladium-109 and yttrium-90, pure beta emitters, have favorable half-lives and energy of beta emission. Yttrium-90 with a half-life of 2.54 days and 2.18 mev beta energy allows lesions of suitable size to be made when it is incorporated in a ceramic sphere.[38] Its half-life also makes it suitable for shipping. Ninety-nine per cent of its energy is deposited in the first 4 mm.[212] Lesions produced in this manner have been found to be spherical and discrete, sharply separated from normal brain by a 0.4- to 0.7-mm zone of transition. No lesions outside of the zones of initial necrosis have been described after prolonged follow-up.

Erosion of ependyma by yttrium-90 seeds that had entered into the lateral ventricle and migration of seeds along necrotic tracts have been reported.[45] Mechanisms for fixing the seed in place and removing it after the desired therapeutic effect have been devised. Other criticisms of the technique are concerned with the fact that 7 to 10 days are necessary before the lesion is fully formed, and even weeks may be necessary to obtain full clinical information, as the resultant edema may last from 10 to 40 days.[38,152,212] When the radioactive source is simply inserted and left in place, the total dose is irretrievably delivered and the extent of necrosis cannot be controlled. Mullan and his associates have reported the use of a 20-mc source of palladium-90 in the form of a wire, which when inserted subcortically produces a lesion of 5 to 6 mm maximum diameter within 90 minutes.[153] No histological extension of the lesion has been seen in experimental animals after the 90-minute period.[152] Temporary insertion of the wire makes it possible to monitor physiological response, and the lesion can be extended or discontinued as necessary. By varying the energy of the source, the duration of exposure, or the method of introduction into the brain, the lesion's size and shape can be accurately controlled.[151]

External Radiation

Leksell and co-workers placed subcortical stereotaxic lesions for the treatment of pain and psychoses by using 280-kv x-rays through the intact skin.[131] Because the high scatter of the low-energy x-rays necessitated a large number of portals through which the radiation had to be administered, it was concluded that the procedure would best be carried out using high-energy particles. In a cyclotron, charged particles can be accelerated and focused upon a specific target. Early work by Tobias and co-workers with 190-mev deuterons demonstrated that this technique could be used for the proportional destruction of neural tissue.[219] In a series of animal experiments, Larsson, Leksell, and Rexed and their colleagues studied the effect of 185-mev proton beams on cerebral tissue.[127,128,132,177] Administering 20,000 rads produced small, well-demarcated lesions that were free of significant hemorrhage. No selective radiation effect or any delayed effects were demonstrated over a three-year period. Nine days were required for the formation of a lesion produced with a dose of 20,000 rads and a 1.5-mm beam. With a wider beam more vascular damage was seen. When a dose greater than 20,000 rads was used, widespread tissue reaction was encountered even with a multiple portal technique. This method has been expanded to limited use in man.[126] In this procedure the patient is rotated and the proton radiation is administered through 16 to 21 portals. In a case of intractable pain in which the spinothalamic tract was irradiated in the midbrain, relief occurred 30 days following irradiation, only to recur within a month. This was found histologically to be the result of a well-demarcated 2- by 4-mm ovoid lesion.[142]

Other investigators have used the end-range of the proton beam, the Bragg peak, in which the ionizing effect is several times as great as elsewhere on the beam.[121,122,143] This appears to be particularly successful in the treatment of pituitary tumors.[120,122] Reports of delayed brain necrosis following the administration of heavy particle radiation are known, but whether this necrosis is frequent and serious enough to prohibit use of this technique has not yet been determined.[10,11,148]

REFERENCES

1. Adey, W. R., Kado, R. T., and Didio, J.: Impedance measurements in brain tissues of animals using microvolt signals. Exp. Neurol., 5:47–66, 1962.
2. Agnoli, A., Eggert, H. R., Zierski, J., Seeger, W., and Kirchoff, D.: Diagnostische Möglichkeiten der positiven Ventrikulographie. Acta Neurochir., 31:227–244, 1975.
3. Albe-Fessard, D., Arfel, G., Guiot, G., Dermone, P., and Guilband, G.: Thalamic unit activity in man. Electroenceph. Clin. Neurophysiol., 25:suppl., 132–142, 1967.
4. Alberts, W. W., Wright, E. W., and Feinstein, B.: An integrated system for brain stimulation and lesion production in human stereotaxic surgery. Confin. Neurol., 35:81–89, 1973.
5. Alberts, W. W., Wright, E. W., Jr., Feinstein, B., and von Bonin, G.: Experimental radiofrequency brain lesion size as a function of physical parameters. J. Neurosurg., 25:421–423, 1966.
6. Alberts, W. W., Wright, E. W., Jr., Levin, G., Feinstein, B., and Mueller, M.: Threshold stimulation of the lateral thalamus and globus pallidus in the waking human. Electroenceph. Clin. Neurophysiol., 13:68–74, 1961.
7. Alberts, W. W., Feinstein, B., Levin, G., Wright, E. W., Darland, M. G., and Scott, E. L.: Stereotaxic surgery for parkinsonism: Clinical Results and stimulating thresholds. J. Neurosurg., 23:174–183, 1965.
8. Amador, L. V., Brunck, H. J., and Wahren, R.: Materials and methods. In Schaltenbrand, G., and Bailey, P., eds.: Introduction to Stereotaxis with an Atlas of the Human Brain. New York, Grune & Stratton, 1959, pp. 3–8.
9. Andy, O. J.: Tremor monitoring for posterior subthalamic placement of lesions in parkinsonism. J. Neurol. Neurosurg. Psychiat., 26:561, 1963.
10. Arnold, A., Bailey, P., and Laughlin, J. S.: Effects of betatron radiation on the brain of primates. Neurology (Minneap.), 4:165–178, 1954.
11. Arnold, A., Bailey, P., Harvey, R. A., Haas, L. L., and Laughlin, J. S.: Changes in the central nervous sytem following irradiation with 23 MeV x-rays from the betatron. Radiology, 62:37–44, 1954.
12. Aronow, S.: The use of radiofrequency power in making lesions in the brain. J. Neurosurg., 17:431–438, 1960.
13. Bagg, H. J.: The action of buried tubes of radium emanation upon normal and neoplastic tissues. Amer. J. Roentgen., 8:536–544, 1921.
14. Bailey, O. T., Boyesen, S., and Campbell, J. B.: Beta radiation of the feline caudate nucleus: Late results. J. Neurosurg., 14:536–542, 1957.
15. Baird, H. W., III, Spiegel, E. A., and Wycis, H. T.: Studies in stereoencephalotomy. IX. The variability in the extent and position of the amygdala. Confin. Neurol., 20:26–36, 1960.
16. Baird, H. W., III, Chavez, M., Adams, J., Wycis, H. T., and Spiegel, E. A.: Studies in stereoencephalotomy. VII. Variations in the position of the globus pallidus. Confin. Neurol., 17:288–299, 1957.
17. Bakay, L., Hueter, T. F., Ballantine, H. T., Jr., and Sosa, D.: Ultrasonically produced changes in the blood-brain barrier. A.M.A. Arch. Neurol. Psychiat., 76:457–467, 1956.
18. Balthasar, K.: Gezielte Kälteschäden in der Grosshirnrinde der Katze. Deutsch. Z. Nervenheilk. 176:173–199, 1957.
19. Barnard, J. W., Fry, W. J., and Brennan, J. F.: Small localized ultrasonic lesions in the white and grey matter of the cat brain. A.M.A. Arch. Neurol. Psychiat., 75:15–34, 1956.
20. Bates, J. V.: Recordings from the thalamus and their value in stereotaxic surgery. J. Neurol. Neurosurg. Psychiat., 29:475, 1966.
21. Beaunis, H.: Note sur l'application des Injections Interstitielles à l'Étude des Fonctions des Centres Nerveux. Paris, Durand, 1868.
22. Benz, R. A., Wycis, H. T., and Spiegel, E. A.: Studies in stereoencephalotomy. XI. Variability studies of the nucleus ventralis lateralis thalami. Confin. Neurol., 20:366–374, 1960.
23. Bertrand, C.: A pneumotaxic technique for producing localized cerebral lesions and its use for the treatment of Parkinson's disease. J. Neurosurg., 15:251–264, 1958.
24. Bertrand, C.: Functional localization with monopolar stimulation. J. Neurosurg., 24:suppl., 403–409, 1966.
25. Bertrand, C.: Personal communication, 1969.
26. Bertrand, C., and Martinez, N.: An apparatus and technique for surgery of dyskinesias. Neurochirurgie, 2:36–46, 1959.
27. Bertrand, C., Martinez, N., and Hardy, J.: Localization of lesions. J. Neurosurg., 24:suppl., 446–448, 1966.
28. Bertrand, C., Hardy, J., Molina-Negro, P., and Martinez, S. N.: Optimum physiological target for the arrest of tremor. Presented at the Third Symposium on Parkinson's Disease at the Royal College of Surgeons of Edinburgh, 22 May, 1968.
29. Bertrand, G.: Personal communication, 1969.
30. Bertrand, G., and Jasper, H.: Microelectrode recording of unit activity in the human thalamus. Confin. Neurol., 26:205–208, 1965.
31. Bertrand, G., Blundell, J., and Musella, R.: Electrical exploration of the internal capsule and neighbouring structures during stereotaxic procedures. J. Neurosurg., 22:333–343, 1965.
32. Bertrand, G., Olivier, A., and Thompson, C. J.: The computer brain atlas: Its use in stereotaxic surgery. Confin. Neurol., 36:312–313, 1973.
33. Bertrand, G., Olivier, A., and Thompson, C. J.: Computer display of stereotaxic brain maps and probe tracts. Acta Neurochir. (Wien), suppl. 21:235–243, 1974.
34. Birg, W., and Mundinger, F.: Computer programs for stereotactic neurosurgery. Confin. Neurol., 36:326–333, 1974.
35. Birg, W., and Mundinger, F.: Calculation of the position of a side-protruding electrode tip in stereotaxic brain operations using a stereotaxic apparatus with polar coordinates. Acta Neurochir. (Wien), 32:83–87, 1975.

36. Bleasel, K., Harrison, J., and Miller, D.: A new approach to stereotaxic localization. Med. J. Aust., *1*:717–722, 1964.

37. Borison, H. L., and Wang, S. C.: Quantitative effects of radon implanted in the medulla oblongata: A technique for producing discrete lesions. J. Comp. Neurol., *94*:33–53, 1951.

38. Boyesen, S., and Campbell, J. B.: Stereotaxic implantation of calibrated Pd¹⁰⁹ and Y⁹⁰ spheres: A technique for producing predictable subcortical lesions in the brains of laboratory animals. Yale J. Biol. Med., *28*:216–224, 1955.

39. Bradley, D. J., Fox, M., and Williams, T. D.: CNS—an on-line program for controlling stereotaxic stimulation within the central nervous system and for recording and analysis of responses in a neurophysiological experiment. Comput. Progr. Biomed., *2*:75–86, 1972.

40. Bravo, E.: Personal communication, 1968.

41. Brierley, J. B., and Beck, E.: The significance in human stereotactic brain surgery of individual variation in the diencephalon and globus pallidus. J. Neurol. Neurosurg. Psychiat., *22*:287–298, 1959.

42. Brodkey, J. S., Miyazaki, Y., Ervin, F. R., and Mark, V. H.: Reversible heat lesions with radiofrequency current. J. Neurosurg., *21*:49–53, 1964.

43. Burton, C. V.: Personal communication, 1968.

44. Burton, C. V., Mozley, J. M., Walker, A. E., and Braitman, H. E.: Induction thermocoagulation of the brain: A new neurosurgical tool. I.E.E.E. Trans. Biomed. Engin., *13*:114–120, 1966.

45. Campbell, J. B., Rossi, H. H., Biavati, M. H., and Biavati, B. J.: Production of subcortical lesions by implantation of radioactive substances. Confin. Neurol., *22*:178–182, 1962.

46. Campbell, R. L., Campbell, J. A., Heimberger, R. F., Kalsbeck, J. E., and Mealey, J.: Ventriculography and myelography with absorbable radiopaque medium. Radiology, *82*:286–289, 1964.

47. Carpenter, M. B., and Whittier, J. R.: Study of methods for producing experimental lesions of the central nervous system with special reference to stereotaxic technique. J. Comp. Neurol., *97*:73–131, 1952.

48. Carreras, M., Mancia, D., Pagni, C. A.: Unit discharges recorded from the human thalamus with microelectrodes. Confin. Neurol., *29*:87–89, 1967.

49. Caruthers, R. P.: An expanding loop encephalotome for use in brain function research. Electroenceph. Clin. Neurophysiol., *24*:590–592, 1968.

50. Clarke, R. H.: Investigation of the Central Nervous System. Part I. Methods and Instruments. Baltimore, Md., Johns Hopkins Press, 1920.

51. Cobble, S. P., and Brackett, C. E.: Changes in the ventricular size during stereotaxic surgery. Amer. J. Roentgen., *95*:890–898, 1965.

52. Coe, J., and Ommaya, A. K.: Evaluation of focal lesions of the central nervous system produced by extreme cold. J. Neurosurg., *21*:433–444, 1964.

53. Colloff, E., Gleason, C. A., Alberts, W. W., and Wright, E. W.: Computer-aided localization techniques for stereotaxic surgery. Confin. Neurol., *35*:65–80, 1973.

54. Cooper, I. S.: Chemopallidectomy: An investigative technique in geriatric parkinsonians. Science, *121*:217–218, 1955.

55. Cooper, I. S.: Parkinsonism—Its Medical and Surgical Therapy. Springfield, Ill., Charles C Thomas, 1961.

56. Cooper, I. S.: Cryogenic cooling and freezing of the basal ganglia. Confin. Neurol., *22*:336–340, 1962.

57. Cooper, I. S.: A cryogenic method for physiologic inhibition and production of lesions in the brain. J. Neurosurg., *19*:853–858, 1962.

58. Cooper, I. S.: Cryogenic surgery of the basal ganglia. J.A.M.A., *181*:600–604, 1962.

59. Cooper, I. S.: Cryothalamectomy—surgical technique. *In* Rand, R. W., Rinfret, A. P., and von Leden, H., eds.: Cryosurgery. Springfield, Ill., Charles C Thomas, 1968, pp. 187–206.

60. Cooper, I. S., and Bravo, G. J.: Chemopallidectomy and chemothalamectomy. J. Neurosurg., *15*:244–250, 1958.

61. Cooper, I. S., and Lee, A. St. J.: Cryostatic congelation: A system for producing a limited controlled region of cooling or freezing of biologic tissues. J. Nerv. Ment. Dis., *133*:259–263, 1961.

62. Cooper, I. S., Gioino, G., and Terry, R.: The cryogenic lesion. Confin. Neurol., *26*:161–177, 1965.

63. Crowell, R. M., Perret, E., Siegfried, J., and Villoz, J. P.: "Movement units" and "tremor phasic units" in the human thalamus. Brain Res., *11*:481–488, 1968.

64. Davies, F. L.: Effect of unabsorbed radiographic contrast media on the central nervous system. Lancet, *2*:747–748, 1956.

65. Davis, F. M., Llewellyn, R. C., and Kirgis, H. D.: Watersoluble contrast myelography using meglumine iothalamate (Conray) with methyl prednisolone acetate (Depo-Medrol). Radiology, *90*:705–710, 1968.

66. Delmas, A., and Pertuiset, B.: Cranio-cerebral Topometry in Man. Location and Variation in Position of Cerebral Subcortical Structures with Special Reference to Neurology, Neurosurgery and Neuroradiology. Springfield, Ill., Charles C Thomas, 1959.

67. Dervin, E., Heywood, O. B., Crossley, T. R., and Dawson, B. H.: The use of a small digital computer for stereotaxic surgery. Acta Neurochir., suppl. *21*:245–252, 1974.

68. Di Chiro, G.: An Atlas of Detailed Normal Pneumoencephalographic Anatomy. Springfield, Ill., Charles C Thomas, 1959.

69. Dieckmann, G., Gabriel, E., and Hassler, R.: Size, form and structural peculiarities of experimental brain lesions obtained by thermocontrolled radiofrequency. Confin. Neurol., *26*:134–142, 1965.

70. Dierssen, G., and Marg, E.: The value of impedance measurements to aid in the localisation in stereotaxic surgery. Confin. Neurol., *26*:407–410, 1965.

71. Doppman, J.: Personal communication, 1969.

72. Edwards, D. J., and Bagg, H. J.: Lesions of the corpus striatum by radium emanation and the

accompanying structural and functional changes. Amer. J. Physiol., *65*:162–173, 1923.

73. Erickson, T. C., and Van Baaren, H. J.: Late meningeal reaction to ethyl iodophenylundecylate used in myelography. Report of a case that terminated fatally. J.A.M.A., *153*:636–639, 1953.

74. Ervin, F. R., and Mark, V. H.: Physiological observations of the human thalamus. Trans. Amer. Neurol. Ass., *84*:94–100, 1959.

75. Ervin, F. R., and Mark, V. H.: Stereotactic thalamotomy in the human. Part II. Physiologic observations on the human thalamus. Arch. Neurol. (Chicago), *3*:368–380, 1960.

76. Eschler, J., Riechert, T., and Umbach, W.: Die Anwendung eines Zielapparates für stereotaktische Operationen in der Mund und Kieferchirurgie als neue technische Möglichkeit. Deutsch. Zahn. Mund. Kieferheilk., *43*:22–29, 1964.

77. Fager, C. A.: Personal communication, 1968.

78. Fairman, D., and Perlmutter, I.: Physiological observations during stereotaxic surgery of the basal ganglia. Confin. Neurol., *26*:299–305, 1965.

79. Feinstein, B.: Electrophysiologic studies of parkinsonism at surgery. Arch. Neurol. (Chicago), *6*:66–67, 1962.

80. Feinstein, B., Alberts, W., Wright, E. W., and Levin, G.: A stereotaxic technique in man allowing multiple spatial and temporal approaches to intracranial targets. J. Neurosurg., *17*:708–720, 1960.

81. Fisher, R.: An experimental evaluation of Pantopaque and other recently developed myelographic contrast media. Radiology, *85*:537–545, 1965.

82. Flamm, E. S., and Van Buren, J. M.: The reliability of reconstructed ventricular landmarks for localization of depth electrodes in man. J. Neurosurg., *25*:67–72, 1966.

83. Fleming, D. G.: A constant current apparatus for the production of electrolytic lesions. Electroenceph. Clin. Neurophysiol., *9*:551–554, 1957.

84. Fry, F. J.: Personal communication, 1969.

85. Fry, F. J., Ades, H. W., and Fry, W. J.: Production of reversible changes in the central nervous system by ultrasound. Science, *127*:83–84, 1958.

86. Fry, W. J.: Use of intense ultrasound in neurological research. Amer. J. Phys. Med., *37*:143–147, 1958.

87. Fry, W. J., and Fry, F. J.: Fundamental neurological research and human neurosurgery using intense ultrasound. I.R.E. Trans. Med. Electronics, ME-7:166–181, 1960.

88. Fry, W. J., Mosberg, W. H., Barnard, J. W., and Fry, F. J.: Production of focal destructive lesions in the central nervous system with ultrasound. J. Neurosurg., *11*:471–478, 1954.

89. Funkquist, B., and Obel, N.: Tonic muscle spasms and blood pressure changes following the subarachnoid injection of contrast media. Acta Radiol., *53*:337–351, 1960.

90. Funkquist, B., and Obel, N.: Effect on the spinal cord of subarachnoid injection of water soluble contrast medium: An experimental study in dogs. Acta Radiol., *56*:449–464, 1961.

91. Gaze, R. M., Gillingham, F. J., Kalyanaraman, S., Porter, R. W., Donaldson, A. A., and Donaldson, R. M. L.: Microelectrode recordings from the human thalamus. Brain, *87*:691–706, 1964.

92. Gildenberg, P. L.: Studies in stereoencephalotomy. VIII. Comparison of the variability of subcortical lesions produced by various procedures. Confin. Neurol., *17*:299–309, 1957.

93. Gildenberg, P. L.: Studies in stereoencephalotomy. X. Variability of subcortical lesions produced by a heating electrode and with Cooper's balloon-cannula. Confin. Neurol., *20*:53–65, 1960.

94. Gillingham, J. F.: Depth recording and stimulation. J. Neurosurg., *24*:suppl., 382–387, 1966.

95. Gillingham, J. F.: Personal communication, 1969.

96. Guiot, G.: Personal communication, 1969.

97. Gybels, J., Kempen, D., Peluso, F., and Van Bael, M.: Computer techniques for tracking penetrating electrodes, plotting two-target trajectories and performing two stage stereotaxic surgery in humans. Confin. Neurol., *36*:302–309, 1974.

98. Hankinson, J., Hudgson, P., Pearce, G. W., and Morris, C. J.: A simple method for obtaining stereotaxic biopsies from the human basal ganglia—a case of cerebral porphyria. Acta Neurochir., suppl. *21*:227–233, 1974.

99. Hardy, J., and Bertrand, C.: Electrophysiological exploration of subcortical structures with microelectrodes during stereotaxic surgery. Confin. Neurol., *26*:201–204, 1965.

100. Harvey, J. P., Jr., and Freiberger, R. H.: Myelography with an absorbable agent. J. Bone Joint Surg., *47-A*:397–416, 1965.

101. Hass, G. M., and Taylor, C. B.: A quantitative hypothermal method for the production of local injury of tissue. Arch. Path., *45*:563–580, 1948.

102. Hassler, R.: Anatomy of the thalamus. *In* Schaltenbrand, G., and Bailey, P., eds.: Introduction to Stereotaxis with an Atlas of the Human Brain. New York, Grune & Stratton, 1959, pp. 230–290.

103. Hassler, R.: Motorische und sensible Effekte umschriebener Reizungen und Ausschaltungen in menschlichen Zwischenhirn. Deutsch. Z. Nervenheilk., *183*:148–171, 1961.

104. Hassler, R., and Riechert, T.: Indikationen und Lokalisationsmethode der gezielten Hirnoperationen. Nervenarzt, *25*:441–447, 1954.

105. Hassler, R., Riechert, T., Mundinger, F., Umbach, W., and Ganglberger, J. A.: Physiological observations in stereotaxic operations in extrapyramidal motor disturbances. Brain, *83*:337–351, 1960.

106. Heimburger, R. F., Kalsbech, J. R., Campbell, R. L., and Mealey, J.: Positive contrast cerebral ventriculography using water-soluble media. J. Neurol. Neurosurg. Psychiat., *29*:281–290, 1966.

107. Hess, W. R.: Die Methodik der lokalisierten Reizung und Ausschaltung subkortikaler Hirnabschnitte, Leipzig, Georg Thieme, 1932.

108. Hoefer, T., Mundinger, F., Birg, W., and Reinke, M.: Computer calculation to localize subcortical targets in plane x-rays for stereotactic neurosurgery. Confin. Neurol., *36*:334–340, 1974.

109. Horsley, V., and Clarke, R. H.: The structure and functions of the cerebellum examined by a new method. Brain, *31*:45–124, 1908.

110. Housepian, E. M., and Pool, J. L.: The accuracy of human stereoencephalotomy as judged by histological confirmation of roentgenographic localization. J. Nerv. Ment. Dis., *130*:520–525, 1960.

111. Housepian, E. M., and Purpura, D. P.: Electrophysiological studies of subcortical-cortical relations in man. Electroenceph. Clin. Neurophysiol., *15*:20–28, 1963.

112. Howland, W. J., Curry, J. L., and Butler, A. K.: Pantopaque arachnoiditis: Experimental study of blood as a potentiating agent. Radiology, *80*:489–491, 1963.

113. Hunsperger, R. W., and Wyss, O. A. M.: Production of localized lesions in nervous tissue by coagulation with high frequency currents. Helv. Physiol. Pharmacol. Acta *11*:283–304, 1953.

114. Hurteau, E. F., Baird, W. C., and Sinclair, E.: Arachnoiditis following use of iodized oil. J. Bone Joint Surg., *36-A*:393–400, 1954.

115. Jasper, H. H., and Bertrand, G.: Thalamic units involved in somatic sensation and voluntary and involuntary movements in man. In Purpura, O. F., and Yahr, M. D., eds.: The Thalamus. New York, Columbia University Press, 1966, pp. 365–384.

116. Jinnai, D.: Cryothalamectomy. Confin. Neurol., *26*:437–440, 1965.

117. Kamm, R. F., and Austin, G.: The use of bony landmarks of the skull for localization of the anterior-posterior commissural line. J. Neurosurg., *22*:576–580, 1965.

118. Kandel, E. I.: Experience with the cryosurgical method in production of lesions of the extrapyramidal system. Confin. Neurol., *26*:306–309, 1965.

119. Kandel, E., and Chebotaryova, N. M.: Conray ventriculography in stereotaxic surgery—experience with 320 operations. Confin. Neurol., *34*:34–40, 1972.

120. Kjellberg, R. N., Nguyen, N. C., and Kliman, B.: Le Bragg Peak protonique en neuro-chirurgie stéréotaxique. Neurochirurgie, *18*:235–265, 1972.

121. Kjellberg, R. N., Koehler, A. M., Preston, W. M., and Sweet, W. H.: Stereotaxic instrument for use with the Bragg peak of a proton beam. Confin. Neurol., *22*:183–189, 1962.

122. Kjellberg, R. N., Shintani, A., Frantz, A. G., and Kliman, B.: Proton-beam therapy in acromegaly. New Eng. J. Med., *278*:689–695, 1968.

123. Laitinen, L. V., and Johansson, G. G.: Locating human cerebral structures by the impedance method. Confin. Neurol., *29*:197–201, 1967.

124. Laitinen, L., Johansson, G. G., and Sipponen, P.: Impedance and phase angle as a locating method in human stereotaxic surgery. J. Neurosurg., *25*:628–633, 1966.

125. Larson, S. J., and Sances, A.: Evoked potentials in man. Neurosurgical applications. Amer. J. Surg., *111*:857–861, 1966.

126. Larsson, B., Leksell, L., and Rexed, B.: The use of high energy protons for cerebral surgery in man. Acta Chir. Scand., *125*:1–7, 1963.

127. Larsson, B., Leksell, L., Rexed, B., and Sourander, P.: Effect of high energy protons on the spinal cord. Acta Radiol., *51*:52–64, 1959.

128. Larsson, B., Leksell, L., Rexed, B., Sourander, P., Mair, W., and Andersson, B.: The high-energy proton beam as a neurosurgical tool. Nature, *182*:1222–1223, 1958.

129. Le Beau, J., Dondey, M., Albe-Fessard, D., Weil, L., and Aleonard, P.: Selective and reversible block of cerebral structures by local cooling. Confin. Neurol., *22*:341–342, 1962.

130. Leksell, L.: Gezielte Hirnoperationen. In Olivecrona, H., and Tönnis, W., eds.: Handbuch der Neurochirurgie, VI. Berlin, Springer-Verlag, 1957, pp. 178–199.

131. Leksell, L., Herner, T., and Lidén, K.: Stereotaxic radiosurgery of the brain. Kungl. Fvsiogvat. Sällsk. Förhandl., *25*:1–10, 1955.

132. Leksell, L., Larsson, B., Andersson, B., Rexed, B., Sourander, P., and Mair, W.: Lesions in the depth of the brain produced by a beam of high energy protons. Acta Radiol., *54*:251–264, 1960.

133. Levin, G.: Electrical stimulation of the globus pallidus and thalamus. J. Neurosurg., *24*: suppl., 415, 1966.

134. Lichtenstein, B.: Abnormal topographical relations of the brain resulting from disease. In Schaltenbrand, G., and Bailey, P., eds.: Introduction to Stereotaxis with an Atlas of the Human Brain. New York, Grune & Stratton, 1959, pp. 65–69.

135. Lilly, J. C., Hughes, J. R., Galkin, T. W., and Alvord, E. C., Jr.: Production and avoidance of injury to brain tissue by electrical current at threshold values. Electroenceph. Clin. Neurophysiol., *7*:458, 1955.

136. Lindblom, K.: Complications of myelography by Abrodil. Acta Radiol., *28*:69–73, 1947.

137. Lindgren, E.: Some aspects on the technique of encephalography. Acta Radiol., *31*:161–177, 1949.

138. Lindgren, E.: Pneumography of the head. In Schinz, H. R., et al., eds.: Roentgendiagnostics. New York, Grune & Stratton, 1952, pp. II: 1637–1686.

139. Lindgren, E., ed.: Röntgenologie; einschliesslich Kontrastmethoden. In Olivecrona, H., and Tönnis, W., eds.: Handbuch der Neurochirurgie, Bd. 2., Berlin, Springer, 1954.

140. Lindstrom, P. A.: Prefrontal ultrasonic irradiation—a substitute for lobotomy. A.M.A. Arch. Neurol. Psychiat., *72*:399–425, 1954.

141. MacIntyre, W. J., Bidder, T. G., and Rowland, V.: The production of brain lesions with electric currents. In Quastler, H., and Morowitz, H. J., eds.: Proceedings of the First National Biophysics Conference, Columbus, Ohio, March 4–6, 1957. New Haven, Conn., Yale University Press, 1959, pp. 723–732.

142. Mair, W., Rexed, B., and Sourander, P.: Histology of the surgical radiolesion in the human brain as produced by high-energy protons. Radiat. Res., *7*:389, 1967.

143. Malis, L. I., Koevinger, R., Kruger, L., and Rose, J. F.: Production of laminar lesions in the cerebral cortex by heavy ionizing particles. Science, *126*:302, 1957.

144. Mark, V. H., and Yakovlev, P. I.: A note on problems and methods in the preparation of a human stereotactic atlas. Including a report of

measurements of the posteromedial portion of the ventral nucleus of the thalamus. Anat. Rec., *121*:745–752, 1955.

145. Mark, V. H., Chiba, T., Ervin, F. R., and Hamlin, H.: The comparison of heat and cold for the production of localized lesions in the central nervous system. Confin. Neurol., *26*:178–184, 1965.

146. Mason, M. S., and Raaf, J.: Complications of Pantopaque myelography: Case report and review. J. Neurosurg., *19*:302–311, 1962.

147. McCaul, J. R.: A method for the localization and production of discrete destructive lesions of the brain. J. Neurol. Neurosurg. Psychiat., *22*:109–112, 1959.

148. McDonald, L. W., Born, J. L., Laurence, J. H., and Lyman, J. L.: Preliminary report on histopathologic changes in brain following heavy-particle irradiation. *In* Semiannual Report on Biology and Medicine, prepared by Donner Laboratory and Donner Pavilion of Lawrence Radiation Laboratory, Berkeley, University of California, 1963, pp. 41–54.

149. Meyers, R., Fry, W. J., Fry, F. J., Dreyer, L. L., Schultz, D. F., and Noyes, R. F.: Early experiences with ultrasonic irradiation of the pallidofugal and nigral complexes in hyperkinetic and hypertonic disorders. J. Neurosurg., *16*:32–54, 1959.

150. Miyazaki, Y., Ervin, F. R., Siegfried, J., Richardson, E. P., and Mark, V. H.: Localized cooling in the central nervous system. Arch. Neurol. (Chicago), *9*:392–399, 1963.

151. Mullan, S.: Observations on deep cerebral "localization" of the tremor of Parkinson's disease. A.M.A. Arch. Neurol., *2*:274–280, 1960.

152. Mullan, S., Harper, P. V., and Gerol, Y.: An experimental study in the use of a rapidly decaying beta source (Pd[109]) in the production of deep cerebral lesions. Amer. J. Roentgen, *84*:108–112, 1960.

153. Mullan, S., Moseley, R. D., and Harper, P. V.: The creation of deep cerebral lesions by small beta ray sources implanted under guidance of fluoroscopic image intensifiers (as used in the treatment of Parkinson's disease). Amer. J. Roentgen., *82*:613–617, 1959.

154. Mullan, S., Mailis, M., Karasick, J., Vailati, G., and Beckman, F.: A reappraisal of the unipolar anodal electrolytic lesion. J. Neurosurg., *22*:531–538, 1965.

155. Mundinger, F., and Potthoff, P.: Messungen im Pneumencephalogramm zur intracerebralen und craniocerebralen Korrelations Topographie bei stereotaktischen Hirnoperationen, unter besonderer Berücksichtigung der stereotaktischen Pallidotomie. Acta Neurochir., *9*:196–214, 1961.

156. Mundinger, F., and Reichert, T.: Ergebnisse der stereotaktischen Hirnoperationen bei extrapyramidalen Bewegunsstörungen auf grund postoperativer und Langzeituntersuchungen. Deutsch. Z. Nervenheilk., *182*:542–576, 1961.

157. Mundinger, F., and Reichert, T.: Die stereotaktischen Hirnoperationen zur Behandlung extrapyramidaler Bewegungsstörungen (Parkinsonismus und Hyperkinesen) und ihre Resultate. Fortschr. Neurol. Psychiat., *31*:1–120, 1963.

158. Mundinger, F., and Riechert, T.: Indikation und Langzeitergebnisse von 1400 uni- und bilateralen stereotaktischen Eingriffen beim Parkinson-Syndrom. Wien. Z. Nervenheilk., *23*:147–177, 1966.

159. Mundinger, F., Riechert, T., and Gabriel, E.: Untersuchungen zu den physikalischen und technischen Voraussetzungen einer dosierten Hochfrequenzkoagulation bei stereotaktischen Hirnoperationen. Zbl. Chir., *85*:1051–1063, 1960.

160. Narabayashi, H.: Discussion des rapports sur les methodes stereotaxiques. *In* Premier Congres International de Neurochirurgie, Bruxelles, 1957, pp. 182–187.

161. Narabayashi, H.: Functional differentiation to and around the ventrolateral nucleus of the thalamus based on experience in human stereoencephalotomy. Johns Hopkins Med. J., *122*:295–300, 1968.

162. Narabayashi, H., and Okuma, T.: Procaine oil blocking of pallidum in cases of athetose double. Psychiat. Neurol. Jap., *54*:672–677, 1953.

163. Narabayashi, H., Shimazu, H., Fujita, Y., Shikaba, S., Nagao, T., and Nagahata, M.: Procaine-oil-wax pallidotomy for double athetosis and spastic states in infantile cerebral palsy. Neurology (Minneap.), *10*:61–69, 1960.

164. Neroth, C. C., Simmons, M., and Marg, E.: Transformation of Horsley-Clarke coordinates for electrode implantation experiments in stereotaxic surgery. Comput. Biomed. Res., *8*:244–253, 1975.

165. Obrador, S., and Dierssen, G.: Cirugía de la región palidal en el síndrome de Parkinson. Técnica personal y resultados immediatos en los seis primeros casos operados. Rev. Clin. Esp., *61*:229–237, 1956.

166. Obrador, S., and Dierssen, G.: Sensory responses to subcortical stimulation and management of pain disorders by stereotaxic methods. Confin. Neurol., *27*:45–51, 1966.

167. Ohye, C., Kubota, K., Hongo, T., Nagao, T., and Narabayashi, H.: Ventrolateral and subventrolateral thalamic stimulation. Motor effects. Arch. Neurol. (Chicago), *11*:427–434, 1964.

168. Ommaya, A. K.: Personal communication, 1969.

169. Ommaya, A. K., and Coe, J.: An experimental appraisal of cryogenic brain lesions in the cat. Confin. Neurol., *26*:185–189, 1965.

170. Organ, L. W., Tasker, R. R., and Moody, N. F.: The impedance profile of the human brain as a localization technique in stereoencephalotomy. Confin. Neurol., *29*:192–196, 1967.

171. Papez, J. W.: Superior olivary nucleus. Arch. Neurol. Psychiat., *24*:1–20, 1930.

172. Peluso, F., and Gybels, J.: Computer calculation of the position of the side-protruding electrode tip during penetration in human brain. Confin. Neurol., *34*:94–100, 1972.

173. Penfield, W., and Jasper, H.: Epilepsy and the Functional Anatomy of the Human Brain. Boston, Little, Brown & Co., 1954.

174. Petty, P. G., and Edsall, G.: Alternating-current electrocoagulation with bipolar electrodes. J. Neurosurg., *26*:399–405, 1967.

175. Rand, R. W., Crandall, P. H., Adey, W. R., Walter, R. D., and Markham, C. H.: Electrophysiologic investigations in Parkinson's dis-

ease and other dyskinesias in man. Neurology (Minneap.), *12*:754–770, 1962.

176. Ranson, S. W.: On the use of the Horsley-Clarke stereotaxic instrument. Psychiat. Neurol. Bl., *38*:534–543, 1934.

177. Rexed, B., Mair, W., Sourander, P., Larsson, B., and Leksell, L.: Effect of high energy protons on the brain of the rabbit. Acta Radiol., *53*:289–299, 1960.

178. Ries, L., and Tytus, J. S.: Rapid freezing: A surgical technique (preliminary report). Bull. Mason Clin., *14*:20–26, 1960.

179. Robinson, B. W., and Tompkins, H. E.: Impedance method for localizing brain structures. An extension of the method. Arch. Neurol. (Chicago), *10*:563–574, 1964.

180. Robinson, B. W., Bryan, J. S., and Rosvold, H. E.: Locating brain structures extensions to the impedance method. Arch. Neurol. (Chicago), *13*:477–486, 1967.

181. Rocamora, R., Aranda, L., Asenjo, A., Chiorino, K., and Donoso, P.: Electrophysiological studies of the thalamic nuclei. Confin. Neurol., *27*:253–257, 1966.

182. Roussy, G.: La Couche Optique. Thèse No. 165, 1–349. Paris, G. Steinheil, 1907.

183. Rowland, V., MacIntyre, W. J., and Bidder, T. G.: The production of brain lesions with electric current. II. Bidirectional currents. J. Neurosurg., *17*:55–69, 1960.

184. Sarkisian, S. S.: Spinal cord pseudotumor: Complication of Pantopaque myelography. U.S. Armed Forces Med. J., *7*:1683–1686, 1956.

185. Schaltenbrand, G., and Bailey, P., eds.: Introduction to Stereotaxis with an Atlas of the Human Brain. New York, Grune & Stratton, 1959.

186. Schaltenbrand, G., and Nürnberger, S.: Radiographic landmarks for stereotactic operations. *In* Schaltenbrand, G., and Bailey, P., eds.: Introduction to Stereotaxis with an Atlas of the Human Brain. New York, Grune & Stratton, 1959, pp. 421–436.

187. Schmiedt, E.: Kraniozerebrale Lagebestimmung des Nucleus dorsomedialis in menschlichen Thalamus. Acta Neurochir., *3*:17–37, 1952.

188. Sem-Jacobsen, C. W.: Depth electrographic stimulation and treatment of patients with Parkinson's disease including neurosurgical technique. Acta Neurol. Scand., *41*:suppl. 13, 365–377, 1965.

189. Siegfried, J.: Panel discussion on utilisation of localized cooling in neurosurgery. Confin. Neurol., *26*:41–44, 1965.

190. Siegfried, J., Ervin, F. R., Miyazaki, Y., and Mark, V. H.: Localized cooling of the central nervous system. I. Neurophysiologic studies in experimental animals. J. Neurosurg., *19*:840–852, 1962.

191. Slaughter, D. G., and Nashold, B. S.: A technique for making thin brain slices for stereotaxic measurements. J. Neurosurg., *29*:302–306, 1968.

192. Smith, M. C.: Cerebral lesions produced by various stereotactic methods. *In* Proceedings of the IV International Congress of Neuropathology. Stuttgart, Georg Thieme Verlag, 1961, Vol. III, pp. 213–217.

193. Smith, M. C.: Location of stereotactic lesions confirmed at necropsy. Brit. Med. J., *1*:900–906, 1962.

194. Smith, M. C.: Pathological changes associated with stereotactic lesions in Parkinson's disease. J. Neurosurg., *24*:suppl., 443–445, 1966.

195. Söderberg, L., Sjöberg, S., and Langland, P.: Neurological complications following myelography with water-soluble contrast medium. Acta Orthop. Scand., *28*:220–223, 1959.

196. Spiegel, E. A.: Methodological problems in stereoencephalotomy. Confin. Neurol., *26*:125–132, 1965.

197. Spiegel, E. A., and Wycis, H. T.: Stereoencephalotomy (Thalamotomy and Related Procedures). Part I. Methods and Stereotaxic Atlas of the Human Brain. New York, Grune & Stratton, 1952.

198. Spiegel, E. A., and Wycis, H. T.: Thalamotomy and pallidotomy for treatment of choreic movements. Acta Neurochir., *2*:417–422, 1952.

199. Spiegel, E. A., and Wycis, H. T.: Stereoencephalotomy. Principles and methods. *In* Premier Congrès International de Neurochirurgie, Bruxelles, 1957, pp. 91–118.

200. Spiegel, E. A., and Wycis, H. T.: Stereoencephalotomy. Part II. Clinical and Physiological Applications. New York, Grune & Stratton, 1962.

201. Spiegel, E. A., Wycis, H. T., and Baird, H. W.: Studies in stereoencephalotomy. I. Topical relationships of subcortical structures to the posterior commissure. Confin. Neurol., *12*:121–133, 1952.

202. Spiegel, E. A., Wycis, H. T., Marks, M., and Lee, A. J.: Stereotaxic apparatus for operations on the human brain. Science, *106*:349–350, 1947.

203. Spiegel, E. A., Wycis, H. T., Szekely, E. G., Soloff, L., Adams, J., Gildenberg, P., and Zanes, C.: Stimulation of Forel's field during stereotaxic operations in the human brain. Electroenceph. Clin. Neurophysiol., *16*:537–548, 1964.

204. Stein, S. N., and Peterson, E. W.: The use of radon seeds to produce deep cerebral lesions. Proc. Soc. Exp. Biol. Med., *74*:583–585, 1950.

205. Strecker: Untersuchungen über die physikalischen Liquorverhältnisse an der Leiche, sowie über das postmortale Quellungsvermögen des Gehirns, mit besonderer Berücksichtigung der Reichardtschen Hirnschwellung. Zbl. Ges. Neurol. Psychiat., *40*:360–362, 1925.

206. Sugita, K., and Doi, T.: The effects of electrical stimulation on the motor and sensory system during stereotaxic operations. Confin. Neurol., *29*:224–229, 1967.

207. Svennilson, E., Torvik, A., Lowe, R., and Leksell, L.: Treatment of parkinsonism by stereotactic thermolesions in the pallidal region. Acta Psychiat. Scand., *35*:358–377, 1960.

208. Sweet, W. H., and Mark, V. H.: Unipolar anodal electrolytic lesions in the brain of man and cat. Arch. Neurol. Psychiat., *70*:224–234, 1953.

209. Szekely, E. G.: Studies in stereoencephalotomy. IV. Variability in the extent of electrolytic lesions. Confin. Neurol., *16*:11–14, 1956.

210. Szekely, E. G., Egyed, J. J., Jacoby, C. G., Moffet, R., and Spiegel, E. A.: High frequency coagulation by means of a stylet electrode under

temperature control. Confin. Neurol., 26:146–152, 1965.

211. Talairach, J., David, M., Tournoux, P., Corredor, H., and Kvasina, T.: Atlas d'Anatomie Stereotaxique. Paris, Masson & Cie, 1957.

212. Talairach, J., Szikla, G., Bonis, A., Bancaud, J., and Schaub, C.: Therapeutic utilization of radio-active isotopes in pituitary surgery. Int. J. Neurol., 5:78–93, 1965.

213. Talairach, J., Szikla, G., Tournoux, P., Prossalentis, A., Bordas-Ferrer, M., Covello, L., Iacob, M., and Mempel, E.: Atlas of Stereotaxic Anatomy of the Telencephalon. Paris, Masson & Cie, 1967.

214. Taren, J. A.: Unusual complication following Pantopaque myelography. J. Neurosurg., 17:323–326, 1960.

215. Taren, J., Guiot, G., Derome, P., and Trigo, J. C.: Hazards of stereotaxic thalamectomy. Added safety factor in corroborating x-ray target localization with neurophysiological methods. J. Neurosurg., 29:173–182, 1968.

216. Tarlov, I. M.: Pantopaque meningitis disclosed at operation. J.A.M.A., 129:1014–1016, 1945.

217. Tasker, R. R., Rowe, I. H., Hawrlyshyn, P., and Organ, L. W.: Proceedings: Computer mapping of human subcortical sensory pathways during stereotaxis. J. Neurol. Neurosurg. Psychiat., 38:408 (Abst.), 1975.

218. Thompson, C. J., and Bertrand, G.: A computer program to aid the neurosurgeon to locate probes used during stereotaxic surgery on deep cerebral structures. Comput. Progr. Biomed., 2:265–276, 1972.

219. Tobias, C. A., Van Dyke, D. C., Simpson, M. E., Anger, H. O., Huft, R. L., and Konett, A. A.: Irradiation of the pituitary of the rat with high energy deuterons. Amer. J. Roentgen., 72:1–21, 1954.

220. Turner, J. W.: A versatile stereotaxic system based on cylindrical coordinates and using absolute measurements. Acta Neurochir., suppl. 21:211–220, 1974.

221. Turner, O. A., Fisher, C. J., and Bernstein, L. L.: Intrathecal sodium diatrizoate. Neurology (Minneap.), 16:230–235, 1966.

222. Umbach, W., and Ehrhardt, K. J.: Micro-electrode recording in the basal ganglia during stereotaxic operations. Confin. Neurol., 26:315–317, 1965.

223. Van Buren, J. M.: The radiographic localization of depth electrodes in the human temporal lobe. In Ramey, E. R., and O'Doherty, D. S., eds.: Electrical Studies on the Unanesthetized Brain. New York, Hoeber Medical Div., Harper & Row, 1960, pp. 177–186.

224. Van Buren, J. M.: Incremental coagulation. In Spiegel, E. A., Barbeau, A., and Doshay, L. J., eds.: Parkinson's Disease. Trends in Research and Treatment. New York, Grune & Stratton, 1965, pp. 155–156.

225. Van Buren, J. M.: A stereotaxic instrument for man. Electroenceph. Clin. Neurophysiol., 19:398–403, 1965.

226. Van Buren, J. M.: Incremental coagulation in stereotactic surgery. J. Neurosurg., 24:suppl., 458–459, 1966.

227. Van Buren, J. M., and Baldwin, M.: Thalamic and cortical representations of the oral and facial area in man. In Bosma, J. F., ed.: Second Symposium on Oral Sensation and Perception. Springfield, Ill., Charles C Thomas, 1970.

228. Van Buren, J. M., and Maccubbin, D. A.: An outline atlas of the human basal ganglia with estimation of anatomical variants. J. Neurosurg., 19:811–839, 1962.

229. Van Buren, J. M., and Borke, R. C.: Variations and Connections of the Human Thalamus. Vol. I. The Nuclei and Cerebral Connections of the Human Thalamus. Vol. II. Variations of the Human Diencephalon. Heidelberg, Springer-Verlag, 1972.

230. Van Den Berg, J., and Van Manen, J.: Graded coagulation of brain tissue. Acta Physiol. Pharmacol. Neerl., 10:353–377, 1962.

231. Walker, A. E.: Stereotactic instrumentation. J. Neurosurg., 24:468, 1966.

232. Walker, A. E., and Burton, C. V.: Radiofrequency telethermocoagulation. J.A.M.A., 197:700–704, 1966.

233. Walsh, L.: The size of the lesion with special reference to patients treated bilaterally. J. Neurosurg., 24:suppl., 440–442, 1966.

234. Walter, R. D., Rand, R. W., Crandall, P. H., Markham, C. H., and Adey, W. R.: Depth electrode studies of thalamus and basal ganglia. Arch. Neurol. (Chicago), 8:388–397, 1960.

235. Waltz, J. M., Riklan, M., Stellar, S., and Cooper, I. S.: Cryothalamectomy for Parkinson's disease. Neurology (Minneap.), 16:994–1002, 1966.

236. Ward, A. A.: Stereotactic instrumentation. J. Neurosurg., 24:468, 1966.

237. Watkins, E. S.: Heat gains in brain during electrocoagulative lesions. J. Neurosurg., 23:319–328, 1965.

238. Wennenstrand, J., del Corral-Gutierrez, J. F., and Sarby, B.: Histologic and volumetric study of intracerebral cold lesions. Acta Neurol. Scand., 43:451–463, 1967.

239. Whittier, J. R., and Mettler, F. A.: Studies on the subthalamus of the rhesus monkey. I. Anatomy and fiber connections of the subthalamic nucleus of Lays. J. Comp. Neurol., 90:281–317, 1949.

240. Wycis, H. T.: A new universal stereoencephalotome (model 6). Confin. Neurol., 35:118–122, 1973.

241. Wycis, H. T., and Gildenberg, P. L.: Further observations on campotomy in various extrapyramidal disorders. In Monographs in Biology and Medicine. New York, Grune & Stratton, 1965, Chapter 20, pp. 134–148.

242. Wyss, O. A. M.: Ein Hochfrequenz-Koagulationsgerät zur reizlosen Ausschaltung. Helv. Physiol. Pharmacol. Acta, 3:437–443, 1945.

243. Yoshida, M., Yanagisawa, N., Shimazu, N., Givre, A., and Narabayashi, H.: Physiological identification of the thalamic nucleus. Arch. Neurol. (Chicago), 11:435–443, 1964.

244. Zervas, N. T.: Eccentric radio-frequency lesions. Confin. Neurol., 26:143–145, 1965.

245. Zervas, N. T., and Kuwayama, A.: Pathological characteristics of experimental thermal lesions, Comparison of induction heating and radiofrequency electrocoagulation. J. Neurosurg., 37:418–422, 1972.

140

ABNORMAL MOVEMENT DISORDERS

DEFINITIONS

The dyskinesias are a group of clinical conditions characterized by involuntary movements of great diversity: choreiform, ballistic, dystonic, tremulous. The classification of these conditions would be most meaningful if based on knowledge of differential pathophysiological substrates. Unfortunately, our knowledge in this area is still fragmentary. Instead, the dyskinesias have been classified descriptively, with compartmentalization of signs and symptoms into arbitrarily named disease entities. A general terminology using operational terms seems more appropriate. Thus the word dyskinesia becomes an appropriate term, arising from the stem *kineo,* meaning "move," for conditions characterized by abnormalities of movement. And "dyskinesia" seems a more appropriate term for these clinical conditions with involuntary movements than another commonly used term, "extrapyramidal diseases." There are many circuits in the central nervous system involved in efferent motor activity; of these, the pyramidal component represents only a small fraction. Thus one would expect that diseases associated with abnormalities of motor control would involve dysfunction of at least some component of the extrapyramidal system. As a result, the term "extrapyramidal diseases" adds little information about these conditions and is less descriptive than the more general rubric "dyskinesias."

The dyskinesias comprise not only abnormal involuntary movements but also, often, associated abnormalities of muscle tonus (rigidity), poverty of voluntary movements (hypokinesia), and impairment of associated movements. These disorders of movement occur in the absence of "true" paralysis (signs of involvement of the pyramidal tracts are usually absent) and in the absence of sensory disturbances. The term dyskinesia therefore includes those syndromes sometimes classified as dystonia musculorum deformans (including that limited dystonia called spasmodic torticollis), choreoathetosis (including Huntington's chorea and Wilson's disease, as well as choreoathetosis due to other causes), cerebellar tumors, and finally the prototype of the group—parkinsonism.

There is some evidence that these conditions should be grouped together under the heading of dyskinesia, not only because of the common clinical feature of involuntary movements but also because there may be some common features in the physiological substrates generating these abnormal movements. Thus the rationale for operative therapy of the dyskinesias may be less concerned with the etiology (e.g., viral encephalitis, birth trauma, genetic traits) or the focal pathological changes than with common alterations of function in circuits controlling movement. Improvement in motor disability following operations may be independent of the cause of the neuronal dysfunction. It is, therefore, important to try to identify common physiological substrates of the dyskinesias, determine how operations modify the motor disability, and formulate models that explain the effectiveness of such treatment. Our knowledge in these areas is greatest for Parkinson's disease, the most common of the dyskinetic clinical syndromes. Our discussion, then,

---

G. A. OJEMANN AND A. A. WARD, JR.

will initially consider parkinsonism, though this is no longer the most common of the dyskinesias treated operatively.

HISTORICAL BACKGROUND

At one time or another, nearly every accessible site in the central and peripheral nervous systems has been approached operatively in an effort to modify the symptoms of patients with severe dyskinesias. Only the highlights of these efforts are recorded here.

Operative therapy for dyskinesias was initially directed primarily toward the relief of the adventitious movements. Parkinson himself had observed that when one of his patients with the "shaking palsy" also suffered a stroke that left him with hemiplegia, the tremor disappeared in the hemiplegic extremities. Built upon this observation, a series of procedures was developed that interrupted the motor system at various levels, providing some degree of relief of the adventitious movements. Shortly after the turn of the century, Sir Victor Horsley resected the precentral gyrus in a boy with hemiathetosis following scarlet fever, achieving dramatic relief of the athetotic movements.[57] In the 1930's, Bucy and his associates acquired considerable experience with unilateral subpial resection of areas 4 and 6 of the cortex in patients with various dyskinesias.[17,18] They found that the choreoathetotic movements, hemiballismus, and the tremor of Parkinson's disease were frequently relieved with this procedure. Parkinsonian rigidity, bradykinesia, "midline" symptoms, and oculogyric crises were unchanged, as was the progression of the disease. The patients were left with mild to moderate hemiplegia, usually being unable to move the individual fingers of the contralateral hand, but as is the case with most of the procedures that interrupt motor systems in a fairly disabled patient, this trade of hemiplegia for a severe motion disorder was usually a therapeutically desirable one. Dystonic movements seemed to respond somewhat less well to cortical resection.

Section of the descending motor pathways at the level of the peduncle was undertaken by a number of investigators who followed Walker.[140] The central third of the peduncle appears to carry the fibers whose destruction modified the tremor of Parkin-

son's disease in approximately 60 per cent of cases, though rarely totally ablating it.[84] Rigidity was unchanged. The patients were left with paresis of varying degree; in some cases the acute postoperative flaccid paralysis resolved in several weeks into remarkably little weakness, which might be less than that seen after cortical resections, with even intact finger function preserved in the opposite extremity. Again, rigidity, "midline" symptoms, and oculogyric crises were unchanged.[140] This procedure also altered hemiballistic, choreoathetoic, and dystonic movements (but not the movements of Huntington's chorea).[63,78,140] Of the procedures for interrupting motor pathways, pedunculotomy is the only one still occasionally performed for dyskinesias.[63,78]

Putnam and Oliver were among those who advocated interruption of the motor pathways at the upper cervical cord level.[100,109] Putnam recommended section of the anterior column for patients with choreoathetosis, beginning the section at the ventral roots and extending it medially from there. This was associated with approximately 40 per cent reduction in power in the ipsilateral extremities. In patients with Parkinson's disease, he recommended section of the dorsal lateral column, which in approximately 50 per cent of cases, produced a reduction in tremor associated with a 30 to 80 per cent reduction in the power of the ipsilateral extremities. Oliver sectioned the entire lateral column, believing that one should have clinical evidence of sensory as well as motor loss in order to get satisfactory relief of the tremor. A group of his patients with this section at the C2 level were tremor-free after more than 10 years. Following lateral column section there was, of course, considerable motor loss in the ipsilateral extremities as well as the usual problems with bladder function after bilateral lesions.

Efforts to relieve symptoms of the dyskinesias by operative interruption of the sensory system did not meet with lasting success. In particular, dorsal rhizotomy, sympathectomy, dorsal column section, and anterolateral cordotomy proved unsatisfactory.[42,106,109]

The development of techniques for operative extirpation of various parts of the basal ganglia ushered in the modern age of operation for dyskinesias. In 1939, Russell Meyers excised the head of the caudate nucleus in a patient with Parkinson's disease and achieved four years of relief of both tremor and rigidity.[81] He followed this with a series of extirpations of different portions of the basal ganglia, finding that removal of the caudate head with an incision in the anterior limb of the internal capsule (extensive enough to produce transient paresis) gave approximately 20 per cent of the parkinsonian patients freedom from tremor and improved another 40 per cent of patients. These patients had no persisting new motor disabilities. Meyers found that an incision placed in the ansa lenticularis by a transventricular approach was even more effective. Following this procedure, the tremor of about 40 per cent of these parkinsonian patients was much improved, and (in contrast to the results of procedures to interrupt the motor system), rigidity was also improved. These procedures however had a relatively high operative mortality rate ranging from 10 to 15 per cent.

This combination of the great risk of open operation with the considerable therapeutic benefit associated with lesions in the basal ganglia provided a major impetus for the application of stereotaxic techniques to man. The equipment for carrying out stereotaxis in animals had been developed in the early part of the twentieth century, starting with the Horsley-Clarke machine intended for cats, developed in 1908.[58] Stereotaxic machines suitable for man were first reported by Spiegel and Wycis in 1947 and demonstrated by Meyers and Hayne and Bailey at about the same time.[85,124] Within the next few years these investigators, along with Talairach, Leksell, and Narabayashi, had placed stereotaxic basal ganglia lesions in patients with motion disorders.[76,90,131] Following Meyer's observations on the efficacy of pallidofugal lesions in altering parkinsonian rigidity and tremor, the globus pallidus or a portion of its outflow system became the most common target for these initial stereotaxic efforts. The improvement in rigidity was especially prominent after this lesion; there was somewhat less improvement in tremor.[47] There followed during the 1950's a flowering of stereotaxic operative technique. A large number of investigators devised a wide variety of machines for directing a probe to a predetermined target by using cranial and especially intracerebral landmarks, and devices for making controlled lesions in the brain (ranging from wax and alcohol to the cryoprobe and leukotome).

More recently, the nucleus ventralis lateralis of the thalamus has become the preferred target for many stereotaxic surgeons. This substitution followed the work of Hassler, who had chosen this as a target area because of its numerous connections to motor and premotor cortex, and also the serendipitous observations of Cooper, who found particularly striking improvement when a planned pallidal lesion was misdirected into the ventral lateral thalamus.[27,51] The thalamic lesion appears to yield greater improvement in tremor, with similar improvement in rigidity, than do pallidal lesions. Although the ventrolateral thalamus has become a standard target for stereotaxic operative procedures for dyskinesias, one of the striking features of the recent history of these operations has been the rather large number of target areas where lesions have produce therapeutically satisfactory results. These include not only the globus pallidus, ventrolateral thalamus, and ansa lenticularis but also the substantia nigra, several targets in Forel's fields caudal to the thalamus, and the dentate nucleus of the cerebellum.[44,54,84,91,125]

With the advent of levodopa therapy, operative treatment for Parkinson's disease has become a rarity. Operation on the ventrolateral thalamus and adjacent targets, however, remains useful in dystonia and intention tremors. Recent years have seen a greater selectivity among these targets in relation to specific symptoms. But the major advance has been nonablative electrical stimulation in dyskinesias. The first technique of this type, surface stimulation of the anterior cerebellar vermis to relieve spasticity, was introduced by Cooper in 1973.[24] The efficacy of that procedure is still being assessed, but the technological advances it represents would seem to open many new possibilities for the operative treatment of abnormal movement disorders.

PHYSIOLOGICAL BASIS OF OPERATION IN THE DYSKINESIAS

Before it is possible to discuss the operative therapy of the dyskinesias meaningfully, it is useful to have a general model of how the central nervous system controls motor activity. Earlier concepts of the physiology of the motor system were those of direct "telephone line" connections from motor cortex to anterior horn cell in the spinal cord to effector muscle unit. Rather discrete movements can be evoked from motor cortex; in fact, under appropriate conditions, precise localization of individual muscle function can be demonstrated in the motor cortex of the monkey.[22] It is clear, however, that such a simple view of nature is not adequate to describe the extraordinary repertoire of complex motor activity seen in man. Rather, the physiology of the motor system seems better explained by adding to such direct cortical control, a second system embodying the principles of servomechanisms. Applied in engineering, these principles have resulted in such goal-seeking devices as thermostats, governors on engines, and most of the control systems of modern aircraft. Servomechanisms utilize the concept of feedback, in which a small amount of the energy of a system is diverted to the regulation of that system. This feedback may be of a positive nature so that as the system runs faster there is a greater input, or it may be negative so that the faster a system runs the more the input to it is decreased. The proper amount of negative feedback tends to keep a system running at a preset speed. A small energy change in the feedback loop can control large energy changes in the primary system; the ratio between these two represents the gain of the system. It is known that when the feedback is adjusted to give great stability the system becomes sluggish and relatively inaccurate in its response. Conversely, when the feedback is adjusted to give great accuracy and rapidity of response the system rapidly approaches a condition of instability.

Accuracy of response and stability of operation thus appear as two absolutely interdependent yet contrary attributes of the feedback system. Nature has been forced to consider this dilemma as feedback systems in living organisms evolved. The process of survival in primates has placed a premium on accuracy and rapidity of phasic movement; if our ancestors had been unable to perform fine finger movement accurately and rapidly they would not have survived. Like all feedback systems, however, our nervous systems have had to pay the price of potential instability in order to achieve these properties. This may be why relatively minor damage in critical circuits can result in a loss of stability of motor control systems with spontaneous oscillation and the resultant shaking palsy that we call parkinsonism.

It is increasingly apparent that motor control is dependent on central processing of sensory information, i.e., on feedback. In addition to simple feedback loops at the segmental levels in the spinal cord, it is clear, motor control involves hierarchies of feedback loops superimposed one on the other that become increasingly complex as one ascends up the central nervous system to the brain stem, cerebellum, thalamus, basal ganglia, and cortex. Since we know most about the detailed synaptic function at the segmental level in the spinal cord, it is logical to discuss these feedback loops before considering the suprasegmental influences on such loops or considering what little is known regarding some of the interacting feedback loops located at higher levels of the central nervous system.

In the ventral horn of the cord are large neurons known as alpha motoneurons that innervate the peripheral striated muscles. These cells are the final common path for driving the power plant. Although higher mammals appear to be able to activate this final common path directly in certain instances, direct activation of the alpha system is useful only for producing gross and often powerful motor activity that usually involves proximal muscle groups. This system cannot generate the fine control required for dexterous motor performance. As is true in engineering, in which fine control of power plants is best achieved by servocontrol, this is achieved in mammals by the gamma system. This loop centers around the muscle spindle, a stretch receptor arranged in parallel with the main muscle mass. The annulospiral endings in this receptor are activated by the passive stretch of the muscle (such as occurs when the knee jerk is elicited by striking the patellar tendon). These endings may also be activated when they are stretched by the active contraction of the polar contractile elements between which the receptor is suspended. These contractile portions of the muscle spindle are innervated from the cord by slowly conducting small motor fibers known as gamma efferents.[75] That this gamma system plays an important role in muscle control is suggested by the fact that one third of the efferent ventral root fibers are in the gamma category. When the sensory elements in the muscle spindle are activated (either by contraction of the gamma-innervated polar contractile elements or by passive stretch of the main muscle mass), their discharge is conducted back to the spinal cord over large, rapidly conducting fibers that project monosynaptically on the alpha motoneuron. Thus, stretch of the spindle generates signals that excite the anterior horn cells of that particular muscle, causing that muscle to contract. This is the myotatic reflex of which the knee jerk is the classic example.

The muscle spindle may be considered to be an exquisite sensing element of a proprioceptive servosystem. It registers the difference in length between the main muscle mass and itself, whereupon the servoloop acts to reduce that difference. Hunt and Eldred and co-workers have shown that there is a heightened gamma efferent discharge that precedes the motoneuron discharge and consequent muscle contraction of spinal and supraspinal reflexes.[38,61] It may be that, when fine motor control is required, orders for "voluntary" motor activity are given to the gamma neurons, and they in turn control the power plant. For that reason, those muscles most involved in dexterous motor activity (such as the intrinsic muscles of the hand) are also those muscles most richly endowed with muscle spindles. Conversely, those muscles over which we have little voluntary control (such as the latissimus dorsi) are very sparsely supplied with muscle spindles.

It is possible to generalize that the suprasegmental control of these local circuits in the cord is characterized by a linked coordinated activity between alpha and gamma motor systems. Motor regulation is achieved by mechanisms of excitation and inhibition for each of the two systems. These functions of brain stem, cerebellum, basal ganglia, and cortex are projected onto segmental mechanisms in the cord, not only over the pyramidal tract but also over nonpyramidal multisynaptic pathways.

It is now possible to apply these concepts to an understanding of the dyskinesias. Of the limited data available, most apply to Parkinson's syndrome. It has been proposed that the pathological alteration of motor control in parkinsonism is the result of an altered alpha-gamma balance characterized by depressed gamma activity and augmented alpha activity.[130]

It is proposed that the lesion in the ventromedial tegmentum that induces a parkinsonian syndrome in monkeys partially interrupts the excitatory circuits, leaving the inhibitory input to the gamma neuron intact.[104,142] The gamma neuron is thus effectively inhibited. The relevant lesion also is postulated to "release" the suprasegmental control of the alpha system, with resultant augmented alpha activity.[130] A state resembling parkinsonism can be produced in monkeys not only by tegmental lesions but also by the intravenous injection of reserpine, which is perhaps the best drug-induced model of the disease.[127] As Steg has shown, this drug-induced animal model is also characterized by inactivity of the gamma efferents while the slow motor units are tonically hyperactive. Both these models not only simulate the clinical signs of parkinsonism but also exhibit the biochemical correlates of the human disease as expressed by reduced dopamine in the striatum.[5,122] Finally, chlorpromazine in appropriate doses also inhibits the gamma system and induces augmented alpha drive.[55,129] That dyskinesias resembling parkinsonism can be produced in some patients receiving large doses of the phenothiazine drugs is well documented.

If the physiological substrate of the dyskinesia in the human consists of an altered alpha-gamma balance characterized by depressed gamma activity and augmented alpha activity, it should be possible to relate the symptoms of bradykinesia, tremor, and rigidity to this substrate.[141] There are pathways from brain that excite the gamma efferent neuron and others that inhibit it. The model proposes that the relevant lesion partially interrupts the excitatory circuit, leaving the inhibitory input to the gamma neuron intact, and that the gamma neuron in the cord therefore has an inhibitory bias. Some confirmation for this proposal is provided by the observations of Jung and Hassler that the Jendrassik reinforcement of deep tendon reflexes is absent in patients with parkinsonism, and that in cases of hemiparkinsonism, it is absent only on the affected side.[66] If the Jendrassik reinforcement response is due to excitation of the gamma system, one might conclude that the ability of patients with parkinsonism to excite their gamma neurons is compromised.[101] This inhibitory bias of the gamma system might account for the bradykinesia exhibited by many patients with dyskinesia. A patient who had lost a major part of the circuits that he normally utilized in fine dexterous movement (via activation of gamma neurons) would have to drive the remaining circuits unusually forcefully to achieve movement at all. Patients with parkinsonism state that enormous effort is often required to induce fine finger movement repetitively and that the circuits tire rapidly. Since the gamma loop is involved maximally in fine movement and minimally in gross movements involving the proximal musculature, one would predict that fine movements would be compromised to a much greater degree. Such is the case.

In addition to the depression of the gamma system, the model also proposes that suprasegmental excitation of the alpha motoneuron is augmented. Rhythmic discharges of single neurons in the thalamus have been recorded in the monkey model of parkinsonism as well as in the human with this disease.[30,48] In both, there is evidence that such rhythmic discharges in some thalamic neurons are related to the generation of the tremor. Since dorsal rhizotomy does not block the tremor in human patients or in the monkey model, it would appear that the tremor in parkinsonism is a consequence of direct pulsed activation of the alpha motoneurons.[105,106]

Finally, the model proposes that the rigidity is also a consequence of increased alpha drive. Since all muscle spindle activity is not abolished but only depressed, it would be expected that the residual spindle input, playing on alpha motoneurons whose activity is increased, should be a factor in the rigidity that is observed. While the alpha rigidity of the ischemic decerebrate cat is not modified by dorsal rhizotomy, Pollock and Davis have shown that dorsal rhizotomy in a patient with parkinsonism resulted in modifications of muscle tone in which the initial decrease in tone after operation was replaced by a "contracture" in flexor muscles at elbow and wrist, which, interestingly, disappeared during sleep.[106] Although further desirable documentation in patients is not available, in experimental parkinsonism induced by drugs the rigidity is related to tonic hyperactivity of slow motor units.[127]

Thus there is modest support for the view that the pathological alteration of motor control in parkinsonism is a result of an altered alpha-gamma balance characterized by depressed gamma activity (accounting for the bradykinesia) and augmented alpha activity (tonic hyperactivity of motoneurons accounting for the rigidity; phasic alpha drive accounting for the tremor).

If this model is relevant, it should be possible to formulate a physiological basis for therapy. One would predict that a part of the imbalance in feedback control would be rectified by restoring circuits that activate the gamma neurons. Obviously, pathways that have been destroyed by disease cannot be replaced. Thus, although it is not possible to increase the activation of the gamma system, it is possible to reduce the inhibitory input on these cells, thereby permitting the remaining excitatory signals to activate these neurons more effectively. One of the major sources of inhibitory input to the gamma system appears to arise in the nucleus ventralis lateralis (VL) of the thalamus according to data obtained in the animal and in man.[128,130] Since one of the major sources of inhibitory input to the gamma system arises in this thalamic nucleus, this may account for the improvement of bradykinesia that follows operative lesions directed at the anterosuperior part of this thalamic target.

It is presumed that therapeutically effective drugs act in the same fashion. As Arvidsson and co-workers pointed out, administration of drugs inhibiting cholinergic transmission or drugs facilitating monoaminergic transmission such as L-dopa will increase gamma neuron activation evoked by dorsal root stimulation.[4] They proposed that this augmentation of gamma activity is a consequence of drug action at the level of the neostriatum. Unfortunately, there are no definitive data at this time regarding the site of action of this therapeutically effective compound. Data that are now appearing, however, suggest that L-dopa has multiple sites of action and also direct actions on spinal neurons. The fact that L-dopa increases gamma neuron activation would be consistent with the model, i.e., this is accomplished by a decrease of inhibitory input as it is also accomplished by stereotaxic lesions in brain.

The classic suprasegmental pathway of the alpha route is the pyramidal tract projecting monosynaptically or, more commonly, through an interneuron on anterior horn cells. Although an anatomically discrete pathway, it is now apparent that the pyramidal tract, strictly defined, represents a relatively small part of the total suprasegmental control of alpha motoneuron activity. It is known that stimulation of either globus pallidus produces facilitation of the alpha motoneuron as monitored by the monosynaptic reflex.[129] This facilitation, or alpha drive, is not blocked by ablation of sensorimotor cortex and may be mediated by direct projections from pallidum to mesencephalic tegmentum.[65,92] Furthermore, stimulation of the contralateral ventrolateral nucleus also facilitates the alpha system, but this is dependent upon the integrity of the sensorimotor cortex. The alpha drive evoked by ventrolateral thalamic or pallidal stimulation is abolished or reversed by barbiturates, which also block the active involuntary movement in most dyskinesias. Utilizing intracellular recording in alpha motoneurons, Sasaki and Tanaka confirmed that activation of the ventrolateral nucleus evokes excitatory postsynaptic potentials in motoneurons, as does excitation of the pyramidal decussation, the reticular formation of the pons and medulla, and the dentate nucleus.[112] Some of these types of alpha drive are rapidly conducted to motoneurons while others are conducted more slowly.

If a part of the disorder of parkinsonism is a consequence of augmented alpha activity, it is not surprising that operative lesions should be beneficial if directed at a target such as the ventrolateral nucleus, which is a principal relay station in the generation of alpha drive. The clinical improvement that may follow the administration of L-dopa would also be consistent with this model, since as Arvidsson and associates have shown, this monoaminergic drug also decreases alpha motoneuron activation.[4]

It is not unreasonable that there should be circuits concentrated in the lateral thalamus that both excite the alpha system and inhibit the gamma system, or that drugs should have similar reciprocal effects. Calma and Kidd, evolving a concept of linked coordinated activity between alpha and gamma motor systems, proposed that motor regulation is achieved by mechanisms of excitation and inhibition for each of the two systems.[20] As in all servosystems, the requirements for accurate control are best met by servoloops containing negative feedback in which the signals inducing muscular movement (alpha system) also retard the gamma system, which is a positive feedback loop at segmental levels of the cord. Thus, negative feedback is provided by recurrent collateral inhibition involving Renshaw cells in the local circuit in the cord, while similar negative feedback is also a property of the suprasegmental control circuits within the brain; in the central nervous system as in the steam engine, activation of the mechanism tends to shut off the power that drives it. Alterations of the balance between positive and negative feedback can lead to pathological activity in physical servosystems, and it is not unreasonable that similar events should occur in biological control systems. In both man and machine, therapy must strive to restore stability in such servoloops.

The physiological basis of the dyskinesias other than parkinsonism is even less well understood. There is some evidence that the active movements that characterize dystonia musculorum deformans and torticollis, as well as the involuntary movements of choreoathetosis or ballism, all share a certain common physiological substrate in which the muscular movements are generated by direct alpha drive and are not modified by dorsal rhizotomy. Clearly the alpha drive may be generated in different ways, as evidenced by the different character of the movements themselves. In the dystonias, abnormal activity generated in circuits involved in postural control are expressed by their suprasegmental input on alpha motoneurons. Somewhat different circuits driving different brain stem circuits may be responsible for the alpha drive characterizing choreoathetosis. An operative lesion directed at circuits generating tonic drive of the alpha system might well modify the dyskinesia, which may account for the improvement in the active component of involuntary movements effected by appropriate lesions of the ventrolateral nucleus in choreoathetosis or the dystonias. Since the thalamic target does not present an opportunity to manipulate the suprasegmental control of the alpha system with great selectivity, one might predict that the effectiveness of thalamotomy in these conditions would be more variable than in parkinsonism.

It is clear that the circuits that are involved in the control of voluntary motor activity in man are complex and poorly understood. As our insight increases, it will become possible to extend the opportunities for operative manipulation of these neuronal systems.

TECHNIQUES OF THALAMIC OPERATIONS FOR DYSKINESIAS

The most common of the surgical treatments for abnormal movement disorders is the stereotaxic placement of lesions in the ventrolateral thalamus or adjacent targets. The techniques for accurately placing these lesions are discussed first; consideration of the individual dyskinesias and the effectiveness of thalamic and other operations in each follows.

A model of the anatomical basis of lateral thalamic operation in the dyskinesias suggests that the thalamic lesion interrupts two systems.[52] One is a pallidofugal system extending from the pallidum via the ansa lenticularis, or directly across the posterior limb of the internal capsule, to the anterior-inferior portion of the ventrolateral thalamus (the portion designated VOA by Hassler) and on to the cortex—particularly area 6. In the model, interruption of this system is considered to provide relief of rigidity. The second system includes fibers from the contralateral cerebellum, principally in the brachium conjunctivum, which pass through the thalamic peduncle into the more posterior parts of the ventrolateral thalamus (the part Hassler designated VOP) and on to area 4 of the cortex. Interruption of this system is associated with alterations in tremor. Both these systems have the common property that the fibers come in beneath the thalamus in the region of the fields of Forel and then turn superiorly and slightly laterally to enter the inferior portions of the ventrolateral (VL) thalamus and fan out into its more superior parts. Lesions that successfully relieve dyskinesias generally fall somewhere in this area. This "area of successful lesions" is surrounded by a number of important structures that must be avoided. Anterolaterally lies the posterior limb of the internal capsule. Posteriorly are the ventroposterior medial and lateral nuclei (VPL, VPM), the main sensory relay nuclei of the thalamus.

Inferiorly lies the subthalamic nucleus and medially, the intralaminar and dorsomedial thalamic nuclei. The anterolateral border of this "area of successful lesions" becomes progressively more medial as one progresses from its more superior to its more inferior portions.

The techniques of stereotaxic operation are discussed in Chapter 139. The importance of using reference points close to the desired target is indicated there: for stereotaxic operations of the thalamus, the landmarks in the area of the third ventricle are generally used as reference points—the midline, the anterior commissure or foramen of Monro, and the posterior commissure and the intercommissural or foramen of Monro–postcommissural line. Despite the use of these nearby reference points, there is still considerable variation among patients in the exact location of a particular anatomical structure such as the nucleus ventralis lateralis. Thus, anatomical coordinates are only used to place a probe in the general area of the desired anatomical structure. The final correction for exact lesion placement in a given patient is made on the basis of local physiological responses. A corollary of this dependence on physiological responses for final lesion placement is that the stereotaxic technique used must have the capacity to systematically probe several sites about the target area selected on anatomical coordinates. To be able to determine physiological responses, it is best to perform these operations under local anesthesia with a minimum of premedication. In older patients, especially those with Parkinson's disease, the authors use only 25 mg of promethazine hydrochloride (Phenergen) and do not supplement this during the operation. For young patients, neuroleptanalgesia with the combination of fentanyl and droperidol (Innovar) has been satisfactory, though this must be carefully titrated so as not to produce lethargy that interferes with reports of physiological responses. With neuroleptanalgesia the authors have performed these operations on children as young as 10 to 12. The loss of many physiological responses when the operation must be done under general anesthesia (as in severe cerebral palsy) significantly increases the risks and decreases the effectiveness of the procedure.

Figures 140–1 and 140–2 show examples

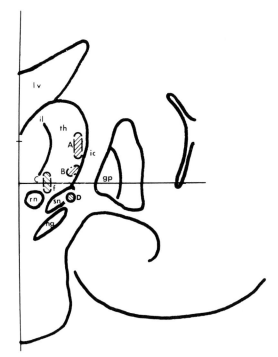

Figure 140–1 Coronal section of thalamus 15 mm posterior to anterior commissure. The mean location of structures with reference to midline, intercommissural line, and anterior commissure are shown. Vertical line is the midline of the third ventricle. Horizontal line is the intercommissural plane. Crossmark on vertical line is 1 cm from origin. lv, lateral ventricle; th, thalamus; il, intralaminar nucleus of thalamus; ic, posterior limb of internal capsule; gp, globus pallidus; rn, red nucleus; sn, subthalamic nucleus; ng, substantia nigra; f, fields of Forel. Thalamic target areas projected onto this section: A, superior ventrolateral nuclear target favored by the authors; B, inferior ventrolateral nuclear target using coordinates from Guiot;[39] C, field of Forel target using coordinates of Spiegel et al.; and D, subthalamic target for tremor described by Bertrand et al.[12,124] (Adapted from Van Buren, J. M., and Borke, R. C.: Variations of the Human Diencephalon. Vol. 2. New York, Springer-Verlag, 1972.)

of several target areas that neurosurgeons have found useful as anatomical guides for the placement of therapeutically successful lesions. These target areas often represent only a first approximation in the placement of a thalamic electrode in the treatment of the dyskinesias. The exact location and size of the thalamic lesions are determined by physiological guides.

The most caudal of these target areas lies immediately beneath the thalamus in Forel's fields. Spiegel and Wycis reported considerable experience with the placement of stereotaxic lesions at this level—a procedure they have called "campotomy."[124] Their average coordinates for

these lesions were: 11 mm anterior to the posterior commissure, 6 to 7 mm lateral on the intercommissural plane; their lesions extended from 2 mm above the intercommissural plane to 2 mm below it, occasionally extending down as far as 4 mm below that plane. In general, lesions at this more caudal level must be smaller than those lying more superiorly within the ventrolateral thalamus.

A second frequently utilized anatomical target for ventrolateral thalamic coagulation lies just above the intercommissural plane in the inferior portions of the ventrolateral thalamus. Guiot has given the average coordinates for the posterior part of this target as: $5/12$ of the intercommissural distance anterior to the posterior commissure, 14.5 mm lateral to the midline of the third ventricle, and 3 mm above the intercommissural plane. Average coordinates for the anterior portion of this target were: 1.5 mm anterior to the midpoint of the intercommissural line, 12.5 mm lateral to the midline, and 2.5 mm above the intercommissural plane.[47]

The authors have often used a target lying more superiorly in the ventrolateral thalamus. At this level of the thalamus the target lies within an area extending from 9 mm posterior to the anterior commissure to 9 mm anterior to the posterior commissure, 6 to 12 mm above the intercommissural plane, and 12 to 15 mm lateral to the midline. An electrode in this target is illustrated in Figures 140–3 and 140–4. Rigidity tends to be benefited by lesions lying in the more anterior portions of this target area, with tremor benefit more prominent with lesions in the more posterior portions. These target areas are most commonly approached from a frontal burr hole, although several stereotaxic surgeons use a posterior approach via a parietal burr hole.[45,47]

The techniques for recording or evoking physiological responses during stereotaxic operations have also been covered in Chapter 139. The physiological guides to lesion placement provide two types of information; responses that indicate the location of one of the structures forming the border of the "area of successful lesions," and information specific to the target area itself.

It will be recalled that the posterior limb of the internal capsule is the anterolateral border of the nucleus ventralis lateralis. The internal capsule has a low threshold to

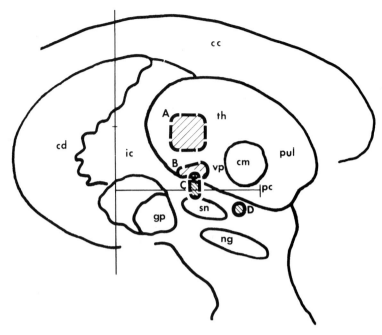

Figure 140–2 Sagittal section 10 mm from midsagittal plane, showing mean location of structures with reference to anterior commissure and intercommissural line. Horizontal line is intercommissural line. Vertical line passes through anterior commissure. Crossmark on vertical line is 1 cm from origin. cc, corpus callosum; ic, internal capsule at genu; cd, head of caudate nucleus; gp, globus pallidus; th, lateral thalamus; vp, nucleus ventralis posterior medalis; cm, nucleus centrum medianum; pul, pulvinar; pc, line of posterior commissure; sn, subthalamic nucleus; ng, substantia nigra. Projection of thalamic target areas onto this section: A, superior ventrolateral nuclear target; B, inferior ventrolateral nuclear target; C, fields of Forel target; D, subthalamic target for tremor. (Adapted from Van Buren, J. M., and Borke, R. C.: Variations of the Human Diencephalon. Vol. 2. New York, Springer-Verlag, 1972.)

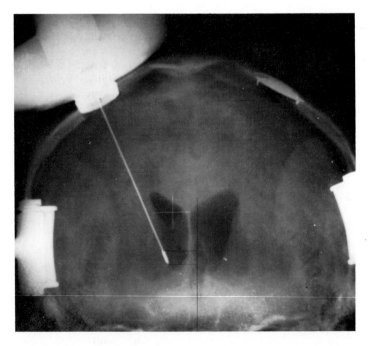

Figure 140–3 Anteroposterior x-ray of a patient with Parkinson's disease undergoing right thalamotomy in which the authors' technique is used. The 1 mm by 5 mm coagulation slug at the end of the electrode is in its initial position in the ventrolateral thalamic target area. The final location of the electrode when a lesion is made will be determined by physiological guides. The frontal portion of the lateral ventricles and the third ventricle have been outlined with air. The fragment of silver clip in the opposite thalamus marks the site of a previous left thalamotomy that resulted in markedly improved function in the right arm and leg.

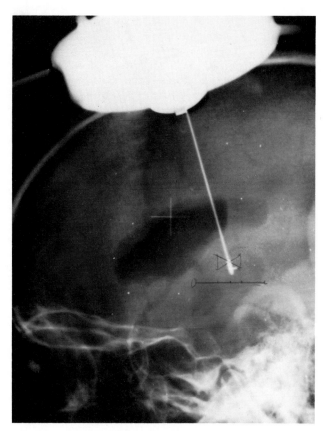

Figure 140–4 Lateral x-ray of the same patient shown in Figure 113–3. The intercommissural line and the thalamic target area have been drawn on the film. The silver clip fragment marking the previous opposite thalamic lesion is again seen.

electrical stimulation, manifest by tonic motor responses in the contralateral extremities (usually arm) or face or both. Considerable information about the distance from the stimulating electrode to the internal capsule can be gained by determining the threshold current for these responses. When the stimulating electrode is within the capsule itself the threshold current is extremely low. As the electrode is located at a progressively greater distance away from the capsule, the threshold increases steadily. Capsular responses can be evoked from an electrode location that will produce satisfactory therapeutic results without paresis, but the threshold current will be quite large. Another technique for determining the distance between the electrode and the capsule is to use a side arm on the electrode such as described by Bertrand.[13] An attempt is then made to find the area where very low-threshold motor responses can be obtained, which would represent the capsule.

The border between the internal capsule and nucleus ventralis lateralis can also sometimes be identified by using microelec-trode recording techniques. Here the absence of unit activity indicates that the electrode is at least in white matter, possibly capsule, and the appearance of unit activity indicates that it is in gray matter. This technique has been most satisfactory when the trajectory of the electrode has passed from thalamus into capsule, as with the posterior approach.[45] Impedance measurements that can distinguish gross differences between pure gray matter and white matter have also been used to indicate the boundary between thalamus and internal capsule.[72]

The nuclei ventralis posterior medialis and lateralis form the posterior boundary of the inferior half of the nucleus ventralis lateralis. The most satisfactory physiological guide to the identification of these nuclei has been the recording of unit responses evoked by peripheral light touch and deep sensation.[47,48,132] The responses to deep sensation may lie in the more anterior portions of this nucleus and indeed may spill over into the posterior inferior portion of the nucleus ventralis lateralis.[8,89] There is the expected somatotopic localization within the nucleus ventralis posterolateralis, with units responding to light touch from the leg being lateral and those from the arm and face more medial.

The ventroposterior medial and lateral nuclei can also be identified by the recording of average evoked responses to transcutaneous nerve shocks. The average evoked response can, however, also be recorded at some distance from these nuclei, perhaps secondary to volume conduction. Hence one must look for the maximal amplitude of the average evoked response if these nuclei are to be accurately located.[74] Stimulation within these thalamic sensory nuclei is associated with localized tingling contralateral dysesthesias that have a very low current threshold. The usefulness of sensory responses to stimulation to localize an electrode is not great. This is true since portions of the ventrolateral thalamus where therapeutically successful lesions can be made also have a low threshold for sensation. The sensory responses from the ventrolateral nucleus, while of a somewhat dysesthetic character, are usually not so discretely localized as those from ventroposterior medial and ventroposterior lateral nuclei.

The inferior portion of this "area of successful lesions," the fields of Forel and the structures immediately beneath this, the subthalamic nucleus, can be identified by the dystonic movements, usually in the contralateral extremities, that can be evoked by electrical stimulation. This area can also be identified by the absence of cortical electroencephalographic responses to stimulation of subthalamic structures, in contrast to the augmenting responses evoked from the ventrolateral nucleus lying immediately superior.[59,89]

The effects of electrical stimulation can also be used to identify structures lying medial to the area of successful lesions. The appearance of respiratory inhibition (usually a prolonged expiration) with electrical stimulation suggests a rather medial placement of the electrode, although this is not an absolute indicator since respiratory inhibition can sometimes be evoked from therapeutically satisfactory sites within the ventrolateral nucleus itself.[113] The phenomenon is evoked at a lower threshold from the left than from the right thalamus.[96] Structures medial to the ventrolateral thalamic nucleus, particularly the intralaminar nucleus, can also be identified by the ability to record recruiting responses from the ipsilateral frontal scalp areas with low-frequency electrical stimulation. High-frequency stimulation of this area has been associated with a flattening of the electroencephalogram and clinical arousal of the patient.[59]

There are a number of physiological responses that are localized to the "area of successful lesions." The portion of the ventrolateral thalamus where a lesion will produce satisfactory therapeutic results shows two effects with electrical stimulation. The first of these is inhibition of the deep tendon reflexes of the contralateral part of the body during stimulation.[129] This alteration in deep tendon reflexes is most easily tested by repetitively evoking the knee jerk. Stimulation within the ventrolateral nucleus produces a diminution in the magnitude of the knee jerk that frequently outlasts the end of the stimulation for a brief period. The effect is best elicited by using small currents at the threshold level. Some care is necessary to differentiate this depression of the knee jerk, on the basis of inhibition of the gamma system, from an apparent depression of the knee jerk that may occur because of muscle tightening. The locations where inhibition of the deep tendon reflexes are evoked with stimulation are those portions of the ventrolateral thalamus where lesions are associated particularly with reductions in bradykinesia and rigidity.

The second localized response that can be evoked with electrical stimulation of the ventrolateral thalamus is production of the patient's usual tremor in the contralateral extremities at the time of stimulation. Very occasionally one sees inhibition of the contralateral tremor with stimulation, particularly if the tremor is very active at the time of stimulation.[89] Either response, driving or inhibition of the tremor, seems to provide about the same localizing information, i.e., that a lesion at the site of stimulation is likely to have a beneficial effect on the tremor.

The effect of local thalamic stimulation on the electroencephalogram recorded from the scalp or cortex can also provide useful data for localizing an electrode to the ventrolateral thalamic nucleus. Low-frequency stimulation is associated with the appearance of a localized augmenting response over the ipsilateral precentral motor and premotor cortex (reflected in the posterior frontal electroencephalographic leads).[59] With stimulation of the more dorsal lateral parts of the ventrolateral nucleus, these responses appear in the medial superior portions of the precentral motor area, and with stimulation of a more medial ventral portion of the nucleus, they are seen in the more inferior lateral portions of the precentral motor area.[89] From the posterior inferior portions of the ventrolateral thalamus, unit activity at frequencies similar to the tremor and uninfluenced by peripheral movements can be recorded.[48] This has been of considerable theoretical interest in determining the mechanism of parkinsonian tremor but, at least at present, has been of little assistance in determining lesion placement.

Those stereotaxic surgeons who utilize a technique involving correction of final lesion placement with physiological parameters usually select several of the physiological guides just mentioned. Several examples illustrate the use of these guides for lesion placement. In the technique of Guiot in which a target point at "B" in Figures 140–1 and 140–2 is approached from posteriorly, the evoked responses to contralateral extremity touch recorded with small electrodes are used as the principal physiological guides.[47,132] As the electrode is advanced along the posterior to anterior trajectory, the unit and electroencephalographic responses to contralateral touch identify the ventroposterior lateral nucleus. Disappearance of these responses identifies the posterior border of the ventrolateral thalamus and the posterior boundary of the lesion. Lateral placement of the lesion is also determined by the somatotopic arrangement of evoked touch responses in the ventroposterior medial and lateral nuclei, and by whether the arm, leg, or face is maximally involved in the contralateral dyskinesia. According to Guiot, with maximal involvement of the leg, the lesion should lie just in front of the area where response is evoked from the fourth and fifth digits of the upper extremity; with maximal involvement of the arm in the dyskinesia, the lesion should lie somewhat more medially in front of the area where responses are obtained from touch of the thumb; and with maximal involvement of the jaw, the lesion should lie in front of the area where touch responses from the tongue are recorded.

In a technique described by Narabayashi, a target at the "B" site in Figures 140–1 and 140–2 is approached from a frontal burr hole.[89] The depth of the electrode along the trajectory is gauged by the topography of the electroencephalographic responses of posterior frontal areas to stimulation in different areas of the nucleus ventralis lateralis. The disappearance of these responses as the electrode is further advanced marks the lower limit of the ventrolateral nucleus. The point at which the patient's usual tremor can be evoked with electrical stimulation marks a satisfactory lesion site. Evoked responses to ulnar nerve stimulation are used to identify the nucleus ventralis posterior lateralis.

In the authors' technique, which approaches a target at "A" in Figures 140–1 and 140–2 frontally, the alterations in deep tendon reflexes and in tremor in response to electrical stimulation within the ventrolateral nucleus are the principal guides to electrode placement. This is augmented by the estimate of the distance from the internal capsule provided by the threshold for contralateral tonic motor responses to electrical stimulation. The lesion is ordinarily placed as laterally as possible without evoking low-threshold contralateral tonic motor responses.

Recently, Bertrand analyzed the effect of different thalamic target areas and observed that in his cases tremor was most often benefited by a subthalamic lesion at the site labeled "D" in Figures 140–1 and 140–2.[12] He places this target under the $8/10$ posterior segment of the intercommissural line, 2 to 4 mm inferior and 13 mm lateral. (The lateral placement in his proportional measurement system, which uses $1/10$ of the intercommissural line as the unit of measure, is 4.5 to 5.5 units lateral.) This target area is roughly triangular, with internal capsule anterolaterally, subthalamic nucleus anteromedially, and lemniscal fibers posteriorly. It is a small target with important structures nearby, so a high degree of precision in placement of the lesion is necessary and the lesion should be small (3 mm or less). Nevertheless, the authors have found this a very effective first choice for a target in situations in which only relief of extremity tremor is necessary. Bertrand uses microelectrode recording as a physiological aid in identifying this target, especially the disappearance of activity identifying the inferior border of the thalamus. The authors have found that electrical stimulation at quite low currents is useful, with low-threshold motor responses indicating too lateral a placement, and low-threshold sensory responses indicating one too posterior. The absence of dystonic or ballistic movements with stimulation gives some assurance that one is well behind the subthalamic nucleus. Tremor is usually driven by stimulation at the target site.

In Chapter 139 the techniques for the creation of reversible lesions are also described. These have proved to be very useful in checking the location of the lesion. Indication of satisfactory lesion placement is improvement in the contralateral dyskinetic symptoms during the reversible lesion.

The techniques of making a permanent lesion are also described in Chapter 139. Generally, lesions should be as small as possible consistent with satisfactory immediate therapeutic results. This not only is likely to reduce the incidence of the complications described in the following section, but in addition, the experience of the authors and others suggests that the most satisfactory long-term relief of tremor is associated with the placement of discrete small lesions rather than large ones in the ventrolateral thalamus. The lesion may be incrementally expanded after a period of observation of some minutes if it does not initially result in optimal therapeutic benefit.

There are only a few studies that directly compare the effectiveness of the different target areas in and around the ventrolateral thalamus in the treatment of specific dyskinetic symptoms.[12,40] The general impression of the authors, however, is that the more anterior and superior target areas are of more benefit for rigidity and bradykinesia, particularly when part of parkinsonism; those in the inferior ventrolateral thalamus are better for athetoid, dystonic, and tremor symptoms, and the subthalamic targets are rather selectively effective for tremor only. Lesions in all these sites are generally more effective for symptoms affecting the extremities than for those involving the face, mouth and tongue, swallowing, and neck or trunk. Such improvement as can be made in dyskinesias involving these latter "midline" structures is usually seen with relatively medial placement of lesions at the various targets.

Avoidance of Complications

The immediate postoperative course following placement of a therapeutically successful thalamic lesion usually includes a period of sleepiness lasting approximately one day. This postoperative lethargy generally is not seen if the patient received 10 mg of dexamethasone as a loading dose prior to thalamotomy and continues to receive 4 mg every six hours during the first two to three days following operation. Similarly, some of the acute side effects of the thalamic lesion—in particular, the speech alterations and confusion—are diminished by dexamethasone therapy. However, those postoperative symptoms that clear with dexamethasone seem to be the same ones that will disappear with the passage of time.

In those patients not treated with dexamethasone, a mild contralateral lower facial paresis for automatic emotional, but not voluntary, movement commonly appears on the first postoperative day and disappears around the third or fourth postoperative day. It is a sign of satisfactory lesion placement.[117]

The acute complications of thalamotomy fall in three general areas. The first can be ascribed to inaccurate placement of the thalamic lesion, e.g., a contralateral hemiparesis may follow coagulation of motor fibers in the posterior limb of the internal capsule. It is, however, apparent that a large and posterior capsular lesion must be made to cause this complication, as studies in man have shown that the motor fibers in the posterior limb of the internal capsule at the thalamic level lie well posterior to the midcommissural coronal plane.[9] Corticobulbar fibers, however, seem to be much closer to the ventrolateral nucleus target. Unilateral damage to these fibers generally produces no symptoms, but bilateral damage can lead to a severe diminution in voice volume and occasionally to aphonia.[11] Placement of the lesions in the ventroposterior medial or lateral nucleus results in a contralateral sensory deficit to pain and touch. On the other hand, dysesthetic sensation as described in the "thalamic syndrome" of Dejerine and Roussy has been rarely reported after thalamotomy even with significant involvement of the ventroposterior medial and lateral nuclei. Similarly, improper placement of the subthalamic lesion in an inferior medial direction may encroach on mesencephalic tectum, causing abnormalities of eye movement.

A second source of complications is the uncontrolled enlargement of the lesion due to local hemorrhage. This is the principal risk in stereotaxic operations, accounting for most of the mortality rate of around 0.5 per cent, and much of the morbidity. Preoperative systolic hypertension predisposes to this complication. It has been the authors' practice to pretreat any patient with a systolic blood pressure greater than 150 mm of mercury with an antihypertensive agent until the blood pressure is under the 150 systolic level. Failure to do this leads to an unacceptably high mortality rate. For those patients who develop systolic hypertension during the course of the operation, the authors have adopted the practice of instituting a trimethaphan (Arfonad) drip prior to making the thalamic lesion and continuing its administration at a level that keeps the blood pressure below a systolic pressure of 150 mm of mercury throughout the remainder of the procedure and the immediate postoperative period. It is seldom necessary to continue the drip much beyond the first few hours postoperatively, as the more relaxed atmosphere of the recovery room and the sleepiness associated with the thalamic lesion generally combine to bring the blood pressure back into a normal range. Not all risk of hemorrhage is confined to the time of placing the lesion; it may also occur within the first several days postoperatively and occasionally even as much as a week or more later. To minimize this risk, the authors have adopted the practice of keeping the patient at bed rest during the first three postoperative days and have had a number of occasions to regret the occasional violation of this routine. Attention to avoiding constipation with attendant straining is important during this period also.

It has been maintained that all the complications of thalamotomy can be ascribed to either misplacement or uncontrolled enlargement of the lesion, and particularly that symmetrical misplacement of the lesions is associated with a very great risk of complications.[47] This view assumes that that portion of the thalamus that must be destroyed in a therapeutically successful lesion subserves no functions other than those related to the motor system and has no fibers related to other functions passing through it. There is, however, some evidence that the same areas of the lateral thalamus are concerned with some higher intellectual functions, including speech and memory, and that if there is sufficient dysfunction elsewhere in those parts of the brain concerned with these activities, significant and occasionally even permanent deficits can follow a satisfactorily placed thalamic lesion.

The role of the ventrolateral thalamus of the dominant hemisphere in language processes is now well described.[94] Although the full extent of this role is not known, the ventrolateral thalamus is involved in those aspects of language that interact with attentional mechanisms, verbal memory, and control of respiration.[95] The medial-central portions of the ventral lateral thalamus and anterior portions of the pulvinar are apparently the most essential areas for these language functions.[93,95,98] It comes as no surprise, then, that ventrolateral thalamotomy seldom improves speech and language, and more often impairs it. Such improvement in speech as is occasionally seen is usually increased voice volume. When this occurs, it is after a first side thalamotomy, usually in the nondominant hemisphere.

Impairments of speech after thalamotomy include decreased voice volume with dysarthria, and dysphasia. Dysarthic decreased voice volume, occasionally so severe as to make the patient aphonic, is most often a complication of bilateral thalamotomies. It is the major complication of bilateral operations, having been reported in as many as 30 per cent of several series.[68,118] It may appear when preoperative speech is normal, but the presence of any degree of speech deficit before operation increases the likelihood of permanent impairment after operation.[10,118] Such impairment is more likely when the first thalamotomy is in the dominant hemisphere and may occasionally follow a unilateral operation on the dominant hemisphere. The diminution of voice volume and the dysarthria are commonly, but not always, transitory, clearing in four to six weeks. But some patients remain permanently aphonic.

Dysphasia is usually manifest by difficulty with object names, often with perseveration. Speech is commonly fluent; occasional jargon may appear, often widely extraneous to the subject of conversation.

Repeating to dictation is usually intact. Thus this language deficit is somewhat different from any of the cortically engendered language deficits.[2,10,94] It rather commonly follows thalamotomy in the dominant hemisphere, and has been reported in 42 per cent of patients in one series.[117] Fortunately, grossly detectable dysphasia is usually transitory, clearing in six weeks or so. Deficits in the verbal components of formal psychological tests, however, can occasionally be detected for many years.

The authors have been interested in techniques for predicting language disturbances during the course of thalamotomy in the dominant hemisphere. When the probe is in the part of the dominant thalamus concerned with language, electrical stimulation (at 60 Hz, 2.5 msec biphasic square wave pulses) during a test of object naming will produce a failure to name with retained ability to speak, the same type of response seen with stimulation of language cortex during naming.[103] The lowest threshold for this effect has been 5 ma (measured between peaks of the biphasic pulses) delivered monopolarly through a low-impedance large (1 by 5 mm) electrode. More frequently 8 to 10 ma must be used; these are current levels similar to those used with cortical language mapping. If disturbances of object naming are evoked at the proposed site of coagulation, it is best to move to another, usually more inferior, placement to minimize the risk of a postoperative language deficit.

Language function in the dominant ventrolateral thalamus seems to be intimately related to short-term verbal memory functions there. As a result, an even more accurate prediction of postoperative language disturbances can be obtained from the effects of intraoperative stimulation on a short-term memory test.[99] Stimulation parameters are the same as for testing for object naming except that the current level need not exceed 4 ma. Short-term verbal memory mechanisms seem to be a global property of the dominant lateral thalamus, so stimulation effects are not specific to a discrete area there, as are stimulation effects on naming. When stimulation during input to memory decreases errors, while the same current at the same site applied during output from memory increases errors and shortens the correct response time, language disturbances are unlikely

after thalamotomy. When these effects are small or absent, both postoperative language and memory disturbance are much more likely and may persist. Under these conditions, the authors generally make only a small lesion or, occasionally, none at all.

In addition to language disturbances, verbal memory deficits also occur immediately after dominant (usually left) thalamotomy.[99] Indeed, verbal memory deficits are among the most common abnormalities found in late follow-up psychological testing of thalamotomy patients.[119] These changes are also more prominant after left side operations. Right thalamic and subthalamic lesions have impaired visuospatial performance and visuospatial memory.[86] The authors have found that the same effect of electrical stimulation during short-term memory tests that predict acute postoperative language disturbances predict the likelihood of these postoperative memory disturbances as well. Others have suggested that the memory disturbance after thalamotomy can be reduced by avoiding damage to the fibers passing from the dorsomedial nucleus across the anterior superior portions of the lateral thalamus.[47]

With the potential impairment of all these higher functions, it is not surprising that IQ often declines somewhat after thalamotomy, and in 7 to 8 per cent or so of patients, this is clinically apparent as disturbed mentation. For this reason, higher intellectual functions should be carefully assessed before thalamotomy, and especially in the old, the procedure should not be undertaken if any noticeable impairment is evident. The severity of the decrease in IQ after thalamotomy is usually less when tested some years after the operation than in the first few months postoperatively, but it does not always return to preoperative levels.[119]

Not all the alterations in motor performance that follow ventrolateral thalamic lesions represent improvement in the patient's dyskinesia. Quite frequently, in the immediate postoperative period the patient does not use the extremity contralateral to the thalamic lesion for habitual activities (such as eating) even when that extremity has been fully relieved of tremor, rigidity, and bradykinesia and is much more facile than the ipsilateral extremity. This apparent neglect of a seemingly useful extremity has also been seen after excision of the caudate head and anterior limb of the internal capsule for dyskinesias.[16] Thus it may be a consequence of the interruption of some of the frontal-thalamic connections. The neglect generally clears in a few weeks.

Disturbances of balance are also relatively common after ventrolateral thalamotomy. Cooper reports an overall incidence of 13 per cent, and a significantly higher incidence after the second of bilateral operations.[23] These, too, are generally transitory, though 4 per cent of Cooper's patients retained some impairment of balance on long-term follow-up. The balance disturbance is most commonly a tendency to lean toward the side of the operation, and it may be associated with some signs of neocerebellar dysfunction in the contralateral extremities. It appears to be more common after lesions in the inferior portions of the ventrolateral nucleus, particularly in the VOP nucleus of Hassler and is probably related to interruption of cerebellar-cortical pathways.

More distressing to both patient and physician is the appearance of hyperkinesias after ventrolateral thalamic lesions. These occurred in 1 to 3 per cent of various series.[23,117] The most common is hemiballismus of the contralateral arm. This is most often—but not always—due to extension of the lesion into a portion of the subthalamic nucleus. Hemiballismus usually, though not invariably, clears in a period of several weeks, during which time the patient is sedated to minimize the hyperkinesia. More rarely, hyperkinesia may take the form of choreoathetotic movements.

Those complications associated with misplacing the lesion can be largely avoided by using careful technique, in particular by using physiological guides to lesion placement rather than relying solely on anatomical landmarks. Complications associated with the uncontrolled enlargement of the lesion related to hemorrhage can in part be controlled through the use of antihypertensive agents both preoperatively and during the procedure if the patient develops systolic hypertension, as well as by a period of bed rest in the immediate postoperative period. Complications related to other functions of the ventrolateral thalamus are somewhat less easily avoided. Making a lesion in only one thalamus at a time and delaying thalamotomy on the other side (if indicated) for six months or more will reduce

all these complications. Minimizing the size of the lesion in the dominant hemisphere, avoiding encroachment on the more posterior-superior aspects of the ventrolateral thalamus, and using some form of intraoperative speech and short-term memory testing prior to making the lesion will diminish complications related to speech and verbal memory. The disturbances of balance are generally of a transitory nature and can be treated expectantly. Perhaps most importantly, complications can be avoided through careful preoperative selection of patients—in particular, by avoiding those with pre-existing language and intellectual impairment.

INDICATIONS AND RESULTS

Parkinson's Disease

The oft-quoted initial passages of James Parkinson's 1817 *Essay on the Shaking Palsy* described the major clinical highlights of the syndrome: "involuntary tremulous motion with lessened muscular power, in parts not in action and even when supported; with a propensity to bend the trunk forwards and to pass from a walking to a running pace: the senses and intellects being uninjured."[102] No two patients with the Parkinson syndrome present exactly the same clinical picture. Most, however, show at least a few signs of tremor, rigidity, and bradykinesia of extremity or midline musculature or both.[56] One patient may present with a marked tremor of one extremity with only minimal rigidity and bradykinesia in that extremity and few other signs; the next patient may exhibit severe bradykinesia of the midline musculature, with monotonic speech, facial masking, festinating gait, and relatively little extremity involvement. The signs and symptoms tend to wax and wane in the same patient. Stress, either emotional or physical, tends to make all the symptoms worse, and they may not return to their original level on removal of the stress.[114]

Tremor is the most frequent initial symptom.[56] It is classically described as occurring at about 3 to 5 cycles per second and having a pill-rolling quality. It tends to be present at rest, is often inhibited when a voluntary action is initiated, but then may reappear with increased vigor as the action continues. A latent tremor may often be brought out by having the patient maintain a limb in an unsupported position, e.g., holding his arms out in front of his chest with index fingers pointing at each other but not quite touching. The tremor is abolished during sleep. Although the tremor is often the most dramatic symptom of Parkinson's disease, it is quite unusual to have a patient who does not show some other sign of parkinsonism, and as a "rule of thumb," tremor alone, without at least a trace of bradykinesia or rigidity in the same or other musculature, is probably not parkinsonism.

The rigidity of the Parkinson syndrome imparts a plastic quality to the muscles when they are passively stretched. Superimposed on this may be the alternating tightening and releasing of the muscle as it is passively stretched that produces the phenomenon known as cogwheeling. This is thought to be due to the superimposition of the muscle tone changes of tremor on the plastic rigidity. Additional useful clinical tests for rigidity include the presence and freedom of arm swing when walking and the freedom of wrist flop when the relaxed forearm is passively flexed and extended.

Associated with rigidity is a tendency for parkinsonian patients to complain of painful muscle cramps in the extremities. The common complaint of severe fatigue is probably also a consequence of the work necessary to overcome the rigidity with each voluntary movement.

Although the presence of rigidity alone can severely interfere with extremity function, relief of the rigidity alone does not necessarily restore facile movement to an extremity. It is evident that there is an independent component of bradykinesia in the Parkinson syndrome. This slowness of movement is particularly noticeable on initiation of a voluntary act; repetitive activity augments the defect. The rates of approximation of the thumb to each finger and of making a fist are measures of upper extremity bradykinesia, while the rate of toe tapping and the freedom of toe wiggling are measures of its presence in the lower extremities. A frequent early manifestation of bradykinesia of the upper extremity is deterioration in handwriting, with progressive diminution in the size of the letters, the so-called micrographia. This usually shows initially in cursive writing while block letter writing is still preserved.

Bradykinesia of the midline musculature produces the picture of en bloc posture and the tendency to freeze in one position and be unable to get started again. Frequent falls are associated with the tendency to freeze.

Among the unusual features of bradykinesia is the patient's ability under some circumstances to carry out a particular action, while under slightly different circumstances exactly the same activity will be impossible. Yakovlev described a patient who could adeptly feed other patients on the ward but was unable to carry out the same movements to feed herself.[145] The bradykinesia can often be dramatically overcome for brief periods, as when the bedridden parkinsonian patient is able to escape fleetly from his burning house. Occasionally one encounters a patient with parkinsonism whose principal kinetic difficulty is restlessness with a feeling of constantly having to move an extremity. This phenomenon, most common in the lower extremities, has been called akathisia.

The distinction between involvement of extremity musculature and midline musculature with parkinsonian symptoms is an important one for the surgeon, for the operative therapy of Parkinson's disease appears to be much more effective for extremity involvement. Midline symptoms include masked facies and the loss of modulation of speech with continued speaking. Speech volume progressively diminishes to a monotone (this defect often being first noticed on the telephone). Inability to protrude the tongue beyond the vermilion border of the lips, and the slow alternating motion of the tongue are signs often associated with speech defects.

The general disturbance of trunk mobility giving a festinating pattern to the gait is also a sign of midline involvement. In a festinating gait, the upper part of the body is bent forward and appears to go faster than the lower. As the patient walks, this difference is accentuated so that he develops the appearance of trying to run after and catch up with his own center of gravity. Additional "midline" signs of Parkinson's disease are the loss of convergence (sometimes clinically manifest by the patient's complaint that he cannot light his cigar), the restriction of upward gaze, and a paucity of blinks. In addition, there may be a tonic inability to open the eyes (blepharoclonus), and episodes of tonic upward deviation of the eyes, the so-called oculogyric crisis. These last two symptoms appear to be particularly common in patients who give a clear history of encephalitis.

Swallowing difficulties are also part of the midline symptom complex. The most common indication of this difficulty (coupled with mask facies) is the inability to clear saliva from the throat and its subsequent draining out through the lips, the so-called sialorrhea. Even in the absence of clinical symptoms of swallowing difficulty it is often possible to demonstrate bradykinesia of the pharyngeal musculature on a barium swallow. The swallowing defect is one of the aspects of parkinsonism that may significantly shorten the patient's life, for occasionally it becomes so severe as to be associated with aspiration pneumonitis.

A number of autonomic changes have also been described in parkinsonian patients, including unusually oily skin with an increase in seborrhea and unusual sweating. Constipation, occasionally with atony of the large bowel, and difficulties with urination (particularly urgency) are not uncommon.

The absence of intellectual deterioration is one of the features emphasized in James Parkinson's original description of the disease. However, one fifth to one sixth of the patients in a number of series appear to have significant intellectual deterioration, particularly in the memory spheres.[107,118] This seems to be somewhat more common in those patients with a previous history of encephalitis but may also be related to drug therapy. A large proportion of these patients show significant depression. Some observers feel that parkinsonian patients have unusually rigid premorbid personalities.[14]

Early cases of Parkinson's disease may be rather difficult to diagnose. Particularly valuable early signs are: the loss of the associated swing of the arms on one or both sides when walking, the loss of the usual semiautomatic movements when sleeping (the patient's spouse may report that he lies unusually still), and the loss of similar movements when sitting (the patient sits with his feet planted squarely under him, unmoving, in the waiting room). In addition, the appearance of the glabellar tap sign (Myerson's reflex) is often an early sign. This response is illicited by tapping over the glabella, usually from behind so that no visual cue is provided. The parkinsonian patient will blink in response to each tap in contrast to the normal patient in whom the blinking rapidly subsides.

Schwab and England pointed out a number of signs that are *not* present in 95 per cent of patients with Parkinson's disease.[114] These include signs of spasticity (although positive Babinski responses are not unknown in the parkinsonian patient), sensory changes, visual field changes, severe pain, and complete loss of bladder function. In particular, seizures are unusually rare in patients with Parkinson's disease.[60]

The diagnosis of Parkinson's disease is a clinical one based on the presence of the aforementioned signs and symptoms. In general, laboratory data contribute little. Efforts have been made to quantitate the clinical signs present in a particular patient at a given time. Some of the machines designed for that purpose have been described in a comprehensive summary.[15] Obviously, this quantitation would be of great value in following patients to determine the efficacy of both operative and medical therapy. Nearly as good data can, however, be more easily obtained by functional tests of the patient's ability: Can he cut meat? Sign checks? Is he able to turn over in bed? Can he button buttons? Can he rise from an overstuffed chair?

Parkinson's syndrome usually has its onset after the age of 50 and is extremely rare below the age of 30. It is a relatively common disease. It is estimated that there are 40,000 new cases per year in the United States and probably an accumulative total of around 300,000 cases at any one time.[118] It is more common in males than in females in a ratio of about one female to every 1.35 males. The course of the disease is variable.[115,116] About 9 per cent of parkinsonian patients have symptoms that involve only the extremities of one side, progress only slowly there, and never spread to the midline or opposite extremities.[116] Another 7 per cent will begin with this form and then have sudden severe progression following some medical catastrophe. Twenty-one per cent have a rapid and malignant form of the disease, while in the remaining majority, the disease slowly but relentlessly progresses, from one side to the other and to midline structures. The details of this progression will vary from patient to patient. Symptoms may start and progress on one side, then begin and progress in midline structures or on the other side while remaining stable on the side of initial appearance, then progress again on that initial side. Two thirds of these patients will, however, be disabled by their disease within 10 years of diagnosis.[56] With onset of the Parkinson syndrome at a younger age, the disease seems to progress more rapidly than with a later onset.

Life span is also shortened. The death rate for the patient with Parkinson's disease was 2.9 times that in age-sex-color matched controls.[56] Pneumonia, and to a lesser extent urinary tract infections, were responsible for most of these additional deaths.

The clinical picture of parkinsonism apparently can be produced by a number of causes. Classically these are given as postencephalitic, atherosclerotic, and idiopathic. Clearly, some patients have the onset of parkinsonian symptoms following a case of Von Economo encephalitis, either immediately or after a delay of from a few months to many years. This association appears to be unique to the Von Economo encephalitis (and possibly particularly to the 1916–1919 epidemic) in that other types of infectious encephalitis have seldom given rise to parkinsonian syndromes as sequelae. On the other hand, atherosclerosis does not seem to be a cause of parkinsonism. The incidence of atherosclerotic disease elsewhere in the body is either normal or lower than normal in patients with Parkinson's disease.[36] Discrete ischemic lesions are not found in cases of parkinsonism, and the few recorded cases of discrete ischemic lesions of the basal ganglia have not been associated with parkinsonian symptoms.[114]

Poskanzer and Schwab presented suggestive evidence that the vast majority of cases of Parkinson's syndrome can be related to the 1916–1919 epidemic of Von Economo encephalitis, and thus the vast majority of cases may really be postencephalitic despite the fact that only about 10 per cent of patients with Parkinson's disease give a history of previous encephalitis.[108] Their evidence was derived from a cohort analysis of the parkinsonian patient population at the Massachusetts General Hospital. They found that the vast number of these patients would have been between ages 5 and 60 in 1919, and this is the age group in which epidemic encephalitis occurred at that time. If this concept is correct (it has been challenged[33]), there should be not only progressive increase in the average age of the patients presenting with Parkinson's disease (thus making them somewhat less suitable candidates for operation), but also a rather abrupt drop in the number of cases about the period 1975 to 1980, with a rapid approach to the pre-1919 incidence of the disease. There is some evidence that this prediction is being borne out.

Since the disease had been observed (though rather infrequently) prior to the early part of the twentieth century, there must also be other causes of the Parkinson syndrome. A very occasional case with the clinical picture of parkinsonism appears to be secondary to some other cause. In their review of this subject, Schwab and England felt that the majority of the associations between parkinsonism and some other disease were just chance associations of one common disease with another.[114] They felt that, although in a few cases the Parkinson syndrome was clearly secondary to another condition, usually there were some unusual signs in these cases that should have tipped off the examiner. There are several case reports in which a Parkinson syndrome has followed a traumatic lesion, usually a severe brain stem injury. A Parkinson syndrome has been reported with parasagittal meningioma, the syndrome abating after removal of the tumor. A number of patients with basal ganglia and midbrain gliomas also demonstrated parkinsonian symptoms, although they usually also had a number of signs not found in the classic Parkinson syndrome. Similarly, patients intoxicated with manganese and carbon monoxide may show a Parkinson syndrome, but these patients, in addition, usually have pyramidal tract signs. The most common cause of secondary parkinsonism is drugs, particularly the phenothiazines and reserpine. The clinical parkinsonian picture that these drugs can produce blends indistinguishably into the picture of "postinfectious" or "idiopathic" parkinsonism.

There is some evidence there may also be familial factors operating in the etiology of Parkinson's syndrome, at least to the extent of producing a tendency for its development. A family history of parkinsonism has been found in as many as one in six patients presenting with Parkinson's syndrome.[70] There may also be some association with a family history of essential familial tremor.

A depletion of dopamine in the brain stem and basal ganglia seems to be the fundamental pathophysiological defect in Parkinson's disease. How this defect arises is not now known, and there may be more than one cause.[7] The vast majority of cases show relatively undramatic pathological abnormalities. In most of them, degeneration of some neurons is noted in a portion of the substantia nigra and is associated with some depigmentation there.[37,50] There may also be neuronal degeneration in the dorsal motor nucleus of the vagus nerve and the hypoglossal nucleus. Lewy bodies, intracellular inclusions with a dark center and clear peripheral zone, are often noticed in basal ganglia neurons as well as occasionally in spinal cord and sympathetic ganglion.[34] These bodies appear to be less common in those patients who have a previous history of encephalitis. Cerebral atrophy is seen about twice as frequently in patients with Parkinson's disease as in controls of the same age, and ventricular enlargement is common (though not necessarily more common than in other people of the same age).[118] Thickening of the pia-arachnoid is also prominent in these patients. A parkinsonian movement disorder associated with dementia and computed tomographic evidence of ventricular enlargement suggests the presence of occult normal-pressure hydrocephalus. This select patient group often shows improvement in both the dyskinesia and the dementia after placement of a cerebrospinal fluid shunt.[130a]

The pathophysiological basis for the progression of parkinsonism also remains unclear. There may indeed be progressive pathological changes in the brain though there is no positive evidence of active inflammation.[3] If this is so, it is hard to account for the observation that focal operative lesions not infrequently produce improvement that is maintained for seemingly indefinite periods, even as the disease progresses in other parts of the same patient. It has also been suggested that the aging process and its attendant neuronal losses superimposed upon the neuronal loss of the previous encephalitic episode may be responsible for the progression. Although this hypothesis accounts well for the progression of parkinsonism in the elderly,

it fails to account readily for similar and often more rapid progression in the relatively young. A third possibility is that the reduced activation of the muscle spindle, as a consequence of the depression of the gamma loop, may lead to progressive atrophic changes in the spindle. Such atrophic changes have been described, though they require further confirmation.[19] If the initial disease process itself is producing secondary changes that are responsible for the symptomatic progression, then early vigorous treatment seems in order.

A few cases of clinical Parkinson's syndrome clearly have a different pathological basis, with rather widespread strial-nigral degeneration.[1]

There really is no differential diagnosis for the combination of tremor, rigidity, and bradykinesia in an adult. Tremor alone and the absence of other signs is more likely to be something else. Essential tremor tends to be familial, faster, and to have a wider amplitude than the parkinsonian tremor; senile tremor tends to be faster, more regular, more likely to occur in voluntary movement, and more likely to involve the head. Juvenile Huntington's chorea may present a picture of rigidity and bradykinesia without tremor or choreic movements, but of course, age here is usually a useful differential point. Occasionally in an adult with Huntington's chorea, rigidity and bradykinesia may be the predominant signs. Those signs coupled with the presence of a strong family history and dementia suggest the diagnosis of Huntington's chorea rather than parkinsonism.

Medical Management

Levodopa is now the mainstay of the medical management of Parkinson's disease. This agent can be given alone or in conjunction with a dopa decarboxylase inhibitor, alpha methyldopa hydrazine (carbidopa), which blocks the peripheral uptake of levodopa, allowing more to enter the brain more rapidly. Levodopa is most effective at relieving rigidity and bradykinesia; relief of tremor generally requires large doses and is often incomplete at the maximum tolerated dose. Both extremity and midline symptoms improve, the former somewhat more rapidly.

In about 5 per cent of patients, levodopa will achieve the same degree of success as the most successful thalamotomies—that is an asymptomatic state. The major side effects of levodopa therapy are nausea and hypotension, which can be handled by adjustment of dosage, and dyskinesias and the "on-off" effect, which are the dose-limiting factors to its use. Dosage should begin at low levels. Giving levodopa with food and spreading dosage throughout the day reduces the nausea, which also is less common with the combination of levodopa and the dopa decarboxylase inhibitor. Dosage is increased—slowly (with levodopa alone) or rapidly (with the decarboxylase inhibitor) —until satisfactory improvement has occurred or dyskinesias appear. The dyskinesias usually involve the face or tongue, often in a choreic pattern, though with wide variations. They seem to be less common in patients who have had previous thalamotomies.[136] Once the dose that produces the dyskinesias is reached, a dose level that provides a suitable balance between the dyskinetic movements and the parkinsonian symptoms is selected. The "on-off" effect, the sudden appearance of general akinesia, lasting from minutes to hours, usually does not occur until the patient has been on levodopa therapy for two to three years. Appearance of these symptoms requires a reduction in dosage. Interestingly, the authors have not encountered the "on-off" effect in their group of postthalamotomy patients receiving levodopa therapy. With the passage of time, the parkinsonian symptoms progress despite continued levodopa treatment, the deterioration often becoming noticeable after five years or so of treatment.[6]

A number of drugs are used as adjuvants to levodopa. Amantadine (Symmetrel) provides modest benefit to many patients with minimal side effects. The anticholinergics also seem to potentiate the effects of levodopa, but with a variety of undesirable side effects: blurred vision, dry mouth, and urinary hesitancy especially. Benzhexol (Artane) is the most widely used of these agents. General medical management of these patients is also most important. They must be kept active. Long periods of confinement in bed or watching television are to be avoided. It is axiomatic that the more a parkinsonian patient does, the better he will be.[39]

Levodopa and thalamotomy appear to be additive in relieving parkinsonian symptoms. Thalamotomy is maximally beneficial for tremor, which levodopa controls with difficulty, while levodopa helps midline symptoms that do not respond to operative intervention. There is one group of patients with Parkinson's disease in whom thalamotomy is probably the primary treatment of choice, those with unilateral disease progressing slowly or not at all, especially if tremor is the major symptom.[97] Thalamotomy is indicated in these patients because of the great probability of its relieving extremity tremor, and the unlikelihood of recurrence of symptoms after many years. In almost all other patients, levodopa is the primary treatment and should receive at least a six months' trial, thalamotomy being reserved for treatment of persisting or recurring extremity symptoms.

Surgical Management

Considerable experience has been gained in the effects of ventrolateral thalamic lesions on Parkinson's syndrome. From this experience it is possible to make definite statements about the probability of relief of a particular parkinsonian symptom by that procedure. The optimal candiate for operation, of course, is one whose Parkinson's disease is characterized by those symptoms that are most likely to be relieved by the operation and in whom no systemic factors are present that increase the general operative risk.

Ventrolateral thalamotomy has produced immediate complete relief of tremor and rigidity in the contralateral extremities in 70 to 90 per cent of patients with unilateral symptoms.[23,118] This relief seems to be more frequent in the upper than lower extremity. Arm movements associated with walking return, and the pain associated with muscle cramping is nearly always relieved. Operations on the right hemisphere appear to be associated with somewhat greater incidence of relief of rigidity than operations on the left hemisphere.

Improvement in tremor and rigidity in extremities ipsilateral to the thalamic lesion is not to be expected, though it does occasionally occur.

When bilateral extremity tremor and rigidity are present, the operation on the second side is not associated with quite as good results as those just quoted for unilateral tremor and rigidity. Relief of tremor and rigidity occurred in about 70 per cent of patients after a second operation, which is about 20 per cent less than those reported to have obtained relief from the first operation in the hands of the same surgeon.[29] There did not appear to be a preferential choice of side for the initial procedure in terms of overall results on tremor and rigidity.

It has become an almost classic dictum in the operative treatment of Parkinson's disease that stereotaxic lesions do not improve bradykinesia. That has not been the authors' experience. The speed of initiating opening and closing of the fist and approximating the thumb to the other fingers appears to be improved, often quite strikingly, in approximately 80 per cent of patients after ventrolateral thalamic lesions, and this improvement is sometimes quite independent of improvement in rigidity and tremor. Improvement in handwriting, which has also been considered to be a good measure of the presence of bradykinesia, is seen much less often, but even here significant improvement may occasionally occur, as illustrated in Figure 140–5.[114] Improvement in the bradykinesia of the musculature involved in pronation and supination of the forearm after thalamotomy has been reported. Quantative tests of fine hand manipulations improve.[136] Occasionally bradykinesia of the foot and toes also improves after contralateral thalamotomy. Some of the difference between the authors' experience and that of others in regard to the effects of ventrolateral thalamotomy on bradykinesia may have to do with the exact location of the lesions within the ventrolateral thalamus, in that the more superior lesions may well be somewhat more efficacious for producing alterations in extremity bradykinesia.

As a general rule the midline symptoms of Parkinson's disease are not benefited by thalamotomy. There are a few exceptions however. Oculogyric crises occasionally improved.[46] Autonomic alterations have been reported to improve, but the presence of significant autonomic symptoms presage a poor long-term result.[23] The seborrheic changes in general are not altered by the operation. Some improvement in facial mobility occasionally occurs. There may be increased voice volume after thalamotomy, but there is usually very little improvement in speech modulation.

The festinating gait does not respond to unilateral thalamic lesions and is sometimes made worse by the disequilibrium that follows bilateral thalamic lesions in approximately 15 per cent of cases.[29] The presence of significant disturbance in swallowing, with the attendant risk of aspiration, contraindicates thalamotomy. Thalamotomy is therefore clearly not indicated for relief of midline symptoms alone, and their presence makes the patient a less suitable candidate for operation, particularly if the extremity disease necessitates bilateral lesions for its relief. Patients with akinesia of midline structures and extremities are not candidates for thalamotomy.

Preoperative evidence of psychological abnormalities generally contraindicates thalamotomy. Even in the absence of evidence of such abnormalities preoperatively, there is a modest incidence of intellectual

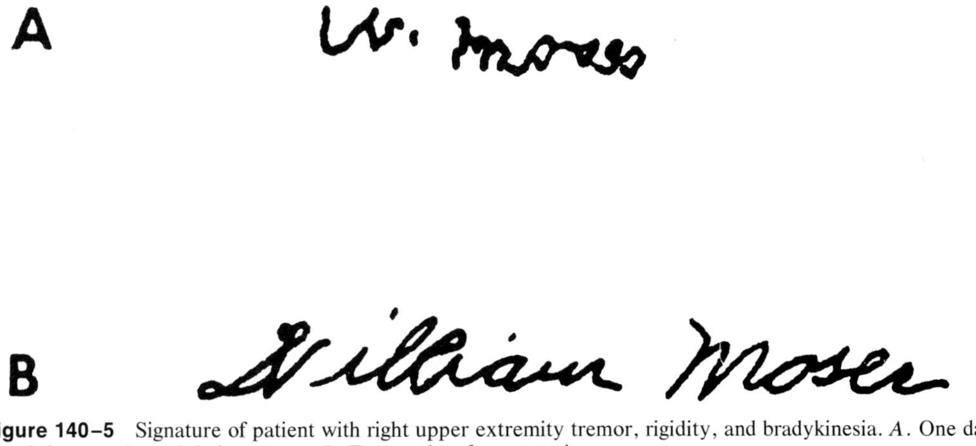

A

B

Figure 140–5　Signature of patient with right upper extremity tremor, rigidity, and bradykinesia. *A.* One day before left ventrolateral thalamotomy. *B.* Ten weeks after operation.

deterioration after thalamotomy, on the order of 5 to 7 per cent.[118] It seems to be a somewhat greater problem after dominant hemisphere lesions, though it is not particularly increased with bilateral lesions. The presence of slow wave abnormalities on the electroencephalogram or atrophy on the CT scan or pneumoencephalogram seems to increase the likelihood of postoperative psychological disturbances, as does advancing age.

A number of systemic factors influence the decision in regard to operative therapy. Hypertension in which the systolic blood pressure is over 150 mm of mercury contraindicates thalamotomy until the hypertension is brought under control. Advancing age increases the risk of postoperative psychological disturbances, with this risk seeming to increase rather sharply after age 65. The operation can clearly be safely done on older people without producing psychological problems, but one must be much more careful in preoperative selection, excluding anyone with a hint of any psychological dysfunction including even mild memory disturbances.

One can construct criteria for the ideal candidate for thalamotomy in cases of Parkinson's disease. This patient's symptoms should be predominantly in the extremities but may be any mix of tremor, rigidity, or bradykinesia, though he will do best if tremor predominates. He will do a little better if the left extremities are involved rather than the right. He should have little or no involvement of midline structures. He will achieve benefit from the operation if he is still relatively functional, and especially if he is still able to work. He will more likely maintain his postoperative improvement if operated on relatively early in the course of his disease. This ideal patient should be less than 65 years old and should have systolic blood pressure of less than 150 mm of mercury. He should have entirely normal intellectual function, especially with reference to recent memory. In such a patient, or even a moderately distant approximation of such an ideal candidate for operation, one could expect relief of the extremity tremor and rigidity in 70 to 90 per cent of instances over the short run. Bradykinesia will not do quite as well. This would be accomplished with an operative mortality rate of about 0.5 per cent and a risk of complications,

previously mentioned, of from 5 to 10 per cent with a higher rate if an operation is necessary on the left hemisphere. Obviously, a variety of factors other than just symptomatic relief enter into a patient's ability to return to work after any particular form of therapy. In a number of reported series, however, generally around one third of patients do so after thalamotomy.[118]

Several studies of the long-term effects of thalamotomy on the symptoms of Parkinson's disease are now available.[110,136,138] Follow-up has often averaged over five years, the maximum being a decade or more. The results of these studies are remarkably similar. Improvement in tremor of the contralateral extremity obtained at operation tends to persist throughout this long follow-up. Improvement in rigidity and bradykinesia of the contralateral extremity tends to be lost with time. "Midline" symptoms progress relentlessly and limit the functional level of many patients. For example, in 1969 or later, before initiating levodopa therapy, the authors reviewed the status of their patients who had undergone thalamotomy in the 1960–1964 period. Thus minimum follow-up was five years, the mean was 6.6 years and the maximum was 10 years. Sixty-nine per cent of those patients who achieved improvement in tremor of the contralateral extremity at the time of thalamotomy had retained at least that degree of improvement at the late follow-up. Only 38 per cent of those with improvement in contralateral extremity rigidity had retained it, as had 39 per cent of those showing improvement in contralateral extremity bradykinesia. Twenty-nine per cent retained overall contralateral extremity function that was at least as good as immediately after operation; 75 per cent retained extremity function that was as good as or better than before thalamotomy. At late follow-up, 26 per cent demonstrated severe "midline" symptoms. The detailed study of Van Buren and co-workers shows similar findings for contralateral extremity function and graphically illustrates the progression of midline symptoms and speech deficits that with passing years lead to major functional impairment.[136] In their series, at about three years after thalamotomy, this functional impairment from midline progression of the Parkinson's disease exceeded the functional improvement in extremity function effected by thalamotomy, and thereafter, their *average* patient functioned less well than before thalamotomy.

Dystonia

The involuntary movements of the dystonias represent a disturbance in the attitude or posture of a segment of, or of the entire body. In contrast to most of the hyperkinesias, this disturbance of attitude is long-lasting, a particular posture being maintained for minutes, occasionally even days. The abnormal posturing is frequently associated with simultaneous contraction of agonist and antagonist musculature, and is often superimposed on normal movements. There are frequently associated abrupt and unpredictable changes in muscle tone.

Dystonic movements occur as the sole manifestation of the syndrome dystonia musculorum deformans; they may also be seen in association with other neurological disturbances as a secondary manifestation from a wide variety of afflictions of the nervous system. These include perinatal brain damage, various degenerative diseases, cerebrovascular disease, encephalitis, meningitis, basal ganglia gliomas, and arteriovenous malformations in the region of the putamen. When the underlying cause is a progressive process, dystonia tends to occur relatively late in the clinical picture.

Dystonia musculorum deformans is a hereditary disease with occasional sporadic manifestations. Dystonia is usually inherited as a dominant trait, although at least one family has been reported in which it follows a recessive pattern.[23,146] Expressivity is variable. Families that carry dystonia also show a high incidence of familial tremor and other dyskinesias. It is particularly common among the Ashkenazi Jews, originally of Southwest Lithuania and Byelorussia, who account for some 56 per cent of all recorded cases of dystonia musculorum deformans.[146] The disease has, however, been seen in all races.

Patients with this disease usually have a history of a normal birth and normal development for the first three years. In two thirds of cases, dystonic symptoms were first manifest by age 15, in some 93 per cent by age 21.[146] The most common age of

onset is between 7 and 10; onset after age 40 is very rare. The nature of the earliest symptom varies with the age of onset. In the 6- to 10-year-old group, the lower extremity is usually first involved. In those who are older at the time of first onset, involvement of axial musculature, including the appearance of torticollis, is a more common first manifestation. The course of the disease is quite variable, tending to be more rapid in the young, in whom it may occasionally progress sufficiently to cause death. The disease not infrequently may be arrested at any stage and very occasionally regresses slightly. In three quarters of patients in one series it had been arrested by age 35. The far-advanced stages of the disease are complicated by the development of fixed postures. Advance of the disease generally occurs by involvement of a new portion of the body rather than by more severe involvement of already affected parts. About a third of patients remain independent, in a similar proportion disability progresses to a wheelchair existence.[77]

Particularly in adults, the disease may affect only a small part of the body. Thus, involvement of only the dominant hand may present as a writer's cramp, and involvement of only the neck muscles as torticollis. (The relationship between torticollis and dystonia is discussed more fully later.) No specific pathophysiological changes have been demonstrated in dystonia musculorum deformans.

Most of the experience with both medical and operative treatment of the dystonias has been in cases of dystonia musculorum deformans. The experience in some cases of secondary dystonia, however, in which the motion disorder represents the chief symptom, suggests that the same principles of treatment apply in all cases with a dystonic dyskinesia. Medical treatment of the dystonias is generally unsatisfactory. Benzhexol (Artane) and diazepam (Valium) are the most useful drugs.

Ventrolateral thalamotomy is the treatment of choice for dystonia. Nearly 70 per cent of patients in the large series reported by Cooper were moderately or markedly improved.[25] Follow-up was at least two years with a mean of 7.9 years. Twelve per cent worsened. In the authors' hands, two thirds of dystonic patients have shown major improvement after thalamotomy, and in one third of the cases, symptomatic relief has been so marked that the patients appear normal. Bilateral operations are usually necessary, both for midline symptoms and bilateral extremity symptoms. Lesions placed on the medial edge of the target area are said to be more effective for midline symptoms. Cooper points out that every symptom of dystonia can on occasion be relieved by thalamotomy. Recurrence of the dystonia, once relieved by thalamotomy, is unusual, but dystonic symptoms do appear in other parts of the body: the ipsilateral extremities, or midline, for example, after a unilateral thalamotomy. Results are generally better in the younger patients, and operation should, of course, be undertaken before contractures develop. Surprisingly, improvement after thalamotomy often comes on rather late. There may be only slight benefit on the operating table, but the symptoms may be entirely gone a month after operation, and the improvement remains at late follow-up. One third of patients in one series continued to improve for six months or more postoperatively.[23] The physiological substrate for this late improvement is unknown.

Complications of thalamotomy in these patients are similar to those in patients with Parkinson's disease, although in the young dystonic patients, large bilateral lesions are generally better tolerated. Dysphonia is the major complication, occurring in 18 per cent of Cooper's series and in about 33 per cent of the authors' series. Although it has been suggested that the second side thalamotomy can be undertaken within a few weeks of the first in these patients, the authors prefer to delay it the full six months.[23]

Torticollis

Spasmodic torticollis is an abnormality of attitude (or posture) confined largely to the head and neck. Occasionally there is associated head tremor or abnormal head movements of an athetotic or myoclonic quality. Torticollis may occur in conjunction with other dyskinesias, particularly dystonia musculorum deformans, choreoathetosis, Huntington's chorea, and occasionally parkinsonism. The following discussion is concerned with torticollis as a relatively isolated dyskinesia.

The average age of onset is 30 to 40, with onset very rare in the first decade. The movements usually start insidiously, and they have a very variable course, rarely regressing, rather frequently becoming static. Although the movements always involve musculature on both sides, involvement may be very asymmetrical so that head rotation is quite common, and there may be associated retroflexion, or anteflexion, lateral flexion or any combination of these. Occasionally the tongue is involved in the abnormal posturing. The movements of torticollis can be markedly influenced by emotion, fatigue, or other stress and different sensory stimuli. As a result, the patient frequently is able to discover a "corrective gesture" that will arrest the movement. This gesture may take a variety of somewhat bizarre forms but often involves placing the hand at a particular point on the chin. Later stages of torticollis frequently are complicated by development of cervical spondylosis and neck pain.

With the head and neck movements being markedly influenced by the patient's emotional state, and the often rather bizarre nature of the corrective gesture that prevents these movements, it is perhaps not surprising that a considerable tradition has developed that torticollis is a psychiatric condition. Present evidence suggests that this is almost never the case. In some cases, the torticollis is clearly secondary to another central nervous system affliction: encephalitis, multiple sclerosis, carbon monoxide poisoning, as well as some of the other dyskinesias mentioned previously. In most cases there is no such history. There is a suggestion, however, that these cases of spasmodic torticollis may be a form of dystonia musculorum deformans confined to the head and neck musculature. A history of dystonia, head tremor, or torticollis in another member of the family is fairly common in patients with torticollis.[23,49] In a number of cases the disease extends beyond the cervical musculature into the trunk or shoulder and clearly has a pattern of dystonia musculorum deformans. Thus, there seems to be a continuum between torticollis, in which the movements are confined strictly to the head and neck, and dystonia, in which the movements extend on down into the trunk and shoulders. When torticollis appears in families with a known history of dystonia musculorum deformans, it tends to appear late (average onset for torticollis is around 25 to 45 years of age in Zeman's series, which is much later than the onset of dystonia in the extremities).[146] This age of onset is the same as that of the isolated cases of spasmodic torticollis and suggests that isolated involvement of the head and neck is a feature of late adult-onset dystonia musculorum deformans.

Torticollis itself is not a fatal disease, and the few reported autopsies showed rather diffuse pathological changes throughout the cortex and basal ganglia, which is fairly typical of many of the hyperkinesias. Thus the exact pathological substrate for torticollis is unknown. Torticollis can, however, be produced in experimental animals with a medially placed mesencephalic tegmental lesion involving the medial reticular formation, the medial longitudinal fasciculus, and the brachium conjunctivum.[41]

The differential diagnosis of torticollis includes an altered head posture secondary to diseases of the upper cervical spine and discs, and tumors. Torticollis is relatively rare under 10 years of age, and abnormal positions of the head and neck in that period are more likely caused by congenital anomalies of the cervical spine or sternocleidomastoid muscle, or possibly are related to a compensatory position for disturbances of extraocular movement, as may sometimes be seen in children with cerebellar tumors.

One of the major problems in evaluating therapy of torticollis is the discrepancy between objective changes in the patient's dyskinesia, and the patient's subjective feelings about his torticollis. Some patients consider improvement that can hardly be demonstrated objectively to be very satisfactory while other patients find even the slightest residual movement of the head and neck totally unsatisfactory.[49] Trial of one or more of the antiparkinsonism medications discussed earlier seems in order in most patients with torticollis. The various atropine derivatives produce relatively little objective change in the torticollis, but in our hands they have occasionally produced very satisfied patients. An occasional patient improves significantly on amantadine. Haloperidol has also been useful in some patients. Levodopa is of little value. Middle ear ionophoresis helps a small number of patients.[35] Integrated electromyographic biofeedback seems to be of more value. Fifty-six per cent of one prospective series showed major improvement initially, although 20 per cent later regressed.[69] Treatment was long and tedious, radiculopathy a frequent complication.

Torticollis is distinguished from the other dyskinesias by having the abnormal movements confined to a local group of muscles in the neck, including the sternocleidomastoid, trapezius, splenius capitis, and other upper pericervical muscles. As a result, operative procedures directed at denervating the muscles responsible for involuntary movements have remained popular in spasmodic torticollis, whereas they are now little used in any of the other dyskinesias. A major problem with these procedures in spasmodic torticollis, however, is that the involvement is bilateral and often extends somewhat beyond the range of muscles that can be denervated.

The most successful and widely used of these peripheral denervating procedures in spasmodic torticollis is anterior rhizotomy of the first three cervical segments bilaterally plus bilateral intradural section of the eleventh cranial nerve at the C1 level.[49,121] On occasion a unilateral section of the anterior root of C4 ipsilateral to the predominantly unilateral sternocleidomastoid and trapezius muscle involvement can be added. Bilateral C4 and lower anterior rhizotomies are, of course, contraindicated because of the danger of compromising function of the diaphragm through the phrenic innervation. Only a unilateral eleventh nerve section is indicated if only one sternocleidomastoid muscle seems to be involved in the torticollis.

The operation is done under general anesthesia in the sitting position through a midline incision with a laminectomy of C1 to C3 and a 1- to 1.5-cm posterior fossa craniectomy enlarged from the foramen magnum. The first anterior cervical root is sometimes identified with difficulty. Identification and severing of the most superior attachment of the dentate ligament will usually expose this root lying between the cord and the intradural entrance of the vertebral artery. Its accurate identification is obviously essential to avoid a C2 to C4 instead of the intended C1 to C3 rhizotomy. When the appropriate roots have been identified, they are sectioned, any small radicular blood vessels crossing the roots being left intact. The eleventh nerve is identified where it crosses the vertebral artery and is sectioned at that level.[49] Higher intradural section of the eleventh nerve—near the jugular foramen—may be indicated if the torticollis includes significant involvement of the trapezius muscle. Postoperatively the patient wears a soft collar for a two- to three-week period when upright, then tapering its use over approximately six weeks. The importance of a physical therapy program to strengthen the muscles of the neck and shoulder following this procedure has been emphasized.[31,49]

The complications of this procedure are limitation of voluntary rotation of the head in slightly over a third, and dysphagia in about a third of the patients. The dysphagia is related to the inability to lift the head while swallowing. It can be overcome by mechanically lifting the head with the hand when swallowing.[31] Almost three quarters of patients have some shoulder paresis, and slightly over half continue to complain of neck pain, though in a significant portion of these it is less than was present preoperatively.[49]

This operation does not completely denervate the sternocleidomastoid and trapezius muscles.[31,49] In part, this is because the bridging anterior rootlets, which may leave the spinal cord at the appropriate segmental level but then pass downward to exit from the dura at a lower level, have not been divided in the anterior rhizotomies that have been done. It has therefore been suggested that if these are still significant contractions in the sternocleidomastoid or trapezius muscles following this procedure, a peripheral eleventh nerve section should then be done, since this will give further denervation of these muscles.

Peripheral section of the eleventh nerve can be undertaken under local or general anesthesia. Incision can be made either parallel to the anterior border of the sternocleidomastoid or transversely in one of the skin creases centered over the anterior border of the sternocleidomastoid in the upper third of the neck. The sternocleidomastoid's anterior border is identified and retracted posteriorly. The nerve is found to lie on the posterior surface of the sternocleidomastoid muscle, sometimes buried within it, from which it travels in the deep cervical fascia extending up toward the transverse process of C2, which can be identified by upward retraction of the digastric muscle. The branch to the sternocleido-

mastoid alone can be separated by mobilizing the nerve from its course within the muscle. In this way the branch to the trapezius muscle can be preserved; or the entire peripheral eleventh nerve can be sectioned just proximal to entry into the sternocleidomastoid muscle.

With this combined approach, that is, anterior cervical rhizotomy from C1 to C3 bilaterally plus usually bilateral eleventh nerve section and later peripheral eleventh nerve section if needed, improvement has been reported in 79 per cent of patients with somewhat less than 10 per cent cured, on the basis of the patients' own estimates.[49] The addition of posterior rhizotomy of the upper cervical roots to the procedure appears to add nothing. Posterior rhizotomy alone may give occasional transient improvement but does not seem to result in permanent improvement in this dyskinesia. Unilateral intradural section of the twelfth cranial nerve at the time of anterior cervical rhizotomy may produce additional improvement when the tongue is involved in the dyskinesia.

Stereotaxic thalamic lesions can also produce relief of spasmodic torticollis. Long-term relief generally requires bilateral lesions, and occasionally no improvement is noted until the second side has been done.[23] Recurrence of torticollis several months postoperatively after initial satisfactory relief is a not infrequent complication. Relief has, however, been produced in 70 to 80 per cent of patients in several reported series.[23,87] Patients with spasmodic torticollis tend to be somewhat better candidates for operation than patients with Parkinson's disease. A significant risk to speech function with bilateral thalamotomies remains, however; in 5 per cent of cases it was lasting.[23,87] Stimulation under local anesthesia can be used as a guide for lesion placement, since in the presence of torticollis, stimulation in the ventrolateral thalamus will evoke the dystonia but such responses are not observed in the absence of torticollis. Stimulation in the region of the fields of Forel is said to evoke movements in the ipsilateral sternocleidomastoid muscle.[111] Stimulation is also useful in making certain that the lesion at the proposed site will not produce speech deficits.

Indeed, several thalamic target areas seem to offer comparable degrees of benefit in torticollis. In Cooper's series, lesions were placed on the medial side of the posterior ventrolateral thalamus.[23] Mundinger and co-workers found a target in the zona incerta, just beneath the thalamus to be most effective.[87] Bertrand has had his best results in torticollis with a lateral ventrolateral thalamic target, just adjacent to the capsule.[11] He indicates that this area is the thalamic portion of a vestibular relay involved in head turning. Microelectrode recording there shows a burst of activity when the patient looks to the side. The coordinates for this site are the $6/10$ block posterior to the anterior commissure on the intercommissural line, the $1/10$ segment above that line, and $5/10$ of the length of that line lateral.[11]

The choice of operative procedure for a particular patient with spasmodic torticollis has not been certainly resolved. In one comparative study, patients treated with thalamotomy did noticeably better than those treated with anterior cervical rhizotomy.[79] If the dystonic process extends beyond the upper cervical musculature, the sternocleidomastoid, and the trapezius muscles, then the stereotaxic approach would seem to be indicated. If the movement seems to be confined to the cervical muscles, then it is probably wisest to start with the anterior cervical rhizotomy and intradural accessory nerve section, coupling this with a peripheral eleventh nerve section if needed. If that fails, bilateral stereotaxic procedures may then be indicated in good-risk patients.

Choreoathetosis, Spasticity, and Cerebral Palsy

Choreic movements are sudden irregular fast jerks, usually of a relatively limited part of the body. Athetosis is characterized by slower, more writhing tonic movements that are differentiated from dystonia by being not quite so slow. These two types of involuntary motions are most commonly seen in the child with cerebral palsy whose injury occurred at or near the time of birth. There are generally widespread pathological changes in the brain in these patients, and they commonly have a mixture of involuntary movement disorders including dystonia, both chorea and athetosis, and in addition show mental disturbances, ataxia, and spasticity, often with attendant contractures. Operative therapy is of little or no benefit for the mental disturbances.[123]

With renewal of interest in operative treatments for the symptoms of cerebral palsy, experience has been gained with a number of procedures: ventrolateral thalamotomy, lesions of the dentate nucleus of the cerebellum, and most recently, long-term electrical stimulation of the anterior cerebellum.

The results obtained with ventrolateral thalamotomy have been quite variable. There is general agreement that only dystonic or choreoathetotic symptoms are helped by this procedure. Spasticity is not helped and may be worse postoperatively. Thus, the only patients with cerebral palsy who appear to be suitable candidates for consideration for thalamic stereotaxic procedures are those in whom the motion disorder predominates, with minimal, if any, spasticity or disturbances of mentation. The ability to evoke the dyskinetic movements with electrical stimulation at the target site remains a useful guide for lesions in patients with choreoathetosis.[71] Narabayashi has reported significant improvement after thalamotomy in 78 per cent of a rather extensive series of children with cerebral palsy.[88] He reports improvement in facial grimacing, leg scissoring, foot inversion, thumb abduction, and shoulder and rectus spasm. He believes that lesions should be placed relatively anteriorly in the ventrolateral thalamus or immediately beneath it in the field of Forel for this condition.[89] Spiegel and associates noted definite improvement in athetotic movements on the side of the body contralateral to lesions in the field of Forel in six cases.[125] Mundinger and co-workers report 18 per cent of 67 choreoathetotic patients notably improved and 32 per cent moderately improved at late follow-up.[87] Nearly all 67 patients were at least moderately improved initially. Other authors have found athetotic movements to be little helped by thalamic lesions; the choreic and dystonic elements, on the other hand, seem to respond better.[23,71,137]

Stereotaxic destruction of a portion of the dentate nucleus has also been of benefit in cerebral palsy. Lesions in the ventrolateral portions of that nucleus seem to give greatest functional improvement. Seigfried places the tip of the electrode at a point 10 mm behind the floor of the fourth ventricle, 5 mm below a line perpendicular to the floor that passes through the fastigium of the fourth ventricle, and 14 mm lateral to the midline.[120] The electrode is oriented in the axis of the nucleus, about 60 degrees to the floor of the fourth ventricle, and 30 degrees to the midline.[91,120] Large lesions should be made. Bilateral lesions may be made at one operation without undue risk. Physiological localization of the target may be obtained by eliciting ipsilateral tonic motor movements, chiefly of axial musculature, with stimulation. Microelectrode recording has been used to identify the borders of the nucleus by the appearance of activity.[120] Results obtained with dentate lesions seem to be a bit better than those obtained with thalamotomy and complications somewhat less. Initially, there is often a reduction in spasticity, though some of this improvement is lost in the following months. Choreoathetosis has improved noticeably, though the improvement is often not evident for some days after operation. That improvement seems to be maintained and may even increase over six months or so. About half the patients seem to achieve significant long-term functional improvement.[43]

Several factors seem to complicate the use of stereotaxic operations in cerebral palsy. There is probably very wide variability in the underlying disease process in these patients, so it is hard to generalize from one patient to another. The severity of the motion disorder is often such that the operations have to be carried out under general anesthesia, which entails loss of many of the physiological guides to localization and resultant greater inaccuracy in lesion placement. Finally, these patients appear to carry a somewhat greater risk of postoperative complications.

Recent experience has suggested that long-term electrical stimulation of the surface of the anterior cerebellar vermis may benefit some patients with cerebral palsy.[28,32,73] In this procedure, a pair of four-contact electrode strips is inserted over the superior surface of the cerebellum, one on each side of the anterior vermis. This is done through a suboccipital craniectomy, usually in the sitting position and under general anesthesia (with the appropriate precautions to avoid air embolism, as detailed elsewhere in this text). The dura is closed tightly around the leads. This is an important step, as spinal fluid dissection along the electrode track has been one of the major complications of this technique. The leads are then passed subcutaneously to a receiver, implanted either over the anterior chest wall or beneath the scalp near the vertex of the head. Postoperatively, the receiver is activated transcutaneously, at 200 Hz, 1 msec pulses, with alternation between electrode strips every eight minutes. Ten volts has been a common setting. Each unit should, however, be individually calibrated with a standard load and current probe before insertion. Effective currents are at present estimated to be in the range of 1.5 to 3.5 ma per electrode pair on the basis of a limited number of short-term measurements.[28,126] Effective levels of stimulation are said to reduce the amplitude of somatosensory evoked potentials by about 50 per cent and to reduce the amplitude of the "H" reflex, allowing some degree of "biocalibration" of an implanted unit.[126,134]

The effectiveness of this procedure in cerebral palsy is still being assessed. The major effect seems to be a reduction of spasticity. Improvement in choreoathetosis is less marked and may be entirely secondary to the changes in spasticity. More than two thirds of the patients in each series reported to date are said to be improved.[28,32,73] Degree of improvement is difficult to assess. On a rating scale, Cooper and associates reported, the best effects of stimulation were a 30 per cent reduction in average spasticity of all limbs compared with preoperative levels and a 19 per cent reduction in athetosis.[28] In that series, patients considered totally dependent decreased from 20 per cent of the group preoperatively to 7 per cent after stimulation, those "relatively independent" increased from 16 per cent to 20 per cent. Improvement in speech was seen less frequently; only half the patients in one series showed any improvement at all, which at best was considered moderate. Best results have been obtained in young patients, in their teens or earlier, who have IQ's above 70 and some evidence of intact muscle function underlying the spasticity. Improvement usually continues for a month or more after stimulation is initiated.

These operations are not without hazard. Mortality rate in one large series is 1 per cent, infection rate 2 per cent. Spinal fluid accumulations around the receiver have been the most common complication, often requiring a second procedure to close the dural leak. Late hydrocephalus has developed in a few patients in several series. A moderate number of patients have complained of headache with stimulation.[26]

The choice of procedures for a patient with cerebral palsy is presently in a state of flux. There is general agreement that all procedures provide greater benefit for younger patients, especially if some evidence of voluntary control of extremities is present and intellectual function is relatively intact. When the clinical picture is dominated by spasticity, cerebellar stimulation seems the most promising approach. When dyskinesias dominate the picture, stereotaxic operations on the thalamus or dentate nucleus are probably indicated. Dentatotomy has the advantage that both sides may be done in one sitting. What, if any, role there is for combinations of these operations in an aggressive approach to the symptoms of cerebral palsy remains to be determined.

Huntington's Chorea

Huntington's chorea is a hereditary condition with onset, usually in mid-adult life, of a diffuse chorea associated with mental deterioration. It is transmitted as an autosomal dominant trait with nearly complete penetrance. The course is progressive. Occasionally the disease may present in a juvenile form with rigidity, seizures, and dementia as the principal features. In either case, the strongly positive family history is a major clue to the diagnosis. The progressive nature of and the presence of mental deterioration in Huntington's chorea have generally contraindicated stereotaxic intervention. A very rare patient with this disease will, however, present with a severe and disabling chorea prior to showing evidence of any mental deterioration, and this patient may very occasionally be benefited by ventrolateral thalamotomy, especially if the chorea is unilateral.

Hemiballism

Hemiballistic movements are gross, violent, ceaseless (while awake) flinging movements particularly of the proximal musculature of the extremities. In its milder form, the movements seem to be indistinguish-able from a hemichorea, while in the more full-blown form, the violence of the movements and the particular involvement of proximal musculature are unique.[23] Hemiballistic movements are frequently associated with lesions of the subthalamic nucleus, but have been occasionally reported in cases in which the subthalamic nucleus is uninvolved; indeed, there is one seemingly valid case report in which hemiballismus followed a lesion in the postcentral gyrus.[23,143] A similar syndrome has been reproduced in animals by destroying approximately 20 per cent of the subthalamic nucleus.[21] An intact pallidum was necessary for production of the movements. In patients, this syndrome most commonly follows local infarction or hemorrhage in the region of the subthalamic nucleus. Its occurrence as a postoperative complication of thalamotomy has already been discussed.

The course of hemiballism is variable—spontaneous recovery occurs, but prolonged debility and death from exhaustion are not uncommon sequelae.[62,82] If the hemiballistic symptoms do not subside within a few weeks, operative therapy should be considered. In contrast to choreoathetosis, hemiballism has been fairly responsive to all types of operative treatment, including cortical excision, pedunculotomy, and cordotomy, as well as stereotaxic basal ganglia operation.[63,82] Ventrolateral thalamotomy contralateral to the involved limb probably is the procedure of choice. Relief can be expected in half the cases with this procedure.[23,87] The more mild "hemichorea" form of hemiballismus appeared to respond even better to ventrolateral thalamic lesions, with 69 per cent of patients in Cooper's series relieved of the hemichorea.[23] The risk of stereotaxic intervention appears to be somewhat greater in patients with hemiballismus than in those with Parkinson's disease.

Myoclonus

In myoclonus, sudden jerks, shorter and more abrupt than in chorea, produce a sudden complex movement, though occasionally involving a single muscle. Myoclonus occurs physiologically in the light stages of sleep. When myoclonus occurs as an involuntary movement disorder, it tends to stop with sleep and to be worsened by stress and voluntary movement. Myoclonus has been associated with pathological changes in rubro-dento-olivary circuitry, with some suggestion from animal studies that medial thalamic lesions may lower the threshold for its appearance.[86] Myoclonus may appear in association with other neurological symptoms, particularly epilepsy, as part of the progressive familial myoclonic epilepsy of Unverricht. Myoclonus may also be secondary to encephalitis and a number of degenerative diseases. Patients with myoclonic jerks associated with epileptiform electroencephalographic changes at the time of the jerk have generally not been considered suitable candidates for stereotaxic treatment. On the other hand, patients with myoclonus without electroencephalographic changes at the time of the jerk, who may also have epilepsy and other electroencephalographic changes, appear to respond as well to operative therapy as do those who have normal electroencephalograms and no history of epilepsy. Myoclonus may also appear in the absence of other neurological symptoms and electroencephalographic changes.

Patients considered for operative therapy for myoclonus have been free of dementia and other evidence of progressive neurological deterioration, and have not had electroencephalographic discharges associated with myoclonic jerks. Relief of myoclonus has followed lesions in the posterior ventrolateral thalamus and in the field of Forel.[53,144] In some cases unilateral lesions, contralateral to the side of major involvement in the jerks, produced bilateral improvement. Appearance of myoclonus ipsilateral to a unilateral lesion has occasionally necessitated a later contralateral lesion. Three quarters of patients achieve major symptomatic relief after thalamotomy.[87]

Palatal myoclonus represents a discrete and definitely separable syndrome in which the myoclonic jerks are much more rapid than in the peripheral muscles and are confined to the oral-pharyngeal-ocular muscles. This syndrome does not seem to have been subjected to operative therapy.

Intention Tremor

Tremor activated by movement—intention tremor—is most common in the upper extremity, particularly in the distal musculature. The movement that precipitates the tremor is usually volitional but may be postural. Occasionally even very slight postural movement may precipitate the tremor. The tremor is most commonly bilateral but often asymmetrical.[23] A constant head tremor and occasional resting tremor are also seen in some of these patients.

The underlying pathological substrate is considered to be the presence of abnormalities in the cerebellum or its efferent tracts, particularly in the dentate nucleus, and in the brachium conjunctivum. Intention tremor may be the predominant symptom in a number of conditions, including residua of encephalitis and trauma, and in cases of multiple sclerosis and Wilson's disease (hepatolenticular degeneration). In these last two conditions there are almost always other associated dyskinesias. In addition, intention tremor may be the sole symptom in a heredofamilial disorder that is somewhat more common in males. About 10 per cent of patients with heredofamilial tremor show some evidence of other dyskinesias.

Regardless of its cause, intention tremor responds well to stereotaxically placed thalamic lesions. However, other manifestations of underlying disease processes obviously may limit the indications for this type of operative intervention. In cases in which the tremor is secondary to multiple sclerosis, operation seems to be indicated in those patients who are completely or seriously incapacitated by the tremor. It had been suggested that patients should be followed for at least a year after the onset of tremor in order to make certain that it will not regress spontaneously.[23] Spasticity, if present, is likely to be made worse by the operation; nystagmus and scanning speech are not likely to be helped.[23,67] Tremor involving the head and neck will require bilateral thalamic lesions.[67] The indications for operative intervention in cases with Wilson's disease are persistence of the disabling tremor after an adequate trial of therapy with BAL and penicillamine, as well as reasonably intact liver function.[23] Tremor in cases of Wilson's disease tends to be coarse, with a flapping quality.

The optimal placement of thalamic lesions appears to be relatively posterior in the ventrolateral thalamus, the posterior edge of the lesion extending just into the ventroposterior lateral nucleus.[23] Electrical stimulation at the therapeutically effective site tends to drive the tremor, particularly if it is relatively inactive, but it may occasionally inhibit very active tremor.[67] The authors have found the subthalamic target described by Bertrand to be an especially useful initial target in intention tremor.[12] That target is identified by the letter "D" in Figures 140–1 and 140–2.

Thalamic operation is more effective in intention tremor than in any of the other dyskinesias. In the heredofamilial form, Cooper noted initial abolition of the tremor in 93 per cent of patients, with a 10 per cent recurrence rate in long-term (5 to 10 years) follow-ups.[23] When intention tremor was secondary to multiple sclerosis, initial relief was obtained in 85 per cent of patients and long-term relief (1 to 8 years) in about 72 per cent.[23,67] Occasionally some ipsilateral improvement as well as the predominant contralateral improvement is noted with these lesions. The patients with the heredofamilial form tend to be better operative candidates than patients with Parkinson's disease and have fewer postoperative complications. The risk of the operation in patients with multiple sclerosis and Wilson's disease depends principally on the associated deficits. Patients with multiple sclerosis also carry an additional risk of having an acute exacerbation of their disease precipitated by thalamotomy. This has been a rather frequent complication in the author's experience. The exacerbation has usually appeared in the second week after operation and has involved visual and spinal cord as well as cerebral symptoms of multiple sclerosis. Carrying these patients on large doses of dexamethazone during the first two weeks after operation seems to prevent this complication.

REFERENCES

1. Adams, R. D., van Bogaert, L., and Van der Eecken, H.: Striato-nigral degeneration. J. Neuropath. Exp. Neurol., 23:584–608, 1964.
2. Allan, C. M., Turner, J. W., and Gadea-Ciria, M.: Investigations into speech disturbances following stereotaxic surgery for parkinsonism. Brit. J. Disord. Commun., 1:55–59, 1966.
3. Alvord, E. C.: Pathology of parkinsonism. In Fields, W. S., ed.: Pathogenesis and Treatment of Parkinsonism. Springfield, Ill., Charles C Thomas, 1958, pp. 161–183.
4. Arvidsson, J., Roos, B. E., and Steg, G.: Reciprocal effects on α and γ motoneurons of drugs influencing monoaminergic and cholinergic

5. transmission. Acta Physiol. Scand., 67:398–404, 1966.
6. Barbeau, A.: Some biochemical disorders in Parkinson's disease—a review. J. Neurosurg., 24:162–164, 1966.
7. Barbeau, A.: The nonsurgical treatment of "Parkinson's disease": a personal view. In Morley, T., ed.: Current Controversies in Neurosurgery. Philadelphia, W. B. Saunders Co., 1976, pp. 419–428.
8. Barbeau, A.: Parkinson's disease: etiological considerations. In Yahr, M., ed.: The Basal Ganglia. New York, Raven Press, 1976, pp. 281–292.
9. Bates, J. A. V.: The electrophysiology of the human thalamus. J. Roy. Coll. Physicians Lond., 1:118, 1967.
10. Beck, E., and Bignami, A.: Some neuro-anatomical observations in cases with stereotactic lesions for the relief of parkinsonism. Brain, 91:589–618, 1968.
11. Bell, D. S.: Speech functions of the thalamus inferred from the effects of thalamotomy. Brain, 91:619–638, 1968.
12. Bertrand, C.: The treatment of spasmodic torticollis with particular reference to thalamotomy. In Morley, T., ed.: Current Controversies in Neurosurgery. Philadelphia, W. B. Saunders Co., 1976, pp. 455–460.
13. Bertrand, C., Martinez, S., Hardy, J., Molina-Negro, P., and Velasco, F.: Stereotaxic surgery for parkinsonism. Progr. Neurol. Surg., 5:79–112, 1973.
14. Bertrand, G.: Stimulation during stereotactic operations for dyskinesias. J. Neurosurg., 24:suppl.:419–428, 1966.
15. Booth, G.: Psychodynamics in parkinsonism. Psychosom. Med., 10:1–14, 1946.
16. Boshes, B., et al.: Signs, symptoms and methods of objective evaluation panel. J. Neurosurg., 24:suppl.:274–338, 1966.
17. Browder, J.: End results following the capsular operation for parkinsonism. Surg. Clin. N. Amer., 28:390–395, 1948.
18. Bucy, P.: Cortical extirpation in the treatment of involuntary movements. Res. Publ. Ass. Res. Ment. Dis., 21:551–595, 1942.
19. Bucy, P.: The surgical treatment of extrapyramidal disease. J. Neurol. Neurosurg. Psychiat., 14:108–117, 1951.
20. Byrnes, C. M.: A contribution to the pathology of paralysis agitans. Arch. Neurol. Psychiat., 15:407–443, 1926.
21. Calma, I., and Kidd, G. L.: The action of the anterior lobe of the cerebellum on alpha motoneurons. J. Physiol., 149:626–652, 1959.
22. Carpenter, M. B., and Mettler, F. A.: Analysis of subthalamic hyperkinesia in the monkey with special reference to ablations of the agranular cortex. J. Comp. Neurol., 95:125–157, 1951.
23. Chang, H. T., Ruch, T. C., and Ward, A. A., Jr.: Topographical representation of muscles in motor cortex of monkeys. J. Neurophysiol., 10:39–56, 1947.
24. Cooper, I. S.: Involuntary Movement Disorders. New York, Hoeber Medical Div. Harper & Rowe, 1969.
25. Cooper, I. S.: Effect of chronic stimulation of anterior cerebellum on neurological disease. Lancet, 1:1321, 1973.

25. Cooper, I. S.: Dystonia: Surgical approaches to treatment and physiologic implications. *In* Yahr, M., ed.: The Basal Ganglia. New York, Raven Press, 1976, pp. 369–384.

26. Cooper, I. S., Amin, I., Upton, A., Riklan, M., Watkins, S., and McLellan, L.: Safety and efficacy of chronic stimulation. Neurosurgery, *1*:203–205, 1977.

27. Cooper, I. S., and Bravo, G. J.: Implications of a five year study of 700 basal ganglia operations. Neurology, *8*:701–707, 1958.

28. Cooper, I., Riklan, M., Amin, I., Waltz, J., and Cullinan, T.: Chronic cerebellar stimulation in cerebral palsy. Neurology, *26*:744–753, 1976.

29. Cooper, I. S. Riklan, M., Stellar, S. Waltz, J. M., Levita, E., Ribera, V., and Zimmerman, J.: A multidisciplinary investigation of neurosurgical rehabilitation in bilateral parkinsonism. J. Amer. Geriat. Soc., *16*:1177–1306, 1968.

30. Cordeau, J. P.: Microelectrode studies in monkeys with postural tremor. Rev. Canad. Biol., *20*:147–157, 1961.

31. Dandy, W. E.: An operation for the treatment of spasmodic torticollis. Arch. Surg., *20*:1021–1032, 1930.

32. Davis, R., Cullen, R., Jr., Flitter, M., Duenas, D., Engle, H., and Ennis, B.: Control of spasticity and involuntary movements. Neurosurgery, *1*:205–207, 1977.

33. DeJong, D.: Parkinson's disease: Statistics. J. Neurosurg., *24*:suppl.:149–158, 1966.

34. Den Hartog, Jager, W. A., and Bethlem, J.: The distribution of Lewy bodies in the central and autonomic nervous systems in idiopathic paralysis agitans. J. Neurol. Neurosurg. Psychiat., *23*:283–290, 1960.

35. Duane, D., and Svien, H.: Preliminary evaluation of labyrinthian supression in the treatment of spasmotic torticollis. Neurology, *22*:399, 1972.

36. Eadie, M. J., and Sutherland, J. M.: Arteriosclerosis in parkinsonism. J. Neurol. Neurosurg. Psychiat., *27*:237–240, 1964.

37. Earle, K. M.: Studies on Parkinson's disease, including x-ray fluorescent spectroscopy of formalin fixed brain tissue. J. Neuropath. Exp. Neurol., *27*:1–14, 1968.

38. Eldred, E., Granit, R., and Merton, P. A.: Supraspinal control of the muscle spindles and its significance. J. Physiol., *122*:498–523, 1953.

39. England, A. C., Jr., and Schwab, R. S.: Parkinson's syndrome. New Eng. J. Med., *265*:785–792, 1961.

40. Fager, C.: Evaluation of thalamic and subthalamic surgical lesions in the alleviation of Parkinson's disease. J. Neurosurg., *28*:145–149, 1968.

41. Foltz, E. L., Knopp, L. M., and Ward, A. A., Jr.: Experimental spasmodic torticollis. J. Neurosurg., *16*:55–67, 1959.

42. Gardner, W. J.: Surgical aspects of Parkinson's syndrome. Postgrad. Med., *5*:107–112, 1949.

43. Garnall, P., Hitchcock, E., and Kirkland, I.: Stereotaxic neurosurgery in the management of cerebral palsy. Develop. Med. Child Neurol., *17*:279, 1975.

44. Gillingham, F. J.: Small localized surgical lesions of the internal capsule in the treatment of the dyskinesias. Confin. Neurol., *22*:385–392, 1962.

45. Gillingham, F. J.: Bilateral stereotactic lesions in the management of parkinsonism. J. Neurosurg., *24*:suppl.:449–457, 1966.

46. Gillingham, F. J., and Kalyanaraman, S.: The surgical treatment of oculogyric crises. Confin. Neurol., *26*:237–245, 1965.

47. Guiot, G., and Derome, P.: The principle of stereotaxic thalamotomy. *In* Kahn, E. A., Crosby, E. C., Schneider, R. C., and Taren, J.: Correlative Neurosurgery. Springfield, Ill., Charles C Thomas, 1969, chap. 18, pp. 376–401.

48. Guiot, G., Hardy, J., and Albe-Fessard, D.: Délimitation précise des structures sous-corticales et identification de noyaux thalamiques chez l'homme par l'electrophysiologie stéréotaxique. Neurochirurgia, *5*:1–18, 1962.

49. Hamby, W., and Schiffer, S.: Spasmodic torticollis: Results after cervical rhizotomy in 50 cases. J. Neurosurg., *31*:323–326, 1969.

50. Hassler, R.: Zur Pathologie der Paralysis agitans und des post-encephalitischen Parkinsonismus. J. Psychol. Neurol., *48*:387–476, 1938.

51. Hassler, R.: The influence of stimulations and coagulations in the human thalamus on the tremor at rest and its physiopathologic mechanisms. *In* Proceedings of the Second International Congress of Neuropathology, London, 1955. Amsterdam, Excerpta Medica Found. pt. 2:637–642.

52. Hassler, R., Mundinger, F., and Reichert, T.: Correlations between clinical and autoptic findings in stereotaxic operations of parkinsonism. Confin. Neurol., *26*:282–290, 1965.

53. Hassler, R., Reichert, T., Mundinger, T., Umbach, W., and Gangelberger, J.: Physiologic observations in stereotaxic operations in extrapyramidal motor disturbances. Brain, *83*:337–350, 1960.

54. Heimberger, R. F., and Whitlock, C. C.: Stereotaxic destruction of the human dentate nucleus. Confin. Neurol., *26*:346–358, 1966.

55. Henatsch, H. D., and Ingvar, D.: Chlorpromazin und Spastizität. Eine experimentelle elektrophysiologische Untersuchung. Arch. Psychiat., *195*:77–93, 1956.

56. Hoehn, M. M., and Yahr, M. D.: Parkinsonism: Onset, progression and mortality. Neurology, *17*:427–442, 1967.

57. Horsley, V.: The Linacre Lecture. The function of the so-called motor area of the brain. Brit. Med., J., *2*:125–132, 1909.

58. Horsley, V., and Clarke, R. H.: The structure and function of the cerebellum examined by a new method. Brain, *31*:45–124, 1908.

59. Housepian, E., and Purpura, D.: Electrophysiological studies of subcortical-cortical relations in man. Electroenceph. Clin. Neurophysiol., *15*:20–28, 1963.

60. Hughes, J. R.: The electroencephalogram in parkinsonism. J. Neurosurg., *24*:suppl.:369–376, 1966.

61. Hunt, C. C.: Reflex activity of mammalian smallnerve fiber. J. Physiol., *115*:456–469, 1951.

62. Hyland, H., and Forman, D.: The prognosis in hemiballism. Neurology, *7*:381–391, 1957.

63. Jane, J. A., Yashon, D., Becker, D., Beatty, R. and Sugar, O.: The effect of destruction of the corticospinal tract in the human cerebral peduncle upon motor function and involuntary movements. J. Neurosurg., 29:581–585, 1968.

64. Jenkins, A. C.: Speech defects following stereotaxic operations for relief of tremor and rigidity in parkinsonism. Med. J. Aust., 1:585–588, 1968.

65. Johnson, T. N., and Clemente, C. D.: An experimental study of the fiber connections between the putamen, globus pallidus, ventral thalamus and midbrain tegmentum in cat. J. Comp. Neurol., 112:83–101, 1959.

66. Jung, R., and Hassler, R.: The extrapyramidal motor system. In Magoun, H. W., et al., eds.: Handbook of Physiology. Baltimore, Md., Williams & Wilkins Co., 1960, vol. 2, pp. 863–927.

67. Krayenbühl, H., and Yasargil, M.: Relief of intention tremor due to multiple sclerosis by stereotaxic thalamotomy. Confin. Neurol., 22:368–374, 1962.

68. Krayenbühl, H., Wyss, O., and Yasargil, M.: Bilateral thalamotomy and pallidotomy as treatment for bilateral parkinsonism. J. Neurosurg., 18:429–444, 1961.

69. Korein, J., and Brudny, J.: Integrated EMG feedback in the management of spasmotic torticollis and focal dystonia: A prospective study of 80 patients. In Yahr, M., ed.: The Basal Ganglia. New York, Raven Press, 1976, pp. 385–424.

70. Kurland, L. T.: Epidemiology, incidence, geographic distribution, genetic considerations. In Fields, W. S., ed.: Pathogenesis and Treatment of Parkinsonism. Springfield, Ill., Charles C Thomas, 1958, pp. 5–49.

71. Laitinen, L.: Short term results of treatment for infantile cerebral palsy. Confin. Neurol., 26:258–263, 1965.

72. Laitinen, L., Johnannson, G., and Sipponew, P.: Impedance and phase angle as a locating method in human stereotaxic surgery. J. Neurosurg., 25:628–633, 1966.

73. Larson, S., Sances, A., Jr., Hemmy, D., and Millar, E.: Physiological and histological effects. Neurosurgery, 1:212–213, 1977.

74. Larson, S. J., and Sances, A. J.: Averaged evoked potentials in stereotaxic surgery. J. Neurosurg., 28:227–232, 1968.

75. Leksell, L.: The action potential and excitatory effects of the small ventral root fibers to skeletal muscle. Acta Physiol. Scand., 10:suppl. 31:1–84, 1945.

76. Leksell, L.: The stereotaxic method and radioscopy of the brain. Acta. Chir. Scand., 10:316–319, 1951.

77. Marsden, C., and Harrison, M.: Idiopathic torsion dystonia. Brain, 97:793–810, 1974.

78. Maspes, P. S., and Pagni, C. A.: Surgical treatment of dystonia and choreoathetosis in infantile cerebral palsy by pedunculotomy. J. Neurosurg., 21:1076–1086, 1964.

79. Meares, R.: Natural history of spasmodic torticollis and effect of surgery. Lancet, 2:149–151, 1971.

80. Meier, M. J., and Story, J. L.: Selective impairment of Porteus Maze test performance after right subthalamotomy. Neurospsychologia, 5:181–189, 1967.

81. Meyers, R.: The modification of alternating tremor, rigidity and festination by surgery of the basal ganglia. Res. Publ. Ass. Res. Nerv. Ment. Dis., 21:602–665, 1942.

82. Meyers, R.: Ballismus. In Vinken, P. J., and Bruyn, G. W., eds.: Handbook of Clinical Neurology. Diseases of the Basal Ganglia. Vol. 6, Amsterdam, North-Holland Pub. Co., 1968–1969, chap. 19, pp. 476–490.

83. Meyers, R.: Discussion of Spiegel et al.: Campotomy in various extrapyramidal disorders. J. Neurosurg., 20:881–882, 1963.

84. Meyers, R.: The surgery of the hyperkinetic disorders. In Vinken, P. J., and Bruyn, G. W., eds.: Handbook of Clinical Neurology. vol. 6, Diseases of the Basal Ganglia. Amsterdam, North-Holland Pub. Co., chap. 33, pp. 844–878, 1968–1969.

85. Meyers, R., and Hayne, R. A.: Tridimensional analysis of deep and superficial structures of the human brain (exhibit). Trans. Amer. Neurol. Ass., 73:175, 1948.

86. Milhorat, T. H.: Experimental myoclonus of thalamic origin. Arch. Neurol., 17:365–378, 1967.

87. Mundinger, F., Reichert, T., and Disselhoff, J.: Long term results of stereotaxic operations on extrapyramidal hyperkinesias (excluding parkinsonism). Confin. Neurol., 32:71–78, 1970.

88. Narabayashi, H.: Stereotaxic surgery for athetosis or the spastic state of cerebral palsy. Confin. Neurol., 22:364–367, 1962.

89. Narabayashi, H., and Kubota, K.: Reconsideration of ventrolateral thalamotomy for hyperkinesias. Progr. Brain Res., 21B:339–349, 1966.

90. Narabayashi, H., and Okuma, T.: Stereotaxic operation (3rd. report)—procaine oil blocking of pallidum in cases of athetose double. Psychiat. Neurol. Jap., 54:672–677, 1953.

91. Nashold, B., and Slaughter, D. G.: Effects of stimulating or destroying the deep cerebellar regions in man. J. Neurosurg., 31:172–186, 1969.

92. Nauta, W. J. H., and Mehler, W. R.: Projections of the lentiform nucleus in the monkey. Brain Res., 1:1–38, 1966.

93. Ojemann, G.: Language and the thalamus: Object naming and recall during and after human thalamic stimulation. Brain Lang., 2:101–110, 1975.

94. Ojemann, G.: Subcortical language mechanisms. In Whitaker, H., and Whitaker, H., eds.: Studies in neurolinguistics. Vol. 1. New York, Academic Press, 1976, pp. 103–138.

95. Ojemann, G.: Asymmetric functions of the thalamus in man. Ann. N.Y. Acad. Sci., 299:380–396, 1977.

96. Ojemann, G., and Van Buren, J.: Respiratory, heart rate and GSR responses from human diencephalon. Arch. Neurol., 16:74–88, 1967.

97. Ojemann, G., and Ward, A.: Present indications for L-dopa and thalamotomy in the treatment of Parkinson's disease. Northwest Med., 70:101–104, 1971.

98. Ojemann, G., and Ward, A.: Speech representa-

tion in ventrolateral thalamus. Brain, *94*:669–680, 1971.

99. Ojemann, G., Hoyenga, K., and Ward, A., Jr.: Prediction of short term verbal memory disturbance after ventrolateral thalamotomy. J. Neurosurg., *35*:203–210, 1971.

100. Oliver, L.: Parkinson's Disease. Springfield, Ill., Charles C Thomas, 1967.

101. Paillard, J.: Réflexes et Régulations d'Origine Proprioceptive Chez l'Homme. Etude Neurophysiologique et Psychophysiologique. Paris, Libraire Arnette, 1955.

102. Parkinson, J.: An Essay on the Shaking Palsy. London, Whittingham & Rowland, 1817.

103. Penfield, W., and Robert, L.: Speech and Brain Mechanisms. Princeton, Princeton University Press, 1959.

104. Poirier, L. J.: Neuroanatomical study of an experimental postural tremor in monkeys. J. Neurosurg., *24*:191–193, 1966.

105. Poirier, L. J., Ohye, C., and Bouchard, R.: Effect of dorsal rhizotomy on postural tremor in the monkey. Physiologist, *12*:329, 1969.

106. Pollock, L., and Davis, L.: Muscle tone in parkinsonian states. Arch. Neurol. Psychiat., *23*:303–311, 1930.

107. Pollock, M., and Hornabrook, R. W.: The prevalence, natural history and dementia of Parkinson's disease. Brain, *89*:429–448, 1966.

108. Poskanzer, D. C., and Schwab, R. S.: Cohort analysis of Parkinson's syndrome. J. Chronic Dis., *16*:961–973, 1963.

109. Putnam, T. J.: The operative treatment of diseases characterized by involuntary movements (tremor, athetosis). Res. Publ. Ass. Res. Nerv. Ment. Dis. *21*:666–696, 1942.

110. Reichert, T.: Stereotaxic surgery for treatment of Parkinson's syndrome. Progr. Neurol. Surg., *5*:1–78, 1973.

111. Sano, K., Yashioka, M., Ogarkiwa, M., Ishijimia, B., Ohye, C., Sekino, H., and Mayanogi, Y.: Central mechanisms of neck movement in the human brain stem. Confin. Neurol., *29*:107–111, 1967.

112. Sasaki, K., and Tanaka, T.: Phasic and tonic innervation of spinal alpha motoneurones from upper brain centers. Jap. J. Physiol., *14*:56–66, 1964.

113. Schaltenbrand, G.: The effects of stereotactic electrical stimulation in the depth of the brain. Brain, *88*:835–840, 1965.

114. Schwab, R. S., and England, A. C., Jr.: Parkinson syndromes due to various specific causes. *In* Vinken, P. J., and Bruyn, G. W., eds.: Handbook of Clinical Neurology. Vol. 6, Diseases of the Basal Ganglia. Amsterdam, North Holland Pub. Co., 1968–1969, chap. 9, pp. 227–247.

115. Schwab, R., England, A., Chafety, M., Timberlake, W., Poskanzer, D., and Tweksbury, H.: A ten year followup of the effect of surgical and medical therapy, training, age and other factors on progression in 100 patients with Parkinson's disease. Scientific Exhibit, American Academy of Neurology, New York, 1962.

116. Scott, R., Brody, J., Schwab, R., and Cooper, I.: Progression of unilateral tremor and rigidity in Parkinson's disease. Neurology, *20*:710–714, 1970.

117. Selby, G.: Stereotaxic surgery for the relief of Parkinson's disease. II. An analysis of the results of a series of 303 patients (413 operations). J. Neurol. Sci., *5*:343–375, 1967.

118. Selby, G.: Parkinson's disease. *In* Vinken, P. J., and Bruyn, G. W., eds.: Handbook of Clinical Neurology. Vol. 6, Diseases of the Basal Ganglia. Amsterdam, North-Holland Pub. Co., 1968–1969, chap. 6, pp. 173–211.

119. Shapiro, D., Sadowsky, D., Henderson, W., and Van Buren, J.: An assessment of cognitive function in postthalamotomy Parkinson patients. Confin. Neurol., *35*:144–166, 1973.

120. Siegfried, J., Esslen, E., Gretener, U., Ketz, E., and Perret, E.: Functional anatomy of the dentate nucleus in the light of stereotaxic operations, Confin. Neurol., *32*:1–10, 1970.

121. Sorenson, B. F., and Hamby, W. B.: Spasmodic torticollis: Results in 71 surgically treated patients. Neurology, *19*:867–878, 1966.

122. Sourkes, T. L.: Effect of brain stem lesions on the concentration of catecholamines in basal ganglia of the monkey. J. Neurosurg., *24*:194–195, 1966.

123. Spiegel, E. A., and Baird, H. W.: Athetotic syndromes. *In* Vinken, P. J., and Bruyn, G. W., eds.: Handbook of Clinical Neurology. Vol. 6, Diseases of the Basal Ganglia. Amsterdam, North-Holland Pub. Co., 1968–1969, chap. 18, pp. 440–475.

124. Spiegel, E. A., Wycis, H. T., Marks, M., and Lee, A. J.: Stereotaxic apparatus for operations on human brain. Science, *106*:349–350, 1947.

125. Spiegel, E. A., Wycis, H., Szekely, E., Adams, J., Flanagan, M., and Baird, H.: Campotomy in various extrapyramidal disorders. J. Neurosurg., *20*:871, 1963.

126. Stances, A., Jr., Larson, S., Myklebust, J., Swiontek, T., Millar, E., Cusick, J., Hemmy, D., Jodat, R., and Ackmann, J.: Studies of electrode configuration. Neurosurgery, *1*:207–212, 1977.

127. Steg, G.: Efferent muscle innervation and rigidity. Acta Physiol. Scand., *61*:suppl. 225:1–53, 1964.

128. Stern, J., and Ward, A. A., Jr.: Inhibition of the muscle spindle discharge by ventrolateral thalamic stimulation. Arch. Neurol., *3*:193–204, 1960.

129. Stern, J., and Ward, A. A., Jr.: Supraspinal and drug modulation of the alpha motor system. Arch. Neurol., *6*:404–413, 1962.

130. Stern, J., and Ward, A. A., Jr.: The relationship of the alpha and gamma motor systems to the efficacy of the surgical therapy of parkinsonism. J. Neurosurg., *20*:185–187, 1963.

130a. Sypert, G., Leffman, H., and Ojemann, G.: Occult normal pressure hydrocephalus manifested by parkinsonism-dementia complex. Neurology (Minneap.), *23*:234–238, 1973.

131. Talairach, J., Hecaen, H., David, M., Monnies, M., and Ajuriaguerra, J. de.: Recherches sur la coagulation thérapeutique des structures sous-corticales chez l'homme. Rev. Neurol., *81*:4–24, 1949.

132. Taren, J., Guiot, G., Derome, P., and Trigo, J.: Hazards of stereotaxic thalamectomy. Added safety factor in corroborating x-ray target lo-

calization with neurophysiological methods. J. Neurosurg., *29*:173–182, 1968.

133. Uno, M., Kukota, K., Ohye, C., Nagao, T., and Narabayashi, H.: Topographical arrangement between thalamic ventrolateral nucleus and precentral motor cortex in man. Electroenceph. Clin. Neurophysiol., *22*:437–443, 1967.

134. Upton, A., and Cooper, I.: Some neurophysiological effects of cerebellar stimulation in man. Canad. J. Neurol. Sci., *3*:237–254, 1976.

135. Van Buren, J. M., and Borke, R. C.: Variations of the Human Diencephalon. Vol. 2. New York, Springer-Verlag, 1972.

136. Van Buren, J., Li, C. L., Shapiro, D., Henderson, W., and Sadowsky, D.: A qualitative and quantitative evaluation of parkinsonians three to six years following thalamotomy. Confin. Neurol., *35*:202–235, 1973.

137. Van Manen, J.: Indications for stereotaxic operations in cerebral palsy. Confin. Neurol., *26*: 254–257, 1965.

138. Van Manen, J.: Long-term results of stereotactic operations for Parkinson's disease. Psychiat., Neurol. Neurochir., *73*:365–374, 1970.

139. Vinken, P. J., and Bruyn, G. W., eds.: Handbook of Clinical Neurology. Vol. 6, Diseases of the Basal Ganglia. Amsterdam, North-Holland Pub. Co., 1968–1969.

140. Walker, A. E.: Cerebral pedunculotomy for relief of involuntary movements: I. Hemiballismus. Acta Psychiat. Neurol., *24*:723–729, 1949.

141. Ward, A. A., Jr.: The function of the basal ganglia. *In* Vinken, P. J., and Bruyn, G. W., eds.: Handbook of Clinical Neurology. Vol. 6, Diseases of the Basal Ganglia. Amsterdam, North-Holland Pub. Co., 1968–1969, chap. 3, pp. 90–115.

142. Ward, A. A., Jr., McCulloch, W. S., and Magoun, H. W.: Production of an alternating tremor at rest in monkeys. J. Neurophysiol., *11*:317–330, 1948.

143. Wilson, S. A. K.: Die Pathogenese der unwillkürlichen Bewegungen mit besonderer Berücksichtigung der Pathologie und Pathogenese der Chorea. Deutsch. Z. Nervenheilk, *108*:4–38, 1929.

144. Wycis, H. T., and Spiegel, E. A.: Campotomy in myoclonia. J. Neurosurg., *30*:708–793, 1969.

145. Yakovlev, P. I.: The central "paradox" of Parkinson's disease. J. Neurosurg., *24*:suppl.: 292–298, 1966.

146. Zeman, W., and Dyken, P.: Dystonia musculorum deformans. *In* Vinken, P., and Bruyn, G., eds.: Handbook of Clinical Neurology. Vol. 6, Diseases of the Basal Ganglia. Amsterdam, North-Holland Pub. Co., 1968–1969, chap. 21, pp. 517–543.

141

NEUROSURGICAL ASPECTS OF EPILEPSY IN CHILDREN AND ADOLESCENTS

The basis for the neurosurgical treatment of epilepsy during childhood and adolescence is multifactorial. Because of the complexities of the epilepsies, both diagnostically and therapeutically, a team effort is required. Participating neurosurgeons need to have specific training and interest in: the preoperative clinical and laboratory studies, the selection of patients for operative treatment, the operative techniques, and the postoperative care and rehabilitation of these children and adolescents. Other members of the group include neurologists, electroencephalographers, neuroradiologists, pediatricians, psychiatrists, neuropsychologists, and social workers.

Convulsive disorders of the newborn, the child, and the adolescent represent a group of the most frequent and challenging disorders known to medicine.* The incidence of seizures in the pediatric population is approximately 7 per cent. With maturation and adulthood this figure drops to 1 per cent.[233] Sixty-seven per cent of cases of epilepsy have had their onset between birth and the age of 19.[289,296]

Repetitive seizures and medications during childhood and adolescence may contribute to behavioral and medical problems that impede or alter normal development of the individual as an independent and productive member of society.[184] Accordingly,

these medical and social factors, coupled with the ability to delineate specific, localized, and resectable epileptogenic lesions, form the basis for the neurosurgical treatment of epilepsy during these years of development. Fortunately, the long-term results of operative treatment may be equal or superior to those of many other more common intracranial operations.

ORIGINS OF OPERATIVE TREATMENT OF EPILEPSY

The treatment of epilepsy has changed according to the current conceptions of the causes of seizures since the beginnings of medicine. Historical aspects of epilepsy are well documented.† In early civilizations, trephinations were practiced for convulsions, allegedly to release or remove supernatural or natural causes. Following his postmortem dissections of epileptics, Boerhaave pointed out that birth trauma as well as a peculiar state of the brain may be present in patients who develop epilepsy.[26] Such ideas brought into being a classification of *idiopathic* and *symptomatic epilepsies*. Pre-Listerian operations for seizures were associated with a mortality rate of over 50 per cent—due mainly to sepsis.

---

* See references 49, 184, 188, 266, 297.

† See references 74, 123, 202, 230, 233, 249, 273, 345, 368.

J. R. GREEN AND A. D. SIDELL

Such procedures were unrewarding until the advent of aseptic techniques and the development of more understanding of cerebral localization during the last quarter of the nineteenth century.

Hughlings Jackson, following intensive study of focal epilepsy between 1864 and 1870, predicted that areas existed in the cerebral cortex that governed movements.[158-161] Electrical stimulation of the cerebral cortex, in animals in 1870 and in man in 1874, confirmed the jacksonian predictions by producing specific movements.[19,94] Jackson formulated concepts that explained paroxysmal seizures of all sorts and considered that the manifestations of epilepsy formed the key to the workings of the nervous system. His statements, "Epilepsy is the name for occasional, sudden, excessive, rapid and local discharge of the gray matter" and "The highly explosive cells of discharging lesions will, on their fulminating discharge, overcome the resistance of, and thus produce excessive discharge of, collateral stable nervous elements" remain pertinent.[159] During the next decade, Jackson and Ferrier continued clinical and laboratory studies of cerebral localization.[86,160] Jackson's first registrar, Gowers, in *Epilepsies and Other Convulsive Disease* stated that operative treatment of focal epilepsy was feasible.[119]

Horsley's first craniotomy at the National Hospital, Queen Square, London, in 1886, was for post-traumatic epilepsy.[148] Horsley demonstrated that in focal epilepsy a point could be found in the cerebral cortex that would give rise to the seizure and that excision of this area was usually followed by cessation of the attacks.[148,149] He later developed subpial resection in order to minimize scar formation following cortical excision and described subpial cortical excision in 1909 ("a vertical incision through the pia mater along the midline of the surface of the convolution, reflecting the pia mater to the sulci on each side and gently separating it to the bottom of the sulci so as to permit of excising the whole depth of the gyrus . . . without any injury to the neighboring gyri").[150]

Foerster and Krause emphasized the importance of reproducing the spontaneous convulsion or aura by electrical stimulation of the cortex rather than relying on charts and anatomical landmarks.[88,180] Foerster and Penfield pioneered in defining the structural basis of traumatic epilepsy and reported their results with radical operations in 1930.[90] The Foerster Institute in Breslau and the Montreal Neurological Institute, which were opened in 1934, were "dedicated to the treatment of sickness and pain and to the study of neurology," having to do, at least in part, with all that might be done for epileptics and all that epilepsy might teach about the brain and mind of man.[244]

The first correlations of clinical epileptic seizures and electroencephalographic studies were published in 1935 by Gibbs, Davis, and Lennox.[108] Electrocorticographic studies in man were initially described by Foerster and Altenburger in the same year and subsequently, in America, in 1939 by Sachs, Schwartz, and Kerr, and in 1941 by Scarff and Rahm and by Penfield and Erickson.[89,246,307,310] The demonstration of hyperirritability of an epileptic area, seen by prolonged afterdischarge in response electrical stimulation, was pointed out later by Walker and co-workers in 1947 as an aid in delineating an epileptogenic focus.[363,372] Electrocorticography has clearly demonstrated that the circatrix itself is inert and that the epileptogenic area is adjacent to this scar.

During the century that has elapsed since Jackson's doctrines were developed, physiological, morphological, and chemical information has added to the growing body of knowledge about the epilepsies and provides the basis for current therapy.

NEUROBIOLOGY OF SEIZURES

Almost any disorder of the body, including the brain, that can significantly alter the morphology, physiology, and chemistry of, and the blood flow to, selected nerve cells within the brain may cause a clinical seizure. The pattern of the clinical seizure will be determined by the site of the epileptogenic area and its synaptic connections.

Morphology

There has been considerable investigation of the mechanisms underlying the epileptogenic focus in the human cortex. Early laboratory models were unable to simulate the fundamental properties of human epilepsy (i.e., the presence of recurrent spontaneous seizures) until the techniques of using alumina cream to create foci in the motor cortices of monkeys were developed.[177,178]

Studies of epileptic neurons in the laboratory and operating room by Ward and associates since 1955 have determined that epileptic foci have the following morphological characteristics: depopulation of neurons with those remaining being smaller than normal, astrocytic gliosis in which the neurons are embedded, striking loss of dendritic spines, and other changes in the dendritic structures as assessed by Golgi stains.[9,375-379,382]

The hypothesis that an active epileptogenic focus continues to undergo pathological changes has been confirmed in the chronically epileptic monkey and in the human.[39,141,312,382] This continuing neuronal degeneration secondary to the frequency and severity of continuing seizures has led Ward to advise that "the prudent strategy would appear to consist of aggressive medical therapy . . . for that period of time necessary to make the judgment in that patient in which a spontaneous remission is not likely to occur. To delay surgical therapy for long periods of time appears to carry the inevitable price of continuing neuronal damage in the vicinity of the focus."[378]

A multiplicity of epileptogenic lesions has been reported, including virtually all the known diseases of the brain. The common denominator in these epileptogenic areas—whether the primary lesion is a neoplasm, cyst, malformation of the brain and of its blood vessels including hamartomas, scars following the healing of penetrating head wounds or abscesses, atrophy and gliosis after brain damage in closed injury, and the effects of hypoxia, ischemia, encephalitis, and meningitis—is the destruction and removal of neurons, impairment of others, occlusion of local vascular networks, and gliosis.

A study of the pathological changes to be found in the brains of patients with chronic epilepsy who had died of natural causes was reported as early as 1825 with observation of induration in the hippocampus in 9 of 18 patients.[32] The importance of this relationship in epilepsy was largely ignored until 1935 when the same condition (*Ammon's horn sclerosis,* the then-current descriptive title) was described at postmortem examination in 36 of 53 cases of epilepsy.[334] Ammon's horn sclerosis was found in slightly more than half the brains examined by Sano and Malamud.[308] Earle, Baldwin, and Penfield provided the experimental data to link injury of the mesial temporal structures with the birth process and to relate this injury to subsequent sclerosis and epilepsy, coining the term "incisural sclerosis."[66] Three years later, in 1956, a study of 40 Falconer's en bloc temporal lobectomies revealed lesions in the mesial structures of the temporal lobe peripheral to Ammon's horn, making it difficult to decide upon the epileptic zone.[46] This led to a new term "mesial temporal sclerosis"—a sclerotic process of the hippocampal structures (uncus, amygdala, and Ammon's horn).[81]

Falconer has summarized evidence to show that mesial temporal sclerosis is an acquired lesion and not an inherited one, although a positive family history was found in about 15 per cent of the cases, indicating a strong genetic factor in those instances. He and his colleagues believe that this lesion is commonly the result of an asphyxial episode in infancy, at birth, with prolonged febrile convulsions or status epilepticus, occurring at a period in life when the hippocampus and other mesial structures are particularly vulnerable to anoxia. The thesis is that the damage caused during infancy subsequently develops into a sclerotic process that becomes the epileptogenic lesion—one of the most common single causes of epilepsy of generalized, psychomotor, or absence types originating during childhood and adolescence. Mesial temporal sclerosis and incisural sclerosis are considered to be the same lesion and based on anoxia from a variety of causes.[70,72-75,77,78,214] Autopsy studies have shown that this lesion is unilateral in about 90 per cent of cases.[81,198] Falconer has reported that mesial temporal sclerosis was the most frequent single lesion in his 250 cases (children and adults) of temporal lobectomy, and the lesions whose excision provided his patients with the best results from the standpoints of relief of epilepsy and improvement in social adaptation. He reported finding hamartomas in 20 per cent of his operations, miscellaneous lesions in 10 to 15 per cent, and equivocal lesions in 20 to 35 per cent.[79]

Brown and the Scheibels, in a morphological study of Crandall's surgical specimens from 29 patients (children and adults) with complex partial seizures found mesial temporal sclerosis in 65 per cent, hamartomas in 18 per cent, miscellaneous lesions in 3 per cent, and no lesions in 14 per cent.[39,312] In a study of procedures for epilepsy in children and adults, Mathieson has recently analyzed 857 epileptogenic lesions of the temporal lobe that were removed by Penfield and associates from 1928 to 1973 of which 35 per cent were "sclerotic temporal atrophy." The smaller percentage was explained by the use of suction rather than en bloc techniques for removal of mesial structures in a number of the patients. Discrete focal lesions were found in 202 patients, poorly circumscribed lesions in 315, anomalies in 2, minor abnormalities in 167, and no pathological condition in 167.[206] Reports concerning epileptogenic lesions of the temporal lobe from other centers, including the authors' own, add no additional information.[125]

Physiology

Kaufman, working under Pavlov and Bectherev in 1912, was probably the first to show that during a seizure abnormal electrical activity arose from the brain and not from the muscles, thus contradicting the work of Gotch and Horsley in England.[35]

The accuracy of Jackson's hypothesis that the epileptic ictus was rapid excessive discharge by gray matter has been directly verified by single unit recordings during the ictal state.[283]

Epileptic Neurons

Epileptic neurons, the foci of abnormal cells that initiate the epileptic discharge, possess the following properties:

Autonomous electrical behavior is due to fewer synaptic endings on dendrites with partial deafferentation and is possible related to circulating chemical substances and spontaneous or excessive discharges.[373,382]

Electrical hyperexcitability, which is not evident in normal cells, is possibly due

circulating chemical substances that promote spontaneous and excessive discharges.[352] Paroxysmal epileptiform discharges of this nature have been demonstrated by the presence of prolonged afterdischarges on direct cortical stimulation and with evoked responses.[59,101,372]

Electrical negativity in relation to the surface of the surrounding cortex is due to a standing partial depolarization of epileptic cell membranes, which causes an increased membrane permeability to depolarizing cations.

Paroxysmal depolarization shifts of their membrane potentials, their action potentials being transmitted via the efferent processes of the epileptic cells, results in epileptic activation of surrounding normal cells and of synaptically related normal cells. The effect of high-frequency synaptic bombardment by the epileptic focus potentiates the firing of normal cells—an essential for the initiation of clinical seizures.[314]

Capability of producing secondary epileptic foci is based on continuous bombardment by the epileptogenic lesion.[153,218,385,386] The development of a mirror focus (a secondary discharging lesion in the homologous hemisphere) and the frequency of bilateral temporal electroencephalographic foci in complex partial seizures support the concept of secondary epileptogenesis.

Epileptic neurons may fire at rates of 200 to 900 per second (normal, 20 per second) during their bursts, which may last from 10 to 40 msec or longer, resulting in disruption of the normal activities of the postsynaptic neuron.[43] Thus, a group of such primary "pacemaker" neurons (those that fire first) in an epileptic focus might be expected to widen the extent of the apparent focus via its synaptic connections to adjacent normal neurons. Pacemaker neurons are intermixed with other neurons whose patterns of firing may vary between normal and epileptic bursts.[394] Data from the monkey model suggest that the epileptic focus contains a spectrum of neurons, including: group 1 or "pacemaker" epileptic neurons, which fire in bursts of 200 to 900 per second, that cannot be modified by sleep or by operant conditioning; and group 2 epileptic cells that fire with lower burst indices and vary from high-frequency burst firing to normal activity, easily conditioned as normal cells; and normal neurons. Group 2 epileptic neurons might represent the potential "critical mass" available for rapid enlargement of a focus necessary to start a spreading, clinical seizure and may have their epileptogenic properties diminished during operant conditioning. Data regarding the therapeutic potential of operant conditioning to control epileptic seizures has, as yet, not been established in an adequate series of patients.[395]

Seizures are precipitated from epileptic neurons as their propagatory burst activity recruits normal cells also to fire in a bursting fashion. Other factors have been identified with the process, such as behavioral arousal and behavioral stress.[393] Alterations of local extracellular potassium ion concentration and other related chemical events in seizures are discussed in the section on chemistry.

The circuits of spread of epileptic discharges depend upon the cells of origin. Preferential pathways from cortical to subcortical structures have been delineated from the frontal granular cortex to the caudate nucleus and dorsomedial thalamic nucleus; the perirolandic cortex to the putamen and the lateral nuclear mass of the thalamus; the temporal cortex to the amygdala, hippocampus, and septum; and the visual striate cortex to the pulvinar and lateral geniculate nucleus of the dorsal thalamus. Temporary episodes of aphasia, apraxia, agnosia, disorientation, illusions in time or place, depression, paranoia, or paralysis may occur with epileptic activity in one or more of these circuits.[263,291,353,373] In addition, continuous interictal firing may modify the otherwise normal functioning of these circuits, resulting in a variety of cognitive and behavioral deficits. If this is so, the goal of therapy should also be to reduce interictal as well as ictal epileptic events, since "interictal firing may not be functionally innocuous."[378]

"Kindling," in which over a period of a few weeks permanent changes in seizure susceptibility can result from repeated, short, daily, initially ineffective stimulation, was reported in 1969.[115] The possibility is real, therefore, that the rate of recurrence of seizures, in man, at one time of life, may influence the long-term prognosis. It has been speculated that "kindling" may account for some aspects of post-traumatic seizures and be the basis for the production of excitable neurons in the vicinity of the

limited number of "epileptic" neurons in the focus, thus producing the critical mass of hyperactive cells that is necessary to induce a clinical seizure.[116] If developing neuronal hyperactivity could be blocked by prophylactic anticonvulsant medications, this sequence could be suppressed. Clinical reports have confirmed this postulate, and a rationale for postoperative anticonvulsant therapy has been established.[378]

The effect of anoxia on the different survival and revival times for particular brain regions was established in 1938.[338] Electrical potentials were found to disappear in the following order from: (1) Ammon's horn and cerebellar gray (2) cerebral cortex, (3) subcortical white matter, (4) corona radiata, (5) caudate nucleus, (6) ventrolateral nucleus of the thalamus, and (7) lateral geniculate body and medulla. Not all nerve cells in the central nervous system are capable of producing clinical epilepsy (e.g., those in the cerebellum, lower brain stem, and spinal cord), but the cerebral cortex, including the hippocampal region and Ammon's horn are potentially epileptogenic in addition to being particularly susceptible to anoxia, injury, neoplasms, vascular changes, and other pathological changes.

As early as 1939, the cerebral blood flow was reported to be increased in the region surrounding the primary epileptic focus in the sensorimotor cortex of monkeys, and in the thalamus, putamen, and globus pallidus.[257] The increased flow during the seizures was measured by a thermocouple method. Subcortical structures in connection with induced epileptic discharges, have been demonstrated to show increased regional cerebral blood flow by the ^{14}C-antipyrine method, although the regional cerebral blood flow method does not permit detailed interpretation of timing or subcortical interactions.[151,285] Interictal neuronal activity is also associated with a local increase of metabolism and cerebral blood flow.[15,152,154] Epileptic seizures are associated with increased metabolism and cerebral blood flow in the nervous tissue associated in the paroxysmal discharge.*

Experimental work has focused on a tight coupling in brain between metabolic changes, blood flow, and electrical dis-

---

* See references 38, 55, 183, 240, 257, 262, 313.

charges in epilepsy, and suggests the possibilities of diagnostic and therapeutic applications.[51,152,355]

Chemistry

Both normal and epileptic neuronal discharges are related to membrane potentials, to the sodium pump mechanisms, and to synaptic transmission.

The neuronal membrane leaks its principal ions in or out of the neuron. Sodium and chloride ions leak in and potassium ions leak out of the membrane in a passive diffusion process. No energy is required. The membrane potential is the equilibrium potential for the ion or ions to which the membrane is permeable at the time. The membrane's capacitance (serving as a capacitor) becomes electrically charged as potassium ion moves downhill along its concentration gradient. The equilibrium potential for potassium ion becomes the potential at which the electrostatic force opposes any further ionic movement, and each ion has a different equilibrium potential. The membrane permeability to a specific ion is determined by the degree of neuronal activity.[117] Calcium ions adjacent to the presynaptic membrane may block sodium and potassium ionic potentials, activate synaptic transmission and epileptic discharge.[187]

The sodium pump, an active process that requires metabolic energy from adenosine triphosphate (ATP) is the mechanism that operates to expel sodium ion outwardly against its concentration gradient to maintain its unequal distribution. This process actually involves a sodium-potassium coupled pump. There is evidence that the pump is electrogenic either to maintain neutrality (one potassium ion in and one sodium ion out), or to create an unequal exchange (such as two potassium ions in and three sodium ions out), thus hyperpolarizing the membrane. This mechanism terminates the seizure discharge.

Synaptic transmission requires selective permeability of the postsynaptic membrane to a specific ion or ions—the permeability change being caused by the release of a transmitter substance by the presynaptic terminal. This induced permeability may have an excitatory or inhibitory effect depending upon the specialization of the postsynaptic function. The summation of these synaptic potentials represents the source of the activities studied by electroencephalography and electrocorticography.

Tower affirms that the locus for the final common set of mechanisms for epileptogenicity is presumably the excitable membrane of the neuron (Fig. 141–1).[350] The stability of the membrane is dependent upon a continuous supply of energy (ATP) and by oxidation of glucose on which the brain is dependent via the cerebral circulation for adequate supplies of oxygen and glucose. Anoxia may depolarize cells and create epileptic seizures. Coincident with or after the onset of seizures there are marked increases in cerebral blood flow, consumption of oxygen and glucose, production by brain of lactic acid, and depletion of tissue levels of oxygen, glucose, and energy-rich phosphates.

Neurotransmitters include gamma-aminobutyric acid (GABA), a mediator of central inhibition acting on postsynaptic effector units, and acetylcholine (ACh), a mediator of central excitation acting on receptor sites in postsynaptic membrane. Generation of sufficient excitatory potential alters the conduction of the membrane for sodium and potassium ions and initiation and propagation of a spike potential along the conducting membrane of the postsynaptic effector cells. This chain of events is self-limiting in that acetylcholine is dissipated by diffusion and especially by hydrolytic inactivation by acetylcholinesterase.

The reactive glial cells (astrocytes) in an epileptogenic focus may be unable to perform the potassium ion–buffering function of normal astrocytes, leading to an accumulation of external potassium ions around the discharging neurons and greater instability of the neuron.[351] "Potassium accumulation" is a proposed hypothesis to account for the transition from an interictal to an ictal seizure discharge.[87] Glutamate decarboxylase (GAD-II), an enzyme that synthesizes gamma-aminobutyric acid from glutamic acid, is widely distributed in the body and is localized in the glial cells of the central nervous system. Therefore, astrogliosis of the epileptic focus may increase its hyperexcitability by both potassium accumulation and a loss of gamma-aminobutyric acid. These concepts add new dimensions to the study of epileptogenic mechanisms, but they require validation.[350] In addition, neurochemical relationships have been es-

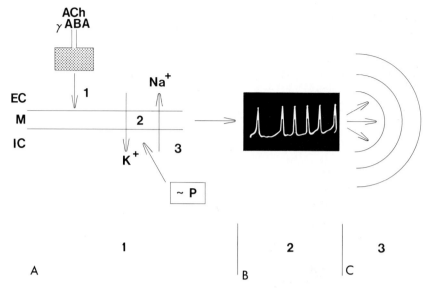

Figure 141–1 Mechanisms of epileptic neuronal activity. *A.* The excitable membrane, M. 1. Neurotransmitters acetylcholine (ACh) and gamma-aminobutyric acid (GABA) impinge on the external aspect of the neuronal membrane, EC. 2. Sodium (Na⁺) and potassium (K⁺) pumps for active, energy dependent transport of sodium ion out of and potassium ion into the cell. 3. Intracellular (IC) mechanisms generate energy in the form of energy-rich phosphates (~P) to fuel the cation transport system. *B.* Initiation of seizure discharges. *C.* Spread of seizure discharges. (Modified from Tower, D. B.: Neurochemistry of epilepsy. *In* Vinken, P. J., and Bruyn, G. W., eds.: Handbook of Clinical Neurology. Vol. 15, The Epilepsies. New York, American Elsevier Publishing Co., 1974, pp. 60–73.)

tablished in relationship to mesial temporal structures and corticosteroids, i.e., an increase of corticosteroids in human plasms and urine is found after stimulation of the amygdala and a decrease after hippocampal stimulation.[305]

CLASSIFICATION OF SEIZURES

Classifications of epilepsies, from the time of Galen, used the term "idiopathic" for all instances of seizures originating in the brain, until Delasiauvé, in 1854, divided the epilepsies as follows: (1) idiopathic or essential—a functional disorder without anatomical cause, (2) symptomatic—associated with a demonstable lesion of the brain, and (3) sympathetic—associated with involvement of the brain secondary to systemic causes.[204]

Gowers, following jacksonian teaching, instigated anatomical, physiological, and pathological inquiries about each seizure patient in order to answer these four questions: "What is the seat of the discharge which thus produces the symptoms of the fit? Is the seat of the discharge the seat of the disease? How far does such discharge explain the symptoms of the attack? What is the nature of the morbid change which causes the discharge?"[119]

Electroencephalography has added a significant dimension to the evaluation and classification of the epilepsies, beginning with correlations based upon paroxysmal cerebral dysrhythmias and progressing to studies related to the location and spread of discharges.[109,163,386]

Penfield and Jasper combined their interest in the surgical treatment of epilepsy, clinical neurophysiology and electroencephalography to develop a seizure classification that placed major emphasis on the anatomical site of the origin of the epileptic discharge. Three categories are included: (1) focal cerebral seizures (those originating in the cerebral cortex), (2) centrencephalic seizures (those originating in subcortical areas), and (3) unlocalized cerebral seizures (those in which the origin of the seizure was unknown [idiopathic] and to be determined).[248]

An attempt to use standardized and specific terms to describe seizures, worked out by Gastaut, has been adopted by the International League Against Epilepsy.[98] In this

TABLE 141-1 INTERNATIONAL CLASSIFICATION OF EPILEPTIC SEIZURES*

PARTIAL SEIZURES (SEIZURES BEGINNING LOCALLY)
Partial seizures with elementary symptoms (generally without impairment of consciousness)
  Motor symptoms (including jacksonian seizures)
  Special sensory or somatosensory symptoms
  Autonomic symptoms
  Compound forms
Partial seizures with complex symptoms (generally with impairment of consciousness; also called temporal lobe or psychomotor seizures)
  Impairment of consciousness only
  Cognitive symptoms
  Affective symptoms
  "Psychosensory" symptoms
  "Psychomotor" symptoms (automatisms)
  Compound forms
Partial seizures secondarily generalized
GENERALIZED SEIZURES (BILATERALLY SYMMETRICAL AND WITHOUT LOCAL ONSET)
  Absences (petit mal)
  Bilateral massive epileptic myoclonus
  Infantile spasms
  Clonic spasms
  Tonic seizures
  Tonic-clonic seizures (grand mal)
  Atonic seizures
  Akinetic seizures
UNILATERAL SEIZURES (OR PREDOMINANTLY SO)
UNCLASSIFIED EPILEPTIC SEIZURES (INCOMPLETE DATA)

* From Gestaut, H.: Clinical and electroencephalographical classification of epileptic seizures. Epilepsia, *11*: 102-113, 1970. Reprinted by permission.

TABLE 141-2 ETIOLOGY OF SEIZURES DURING CHILDHOOD*

CAUSES OF SEIZURES
Infections
  Intracranial (meningitis, encephalitis, abscess)
Systemic (febrile, toxic)
Trauma
  Reversible physiological change
  Structural brain insult
  Hematoma (subdural and epidural)
Fluid and electrolyte imbalance
  Related to systemic disease
  Iatrogenic
Metabolic disorders
  Hypoglycemia
  Hypocalcemia
  Rare disorders of amino acid or carbohydrate metabolism
  Rare genetically determined enzyme deficiency
Anoxia
  Paranatal problems
Drugs and toxins
Congenital malformations
  Neurocutaneous abnormalities
  Hamartomas
  Other structural malformations
Neoplasms
Cardiovascular problems
  Vasculitis
  Stroke (acute infantile hemiplegia)
  Vascular malformation
DISORDERS THAT SIMULATE SEIZURES
Nocturnal episodes (night terrors, nightmares, somnambulism, talking and other vocalizations)
Syncope (vasogenic, cardiogenic)
Migraine
Apneic episodes (infants)
Breath holding
Temper tantrums
Paroxysmal vertigo
Movement disorders
Posturing (opisthotonus) associated with abrupt changes in intracranial pressure or brain stem dysfunction.

* Adapted from Greer, M., and Andriola, M. R.: Convulsive disorders of childhood. *In* Thompson, R. A., and Green, J. R., eds.: Pediatric Neurology and Neurosurgery. Jamaica, N.Y., Spectrum Publications, 1977, 1978.

classification the term "partial" is used instead of the word "focal." Obviously, the current state of knowledge is such that classifications of seizures will continue to change, but current medical literature suggests increasing use of the International Classification (Table 141-1).

CAUSES OF THE EPILEPSIES

With appropriate investigation and follow-up studies, definable causes can be found to account for the majority of seizures in infancy, childhood, and adolescence. The most likely etiology is suggested by the age of the patient at the time of the onset of the first fit. Approximately 67 per cent of cases of epilepsy occur prior to the beginning of the second decade of life.[289,299]

The causes of seizures during childhood include nine major categories—infections, trauma, fluid and electrolyte imbalance, metabolic disorders, anoxia, drugs and toxins, congenital malformations, neoplasms, and cardiovascular problems—and

there are nine additional disorders that must be ruled out (Table 141-2).[134]

The true incidence of seizures during the newborn period is unknown. Most neonatal seizures are due to metabolic causes (almost 75 per cent). In the newborn infant, seizures are the most common indication of anoxia, which may be due to a traumatic birth, premature separation of the placenta, prolonged labor, or inability to initiate respiration.*

A retrospective comparison of birth records of 101 patients with focal epilepsy and 208 control subjects with nonfocal epilepsy suggested that a more liberal attitude toward caesarean section would be justified

* See references 49, 54, 147, 266, 296, 297, 359.

in cases of breech presentation, prematurity, toxemia, and other hypertensive disorders.[346] Hypertension was the only maternal disorder that correlated with cerebral lesions in the child.

A review of the records of 153 infants weighing 2500 gm or less admitted consecutively to a newborn intensive care unit revealed 31 (20.2 per cent) with seizures, and there were 28 (90 per cent) deaths among these infants, in 27 of whom (87 per cent) a diagnosis of intraventricular hemorrhage was made. In comparison, only 21 of 122 (17 per cent) of patients without seizures died. Anticonvulsant medication had little effect on clinical seizure activity or outcome.[318]

The relationships in the newborn, infants, children, and adolescents with such vascular problems as congenital heart disease, subdural hematoma, Sturge-Weber syndrome, arteriovenous malformation, infantile hemiparesis, and vascular disorders of childhood including familial hemiplegic migraine and some syncopal attacks in connection with anoxia and seizures are established.[288]

Prolonged febrile seizures of infancy and childhood may cause brain damage and later afebrile seizures.[185] Two to five per cent of children experience at least one febrile seizure in their early years. The first febrile seizure usually occurs between 6 months and 3 years in 93 per cent of these children.[216] In a study of 1706 children who had experienced at least one febrile seizure, it was found that epilepsy developed by 7 years of age in 2 per cent, and another 1 per cent had at least one later afebrile seizure that did not meet the definition of epilepsy. In children whose neurological or developmental status was suspect or abnormal before any seizure and whose first seizure was complex (longer than 15 minutes, multiple, or focal), however, epilepsy developed at a rate 18 times as high as in children with no febrile seizures. Prior neurological and developmental status and the characteristics of the first febrile seizure are important predictors of epilepsy after febrile seizures.[227] Ounsted, in personal observation of a series of 438 infants with febrile convulsions, noted that 33 (8 per cent) died in convulsions and 125 (30 per cent) developed drug-resistant habitual seizures.[236] It is the contention of Falconer that a prolonged febrile convulsion in infancy (of the order of 30 minutes or more) may lead to hypoxic changes in such structures as the hippocampus, amygdala, and parahippocampal gyrus, which result in mesial temporal sclerosis. This lesion, in turn, frequently becomes a cause of habitual temporal lobe epilepsy in children, adolescents, and adults, and is commonly unilateral.[78]

Epilepsy occurring soon after injury (early epilepsy) and seizures that occur after the first week (late epilepsy) need to be considered separately.

Early epilepsy is more common after serious injuries (linear fracture, depressed fracture, acute intracranial hematoma, focal signs, or post-traumatic amnesia of more than 24 hours). Children under 5 years are more prone to post-traumatic epilepsy, even with mild injuries, than are older children or adults. The overall rate at which children under 5, including those with mild injuries, develop seizures is about 10 per cent; it is 17 per cent for infants under 1 year, excluding those with birth injuries.[144,165] The first (sometimes the only) early fit occurs within 24 hours of injury, in almost half the cases in the first hour, in nonmissile injuries. Epilepsy more often begins on the first day after depressed fracture and in children. More than one seizure occurs in the first week in 65 per cent of patients with early epilepsy, with status epilepticus in 10 per cent (but in 20 per cent of children under the age of 5). The occurrence of a fit in the first week after injury is not an indication for any particular action, unless there are other features suggestive of an intracranial complication (a third of patients with early epilepsy have acute hematoma—usually subdural or intracerebral). The ultimate significance of early epilepsy is that it greatly increases the risk of epilepsy developing in the future.

Late epilepsy is likely to continue in patients with seizures occurring after one week following head trauma. About 60 per cent of patients who develop late epilepsy have their first fit within one year after injury. Late epilepsy after nonmissile injuries is focal in 40 per cent of cases, and almost half of these focal seizures are of the temporal lobe type. The patient's age is relatively unimportant as far as late epilepsy is concerned, unlike early epilepsy. The overall rate for all patients with nonmissile injuries admitted to the hospital is about 5 per cent.[165]

These findings illustrate variations from the pattern of post-traumatic epilepsy in adults.[362]

Patients with all types of epilepsy, generalized or focal, including those with febrile seizures, demonstrate a common genetically controlled disposing factor, but this decreases in importance with age.[76,213,292,369]

CLINICAL DIAGNOSIS

Clinical diagnosis of epileptic seizures in an infant, child, or adolescent requires: (1) determination of the anatomical origin and physiological spread of the clinical seizure based upon history, observation, and electroencephalography; and (2) conceptualization of the most probable pathological cause of the seizures, depending upon history, examination, and laboratory and neuroradiological studies.

Localization of the Epileptogenic Area

History

The single most important prerequisite to a diagnosis is a thorough history taken not only from the parent but also from the child and from an observer of the seizures. The physician usually will not be able to witness an attack, and hospitalization for this purpose is frequently nonproductive except in severe seizure disorders. The observer, often the parent, is able to provide an objective description of the seizure pattern. The child usually is able to report the warning of the seizure (the aura), but may lose consciousness or memory and be unable to relate other events of the seizure except that he was incontinent of urine or feces, bit his tongue, had a time lapse, or found himself at a distance from where he was at the time of the aura. Partial (focal) seizures with both simple (jacksonian) and complex (psychomotor) symptoms may occur nocturnally and present as generalized convulsions (grand mal) only. Likewise, seizures may originate in silent portions of the cerebral cortex, such as the frontal region, and simulate generalized seizure disorders.

From birth until the age of 15 days, the newborn's brain, being very excitable, is still usually incapable of discharging in its entirety—which results, therefore, in partial attacks with neuronal discharges that arise erratically from one or several parts of one or both hemispheres. The seizures are usually localized brief tonic or clonic convulsions with unstable electroencephalographic patterns—the origin of the term "erratic seizures of the newborn."

From the age of about 15 days to 2 years, the brain remains hyperexcitable but increasingly capable of discharging through one or both hemispheres—and most seizures are unilateral or generalized. The epilepsies of infancy are most frequently unilateral seizures that may be continuous (unilateral status epilepticus of infancy) and result in hemispheral lesions that produce permanent hemiplegia and residual organic epilepsy. Generalized seizures occur less commonly during infancy and usually consist of tonic attacks or infantile spasms. Partial seizures are rarer still and almost always consist of epigastric, abdominal, salivary, or masticatory attacks of temporal lobe origin—indicative of both the site of predilection of paranatal ischemic lesions (mesial temporal sclerosis) and the inability of the immature brain to elaborate, as yet, complex psychosensory or psychomotor manifestations.

After the age of 2 or 3, the brain becomes less excitable and there is an appreciable decrease in the incidence of epileptic seizures, especially those seizures due to genetic or metabolic factors, including febrile seizures. The most frequent generalized attacks are tonic-clonic seizures, absences, clonic seizures, atonic seizures, or combinations. During early childhood unilateral seizures are common, but are rare after 5 or 6 years of age, and there is an associated diminution in the tendency to status epilepticus. Partial seizures are still rare during childhood, but at this age the brain is capable of producing psychosensory and psychomotor symptoms and these become increasingly complex between the years of childhood and late adolescence.

After puberty, and with brain maturation, tonic-clonic seizures, generalized from the start, are seen occasionally, and partial seizures, either alone or with secondary generalization, are much more frequent.[188]

Clinical seizure patterns have been well described.* The first symptom of the seizure may suggest the locus of the epileptogenic area and whether it is in the cerebral cortex or is subcortical. The many variables of this generalization, particularly in infancy and childhood, require localization by means of electroencephalographic and neuroradiological techniques.

Electroencephalography

Electroencephalography provides the only available method to demonstrate specific neuronal dysfunction directly as the basis for the clinical seizure. It is generally recognized that the recording of a focal onset of the spontaneous ictal event itself is the ideal means of identifying the site or origin of an attack. The second best localizing

and diagnostic evidence is the stable, localized interictal epileptic discharge on the electroencephalogram.[67a] Such interictal discharges provide direct and essential evidence of neuronal dysfunction of an epileptiform type. This is valuable diagnostically if evaluated serially and critically. At the present time, there is no specific study that correlates long-term clinical results following operation with electroencephalographic localization obtained by analysis of interictal recordings in comparison with ictal recordings. It has been noted with both methods that excision of the epileptogenic focus on the basis of either ictal or interictal abnormalities may not result in cessation of habitual seizures.[47,113,369] Epileptic discharges that originate in subcortical and even cortical areas may or may not be evident with routine scalp electroencephalographic studies (Fig. 141–2).†

* See references 14, 49, 84, 89, 99, 104, 108, 120, 126, 184, 187, 188, 212, 230, 233, 243, 246, 249, 250, 254.

† See references 16, 17, 36, 37, 41, 55, 374.

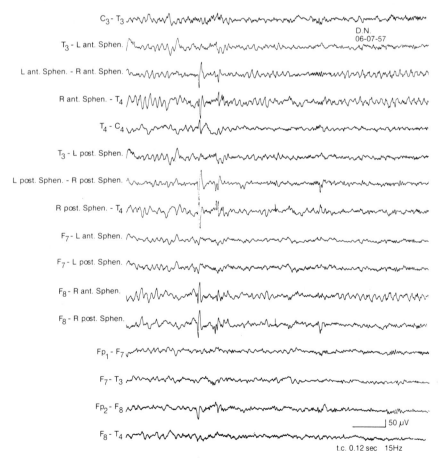

Figure 141–2 Spike discharge from right inferior mesially situated sphenoidal electrode. There is no evidence of spread to cortical surface.

Electroencephalographic localization of epileptic discharge has developed remarkably since the early clinical correlations in man.[*] Among the contributions to electroencephalography are discovery of the diagnostic and localization value of sleep, and the report of localization of abnormalities in the anterior temporal area or areas in the majority of patients with psychomotor epilepsy during drowsiness and sleep.[104,105] Stereotaxically placed depth electrodes have been used for recording epileptic discharges from subcortical regions, as have sphenoidal electrodes to record more directly from the mesial structures of the temporal lobe.[†] A systematic study and therapy program has utilized stereoencephalography (SEEG) with electrodes implanted at the time of testing.[340–343] Single-neuron recordings have been made in animals and man.[186,283,375–379] It was found that electrical stimulation of the cerebellar cortex could stop a seizure that was induced by a 6-volt cerebral stimulation and that this property of cerebellar inhibition could also be demonstrated by cooling and ablation, and that electrical stimulation of the hippocampal region could localize epileptic discharges in temporal lobe automatisms in man.[34,65,85,234] The carotid amobarbital test has been used to ascertain lateralization of speech and to aid in the localization and lateralization of epileptic discharges.[97,301,361] Semipermanent stereotaxically implanted electrodes have been used to determine electrophysiological and clinical correlations of initiation and spread of epileptic discharges and seizure patterns.[37,41,55,58,374] The application of multichannel computer telemetry has further refined localization and the tracing of transmission of seizure discharges, and has been combined with videotaping of clinical seizure patterns.[‡] Finally, the implantation of an extradural array of electrodes with the patient under anesthesia for the recording of sensory evoked responses makes it possible to identify the sensorimotor cortex, and electrical stimulations and later recordings can be used to delineate the boundaries of the epileptogenic area for cortical excision.[118] This tactic is applicable to children and less cooperative patients, particularly for identification of epileptogenic lesions of the convexity of the cerebrum.

Comprehensive appraisal by Gloor of interictal and ictal electroencephalographic recordings for localizing and lateralizing the epileptogenic area may be summarized as follows:

1. If clinical localization derived from the observation of spontaneous seizures by trained observers is clear and congruent with electroencephalographic localization of interictal abnormalities, operative therapy can be recommended, particularly if radiological and psychological examinations concur with this localization.

2. If the interictal electroencephalogram and clinical, radiological, and psychological data concur in their main localizing significance, yet if one portion of the data indicates involvement of an additional part of the brain, the therapeutic results may be less than optimal. In such an instance, or if lateralization on clinical grounds is uncertain, one should attempt to record a seizure in order to confirm the localizing and lateralizing evidence provided by the interictal electroencephalogram. If this evidence cannot be obtained, the decision to proceed with operative therapy must be carefully weighed with all other factors.

3. Ictal electroencephalograms provide the best diagnostic evidence of the location of the patient's epileptogenic area, but may be elusive because spontaneous seizures are intermittent and unpredictable. Focal epileptic attacks can rarely be provided at will, and ictal seizure records may be obscured by muscle artifacts. Not all of the cerebral cortex is available to conventional scalp recordings, and there may be doubt that all the seizures consistently originate from the same cerebral region.

4. The accuracy and value of ictal recordings may be increased by several tactics, including: (1) prolonged recordings, including the use of sphenoidal electrodes in patients with temporal lobe epilepsy; (2) precipitation of seizures with activating stimuli known by the patient or by the intravenous injection of pentylenetetrazol; (3) telemetric recordings, which, because they overcome many of the difficulties inherent in prolonged recordings, provide freedom of movement and can multiplex a large number of channels onto one carrier track on a tape recorder; (4) patient-monitoring

---

[*] See references 107, 109, 110, 162, 163, 248, 298.

[†] See references 1, 22, 237, 248, 260, 301, 322, 364, 371, 374.

[‡] See references 3, 55, 155–157, 336, 374.

systems with or without computer assistance; and (5) depth electrode recording through stereotaxically implanted electrodes.[113]

It is usually, but not always, possible to obtain localizing and lateralizing electroencephalograms in epileptic patients who are being studied prior to the decision to operate by means of simple activation or special recording procedures to bring out a latent interictal or ictal focal abnormality.[385] Such procedures include (1) sleep recordings, (2) withdrawal of anticonvulsant drugs, (3) studies with sphenoidal and nasopharyngeal electrodes, (4) photic stimulation and hyperventilation, and (5) intravenous methohexital (Brevital) or pentylenetetrazol (Metrazol) tests.

Sleep Recordings

First described as useful for activating interictal and ictal epileptiform abnormalities of all types, sleep recordings are particularly helpful in partial epilepsies with complex symptoms (psychomotor, temporal lobe, limbic types).[48,104] Natural sleep can usually be obtained for prolonged recordings by sleep-deprivation the night before the examination. Secobarbital (Seconal), 100 mg with or without chloropromazine, is effective if necessary. If diagnostic recordings are not obtained, medications may be withdrawn and the study may be repeated.

Withdrawal of Anticonvulsant Drugs

Drug withdrawal is done gradually in the hospital (unless the patient is prone to status epilepticus). Controlled study has shown that withdrawal of medication results in specific focal activation in only 25 per cent; complex activation with wide spread of the initial "on-medication" focus or appearance of additional independent epileptogenic foci in 29 per cent; nonspecific activation (bursts of either bilaterally synchronous and frontally dominant spike and waves, triphasic waves, or smaller amplitude rapid and diffuse spike-wave complexes) in 63 per cent; and no effect in 20 per cent of the patients.[192] There appears to be no association between the type of effect and the topography of the "on-medication" focus, the duration of therapy, the type of anticonvulsant used,

the suspected underlying cause, or the median age when the medication was withdrawn. "Off-medication" recordings appear to be of greatest value in patients with partial seizures whose electroencephalograms reveal either minimal or no epileptiform discharges.

Sphenoidal Electroencephalograms

Recordings made with sphenoidal electrodes were first described in 1951.[260] They are particularly useful in the evaluation of patients with complex partial seizures (psychomotor epilepsy) because the mesial temporal structures are not directly accessible to recording from the scalp. Sphenoidal recordings during drowsiness and sleep may reveal definite epileptiform abnormality, provide lateralization, or disclose an unsuspected focal discharge responsible for the triggering of generalized, bilateral synchronous spike and wave discharges.*

Nasopharyngeal Electroencephalograms

This technique was first described in 1938.[137] Analyses, in a videotape study of 76 attacks in 14 epileptics have shown two types of psychomotor attacks: (1) a sequence from an initial motionless stare, stereotyped movements, and reactive automatisms during impaired consciousness; and (2) a less common sequence starting with stereotyped and reactive automatisms. Focal temporal or lateralizing features were common with the first type, but there were only diffuse electrical changes in the second type.[68] Nasopharyngeal and sphenoidal electrodes are located in the immediate vicinity of the uncinate area of the temporal lobe. The nasopharyngeal electrodes are placed 2 to 2.5 cm more mesially and anteriorly than the sphenoidal electrodes. They are also farther from the amygdaloid complex and closer to the proximal orbital surfaces of the frontal lobes than the sphenoidal electrodes.[301]

---

* Secondary bilateral synchrony, i.e., generalization of epileptiform discharge secondary to focal epileptiform activity may also be evaluated by means of stereotaxic depth electrode explorations, and tests with intracarotid amobarbital, pentylenetetrazol, and intravenous thiopental.[191,249,351]

Methohexital and Pentylenetetrazol Activation

Intravenous methohexital (Brevital) and pentylenetetrazol (Metrazol) may also be used to activate ictal abnormalities.[114,172,303] Methohexital in subanesthetic or anesthetic doses may bring out epileptiform abnormalities but may have no real advantage over conventional sleep activation.[48,348] Intravenous pentylenetetrazol, introduced in 1947, is useful to demonstrate ictal abnormalities, but it is not certain that the drug activates the epileptogenic mechanism responsible for the patient's spontaneous seizures.[172]

Depth Electrode Implantation

In the evaluation of ictal and interictal EEG abnormalities and the propagation of seizure discharges, implantation of depth electrodes has added an important dimension to the understanding of the pathophysiology of the epilepsies and the care of selected patients.[10,22,330a] The most obvious candidates for depth electrode studies are patients with bitemporal foci in whom the side of the seizure onset cannot be determined in spite of repeated scalp and sphenoidal electroencephalographic recordings serially and for prolonged periods, including sleep records. Other foci on the medial or orbital surfaces of the cerebral cortex, inaccessible to direct scalp recordings, also lend themselves to stereotaxic exploration. Depth electrode investigations should not

be undertaken lightly. Though the risk is statistically small, the implantation of multiple electrodes in the brain can result in infection and hemorrhage immediately and potential minimal brain damage in the future. At present, there is no evidence of untoward effects from multiple long-term implantations that have been followed for a fairly long time. The complications of immediate infection and hemorrhage are remarkably few. Methods of depth electrode implantation are discussed in the work of Angeleri, Bancaud, and Crandall and their associates; Gloor; Rossi; Talairach and associates; and Walker.* The method of Babb and Crandall is depicted in Figure 141–3.[10]

Determination of the Pathological Cause of the Seizures

The pathological causes of seizures are suggested by the age of the patient and the circumstances at the time of the first seizure. *A detailed history is essential.* The causes and the form and structure of epileptic foci have been discussed in earlier sections of this presentation.

Physical and Neurological Examinations

In epileptic infants, children, and adolescents, examinations may reveal abnormali-

---

* See references 8, 10, 16, 17, 55, 58, 112, 113, 300, 340, 343, 364.

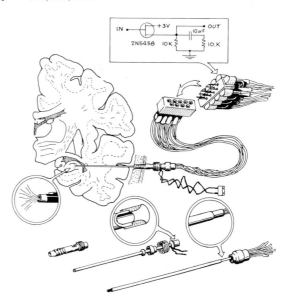

Figure 141–3 Schematic illustration of the components for microelectrode implantation and recording. (From Babb, T. L., and Crandall, P. H.: Epileptogenesis of human limbic neurons in psychomotor epileptics. Electroenceph. Clin. Neurophysiol., *40*:225–243, 1976. Reprinted by permission.)

ties: (1) when there is underlying cerebral disease, (2) when the examination is made shortly after a seizure has occurred, (3) when cerebral dysfunction results from recurrent seizures, and (4) when anticonvulsant medications cause toxic or allergic manifestations.

Absence of neurological abnormality on examination does not rule out an underlying lesion. If abnormal findings are elicited, a diagnosis of symptomatic rather than idiopathic epilepsy is favored—assuming that the lesion responsible for the findings and for the seizures is the same. Hemiparesis, hemiatrophy, and seizures are suggestive of a lesion of the contralateral hemisphere, e.g., a porencephalic cyst. Aphasia, hemianopia, and mental retardation may or may not be associated but must be documented. Facial asymmetry may be a useful sign in the lateralization of temporal lobe epilepsy.[284]

General physical examination may reveal cutaneous manifestations of epileptogenic lesions of the brain, such as the port-wine stain on the face associated with Sturge-Weber syndrome, the adenoma sebaceum of tuberous sclerosis, or the café au lait spots of neurofibromatosis. Signs of decreased consciousness, stiffness of the neck, and elevated temperature may suggest encephalitis, meningitis, or abscess as the cause of the seizure disorder. An enlarging head in an infant and signs of increased intracranial pressure may be associated with seizures and require appropriate studies to ascertain the cause.

Neuropsychological Testing

Psychological testing is a valuable extension of the neurological examination for the diagnosis of epilepsy in patients with suspected cerebral involvement as well as for defining the specific nature and degree of impairment of higher- and lower-level cerebral functions in patients with confirmed cerebral lesions.[326] Selection of appropriate tests should proceed from two basic principles. The tests should (1) include a standardized and objective measure of a broad range of language, verbal and nonverbal reasoning, and auditory and visual memory functions, since premorbid measures are usually lacking; and (2) should permit differentiation of the sensory and motor modalities involved in perception and execution of the task (lower-level functions) from the mental and cognitive processes (higher-level functions) they were designed to measure.

Milner utilizes the Wechsler Intelligence Scale for Children and stories more appropriate to a child's interests and vocabulary, instead of the prose passages of the Memory Scales, to test verbal memory for normal children below the age of 11 and for older children who are retarded.[217] The Rey-Osterrieth figure can still be used to test memory for visual patterns. It has been found that alert 7-year-old children can perform the Wisconsin Card Sorting Test well, and that between the ages of 6 and 10 sensory testing should probably be limited to pressure sensitivity and two-point discrimination of the hands. Since 1950, 955 patients with focal seizures, children and adults, have been studied psychologically before and after operation at the Montreal Neurological Institute. The importance of this work to the neurosurgeon and the patient is illustrated by the following observations:

1. In patients whose focal seizures are attributable to an early static lesion, the preoperative IQ reflects in part the severity of the original injury.

2. Preoperative test findings indicate that whatever interfering effect the focal lesion may have must be quite stable. Repeated IQ testing years apart demonstrates only minor and insignificant changes from one examination to another.

3. Clues to lateralization of a focal lesion can be sought preoperatively in the difference between the Verbal IQ (based on verbal and numerical tasks) and the Performance IQ (based on spatial and other perceptual tasks).

4. Specific effects of focal cortical lesions may be elicited, such as disturbances of verbal memory function with lesions of the left temporal lobe and of perceptual and memory function with lesions of the right temporal lobe, amnesia in bilateral lesions of the hippocampus, impairment of card-sorting ability after dorsolateral frontal lobe lesions and of word fluency after lesions of the left frontal lobe, and quantitative changes in sensory discrimination on the hand in lesions of the postcentral gyrus.

5. Preoperative testing of speech and memory by means of intracarotid amobarbital (Amytal) injection has added security

to the determination of lateralization of these functions.

Psychiatric and Social Service Evaluation

An association between behavior and epilepsy has been noted for centuries. The spectrum spreads from no abnormality to total disability because of assaultive, destructive, psychoneurotic, or psychotic actions. If such problems appear to be present to the consultants who are evaluating the child or adolescent with seizures, psychiatric evaluation, including a social service survey, is imperative. Should the patient become a candidate for operative treatment, such information and support is essential to having a cooperative patient and family in the hospital and at home, and will enhance the opportunities for rehabilitation.

Laboratory Studies

Laboratory tests are directed toward uncovering the cause of the seizures.

In the infant and young child, blood counts, platelet counts, serial hematocrit determinations, urinalysis, analysis of blood chemistry, electrolyte values, cultures for sepsis, assay of blood and urine amino acids, lumbar puncture, screening for intrauterine infections (e.g., toxoplasmosis, syphilis, cytomegalic inclusion disease, rubella, herpes), and subdural taps in patients who have a history of birth trauma or in whom transillumination is positive or who have a tense fontanelle or a rapidly enlarging head are among the possibilities. Laboratory investigation in the older child or adolescent should also include blood counts, evaluation of blood chemistry, electrolyte determinations, and cerebrospinal fluid study if the diagnosis is in doubt.

Neuroradiological Examinations

In epileptic patients, neuroradiological examinations are indispensible for evaluating the cause of seizures. The studies include one or more of the following procedures: (1) plain radiographs of the skull (for evidence of increased intracranial pressure, pineal shift, abnormal calcifications, asymmetry of the skull, or depressed fracture); (2) radionuclide brain scans (for arteriovenous malformation, tumor, subdural hematoma, and areas of disruption of the blood-brain barrier); (3) computed tomography, illustrated in Figure 141–4 (for evaluating ventricular size and noting cerebral atrophy, tumors, hemorrhage, intraventricular lesions, and temporal horn atrophy or tumor); (4) cerebral angiography, as shown in Figure 141–5 (for vascular problems, tumor abscess, subdural hematoma); and (5) pneumoencephalography and ventriculography (used less commonly since the advent of CT scanning but sometimes providing the best information regarding the cerebrospinal fluid pathways).

Frequently all these studies are normal and yet an epileptogenic lesion is found at operation. Excellent reviews of the radiology of epilepsy have been made. [45,208] Computed tomographic scanning in 50 consecutive unselected patients referred to a neurological practice for evaluation of focal epilepsy demonstrated structural lesions in 35.3 per cent (porencephalic cysts in six patients, diffuse cerebral atrophy in five, cerebral hemiatrophy in three, focal cortical atrophy in two, neoplasms in two, hydrocephalus in one, and cerebellar hypoplasia in one).[27] The conclusion is that the

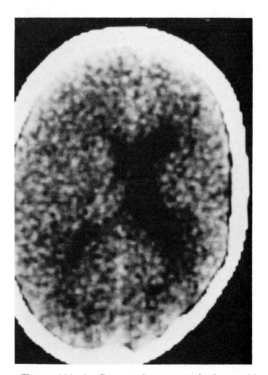

Figure 141–4 Computed tomogram in 5-year-old boy with infantile hemiplegia on left, preservation of visual fields, medically refractory seizures, and behavioral outbursts.

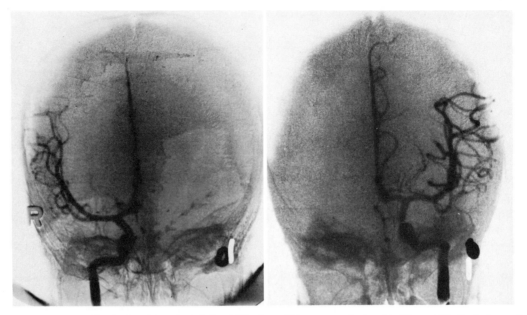

Figure 141–5   Cerebral angiography (of the child whose CT scan was depicted in Figure 141–4) via femoral catheterization disclosing small right hemicranium and widening of the U-loop compatible with the diagnosis of an atrophic right cerebral hemisphere.

CT scan is useful for both outpatient and inpatient evaluation of epileptic patients.

A recent report has described neuroradiological localization of ictal and interictal epileptic foci on the cerebral convexity by means of regional cerebral blood flow studies following intracarotid injection of ^{133}xenon and utilizing a computer-assisted gamma camera system with 254 detectors.[152] This work is in the process of development.

MEDICAL TREATMENT

Drug therapy has the goal of controlling the abnormal discharge of epileptic neurons without interfering with their normal function. The objective in the treatment of the epileptic infant, child, or adolescent is complete control of seizures, or a reduction in their frequency so that they no longer interfere with physical, mental, and social well-being. Unfortunately all drugs have some undesirable side effects.[258]

Patients with recurrent seizures should be treated as soon as the diagnosis is established. Antiepileptic drugs, however, have no value in the prevention or treatment of breath-holding syncopal or tetanic spells of the infant, or hysterical or syncopal or migrainous attacks that simulate seizures in the young child or adolescent.

Neonatal Seizures

The medical treatment of neonatal seizures consists of correcting the cause of the attacks, if possible.[266] Possible causes include metabolic disorders (hypoglycemia, hypocalcemia, hypomagnesemia, pyridoxine dependency, hyponatremia and hypernatremia, aminoaciduria, drug withdrawal, and kernicterus), infection (meningitis, sepsis, and encephalitis from intrauterine infection), perinatal anoxia, intracranial birth injury, and congenital anomalies. The treatment of status epilepticus in the neonate consists of: (1) establishment of adequate airway and oxygenation, (2) spinal tap to rule out meningitis, (3) blood chemistry and electrolyte determinations, (4) administration of intravenous fluids (glucose, 5 to 10 ml of 20 to 30 per cent solution; pyridoxine, 25 to 50 mg given intravenously; and if no response, magnesium sulfate, 2 to 3 per cent solution, 2 to 6 ml intravenously), and electrocardiographic monitoring. (5) If the seizures do not respond to this management, they must be stopped with either phenobarbital (5 to 15 mg per kilogram over several minutes) or diazepam (Valium; 0.2 to 1 mg slowly intravenously) but not both because of drug synergy and respiratory depression, and (6) control must be maintained with phenobarbital intramuscularly once the seizures have been stopped.[330]

The cause of the seizures and the promptness and adequacy of the therapy will determine the prognosis for the neonate with seizures. A long-term clinical, pathological, and electroencephalographic study of 137 full-term babies with neonatal seizures followed to the age of 4 found that 50 per cent were normal, 30 per cent had serious neurological sequelae, and 20 per cent had died.[294] A similar study of 278 infants with neonatal seizures showed that 53 per cent were normal, 24 per cent had serious neurological sequelae, and 23 per cent died. Deaths that occurred during the first three months were due to cerebral hemorrhage in 26, cerebral edema in 16, and malformation in 3. Neurological sequelae in this series included "cerebral palsy" in 37, mental retardation in 17, mental retardation and seizures in 14, and seizures in 5 children.[235]

Studies of factors inducing seizures in the first 10 days of life and their relative frequency, as determined by autopsy, indicate that birth injury, particularly subdural hemorrhage and intraventricular hemorrhage, is the most common cause of death.[54,147]

The neurosurgeon's role in the care of neonatal seizures is to treat subdural hematoma, cerebral edema, intraventricular hemorrhage, and developmental anomalies appropriately and promptly, recognizing the need for both intensive neonatal care and possible neurosurgical care later in life.

Febrile Seizures

Medical treatment of febrile seizures consists of treating systemic infection, if present, of ruling out meningitis by lumbar puncture, and of ending the seizure as quickly as possible in order to prevent irreversible brain damage. To stop the seizure, diazepam (Valium; 0.1 mg per kilogram of body weight with a maximum of 10 mg) is given parenterally.[330] Respiratory depression can occur with diazepam, especially if the child is already receiving phenobarbital. Abrupt termination of the febrile convulsion is the goal in order to prevent the sequelae of temporal lobe epilepsy. Prophylactic phenobarbital, 5 mg per kilogram per day to maintain blood levels in the range of 15 μg per milliliter will prevent febrile seizures in 96 per cent of children so treated. The following regimen has been suggested: Phenobarbital, 2 mg per kilogram at bedtime during the first week, with the addition of 1 mg per kilogram each week until a therapeutic dose of 5 mg per kilogram is reached. Medications should be continued until the child is 4 to 5 years of age and has had at least one seizure-free year. The medication can then be tapered off over a three-month period.[330] Diphenylhydantoin does not appear to protect against single febrile seizures.

The efficacy of anticonvulsants in the prevention of recurrences of febrile seizures remains controversial—with respect to both the benefits and the risks. It may be reasonable to consider long-term therapy for only the minority of children with febrile convulsions who are in special jeopardy, or who have had two or three such episodes.[227]

Afebrile Seizures

Preventive treatment of children with open or closed head injury has been developed on the basis of individual selection. A recent review has indicated that anticonvulsant medications, if begun soon enough, can be effective in reducing the incidence of late post-traumatic epilepsy.[268] A survey of attitudes toward preventive treatment of post-traumatic epilepsy found that only a minority of patients with head injuries are so treated because of the uncertainty about which patients are at risk—and how great the likelihood of epilepsy really is.[269] Jennett and Van de Sande point out the difficulty of application of preventive treatment within the first hours after injury, since patients may not enter the high-risk group until they have developed an early seizure or an acute intracranial hematoma. Thus, early epilepsy, depressed fracture, and acute intracranial hematoma each increases the risk of late epilepsy significantly. Prolonged post-traumatic amnesia is associated with higher risk in those patients with evidence of focal brain damage but does not increase the risk of epilepsy if depressed fracture, acute hematoma, or focal brain damage is not present. The electroencephalogram is not helpful in predicting the risk of late epilepsy and does not provide definitive correlations, whether normal or abnormal.[166] The effect of combinations of factors is emphasized by a study of compound depressed fractures. Post-traumatic amnesia of duration greater than 24 hours and gross focal brain damage together carry the highest risk of post-traumatic epilepsy. It is the authors' policy to treat such patients prophylactically. With this exception, other children with head injuries are usually not given anticonvulsant medications unless a seizure occurs. If medication is started, it is continued for a minimum of one year.

Medical treatment of afebrile seizures should follow several established therapeutic principles:

1. Select as the drug of first choice the one best suited for the seizure type and the one with the most acceptable potential toxicity (Table 141–3). New drugs are needed and are under investigation.[205,259] Sodium

TABLE 141–3 DRUGS FOR TREATMENT OF AFEBRILE SEIZURES

GENERALIZED SEIZURES (BILATERALLY SYMMETRICAL, WITHOUT LOCAL ONSET)
Tonic-clonic seizures (grand mal)
  In order of preference:
    Phenobarbital
    Diphenylhydantoin (Dilantin)
    Primidone (Mysoline)
    Carbamazepine (Tegretol)
    Mephenytoin (Mesatoin)
    Mephobarbital (Mebaral)
Absences (petit mal)
  In order of preference:
    Ethosuximide (Zarontin)
    Clonazepam (Clonopin)
    Trimethadione (Tridione)
    Paramethadione (Paradione)
    Methsuximide (Celontin)
Myoclonic seizures
  Akinetic—minor motor seizures
    Clonazepam (Clonopin)
    Diazepam (Valium)
    Primidone (Mysoline)
    Ketogenic diet
    ACTH or corticosteroids
  Infantile spasms
    Nitrazepam (Mogadon)
    Clonazepam (Clonopin)
    Diazepam (Valium)
    ACTH or corticosteroids
PARTIAL SEIZURES (SEIZURES BEGINNING LOCALLY—FOCAL SEIZURES)
With elementary symptoms (generally without impairment of consciousness)
  Diphenylhydantoin (Dilantin)
  Primidone (Mysoline)
  Phenobarbital
With complex symptoms, generally with impairment of consciousness (temporal lobe and psychomotor epilepsy)
  Diphenylhydantoin (Dilantin)
  Carbamazepine (Tegretol)
  Primidone (Mysoline)
  Phenobarbital
  Mephobarbital (Mebaral)
  Phenacemide (Phenurone)

dipropylacetate (Depakene or DPA) is reported to be the most promising of the new drugs because of its wide spectrum of effectiveness and few side effects.[319]

2. Increase the drug of choice until seizures are controlled or the child becomes intoxicated. If seizure control is improved but incomplete, the drug of second choice is added and its dosage is slowly increased. Drug dosage should be altered slowly and not more frequently than every five to seven days.

3. Monitor blood or salivary drug levels in patients whose seizures are not responding or who become intoxicated.[182,207] The monitoring of blood levels has increased the safety and effectiveness of drug therapy. This tactic facilitates individualization of the dosage regime and detection of irregular intake, and identifies the responsible agents in patients who are receiving multiple drugs and who become intoxicated. Salivary anticonvulsant drug concentrations, as reported in 1974, have been shown to be equivalent to those of cerebrospinal fluid, providing a direct measurement by a noninvasive method of biologically free drugs.[25]

4. Anticonvulsant drugs should be withdrawn gradually, in order to avoid precipitating status epilepticus.

Medications, singly and in combination, and dosages must be adjusted according to the needs of the patient (Table 141–4).[64,339]

Phenobarbital is usually prescribed in two divided doses of 5 mg per kilogram per day with an average effective dose of 2 to 3 mg per kilogram per day in 10- to 20-kg children and 2 mg per kilogram in larger children. The desired blood serum level for control of seizures is 10 to 15 μg per milliliter, with signs of intoxication appearing at 35 μg per milliliter.

Diphenylhydantoin (Dilantin) is usually prescribed in two divided doses of 5 to 10 mg per kilogram per day with an average effective dose of 5 to 10 mg per kilogram per day. The desired blood serum level for control of seizures is 10 to 20 μg per milliliter (optimal at 18 μg per milliliter), with signs of intoxication appearing at 15 to 30 μg per milliliter (nystagmus), 30 μg per milliliter (ataxia), and 40 μg per milliliter (lethargy, ataxia, nystagmus).

Primidone (Mysoline) is started at a dosage of 50 mg per day. The average effective dosage is 150 to 500 mg per day.

Carbamazepine (Tegretol) is started at a

TABLE 141–4 PROTEIN BINDING, METABOLIC HALF-LIFE (T½), RECOMMENDED STARTING DOSAGES AND THERAPEUTIC RANGES FOR FREQUENTLY PRESCRIBED ANTICONVULSANTS

DRUG	FRACTION OF DRUG BOUND TO PROTEIN IN SERUM	METABOLIC HALF-LIFE (hr)	RECOMMENDED DOSAGE RANGE (mg/kg/day)	THERAPEUTIC RANGE (μg/ml)
Phenobarbital	0.5–0.6	Note below	1–5	10–20
Primidone (Mysoline)	0.03	3.3–12.5	10–15	6–10
Diphenylhydantoin (Dilantin)	0.9	Note below	4–8	5–20
Ethosuximide (Zarontin)	0–0.1	24–60	20–35	40–100
Trimethadione (Tridione)	0	0.5	15–20	
Diazepam (Valium)	0.96	24–53	0.12–2	
Clonazepam (Clonopin)		22–38	0.03–0.05	0.013–0.072
Carbamazepine (Tegretol)	0.8	16–40	10–30	2–12

Note: Variation of metabolic half-life (T½) of anticonvulsants with age

	Phenobarbital	Diphenylhydantoin	Ethosuximide
>15 yr	64–141 hr	22 + 9	24–60
1–15 yr	37–73	46–66	24–30
1–12 mo	47 ± 8	2–6.9	
0–1 mo	63–98	60	

* From Dodson, W. E., Prensky, A. L., DeVivo, D. C., Goldring, S., and Dodge, P. R.: Management of seizure disorders. Selected aspects. Part I, J. Pediat., 89:527–540, Reprinted by permission.

dosage of 100 mg per day. Average effective dosages are 200 to 800 mg per day in children over 6 and 100 mg per day in children under 6.

Mephenytoin (Mesantoin), 100 mg three times a day, is used for children 6 years old and over.

Ethosuximide (Zarontin), 250 mg two or three times a day, is prescribed for children.

Trimethadione (Tridione) may be prescribed in doses of 300 mg twice a day up to 600 mg three times a day for children.

Diazepam (Valium) is used in doses of 5 to 30 mg per day.

Clonazepam (Clonopin), 0.05 mg per kilogram per day, is given two or three times per day, with increases by one dose every five to seven days, until seizures are controlled, or up to 0.25 μg per kilogram per day.

Diphenylhydantoin (Dilantin) and primidone (Mysoline) is often the best combination in patients with psychomotor attacks. Carbamazepine (Tegretol) has gradually become the drug of first choice of many clinicians for children with complex partial (psychomotor) and focal motor seizures.[96] If the child has both major (grand mal) and minor (petit mal) seizures, phenobarbital may control both types or may require supplementation by ethosuximide (Zarontin). Diphenylhydantoin (Dilantin) should not be used in such a problem because this drug increases the frequency of petit mal attacks. The potential dangers of each of the drugs mentioned have repeatedly been described in the literature.

Prolonged Seizure Activity

Prolonged seizure activity of acute onset in infants and children has been defined in four categories: *Status epilepticus* (repeated or persistent clonic, hemiclonic, or, rarely, tonic convulsions, usually lasting one hour, during which time the patient never regains consciousness), *serial seizures* (frequent, generalized, focal, or multifocal convulsions occurring during the course of an acute insult to the brain in which the patient may revert to his pre-existing level of consciousness between seizures), *epilepsia partialis continua* (continuous clonic movements lasting for days, weeks, or longer, but limited to a discrete part of the body and usually not associated with a change in the level of consciousness), and *absence status* (sustained clouding of consciousness with minimal stereotyped movements or no abnormal motor activity).[64] Treatment involves control of seizures, preservation of the patient's vital functions, and diagnosis and treatment of the underlying disease. Therapy is discussed by category of prolonged seizure activity.

Therapy in status epilepticus and frequent serial seizure activity consists of a number of measures: (1) maintenance of airway, oxygenation, and blood pressure;

(2) blood chemistry and electrolyte determinations; (3) intravenous administration of 10 per cent glucose solution in Isolyte M (limited to 1200 ml per day) and monitoring of output by indwelling catheter; (4) intravenous dexamethasone if intracranial pressure is increased (initial dose 2 to 6 mg depending on the weight of the child, followed by 1 to 4 mg every six hours), and addition of mannitol (1 gm per kilogram body weight over a 20- to 30-minute period) if elevation of intracranial pressure is threatening; (5) control of hyperthermia by vigorous sponging; and (6) intravenous diazepam (Valium; 0.25 mg per kilogram over a two-minute period, maximum of 10 mg as an initial dose). The response is usually apparent within five minutes or sooner. If there is no response and if there has been no change in respiratory or cardiovascular function, a second injection of 0.5 mg per kilogram is given (a maximum dose or 15 mg) over a two-minute period. A third injection of 0.5 mg per kilogram (maximum dose of 20 mg) may be given 20 to 30 minutes later in the absence of adverse reaction to the second. Diazepam should not be used further if not effective. Intravenous diphenylhydantoin, rectal paraldehyde, and phenobarbital are alternatives. General anesthesia is rarely needed. Intravenous diphenylhydantoin (13 mg per kilogram of body weight) has been reported to be a safe, effective means of rapidly achieving therapeutic plasma levels and stopping seizure activity in status epilepticus.[388] Sodium phenobarbital is believed by Menkes to be the drug of choice for status epilepticus.[212] The initial dose of 10 mg per kilogram is administered subcutaneously. If seizures do not subside in 20 to 30 minutes, intramuscular paraldehyde (1 ml per year of age, not exceeding 5 ml) is given. If this fails, a second dose of sodium phenobarbital (10 mg per kilogram) is injected subcutaneously. If these measures are ineffective, an anesthesiologist is called to provide ether anesthesia. (7) Oral anticonvulsants are resumed upon recovery. The usual cause of status epilepticus is the failure of the patient to comply with an oral medication schedule.

In epilepsia partialis continua, the patient is alert, and often one or more doses of diazepam intravenously will permanently stop the seizure. Resumption of adequate levels of diphenylhydantoin and phenobarbital is essential. Determination of the nature of the focal abnormality responsible for the seizures is important.

In absence status, it is essential to decide whether the cause is petit mal or a focal disorder such as psychomotor status.[5] Treatment consists of intravenous diazepam in a dosage of 0.25 mg per kilogram to a maximum of 10 mg given over a two-minute period. An increase in the oral dose of ethosuximide (Zarontin) or trimethadione (Tridione) to achieve therapeutic serum levels may prove effective.[8] Intravenous diphenylhydantoin or phenobarbital in doses of 5 to 10 mg per kilogram may be effective in absence status arising from the temporal lobe (psychomotor status).

Prognosis

Studies of the clinical efficacy of marketed antiepileptic drugs provided the estimate that seizures are completely controlled in more than 50 per cent of patients with epilepsy and that, in another 30 to 40 per cent, the results are improved with additional drugs, although not without some side effects.[50] An overall picture that has emerged from the literature is that complete seizure control is achieved for two years in 30 to 37 per cent of patients, but this figure drops to 20 per cent at five years and 10 per cent at 10 years.[286,287] An investigation of prognosis following withdrawal of antiepileptic drugs after four years of complete seizure control in 148 children who were followed for 5 to 12 years after withdrawal found a consistent relapse rate of 20 to 40 per cent.[146]

A growing number of long-term complications of drug therapy, especially with the older drugs, are being recognized, such as folate deficiency in some 50 per cent of patients, vitamin D deficiency in 33 per cent, peripheral neuropathy in 10 to 20 per cent; and changes in connective tissue, liver, endocrine, immunological, and mental functions are more common than previously supposed.[286,287]

A seizure disorder with an onset early in life carries with it a high risk of associated low intelligence regardless of cause. In addition, according to Rodin, the IQ tends to rise if the patient achieves a remission for at least two years. The presence of anoxia and cyanosis during convulsions has been related to learning problems. Rodin computed that 1.3 per cent of epileptic patients die annually—a rate that is five times as great as the age-adjusted national death rate. He concludes that the "operative results for temporal lobe epilepsy seem to be definitely superior to medical treatment.[292] Kiørboe has documented that the chance of becoming seizure-free is dependent upon the seizure pattern, the likelihood with generalized seizures being almost twice that with psychomotor seizures.[174]

There is considerable discrepancy in the literature regarding the mortality rates for epileptics. Livingston found no difference in life expectancy apart from an excessive mortality rate in the group with brain damage.[187,188] Jüül-Jensen reported a death rate among epileptics to be 200 per cent higher than normal.[169]

These considerations emphasize the unsatisfactory state of the present drug treatment of epilepsy. Far more needs to be known about the effects of lifelong consumption of these drugs, a matter currently under scrutiny.[287]

OPERATIVE TREATMENT

From the foregoing discussions it is obvious that epileptic infants, children, and adolescents require optimal care, and if a normally productive and independent life cannot be provided by medical management, that neurosurgical treatment be considered. Some epileptologists consider that 95 per cent of epileptic disorders are the result of a focal brain lesion and that possibly 5 per cent may be offered an operation.[364]

Children with chronic epilepsy are faced with many problems that make it difficult, if not impossible, to become independent and productive.[169,170] Aggressive outbursts, learning difficulties because of heavy medications, difficulty in being accepted by schoolmates and employers and the public are among the obstacles. In addition, the current physiological evidence of the continuation of pathological changes in an active epileptogenic focus, of "kindling," and of secondary epileptogenesis make it an obligation to evaluate children and adolescents with seizures persistently to insure that they are truly under medical control that does not preclude normal living.[60,124,132]

Indications for Cortical Resections

Criteria for the selection of patients for neurosurgical intervention by means of cortical resection have gradually evolved from a number of sources.* They consist of the following considerations:

1. The clinical seizure pattern should indicate a discharging lesion in a localized, operatively accessible area of the brain—gyrus, lobe, or hemisphere.

2. Serial electroencephalograms, supplemented by special studies, should localize this epileptogenic area. There is some variation in opinions regarding the extent to which special studies should be utilized, such as sphenoidal EEG recordings during sleep, carotid-amobarbital-metrazol electroencephalograms and angiographic examinations, and short- or long-term implanted electrode studies with radiotelemetry. It is essential that the localization is stable.

3. A cortical lesion should be suggested by the clinical and laboratory evidence as the cause of the seizures.

4. It must have been demonstrated that intensive and methodical treatment with anticonvulsant drugs, verified by adequate blood levels of the drugs used, are inadequate to stop the seizures and to provide the patient with normal and productive home, school, and job adjustment.

5. The patient's physical status must be such that a major operative procedure can be undergone without undue risk. His preoperative mental state should be documented, and his intelligence should be adequate to allow a relatively normal life if the seizures and medications can be eliminated or significantly reduced. An IQ of less than 60 is usually a contraindication.

6. Children and adolescents (like adults), if more than 10 years of age, must be completely willing to cooperate for the diagnostic procedures and the operation if they are to be performed under local anesthesia successfully. General anesthesia, however, is adaptable in many operaions for epilepsy in children and adolescents, including hemicorticectomy and temporal lobectomy, and results have been excellent.

---

* See references 14, 33, 56, 64, 76, 82, 121, 122, 135, 139, 211, 230, 241, 249, 261, 279, 280, 288, 300, 358, 366, 369.

Neurosurgical Hypothesis for Cortical Excision

The pioneers of the surgical treatment of epilepsy (Horsley, Foerster, Sachs, Penfield, Rowe and Watts, Furlow, German, and Tönnis, among others) operated primarily to remove scars, which were believed to be the cause of chronic focal epilepsy.[*] For localization of the lesion, they were dependent upon the clinical seizure patterns elicited with stimulating electrodes.[90] With the development of electrocorticography, the presumptive role of the scar in the production of epilepsy was modified to include the adjacent cortex.[162,363,370] Delineation of this epileptogenic area of abnormal cortex became possible by means of corticograms that demonstrated localized hyperirritability (spontaneous abnormal discharges and prolonged afterdischarges following stimulation) in addition to the classic methods with electrical stimulation.

A continuing analysis and study of patients operated on since 1928 by Penfield and his associates and successors has contributed the current neurosurgical hypothesis for cortical resection in the treatment of focal epilepsy.[244,272,273,277] The hypothesis: (1) small, discrete epileptogenic foci are rare; (2) the great majority of patients have epileptogenic areas of considerable extent with the region of lowest threshold giving the local sign to the attack pattern; (3) the success in stopping the seizure is correlated with the completeness of excision of epileptogenic cortex, and (4) failures of operative resection, related to excisions of only the restricted focus of lowest seizure threshold, may frequently be converted to successes with reoperation and complete excision of the epileptogenic area.

This hypothesis seems to be supported by particularly good results with patients having hemicorticectomy and temporal lobectomy, poorer results with other excisions unless all surrounding epileptogenic cortex is removed, which is more difficult, and the relatively inconsistent and less permanent results with stereotaxic lesions.

Reports indicate that resection of the temporal lobe is now the most frequent procedure in the operative treatment of epilepsy.[†] Approximately 10 per cent of Penfield's pioneering operations for focal epilepsy were directed toward the temporal lobe during the 1930's and early 1940's, although the role of the temporal lobe in seizures with hallucinatory and illusional content with or without automatisms had been well described.[248,277] Additional attention was directed to the temporal lobe in the late 1940's by the electroencephalographic localization and lateralization of the lesion in the anterior temporal region in the majority of patients with psychomotor epilepsy and the excisions of anterior temporal cortex based upon that localization, even in patients with associated psychiatric problems.[105] The procedures were done under general anesthesia, thus adding new dimensions to the operative treatment of epilepsy.[12] During the past two decades, operations for temporal lobe epilepsy at the Montreal Neurological Institute have increased to two thirds or more of all cortical resections for focal epilepsy due to nontumoral epileptogenic lesions.[277] The authors' experience, spanning the years since 1948, includes 145 operations for epileptogenic lesions in children and adults. One hundred and seven (73.8 per cent) were temporal lobectomies; and of 50 operations during childhood and adolescence, 32 (64 per cent) were temporal lobectomies.[124,132]

An understanding of the relationships between behavior and epilepsy is essential to the discussion of the surgical aspects of epilepsy during childhood and adolescence.

Epilepsy, Behavior Abnormalities, and Operative Therapy

Behavioral aspects of epilepsy have been recognized for centuries, and the social problems associated with seizures have enhanced the very real hazards to a productive and independent way of life for many individuals who are so afflicted.[169,170,380] Hippocrates began the destruction of the ancient concepts of "the falling sickness" when he laid down the principle that epilepsy was due to natural causes. Hughlings Jackson's theory, which accounted for all kinds of seizures as well as insanity on the basis of neurological abnormalities, marked the beginning of the modern era.[345]

The mentality of epileptic patients, like the mentality of the general population, may range from the genius to the imbecile.

---

[*] See references 88, 95, 102, 148, 239, 304, 306, 349.

[†] See references 56, 60, 67, 79, 132, 230, 273, 277, 367, 369, 374.

Impairment of mentality is encountered in only a minority of persons subject to seizures. Such "epileptic deterioration" is due to one or more of five possible causes: (1) a genetic influence, (2) an organic abnormality of the brain; (3) epilepsy itself—either the epileptic discharges (with or without concomitant symptoms), the convulsions, or the pathological sequelae of a seizure, ranging from a thrombosed artery to a cracked skull; (4) sociopsychological isolation and repression; or (5) drug intoxication with anticonvulsant medications.[184]

Considerable advances have been made in elucidation of the functional relationships of the various regions of the brain in the processes of consciousness. The reticular formation, by way of ascending sensory influences and descending cortical projections with neural integration at a high level, is concerned with sleep and wakefulness. New developments in exploring the involvement of the reticular core in conditioned learning are particularly essential to an understanding of behavior.[2,195] The hippocampal regions of the temporal lobes are involved in the process of arousal, receiving projections from the reticular formation through the fornices and responding to all alerting stimuli with slow 2- to 5-Hz waves resembling those seen in temporal areas of emotionally immature and psychopathologically aggressive patients. Behavioral changes have been well documented following lesions and ablations of the temporal lobe.[2,367] The importance of the mesial structure of the temporal lobe for the regulation of sexual behavior was first demonstrated in monkeys with bilateral temporal ablations.[175] Hyposexuality has been reported in more than half of patients with temporal lobe epilepsy if the illness is of considerable duration and severity, but is rare in other types of epilepsy.[24,100,367]

Psychiatric abnormalities, which in their milder forms are classified as personality disorders and in more severe forms as psychoses, are common complications of complex partial seizures (also called psychomotor, temporal lobe, and limbic epilepsy).[262] If convulsions are not a part of the seizure pattern it is not uncommon to have psychiatric diagnoses made, such as neurosis, hysteria, psychopathic personality, paranoia, or schizophrenic or manic-depressive psychosis; and an increase in the dosage of anticonvulsants usually has no effect on the psychiatric symptoms.[40,106,244] Electroencephalographic studies are required to differentiate ictal and nonictal psychiatric disorders.[107,111,316] As long as the spike discharges remain focal in the temporal lobe they are not immediately associated with symptoms or disordered behavior—the clinical manifestations of psychomotor epilepsy develop when the discharge spreads.[55,107] A discharging epileptogenic lesion may be even more disturbing to the patient than a destructive lesion of comparable size. It is an attractive hypothesis to relate continuing behavioral abnormalities in man to irritative lesions of the temporal lobe within the limbic system in that the limbic system has been implicated in the elaboration of behavior and emotion.* The failure to diagnose tumors within the limbic system, particularly in the temporocingulate and third ventricular regions, until late usually occurs because initially many of these patients present with severe psychiatric problems.[196,197] Tumors of the dominant temporal lobe also show a stronger tendency to produce mental impairment than do tumors in the opposite temporal lobe.[23]

Mental disturbances and temporary psychoses may follow a series of focal cerebral seizures, particularly when the focus of discharge is in the intermediate frontal and temporal regions.[20,40,47,293,321] Behavioral abnormalities and memory loss are more frequently associated with a long history of temporal lobe seizures than with those that arise in other areas, and an increase in such difficulties occasionally may constitute a postoperative complication of radical ablation in the temporal region.[23,249] In the recall of experience, the hippocampi play an indispensable role in memory, voluntary or automatic, a requirement for routine recognition and interpretation. Either hippocampus can carry out this function in the absence of the other, but loss of both hippocampi creates loss of memory.†

Several studies have failed to observe any characteristic behavior in psychological abnormalities that separates those patients with temporal lobe epilepsy from those with other epilepsies.[138,215,325,335] Stevens suggests that factors of age distribution and the selection of patients from psy-

---

* See references 18, 103, 111, 145, 176, 193, 194, 238, 265, 294, 295, 337, 380, 384.

† See references 245, 251, 252, 317, 320, 367.

chiatric populations have led to the untenable conclusion of specificity of psychological abnormalities with temporal lobe epilepsy. Her conclusion is that interictal behavioral disturbances and psychoses in patients with all forms of epilepsy most commonly are postictal events, and that the most successful treatment for the psychiatric symptoms associated with epilepsy is the abolition of seizures by appropriate medical and surgical treatment.[335]

Psychical responses to electrical stimulation of the temporal lobe were first observed by Penfield in 1931. A patient who was being operated upon under local anesthesia told him that she was reliving an experience. Since then, other psychical seizures in response to electrical stimulation of the temporal lobe structures have been described, including those that are experiential (psychical hallucinations, auditory or visual phenomena, "flash-back"), interpretative (psychical illusions, déjà vu phenomena, fear, and the like), and amnesic (automatisms, psychomotor confusion).*

The concept that epileptic cortex may act as a source of noxious influences on the functioning and the evolution of normal brain was developed by Penfield in connection with the operative treatment of epilepsy. Progressive mental retardation, seizures, and infantile hemiplegia, and progressive intellectual and behavioral abnormalities and temporal lobe seizures in adults are deemed to be the results of such epileptogenic foci.[241]

Bailey added a new dimension to the operative treatment of epilepsy in 1946. He introduced limited temporal excision under general anesthesia in patients with psychomotor epilepsy and personality disorders or psychoses, localizing the epileptic discharge by means of electroencephalography and electrocorticography. The mesial temporal lobe structures were not excised in these patients, and yet some of them became normal with respect to their seizures and aggressiveness, but not to their psychoses.[12] The procedure was further developed in patients in a mental institution.[127-129] In these patients with psychomotor epilepsy and psychiatric symptoms, the mesial temporal structures were resected if electrocorticographic and depth electrode recordings revealed them to be

epileptogenic. Reversal of an "epileptic psychosis" that had necessitated confinement of the patient in a disturbed ward for most of a five-year period prior to operation was reported. This patient has been independent and productive during the 28 years since the procedure.[120] Atrophic and sclerotic consistency of mesial temporal structures was observed in some of these patients, and individuals with marked affective behavioral changes, including hostility, assaultiveness, and aggressivity, were normalized or improved in accordance with seizure control. The majority of patients with psychoses, psychopathic personalities, or addiction, however, did poorly, with few exceptions.[11,127,319]

A combined report to the American Association for Research in Nervous and Mental Disease in December 1951, based upon experiences with 36 excisions sparing mesial temporal structures and 28 excisions including 17 resections of mesial temporal epileptogenic structures, included this statement: "Psychiatric abnormalities are no longer considered to be a surgical contraindication—in fact, it appears that anterior temporal lobectomy in selected patients offers considerable chance of psychiatric improvement, more mental alertness, conative drive, and continuing integration and social adjustment."[13] A follow-up report five years later, in December 1956, regarding 43 institutionalized psychomotor epileptics indicated full rehabilitation of two and worthwhile rehabilitation of three of nine psychotic patients following temporal lobectomy. Two additional points were emphasized: (1) mesial temporal structures need not be removed routinely to obtain excellent clinical rehabilitation of patients with psychomotor epilepsy—such excisions being done if electrocorticographic and depth electrode studies determined epileptogenicity therein, and (2) "surgical excision of a well-localized focus of epileptogenic tissue should not be postponed until the behavior becomes irreversibly changed."[133]

Three types of psychoses (acute confusional, paranoid, and schizophrenic) were described among the 12 patients who underwent temporal lobectomies in Falconer's first 100 operations for temporal lobe epilepsy. Two successful results were reported as well as the finding of more hamartomas than any other lesion in this group

---

* See references 84, 221, 242, 253, 381.

of patients.[324] In another study, mesial temporal sclerosis was found in three of five operative specimens obtained from psychotic patients with psychomotor epilepsy who had become independent and self-supporting following the operation.[122]

Pathological aggressiveness is the most common behavioral abnormality associated with complex partial seizures during childhood and adolescence.* It has been observed that a state of amygdaloid excitability is present in such patients to a much greater degree than in patients with seizures but without aggressive behavior. It is this degree of amygdaloid excitability that may account for the symptoms of aggression when transmitted to septohypothalamic structures to which the amygdala strongly projects and from which aggression can be readily elicited.[6,199,201] The hypothesis is that a chronic state of increased amygdaloid excitability serves as the neural substrate underlying aggressive behavior in patients with psychomotor epilepsy, and such behavioral abnormality can represent clinical manifestations of a seizure as well as an interictal event.[6]

Operation to eliminate or reduce seizures and the need for medication to assist young patients in their struggle from a life of dependency to the responsibilities of a productive and independent person is best undertaken during childhood or adolescence, once the epileptogenic area has been defined and medical measures have been determined to be unsuccessful. This thesis has been re-emphasized during the past two decades.† Behavioral abnormalities associated with epileptic seizures, particularly aggressivity, assaultiveness, and postictal confusional psychoses are usually benefited along with the epilepsy following appropriate operative procedures. If the patient is also severely schizophrenic or paranoid, however, he will probably remain so.[31,324]

Operative Procedures

Two of the most commonly utilized and most effective operative procedures for drug-resistant epilepsy during childhood and adolescence are temporal lobectomy and hemicorticectomy. Therefore, these procedures are described and other procedures, which require similar preparations and techniques, are discussed briefly. Stereotaxic procedures applicable to epileptic patients are described in Chapters 139 and 143 of this text. The identification of sensorimotor cortex by means of sensory-evoked responses and the use of an extradural electrode array to delineate the boundaries of the epileptic focus are discussed in Chapter 142.

Temporal Lobectomy in Children and Adolescents

Preoperative Preparation

Anticonvulsant medications are maintained unless it has been previously determined that it is impossible to obtain precise electroencephalographic localization without reduction or withdrawal of these drugs. Dexamethasone is given orally for 24 to 48 hours preoperatively, intravenously during the procedure, and by mouth postoperatively for four days.[281] The dosage varies with the weight of the patient (2 to 4 mg per day orally and 5 to 10 mg per day intravenously). Prophylactic antibiotics are prescribed, commencing with the craniotomy. Cephalothin (Keflin) in dosage of 1 to 2 gm is given intravenously daily for four days, commencing with anesthesia. A sedative such as secobarbital, 50 to 100 mg, is given the night before operation and is repeated an hour before the operation begins.

Anesthesia

Since sleep is one of the most effective means to activate electroencephalographic abnormality and because children and adolescents below the age of 14 or 15 and those who have episodic behavior outbursts may be unreliable and uncooperative under local anesthesia, general anesthesia is advisable for these patients. With general anesthesia it is still possible to use electrical stimulation to identify prolonged afterdischarges, a frequent finding in the epileptogenic area, but it is not possible to reproduce the patient's aura of the attack or to map out the cerebral cortex adequately. Electrocorticography is useful under these conditions in the evaluation of the temporal cortex, including the hippocampus, and is supple-

---

* See references 60, 83, 132, 198, 315.
† See references 60, 61, 77, 79, 83, 124, 277, 319–321, 358.

mented with depth electrode studies, if not diagnostic.

Procedures for anesthesia are as follows:*

General anesthesia alternative techniques include: (1) sodium thiopental (Pentothal), nitrous oxide, oxygen, tubocurarine; (2) nitrous oxide, oxygen, halothane (Fluothane); or (3) droperidol (Inapsine), fentanyl (Sublimase), nitrous oxide, oxygen, and tubocurarine.

The level of anesthesia should be lightened before electrocorticography. Nitrous oxide may have a prolonged depressant effect on epileptic pattern, and should be discontinued before recording.

The neuromuscular blocking effect of curare must be reversed if motor stimulation is anticipated. Complete reversal may be confirmed by the anesthesiologist's use of a peripheral nerve stimulator.

Small doses (0.5 to 1.0 mg per kilogram) of sodium thiopental or methohexital sodium (Brevital) may be used during electrocorticography.

General principles that are important in anesthesia for intracranial surgery are applicable.

Local anesthesia requires: (1) careful preoperative preparation of the patient by both surgeon and anesthesiologist to reduce anxiety and to make the patient aware of what will be expected of him. (2) The agents used are tetracaine (Pontocaine) or bupivacaine (Marcaine), long-acting local anesthetics. These agents are used with epinephrine (low concentration 1:200,000 to 1:400,000) to reduce bleeding. (3) Sedation is achieved with droperidol (Inapsine) and fentanyl (Sublimaze), initially as the combination Innovar; then fentanyl is given alone. Verbal encouragement, attention to positioning, and padding of pressure points are among the responsibilities of the anesthesiologist and are all important in making the patient relaxed and comfortable. (4) Other adjuncts include the usual monitoring devices, padded light restraints on the patient's arms, low-flow oxygen via nasal catheter, suction apparatus available (the patient occasionally vomits during stimulation). (5) The anesthesiologist should be familiar with the patient's usual aura and seizure pattern. (6) The level of sedation should be one that achieves a relaxed and comfortable patient who is able to respond to commands and interpret sensations, both normal and abnormal, during stimulation. Speech and motor function (i.e., hand grip, leg movement) are repeatedly checked during resection. (7) Following excision of the epileptogenic focus and final recordings, the level of sedation may be deepened, or general anesthesia may be instituted if necessary. Additional infiltration of local anesthetic may also be necessary. It is fortunate that this is possible because of the numbers of patients who cannot tolerate long procedures under local anesthesia.

Scalp Incision, Osteoplastic Craniotomy, and Exposure

After preparation of the skin, scalp and reference electrodes are applied under sterile conditions by the electroencephalographer. The skin incision is marked out on the scalp with gentian violet, commencing at the level of the zygoma, 1 cm anterior to the tragus of the ear, and then drawn perpendicularly from the zygoma for 2 to 3 cm, then anteriorly to the hairline to a point 2 to 3 cm lateral to the midline, curving directly posteriorly to the postrolandic area, and then inferiorly to end just above the mastoid process. Subgaleal infiltration of this line is then made with 0.5 per cent procaine (if general anesthesia is being used) or 0.15 per cent tetracaine (Pontocaine) (if local anesthesia has been decided upon) with epinephrine. Towel and plastic drapes are applied to the head, and draping is completed in such a way that the patient's face, body, and extremities are visible to the anesthetist.

The initial skin incision commences at the level of the zygoma, goes through the galea, and is continued in limbs to completion as marked out. Hemostasis is obtained with electrocoagulation and with Michel or Raney clips. The anterior portion of the temporal scalp is undermined and retracted anteriorly. The temporal fascia is opened vertically in its most anterior portion. The anterior portion of the temporal muscle is retracted from the field by means of fishhook retractors. Trephination with an air-powered drill is made anteriorly in the squamous portion of the temporal bone,

---

* Dr. Lisa Wilkinson, Chairman, Division of Neuroanesthesia, Barrow Neurological Institute, describes her methods in this section.

notching the posterior portion of the opening for a distance of about 2 cm. Hemostasis is maintained with electrocoagulation and bone wax. The second trephination is placed in the midfrontal convexity, the third and fourth in precentral and postcentral regions 2 to 3 cm lateral to the midline, and the fifth, immediately above the ear, notching this hole for a distance of about 2 cm in the direction of the first trephination. All except the two low temporal holes are connected by means of a Gigli saw (which the authors prefer over power tools to avoid settling in of the flap and palpable ridging in the scalp postoperatively). The bone flap is turned and hinged on temporal muscle. Hemostasis is maintained. The remaining temporal bone, exposed with a broad-ended periosteal elevator, is removed to the floor of the middle fossa and anteriorly to the pterion. Drill holes are made midway between trephinations (except inferiorly); 2-0 nylon sutures are placed through each drill hole and held in individual hemostats preparatory to closure. No. 3-0 Tevdek dural stay-sutures are then tied through the drill holes to obviate epidural bleeding during or following the procedure. The skull clamp of the post of the Grass cortical electrode assembly is then placed and screwed tightly to the midportion of the medial aspect of the frontal bone. After the bone edges and periphery are walled off with large cottonoid packs, the dura is opened, hinged medially, and covered with a moist Telfa sponge. Linear cuts are made in the dura, antero- and posteroinferiorly, to expose the lateral surface of the temporal lobe. The dural edges are tented with 3-0 Tevdek sutures in order to obtain maximum exposure. This approach provides optimal exposure of the lateral surface of the temporal lobe, including its pole, as well as an equal amount of frontal and parietal convexity. The authors have also found it exceedingly useful for the operative management of other lesions along the sphenoid wing.

Electrocorticography

During 26 years and 122 additional electrocorticographic studies of the temporal and surrounding structures since the authors' method of electrocorticography in psychomotor epilepsy was published, the basic tactics have continued to be useful.[128]

A photograph and an operative sketch (utilizing brain maps) are made to document the anatomy and the pathological changes, and for orientation of electrode placements and the responses to electrical stimulation (if used).[255]

The Grass electrode assembly with its 18 cotton wick electrodes is secured to the post (Fig. 141–6). It usually requires two or three placements of the electrodes, gyrus by gyrus, separated by intervals of 5 to 10

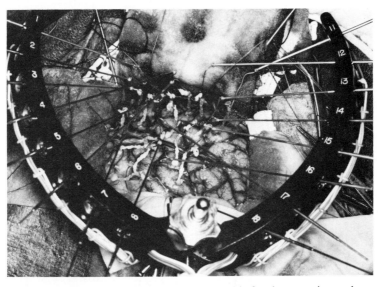

Figure 141–6   Grass cortical electrode assembly for electrocorticography.

mm to obtain a study of the exposed fronto-temporoparietal cortex. The electroencephalographer and neurosurgeon collaborate on the orientation of the electrodes and on the cortical recordings. A 16-channel Grass electroencephalograph (Model 6) located in a monitoring room, immediately adjacent and with audiovisual communication capability for all concerned, is connected via a conduit to a floor plug at the head end of the operating table. Scalp, cortical, reference, and ground leads are appropriately inserted into a junction box, which is connected to the system. An adequate study to determine epileptiform activity from the exposed cortex usually requires 20 to 40 minutes. A moderate increase in depth of anesthesia, like sleep, will frequently activate abnormalities if they are not evident during lighter planes of consciousness. In the great majority of patients who have been selected for possible temporal lobectomy, high-amplitude, sharp spike discharges will be encountered in the anterior 2 to 3 cm of the first and second temporal convolutions. Through the earlier years multilevel depth electrodes were routinely inserted into the mesial temporal structures to trace the localization of these discharges.[127,128] Because of a direct correlation between amygdaloid discharges and anterior temporal discharges of the type described, the use of depth electrodes has been discontinued when epileptiform cortical localization is definite in this location and the amygdaloid complex is included in the lobectomy. If electrocorticography is not diagnostic or if multicentric epileptiform activity is evident, two additional tactics may be helpful. One technique is to insert flexible wire electrodes on the orbital surface of the frontal lobe and on the inferior surface of the temporal lobe including the hippocampal gyrus. The other method is to utilize depth electrodes. The depth electrode is inserted perpendicularly into the second temporal convolution 3 cm from the temporal pole for a distance of 3 to 3.5 cm. This places the deepest ring of the depth electrode in the amygdaloid nucleus. These techniques of electrocorticography have been used successfully to localize the epileptogenic area and to confirm the preoperative diagnosis with a high degree of reliability in anesthetized patients. Areas of abnormality are designated by sterile number tags on the cortex, recorded, photographed, and identified on the brain map.

Electrical Stimulation

Electrical stimulation has been a useful technique in operations for epilepsy since the beginning of the modern era of neurological surgery. It has been performed to identify motor, sensory, and speech areas, to reproduce the patient's aura or seizure, and to determine cortical hyperirritability by eliciting localized prolonged afterdischarges. In order to obtain all the advantages of electrical stimulation, the operation must be done under local anesthesia. Very light anesthesia can be used for the painful part of the procedure, however, and the patient then is allowed to awaken to respond to electrical stimulation. He must be old eough to cooperate, usually 13 to 14 years or older, and be psychiatrically stable. Accordingly, some centers prefer not to accept patients who do not fulfill these criteria. It is possible, fortunately, for electrical stimulation to be useful in many anesthetized patients for all of its purposes except the reproduction of the aura of the seizure and the complete delineation of the central sulcus. This disadvantage is rarely important enough in complex partial seizures or in infantile hemiplegia to contraindicate treatment under appropriate general anesthesia.

The parameters of electrical stimulation may be varied in order to obtain satisfactory responses. Two-millisecond square wave pulses with a 60 per second frequency will usually provide the desired physiological responses. The initial stimulation is begun at 1 volt or 0.5 ma and gradually increased four- or fivefold, if necessary, to obtain responses. It is essential that several minutes elapse between stimulations. Cortical recordings are done during the stimulation procedures.

Anatomical landmarks and clinical and physiological responses are recorded by means of sterile letter tags on the cortex and notation on the brain map.

Temporal Lobectomy

Although temporal lobectomy for temporal lobe or psychomotor seizures was described earlier, the most complete early descriptions of two effective methods of temporal lobectomy for the treatment of "temporal lobe seizures" were published in 1952 and 1953.[12,127,219,247] The technique of subtotal temporal lobectomy described by

Penfield and Baldwin, utilizing local anesthesia and purposefully excluding patients with disabling behavioral disorders, has been further developed, particularly by Rasmussen and Van Buren and co-workers.[245,277,358] The technique of en bloc resection of the temporal lobe described by Falconer, performed under general anesthesia and used even for patients with disabling psychiatric problems, has also enabled pathologists to ascertain more fully the common pathological substrates of complex partial epilepsy.[69,75] Walker's technique for temporal lobectomy spares the first temporal convolution and excises the amygdala and rostral hippocampus so that ablation along the floor of the middle fossa measures 5 to 6.5 cm in both right and left hemispheres.[365] Niemeyer described transventricular amygdalohippocampectomy.[228] Morris suggested removal of the uncus, hippocampus, and amygdala without electrocorticography.[220]

It should be mentioned that the excellent description of temporal lobectomy in Kempe's *Operative Neurosurgery* was intended for the operative treatment of neoplasms and not as a technique for temporal lobe epilepsy.[173] The procedure described in the following text for treatment of epilepsy is also applicable to neoplasms.

The first step in the procedure is to cover the exposed cerebral cortex with Telfa, except for the portion of the temporal lobe that is to be resected. The measurements for the excision are: 3 to 5 cm from the temporal pole along the first temporal convolution on the nondominant side, usually the right side, or 3 to 4 cm in the same plane on the dominant side, usually the left side, if the epileptogenic region has been determined to be on that side. The posterior limit of the resection is usually the vein of Labbé. The distance from the temporal pole along the third temporal convolution is usually about 1 cm greater than along the first temporal convolution. The central fissure at the sylvian fissure is usually immediately superior to Heschl's gyrus, and excision on the dominant side is placed no closer than 1 cm from these structures to avoid verbal and auditory agnosia. If possible, the first temporal convolution on the dominant side of the brain should be preserved. The amount of resection varies appropriately with the patient's age and the electrocorticographic localization. The exposed brain is kept moist with saline solution during the excision.

The pia-arachnoid of the first temporal convolution is coagulated with fine bipolar forceps, under low magnification (loupes), and opened with a No. 11 scalpel blade, the incision commencing 3 to 5 cm from the temporal pole and 2 to 3 mm from the sylvian veins. Following bipolar coagulation of bleeding veins and clipping of small arteries, the pia-arachnoid is then opened with scissors. The cortex and white matter of the superior temporal convolution are gently removed superiorly with a small suction tip, exposing and preserving the pia-arachnoid on the medial surface and exposing the insula. The dissection is carried anteriorly to the temporal pole and then downward toward the floor of the middle fossa. The pterional process of the sphenoid bone, which grooves the anterior portion of the sylvian fissure, is a major landmark for identifying and separating frontal and temporal cortex. As the temporal pole is separated from sylvian veins and arteries, these structures are electrocoagulated and clipped on the temporal side. With the fine suction tip and bipolar coagulation, the exposure is continued into the uncal region. The dissected area is then covered with sponges on strings. The temporal lobe is transected posteriorly by means of bipolar coagulation and clips for hemostasis, scissors to cut the pia-arachnoid and vessels, and a fine suction tip to traverse cortex and white matter to the inferior surface posteriorly. From this point, the lobectomy is angled forward about 30 degrees so as to aim just posterior to the tip of the temporal horn of the ventricle. At this point in the operation the temporal lobe has been removed from the insula and middle cerebral vessels, and the physiologically important mesial temporal structures with subcortical connections remain. The inferior portion of the semicircular sulcus of the insula is exposed. This exposure is made slowly, gently, and with minimal retraction of middle cerebral vessels, because of the potential for "manipulation hemiplegia."[256]

Completion, including the extent of lobectomy, depends upon preoperative and operative localization studies. The mesial temporal structures (uncus, amygdala, hippocampus), if not epileptogenic, are left intact, making possible a reduction of operative risks of injury to the optic radiation and "manipulation hemiplegia," and the lobectomy is completed by extending the posterior end of the excision forward to join the anterior portion in the uncal region, the cut being superficial to the amygdala and temporal horn and lateral to the hippocampus.[91,256] If the mesial temporal structures are epileptogenic, as is usually the case, the surgeon has two options, with variations according to the pathological findings, regarding tactics to complete the lobectomy. They are either subpial suction removal of the uncus, amygdala, and sometimes a portion of the hippocampus; or en bloc excision of the mesial temporal structures. With mesial temporal sclerosis the structures are atrophic and more amenable to en bloc excision than if fibrotic from inflammation or trauma. Magnification of the procedure 6 to 10 times adds to the precision of the dissection.

SUBPIAL REMOVAL OF MESIAL TEMPORAL STRUCTURES BY SUCTION. The mesial temporal structures, having been exposed laterally, are opened. The tip of the temporal horn of the ventricle, the pes hippocampus, and the amygdaloid nucleus are visualized. It has been the authors' experience that visual pathways are not involved if 1 cm or less of the anterior portion of the temporal horn, including the amygdaloid nucleus, is removed. The temporal stem is transected, and the lobectomy is completed by utilizing suction, electrocoagulation, and clips. The hippocampus, amygdala,

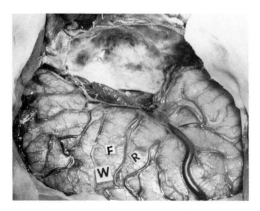

Figure 141–7 Temporal lobectomy—4.5 cm from temporal tip along the superior temporal convolution, 1.5 cm of temporal horn, including amygdaloid complex, uncus, and anterior hippocampus. Note pia-arachnoid covering the insula and oculomotor nerve, which is the white structure adjacent to the incisura of the tentorium.

and uncus are removed by means of subpial suction dissection—sparing the pia-arachnoid across the edge of the tentorium. The structures adjacent to the midbrain, including the occulomotor nerve, are all visible through the pia-arachnoid. Hemostasis is obtained by means of electrocoagulation and clips.

EN BLOC LOBECTOMY. In this procedure the lobectomy is completed by extending the incision through the mesial portion of the hippocampus approximately 1 to 2 cm from the lip of the temporal horn, peeling off the mesial structures with the remainder of the anterior portion of the temporal lobe in one piece, and sparing the pia-arachnoid structures that cover the edge of the tentorium (Fig. 141–7).

Postexcision Electrocorticography

The cortical electrodes are placed on the insula, on the cut edge of the hippocampus and temporal stem as well as on frontotemporal cortex surrounding the lobectomy and on the more distant parietal cortex. If residual epileptiform activity is encountered and if further excision is feasible without apparent risk of causing neurological deficit (frontal, temporal, and hippocampal structures) such additional resection is done in order to obtain recordings without any evidence of seizure discharges, if possible. Although its prognostic significance is not entirely reliable, postexcision electrocorticography is more informative than any other tactic available currently.[67] Spike discharges from the insula, however, do not warrant further excision because of potential complications, including "manipulation hemiplegia," and because it has been observed that the final outcome of seizure control is not affected by retaining the insula under such circumstances.[256,322]

Closure of Dura, Bone, and Scalp

Following meticulous hemostasis, a watertight dural closure is made with running 4-0 Tevdek suture material. A No. 12 Robinson rubber catheter is run from the extradural space in the anterior temporal region, through the posterior parietal burr hole, and exteriorized by means of a stab wound in the skin approximately 1 to 2 cm peripheral to the incision. Drill holes are placed equidistant between burr holes in the flap.

The bone flap is returned to its normal position and tied tightly to the skull with 2-0 nylon sutures through the matching drill holes. Temporal muscle and fascial layers are closed separately with interrupted 3-0 Tevdek sutures, the galea with interrupted 4-0 Tevdek sutures, and the skin with running-locked 4-0 nylon suture material. A nylon suture is placed across the skin of the stab wound to anchor the drainage tube. Head dressings are secured with the drainage tube making its exit in the parietal region. The junction between the cheek and dressing is sealed tightly with paper tape to prevent exposure of the temporal limb of the incision during the restless period. Extubation is done, if general anesthesia is used. The patient is transferred to the recovery room, where vital signs are monitored and the extradural drainage tube is connected to a sterile bottle and Stedman pump.

Postoperative Care

Cephalothin (Keflin), dexamethasone, diphenylhydantoin and phenobarbital (Luminal R sodium) are given parenterally. Intravenous fluids are limited to 750 to 1500 ml for the first two days.

Seizures may occur during the postoperative period but are usually of a different pattern than preoperatively and do not indicate the prognosis for ultimate recovery any more than does freedom from attacks during this period. The extradural drain is removed in 24 to 48 hours, depending upon the amount of drainage. Progressive increases in diet and ambulation are begun after 48 to 72 hours. The sutures are removed on the seventh postoperative day, and a protective dressing is maintained for another week. Dexamethasone is tapered, beginning on the third postoperative day, and is discontinued by the time the patient leaves the hospital—usually on the eighth to twelfth postoperative day. Unless the patient has reacted poorly to diphenylhydantoin and phenobarbital in the past, these medications are continued: diphenylhydantoin in divided doses of 200 to 300 mg, and 50 to 100 mg of phenobarbital on retiring. Carbamazepine (Tegretol) or primidone (Mysoline) may be substituted in comparable maintenance doses. The patients are reevaluated in the office monthly for three months, then every three months for the first year—if feasible. If no seizures or warnings of seizures have occurred during a period of two to three years since leaving the hospital and if the electroencephalogram shows no or minimal epileptiform activity, the anticonvulsant medications are gradually withdrawn over a period of six months. In the authors' experience, the majority of patients require medications in reduced amounts either because of abnormal electroencephalographic recordings, warnings of seizures, occasional seizures, or personal anxiety. If seizures recur or if surgical complications have occurred, the plan as outlined is modified to treat the needs of the patient.

The child or adolescent is encouraged to complete his education and to obtain productive employment as soon as conditions warrant. These goals are the primary purposes of neurosurgical care.

Risks

The risk for a particular patient cannot be given in advance; however, the following experience gives some general guidelines. An adequate follow-up of 28 patients from among 32 children and adolescents treated from 1949 through 1973 provides the information that there were: (1) no operative deaths; (2) no hematomas; (3) one *Staphylococcus aureus* wound infection, which responded to antibiotics in three weeks; (4) 10 instances of "aseptic meningitis" due to blood in the ventricles; associated with a febrile course for 3 to 10 days; (5) three patients with transitory (six hours to 10 days) "manipulation hemiplegia;" (6) one adolescent with permanent left hemiparesis and left homonymous hemianopia; (7) one child with a partial Klüver-Bucy syndrome; and (8) four patients with upper quadrantic homonymous visual field defects.[124,132,175]

The prevention of neurosurgical infections is multifactorial, and the length of the procedures for epilepsy may increase the risk slightly.[131] The rate of 1 patient in 32 (3 per cent) is, however, higher than the average for craniotomy (2.6 per cent) on the general neurosurgical service, and slightly higher than that reported by Rasmussen. It appears that the techniques used for hemostasis have practically eliminated the postoperative complication of hematoma, but the patient and family should be told that it is a possibility. It is difficult, if not impossible, to completely avoid getting blood into the ventricular system when the tip of the temporal horn is resected. This ventricular blood has caused "aseptic meningitis" and transient febrile problems in 10 of 32 patients (31 per cent). Fortunately this complication has not prolonged the period of hospitalization.

The most worrisome risk of temporal lobectomy is that of "manipulation hemiplegia." This is considered to be caused by manipulation or retraction of the middle cerebral artery branches on the insula or removal of the insular cortex.[256,316] Utilizing a technique described in 1961, Rasmussen has encountered no instance of persistent hemiparesis or of dysphasia.[256] In the authors' series of young patients, this complication occurred in four patients, cleared completely in six hours to 10 days in three patients, and in one 14-year-old girl in 1954, was followed by a very mild left hemiparesis. Thus, the incidence of residuals from this complication in their series of children and adolescents is 3 per cent. In addition to the techniques already described to prevent manipulation hemiplegia, micro-operative dissection of the mesial temporal structures and, most recently, monitoring of regional cerebral blood flow of the middle cerebral artery on the low frontal cortex may prove to add a measure of security.[44] An experience with a thermal diffusion blood flow probe, under development in the authors' research laboratories, has been impressive in this regard. As the hippocampal attachment of the temporal lobe was being gently detached to complete the temporal lobectomy, the cortical blood flow in the low frontal region in the distribution of the middle cerebral artery was noted to drop from 90 ml per 100 gm of tissue per minute (a flow rate that had been stable during the preceding hour) to 50 ml per 100 gm of tissue per minute. The resection was stopped, and a sponge soaked with papaverine was applied to the vessels in the area of dissection. Gradually during the next 10 minutes the cortical blood flow returned to 95 ml per 100 gm of tissue per minute, the lobectomy was completed, the blood flow remained stable, and the patient had no neurological deficit following the procedure. This tactic may reduce the risks of "manipulation hemiplegia" and possibly may be useful in mapping out epileptic foci. Studies are in progress in these areas.

Upper quadrantic visual field defects do not become significant handicaps and are rarely noticed by the patient. Four of thirty-two patients (12.4 per cent) had this defect. In each instance the resection included 1.5 to 2 cm of the tip of the temporal horn. This type of visual defect was not observed when less than this amount of temporal horn was excised with the amygdala. A full homonymous hemianopia and a partial hemiparesis resulted in the patient who had a resection 3 cm posterior to the tip of the temporal horn.

One patient was 16 years of age when committed to a state mental institution in 1949 because of seizures and psychotic behavior. Although bitemporal anterior temporal epileptiform activity was constant, maximal on the right side, he responded to neither right anterior temporal lobectomy nor to left anterior temporal lobectomy. The mesial temporal structures were spared in both operations and yet a modified Klüver-Bucy syndrome with oral tendencies and loss of fear reactions appeared.[175,347] Subsequently, the patient died. In the modern era, he would have been studied with implanted electrodes and possibly would be treated by means of bilateral stereotaxic amygdalotomy.

Psychological deficits are usually either nonexistent or minimal following temporal lobectomy in children except in cases of extended resections or complications. These abnormalities rarely interefere with the rehabilitation of patients.

Results

Recently, three centers have published reports on the operative treatment of epilepsy during childhood and adolescence.* All agree that the quality of long-term results of operative treatment in this age population is even better than has been achieved with adults. Other reports regarding operative therapy include a few children and adolescents but make no differentiation according to age.

Davidson and Falconer report that their best results in achieving relief of seizures and normalization of behavior occurred when mesial temporal sclerosis was encountered in the epileptogenic area. A history of febrile convulsions during infancy was elicited in 18 of 22 patients with mesial temporal sclerosis, in one patient with both

---

* See references 60, 61, 124, 132, 278.

mesial temporal sclerosis and a hamartoma, and in none of the patients with hamartomas alone or with nonspecific pathological changes (one patient with viral encephalitis).[60]

The reporting of results regarding seizure control has not been uniform in various publications, except within a given institution. The London group reports that 31 of 40 patients (77 per cent) are seizure-free or about seizure-free following temporal lobectomy.[60,61] The Montreal group reports 53 of 72 patients (73 per cent), as shown in Table 141–5, and the Phoenix group reports 26 of 32 patients (81 per cent) to be seizure-free after temporal lobectomy. It must be remembered that the Montreal series dates back to 1936, prior to the recognition of the need to resect the region of the amygdala in most operations. The Phoenix series has also indicated the favorable relationship of mesial temporal sclerosis and seizure control following temporal lobectomy. This type of pathologic condition was found in 24 of 32 patients and in 24 of the 26 patients who are now either seizure-free or almost so with a marked reduction of medications. Crandall states that the University of California, Los Angeles, group has had three patients below 15 years of age and more than 25 patients in the age group between 15 and 24. Follow-up studies on these patients following temporal lobectomy indicated that ''the rehabilitation of persons with epilepsy in that age group was very much easier and the end results better than in those older than this category.''[57]

Behavioral abnormalities may also be modified by temporal lobectomy if seizures are eliminated or greatly minimized so that anticonvulsant medications can be significantly reduced. Disturbing aggressiveness was noted in all except one patient in the London series.[60] This aspect of their behavior became normal in 20 patients and was much improved in 6 others, thus giving a significant improvement in 65 per cent. Seventeen of these patients were found to have mesial temporal sclerosis. The authors' experience is similar. Thirteen of the twenty-eight children and adolescents were normal, eleven were assaultive and aggressive, three were mentally retarded, and one showed emotional instability. Following temporal lobectomy the normal patients remained normal. Seven of the eleven aggressive and assaultive patients became normal, and two were significantly improved. The one patient with emotional instability was significantly improved. In this series, 80 per cent of the abnormal patients became normal or had significant improvement. These experiences confirm Rasmussen's statement about temporal lobectomy in all age groups: ''The patient who has episodic, aggressive behavior in addition to temporal lobe epilepsy sometimes gets fairly good results from the standpoint of his aggressive behavior. But the more con-

TABLE 141–5   RESULTS OF CORTICAL EXCISION IN TEMPORAL LOBE EPILEPSY*

	NUMBER OF PATIENTS			
Seizure-free discharge	18 (25%)	31 (43%)		
Became seizure-free after some early attacks	13 (18%)		53 (73%)	72 with follow-up data of 2 to 30 yr
Free 3 to 17 years then rare or occasional attacks	8 (11%)	22 (30%)		
Marked reduction of seizure tendency	14 (19%)			
Moderate or less reduction of seizure tendency	19 (26%)			median 12 yr
Inadequate data	5			
Total	77			

* Children (age 4 through 15 years) with nontumoral lesions were operated upon from 1936 through 1973. (From Rasmussen, T.: Temporal lobe epilepsy—surgical aspects. Reprinted by permission from Table VI, page 149 in Topics in Child Neurology by Michael E. Blaw, Isabelle Rapin and Marcel Kilbourne (eds). Copyright 1979, Spectrum Publications, Inc., New York.)

tinuous the aggressive behavior, the more it becomes in effect a continuing paranoid psychosis rather than episodic rage reactions limited in time, the less likelihood is that the behavior is going to be benefited by temporal lobe removal."

Social and economic rehabilitation of children and adolescents following temporal lobectomy is the final item to be considered in the assessment of results.[140,344] Of 28 patients followed for 4 to 34 years, 82 per cent are now independent and self-supporting. Two patients died during this period, one from an astrocytoma and the other from pulmonary tuberculosis, and two patients were retarded. These four patients were precluded from becoming independent and self-supporting.[124,132] These results are generally superior to those obtainable with operative treatment of many more common neurosurgical problems and also to the medical therapy of temporal lobe epilepsy.

Hemicorticectomy in Children and Adolescents

The terms "hemicorticectomy" and "subtotal hemicorticectomy" describe the operative procedures for children with intractable seizures, behavior disturbances, spastic hemiparesis, and hemiatrophy due to gross atrophy of the contralateral brain more accurately than the term "hemispherectomy" in that the line of excision excludes the basal ganglia. Hemispherectomy was first performed in 1938 by McKenzie, but was established as a useful procedure in the modern sense by Krynauw, Penfield, Cairns and Davidson, and Obrador.[42,181,210,241,231]

Scalp Incision, Osteoplastic Craniotomy, and Exposure

Following preparation of the scalp, the scalp incision is marked with gentian violet. This begins at the level of the zygoma 1 cm anterior to the tragus of the ear, is curved to the hairline anteriorly, ending 2 cm anterior to the hairline at the midline, and then reversed posteriorly along the midline to a point 2 cm above the external occipital protuberance, thence laterally to the base of the mastoid process. After draping, local anesthetic is infiltrated in the subgaleal layer beneath the skin markings, and trephinations are made to outline the margins of the cerebrum at intervals of 3 to 4 cm and connected by means of saw guides and Gigli saws. After adequate notching of the temporal trephinations toward one another, the large bone flap is turned on a hinge of temporal muscle. The squamous portion of the temporal bone is rongeured to the floor of the middle fossa. Drill holes and sutures are placed in preparation for tying down the flap and suturing the dura to these sites or wherever extradural bleeding is apparent, techniques described earlier for temporal lobectomy. The dura is opened, hinged toward the sagittal sinus and toward the lateral sinus, cut where necessary to expose the lateral convexity of the cerebrum, and retracted to the bone and sinuses by means of temporary stay sutures to maximize exposure (Fig. 141–8).

Electrocorticography and Electrical Stimulation

The localizing methods described earlier usually delineate multifocal epileptiform

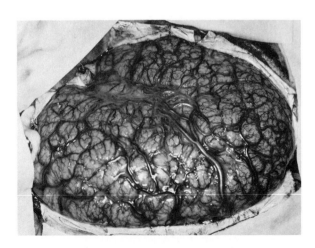

Figure 141–8   Exposure required for hemicorticectomy.

activity and also a lobe or lobes with minimal or no abnormality. Systematic stimulation of the cerebral cortex assists in defining zones of electrical hyperirritability with afterdischarges as well as anatomical orientation. If the visual fields are intact and preoperative electroencephalographic studies have shown minimal abnormalities in the occipital area, and these findings are confirmed by electrocorticography and electrical stimulation, the occipital lobe and the posterior cerebral circulation should be preserved. Preservation of a small portion of the hemisphere appears to prevent the complications of superficial cerebral hemosiderosis.[271,274] Preservation of a portion of the cortex usually means leaving in situ the frontal or occipital pole or occasionally the upper central parasagittal region, depending on which area is the least epileptogenic.

Hemicorticectomy

1. The middle cerebral artery is doubly clipped and divided just distal to the small perforating vessels in the area of the limen insulae. The approach, similar to that for an aneurysm of the middle cerebral artery, is made more precise by the magnification and illumination provided by the operating microscope. It is necessary to coagulate and divide the bridging veins of the temporal pole in order to open the medial part of the sylvian fissure to expose the sphenoidal portion of the middle cerebral artery. Caution not to injure the small perforating arteries is fundamental in avoiding undesirable complications.

2. The bridging veins, on the inferior surface of the temporal lobe, including the vein of Labbé, are electrocoagulated and divided. The temporal lobe is elevated gently in order to expose the edge of the tentorium. The arachnoid over the cerebral peduncle is opened, and the posterior cerebral artery is double clipped and then divided. In the event that the child has normal visual fields and minimal epileptiform activity in the occipital area, the posterior cerebral artery and the visual radiation, including the occipital lobe, are preserved.

3. The bridging veins from the frontal convexity to the longitudinal sinus are coagulated and divided. Gentle retraction of the medial aspect of the frontal lobe exposes the corpus callosum and the anterior cerebral artery. The opposite anterior cerebral artery is protected with great care. The anterior cerebral artery is then double clipped and divided at the genu of the corpus callosum. The approach is similar to that for an aneurysm or tumor of this region. The frontal lobe is now dissected and retracted laterally from the genu of the corpus callosum. The frontal lobe is lifted up carefully from the anterior fossa, making it possible to coagulate and dissect the orbital portion of the frontal lobe about 1.5 cm in front of the optic chiasm. The cut is carried laterally to join the one exposing the sylvian vessels, exposing the temporal lobe.

4. The remaining bridging veins to the longitudinal sinus are coagulated and divided. The medial surface of the cerebrum is retracted laterally in a gentle fashion across the corpus callosum. The corpus callosum is dissected laterally, by means of electrocoagulation and suction, to expose the superolateral aspect of the lateral ventricle. This line of resection is then continued lateral to the basal ganglia through the white matter to the insular cortex where the middle cerebral artery was divided. Cottonoid packing on a string is placed over the foramen of Monro to shield the third ventricle from blood. If the occipital lobe, including the visual pathways, is to be preserved, these areas are excluded from the dissection. If not, the dissection is carried posteriorly and laterally to the posterior portion of the tentorial edge to the point where the posterior cerebral artery was divided. The mesial aspects of the temporal lobe are the attachments that now remain.

5. In the event that the patient already has a homonymous hemianopia, as is usually the case, the hippocampal gyrus and remaining attachments of the hemisphere are removed, and the hemicorticectomy is complete.

If the visual field is to be preserved, however, the posterior cerebral artery, the occipital lobe, and the hippocampal structures 1.5 cm posterior to the tip of the temporal horn must be excluded from the subtotal hemicorticectomy. In a recent operation a thermal diffusion probe, under development by Carter, White and Atkinson, recorded hyperemia (118 to 140 ml per 100 gm of tissue per minute) in areas of electrocorticographic epileptiform activity and low-normal regional cerebral blood flow (61.5 ml per 100 gm of tissue per minute) in the occipital lobe from which minimal cortical

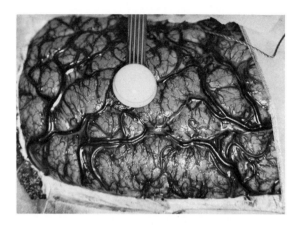

Figure 141–9   Thermal diffusion regional cerebral blood flow probe currently under investigation in epileptic foci and cortical resections. (From Carter, L. P., White, W. L., and Atkinson, J. R.: Regional cerebral blood flow at craniotomy. Neurosurgery, 2:223–229, 1978. Reprinted by permission.)

dysrhythmia was observed (Fig. 141–9).[44] The five-year-old child who was being operated on had normal visual fields. The operation spared the posterior circulation and visual radiation, and postresection regional blood flow in the occipital cortex was 115 ml per 100 gm per minute. The instrumentation for measurement of regional cerebral blood flow and its diagnostic and therapeutic applications in the surgical management of epilepsy are still in the early developmental phases.

6. The choroid plexus of the lateral ventricle is removed, meticulous hemostasis is obtained, and the ventricle and operative field are irrigated with bacitracin solution. A watertight dural closure is made.

7. An extradural drainage tube is led through a stab wound 2 cm peripheral to an occipital trephination. Drill holes are made in the bone flap, equidistant between the trephinations, and in the center of the flap. Dural sutures are placed in the center of the dural exposure and led through the central drill holes in the bone flap. The bone flap is tied down with 2-0 nylon sutures across the adjoining drill holes, and the central part of the dura is tented against the bone flap by tying the central dural suture. The remainder of the closure, the dressings, and the connection of the drainage tube to a sterile bottle and Stedman pump are as described for temporal lobectomy.

Other techniques for hemispherectomy, hemicorticectomy, subtotal or total, have been reported to provide excellent results.*

---

* See references 92, 93, 173, 274, 368, 383, 391.

Postoperative Care

With a few exceptions the postoperative care of a patient following hemicorticectomy is the same as that for temporal lobectomy. The removal of the large cortical segment and the wide exposure of the lateral ventricle almost invariably create aseptic meningitis due to blood in the ventricular system. Drainage of 20 to 30 ml of cerebrospinal fluid by daily lumbar punctures appears to reduce the symptoms and duration of aseptic meningitis.

Risks

The operative mortality rate is higher for hemispherectomy than for temporal lobectomy, but still comparatively low, 2 per cent in experienced hands.[274,391] In smaller series of patients, mortality rates of 25 per cent (2 of 8 patients), 16.66 per cent (1 to 6), and 0 per cent (0 per cent of 18 patients) have been reported.[93,124,354] The cause of the single operative fatality in the authors' series was massive central neurogenic pulmonary edema. Neurogenic pulmonary edema has been described previously in sudden severe increased intracranial pressure, the triggering mechanism of hypothalamic compromise.[179] Reviews of over 500 cases of hemispherectomy for infantile hemiplegia show a relatively low mortality rate (about 7 per cent), the proportions of left and right hemispherectomy being approximately equal.[327]

Superficial cerebral hemosiderosis may affect a fourth to a third of these patients who are followed for more than five years.[271,276,390] This condition results from jolts to the head, coughing, and other injuries, which may be minor, that cause a gradual seepage of erythrocytes into the cavity.[235,390] There is an accumulation of iron and protein in the fluid, granular ependymitis and thickening of the leptomeninges develop, and the aqueduct of Sylvius or the foramen of Munro may gradually become stenosed. The syndrome of superficial cerebral hemosiderosis develops insidiously and proceeds from neurological deterioration and evidence of intracranial pressure to death. The cavity becomes coated with a vascular granular membrane similar to that of a chronic subdural hematoma, which may require shunting, removal, or both. This complication accounted for 15 deaths in 50 hemispherectomies in the London series.[390] Nine of twenty-seven hemispherectomy patients at the Montreal Neurological Institute developed this complication after being neurologically stable for periods of $4^{1}/_{2}$ to 20 years after operation.[271] The nine patients were treated with ventriculoatrial shunts, with long-term success in four and subsequent death in five. Rasmussen reports that preservation of a small portion of the hemisphere seems to have prevented this complication in 48 patients who had removal of at least three lobes of the brain between 1937 through 1972 for criteria similar to those used for total hemispherectomy.[276] Since 1968, the Montreal Neurological Institute policy has been to preserve a small portion of the least epileptogenic region of the damaged hemisphere in patients who would have had total hemispherectomy. The authors support this idea and have also had the experience of having the patient need a shunt in the first few weeks following operation. The ventriculoperitoneal shunt system is preferred.

Results

Hemispherectomy, possibly because it is the most radical operation for epilepsy with the least chance of leaving significant epileptogenic tissue, has proved to be one of the most successful procedures except for those few patients who succumb from the operation or develop hydrocephalus (which may be preventable in most patients). Results are evaluated on the basis of the effects of the procedure on epilepsy, behavior, and motor function.

EPILEPSY. Freedom from seizures or significant improvement of seizures following hemispherectomy has been reported in a high percentage of patients in a number of series. The specific numbers are 85 per cent (23 out of 29 patients) with hemispherectomy and 70 per cent (28 of 40 patients) with subtotal hemispherectomy, 82 per cent (28 of 34 patients), 80 per cent (number of patients not given), 100 per cent (8 of 8 patients), 87.5 per cent (7 of 8 patients), and 80 per cent (4 of 5 patients).* The majority of these patients continued to take anticonvulsant medications, but in reduced dosages. Electrical changes occur after hemispherectomy and correlate with these results.[203]

BEHAVIOR. Improvement in the mental sphere following hemispherectomy for intractable seizures in infantile hemiplegia presupposes, and is dependent upon, the integrity of the remaining hemisphere and its ability to function normally once it has been released from abnormal influences from the pathological side.[181,241,381,391] Accordingly, the better the original substrate for behavior of a child or adolescent, the better are the chances for achievement following operation.

Initially studies reported no apparent differences after removal of a right versus a left hemisphere that had been damaged in early life, but later studies[209] have suggested that the procedure results in limitation of developmental potential of language and nonlanguage functions and that "transfer of intellectual faculty from one hemisphere to another may be incomplete, as it is for somatic functions."[209] The implicit assumption that the remaining hemisphere is intact, however, is often incorrect and may result in misleading conclusions.[326,327] It is still not known how early differentiation between hemispheres arises, whether before birth or after.

The left hemisphere is dominant for speech in 95 per cent of right-handed patients and in about 66 per cent of all left-handed individuals. The dominance of the left hemisphere for speech appears to be inherited.[291] The absence of aphasia following left or right hemispherectomy for infan-

---

* See references 93, 124, 132, 135, 274, 276, 354, 391.

tile hemiplegia has been explained on the basis that "at birth the two hemispheres are virtually equipotential in regard to the acquisition of language and that dominance may be readily shifted in consequence to early brain injury."[396] Improvements or development of language or mental functions following left or right hemispherectomy for infantile hemiplegia have been cited as evidence that the hemisphere removed was the "nondominant" one.[92,181,231,241]

Behavioral disorders, which may become progressively more disabling, consist of mental retardation or explosive, impulsive, aggressive, assaultive outbursts. Following hemispherectomy, the majority of patients become normal or improve. Behavioral disorders were abolished in 93 per cent, and psychological improvement occurred in nearly 50 per cent.[391] Similar findings have been reported by others.* In the authors' series, five patients with long-term follow-up were significantly improved, according to psychiatric, neuropsychological, and family assessments. Development of above-normal language and intelligence 20 years after left hemispherectomy has been reported.[338]

MOTOR FUNCTION. Hemispherectomy does not add further neurological deficit in those cases in which the atrophy is extensive and severe. Sufferers from severe hemiplegia are sometimes benefited by complete ablation of the abnormal rolandic-sensorimotor cortex, which has eliminated seizures and decreased spasticity. A patient who already has no control of the hand for delicate movements retains preoperative movement of the arm and may obtain considerable lessening of the spasticity that hampers those movements of which he is otherwise capable if the damage is extensive and occurred early in life. Following hemicorticectomy, movement is controlled by subcortical mechanisms.[92,241]

Other Cortical Resections in Children and Adolescents

Epileptogenic lesions of childhood and adolescence, amenable to operation, are most commonly located in the temporal lobe; next most commonly in the frontal lobe, in the central (sensorimotor) region, and in the parietal lobe; and most rarely in the occipital lobe. Rasmussen's reports are

---

* See references 93, 124, 132, 136, 271, 353, 383.

the most comprehensive and extensive of the publications on the subject of the operative treatment of extra–temporal lobe epilepsy. In his series, 42 patients, 1 to 15 years of age, had frontal lobe epilepsy. Eradication of or significant improvement of seizures occurred in 55 per cent. Twenty-nine patients, 2 to 15 years of age, had central (sensorimotor) epilepsy, and excellent results occurred in 57 per cent. Twenty patients up to 15 years of age had parietal lobe epilepsy, and 59 per cent of them obtained excellent seizure control. In the few patients with epileptogenic lesions in the occipital lobe, the success rate for operation was 68 per cent.[275] It is apparent that, although these results are good, seizure control is even better after temporal lobectomy and, especially, hemicorticectomy.

Birth trauma, postnatal trauma, postinflammatory brain scarring, miscellaneous lesions such as tuberous sclerosis, Sturge-Weber disease, hamartomas, scarring from previous craniotomies for a variety of disorders, tumors, and arteriovenous malformations were found as epileptogenic lesions. In about 20 per cent of the cases, the lesion was disclosed only at operation despite complete and serial neuroradiological studies. No pathological condition was found in about an equal number of patients.[274]

The patients in whom no lesion can be demonstrated and localized preoperatively are particularly challenging. This limitation makes it difficult to precisely localize and excise the epileptogenic area without creating neurological deficits of disabling proportions, i.e., aphasia, agnosia, apraxia, paresis, and the like. This difficulty accounts for the somewhat poorer results with operative excision in these patients.

Intra-carotid amobarbital (Amytal)–pentylenetetrazol (Metrazol) electroencephalographic testing usually is not possible in children below the age of 12 or 13 because of the patience and cooperation required for this lengthy study.[97,114,301,303] It is of great value in adolescents and adults, particularly to determine whether a unilateral cortical focus is responsible for bilaterally synchronous epileptiform activity. The Lombroso-Erba Pentothal activation test, an indirect method of differentiating secondary and primary bilateral synchrony in the electroencephalogram and diffuse multifocal epileptiform processes, may be used successfully in young children and adolescents.[191]

The information to be obtained by electrical stimulation studies during the operation is essential in patients in these categories. Accordingly, children below the ages of 12 or 13 are given secobarbital the evening before operation and one hour preoperatively. Atropine is also given one hour preoperatively. Light anesthesia and topical anesthesia to the throat and trachea are given before endotracheal intubation. Intermittently administered methohexital, fentanyl, and compressed air with oxygen are used to maintain light sleep. Local infiltration of the scalp with tetracaine (Pontocaine) then makes it possible to use a minimal amount of anesthetic agent and to obtain epileptiform activity on electrocorticography and responses on electrical stimulation. Adolescents, with appropriate motivation and explanation, can usually be operated on entirely with local anesthesia.

The operative tactics of adequate exposure, electrocorticography, electrical stimulation, and cortical excision utilizing the subpial dissection of Horsley are well standardized. A method employing implantation of an extradural electrode array under general anesthesia in children, adolescents, or adults in the first stage; identification of the sensorimotor cortex by means of sensory evoked potentials; prolonged recordings under close observation to identify the source of epileptiform discharges in relationship to this matrix of electrodes; and excision of the epileptiform area at a second stage has been introduced recently.[118] This method is of interest, particularly in this group of patients, even though it does not sample the medial or inferior surfaces of the brain.

The best results with operative treatment of lesions of the extratemporal convexity have been with excision of epileptogenic atrophic gyri within porencephalic cysts during adolescence.[124,132] Since epilepsy is perhaps the most important neurological symptoms in the Sturge-Weber syndrome, radical excision of the vascular malformation has been attempted in order to eliminate the seizures.[71,130,229,274] Because of the great variations in the clinical syndromes in these cases the surgical problems are complicated. Some patients do excellently for a period of years following operation and then gradually deteriorate.[130] Maximal removal of the epileptogenic areas (lobectomies, subtotal hemicorticectomies), including the angiomatous area, is necessary to obtain successful results.[71,282]

Indications for Other Operative Procedures

In the event that a child or adolescent is disabled by chronic seizures and does not satisfy the criteria with respect to localization and lateralization for cortical excision, lobectomy, or hemicorticectomy, consideration should be given to the indications for other methods.

Stereotaxic Operations

Stereotaxic amygdalotomy is a particularly useful procedure for children and adolescents with medically-resistant psychomotor epilepsy associated with aggressive behavior and bitemporal epileptogenic areas.* Although the decrease in seizures and the rate of rehabilitation are generally inferior to the results of standard temporal lobectomy, the risks and complications of medial temporal stereotaxic lesions are few in most reports. Three types of patients have been suggested as candidates for this procedure: (1) Patients with bitemporal foci in whom the issue is to be solved by depth electrodes (a stereotaxic lesion may be placed in the amygdala or one of the other medial temporal structures by way of an already implanted electrode in the worst side; if the stereotaxic lesion fails to control the seizures successfully, depth electrode studies and possibly temporal lobectomy can follow), (2) patients with bitemporal electrical foci and without any lateralization with any tactic, and (3) patients who have recurrent seizures emanating from the contralateral medial temporal region following temporal lobectomy.[232] Such lesions do not seem to create the major neuropsychological memory deficits that have been associated with bilateral hippocampal lesions or temporal lobectomy, if they are confined to the amygdala or fornix and are staged.[217,252,317] Bilateral hippocampal and hippocampal gyrus stereotaxic lesions,

---

* See references 1, 6, 7, 21, 33, 143, 199, 200, 223–226, 267, 315, 341, 357, 364.

however, may not be quite so safe in this regard.[224]

Other stereotaxic procedures involving the internal capsule, pallidum, putamen, ventral anterior nucleus, ventral lateral nucleus, centromedian nucleus, internal medullary lamina, fields of Forel, hypothalamus, cingulum, corpus callosum, and fornix have been performed for a variety of seizure disorders during the past 20 years with a few good results.*

Chronic Cerebellar Stimulation

The concept of long-term cerebellar stimulation to induce Pürkinje cell inhibition prosthetically and to modify abnormal neurological activity, including epileptic discharges, was applied clinically in 1972.[52] Results of these studies and stimulations in 15 patients were reported by Cooper and associates in 1976. There were excellent results in three patients, some reduction of seizures in seven other patients, and no help to the remaining five patients.[53] This procedure may be used in generalized seizures or in patients with bitemporal epileptic foci.

Commissurotomy

Operative division of the commissural pathways in the corpus callosum to control convulsions was first reported by Van Wagenen and Herren in 1940.[360] It was further developed by Bogen and associates and by Wilson and associates.[28–30,333,389] A wide variety of disconnection deficits are apparent on special testing even though these patients have generally benefited from the standpoint of seizure control and present an essentially normal appearance. This procedure may be considered in desperate problems with the hope of confining the seizures to one side, preserving consciousness during the attack, providing warning so that the patient may take precautionary or control measures at the onset of the seizure, and eliminating the commissural contribution to mutual re-enforcement of seizures

during the generalized phase, especially during status epilepticus.

OVERVIEW

There is a growing recognition of the real and potential hazards of long-term drug therapy in the epilepsies and of the suboptimal results with respect to normal education and working capabilities of epileptic children and adolescents.

Each seizure increases the risk of irreparable neuronal damage. If it becomes apparent that epilepsy in a child or adolescent is not completely controlled and he is not able to function in a normal fashion, a thorough investigation of the cause and localization of his seizure disorder is indicated.

The operative treatment of epilepsy requires a team effort. It is doubtful that its results will ever be 100 per cent successful, any more than those of other major neurosurgery. Better methods of case selection, improved diagnostic tactics, new and improved operative techniques, and more comprehensive rehabilitation services are factors that should improve the prognosis for epileptic children and adolescents.

The results of operative treatment of epilepsy in the childhood and adolescent period of life are gratifying from the standpoints of seizure control, improvement of behavioral abnormalities, and social and economic rehabilitation. There seems to be no significant difference in the quality and number of rehabilitated patients whether the operative procedures are done with local anesthesia or general anesthesia or whether aggressive and assaultive behavior were present prior to operation. The essential elements in successful operative treatment are related to the selection of patients and the adaptation of the optimal operative procedure, anesthesia, and aftercare for each individual child or adolescent.

---

* See references: internal capsule, 164, 171, 222; pallidum, 311, 332, 392; putamen, 63; ventral anterior nucleus, 222, 340; ventral lateral nucleus, 222; centromedian nucleus, 171, 222; internal medullary lamina, 142, 222, 332; fields of Forel, 167, 168, 222; hypothalamus, 309; cingulum, 62; corpus callosum, 311; fornix, 142, 356.

REFERENCES

1. Adams, J., and Rutkin, B.: Treatment of temporal lobe epilepsy by stereotactic surgery. Confin. Neurol., *31*:80–85, 1969.
2. Adey, W. R.: The neuroanatomical basis of mental disorder. Aust. Ann. Med., *5*:153–162, 1956.
3. Adey, W. R., Hanley, J., Kado, R. T., and Sweizig, J. R.: A multichannel telemetry system for

EEG recording. Proc. Symp. Biomed. Eng., Marquette Univ., *1*:36–39, 1966.

4. Ajmone-Marsan, C., and Zwin, L. S.: Factors related to the occurrence of typical paroxysmal EEG records of epileptic patients. Epilepsia, *11*:361–381, 1970.

5. Andermann, F., and Robb, J. P.: Absence status. A reappraisal following review of thirty-eight patients. Epilepsia (Amst.), *13*:177, 1972.

6. Andy, O. J., and Jurko, M.: The human amygdala: Excitability state and aggression. *In* Sweet, W. H., Obrador, S., and Martin-Rodriguez, J. G., eds.: Neurosurgical Treatment in Psychiatry, Pain, and Epilepsy. Baltimore, London, Tokyo, University Park Press, 1977, pp. 417–427.

7. Andy, O., Jurko, M. F., and Hughes, J. R.: Amygdalotomy for bitemporal lobe seizures. Southern Med. J., *68*:743–748, 1975.

8. Angeleri, F., Ferro-Milone, F., and Parigi, S.: Electrical activity and reactivity of the rhinencephalic, pararhinencephalic, and thalamic structures: Prolonged implantation of electrodes in man. Electroenceph. Clin. Neurophysiol., *16*:100–129, 1964.

9. Atkinson, J. R., and Ward, A. A., Jr.: Intracellular studies of cortical neurons in chronic epileptogenic foci in the monkey. Exp. Neurol., *10*:285, 1964.

10. Babb, T. L., and Crandall, P. H.: Epileptogenesis of human limbic neurons in psychomotor epileptics. Electroenceph. Clin. Neurophysiol., *40*:225–243, 1976.

11. Bailey, P.: Surgical treatment of psychomotor epilepsy: Five year follow-up. Southern Med. J., *54*:299–301, 1961.

12. Bailey, P., and Gibbs, F. A.: The surgical treatment of psychomotor epilepsy. J.A.M.A., *145*:365–370, 1951.

13. Bailey, P., Green, J. R., Amador, L., and Gibbs, F. A.: Treatment of psychomotor states by anterior temporal lobectomy. Proc. Ass. Res. Nerv. Ment. Dis., *31*:341–346, 1953.

14. Baldwin, M., and Bailey, P.: Temporal Lobe Epilepsy. Springfield, Ill., Charles C Thomas, 1958.

15. Baldy-Moulinier, M., Arias, L. P., and Passouant, P.: Hippocampal epilepsy produced by Ouabain. Eur. Neurol., *9*:333–348, 1973.

16. Bancaud, J.: Physiopathogenesis of generalized epilepsies of organic nature (stereo-electroencephalographic study). *In* Gastaut, H., Jasper, H., Bancaud, J., and Waltregny, A., eds.: Physio-pathogenesis of the Epilepsies. Springfield, Ill., Charles C Thomas, 1969.

17. Bancaud, J., Talairach, J., et al.: La stéréo électroencéphalograph dans l'épilepsie. Informations neurophysiopathologiques apportées par l'investigation fonctionelle stéréotaxique. Paris, Masson, 1965.

18. Bard, P.: The central representation of the sympathetic nervous system as indicated by certain physiologic observations. Arch. Neurol. Psychiat., *22*:230–246, 1929.

19. Bartholow, R.: Experimental investigations in the functions of the human brain. Amer. J. Med. Sci., *67*:305–313, 1874.

20. Bartlett, J. E. A.: Charonic psychosis following epilepsy. Amer. J. Psychiat., *114*:338–343, 1957.

21. Bhatia, R., and Kollevald, T.: A follow-up study of 91 patients operated upon for focal epilepsy. Epilepsia (Amst.), *17*:61–66, 1976.

22. Bickford, R. G.: The application of depth electrography in some varieties of epilepsy. Electroenceph. Clin. Neurophysiol., *8*:526–527, 1956.

23. Bingley, T.: Mental symptoms in temporal lobe epilepsy and temporal lobe gliomas. Acta Psychiat. Neurol. Scand., *33*:suppl. 120:1–151, 1958.

24. Blumer, D., and Walker, A. E.: Sexual behavior in temporal lobe epilepsy, Arch. Neurol. (Chicago), *16*:37–43, 1967.

25. Bochner, F., Hooper, W., Sutherland, J. M., et al.: Diphenylhydantoin concentrations in saliva. Arch. Neurol. (Chicago), *31*:57–59, 1974.

26. Boerhaave, H.: Praelectiones academicae de morbis nervorum quas ex auditorum manuscriptis collectas edi curavit Jacobus van Eems. Francofurti and Lipsiae: Sumptibus Societatis. Vol. 2. 1762, pp. 285–702.

27. Bogdanoff, B. M., Stafford, C. R., Green, L., and Gonzalez, C. F.: Computerized transaxial tomography in the evaluation of patients with focal epilepsy. Neurology (Minneap.), *25*: 1013–1017, 1975.

28. Bogen, J. E., and Vogel, P. J.: Cerebral commissurotomy in man. Preliminary care report. Bull. Los Angeles Neurol. Soc., *27*:169–172, 1962.

29. Bogen, J. E., and Vogel, P. J.: Neurological status in the long-term following complete cerebral commissurotomy. *In* Michel, F., and Schott, B., eds.: Lés syndromes dé disconnexion calleuse chéz l'homme. Hop. Neurol., Lyon, 1975.

30. Bogen, J. E., Sperry, R. W., and Vogel, P. J.: Commissural section and the propagation of seizures. *In* Jasper, H. H., Ward, A. A., Jr., and Pope, A., eds.: Basic Mechanisms of the Epilepsies. Boston, Little, Brown & Co., 1969.

31. Bouchard, G.: Behavioral and psychiatric problems in epilepsy. *In* Sweet, W. H., Obrador, S., and Martin-Rodriquez, J. G., eds.: Neurosurgical Treatment in Psychiatry, Pain, and Epilepsy. Baltimore, London, Tokyo, University Park Press, 1977, pp. 539–551.

32. Bouchet and Cazauvieihl: De l'épilepsie considerée dans ses rapports avec l'alienation normale. Arch. Gen. Med., Paris, *9*:510, 1825.

33. Branch, C. L.: Operative treatment of epilepsy. *In* Youmans, J. R., ed.: Neurological Surgery. Philadelphia, London, Toronto, W. B. Saunders Co., 1973, pp. 1868–1880.

34. Branch, C. L., Milner, B., and Rasmussen, T.: Intracarotid Sodium Amytal for the lateralization of speech dominance: Observations in 123 patients. J. Neurosurg., *21*:399–405, 1964.

35. Brazier, M. A. B.: Historical introduction: The role of electricity in the exploration and elucidation of the epileptic seizure. *In* Brazier, M. A. B., ed.: Epilepsy: Its Phenomena in Man. UCLA Forum in Medical Sciences, No. 17. New York, Academic Press, 1973, pp. 1–9.

36. Brazier, M. A. B.: Electrical seizure discharges within the human brain: The problem of spread. *In* Brazier, M. A. B., ed.: Epilepsy: Its Phenomena in Man. New York and London, Academic Press, 1973, pp. 153–170.

37. Brazier, M. A. B., Crandall, P. H., and Brown, W. J.: Long term follow-up of EEG changes following therapeutic surgery for epilepsy. Electroenceph. Clin. Neurophysiol., *38*:495–506, 1975.

38. Broderson, P., Paulson, O. B., Bolwig, T. T., et al.: Cerebral hyperemia in electrically induced epileptic seizures. Arch Neurol. (Chicago), *28*:334–338, 1973.

39. Brown, W. J.: Structural substrate of seizure foci in the human temporal lobe. A combined electrophysiological optic microscopic and ultrastructural study. *In* Brazier, M. A. B., ed.: Epilepsy, Its Phenomena in Man. New York and London, Academic Press, 1973, pp. 339–374.

40. Bruens, J. H.: Psychosis in epilepsy. *In* Vinken, P. J., and Bruyn, G. W., eds.: Handbook of Clinical Neurology, Vol. 15, The Epilepsies. Amsterdam, North-Holland Publishing Co.; New York, American Elsevier Publishing Co., Inc., 1974, pp. 593–610.

41. Buser, P., Bancaud, J., and Talairach, J.: Depth recordings in man in temporal lobe epilepsy. *In* Brazier, M. A. B., ed.: Epilepsy: Its Phenomena in Man. New York and London, Academic Press, 1973, pp. 67–98.

42. Cairns, H., and Davidson, M. A.: Hemispherectomy in the treatment of infantile hemiplegia. Lancet, *2*:411–415, 1951.

43. Calvin, W. H.: Synaptic summation and repetitive firing mechanisms: Input-output theory for the recruitment of neurons into epileptic bursting firing patterns. Brain Res., *39*:71–94, 1972.

44. Carter, L. P., White, W. L., and Atkinson, J. R.: Regional Cerebral Blood Flow at Craniotomy. (Presented at annual meeting of the American Association Neurological Surgeons, Toronto, April, 1977.)

45. Castorina, G., and McCrae, D. L.: Radiological findings in temporal lobe epilepsy of non-tumoral origin. Acta Radiol. (Stockholm), *1*:541–557, 1963.

46. Cavanaugh, J. B., and Meyer, A.: Aetiological aspects of Ammon's horn sclerosis associated with temporal lobe epilepsy. Brit. Med. J., *2*:1402–1403, 1956.

47. Cazzullo, C. L.: Psychiatric aspects of epilepsy. Int. J. Neurol., *1*:53–65, 1959.

48. Celesia, G. G., and Paulsen, R. E.: Electroencephalographic activation with sleep and methohexital. Arch. Neurol. (Chicago), *27*:361–363, 1972.

49. Chao, L. H. C., Druckman, R., and Kellaway, P.: Convulsive Disorders in Children. Philadelphia and London, W. B. Saunders Co., 1958, pp. 151.

50. Coatsworth, J. J., and Penry, J. K.: Clinical efficacy and use. *In* Penry, J. K. and Schmidt, R. P., eds.: Antiepileptic Drugs. New York, Raven Press, 1972, pp. 87–96.

51. Collins, R. C., Kennedy, C., Sokoloff, L., and Plum, F.: Metabolic anatomy of focal motor seizures. Arch. Neurol. (Chicago), *33*:536–542, 1976.

52. Cooper, I. S.: Effect of chronic stimulation of anterior cerebellum on neurologic disease. Lancet, *1*:1321, 1973.

53. Cooper, I. S., Amin, I., Riklin, M., Waltz, J. M., and Poor, T. P.: Chronic cerebellar stimulation in epilepsy. Arch. Neurol. (Chicago), *33*:559–570, 1976.

54. Craig, W. S.: Convulsive movements occurring in first 10 days of life. Arch. Dis. Child., *35*: 336–344, 1960.

55. Crandall, P. H.: Developments in direct recordings from epileptogenic regions in the surgical treatment of partial epilepsies. *In* Brazier, M. A. B., ed.: Epilepsy: Its Phenomena in Man. New York and London, Academic Press, 1973, pp. 287–310.

56. Crandall, P. H.: Neurosurgical management of the epilepsies. Postoperative management and criteria for evaluation. Advances Neurol., *8*:265–279, 1975.

57. Crandall, P. H.: Personal communication, 1977.

58. Crandall, P. H., Walter, R. D., and Rand, R. W.: Clinical applications of studies in stereotactically implanted electrodes in temporal lobe epilepsy. J. Neurosurg., *20*:820–840, 1963.

59. Daube, J. R.: Sensory precipitated seizures: A review. J. Nerv. Ment. Dis., *141*:524–539, 1966.

60. Davidson, S., and Falconer, M. A.: Outcome of surgery in forty children with temporal lobe epilepsy. Lancet, *1*:1260–1263, 1975.

61. Davidson, S., Falconer, M. A., and Stroud, C. E.: The place of surgery of epilepsy in childhood and adolescence: A preliminary report in 13 cases. Develop. Med. Child. Neurol., *14*: 796–803, 1972.

62. Diemath, H., Heppner, F., Enge, S., and Lechner, H.: Die stereotaktische vordere Cingulotomie bei therapieresistenter generalisierter Epilepsie. Confin. Neurol., *27*:144, 1966.

63. Dierssen, G.: Discussion of Wycis, Baird, and Spiegel, Ref. 391.

64. Dodson, W. E., Prensky, A. L., DeVivo, D. C., Goldring, S., and Dodge, P. R.: Management of seizure disorders. Selected aspects. Part I, J. Pediat., *89*:527–540; Part II, J. Pediat., *89*:693–703, 1976.

65. Dow, R. S., Fernandez-Guardiola, A., and Manni, E.: The influence of the cerebellum on experimental epilepsy. Electroenceph. Clin. Neurophysiol., *14*:383–398, 1962.

66. Earle, K. M., Baldwin, M., and Penfield, W.: Incisural sclerosis and temporal lobe seizures produced by hippocampal herniation at birth. Arch. Neurol. Psychiat., *69*:27–42, 1953.

67. Engel, J., Jr., Driver, M., and Falconer, M. A.: Electrophysiological correlates of pathology and surgical results in temporal lobe epilepsy. Brain, *98*:129–156, 1975.

67a. Engel, J., Jr., Rausch, R., Lieb, J. P., Kubl, D. E., and Crandall, P. H.: Correlation of criteria used for localizing epileptic foci in patients considered for surgical therapy of epilepsy. Ann. Neurol. 9:215–224, 1981.

68. Escueta, A. V., Kunze, V., Waddell, G., Boxley, J., and Nadel, A.: Lapse of consciousness and automatisms in temporal lobe epilepsy: A videotape analysis. Neurology (Minneap.), *27*: 144–155, 1977.

69. Falconer, M. A.: Discussion on the surgery of temporal lobe epilepsy. Surgical and pathological aspects. Proc. Roy. Soc. Med., *46*:971–975, 1953.

70. Falconer, M. A.: The surgical treatment of temporal lobe epilepsy. Neurochirurgica, *8*:161–172, 1965.

71. Falconer, M. A.: Personal communication, 1977.

72. Falconer, M. A.: The significance of mesial temporal sclerosis (Ammon's horn sclerosis) in epilepsy. Guy's Hosp. Rep., *117*:1–12, 1968.

73. Falconer, M. A.: The significance of surgery for temporal lobe epilepsy in childhood and adolescence. J. Neurosurg., *33*:233–238, 1970.

74. Falconer, M. A.: The pathological substrate of temporal lobe epilepsy. Guy's Hosp. Rep., *119*:47–60, 1970.

75. Falconer, M. A.: Anterior temporal lobectomy for epilepsy. *In* Logue, V., ed.: Operative Surgery. Vol. 14, Neurosurgery. London, Butterworths, 1971, pp. 142–149.

76. Falconer, M. A.: Genetic and retarded aetiological factors in temporal lobe epilepsy. Epilepsia, *12*:13–31, 1971.

77. Falconer, M. A.: Place of surgery for temporal lobe epilepsy during childhood. Brit. Med. J., *2*:631–635, 1972.

78. Falconer, M. A.: Febrile convulsions in early childhood. Brit. Med. J., *3*:292, 29 July 1972.

79. Falconer, M. A.: Reversibility by temporal-lobe resection of the behavioral abnormalities of temporal-lobe epilepsy. New Eng. J. Med., *289*:451–455, 1973.

80. Falconer, M. A., and Wilson, P. J. E.: Complications related to delayed hemorrhage after hemispherectomy. J. Neurosurg., *30*:413–426, 1969.

81. Falconer, M. A., Serafetinides, E. A., and Corsellis, J. A. N.: Etiology and pathogenesis of temporal lobe epilepsy. Arch. Neurol. (Chicago), *10*:233–248, 1964.

82. Falconer, M. A., Hill, D., Meyer, A., and Wilson, J. L.: Clinical, radiological, and EEG correlations with pathological changes in temporal lobe epilepsy and their significance in surgical treatment. *In* Baldwin, M., and Bailey, P., eds.: Temporal Lobe Epilepsy. Springfield, Ill., Charles C Thomas, 1958, pp. 396–410.

83. Falconer, M. A., Pond, D. A., Meyer, A., and Woolf, A. L.: Temporal lobe epilepsy with personality and behavior disorders caused by unusual calcifying lesions. J. Neurol. Neurosurg. Psychiat., *16*:234–244, 1953.

84. Feindel, W.: Temporal lobe seizures. *In* Vinken, P. J., and Bruyn, G. W., eds.: Handbook of Clinical Neurology. Vol. 15, The Epilepsies. Amsterdam, North Holland Publishing Co., 1974.

85. Feindel, W., and Penfield, W.: Localization of discharge in temporal lobe automatisms. Arch. Neurol. Psychiat., *72*:605–630, 1954.

86. Ferrier, D.: Experimental researches in cerebral physiology and pathology. West Riding Lunatic Asylum Med. Rep., *3*:30–96, 1873.

87. Fertziger, A. P., and Ranck, J. B., Jr.: Potassium accumulation in interstitial space during epileptiform seizures. Exp. Neurol., *26*:571–585, 1970.

88. Foerster, O.: Zur Pathogenese und chirurgischen Behandlung der Epilepsie. Zbl. Chir., *52*:531–549, 1925.

89. Foerster, O., and Altenburger, H.: Electrobiologische Vorgänge an der menschlichen Hirnrinde, Deutsch. Z. Nervenheilk., *135*:277–288, 1935.

90. Foerster, O., and Penfield, W.: The structural basis of traumatic epilepsy and results of radical operation. Brain, *53*:99–119, 1930.

91. French, L. A.: The significance of small field defects in the region of the vertical meridian. J. Neurosurg., *19*:522–528, 1962.

92. French, L. A., and Johnson, R. D.: Observations on the motor system following cerebral hemispherectomy. Neurology (Minneap.), *5*:11–14, 1955.

93. French, L. A., Johnson, D. R., and Adkins, G. H.: Cerebral hemispherectomy for intractable seizures. A long-term follow-up. J. Lancet, *81*:58–65, 1961.

94. Fritsch, G., and Hitzig, E.: Über die elektrische Erregbarkeit des Grosshirns. Arch. Anat. Physiol. Wissensch. Med., *37*:300–332, 1870.

95. Furlow, L. T.: Subpial resection of the cortex of focal epilepsy. Further observations. J.A.M.A., *111*:2092–2095, 1938.

96. Gamstorp, I.: Treatment with carbamazepine: Children. Advances Neurol., *11*:237–248, 1975.

97. Garretson, H., Gloor, P., and Rasmussen, T.: The effect of intracarotid amobarbital and mettrazol test for the study of epileptiform discharge in man: A note on its technique. Electroenceph. Clin. Neurophysiol., *21*:607–610, 1966.

98. Gastaut, H.: Clinical and electroencephalographical classification of epileptic seizures. Epilepsia, *11*:102–113, 1970.

99. Gastaut, H., and Broughton, R.: Epileptic Seizures. Clinical and Electrographic Features, Diagnosis and Treatment. Springfield, Ill., Charles C Thomas, 1972.

100. Gastaut, H., and Collomb, H.: Étude du comportement sexuel chéz les épileptiques psychomoteurs. Ann. Medicopsychol. (Paris), *112*:657–696, 1954.

101. Gastaut, H., and Tasinari, C. A.: Triggering mechanisms in epilepsy. The electroclinical point of view. Epilepsia, *7*:85–138, 1966.

102. German, W. J.: Epileptogenic cortical scars. Results of surgical removal. Arch. Neurol. Psychiat., *41*:73–81, 1939.

103. Geschwind, N.: Effects of temporal-lobe surgery on behavior. Editorial. New Eng. J. Med., *289*:480–481, 1973.

104. Gibbs, E. L., and Gibbs, F. A.: Diagnostic and localizing value of EEG studies in sleep. Proc. Ass. Res. Nerv. Ment. Dis., *25*:366–376, 1946.

105. Gibbs, E. L., Gibbs, F. A., and Fuster, B.: Psychomotor epilepsy. Arch. Neurol. Psychiat., *60*:331–339, 1948.

106. Gibbs, F. A.: Ictal and non-ictal psychiatric disorders in temporal lobe epilepsy. J. Nerv. Ment. Dis., *113*:522–528, 1951.

107. Gibbs, F. A.: Abnormal electrical activity in the temporal regions and its relationship to abnormalities of behavior. Res. Publ. Ass. Res. Nerv. Ment. Dis., *36*:278–294, 1958.

108. Gibbs, F. A., and Stamps, F. W.: Epilepsy Handbook. Springfield, Ill., Charles C Thomas, 1958.

109. Gibbs, F. A., Davis, H., and Lennox, W. G.: The electroencephalogram in epilepsy and in conditions of impaired consciousness. Arch. Neurol. Psychiat., *34*:113–148, 1935.

110. Gibbs, F. A., Gibbs, E. L., and Lennox, W. G.:

Epilepsy: A paroxysmal cerebral dysrhythmia. Brain, *60*:377–388, 1937.

111. Glaser, G. H.: The problem of psychosis in psychomotor temporal lobe epileptics. Epilepsia, *5*:271–278, 1964.

112. Gloor, P.: Neurophysiological bases of generalized seizures termed centrencephalic. *In* Gastaut, H., Jasper, H., Bancaud, J., and Waltregny, A., eds.: The Physiopathogenesis of the Epilepsies. Springfield, Ill., Charles C Thomas, 1969, pp. 209–236.

113. Gloor, P.: Contributions of electroencephalography and electrocorticography to the neurosurgical treatment of the epilepsies. Advances Neurol., *8*:59–105, 1975.

114. Gloor, P., Rasmussen, T., Altuzarra, A., and Garretson, H.: Role of the intra-carotid amobarbital-pentylenetrazol test in the diagnosis and surgical treatment of patients with complex seizure problems. Epilepsia, *17*:15–31, 1976.

115. Goddard, G. B., McIntyre, D. C., and Leech, C. K.: A permanent change in brain function resulting from daily electrical stimulation. Exp. Neurol., *25*:295–330, 1969.

116. Goldensohn, E. S., and Ward, A. A., Jr.: Pathogenesis of epileptic seizures. *In* Tower, D. B., ed.: The Nervous System. Vol. 2, The Clinical Neurosciences. New York, Raven Press, 1975, pp. 249–260.

117. Goldring, S.: Pathophysiology of epileptic discharge. *In* Neurological Pathophysiology. New York, London, Toronto, Oxford University Press, 1974, pp. 155–167.

118. Goldring, S.: *In* Dodson, W. E., Prensky, A. L., DeVivo, D. C., and Goldring, S.: Management of seizure disorders: Selected aspects. Part II. J. Pediat., *89*:693–703, 1976.

119. Gowers, W. R.: Epilepsy and Other Convulsive Disorders: Their Causes, Symptoms, and Treatment. London, J. A. Churchill, 1881.

120. Gowers, W. R.: A Manual of Diseases of the Nervous System. 3rd Ed. Philadelphia, P. Blakiston's Son & Co., 1899–1903.

121. Green, J. R.: Indications for surgical therapy in epilepsy. Arizona Med., *8*:21–27, 1951.

122. Green, J. R.: Temporal lobectomy, with special reference to selection of epileptic patients. Presbyterian–St. Luke's Hospital Alumni Foundation Lecture. J. Neurosurg., *26*:584–593, 1967.

123. Green, J. R.: The surgery of focal epilepsy. *In* Mark, V., ed.: Practice of Surgery. Hagerstown, Md., Harper & Row, 1971, pp. 1–32.

124. Green, J. R.: Percival Bailey Oration: Surgical treatment of epilepsy during childhood and adolescence. Surg. Neurol., *8*:71–80, 1977.

125. Green, J. R., and Scheetz, D. G.: Surgery of epileptogenic lesions of the temporal lobe. Arch. Neurol. (Chicago), *10*:135–148, 1964.

126. Green, J. R., and Steelman, H. F.: Epileptic Seizures. Baltimore, Williams & Wilkins Co., 1956.

127. Green, J. R., Duisberg, R. E. H., and McGrath, W. B.: Focal epilepsy of psychomotor type. A preliminary report of observations on effects of surgical therapy. J. Neurosurg., *8*:157–172, 1951.

128. Green, J. R., Duisberg, R. E. H., and McGrath, W. B.: Electrocorticography in psychomotor epilepsy. Electroenceph. Clin. Neurophysiol. *3*:293–299, 1951.

129. Green, J. R., Duisberg, R. E. H., and McGrath, W. B.: Results of 100 craniotomies at the Arizona State Hospital. Arizona Med., *9*:33–38, 1952.

130. Green, J. R., Foster, J., and Berens, D. L.: Encephalotrigeminal angiomatosis (Sturge-Weber syndrome). Amer. J. Roentgen., *64*:391–398, 1950.

131. Green, J. R., Kanshepolsky, J., and Turkian, B.: Incidence and significance of central nervous system infection in neurosurgical patients. Advances Neurol., *6*:223–228, 1974.

132. Green, J. R., Sidell, A. D., and Walker, M. L.: Neurosurgery of epilepsy in childhood and adolescence, with comments about 50 patients. *In* Thompson, R. A., and Green, J. R., eds.: Pediatric Neurology and Neurosurgery. Jamaica, N.Y., Spectrum Publications, 1978.

133. Green, J. R., Steelman, H. F., Duisberg, R. E. H., McGrath, W. B., and Wick, S. H.: Behavior changes following radical temporal lobe excision in the treatment of focal epilepsy. Res. Pub. Ass. Res. Nerv. Ment. Dis., *36*:295–315, 1958.

134. Greer, M., and Andriola, M. R.: Convulsive disorders of childhood. *In* Thompson, R. A., and Green, J. R., eds.: Pediatric Neurology and Neurosurgery. Jamaica, N.Y., Spectrum Publications, 1978.

135. Griffith, H. B.: Cerebral hemispherectomy for infantile hemiplegia. Ann. Roy. Coll. Surg. Eng., *41*:183–201, 1967.

136. Griffith, H., and Davidson, M.: Long-term changes in intellect and behavior after hemispherectomy. J. Neurol. Neurosurg. Psychiat., *29*:571–576, 1968.

137. Grinker, R. R.: Method for studying and influencing corticohypothalamic relations. Science, *87*:73–74, 1938.

138. Guerrant, J., Anderson, W. W., Fischer, A., Weinstein, M. R., Jaros, R. M., and Deskins, A.: Personality in Epilepsy. Springfield, Ill., Charles C Thomas, 1962.

139. Guillaume, J., Mazars, G., and Mazars, Y.: Surgical indications in so-called "temporal epilepsy." Rev. Neurol. (Paris), *88*:461–501, 1953.

140. Hamlin, H., and Delgado, J. M. R.: Case Report. Juvenile psychomotor epilepsy and associated behavior disorder—20-year follow-up of temporal lobectomy. *In* Sweet, W. H., Obrador, S., and Martin-Rodriquez, J. G., eds.: Neurosurgical Treatment in Psychiatry, Pain, and Epilepsy. Baltimore, London, Tokyo, University Park Press, 1977, pp. 569–571.

141. Harris, A. B.: Degeneration in experimental epileptic foci. Arch. Neurol. (Chicago), *26*:434–449, 1972.

142. Hassler, P., and Riechert, T.: Über einer Fall von doppelseitiger Fornicotomie bei sogenaunter temporales Epilepsie. Acta Neurochir., *5*:330–340, 1957.

143. Heimburger, R. F., Whitlock, C. C., and Kalsbeck, J. E.: Stereotaxic amygdalotomy for epilepsy with aggressive behavior. J.A.M.A., *198*:741–745, 1966.

144. Hendrick, E. B., and Harris, L.: Post-traumatic epilepsy in children. J. Trauma, 8:547–556, 1968.

145. Herrick, C. J.: The functions of the olfactory parts of the cerebral cortex. Proc. Nat. Acad. Sci., 19:7–14, 1933.

146. Holowach, J., Thurston, D. L., and O'Leary, J.: Prognosis in childhood epilepsy. New Eng. J. Med., 286:169–174, 1972.

147. Hopkins, I. J.: Seizures in the first week of life. A study of aetiological factors. Med. J. Aust., 2:647, 1972.

148. Horsley, V.: Brain surgery. Brit. Med. J., 2:670–675, 1886.

149. Horsley, V.: The origin and seat of epileptic disturbance. Brit. Med. J., 1:693–696, 1892.

150. Horsley, V.: On the technique of operations on the central nervous system. Brit. Med. J., 2:411–423, 1906.

151. Hosokawa, S., Yamashita, Y., Ueno, H., and Caveness, W. F.: Regional cerebral blood flow pattern in subcortical propagation of focal seizures in newborn monkeys. Ann. Neurol., 1:225–234, 1977.

152. Hougaard, K., Oikawa, T., Sveinsdottir, E., Skinkøj, E. Ingvar, H., and Lassen, N. A.: Regional cerebral blood flow in focal cortical epilepsy. Arch. Neurol. (Chicago), 33:527–535, 1976.

153. Hughes, J. R.: Bilateral EEG abnormalities on corresponding areas. Epilepsia, 7:44–52, 1966.

154. Ingvar, D. H.: rCBF in focal cortical epilepsy. In Langfitt, T. W., McHenry, L. C., Reivich, M., et al., eds.: Cerebral Circulation and Metabolism. New York, Heidelberg, Berlin, Springer-Verlag, 1975, pp. 361–364.

155. Ives, J. R., Gloor, P., Rasmussen, T., Olivier, A.: Preliminary report on epileptic patients whose spontaneous seizures were recorded during their routine work-up as seizure surgery candidates. Proc. Amer. EEG Soc., Miami, Florida, June 22–24, 1977.

156. Ives, J. R., Thompson, C. J., Gloor, P., Olivier, A., and Woods, J. F.: Multichannel telemetry-computer monitoring of epileptic patients. In Biotelemetry II. Second International Symposium. Karger, Basel, 1974.

157. Ives, J. R., Thompson, C. J., Gloor, P., Olivier, A., and Woods, J. F.: The on-line computer detection and recording of spontaneous temporal lobe epileptic seizures with implanted depth electrodes via a radio-telemetry link. EEG J. 37:205, 1975. (Abstract)

158. Jackson, J. H.: Unilateral epileptiform seizures beginning by a disagreeable smell. Med. Times Gaz., 2:168, 1864.

159. Jackson, J. H.: On the anatomical, physiological, and pathological investigation of the epilepsies. West Riding Lunatic Asylum, Med. Rep., 3:315–339, 1873.

160. Jackson, J. H.: Croonian lectures on evolution and dissolution of the nervous system. Brit. Med. J., 1:591–593, 660–663, 703, 707, 1884.

161. Jackson, J. H.: Selected Writings of John Hughlings Jackson. Vol. 1, On Epilepsy and Epileptiform Convulsions. London, Hodder & Stoughton, Ltd., 1931.

162. Jasper, H. H.: Electrocorticograms in man. Electroenceph. Clin. Neurophysiol., suppl., 2:16–29, 1949.

163. Jasper, H. H., and Kershman, J.: Electroencephalographic classification of the epilepsies. Arch. Neurol. Psychiat., 135:690–741, 1942.

164. Jelsma, R., Bertrand, C., Martinez, S., and Molina-Negro, P.: Stereotaxic treatment of frontal lobe and centrencephalic epilepsy. J. Neurosurg., 39:42–51, 1973.

165. Jennett, B.: Post-traumatic epilepsy. In Vinken, P. J., and Bruyn, G. W., eds.: Handbook of Clinical Neurology. Vol. 24, Injuries of the Brain and Skull, Part II. Amsterdam, Oxford, North-Holland Publishing Co.; New York, American Elsevier Publishing Co., Inc., 1976, pp. 445–454.

166. Jennett, B., and Van de Sande, J.: EEG prediction of post-traumatic epilepsy. Epilepsia, 16:251–256, 1975.

167. Jinnai, D.: Clinical results and significance of Forel-H-tomy in the treatment of epilepsy. Confin. Neurol., 27:129–136, 1966.

168. Jinnai, D., and Mukawa, J.: Forel-H-tomy in the treatment of epilepsy. Confin. Neurol., 32:307–315, 1970.

169. Jüul-Jensen, F.: Epilepsy: A Clinical and Social Analysis. Copenhagen, Munksgaard Press, 1963.

170. Jüül-Jensen, P.: Social prognosis. In Vinken, P. J., and Bruyn, G. W., eds.: Handbook of Clinical Neurology. Vol. 15, The Epilepsies. Amsterdam, North-Holland Publishing Co.; New York, American Elsevier Publishing Co., Inc., 1974, pp. 800–814.

171. Kalyanaraman, S., and Ramamurthi, B.: Stereotaxic surgery for generalized epilepsy. Neurol. India, 18:suppl.:34–41, 1970.

172. Kaufman, I. C., Marshall, C., and Walker, A. E.: Activated electroencephalography. Arch. Neurol. Psychiat., 58:533–549, 1947.

173. Kempe, L. G.: Operative Neurosurgery. Vol. 1. New York, Springer-Verlag, 1968, pp. 180–189 (Hemispherectomy) and pp. 190–195 (Temporal lobectomy).

174. Kiørboe, E.: Medical prognosis in epilepsy. In Vinken, P. J., and Bruyn, G. W., eds.: Handbook of Clinical Neurology. Vol. 15, The Epilepsies. New York, American Elsevier Publishing Co., Inc., 1974, pp. 783–799.

175. Klüver, H., and Bucy, P. C.: Preliminary analysis of functions of the temporal lobes in monkeys. Arch. Neurol. Psychiat., 42:979–1000, 1939.

176. Knox, S. J.: Epileptic automatism and violence. Med. Sci. Law, 8:96–104, 1968.

177. Kopeloff, L. M., Barrera, S. E., and Kopeloff, N.: Recurrent convulsive seizures in animals produced by immunologic and chemical means. Amer. J. Psychiat., 98:881, 1942.

178. Kopeloff, L. M., Chusid, J. C., and Kopeloff, N.: Epilepsy in Macacca mulatta after cortical or intracerebral alumina. Arch. Neurol. Psychiat., 74:523, 1955.

179. Kosnik, E. J., Paul, S. E., Rossel, C. W., and Sayers, M. P.: Central neurogenic pulmonary edema: With a review of its pathogenesis and treatment. Child's Brain, 3:37–47, 1977.

180. Krause, F.: Surgery of the Brain and Spinal Cord Based on Personal Experiences. Transl. by H.

Haubold and M. Thorek. New York, Rebman Co., 1909–1912.

181. Krynauw, R. A.: Infantile hemiparesis treated by removing one cerebral hemisphere. J. Neurol. Neurosurg. Psychiat., *13*:243–267, 1950.

182. Kutt, H., and Penry, J. K.: Usefulness of blood levels of antiepileptic drugs. Arch. Neurol. (Chicago), *31*:283–288, 1974.

183. Lassen, N. A., and Ingvar, D. H.: Clinical relevance of cerebral blood flow measurements. II. Focal cortical epilepsy. *In* Krayenbuhl, H., et al., eds.: Advances and Technical Standards in Neurosurgery. Vol. 4, Wein, New York, Springer-Verlag, 1977, pp. 5–8.

184. Lennox, W. G., and Lennox, M. A.: Epilepsy and Related Disorders. Vol. 2. Boston, Toronto, Little, Brown & Co., 1960.

185. Lennox-Buchtal, M.: Febrile convulsions. *In* Vinken, P. J., and Bruyn, G. W., eds.: Handbook of Neurology. Vol. 15, The Epilepsies. Amsterdam, North-Holland Publishing Co.; New York, American Elsevier Press, 1974, pp. 246–263.

186. Li, C. L., and Jasper, H.: Microelectrode studies of the electrical activity of the cerebral cortex of the cat. J. Physiol. (London), *12*:117–140, 1953.

187. Livingston, S.: Living with Epileptic Seizures. Springfield, Ill., Charles C Thomas, 1963.

188. Livingston, S.: Comprehensive Management of Epilepsy in Infancy, Childhood and Adolescence. Springfield, Ill., Charles C Thomas, 1972, pp. 378–405.

189. Llinas, R. R.: Synaptic transmission and organization of the nervous System. Proc. Soc. of Neurol. Surgeons, Rochester, Minnesota, June 1, 1977.

190. Lombroso, C. T.: Seizures in the newborn period. *In* Vinken, P. J., and Bruyn, G. W., eds.: Handbook of Neurology. Vol. 15, The Epilepsies. Amsterdam, North-Holland Publishing Co., New York, American Elsevier Press, 1974, pp. 189–218.

191. Lombroso, C. T., and Erba, G.: Primary and secondary bilateral synchrony in epilepsy. A clinical and electroencephalographic study. Arch. Neurol. (Chicago), *22*:321–334, 1970.

192. Ludwig, B. I., and Ajmone-Marsan, C.: EEG changes after withdrawal of medications in epileptic patients. Electroenceph. Clin. Neurophysiol., *39*:173–181, 1975.

193. MacLean, P.: Some psychiatric implications of physiological studies on fronto-temporal portion of the limbic system. Electroenceph. Clin. Neurophysiol., *4*:407–418, 1952.

194. MacLean, P. D.: The limbic system ("visceral brain") and emotional behavior. Arch. Neurol. Psychiat., *73*:130–134, 1955.

195. Magoun, H. W.: The Waking Brain. Springfield, Ill., Charles C Thomas, 1958.

196. Malamud, N.: The epileptogenic focus in temporal lobe epilepsy from a pathological standpoint. Arch. Neurol. (Chicago), *14*:190–195, 1966.

197. Malamud, N.: Psychiatric disorder with intracranial tumors of limbic system. Arch. Neurol. (Chicago), *17*:113–123, 1967.

198. Margerison, J. H., and Corsellis, J. A. N.: Epilepsy and the temporal lobes: A clinical, electroencephalographic and neuropathological study of the brain in epilepsy, with particular reference to the temporal lobes, Brain, *89*:490–530, 1966.

199. Mark, V. H., and Sweet, W. H.: The role of limbic brain dysfunction in aggression. Res. Publ. Ass. Res. Nerv. Ment. Dis., *52*:186–200, 1974.

200. Mark, V. H., Sweet, W. H., and Ervin, F. R.: The effect of amygdalotomy on violent behavior in patients with temporal lobe epilepsy. *In* Hitchcock, E., Laitinen, L., and Vaernet, K., eds.: Psychosurgery. Springfield, Ill., Charles C Thomas, 1972, pp. 139–155.

201. Mark, V. H., Erwin, F. R., Sweet, W. H., and Delgado, J.: Remote telemeter stimulation and recording from implanted temporal lobe electrodes. Confin. Neurol., *31*:86–93, 1969.

202. Marshall, C.: Surgery of epilepsy and motor disorders. *In* Walker, A. E., ed.: A History of Neurological Surgery. Baltimore, Williams & Wilkins Co., 1951, pp. 288–300.

203. Marshall, C., and Walker, A. E.: The electroencephalographic changes after hemispherectomy in man. Electroenceph. Clin. Neurophysiol., *2*:147–156, 1950.

204. Masland, R. L.: The classification of the epilepsies. *In* Vinken, P. J., and Bruyn, G. W., eds.: Handbook of Clinical Neurology. Vol. 15, The Epilepsies. New York, American Elsevier Publishing Co., Inc., pp. 1–29.

205. Masland, R. L.: Epilepsy commission favors quicker use of drug to control seizures. J.A.M.A., *237*:2021–2022, 1977.

206. Mathieson, G.: Pathology of temporal lobe foci. Advances Neurol., *11*:163–185, 1975.

207. McAuliffe, J. J., Sherwin, A. L., Leppik, I. E., Fayle, S. A., and Pippenger, C. E.: Salivary levels of anticonvulsants: A practical approach to drug monitoring. Neurology (Minneap.), *27*:409–413, 1977.

208. McCrae, D. L.: Radiology in epilepsy. *In* Vinken, P. J., and Bruyn, G. W., eds.: Handbook of Clinical Neurology. Vol. 15, The Epilepsies. New York, American Elsevier Publishing Co., Inc., 1974, pp. 533–558.

209. McFie, J.: The effects of hemispherectomy on intellectual functioning in cases of infantile hemiplegia. J. Neurol. Neurosurg. Psychiat., *24*:240–249, 1961.

210. McKenzie, K. G.: The present status of a patient who had the right cerebral hemisphere removed. J.A.M.A., *111*:168, 1938.

211. McNaughton, F. L., and Rasmussen, T.: Criteria for selection of patients for neurosurgical treatment. Advances Neurol., *8*:37–48, 1975.

212. Menkes, J. H.: Textbook of Child Neurology. Philadelphia, Lea & Febiger, 1974.

213. Metrakos, K., and Metrakos, J. D.: Genetics of epilepsy. *In* Vinken, P. J., and Bruyn, G. W., eds.: Handbook of Clinical Neurology. Vol. 15, The Epilepsies. New York, American Elsevier Publishing Co., Inc., 1974, pp. 429–439.

214. Meyer, A., Falconer, M. A., and Beck, E.: Pathological findings in temporal lobe epilepsy. J. Neurol. Neurosurg. Psychiat., *17*:276–285, 1954.

215. Mignone, R. J., Donnelly, E. F., and Sadowsky,

D.: Psychological and neurological comparisons of psychomotor and non-psychomotor epileptic patients. Epilepsia, *11*:345–359, 1970.

216. Millechap, J. G., Madsen, J. A., and Aledort, L. M.: Studies in febrile seizures. V. Clinical and electroencephalographic study in unselected patients. Neurology (Minneap.), *10*:643, 1960.

217. Milner, B.: Psychological aspects of focal epilepsy and its neurosurgical management. Advances Neurol., *8*:299–321, 1975.

218. Morrell, F.: Secondary epileptogenic lesions. Epilepsia, *1*:538–560, 1959.

219. Morris, A. A.: The surgical treatment of psychomotor epilepsy. M. Ann. D.C., *19*:121–131, 1950.

220. Morris, A. A.: Temporal lobectomy with removal of uncus, hippocampus and amygdala. Arch. Neurol. Psychiat., *76*:479–496, 1956.

221. Mullan, S., and Penfield, W.: Illusions of comparative interpretation and emotion. Arch. Neurol. Psychiat., *81*:269–284, 1959.

222. Mullan, S., Vailati, G., Karasick, J., and Mailis, M.: Thalamic lesions for the control of epilepsy. Arch. Neurol. (Chicago), *16*:277–285, 1967.

223. Narabayashi, H.: Discussion of Vaernet, K.: Stereotaxic amygdalotomy in temporal lobe epilepsy. Confin. Neurol., *34*:182, 1972.

224. Narabayashi, H., and Mizutani, T.: Epileptic seizures and stereotaxic amygdalotomy. Confin. Neurol., *32*:289–297, 1970.

225. Narabayashi, H., Nagao, T., Saito, Y., Yoshida, M., and Nagahata, M.: Stereotaxic amygdalotomy for behavior disorders. Arch. Neurol. (Chicago), *9*:1–16, 1963.

226. Nashold, B., Flanigin, H., Wilson, W., and Steward, B.: Stereotactic evaluation of bitemporal epilepsy with electrodes and lesions, Confin. Neurol., *35*:94–100, 1973.

227. Nelson, K. B., and Ellenberg, J. H.: Predictors of epilepsy in children who have experienced febrile seizures. New Engl. J. Med., *295*:1029–1033, 1976.

228. Niemeyer, P.: The transventricular amygdalo-hippocampectomy in temporal lobe epilepsy. *In* Baldwin, M., and Bailey, P., eds.: Temporal Lobe Epilepsy. Springfield, Ill., Charles C Thomas, 1958, pp. 461–482.

229. Norlén, G.: The surgical treatment of Stürge-Weber's disease. Neurochirurgia, *1*:243–255, 1959.

230. Northfield, D. W. C.: Surgical treatment of epilepsy. *In* Northfield, D. W. C.: The Surgery of the Central Nervous System. Oxford, London, Edinburgh, Melbourne, Blackwell Scientific Publications, 1973, pp. 537–514.

231. Obrador, A. S.: Hemisferectomía en el tratamiento de las convulsiones de la hemiplegía infantil por hemiatrofía cerebral. Arq. Neuropsiquiat. (S. Paulo), *9*:191–197, 1951.

232. Ojemann, G. A., and Ward, A. A., Jr.: Stereotactic and other procedures for epilepsy. Advances Neurol., *8*:241–263, 1975.

233. O'Leary, J. L., and Goldring, S.: Science and Epilepsy. Neuroscience Gains in Epilepsy Research. New York, Raven Press, 1976.

234. Olivier, A., Gloor, P., and Ives, J.: Stereotaxic seizure monitoring with bitemporal epilepsy:

Indications, technique and results. Proceedings, American Association of Neurological Surgeons. Toronto, April 1977.

235. Oppenheimer, D. R., and Griffith, H. B.: Persistent intracranial bleeding as a complication of hemispherectomy. J. Neurol. Neurosurg. Psychiat., *29*:229–240, 1966.

236. Ounsted, C.: *In* Recent Advances in Paediatrics, edited by Gairdner, D., and Hull, D., 4th Ed. London, Churchill, 1971.

237. Pampiglione, G., and Kerridge, J.: EEG abnormalities from the temporal lobe studied with sphenoidal electrodes. J. Neurol. Neurosurg. Psychiat., *19*:117–119, 1956.

238. Papez, J. W.: A proposed mechanism of emotion. Arch. Neurol. Psychiat., *38*:725–743, 1937.

239. Penfield, W.: Epilepsy and surgical therapy. Arch. Neurol. Psychiat. *36*:449–484, 1936.

240. Penfield, W.: The circulation of the epileptic brain. Res. Publ. Ass. Res. Nerv. Ment. Dis., *18*:605–637, 1937.

241. Penfield, W.: Ablation of abnormal cortex in cerebral palsy. J. Neurol. Neurosurg. Psychiat., *15*:73–78, 1952.

242. Penfield, W.: The Twenty-Ninth Maudsley Lecture: The role of the temporal cortex in certain psychical phenomena. J. Ment. Sci., *100*:451–465, 1955.

243. Penfield, W.: The excitable cortex in conscious man. Fifth Sherrington Lecture. Springfield, Ill., Charles C Thomas, 1958.

244. Penfield, W.: Introduction: The physiology of epilepsy. Advances Neurol., *8*:1–9, 1975.

245. Penfield, W., and Baldwin, M.: Temporal lobe seizures and the technique of subtotal temporal lobectomy. Ann. Surg., *136*:625–634, 1952.

246. Penfield, W., and Erickson, T. C.: Epilepsy and Cerebral Localization. Springfield, Ill., Charles C Thomas, 1941.

247. Penfield, W., and Flanigin, H.: Surgical treatment of temporal lobe seizures. Arch. Neurol. Psychiat., *64*:491–500, 1950.

248. Penfield, W., and Jasper, H. A.: Electroencephalography in focal epilepsy. Trans. Amer. Neurol. Ass., *66*:209–211, 1940.

249. Penfield, W., and Jasper, H.: Epilepsy and Functional Anatomy of the Human Brain. Boston, Little, Brown & Co., 1954.

250. Penfield, W., and Kristiansen, K.: Epileptic Seizure Patterns. Springfield, Ill., Charles C Thomas, 1951, pp. 537–574.

251. Penfield, W., and Mathieson, G.: Memory: Autopsy findings and comments on the role of the hippocampus in experiential recall. Arch. Neurol. (Chicago), *31*:145–154, 1974.

252. Penfield, W., and Milner, B.: Memory deficit produced by bilateral lesions in the hippocampal region. Arch. Neurol. Psychiat., *79*:475–497, 1958.

253. Penfield, W., and Perot, P.: The brain's record of auditory and visual experience. Brain, *86*:595–696, 1963.

254. Penfield, W., and Rasmussen, T.: The Cerebral Cortex of Man. A Clinical Study of Localization of Function. New York, Macmillan Co., 1950.

255. Penfield, W., and Steelman, H.: The treatment of

focal epilepsy by cortical excision. Ann. Surg., *126*:740–761, 1947.

256. Penfield, W., Lende, R. A., and Rasmussen, T.: Manipulation hemiplegia. An untoward complication in the surgery of focal epilepsy. J. Neurosurg., *18*:760–766, 1961.

257. Penfield, W., Von Santha, D., and Cipriani, A.: Cerebral blood flow during induced epileptiform seizures in animals and man. J. Neurophysiol., *2*:257–267, 1939.

258. Penry, J. K.: Medical treatment of convulsive disorders. *In* Tower, D. B., ed.: The Nervous System. Vol. 2, The Clinical Neurosciences. New York, Raven Press, 1975, pp. 267–275.

259. Penry, J. K.: *Cited in* Epilepsy commission favors quicker use of drug to control seizures. J.A.M.A., *237*:2021–2022, 1977.

260. Pertuiset, B., and Capdevielle-Arfel, G.: Deux techniques particulières d'exploration basale. Les électrodes sphéno-ptérygoidiennes et orbitaires. Rev. Neurol. (Paris), *84*:605–612, 1951.

261. Petit-Dutaillis, D., Christophe, J., Pertuiset, B., and Dreyfus, B. C.: Indications for and results of cortical excision in temporal epilepsy. Sem. Hôp. Paris, *29*:1–10, 1953.

262. Plum, F., Posner, J. B., and Troy, B.: Cerebral metabolism and circulatory responses to induced convulsions in animals. Arch. Neurol. (Chicago), *18*:1–13, 1968.

263. Poggio, G. F., Walker, A. E., and Andy, O. J.: The propagation of afterdischarge through subcortical structures. Arch. Neurol. Psychiat., *75*:350–361, 1956.

264. Pond, D. A.: Epilepsy and personality disorders. *In* Vinden, P. J., and Bruyn, G. W., eds.: Handbook of Clinical Neurology. Vol. 15, The Epilepsies. Amsterdam, North-Holland Publishing Co.; New York, American Elsevier Publishing Co., Inc., 1974, pp. 576–592.

265. Pool, J. L.: The visceral brain of man. J. Neurosurg., *11*:45–63, 1954.

266. Prichard, J. S.: The character and significance of epileptic seizures in infancy. *In* Kellaway, P., and Petersen, I., eds.: Neurological and Electroencephalographic Correlative Studies in Infancy. New York, Grune & Stratton, Inc., 1964.

267. Ramamurthi, B.: Stereotaxic surgery in temporal lobe epilepsy. Neurol. India, *18*:suppl.1:42–45, 1970.

268. Rapport, R. L., and Prensky, J. K.: Pharmacologic prophylaxis of post-traumatic epilepsy. Epilepsia, *13*:295–304, 1972.

269. Rapport, R. L., and Prensky, J. K.: A survey of attitudes towards the pharmacological prophylaxis of post-traumatic epilepsy. J. Neurosurg., *38*:159–166, 1973.

270. Rapport, R. L., II, Ojemann, G. A., Wyler, A. R., and Ward, A. A., Jr.: Surgical management of epilepsy. West. J. Med., *127*:185–189, 1977.

271. Rasmussen, T.: Postoperative superficial hemosiderosis of the brain, its diagnosis, treatment and prevention. Trans. Amer. Neurol. Ass., *98*:133–137, 1973.

272. Rasmussen, T.: Cortical excision for medically refractory focal epilepsy. *In* Harris, P., and Maudsley, C., eds.: The Natural History and Management of Epilepsy. Edinburgh, Churchill Livingstone, 1974.

273. Rasmussen, T.: Surgical treatment of epilepsy. *In* Tower, D. B., ed.: The Nervous System. Vol. 2, The Clinical Neurosciences. New York Raven Press, 1975, pp. 277–286.

274. Rasmussen, T.: Cortical resection in the treatment of focal epilepsy. Advances Neurol., *8*:139–154, 1975.

275. Rasmussen, T.: Surgery of frontal lobe epilepsy. Advances Neurol., *8*:197–205, 1975.

276. Rasmussen, T.: Surgery for epilepsy arising in regions other than the temporal and frontal lobes. Advances Neurol., *8*:207–226, 1975.

277. Rasmussen, T.: Surgical treatment of patients with complex partial seizures. Advances Neurol., *11*:415–449, 1975.

278. Rasmussen, T.: Personal communication and table of results of cortical excision in childhood and adolescent temporal lobe epilepsy. Presented at Pediatric Congress, Toronto, October, 1975. Jamaica, N.Y., Spectrum Publications, 1978.

279. Rasmussen, T., and Branch, C. L.: Temporal lobe epilepsy: Indications for and results of surgical therapy. Postgrad. Med. J., *31*:9–14, 1962.

280. Rasmussen, T., and Gossman, H.: Epilepsy due to gross destructive brain lesions. Neurology (Minneap.), *13*:659–669, 1963.

281. Rasmussen, T., and Gulati, P. R.: Cortisone in the treatment of postoperative cerebral edema. J. Neurosurg., *19*:535–544, 1962.

282. Rasmussen, T., Mathieson, G., and Leblanc, F.: Surgical therapy of typical and a forme fruste variety of the Sturge-Weber syndrome. Arch. Suisses Neurol. Neurochir. Psychiat., *111*:393–409, 1972.

283. Rayport, M.: The jacksonian hypothesis: An appraisal in the single unit recording in focal epileptogenic gray matter in man. Proc. Rudolf Virchow Med. Soc. N.Y., suppl., *26*:301–324, 1968.

284. Remillard, G. M., Andermann, F., Rhi-Sausi, A., and Robbins, N. M.: Facial asymmetry in patients with temporal lobe epilepsy. A clinical sign useful in the lateralization of temporal epileptogenic foci. Neurology (Minneap.), *27*:109–114, 1977.

285. Reivich, M., Jehle, J., Sokoloff, L., et al.: Measurement of regional cerebral blood flow with antipyrine-^{14}C in awake cats. J. Appl. Physiol., *27*:296–300, 1969.

286. Reynolds, E. H.: Chronic antiepileptic toxicity: A review. Epilepsia, *16*:319–352, 1975.

287. Reynolds, E. H.: Unsatisfactory aspects of the drug treatment of epilepsy. Editorial. Epilepsia, *17*:xiii–xv, 1976.

288. Rhoton, A. L., and Groover, R. V.: The surgical treatment of epilepsy. Surg. Clin. N. Amer., *49*:1021–1032, 1969.

289. Robb, P.: Focal epilepsy: The problem, prevalence, and contributing factors. Advances Neurol., *8*:11–22, 1975.

290. Robb, P., and McNaughton, F.: Vascular disease. *In* Vinken, P. J., and Bruyn, G. W., eds.: Handbook of Clinical Neurology. Vol. 15, The Epilepsies. New York, American Elsevier Publishing Co., 1974, pp. 302–305.

291. Roberts, L.: Aphasia, apraxia, and agnosia in abnormal states of cerebral dominance. *In* Vin-

ken, P. J., and Bruyn, G. W., eds.: Handbook of Clinical Neurology. Vol. 4. New York, John Wiley, 1969, pp. 312–326.

292. Rodin, E. A.: The Prognosis of Patients with Epilepsy. Springfield, Ill., Charles C Thomas, 1968.

293. Rodin, E., and DeJong, R. P.: Relationship between certain forms of psychomotor epilepsy and schizophrenia. Arch. Neurol. Psychiat., 7:449, 1957.

294. Rodin, E. A., and Gonzalez, S.: Hereditary components in epileptic patients, EEG family studies. J.A.M.A., 198:221, 1966.

295. Rose, A. A.: Psychomotor epilepsy and the role of emotions in the convulsive disorders. A review and a suggestion for treatment. In Green, J. R., and Steelman, H. F., eds.: Epileptic Seizures. Baltimore, Williams & Wilkins Co., 1956, pp. 50–62.

296. Rose, A. L., and Lombroso, C. T.: Neonatal seizure states: A study of clinical, pathological and electroencephalographic features in 137 full-term babies with long-term follow-up. Pediatrics, 45:404–425, 1970.

297. Rose, S. W., Penry, J. K., Markush, R. E., et al.: Prevalence of epilepsy in children. Epilepsia, 14:133–152, 1973.

298. Roseman, E.: The epileptic in the Army. Amer. J. Psychiat., 101:349–354, 1944.

299. Ross, E. M.: Convulsive disorders in British children. Proc. Roy. Soc. Med., 66:763–704, 1973.

300. Rossi, G. F.: Considerations on the principles of surgical treatment of partial epilepsy. Brain Res., 95:395–402, 1975.

301. Rovit, R., Gloor, P., and Rasmussen, T.: Intracarotid amobarbital in epileptic patients. Arch. Neurol. (Chicago), 5:606–626, 1961.

302. Rovit, R. L., Gloor, P., and Rasmussen, T.: Sphenoidal electrodes in the electroencephalographic study of patients with temporal lobe epilepsy. An evaluation. J. Neurosurg., 2:151–158, 1961.

303. Rovit, R., Rasmussen, T., Garretson, H., and Maroun, F.: Fractional intra-carotid Metrazol injection. A new diagnostic method in the electroencephalography. Electroenceph. Clin. Neurophysiol., 17:322–327, 1964.

304. Rowe, S. N., and Watts, J. W.: Traumatic epilepsy with cortical scar. Diagnosis and results in 20 cases. Med. Ann. D.C., 5:298–301, 1936.

305. Rubin, R. T., Mandell, A. J., and Crandall, P. H.: Corticosteroid responses to limbic stimulation in man. Localization of stimulus sites. Science, 153:767–768, 1966.

306. Sachs, E.: The subpial resection of the cortex in the treatment of Jacksonian epilepsy (Horsley operation) with observations on areas 4 and 6. Brain, 58:492–523, 1935.

307. Sachs, E., Schwartz, H. G., and Kerr, A. S.: Electrical activity of the exposed human brain. Trans. Amer. Neurol. Ass., 65:14–17, 1939.

308. Sano, K., and Malamud, N.: Clinical significance of sclerosis of the cornu Ammonis: Ictal "psychic phenomena." Arch. Neurol. Psychiat., 70:40–53, 1953.

309. Sano, K., Mayanaji, Y., Sekino, H., Ogashiwa, M., and Ishijima, B.: Results of stimulation and destruction of the posterior hypothalamus in man. J. Neurosurg., 33:689–707, 1970.

310. Scarff, J. E., and Rahm, W. E., Jr.: The human

electrocorticogram. A report of spontaneous electrical potentials obtained from the exposed human brain. J. Neurophysiol., 4:418–426, 1941.

311. Schaltenbrand, G., Spuler, H., Nadjimi, M., Hopf, H., and Wahren, W.: Die stereotaktische Behandlung der Epilepsien. Confin. Neurol., 27:111–113, 1966.

312. Scheibel, M. E., and Scheibel, A. B.: Hippocampal pathology in temporal lobe epilepsy, a Golgi survey. In Brazier, M. A. B., ed.: Epilepsy: Its Phenomena in Man. New York, Academic Press, 1973, pp. 311–337.

313. Schmidt, C. F., Kety, S. S., and Pennes, H. H.: The gaseous metabolism of the brain of the monkey. Amer. J. Physiol., 143:33–52, 1945.

314. Schmidt, R. P., and Wilder, B. J.: Epilepsy. Contemporary Neurology Series No. 18, Philadelphia, F. A. Davis Co., 1968.

315. Schwab, R., Sweet, W., Mark, V., Kjellberg, R., and Ervin, F.: Treatment of intractable temporal lobe epilepsy by stereotactic amygdala lesions. Trans. Amer. Neurol. Ass., 90:12–19, 1965.

316. Scott, D. F.: Psychiatric aspects of epilepsy. Postgrad. Med. J., 44:319–326, 1968.

317. Scoville, W. B., and Milner, B.: Loss of recent memory after bilateral hippocampal lesions. J. Neurol. Neurosurg. Psychiat., 20:11–21, 1957.

318. Seay, A. R., and Bray, P. F.: Significance of seizures in infants weighing less than 2500 grams. Arch. Neurol. (Chicago), 34:381–382, 1977.

319. Serafetinides, E. A.: Aggressiveness in temporal lobe epileptics and its relationship to cerebral dysfunction and environmental factors. Epilepsia, 6:33–42, 1965.

320. Serafetinides, E. A., and Falconer, M. A.: Some observations on memory impairment after temporal lobectomy for epilepsy. J. Neurol. Neurosurg. Psychiat., 25:251–255, 1962.

321. Serafetinides, E. A., and Falconer, M. A.: The effects of temporal lobectomy in epileptic patients with psychosis. J. Ment. Sci., 108:584, 1962.

322. Silfenius, H., Gloor, P., and Rasmussen, T.: Evaluation of insular ablation in surgical treatment of temporal lobe epilepsy. Epilepsia, 5:307–320, 1964.

323. Simon, D., and Penry, J. K.: Sodium di-N-propylacetate (DPA) in the treatment of epilepsy: A review. Epilepsia, 16:549–573, 1975.

324. Slater, E., Beard, A. W., and Glithero, E.: The schizophrenia-like psychoses of epilepsy. Brit. J. Psychiat., 109:95–150, 1963.

325. Small, J. G., Milstein, V., and Stevens, J. R.: Are psychomotor epileptics different? A controlled study. Arch. Neurol. (Chicago), 7:187–194, 1962.

326. Smith, A.: Certain hypothesized hemispheric differences in language and visual function in human adults. Cortex, 2:109, 1965.

327. Smith, A.: Dominant and nondominant hemispherectomy. In Smith, W. L., ed.: Drugs, Development and Cerebral Function. Springfield, Ill., Charles C Thomas, 1972, pp. 37–68.

328. Smith, A.: Neuropsychological testing in neurological disorders. Advances Neurol., 7:49–110, 1975.

329. Smith, A., and Sugar, O.: Development of

above-normal language and intelligence 21 years after left hemispherectomy. Neurology (Minneap.), 25:813–818, 1975.

330. Solomon, G. E., and Plum, F.: Clinical Management of Seizures: A Guide for the Physician. Philadelphia, London, Toronto, W. B. Saunders Co., 1976.

330a. Spencer, S. S. Depth electroencephalography in selection of refractory epilepsy for surgery. Ann. Neurol., 9:207–214, 1981.

331. Spiegel, E. A., and Wycis, H. T.: Thalamic recordings in man with special reference to seizure discharges. Electroenceph. Clin. Neurophysiol., 2:23–27, 1950.

332. Spiegel, E., Wycis, H., and Baird, H.: Subcortical mechanisms in convulsive disorders. In Spiegel, E., and Wycis, H., eds.: Stereoencephalotomy. Part II. New York, Grune & Stratton, 1962.

333. Sperry, R. W., Gassaniga, M. S., and Bogen, J. E.: Interhemispheric relationships: The neocortical commissures; syndromes of hemisphere disconnection. In Vinken, P. J., and Bruyn, G. W., eds.: Handbook of Clinical Neurology. Vol. 4. Amsterdam, North-Holland Publishing Co., 1969, pp. 273–290.

334. Stauder, H. K.: Epilepsie und Schläfenlappen. Arch. Psychiat. Nervenkr., 104:181, 1935.

335. Stevens, J. R.: Psychiatric implications of psychomotor epilepsy. Arch. Gen. Psychiat., 14:461–477, 1966.

336. Stevens, J. R.: Localization of epileptic focus by protracted monitoring of EEG by radiotelemetry. Epilepsia, 10:420, 1969. (Abstract)

337. Stevens, J. R.: Interictal clinical manifestations of complex partial seizures. Advances Neurol., 11:85–112, 1975.

338. Sugar, O., and Gerard, R. W.: Anoxia and brain potentials. J. Neurophysiol., 1:558–572, 1938.

339. Svensmark, O., and Buchthal, F.: Diphenylhydantoin and phenobarbital. Amer. J. Dis. Child., 108:82, 1964.

340. Talairach, J.: Destruction du noyau ventral antérieur thalamique dans le traitement des maladies mentales. Rev. Neurol. (Paris), 87:352–357, 1952.

341. Talairach, J., and Szikla, G.: Destruction partielle amygdalohippocampique par l'yttrium 90 dans le traitment de certaines épilepsies à expression rhinencéphalique. Neurochirurgie, 11:233–240, 1965.

342. Talairach, J., De Ajuriguerre, J., and David, M.: Études stéréotaxiques et structures encéphaliques profondes chez l'homme. Presse Med., 28:605–609, 1952.

343. Talairach, J., Szikla, G., Tournoux, P., Prossalentis, A., Bordas-Ferer, M., Jacob, M., and Menpel, E.: Atlas d'Anatomie Stéréotaxique du Téléncephale. Paris, Masson, 1967.

344. Taylor, D. C., and Falconer, M. A.: Clinical, socioeconomic and psychological changes after temporal lobectomy for seizures. Brit. J. Psychiat., 114:1247–1261, 1968.

345. Temkin, O.: The Falling Sickness. Baltimore, The Johns Hopkins Press, 1945.

346. Tervila, L., Huhmar, E. O. T., and Krofkors, E.: Cerebral birth injury as a cause of epilepsy. Ann. Chir. Gynaec., Fenniae, 64:118–122, 1975.

347. Terzian, H., and Ore, G. D.: Syndrome of Klüver and Bucy reproduced in man by bilateral removal of temporal lobes. Neurology (Minneap.), 5:373–380, 1955.

348. Tomlinson, B. E., and Walton, J. N.: Superficial hemosiderosis of the central nervous system. J. Neurol. Neurosurg. Psychiat., 27:332–339, 1964.

349. Tönnis, W.: Die Behandlung der posttraumatischen Spätepilepsie, Zbl. Neurochir., 4:240–241, 1939.

350. Tower, D. B.: Neurochemistry of epilepsy. In Vinken, P. J., and Bruyn, G. W., eds.: Handbook of Clinical Neurology. Vol. 15, The Epilepsies. New York, American Elsevier Publishing Co., Inc., 1974, pp. 60–73.

351. Trachtenberg, M. C., and Pollen, D. A.: Neurogia: biophysical properties and physiological function. Science, 167:1248–1252, 1970.

352. Tükel, K., and Jasper, H.: The electroencephalogram in parasagittal lesions. Electroenceph. Clin. Neurophysiol., 4:481–494, 1952.

353. Udvarhelyi, G. B., and Walker, A. E.: Dissemination of acute focal seizures in the monkey. Arch. Neurol. (Chicago) 12:333–356, 1965.

354. Ueki, K.: Hemispherectomy in the human being with special reference to the preservation of function. Progr. Brain Res., 21:285–338, 1966.

355. Ueno, H., Yamashita, Y., and Caveness, W. F.: Regional cerebral blood flow pattern in focal epileptiform seizures in the monkey. Exp. Neurol., 47:81–96, 1975.

356. Umbach, W.: Long-term results of fornicotomy for temporal epilepsy. Confin. Neurol., 27:121–123, 1966.

357. Vaernet, K.: Stereotaxic amygdalotomy in temporal lobe epilepsy. Confin. Neurol., 34:176–180, 1972.

358. Van Buren, J. M., Ajmone-Marsan, C., Mutsuga, N., and Sandowsky, D.: Surgery of temporal lobe epilepsy. Advances Neurol., 8:155–196, 1975.

359. Van den Berg, B. J., and Yereshalmy, J.: Studies on convulsive disorders in young children. I. Incidence of febrile and nonfebrile convulsions by age and other factors. Pediat. Res., 3:298–304, 1969.

360. Van Wagenen, W., and Herren, R.: Surgical division of commissural pathways in the corpus callosum. Arch. Neurol. Psychiat. 44:740–759, 1940.

361. Wada, J., and Rasmussen, T.: Intracarotid injection of Sodium Amytal for the lateralization of speech dominance. Experimental and clinical observations. J. Neurosurg., 17:266–282, 1952.

362. Walker, A. E.: Posttraumatic Epilepsy. Springfield, Ill., Charles C Thomas, 1949.

363. Walker, A. E.: Electrocorticography in epilepsy. A surgeon's appraisal. Electroenceph. Clin. Neurophysiol., 2:suppl. 2:30–37, 1949.

364. Walker, A. E.: Stereotaxic methods for the study of subcortical activity in epilepsy. Confin. Neurol., 22:17–222, 1962.

365. Walker, A. E.: Temporal lobectomy. J. Neurosurg., 26:642–649, 1967.

366. Walker, A. E.: Surgical treatment for epilepsy. In Livingston, S., ed.: Comprehensive Management of Epilepsy in Infancy, Childhood and

Adolescence. Springfield, Ill., Charles C Thomas, 1972, pp. 406–436.

367. Walker, A. E.: Man and his temporal lobes. John Hughlings Jackson Lecture. Surg. Neurol., 1:69–79, 1973.

368. Walker, A. E.: Surgery for epilepsy. In Vinken, P. J., and Bruyn, G. W., eds.: Handbook of Clinical Neurology. Vol. 15, The Epilepsies. New York, American Elsevier Publishing Co., Inc., 1974, pp. 739–757.

369. Walker, A. E.: Critique and perspectives. Advances Neurol., 8:333–350, 1975.

370. Walker, A. E., Lichtenstein, R. S., and Marshall, C.: A critical analysis of electrocorticography in temporal lobe epilepsy. Arch. Neurol. (Chicago), 2:172–182, 1960.

371. Walker, A. E., and Marshall, C.: The contribution of depth recording to clinical medicine. Electroenceph. Clin. Neurophysiol., 16:88–99, 1964.

372. Walker, A. E., Marshall, C., and Beresford, E. N.: Electrocorticographic characteristics of the cerebrum in posttraumatic epilepsy. Res. Publ. Ass. Res. Nerv. Ment. Dis., 26:502–515, 1947.

373. Walker, A. E., Poggio, G. F., and Andy, O. J.: Structural spread of cortical induced epileptic discharge. Neurology (Minneap.), 6:618–621, 1956.

374. Walter, R. D.: Tactical considerations leading to surgical treatment of limbic epilepsy. In Brazier, M. A. B., ed.: Epilepsy: Its Phenomena in Man. New York and London, Academic Press, 1973, pp. 99–120.

375. Ward, A. A., Jr.: The epileptic neuron. Epilepsia, 2:70–80, 1961.

376. Ward, A. A., Jr.: The hyperirritable neuron—epilepsy. In Rodahl, K., and Issekutz, B. J., eds.: Nerve as a Tissue. New York, Harper & Row, 1966, pp. 379–411.

377. Ward, A. A., Jr.: The epileptic neuron: Chronic foci in animals and man. In Jasper, H. H., Ward, A. A., Jr., and Pope, A., eds.: Basic Mechanisms of the Epilepsies. Boston, Little, Brown & Co., 1969, pp. 263–268.

378. Ward, A. A., Jr.: Theoretical basis for epilepsy surgery. Advances Neurol., 8:23–25, 1975.

379. Ward, A. A., Jr., and Thomas, L. B.: The electrical activity of single units in the cerebral cortex of man. Electroenceph. Clin. Neurophysiol., 7:135–136, 1955.

380. Weil, A. A.: Ictal depression and anxiety in temporal lobe disorders. Amer. J. Psychiat., 113:149–157, 1965.

381. Weingarten, S. M., Cherlow, D. G., and Halgren, E.: Relationship of hallucinations to depth structures of the temporal lobe. In Sweet, W. H., Obrador, S., and Martin-Rodriquez, J. G., eds.: Neurosurgical Treatment in Psychiatry, Pain, and Epilepsy. Baltimore, London, Tokyo, University Park Press, 1977, pp. 553–568.

382. Westrum, L. E., White, L. E., and Ward, A. A., Jr.: Morphology of the experimental epileptic focus. J. Neurosurg., 21:1035, 1965.

383. White, H. H.: Cerebral hemispherectomy in the treatment of infantile hemiplegia. Confin. Neurol., 21:1–50, 1961.

384. White, L. E., Jr.: A morphologic concept of the limbic lobe. Int. Rev. Neurobiol., 8:1–34, 1965.

385. Wilder, B. J.: Electroencephalographic activation in medically intractable epileptic patients: Activation technique including surgical follow-up. Arch. Neurol. (Chicago), 25:415–426, 1971.

386. Wilder, B. J., and Schmidt, R. P.: Propagation of focal paroxysmal activity in the Macaca mulatta at birth and at 24 months. Brain, 96:757–764, 1973.

387. Wilder, B. J., King, R. L., and Schmidt, R. P.: Cortical and subcortical epileptogenesis in monkeys. Neurology (Minneap.), 17:282, 1967. (Abstract)

388. Wilder, B. J., Ramsay, R. E., Willmore, L. J., Feussner, G. F., Perchalski, R. J., and Schumate, J. B., Jr.: Efficacy of intravenous phenytoin in the treatment of status epilepticus: Kinetics of central nervous system penetration. Ann. Neurol., 1:511–518, 1977.

389. Wilson, D. H., Reeves, A., Gazzaniga, M., and Culver, C.: Commissurotomy for control of intractable seizures. Neurology (Minneap.), 27:708–715, 1977.

390. Wilson, P. J.: Complications related to delayed hemorrhage after hemispherectomy. J. Neurosurg., 30:413, 1969.

391. Wilson, P. J.: Cerebral hemispherectomy for infantile hemiplegia. A report of 50 cases. Brain, 93:147–180, 1970.

392. Wycis, H., Baird, H., and Spiegel, E.: Long-range results following pallidotomy and pallido-amygdalotomy in certain types of convulsive disorders. Confin. Neurol., 27:114–120, 1966.

393. Wyler, A. R.: Epileptic neurons during sleep and wakefulness. Exp. Neurol., 42:593–608, 1974.

394. Wyler, A. R., and Fetz, E. E.: Behavioral control of firing patterns of normal and abnormal neurons in chronic epileptic cortex. Exp. Neurol., 42:448–464, 1974.

395. Wyler, A. R., Fetz, E. E., and Ward, A. A., Jr.: Effects of operantly conditioning epileptic unit activity on seizures frequencies and electrophysiology of neocortical experimental foci. Exp. Neurol., 44:113–125, 1974.

396. Zangwill, O. L.: Cerebral Dominance and Its Relation to Psychological Function. Edinburgh, Oliver and Boyd, 1960.

142

NEUROSURGICAL ASPECTS OF EPILEPSY IN ADULTS

Epilepsy afflicts about 1 per cent of the American population. Of these cases, 25 per cent are difficult to control with anticonvulsant medication, and 10 per cent, or about 200,000 individuals, are resistant to medical management. It is in this group that some patients are found who have focal brain damage as the cause of their seizures and can benefit from surgery. Such patients may have had a birth injury, head trauma, infection, brain hemorrhage, or thrombosis of a major cerebral artery. When the seizures originate in the temporal lobe there is frequently a history of a prolonged febrile convulsion in infancy, and the pathological change usually is restricted to the medial temporal lobe (so-called mesial sclerosis). In patients in whom the insult occurred in infancy, with widespread injury throughout one hemisphere, there may be a hemiplegia in addition to seizures—infantile hemiplegia. Occasionally a cryptic tumor, vascular anomaly, or other lesions are discovered as the cause of the epilepsy.

RATIONALE OF OPERATIVE TREATMENT

Of itself, epilepsy is infrequently a threat to life as is, for instance, a progressively growing brain tumor. With seizures alone there is always hope that an effective new drug will emerge. Thus, in most patients with epilepsy that is difficult to control, operative treatment is delayed for several years while available antiepileptic drugs are tried in different combinations to achieve adequate seizure control. In children there is also the possibility that the seizures will diminish in frequency or disappear with age. However, frequent convulsions over extended intervals and reduced mental activity, in part due to excessive doses of antiepileptic agents, may make an adult dependent on his family or society, and a child uneducable. Thus, in some epileptics with uncontrolled seizures the time comes when the quality of life, present and future, must be weighed against both the operative risk and the probability that the operation can effect seizure control.

Operative management of intractable epilepsy is usually employed in patients who have seizures that arise invariably from a circumscribed area of one side of the brain —focal epilepsy. Less commonly, patients with intractable *generalized* seizures have been managed with procedures that interrupt neuronal pathways along which the seizure activity spreads, e.g., division of the corpus callosum. More recently operations attempting to suppress seizures by control of neural transmission (electrical stimulation of the cerebellum) have been tried.[4]

In operations for focal epilepsy, excision of brain that does not harbor a progressively growing lesion and frequently appears normal on visual inspection may seem to be a drastic step. In reality, however, one is careful to remove tissue that

S. GOLDRING

serves no important purpose and that exerts an adverse influence that is expressed in repeated convulsions. Because the seizure activity does not arise from the lesion itself, but from the adjacent epileptogenic cortex, this marginal tissue must be removed. It may seem paradoxical that operative excision, which of itself produces focal brain damage and glial scarring, should act to prevent the development of convulsions. In cases in which the epileptogenic cicatrix is a *residuum* of a previous *open* head injury or brain abscess, the paradox may be explained by the histological features of the scars. They frequently harbor both mesenchymal and glial elements, and the former are thought by some to be more epileptogenic, although data in support of this thesis are not compelling. In any case we lack a full explanation of the epileptogenicity of pathological scars, compared with the relatively weak epileptogenic effect of an operative cicatrix.

EVALUATION FOR OPERATION

The most critical and specialized aspect of surgical management of epilepsy is the accumulation of evidence establishing that the clinical seizure arises from a single focus in a functionally silent area of the brain. The evidence for a focal origin of seizures comes from the sequence of the motor, sensory, and behavioral manifestations that the patient experiences. For example, the attack may commence with twitching of the left thumb and then spread to involve the entire left side. This type of attack would indicate a focus with an origin in the thumb area of the right prerolandic motor cortex. If the patient develops a blank stare, loses contact with his surroundings, and fumbles with his clothes, this behavioral feature of a psychomotor seizure suggests an origin of the seizure in one or the other temporal lobe.

Electroencephalography

Given a history of a focal onset, an electroencephalographic (EEG) confirmation of an abnormal focus is highly desirable, but is not essential before proceeding with operative treatment. In some cases routine elec-

troencephalograms, even a series of them, will not provide information as to the location of the focus of origin. Recordings from the scalp often fail to reveal abnormal activity that comes from the depth of the brain. One example of this failure is in mesial sclerosis of temporal lobe epilepsy. Another is that routine tracings may fail to localize a seizure focus, even when it is located near the brain's surface. In both instances, various means of activating latent abnormalities of a seizure focus are used. Recording with nasopharyngeal or sphenoidal electrodes during sleep, either natural or induced by barbiturate, is especially useful in temporal lobe epilepsy. In other forms, intravenous injection of pentylenetetrazol (Metrazol) is sometimes helpful in activating the electrical seizure focus.

In some subjects who have generalized seizures and show a diffusely disordered electroencephalogram, the seizures have nevertheless been proved to have a focal origin, usually in the frontal lobe.[29] In those instances, injections of an anesthetic agent into a single carotid artery will abolish the electrical activity on both sides if injected on the side containing the focus. When the anesthetic is injected into the carotid supplying the innocent hemisphere, only the abnormal activity on that side will be affected.[11,31]

A similar method is used to determine the dominant hemisphere for speech. The test utilizes the intracarotid injection of sodium amobarbital. Dominant-side injections produce transient loss of the ability to speak in addition to paresis of the contralateral limbs.[41]

Radiological Imaging Procedures

A complete radiological examination is required to determine whether a tumor or vascular malformation underlies the epilepsy. The survey includes skull films, radionuclide brain scan, computed tomography (CT) cerebral arteriography, and pneumoencephalography. All these examinations, however, usually show either no abnormality or only evidence of a cicatrix, atrophy, or porencephalic cyst. When the radiological procedures are normal, the brain may also appear normal at the time of operation. But if an epileptogenic focus can be defined and excised, subsequent histological examination will usually reveal a specific pathological process.

OPERATIVE MANAGEMENT

Excision of Epileptogenic Focus

Intraoperative Electrocorticography for Localization of Focus

The operative procedure used most commonly was developed by Penfield and Jasper at the Montreal Neurological Institute.[26,27] It requires that the procedure be carried out under local anesthesia. General anesthesia is avoided because it suppresses both electroencephalographic seizure activity and the motor responses to electrical stimulation of the cortical surface, both of which are used to identify the sensorimotor region. In addition, production of an afterdischarge (locally recorded seizure activity sustained after the cessation of focal electrical stimulation) is suppressed by general anesthesia. Afterdischarge can be a significant indicator of epileptogenicity when accompanied by the partial seizure with which the naturally occurring convulsions begin. After the limits of cortex to be removed are mapped, the involved tissue is excised. Electrical recordings are repeated along the margins of removal, seeking residue of epileptogenic tissue. If abnormal activity still persists there, these areas are excised also if they do not encroach upon the source of an important cortical function.

Rasmussen analyzed the results of operation for treatment of focal epilepsy (other than that originating in the temporal lobe) in 1145 patients who had been followed for 2 to 48 years. *Sixty-four per cent of them had complete or nearly complete elimination of their seizures.*[28]

Operative management of epilepsy has certain limitations, however. Not all patients can undergo an operation under local anesthesia with the necessary degree of cooperation, and this is especially true in children. Furthermore, it has become increasingly clear that the most reliable evidence for localizing an epileptogenic focus is that which is obtained in electrical recordings made during a *spontaneous* convulsion.[5,6,24,37,45] During an operation abnormal interictal electrical discharges may be unreliable, whether they occur spontaneously or are induced by electrical stimulation. Even an afterdischarge associated with the partial seizure from which the clinical convulsion develops sometimes provides erroneous localization. Furthermore, the partial seizure may spread rapidly into a generalized one, an event that is undesirable during operation. As a result, it is preferable to use *extraoperative* recording with indwelling electrodes for the precise localization of epileptogenic foci.

Extraoperative Electrocorticography for Localization of Focus

Epidural Surface Electrode Arrays in Focal Cortical Epilepsy

The important features of the procedure are: (1) all operative manipulation is performed under general, rather than local, anesthesia; (2) the sensorimotor region is readily identified in the anesthetized patient by recording cortical sensory evoked responses; and (3) the epileptogenic focus is localized by *extraoperative* electrocorticography (ECG) via indwelling electrode arrays during spontaneously occurring seizures. In cases in which an epileptogenic focus in other than the medial temporal lobe is suspected, a craniotomy is performed under general endotracheal anesthesia, and the brain is exposed and inspected. As mentioned earlier, it may be difficult to identify the important area of sensorimotor control by electrical stimulation of the cortex because general anesthesia raises the threshold for eliciting movements produced by cortical stimulation. This problem has been overcome by recording, with a special purpose computer, the average evoked cortical responses to somatosensory stimulation. In both the *anesthetized* and awake states only the *sensory and motor gyri* generate an electrical response to stimulation of the contralateral median nerve, and stimulation of the ipsilateral median nerve is ineffective.[13,17,36] These studies are the basis for using evoked responses for routine identification of the sensorimotor region. The method is as follows: A Silastic template holding nine linearly oriented electrodes, each separated from the next by a distance of 1.5 cm, is placed on the cortical surface in a plane parallel to the midline (Fig. 142–1). Simultaneous records are made from each adja-

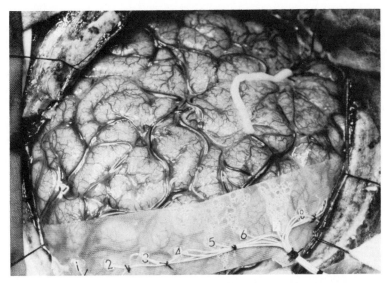

Figure 142–1 Linear electrode array for recording somatosensory evoked responses. An electrode contact underlies each number. Recordings are made simultaneously from each adjacent pair of electrodes (1–2, 2–3, . . .) while the median nerve is electrically stimulated transcutaneously at the wrist. Midline is at bottom and anterior is to the right. The recordings in this patient identified the gyrus underlying electrode No. 5 as the somatosensory gyrus (see text and Figure 142–2).

cent pair of electrodes (i.e., 1–2, 2–3, 3–4, . . .) while the contralateral median nerve at the wrist is stimulated transcutaneously with electrical stimuli. The computer stores the epoch of electrical activity following each stimulus. After approximately 25 stimuli, delivered at a frequency of one per second, the computer adds the epochs. The spontaneous brain waves that are of random occurrence do not add significantly, while the evoked responses having a con-

sistent polarity and latency summate, becoming clearly exposed above the background rhythm (Fig. 142–2). The face area can be similarly identified (Fig. 142–3). Even in patients under local anesthesia, this method of localization has proved to be a quicker method of identifying the sensorimotor region than using electrical stimulation of the cortical surface to produce movement. After identification of the sensorimotor region, the dura is closed and a

Figure 142–2 Simultaneous recordings made from each adjacent electrode pair shown in Figure 142–1. The only traces that show a significant response are those derived from electrode combinations 4–5 and 5–6. The following observations establish the area underlying electrode No. 5 as the somatosensory hand area: (1) No. 5 is common to both electrode combinations, (2) a response is not seen in the recordings in which electrodes No. 4 and No. 6 are each paired with an electrode other than No. 5 (i.e., 3–4 and 6–7), (3) the polarity of the responses recorded from these two adjacent pairs of electrodes is reversed. Cal., 12.5 μv; 18 msec.

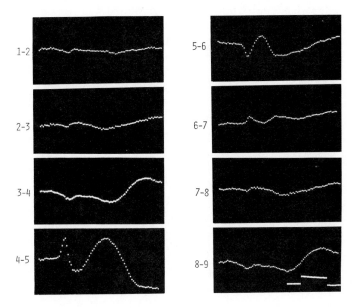

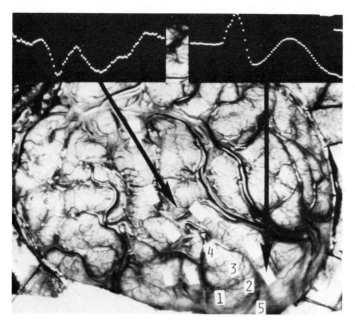

Figure 142–3 Identification of somatosensory hand and face areas. Midline is at bottom; anterior is to the left. Obliquely directed arrow identifies the face area, the other arrow identifies the hand area. Cal., 20 μv; 19 msec. After these responses were recorded, anesthesia was lightened and electrical stimulation of cortical surface was carried out at all sites underlying the tickets. No motor responses were obtained with stimuli applied to areas underlying the blank tickets. Hand and arm movements were obtained from areas beneath tickets 1 to 5. No facial movements were produced. The recorded evoked responses were the only means of showing the boundary between the domains of the face and upper extremity. This is the author's usual experience in patients under general anesthesia.

quasi-rectangular Silastic template holding about 24 electrodes is sewn in epidurally (Fig. 142–4). The electrodes are arranged in rows with interelectrode distances of 1.5 cm and 2 cm in the sagittal and coronal planes respectively. The electrode template spans the suspected area of epileptogenicity, the surrounding area, and the sensorimotor region. The remainder of the closure is completed and recordings are begun on the following day. The subject rests quietly without discomfort, and electroencephalographic and motor activity are recorded continuously and displayed side by side on the split screen of a television monitor. The

recordings are taped and provide the additional opportunity for replays of any seizures that occur. The simultaneous recording of electrical and motor activity is necessary to determine accurately which cortical area shows the first sign of abnormal activity in the moments preceding the onset of a convulsion, which is the information that is necessary for localizing the epileptogenic focus. Evoked responses can be recorded and the cortex can be stimulated through the epidural electrodes. If the recordings are from the dominant hemisphere, electrical stimulation through the recording electrodes is also used to deter-

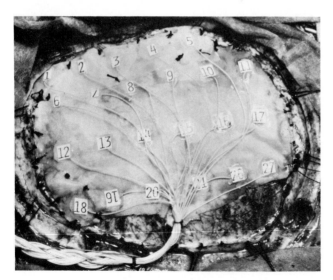

Figure 142–4 Surface electrode array sewn in epidurally. Each number overlies an electrode contact. Midline is at bottom, anterior is to the left. Bundle of lead wires (*bottom*) serves as an epidural drain. When the dura is being opened, the incision is made around the entire circumference of the exposed dura. This is done to minimize the development of epidural clot, which could attenuate the recorded electrical activity. Photograph was taken at the time of secondary craniotomy and shows no appreciable clot underlying the electrode array.

mine the boundaries of the area controlling speech. Thus, all the techniques used in localizing an epileptogenic focus during an open operative procedure under local anesthesia can be performed by recording (and sometimes stimulating) epidurally with the indwelling electrode arrays. In addition, the recordings can be made leisurely, free from the usual stresses of the operative procedure. Finally, the opportunity to record the electroencephalogram during a spontaneous clinical seizure, or if necessary, an activated one, is markedly enhanced.

Since the majority of these patients have at least several seizures a day, recording with the surface electrode arrays usually continues for 24 to 48 hours. Such recording of spontaneous convulsion during routine daily activities is facilitated by the use of radiotelemetry for continuous monitoring. If the observations localize the boundaries of a single epileptogenic focus, then that brain tissue is excised at a secondary craniotomy; if not, the surface electrode array is removed and the operative wound is closed.

The following case illustrates the application and advantages of epidural surface electrode arrays for localizing an epileptogenic focus with extraoperative electrocorticography.

The patient was a 20-year-old man who had intractable seizures occurring three to five times a month for 11 years. The ictus was ushered in by a visual aura—vision "goes out" with a flickering traveling from left to right, and head and eyes turn to right—followed usually by a tonic-clonic convulsion. In such a patient the occurrence of a spontaneous seizure during intraoperative electrocorticography is unlikely and undesirable, and one must rely on spontaneous spiking and appearance of afterdischarge in response to electrical stimulation to localize the focus. Observations in this patient will demonstrate that: (1) seizure discharge produced by electrical stimulation may provide *false localization* of the epileptogenic focus; (2) recording during the clinical seizure from which the patient is incapacitated is of utmost importance; and (3) using extraoperative electrocorticography, one can safely activate seizures, even generalized ones, to localize the epileptogenic focus.

Under general anesthesia a craniotomy was performed and an epidural surface electrode array was inserted. Because the seizures began with a visual aura the electrode array was positioned posteriorly (Fig. 142–5). During two days of extraoperative recording, the patient failed to have a seizure. Epidural electrical stimulation via each of the recording electrodes at a stimulus strength that was just adequate for producing a hand movement when applied over motor cortex failed to elicit the patient's clinical seizure. From two adjacent electrodes overlying the posterior temporal region, however, an afterdischarge was readily produced and was accompanied by confusion and receptive dysphasia. That is, a seizure was produced, but it was not the patient's symptomatic seizure, and he had never experienced such an episode before (Fig. 142–6). Next pentylenetetrazol (Metrazol) activation was used. After receiving a total of 200 mg (50 mg every 30 seconds) the patient reported his visual aura, the head and eyes turned to the right, and a generalized seizure followed. The activated seizure was identical to the patient's spontaneously occurring clinical seizure. It was ushered in by electrical seizure activity appearing in electrodes

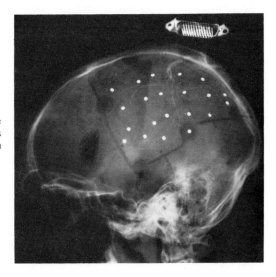

Figure 142–5 Lateral skull x-ray showing electrode contacts of epidural surface electrode array. Lead wires from each electrode are collected into a bundle, which exits at burr hole site and serves as epidural drain.

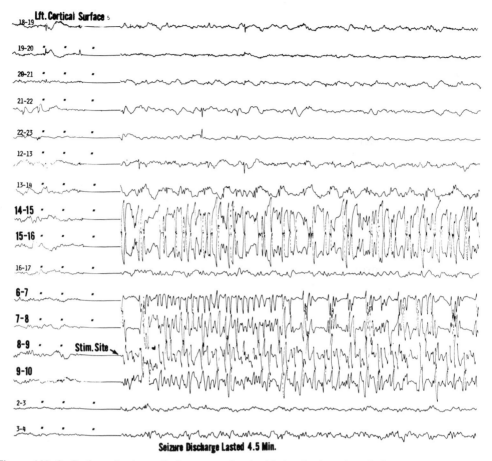

Figure 142–6 Prolonged seizure discharge associated with dysphasia and confusion produced by electrical stimulation via recording electrodes 8 and 9 of the surface electrode array. The patient had never experienced such a seizure before. Stimulus intensity was just sufficient to produce hand movement when applied to motor cortex. The stimulus was applied in the posterior temporal area and spread to adjacent sites in the immediately surrounding posterior temporal and parietal regions (14–15, 15–16, 6–7, 7–8, 9–10). Electrical stimulation via all the epidural recording electrodes other than 8 and 9 failed to produce any significant afterdischarge. The only behavioral responses were movements, and there were paresthesias in the right upper extremity and face when stimuli were applied to electrodes in the sensorimotor area.

overlying *occipital* cortex sites where electrical stimulation had failed to generate either afterdischarge or clinical seizure (Fig. 142–7).

The resected tissue showed reactive gliosis. Postoperatively, the patient has been seizure-free for one and one-half years.

It is doubtful that the correct localization of the epileptogenic focus in this patient could have been accomplished by the usual method of intraoperative electrocorticography under local anesthesia.

During the 10 years from 1966 to 1977, 92 patients with intractable epilepsy have been managed by the author. Of these, 29 have been evaluated with extraoperative electrocorticography using epidural surface electrode arrays. In 24 the recordings were con-

sidered to identify an epileptogenic focus and led to excision of the area that was suspect. Eighteen of these patients have been followed for one to six years after operation. Eleven, or 61 per cent, have had a good result defined as either (1) complete cessation of seizures; (2) reduction in seizure frequency that permitted employment or educability, neither of which were possible before operation; or (3) reduction in seizure frequency that prevented institutionalization. The results are made more significant by the fact that the majority of these 15 patients were experiencing between 6 and 50 seizures daily. In all but one of the patients who had excision of an epileptogenic focus, microscopic examination of the removed tissue identified a lesion.

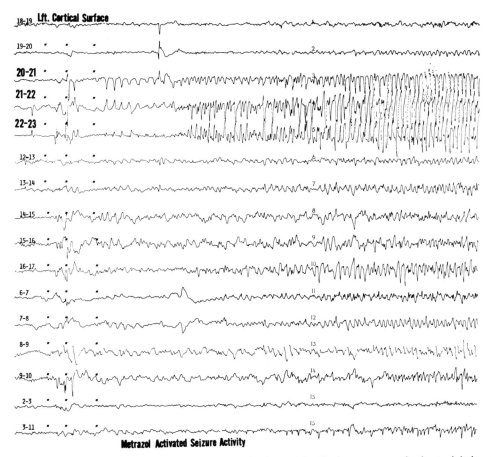

Figure 142–7 Pentylenetetrazol (Metrazol)-activated seizure. The discharge appears in the occipital region underlying electrodes 21, 22, and 23. Electrical stimulation at these sites failed to produce afterdischarge or any behavioral response. This Metrazol-activated seizure was identical to the clinical seizures from which the patient suffered.

Depth Electrodes in Temporal Lobe Epilepsy

This seizure disorder is the commonest variety of epilepsy treated by the neurological surgeon. In about 50 per cent of patients with temporal lobe epilepsy, Sommer's sector of Ammon's horn shows gliosis and loss of neurons. This pathological change, called mesial temporal sclerosis, is the most common single lesion to be found postmortem in the brains of epileptics who die of unrelated disease.[10]

A temporal lobe seizure may consist of only a brief loss of orientation and lapse of consciousness; or the episode may last longer and be accompanied by automatic behavior such as chewing, fumbling with clothes, walking or running aimlessly, phrasing incoherent speech, or performing aggressive and asocial acts. For these events the subject is amnesic. Less frequently, the seizure consists of or includes perceptual illusions (objects looking brighter, larger, or smaller; sounds seeming louder; a déjà vu recall of what is past and very familiar). Vague feelings of impending doom, fear, or unreality also may arise; and for many of these experiences there is recall. Finally, a seizure may have hallucinatory aspects. These may include odors, sights, or sounds, or combinations of visual and auditory perceptions.

Penfield and Flanigin, Bailey and Gibbs, and Green, Duisberg, and McGrath were among the first to remove parts of the temporal lobe to alleviate such seizures.[1,15,25] Bailey and Gibbs resected the laterally placed temporal gyri, the resections being based on electroencephalographic findings.[1] Penfield and Flanigin introduced the operation of temporal lobectomy now elected most frequently, a resection that includes the medially placed amygdala and hippocampus.[42]

In the currently used procedure, 4 to 6 cm of the anterior temporal lobe is removed. Since the actual focus usually lies deep in the medial inferior region of the lobe, the resection may include brain tissue not involved in the epileptogenic process. Such a liberal resection is permissible, since the region involved is relatively silent insofar as known brain functions are concerned. Milner has shown that in the nondominant hemisphere such removals have little effect on mentation, except that they reduce understanding of pictures.[20] A corresponding resection within the dominant hemisphere is associated with word recall difficulties. These losses are of debatable significance in any case, because in temporal lobe epileptics they usually exist before a lobe's removal.

Falconer has emphasized the importance of asphyxia during infancy as a cause of mesial sclerosis.[8-10] The episodes of asphyxia occur in conjunction with status epilepticus, febrile convulsions, severe infections, and head injury. His results with anterior temporal lobectomies are similar to those reported from the Montreal Neurological Institute. *Relief from attacks was recorded in 62 per cent of subjects followed 2 to 12 years after operation.*

About 50 per cent of Falconer's patients had a history of episodes of aggression, neuroticism, or even psychosis, and this is true in the experience of others. A lucid description of such deviation from normal behavior is given by Walker.

These interpersonal aberrations are continuously manifested by withdrawal, seclusiveness, anxiety, paranoia, insecurity, fanatic pseudoreligiosity, or paroxysmal outbursts of temper, which lead to a personality label of queer. One of the most frequently encountered behavioral deviations is a modification of aggression expressed in all modalities of conduct. In temporal lobe epilepsy, aggressivity is typically impulsive irritable behavior, characterized by relatively unmotivated, paroxysmal outbursts of episodic anger, abusiveness or assaultiveness, quite in contrast with the patient's usual behavior. Between those outbursts, the individual usually is good-natured. Close associates often can recognize the dysphoric moods characterized by increasing irritability and hypersensitivity, lasting hours or days, which may herald an outburst of anger or a seizure. After such an episode, the ir-

ritable patient regains his normal more pleasant disposition.[43]

In both Falconer's and Walker's experiences, the majority of subjects whose epilepsy was relieved by operation also showed marked lessening of aggressive behavior after the procedure. Walker also noted a similar salutary effect of operation on the hyposexuality that characterized about 70 per cent of his patients with intractable temporal lobe epilepsy. Before operation they had little or no heterosexual interest or outlet. Afterward sexual drive improved in about one third, the improvement correlating positively with relief from psychomotor seizures. In neither Falconer's or Walker's subjects was operation done because of the existence of a behavior disorder, but solely for the relief of seizures. This is also the author's practice.

In patients with typical psychomotor seizures, a consistent unilateral temporal spike focus on repeated routine electroencephalographic examinations, and radiological evidence of temporal lobe abnormality (dilated temporal horn or calcification) on the side of the electrical focus, a standard anterior temporal lobe resection may be performed with or without *intraoperative* electrocorticography and a good result may be anticipated. Since the epileptogenic focus frequently is not located in the lateral temporal cortex, however, routine electroencephalograms may be normal. Also, recordings with nasopharyngeal leads may show independent spiking from both temporal lobes, and radiological information may be inadequate to indicate the involved lobe. In such patients *extraoperative* recording with indwelling depth electrodes during spontaneous clinical seizures is of great value in deciding whether the seizures originate in one or the other of the temporal lobes or from both. Electroencephalographic recordings with sphenoidal leads either during spontaneous seizures or during thiopental activation, or both, may also be used to localize the side of seizure origin.[10,11] An extraoperative electrocorticogram with indwelling electrodes, however, is superior for localizing the abnormal discharges and is not as readily contaminated by movement artifact.

Before proceeding with an operation, special consideration must be given to a patient who shows abnormal electrical discharges that arise independently from both temporal lobes but in whom seizures can only be shown to begin in one lobe. In such a case both temporal lobes may harbor a lesion (e.g., mesial sclerosis) and unilateral resection of either temporal lobe carries the same risk as a bilateral one; that is, the possibility of marked impairment of memory. Thus, it is important to evaluate preoperatively the effect of inactivating either temporal lobe. This evaluation can be done by injecting sodium amobarbital (Amytal) into one carotid artery and giving the patient a simple memory test before the hemiparesis has cleared, or before the speech has largely returned if the injection is on the dominant side. Failure to recall the test items indicates that the patient's memory function could be impaired if the anterior temporal lobe contralateral to the side of injection were removed.[20,21]

The following case illustrates the value of extraoperative electrocorticography with indwelling electrodes in cases of temporal lobe epilepsy in which independent spiking occurs in both temporal lobes.

A 25-year-old woman began to experience psychomotor seizures at age 16. Repeated awake electroencephalograms were mildly paroxysmal and nonfocal (Fig. 142–8). Sleep electroencephalograms with nasopharyngeal leads showed right mesial temporal spiking. Radiographic studies were normal except for minimal dilatation of the left temporal horn. Recording with indwelling electrodes revealed independent spiking from both medial temporal lobes in the region of the anterior hippocampus (Fig. 142–9). Also, several 30-second to two-minute runs of electrical seizure discharge were recorded independently from each temporal lobe (Fig. 142–10). These recordings had no clinical concomitant. However, when recordings were made during spontaneous clinical seizures (six in all), the seizure activity always started in the *right* medial temporal lobe, spread to the right frontal cortex and then to the left medial temporal region and left frontal cortex (Fig. 142–11). The patient underwent a right anterior temporal lobectomy, and histological examination revealed mesial sclerosis.

Epidural Surface Electrode Arrays in Epilepsy Associated with Infantile Hemiplegia

Victims of this affliction either are born with complete paralysis of one side of the body or acquire the defect in infancy. Later they may develop epilepsy, and frequently

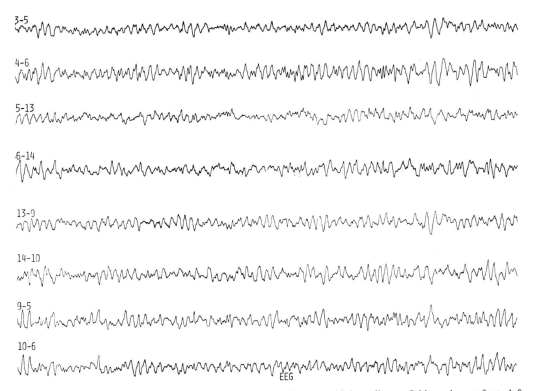

Figure 142–8 Nonfocal electroencephalogram in a case of temporal lobe epilepsy. Odd numbers refer to left side, even ones to corresponding electrode locations on right side. From top down, electrode locations in each adjacent pair of traces are: frontocentral, frontotemporal, temporal-occipital, and occipital-central.

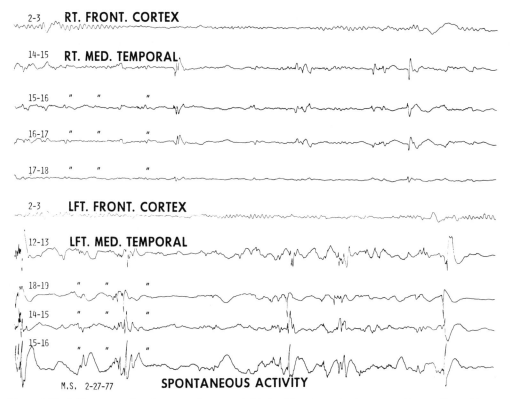

Figure 142–9 Extraoperative electrocorticogram with indwelling electrodes in temporal lobe epilepsy (the same case as Figure 142–8). Records show independent spiking in both medial temporal lobes. The medial temporal lobe traces are bipolar records made at sequential depths in the region of the amygdala.

they show mental retardation or asocial behavior. The asocial behavior of the infantile hemiplegic is usually characterized by episodic, aggressive outbursts and unprovoked temper tantrums. The convulsions are usually focal in origin, later becoming generalized, but may be generalized from the start. Psychomotor seizures also occur. The unique feature is a pathological process that is limited to one hemisphere, which is shrunken and has large areas of neuron replacement by reactive glial tissue and cystic lesions that may or may not communicate with the ventricular system.

The causes are various: birth injury, occlusion of a major cerebral artery, hemorrhage, trauma, and focal infection. In some instances the etiology remains unknown. The badly deteriorated hemisphere serves no purpose. All useful motor and mental activities have to be controlled from the uninvolved half of the brain. Furthermore, the damaged hemisphere is not simply a missing one. Rather its remaining action is expressed adversely in repeated convulsions and episodic abnormalities in behavior. It is

because the hemisphere contributes nothing that is useful and much that is injurious to brain and mind that the radical procedure of hemispherectomy has proved to be an effective means of treatment.

In 1938, McKenzie performed the first hemispherectomy in a young woman who had spastic hemiplegia and intractable convulsions that stemmed from a severe childhood head injury.[19] His lead was not followed, however, until 1950, when Krynauw reported excellent results in 12 infantile hemiplegics in whom he performed a hemispherectomy for intractable seizures.[18] Thereafter, others began to perform hemispherectomies in similar patients. Review of large series of cases shows that following hemispherectomy, 82 per cent of the patients either had no further seizures or showed a substantial reduction in the number of attacks and their severity.[46,48] Improvement in behavior has been equally gratifying. Ninety-three per cent showed disappearance or marked improvement of abnormal behavior. The aggressive episodes ceased. In a significant number the

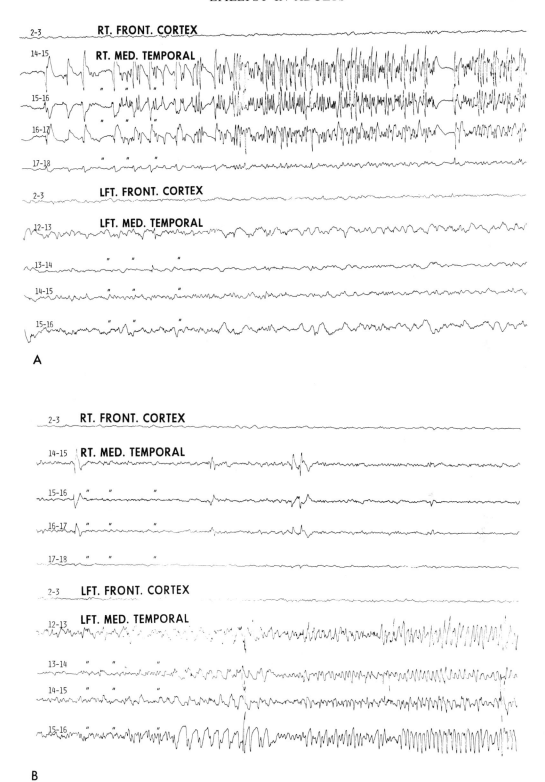

Figure 142–10 Two runs of electrical seizure discharge recorded independently from each temporal lobe in the same case shown in Figures 142–8 and 142–9. These recordings had no clinical concomitant. *A*. Right medial temporal spontaneous seizure activity (130 seconds' duration without a clinical seizure). *B*. Left medial temporal spontaneous seizure activity (90 seconds' duration without a clinical seizure). Each trace was made with bipolar electrodes at sequential depths in the region of the amygdala.

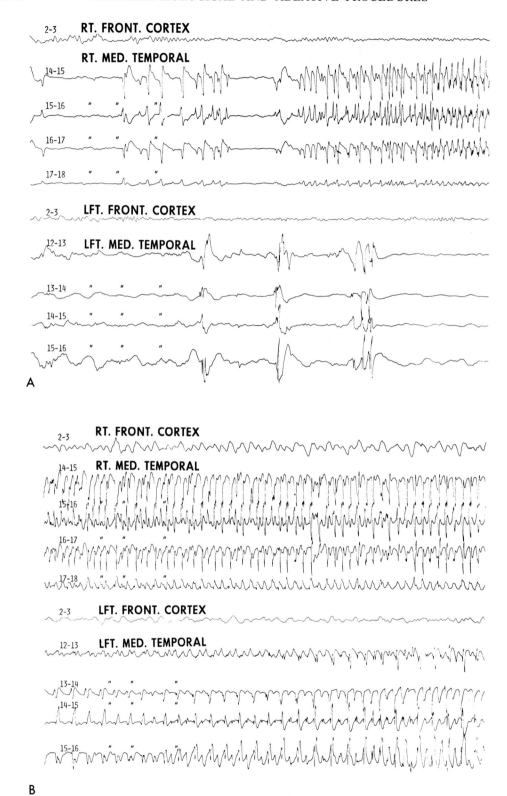

Figure 142–11 Spontaneous clinical seizure in the same case as Figure 142–8, 142–9, and 142–10. *A*. Seizure activity begins in right medial temporal lobe and spreads to left medial temporal lobe and both frontal cortices. *B*. Forty seconds after onset. Medial temporal lobe traces are bipolar records made at sequential depths in the region of the amygdala.

IQ improved, and some subjects became educable. There are examples, admittedly not many, of those who have completed a college education after having had such a hemispherectomy. The improvement in intellectual functions is directly attributable to the cessation of seizures and the reduction or elimination of excessive amounts of anticonvulsant medications.

In a large number of patients it is the left hemisphere that is involved. Even though the left side is usually dominant for speech, that function is not affected because the damage was done prior to the time that the individual learned to talk, and during early infancy either hemisphere can develop into the primary repository for speech function. It is of added significance that one third of subjects also show improved motor function on the paralyzed side, owing in all probability to lessening of the disabling hypertonicity of the paralyzed limbs. In other words, the rigidity of the affected arm and leg lessens, and their gross movements, at least, are more readily achieved. In walking, the affected leg moves more freely, and arm movements are accomplished with less difficulty. Inability to perform single-finger movements persists, but many of the patients come to open and close the hand, whereas previously the spastic hand was held in a tightly clenched fist.

Many such subjects have now been followed for 10 to 20 years after hemispheric removal. In the majority, the results are lasting and excellent, but in about one quarter of them neurological deterioration and hydrocephalus develop late—as long as 5 to 20 years after operation. Minor head trauma and even coughing are believed to cause repeated episodes of bleeding into the large cavity created by the hemispherectomy. The dead space also predisposes to major shifts in position of the brain stem and the remaining hemisphere, which can cause kinking of the aqueduct. The fluid within the cavity acquires a high protein and iron content, which gives rise to thickening of the leptomeninges and a granular ependymitis with cystic degeneration beneath the leptomeninges and ependyma (hemosiderosis). The granular ependymitis can occlude the aqueduct and cause hydrocephalus. Because of these factors, it is preferable to perform, when possible, an incomplete hemispherectomy, leaving behind one or more lobes that do not appear involved in the pathological process.[30] In this effort the extraoperative electrocorticogram is of great value. Based on the recordings with epidural surface electrode arrays, resections can be limited to only those areas that are shown to be involved in the clinical seizure. Three patients with infantile hemiplegia who have had limited resections based on extraoperative electrocorticography have been followed for one, two, and three years, and remain free of seizures.

Procedures Directed Toward Prevention of Seizure Spread

Those who have studied human epilepsy prior to operation through use of implanted recording electrodes have repeatedly observed localized seizure discharges that occur unaccompanied by clinical manifestations (see Fig. 142–10). Such an abnormal discharge probably occurs in a functionally silent area of the brain, and the clinical seizure becomes manifest as it spreads to involve a discrete critical region. This finding suggests that an alternative method of dealing with drug-resistant epilepsies might be the interruption of paths of preferential spread of seizure discharge. Such an approach would be especially useful in those cases of intractable epilepsy in which no epileptogenic focus can be demonstrated, or in which it is ill-defined or located in a vital area where an operative resection would represent a calculated risk of some magnitude.

Callosal Section and Anterior Commissurectomy

Such a rationale prompted Van Wagenen and Herren to section the corpus callosum in patients with generalized convulsions.[40] Some of Van Wagenen's subjects improved, but the beneficial results were not sufficiently convincing to prompt more than occasional use of callosal section for operative treatment of intractable epilepsy. One of the larger experiences with this procedure has been reported by Bogen, Sperry, and Vogel.[3] In addition to dividing the corpus callosum, they disconnected the anterior commissure. Of 10 subjects in whom "generalized" convulsions had been occurring with great and increasing frequency before operation, the seizures were largely abolished, in nine cases, during a two- to seven-year follow-up.

Of special interest is the minor nature of the functional impairment that is caused by a total cerebral commissurectomy, although special psychological tests have revealed that disconnecting the cerebral hemispheres does have effects on the highest level of function. An example is the inability of blindfolded, right-handed subjects to name objects placed in the left hand, information regarding size, shape, and texture of the object felt with that hand being registered only in the right hemisphere. The commissurectomy prevents such information from being transferred to the dominant left hemisphere, a prerequisite for verbal recognition of the object that is held. More recently, Bogen and Wilson and their co-workers have spared the splenium and limited the section to the anterior corpus calosum and anterior commissure.[14,47] With such limited sections, the disconnection syndrome does not appear to develop. At present it is uncertain whether limited section of the corpus callosum with or without section of the anterior commissure will prove as effective for seizure control as is total section of the corpus callosum and anterior commissure.[47]

Stereotaxic Lesions

Some paths that spread from an epileptic focus lie within the brain's interior and cannot be approached directly by operation without excessively damaging the brain. Deep strategic sites can, however, be reached by stereotaxic techniques.[23]

First to use the stereotaxic technique in treating intractable seizures were Spiegel and Wycis. In 1948, they reported on two patients with drug-resistant petit mal epilepsy treated by this method.[34,50] The electrode tips had been guided stereotaxically to the center of the thalamus. Spiegel and Wycis noted that their choice of the target was influenced by animal studies of Jasper and Droogleever-Fortuyn, who showed that episodes resembling petit mal and grand mal could be initiated in freely moving cats by electrical stimulation of the medial thalamus.[15a] Spiegel and Wycis used direct current to coagulate the tissue in the immediate neighborhood of their electrode tips. The results were inconclusive, and no further

lesions were made there. But in 1958 they reported on an additional group of patients in whom lesions were made in the globus pallidus, either singly or in combination with lesions in the amygdala.[35] Earlier experimental studies by Walker had demonstrated preferential spread of seizure discharge from cerebral cortex to the globus pallidus as well as to other subcortical nuclei, and this prompted the Spiegel-Wycis choice of the pallidum as a site for interruption.[7,44] The subjects selected had both salaam and grand mal attacks. They were observed for many years after undergoing the operation.[49] The results are somewhat difficult to evaluate, but it appears that the salaam attacks were favorably influenced in 6 of 10 patients who exhibited such seizures. All six were freed of such attacks or had only sporadic occurrences after operation.

Other surgeons have placed lesions in the thalamus, posterior internal capsule, or subthalamus.[23] The reports are few in number, and each series of patients is small. The follow-up intervals are also too short to permit a conclusive statement concerning the percentage of successes. One of the larger series of stereotaxic lesions is that of Jinnai, who made lesions in the subthalamus for both generalized and focal epilepsy, exclusive of temporal lobe epilepsy.[16] Of 43 subjects who had been followed for one to nine years, 12 showed complete relief from seizures, and 7 were improved. Of those relieved completely, four had had generalized seizures. Lesions in the subthalamus have not proved effective in treating temporal lobe epilepsy.

Temporal lobe seizure problems have also been managed stereotaxically by placing lesions in the amygdala or fornix and anterior commissure. The reason these limited, targeted destructions have been effective is probably that expressed by Walker, who says that "the preferential pathways for discharge from the temporal cortex are the amygdala and hippocampus and from these medial structures to mesencephalic and diencephalic centers, whereby the external manifestation of the epileptic discharge is mediated."[43] The fact that only small areas of brain have to be destroyed in this instance would render it the obvious procedure of choice if it were as effective as removal of the entire anterior temporal lobe. Yet, the results, so far, do not appear to be as enduring as those that follow anterior temporal lobectomy. Nevertheless, stereotaxic amygdalectomy may prove to have a place in managing some cases of temporal lobe epilepsy, especially those complicated by independent epileptogenic foci in the two temporal lobes. In contrast to bilateral temporal lobectomy, bilateral amygdalar lesions have not been followed by memory impairment.

Procedures Directed Toward Modifying Neural Transmission

Earlier anatomical and physiological studies showing cerebellar cortex to have a modulating effect on motor function prompted Cooper to employ long-term cerebellar stimulation to suppress seizures.[4] The electrodes are implanted on the surface of the anterior and posterior lobes of the cerebellum, and stimulation is accomplished by transcutaneous inductive coupling of the electrodes with a small stimulator that the patient wears. Ten of fifteen patients so treated and followed up to three years were considered improved. Van Buren and co-workers, however, in a rigorously controlled study of five patients, found that cerebellar stimulation had no effect on seizure frequency.[39] More time and experience is needed before this method of management can be assessed conclusively.

REFERENCES

1. Bailey, P., and Gibbs, F. A.: Surgical treatment of psychomotor epilepsy. J.A.M.A., 145:365–370, 1951.
2. Bancaud, J., Angelergues, R., Bernouilli, A., Bonis, A., Bordas-Ferrer, M., Bressen, M., Buser, P., Covello, L., Morel, P., Szikla, G., Takeda, A., and Talairach, J.: Functional stereotaxic exploration (SEEG) of epilepsy. Electroenceph. Clin. Neurophysiol., 28:85–86, 1970.
3. Bogen, J. E., Sperry, R. W., and Vogel, P. J.: Commissural section and propagation of seizures. In Jasper, H. H., Ward, A. A., Jr., and Pope, A., eds.: Basic Mechanisms of the Epilepsies. Boston, Little, Brown & Co., 1969.
4. Cooper, I. S., Amin, I., Riklan, M., Waltz, J. M., and Poon, T. P.: Chronic cerebellar stimulation in epilepsy. Arch. Neurol. (Chicago), 33:559–570, 1976.
5. Crandall, P. H.: Developments in direct recordings from epileptogenic regions in the surgical treatment of partial epilepsies. In Brazier, M. A. B. ed.: Epilepsy: Its Phenomena in Man. New York and London, Academic Press, 1973, pp. 288–309.
6. Dodson, W. E., Prensky, A. L., DeVivo, D. C., Goldring, S., and Dodge, P. R.: Management of seizure disorders: Selected aspects. Part II. J. Pediatr., 89:695–703, 1976.
7. Faeth, W. H., Walker, A. E., and Warner, W. A.: Experimental subcortical epilepsy. Arch. Neurol. Psychiat., 75:548–562, 1956.
8. Falconer, M. A.: Surgical treatment of temporal lobe epilepsy. New Zeal. Med. J., 66:539–542, 1967.
9. Falconer, M. A.: Mesial temporal (Ammon's horn) sclerosis as a common cause of epilepsy. Aetiology, treatment, and prevention. Lancet, 2:767, 1974.
10. Falconer, M. A., and Taylor, D. C.: Surgical treatment of drug-resistant epilepsy due to mesial temporal sclerosis. Etiology and significance. Arch. Neurol. (Chicago), 19:353–361, 1968.
11. Gloor, P.: Contributions of electroencephalography and electrocorticography to the neurosurgical treatment of the epilepsies. Advances Neurol., 8:59–105, 1975.
12. Goldring, S.: The role of prefrontal cortex in grand mal convulsion. Arch. Neurol. (Chicago), 26:109–119, 1972.
13. Goldring, S., Aras, E., and Weber, P. C.: Comparative study of sensory input to motor cortex in animals and man. Electroenceph. Clin. Neurophysiol., 29:537–550, 1970.
14. Gordon, H. W., Bogen, J. E., and Sperry, R. W.: Absence of deconnexion syndrome in two patients with partial section of the neocommissures. Brain, 94:327–336, 1971.
15. Green, J. R., Duisberg, R. E. H., and McGrath, W. B.: Focal epilepsy of psychomotor type; a preliminary report of observations on effects of surgical therapy. J. Neurosurg., 8:157–172, 1951.
15a. Jasper, H. H., and Droogleever-Fortuyn., J.: Experimental studies on the functional anatomy of petit mal epilepsy. Ass. Res. Nerv. Ment. Dis. Proc., 26:272–298, 1947.
16. Jinnai, D.: Clinical results and the significance of Forel-H-tomy in the treatment of epilepsy. Confin. Neurol., 27:129–136, 1966.
17. Kelly, D. L., Jr., Goldring, S., and O'Leary, J. L.: Average evoked somatosensory responses from exposed cortex of man. Arch. Neurol. (Chicago), 13:1–9, 1965.
18. Krynauw, R. A.: Infantile hemiplegia treated by removing one cerebral hemisphere. J. Neurol. Neurosurg. Psychiat., 13:243–267, 1950.
19. McKenzie, K. G.: The functional responses of the sympathetic nervous system of man following hemidecortication. J. Neurol. Psychiat., 2:313–322, 1938.
20. Milner, B.: Psychological defects produced by temporal lobe excision. Ass. Res. Nerv. Ment. Dis., 26:244–257, 1958.
21. Milner, B., Branch, C. L., and Rasmussen, T.: Study of short-term memory after intracarotid injection of Sodium Amytal. Trans. Amer. Neurol. Ass., 87:224–226, 1962.
22. Mullan, S., Vailati, G., Karasick, J., and Mailis, M.: Thalamic lesions for the control of epilepsy. A study of 9 cases. Arch. Neurol. (Chicago), 16:277–285, 1967.
23. Ojemann, G. A., and Ward, A. A., Jr.: Stereotactic and other procedures for epilepsy. Advances Neurol. 8:241–263, 1975.

24. O'Leary, J. L., and Goldring, S.: Science and Epilepsy: Neuroscience Gains in Epilepsy Research. New York, Raven Press, 1976.
25. Penfield, W., and Flanigin, I. T.: Surgical therapy of temporal lobe seizures. Arch. Neurol. Psychiat., *64*:491–500, 1950.
26. Penfield, W., and Jasper, H.: Epilepsy and the Functional Anatomy of the Human Brain. Boston, Little, Brown & Co., 1954.
27. Rasmussen, T.: Surgical therapy of focal epilepsy. *In* Critchley, M., O'Leary, J. L., and Jennett, B., eds.: Scientific Foundations of Neurology. Philadelphia, F. A. Davis & Co., 1972, pp. 101–107.
28. Rasmussen, T.: Cortical resection in the treatment of focal epilepsy. Advances Neurol., 139–154, 1975.
29. Rasmussen, T.: Surgery of frontal lobe epilepsy. Advances Neurol., 197–206, 1975.
30. Rasmussen, T.: Surgery for epilepsy arising in regions other than the temporal and frontal lobes. Advances Neurol., 207–226, 1975.
31. Rovitt, R. L., Gloor, P., and Rasmussen, T.: Intracarotid amobarbital in epilepsy. Arch. Neurol. (Chicago), *5*:606–626, 1961.
32. Rovitt, R. L., Gloor, P., and Rasmussen, T.: Sphenoid electrodes in the electrographic study of patients with temporal lobe epilepsy. J. Neurosurg., *18*:151–158, 1961.
33. Schwab, R. S., Sweet, W. H., Mark, V. H., Kjellberg, R. N., and Ervin, F. R.: Treatment of intractable temporal lobe epilepsy by stereotactic amygdala lesions. Trans. Amer. Neurol. Ass., *90*:12–19, 1965.
34. Spiegel, E. R., and Wycis, H. T.: Thalamic recordings in man with special reference to seizure discharges. Electroenceph. Clin. Neurophysiol., *2*:23–27, 1950.
35. Spiegel, E. A., Wycis, H. T., and Baird, H. W., III.: Pallidotomy and pallidoamygdalotomy in certain types of convulsive disorders. Arch. Neurol. Psychiat., *80*:714–728, 1958.
36. Stohr, P. E., and Goldring, S.: Origin of somatosensory evoked scalp responses in man. J. Neurosurg., *31*:2:117–127, 1969.
37. Talairach, J., and Bancaud, J.: Lesion, "irritative" zone and epileptogenic focus. Confin. Neurol., *27*:91–94, 1966.
38. Van Buren, J. M., Ajmone-Marsan, C., and Mutsuga, N.: Temporal-lobe seizures with additional foci treated by resection. J. Neurosurg., *43*:598, 1975.
39. Van Buren, J. M., Wood, J. H., Oakley, J., and Hambrecht, F.: Preliminary evaluation of cerebellar stimulation by double-blind stimulation and biological criteria in the treatment of epilepsy. J. Neurosurg., *48*:407–416, 1978.
40. Van Wagenen, W. P., and Herren, R. Y.: Surgical division of commissural pathways in the corpus callosum. Relation to spread of an epileptic attack. Arch. Neurol. Psychiat., *44*:740–759, 1940.
41. Wada, J., and Rasmussen, T.: Intracarotid injection of sodium Amytal for the lateralization of cerebral speech dominance. Experimental and clinical observations. J. Neurosurg., *17*:226–282, 1960.
42. Walker, A. E.: Temporal lobectomy. J. Neurosurg., *26*:642–649, 1967.
43. Walker, A. E.: Man and his temporal lobes. Surg. Neurol., *1*:69–79, 1973.
44. Walker, A. E., Poggio, G. F., and Andy, O. J.: Structural spread of cortically-induced epileptic discharges. Neurology (Minneap.) *6*:616–626, 1956.
45. Walker, R. D.: Tactical considerations leading to surgical treatment of limbis epilepsy. *In* Brazier, M. A. B., ed.: Epilepsy: Its Phenomena in Man. New York and London, Academic Press, 1973, pp. 99–119.
46. White, H. H.: Cerebral hemispherectomy in the treatment of infantile hemiplegia. Confin. Neurol., *21*:1–50, 1961.
47. Wilson, D. H., Reeves, A., Gazzaniga, M., and Culver, C.: Forebrain commissurotomy for the relief of intractable seizures. Neurology. (Minneap.), *27*:708–715, 1977.
48. Wilson, P. J. E.: Cerebral hemispherectomy for infantile hemiplegia. A report of 50 cases. Brain., *93*:147–180, 1970.
49. Wycis, H. T., Baird, H. W., and Spiegel, E. A.: Long range results following pallidotomy and pallidoamygdalotomy in certain types of convulsive disorders. Confin. Neurol., *27*:114–120, 1966.
50. Wycis, H. T., Lee, A. J., and Spiegel, E. A.: Simultaneous records of thalamic and cortical (scalp) potentials in schizophrenics and epileptics. Confin, Neurol., *45*:264–272, 1949.

143

NEUROSURGICAL ASPECTS OF PRIMARY AFFECTIVE DISORDERS

In 1935, Fulton and Jacobsen reported the experimental production—and relief—of disabling neuroses in chimpanzees by making lesions in their frontal lobes.[23] Moniz was impressed by the potential for treatment of human mental disorders and persuaded his neurosurgical colleague Lima to make bilateral frontal lesions in the white matter in a series of disabled mental patients.[46] Their results encouraged the psychiatrist Freeman and the neurosurgeon Watts to develop the technique for making extensive bilateral sections of the frontal lobe white matter, usually in the coronal plane of the midfrontal region.[24] This simple low-risk procedure proved to be sufficiently helpful to enough patients incapacitated by their psychoses to be performed, in the decade and a half from 1940 to 1955, on many thousands of patients throughout the world. In 1949 Moniz was awarded the Nobel prize "for his discovery of the therapeutic value of prefrontal leucotomy in certain psychoses."[67] At that time, there was little other therapy to offer to such patients, a fact of which sight is often lost by the vitriolic critics of these operations.[58] The critical voices became more and more strident in the 1970's. By that time the operations involving extensive bilateral sections of the frontal lobe white matter, against which they were inveighing, had already become rare. Indeed, the original Freeman-Watts procedure had long since been replaced by the making of progressively smaller zones of destruction in the medial parts of the anterior frontal white matter. There has been a stepwise reduction in the amount of white matter that need be destroyed for a good therapeutic result. This reduction has been accompanied by the pragmatic decision to concentrate the lesions in various parts of the limbic system's representation in the frontal lobes. The tactic has resulted in a major reduction to virtual elimination of the adverse side effects of the procedures, while their efficiency in ameliorating the disabling symptoms has suffered but little.

Operations for treatment of psychiatric disorders have had several labels. Freeman and Watts call them psychosurgery.[24] The longer term "psychiatric surgery" has been adopted by some surgeons in the field. It should, however, be noted that one operates on psychiatric patients—not on the psyche or the mind. It is more accurate to speak of operative procedures performed for psychiatric disorders.

ERAS OF OPERATIONS FOR PSYCHIATRIC DISORDERS

The first era was that of the extensive operation, usually a unilateral or bilateral anterior lobotomy. The second era was that in which less extensive operations were done. These operations usually involved division of one half to one quarter of the frontal white fibers in the coronal plane near the anterior tip of the lateral ventricles. The third era saw the development of stereotaxic, or small-lesion, operations of various types.

W. H. SWEET

Era of Extensive Operations

The original operations usually were bilateral, since even extensive unilateral anterior frontal lobectomies produced only modest changes both in lower primates and in many patients. The so-called standard operation consisted of making a pair of small openings in skull and dura over the superolateral surface of each frontal lobe in the coronal plane of the anterior tips of the lateral ventricles. The great majority of the white fibers in this plane were then divided blindly with a spatula or under direct vision with suction and cautery.[24,53] The small percentage of direct operative complications of either type of approach plus initial favorable appraisals of the total results led to widespread adoption of this therapy. The general verdict shifted to uneasiness and then disapproval as discouraging percentages of permanent sequelae were reported. Two widely quoted studies (but with only late retrospective controls), those of Robin in Britain and of McKenzie and Kaczanowski in Canada, were especially influential.[41,55] These two reports were, however, eclipsed by the huge and only prospectively controlled analysis of such operations performed at six hospitals of the United States Veterans Administration. Of their 373 patients, all but 12 were schizophrenics. About half, 185, were controls matched in advance as closely as possible with those subjected either to the standard operation of extensive bilateral anterior frontal lobotomy (140 patients) or to the division of about one third of the white fibers in the same coronal plane, a bimedial lobotomy (26 patients). Unusually complete initial appraisals were succeeded by equally intensive and protracted follow-ups, resulting in seven reports, the last by Ball, Klett, and Gresock. The appraisals continued for five years after the last operations were done in 1952. A higher percentage of operatively treated patients than of controls could be discharged from the hospital. Both the community adjustments of those discharged and the performance of those still hospitalized were better in the group with the operation. The more beneficial results after both the standard and the bimedial operation were significant at the 0.05 level of confidence.[7] These results of 25 years ago are cited as evidence that there is inadequate factual support for the wave of condemnation that swept this country and Japan in the 1970's based on the alleged "mutilating" results of the extensive operations performed more than 20 years before.

The use of chlorpromazine started in 1952, and by the middle and late 1950's this and other ataractic or psychotropic drugs had proved sufficiently effective to replace extensive lobotomy. Operative treatment of psychiatric problems virtually ceased in the United States.

Era of Less Extensive Operations

In the second phase in the evolution of operations for psychiatric disorders, vastly fewer patients were treated by this modality. It was largely British, Canadian, and Australian psychiatrists who not only acknowledged that some of their patients were failures on psychiatric-pharmacological management but referred these small numbers of intractably disabled patients for operation. In the bimedial leucotomy, about one third as many white fibers are divided as in a "standard" lobotomy. The other common operation was division of only the lower medial frontal white quadrants. In a number of the British reports the results were compared with a retrospectively matched control series of patients who were not operated on. Despite the fact that in several of the series no control subjects could be found as severely disabled preoperatively as some of those treated by operation, the group that had the operations fared better than those who continued on medical management.[39,74] Sustained adverse personality or other deficits became infrequent; the mortality rate dropped to the 0.5 to 2 per cent range, and the majority of patients with affective disorders were significantly improved. The disabling types of behavior most likely to be alleviated were, and remain, the phobias, tension states, anxieties, and depressions. Even when these symptomatic components were present in certain schizophrenics—the so-called pseudoneurotic variety—they were likely to be improved. In obsessive-compulsive neurotics the results were less favorable, and for the hallucinatory and paranoid features of schizophrenia they were even less so. The best candidates, as epitomized by Arnot in 1949, remained those in a "fixed state of tortured self concern."[3] The more convincing publications described: (1) long-term follow-ups in which social workers investigated home, social, and work adjustments of the patients; (2) use of objective rating scales for performance in many categories; and (3) appraisal by individuals who did not know which treatments were given. Typically about two thirds of these disabled patients with affective psychoses had excellent to satisfactory results, returning to full or almost full working capacity. It became apparent that those patients who had concerned family members willing to be maximally supportive over the long term had a better chance to achieve sustained improvement. Indeed, Tucker believes that a virtual prerequisite to a good result is a responsible, helpful relative.[76] Older patients did about as well as the younger ones, and the result in a given individual tended to improve with the passage of time, although recurrences also took place.

As one reads the uninterrupted succession of favorable reports from many quarters of the globe and emanating from major responsible psychiatric services, one is amazed that more of the patients in whom protracted medical management had failed were not submitted to operation. One reason may be that, as Hohne and Walsh point out, "those who have had the operation are not likely to broadcast the fact," unlike many recipients of other types of operation.[27] The occasional but not inconsequential adverse changes in personality type and behavior related to these operations have been characterized by the psychologist Walsh, who studied 250 patients treated by open orbitomedial leucotomy. There was improvement in all but one of the scales of the Minnesota Multiphasic Personality Inventory, the widely used MMPI. The standardized intelligence tests such as the Wechsler scales showed no change postoperatively.[80] The specially devised tests of Lhermitte and co-workers, of Luria, and of Milner, however, brought out subtle deterioration in the areas of ability to make the preliminary analysis to solve complex problems, ability to use information from errors to modify ongoing behavior, and inflexibility in conceptual behavior.[34,36,43]

Another undesirable feature of the bimedial open operations and to a lesser extent of those in the lower medial quadrants has been the long time for rehabilitation. Thus the Lopez-Ibors reported that although 57 per cent of their patients had complete remission and 22 per cent were greatly improved, about a year of rehabilitation was required. They had followed up 75 patients with obsessive and phobic compulsive neuroses after bimedial operations done between 1951 and 1969.[35]

Post and co-workers reported that their bimedial leucotomies produced undesirable postoperative effects that were troublesome to the patient or relatives in 21 per cent of the patients and serious in 8 per cent. On the positive side was the recovery by 67 per cent of their 64 patients to full or almost full working capacity after long illness — in most cases more than five years.[54]

Era of Stereotaxic, or Small-Lesion, Operations

During the 1960's several neurosurgeons sought further to reduce the adverse effects of operations for psychiatric disorders by decreasing the size of the lesion and maximally avoiding the cortical gray matter in order to minimize any tendency to seizures.*

Rationale for Selection of Site to Destroy

Since the affective disorders have yielded the best results after destruction of some part of the frontal lobes, that part of the brain presumably related to control of emotions has been arbitrarily selected as the main target zone. The white fibers almost encircling the corpus callosum and lying in or deep to the gyrus cinguli have been shown in animal studies to include major pathways in the cerebrum for expression of emotion. The "limbic system," that portion of the brain perhaps primarily concerned with this function, includes not only these fiber tracts but also the amygdala and hippocampus in the cerebral hemispheres as well as deeper nuclei in thalamus and hypothalamus. Early in the history of operations for psychiatric disorders it was suggested that the inferior part of the thalamo-

---

* See references 9, 13, 14, 18, 21, 31, 33, 40, 45, 49, 68, 79.

frontal radiation was an appropriate target for transection.[22] The medial part of this tract connects two components of the limbic system, the magnocellular part of the dorsomedial nucleus of the thalamus and the medial half of the cortex on the orbital surface of the frontal lobe (Fig. 143–1). More recently pathways have been described arising from the entire circumference of the gyrus cinguli and projecting to the granular neocortex of the frontal lobes.[42,51] Reciprocal pathways extend from these back to the gyrus cinguli; the two components of the projections are indicated by the forward and backward arrows in Figure 143–1. Nauta points out that this enables the frontal cortex to modulate activity in the limbic system, partly on the basis of data it receives therefrom.[51,52] Another pathway from neocortex to limbic structure, that from orbital cortex to uncus,

has recently been described by van Hoesen and colleagues.[78] If one assumes that emotional control mechanisms are disturbed in an affective psychosis, one might equally well decide that any lesion here could only make a bad matter worse and that the lesion had better be elsewhere. In fact, however, several components of the limbic system have proved to be safe and often successful targets. Lesions are being made in the white matter deep to the gyrus cinguli above or in front of the corpus callosum, in the coronal planes of the tips of the ventricular frontal horns, or below the heads of the caudate nuclei in front of the substantia innominata. That cluster of nuclei called the amygdala at the anterior tips of the temporal horns is also a target. In the present state of ignorance about the mechanisms for normal control of emotions and even greater ignorance of the mechanisms in-

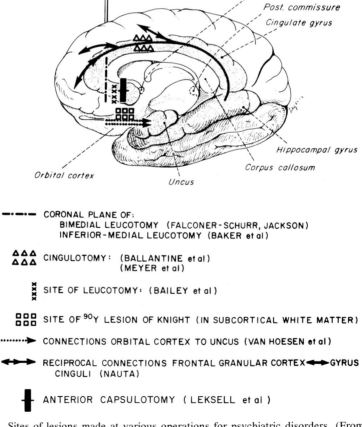

Figure 143–1 Sites of lesions made at various operations for psychiatric disorders. (From Sweet, W. H.: *In* Brady, J. P., and Brodie, H. K. H., eds.: Controversy in Psychiatry. Philadelphia, W. B. Saunders Co., 1978. Reprinted by permission.)

volved in affective or other psychoses, it probably is presumptuous to contend that anything approaching a pathophysiological rationale is available for selecting the targets. Hence it is all the more reasonable to assess the patients and what is done to them with all the precision that is possible.

Techniques

Stereotaxic introduction of electrodes to make a heat lesion at radiofrequency, of cryoprobes, or of beta-emitting 90yttrium seeds has had extensive trial.* The least expensive and the most controllable of the three methods uses electrodes for radiofrequency heat lesions. Beta-emitting seeds, though they make their lesion at a very gradual, safe rate, have been reported in rare instances to migrate to undesirable positions such as the hypothalamus.[17a] A neurosurgical service is already likely to use radiofrequency heating for production of lesions elsewhere, and hence to be experienced with the method. The largest series, however, 750 patients operated on for psychiatric disorders, were treated by Knight and colleagues, who used two rows of 90yttrium beads placed on each side in the posterior medial orbital white matter below the heads of the caudate nuclei—a "subcaudate tractotomy," as illustrated in Figure 143–1.[25,28,29,68] Talairach's service also makes the lesions with beads of 90yttrium.[16] In most other significant series of these operations, electrodes transmitting current at radiofrequencies (RF) were used to create a heat lesion. After making tiny parasagittal openings, one on each side of the frontal area of the skull, the surgeon injects enough air, about 20 cc, into one lateral ventricle to show the anterior parts of the first three ventricles. This suffices for orientation if his target is either in the cingulum or the subcaudate white matter. If the amygdala is his target the temporal horn must be shown. The usual electrode is a cylinder about 1 cm high with a diameter of 1 mm. When one uses this as a monopolar electrode with a ground placed subcutaneously, the lesion tends to be a cylinder about 12 mm high and 10 mm in diameter.

Following the lead of Leksell, two groups of Swedish psychiatrists and neurosur-

geons have made lesions in the anterior part of the internal capsule at a region of convergence of fibers connecting the cortex of the anterior frontal lobe with the thalamus.[13] Leksell introduces electrodes into the brain in the coronal plane, a pair on each side and 6 mm apart (Fig. 143–2). The coordinates are: coronal plane, 17 mm anterior to anterior commissure; horizontal plane, 0 mm relative to line joining anterior and posterior commissures; sagittal plane, 20 mm lateral to midline. Each bipolar radiofrequency lesion is an ellipsoidal cylinder about 20 mm high with a major axis of 8 mm.

The sites of the radiofrequency lesions are ascertainable not only from the radiographs showing both the electrodes and the ventricles but also from the computed tomographic scans (Figs. 143–3 and 143–4).

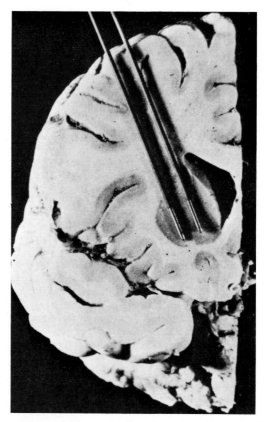

Figure 143–2 Type and site of bipolar electrodes for Leksell's anterior capsulotomy. (From Bingley, T., Leksell, L., Myerson, B. A., and Rylander, G.: Stereotactic anterior capsulotomy in anxiety and obsessive-compulsive states. *In* Laitinen, L. V., and Livingston, K. E., eds.: Surgical Approaches in Psychiatry. Baltimore, University Park Press, 1974. Reprinted by permission.)

---

* See references 8, 9, 13, 14, 16, 18, 21, 25, 31, 33, 38, 40, 45, 47, 56, 57, 61, 65, 68, 79, 81.

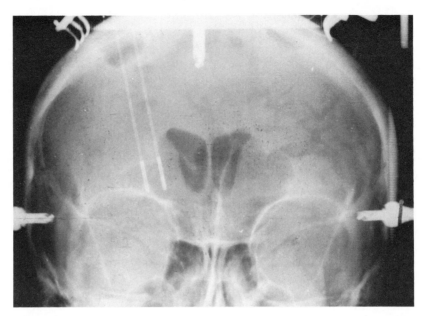

Figure 143–3 Radiographic appearance of electrodes in coronal plane 17 mm anterior to anterior commissure for Leksell's anterior capsulotomy. (From Bingley, T., Leksell, L., Myerson, B. A., and Rylander, G.: Stereotactic anterior capsulotomy in anxiety and obsessive-compulsive states. *In* Laitinen, L. V., and Livingston, K. E., eds.: Surgical Approaches in Psychiatry. Baltimore, University Park Press, 1974. Reprinted by permission.)

Results

The widespread recognition in several European countries of the value of operative treatment of psychiatric disorders in appropriately selected cases has led to three world congresses on the subject being held there.[26,32,73] The proceedings of all three congresses were published as books. Yet, in the early 1970's, public uneasiness in the United States concerning "psycho-

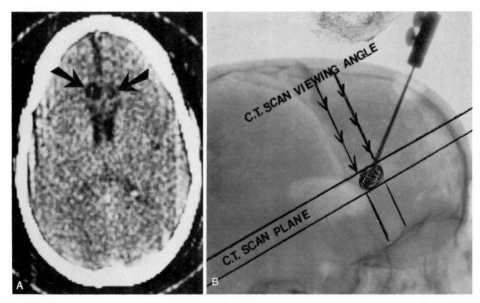

Figure 143–4 *A.* Computed tomography (CT scan) depicting bilateral cingulate lesions. *B.* Lateral air study with superimposed diagram showing that tilt from horizontal plane of CT scan obscures the fact that lesions are actually superior and 1 cm posterior to tips of frontal horns of lateral ventricles. (From Ballantine, H. T., Levy, B. S., Dagi, T. F., and Giriunas, I.: Cingulotomy for psychiatric illness: Report of 13 years' experience. *In* Sweet, W. H., Obrador, S., and Martin-Rodriguez, J., eds.: Neurosurgical Treatment in Psychiatry, Pain and Epilepsy. Baltimore, University Park Press, 1974. Reprinted by permission.)

surgery" led to the inclusion in the National Research Act of a mandate to investigate it. The newly created National Commission for the Protection of Human Subjects of Biomedical and Behavioral Research was directed to "evaluate the need for it, and recommend policies defining the circumstances (if any) under which its use may be appropriate."[50] Critics of operations for psychiatric disorders have contended that their risks are great, especially so because the procedures are irreversible, and that data concerning results are inconclusive and contradictory. They also contend that these operations have been used selectively *against* [sic] blacks, women, other minorities, and institutionalized persons as a social or political tool to control dissidence.[50] Neurosurgeons doing these operations have been denounced as "the tools of imperialistic capitalism." This is the theme of numerous statements issued as typewritten sheets by the Boston Area Medical Challenge Clubs, composed of members and friends of the revolutionary communist Progressive Labor Party. The allegations that the operations are used or will be used for other than bona fide therapy are ridiculous, and compelling arguments against these allegations are presented in the report of the previously mentioned National Commission. Physicians in the Western world do not use their treatment modalities of any sort for any other primary purpose than to try to help the individual patient.

Because of the resistance to these operations that was developing, especially in the United States and Japan, the contributors to the Fourth World Congress of Psychiatric Surgery in Madrid in 1975 were urged to present maximal documentation of their preoperative studies and protracted postoperative detailed follow-ups. The resulting volume, published early in 1977, is the most comprehensive summary available of experience around the world.[73] In the course of a personal search leading to the publication of a review in 1973 as well as the search entailed in being program chairman and an editor of the proceedings of the Madrid congress, the author found that every article describing the limited forms of frontal leucotomy for psychiatric disease came to the conclusion without a single exception that the procedure gave useful results for most of the medically intractable cases of

psychosis treated—this at the price of almost no deaths and little morbidity.[70] Would that the same could be said about more branches of neurological surgery! Incidentally, in many earlier articles this accolade was not given to the original types of extensive frontal leucotomy.

As Walsh and others have emphasized, it is certain types of symptoms rather than whole diagnostic or nosological groups that are likely to be responsive to this operation.[80] Phobias, anxieties, depressions, obsessive compulsions, and the affective ("pseudoneurotic") components of schizophrenia are the types of behavior most likely to be improved. The author has noted that their common denominator is *stereotypy of an excessive and futile emotional response*. This seems also to characterize those among the patients with intractable chronic pain who are likely to be relieved of their suffering by the same kind of operation.

Cingulotomy

Ballantine and his colleagues did 308 stereotaxic anterior operations in 204 psychiatric patients in the 13 years ending September 1975. Their disease had disabled these patients for from 2 to 35 years with an average of 10 years.[9]

No deaths and *no* serious complications related to the operation had occurred in this series at the time of the report or in the subsequent seven years. There have been almost no postoperative seizures; only three of the patients take diphenylhydantoin (Dilantin), on which drug they are seizure-free. The intractable symptoms leading to operation were all in the affective category already described. About 80 per cent of 84 carefully reappraised patients remained significantly improved as evaluated by themselves, their relatives, their physicians, and the authors of the report. Only half the patients who were to derive significant benefit from the operation had done so within two months, but by two years 95 per cent of those who were to improve significantly had done so. The percentage of significantly improved patients remained stable in surveys conducted by the authors in 1970 and 1975—respectively 78 and 77 per cent.[8,9] There was much variation in the status of individual patients, however, some becoming better and others worse.

Martin, McElhaney, and Meyer performed an extensive battery of psychological tests before and after operation on their 62 psychiatric patients. Included in their group was an unusually high percentage of patients with schizophrenia—29, or 47 per cent, whose primary symptom was anxiety. Even in this group, 13 had excellent and 7 had moderate improvement—the same percentage in the excellent category as for the whole series (Table 143–1). The mean IQ increased in every patient, in one by 33 points and in another by 28 points. In agreement with Ballantine and other workers, they found that if the first lesions yielded only inadequate or transient improvement, a second pair of lesions 18 months or so later had a good chance of achieving a favorable result.[40]

In another study that involved six patients with intractable psychiatric disorders, Levin and co-workers found subtle reductions in cognitive function in two patients. They also noted that previous treatments with psychotropic drugs and electroshock, and perhaps the disease itself, may produce subnormal test scores preoperatively.[33] Clearly the assumption of intact cerebral function in these patients may be wrong.

Subcaudate Tractotomy

The largest series of patients with small lesions made stereotaxically was started by Knight in the early 1960's. He implanted

TABLE 143–1 RESULTS OF BILATERAL CINGULOTOMY*

RESULTS OF OPERATION

| | Improvement | | | |
	Excellent	Moderate	Slight	No Change
Number of patients	29	14	11	8
Per cent	47	22	18	13

(The results were also "excellent" in 6 other patients—all classified as alcoholics.)

PSYCHOLOGICAL TESTS AFTER CINGULOTOMY

| | | Minnesota Multiphasic Personality Inventory | | | |
	Mean IQ	Depression	Hostility	Anxiety	Schizophrenia
Preoperatively	96.2	88	72	83	82
Postoperatively	103.5	77	61	70	71

* Data from Martin, W. L., McElhaney, M. L., and Meyer, G. A.: Stereotactic cingulotomy: Results of psychological testing and clinical evaluation preoperatively and postoperatively. In Sweet, W. H., et al., eds.: Neurosurgical Treatment in Psychiatry, Pain and Epilepsy. Baltimore, University Park Press, 1977, pp. 381–386.

[90]yttrium beads, which emit beta particles. Groups of psychiatrists and social workers have repeatedly assessed the results in those 750 patients who have been studied for a minimum of two and a half years after operation.[25,28,29,68] The figures in Table 143–2 incorporate the results of reports

TABLE 143–2 RESULTS OF STEREOTAXIC SUBCAUDATE TRACTOTOMY WITH [90]YTTRIUM*

| DISORDER | NUMBER OF PATIENTS | CATEGORY | | | | | PER CENT WELL | PER CENT IMPROVED |
		I	II	III	IV	V		
Obsession	38	14	5	9	9	1	50	74
Anxiety	70	21	13	16	20	0	49	71
Depression	153	58	37	34	24	0	62	84
Schizophrenia	9	0	0	4	5	0	0	44
Total	270							

Definition of categories:
    Category I—requires no treatment, asymptomatic
    Category II—requires no treatment, minor symptoms
    Category III—improved but symptomatic enough to require treatment
    Category IV—unchanged
    Category V—worse

* Outcome after 2½ years. Data from Knight, G. C.: Bifrontal stereotactic tractotomy: An atraumatic operation of value in the treatment of intractable psychoneurosis. Brit. J. Psychiat., 115:257–266, 1969; Further observations from an experience of 660 cases of stereotactic tractotomy. Postgrad. Med. J., 49:845–854, 1973; Göktepe, E. O., Young, L. B., and Bridges, P. K.: A further review of the results of stereotactic subcaudate tractotomy. Brit. J. Psychiat., 126:270–280, 1975; Ström-Olsen, R., and Carlisle, S.: Bifrontal stereotactic tractotomy: A followup study of its effects on 210 patients. Brit. J. Psychiat., 118:141–154, 1971.

from 1971 and 1975. The patients in categories I and II require no treatment; those in I are asymptomatic, and those in II have minor symptoms. Patients in category III are improved but symptomatic enough to require treatment; those in IV are unchanged, and those in V are worse. A particularly comprehensive appraisal of home and work adjustments was aided by interviews with relatives, who complained of the development of undesirable personality traits—none of which was socially disabling—in only 7 per cent of the patients.

Combined Cingulotomy and Subcaudate Tractotomy

A convincing series of papers has emerged under the aegis of the psychiatrist Kelly. His group reported on 120 patients in whom inferior posterior medial frontal lesions were made.[45] These lesions usually were combined with cingulate lesions or, in a few patients, with lesions in the genu of the corpus callosum, as advocated by Laitinen and by Vilkki.[79] Using the same categories for their clinical rating as those in Table 143–2, they have compared their results at six weeks in their first 66 consecutive patients with those at 16 months (Table 143–3). The ratings, made independently by the medical staff members, take into account the appraisals of other relevant members of the staff such as nurses and occupational therapists. The *least* favorable rating was used in the statistical compilation. Table 143–3 reveals that the good results are not only maintained, they are a trifle improved at 16 months over the six-week rat-

ings. Noteworthy is the high percentage of betterment in the obsessional neurotics and schizophrenics. In the former category the patients appear to have done better than those with either cingulotomy or subcaudate tractotomy alone. The schizophrenics were selected for operation on the basis of marked affective components in their illnesses. Despite the more extensive destruction, adverse personality changes did not occur, even in the schizophrenics. In addition to standard psychometric and physiological studies, a variety of special rating scales were used for the attempted quantitative measurement of anxiety, depression, "neuroticism," hysteria, and obsessions. Full details are given of the degrees of improvements in these measures in the various types of patient.[45] The lack thus far of standardized methods of appraisal has made it difficult to compare the effects of lesions at different sites—or combinations thereof—as performed in different centers.

Capsulotomy

A bilateral anterior capsulotomy was proposed and tried out by Leksell in many types of mental illness during the early 1950's (cf. Fig. 143–2). It was found to be particularly favorable for the obsessive-compulsive patients; hence a study of the procedure confined to this group was resumed about 10 years ago. The results described have been supplemented by performance and personality appraisals under the leadership of Rylander.[14] Since the 1930's his analyses of the effects of cerebral

TABLE 143–3 STEREOTAXIC SMALL LESIONS IN LOWER MEDIAL QUADRANTS AND ANTERIOR CINGULUM*

		CLINICAL RATINGS									
		6 Weeks					26 Months				
		Categories[a]				Per Cent Improved	Categories[a]				Per Cent Improved
DISORDER	NUMBER OF PATIENTS	I	II	III	IV–V		I	II	III	IV–V	
Obsession	27	1	14	8	4	85	7	11	6	3	89
Anxiety	15	1	3	4	7	53	3	1	6	5	66
Depression	9	3	3	3	0	100	3	2	2	2	78
Schizophrenia	7	0	2	4	1	86	0	4	2	1	86

[a] Categories defined as in Table 143–2. The results in 8 other patients in 6 other diagnostic categories are also given in the original table of the authors.

* Adapted from Mitchell-Heggs, N., Kelly, D., and Richardson, A. E.: Stereotactic limbic leucotomy: Clinical, psychological and physiological assessment at 16 months. *In* Sweet, W. H., et al., eds.: Neurosurgical Treatment in Psychiatry, Pain and Epilepsy. Baltimore, University Park Press, 1977, pp. 367–379.

lobectomies have been models of thoroughness. He was also one of the first to point out the major personality alterations that might occur after extensive bilateral lobotomies, quoting the relatives of some of these patients as finding them so changed that they had "lost their souls."[59] His clinical observations and objective tests before and after capsulotomy, however, brought to light "no evidence of any intellectual reduction or adverse personality changes."[60] Indeed, he noted two patients, in one of whom scientific and in the other, artistic, creative ability *had been restored*. Moreover, as he had already emphasized in 1948, patients with obsessive-compulsive neuroses have such intact personalities on other scores that they are particularly suitable for uncovering modest deficits related to cerebral deterioration.[59] Table 143–4 summarizes the results of his group in their 35 patients.

Anterior capsulotomy has been used by Kullberg and the Lopez-Ibors.[31,35] The former worker compared the results of this operation with those of anterior cingulotomy on the basis of 13 operations in each group of patients. Only those disabled by obsessive-compulsive or anxiety states were treated by operation. The sequelae and results are given in Table 143–5. More capsulotomized patients had longer-lasting, though transient, psychic sequelae; this was the price they paid for being much better at late follow-up than those patients who had had cingulotomy. The Lopez-Ibors followed six patients for up to two years after anterior capsulotomies. These psychiatrists were so impressed with the results that they have requested this operation exclusively in their 67 patients operated upon since 1969. Of these, 57 had obsessive neuroses.

TABLE 143–4 STEREOTAXIC ANTERIOR CAPSULOTOMY IN OBSESSIVE-COMPULSIVE NEUROSIS*

RESULTS IN 35 CASES
Duration of illness 4–25 years—Mean 17 years
Duration of postoperative follow-up 4–55 months—
   Mean 35 months
Status of patient
   Symptom-free   16
   Much improved   9
   Slightly improved   10

PRE-OPERATIVE STATUS	NUMBER OF PATIENTS	POSTOPERATIVE STATUS		
		Inca-pacitated	*Partly Working*	*Fully Working*
Incapacitated	24	4	14	6
Partly working	8		3	5
Fully working	3			3

* Data from Bingley, T., Leksell, L., Myerson, B. A., and Rylander, G.: Long-term results of stereotactic anterior capsulotomy in chronic obsessive-compulsive neurosis. *In* Sweet, W. H., et al., eds.: Neurosurgical Treatment in Psychiatry, Pain and Epilepsy. Baltimore, University Park Press, 1977, pp. 287–299.

TABLE 143–5 CAPSULOTOMY VERSUS CINGULOTOMY*

	Capsulotomy (13 operations)			Cingulotomy (13 operations)		
TRANSIENT PSYCHIC SEQUELAE						
Confusion						
Few days	3			2		
1 to 3 weeks	2			0		
Affective deficit						
1 to 2 weeks	5			2		
3 to 4 weeks	2			0		

BEHAVIORAL STATUS AT END OF 1- TO 9-YEAR FOLLOW-UP

	Obsession	Anxiety	Total	Obsession	Anxiety	Total
Excellent	1	3	4	0	2	2
Good	2	0	2	0	1	1
Moderate	2	2	4	0	1	1
Slight change or none	3	0	3	3	6	9

* Data from Kullberg, G.: Differences in effect of capsulotomy and cingulotomy. *In* Sweet, W. H., et al., eds.: Neurosurgical Treatment in Psychiatry, Pain and Epilepsy. Baltimore, University Park Press, 1977, pp. 301–308.

Evaluations of Operations for Psychiatric Disorders

The foregoing brief abstracts of recent reports do not include 12 of those given in Madrid on small-lesion operations for psychiatric disorders. The most extensive presentations in one volume of preoperative and postoperative studies of patients having such operations are found in the Proceedings of the Fourth World Congress of Psychiatric Surgery held in Madrid in 1975.[73]

Three more publications deserve special mention. They describe work that was concerned with "psychosurgery" and was performed under contracts let by the United States National Commission for the Protection of Human Subjects of Biomedical and Behavioral Research. Valenstein, a professor of psychology, was given the task of evaluating the literature in English. He found 153 articles published between 1971 and 1976 concerning operations done for psychiatric disorders that were written by persons having direct contact with patients or their medical records. These reports along with his 476 other references on related aspects of the subject constitute a valuable reference source.[77] His summary of what the literature says is in line with the content of this chapter. He judges the literature in the field "to be low in scientific merit," however. Whether this is true is not germane to the problem in hand. A single superbly executed study that reaches an unequivocal conclusion suffices to make its point. The several well-documented studies, cited earlier in this chapter, of the value of small medial frontal lesions in the white matter in the treatment of disabling affective psychiatric disorders have been convincing to many reasonable people. The number of other communications in which flaws can be demonstrated is irrelevant. The type of analysis on which Valenstein, who is not a clinician, based his conclusion deserves scrutiny. He gave a top rating of "1" to studies that had matched control groups, used objective tests, evaluated patients for an adequate period, analyzed data statistically, employed independent testers, and did not confound any relevant variables (e.g., drug treatment, support from family or friends, and the like). As an example of this last-named fault he cited this statement

from the Swedish study on anterior capsulotomy to which Rylander contributed:

> The importance of an intensive and long-lasting post-operative rehabilitation in conjunction with psychosurgical treatment cannot be over-rated. The fact that this was given to virtually all our patients is presumably a contributing factor to the favorable long-term results.[14]

In the view of many observers, it would be poor judgment not to take the fullest advantage of whatever impetus to recovery an operation might give; hence the author would hope that this criterion of Valenstein's would never be met. It is also worth noting that if an operation for psychiatric disorders is to be used only when every other treatment has been exhausted, then it would never be ethically permissible to withhold the operation once one had decided that this was the only therapy with any hope of success; hence there could not be matched control groups. Finally, with respect to the use of independent testers, one must note that the cost of the testers should be borne from sources independent of the responsible physicians and their patients—a requirement that can rarely be met.

The requirement for independent testers was met in two studies. Two groups, each under the primary direction of psychologists, were given contracts for objective evaluation of patients who had been operated on with whom they had never had any previous association. One group, that of Teuber, Corkin, and Twitchell, studied 34 patients submitted to cingulotomy by Ballantine. The examination protocol for these 34 patients included two dozen psychological tests. Only 18 of the patients had the same extensive preoperative testing as all 34 had after operation.[75] It should be noted that Teuber is distinguished for his development of tests to detect occult defects in performance related to small lesions in the human brain. With this background of expertise plus Teuber's bias against operations for psychiatric disorders, it is significant that these investigators found "no lasting effects of the cingulotomy in the 24 behavioral tasks sampled in our study," and they described themselves as "baffled in our current attempts at detecting any specific effects of the cingulate lesions."[75] In fact the IQ ratings of all patients tested preoperatively and then a second time more than four months after operation showed significant *rises* (italics added) in Full-Scale, Verbal, and Performance IQ ratings.[75] Likewise, more general types of appraisal of life-history data and interview material failed to disclose any obvious "costs" of the intervention. There were no evident increase in marital instability, no alteration in sexual activity according to patients and their spouses, and a slight gain in employment after operation; and "all (except two cases of borderline schizophrenia) insisted that they were still capable of appropriate depth of feeling (such as anguish after a bereavement)."[75] The results varied with the type of patient. Of 11 patients with primary complaints of chronic pain along with some depression, 9 had complete or nearly complete relief from pain that had lasted for many years or even decades in some. None of these patients required a repeat cingulotomy. Four of them who had been addicted to opiates or related drugs could discontinue these medications without withdrawal symptoms. Of seven

patients complaining primarily of depression, five had full or partial relief; two were not helped at all. The four obsessive-compulsive patients were unimproved. A heterogenous group of 11 cases ranging from severe anxiety to borderline schizophrenia had the most varied outcomes.

The second group of patients were studied by Mirsky and Orzack. These investigators conducted postoperative studies of 27 patients upon whom three types of operation had been done, each type by a different neurosurgeon. The three types of operation were: orbital undercutting, an open operation in which the white fibers above the medial part of the orbital cortex are divided under direct vision, as shown in Figure 143–5; a multitarget procedure in which an anterior cingulate, a preinnominate (subcaudate), and an amygdalar lesion are made on each side, illustrated in Figure 143–6; and ultrasonic irradiation of the white matter in the lower medial quadrant of the frontal lobes anterior to the ventricles, as diagrammed in Figure 143–7. Psychiatrists,

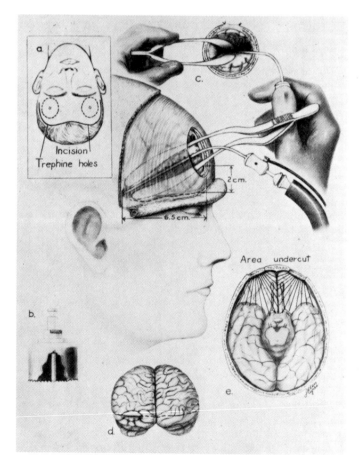

Figure 143–5 Site and instruments for Scoville's orbital undercutting procedure. *a.* Diagram of sites of trephine openings. *b.* Cutaway diagram of trephining tool to show central metal pin that stabilizes the cutting edge. *c.* The surgeon's view through the trephine opening in skull and the incision into brain. (From Scoville, W.: *In* Laitinen, L., and Vaernet, K., eds.: Psychosurgery. Springfield, Ill., Charles C Thomas, 1972. Reprinted by permission.)

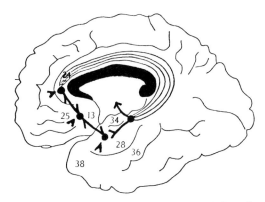

Figure 143–6 Diagram of the three lesions in Brown's multitarget operation: (1) anterior cingulum, (2) preinnominate subcaudate area, and (3) amygdala. Arrows point to lesion sites; numbers are of Brodmann's areas. (From Mirsky, A. F., and Orzack, M. H.: *In* National Commission for the Protection of Human Subjects of Biomedical and Behavioral Research: Appendix Psychosurgery. U.S. Department of Health, Education and Welfare Publication No. (OS)77-0002, 1977.)

psychologists, social workers, neurologists, neurophysiologists, and electroencephalographers conducted the intensive studies. They were performed also on eight control subjects matched as well as possible under the time constraints of the contract for the study. The majority of the scores in the tests administered showed no significant differences between the control group and the patients who were operated on. The exception was a category test in which those who had had operations made more perseverative errors as they at-

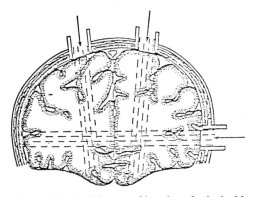

Figure 143–7 Diagram of location of principal lesions—anterior to frontal horns of ventricles—in Lindstrom's ultrasonic radiation procedure. (From Mirsky, A. F., and Orzack, M. H.: *In* National Commission for the Protection of Human Subjects of Biomedical and Behavioral Research: Appendix Psychosurgery, U.S. Department of Health, Education and Welfare Publication No. (OS)77-0002, 1977.)

tempted to shift from one category to another (the Wisconsin Card Sorting Test).[44] This difference from the control subjects and from the patients who had cingulotomies may have been related to the fact that these patients presumably had more destruction of frontal lobe white matter than those studied by Teuber and associates. The Teuber group had also used the same Wisconsin Card Sorting Test. The clinical outcome was "very favorable" in 14 of the 27 patients studied by Mirsky and Orzack, and there was moderate improvement in 7 more, i.e., 78 per cent of the total showed moderate to marked improvement.

The postoperative complications found by the two groups were also minor—they consisted of seizures in three patients with no prior history thereof and none of brain injury. One patient had only one seizure, another had three in the postoperative months, and the seizures in the third patient were controlled with continued anticonvulsant medication.

The full reports of all three contracting groups have been published as the Appendix to the Report and Recommendations of the National Commission.[44,75,77] One major value of the two studies of patients is that they confirm in a striking way the statements in the reports of numerous larger series already cited regarding the need to secure adequate informed consent. Also they confirm the minor nature of the deficits and complications following the small lesions in medial frontal white matter. Furthermore, the clinical results are encouraging because the operations were performed only as a last resort after all other reasonable forms of therapy had failed. Statements made by the original reporters in all the articles cited in this chapter were confirmed by the Teuber and Mirsky groups for the patients they studied. The emphatic phrases of the Teuber report were:

The operation added its effects not only to those of a persistent illness that preceded it, but to the cumulative impact of the massive earlier treatment efforts, which by themselves seemed to be interfering with certain higher functions, and often to an extent where it appeared futile to expect that the effect of [surgery] as such might have become discernible, within the welter of other handicaps that already weighed upon the patients.[75]

The Teuber group's study is of major importance in still another respect, namely its finding with respect to electroconvulsive therapy (ECT). Patients whose preoperative treatments

. . . had included ECT were inferior to normal control subjects and to patients who had been spared ECT, and this inferiority was apparent on the following measures: verbal and nonverbal fluency, delayed alternation performance, tactual maze learning, continuous recognition of faces and houses, and identification of famous public figures. In some cases, the degree of deficit was related to the number of ECT received, patients who had been given more than 50 ECT being significantly worse than those who had sustained fewer than 50.[75]

Corkin and colleagues are continuing these studies; the number of patients they assessed both before and after operation has risen from 18 to 41. Four patients have been added who had responded favorably to massive doses of electroshock therapy and were therefore not treated by operation. These four patients seemed to be as impaired on some tests as those cingulotomy patients who had received more than 40 electroshock treatments.

The two studies of the Teuber and Mirsky groups cost the United States taxpayers $300,000. Their total independence from the original physicians, however, and their thoroughness make them well worth it. They demonstrate by their close agreement with the final conclusions of the whole range of reports from around the world that in general one can place reliance on the honesty of the medical profession and this crucial feature of the system in which they work. Namely, a physician such as a psychiatrist refers a patient to a surgeon with no remuneration to the referring doctor for so doing. This gives the patient a built-in further assurance that the referral is made because of genuine belief that the patient will benefit. Indeed, if he does improve enough, the referring physician may lose the income from the otherwise continuing medical treatment.

Two other allegations about operative procedures for psychiatric disorders merit examination. The first is that the lesions are irreversible because of the apparent inability of neuron cell bodies to undergo mitosis in the mature nervous system. While the logical premise that this system should have a stable fundamental organization appears to be related to this characteristic, the central nervous system is by no means devoid of reparative mechanisms. Much of the present knowledge in this field has been summarized by Schneider.[63] Suffice it to say that new, functional synapses form in anomalous locations after certain lesions in both the developing and the mature mammalian brain, and that the normal dendrites and axons of the normal brain appear to be in a rapidly changing dynamic state related to adaptation and learning. From the practical standpoint of the results of destructive neurosurgical procedures, this reparative capacity may be more of a hindrance than a help. Thus, even in that relatively less plastic structure than brain, the spinal cord, the cutaneous analgesia to pinprick is often maintained for only one or a few years after transection of most of one anterior quadrant—the well-established operation, "cordotomy" for pain. In fact, White and Sweet found this to be the case in about half the 47 patients followed for 1 to 32 years.[81]

A second criticism of operative treatment for psychiatric disorders is that, regardless of where the lesion is made in the frontal lobes, the percentage of good results is about the same. It is true that there is a lack of quantitative measures of proved validity of such factors as anxiety, depression, and compulsions; moreover, the scales that are available are used infrequently. Hence, there is need for good data pertaining to which type of lesion most benefits which symptom. The best indication is that anterior capsulotomy is more likely to benefit obsessive-compulsive disorders than either supracallosal cingulotomy or inferior posteromedial frontal leucotomy. Lesions at both of these latter sites in the hands of Kelly's group have, however, been about as effective as anterior capsulotomy.[45]

Verification of Sites of Lesions

Because of the virtual absence of deaths from the operation, there is a dearth of postmortem data to prove the sites of the lesions. There are fragmentary reports that are relevant, however. Thus Corsellis studied the brains of eight older patients who died late postoperatively of causes unrelated to a subcaudate tractotomy with ^{90}yttrium beads. The lesions in the four patients who had recovered or improved were in the intended position, but in the four patients whose illness was unchanged the beads and hence the lesions were too far forward and

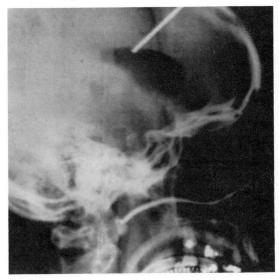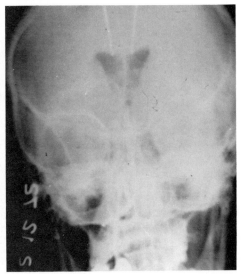

Figure 143–8 Anterior cingulotomy: Site of electrodes to insure destruction of inferior cingulate fibers. (From Ballantine, H. T., Levy, B. S., Dagi, T. F., and Giriunas, I.: Cingulotomy for psychiatric illness: Report of 13 years' experience. *In* Sweet, W. H., Obrador, S., and Martin-Rodriguez, J., eds.: Neurosurgical Treatment in Psychiatry, Pain and Epilepsy. Baltimore, University Park Press, 1974. Reprinted by permission.)

too far lateral on one or both sides.[68] Evans studied the brains of two depressed patients who failed to improve and committed suicide after open leucotomy. The planned division of the thalamofrontal radiations had not been achieved in either of them.[20] Conversely a late postmortem study after a clinically and anatomically successful orbital leucotomy revealed the appropriate degeneration in the medial part of the dorsomedial nucleus of the thalamus.[69] Ballantine and colleagues carefully restudied the radiographs for electrode placement in their operations. They found that in some of their patients, all of the first cingulotomy lesions must have lain superior to the roof of the lateral ventricle, as shown in the lateral view of an air study, with sparing of the inferior cingulate fibers (Fig. 143–8). When at reoperation new deeper lesions were placed to include all of the cingulum and some of the fibers of the corpus callosum, the numbers with useful improvement rose from 53 to 80 per cent.[8,9]

NEED FOR PSYCHIATRIC SURGERY

The vociferous criticisms of operative treatment for psychiatric disorders have understandably reduced its use. There were only circa 308 to 343 such operations performed per annum in the years 1971 to 1973

in the United States, whereas in the United Kingdom there were about 200 to 300 such operations per year. Translated into per capita rates, operations for psychiatric disorders are done in the United Kingdom at over twice, and in Australia at about thrice, the rate in the United States.[77] If the present criteria for these operations were to be universally applied in Britain, the Research Committee of the Royal College of Psychiatrists estimates, the operation would be considered for perhaps 800 to 1000 patients per year.[10] Thus it would appear that this form of treatment may be significantly underutilized in both countries. Accordingly, it has seemed useful to document more precisely than would otherwise have been necessary the bases for such procedures in order to strengthen the hands of neurosurgeons willing to develop the requisite expertise to do this work.

OPERATIONS FOR OTHER BEHAVIORAL DISORDERS

There remain for consideration other less-well-studied indications for various forms of operations for psychiatric problems. The most common of these is dangerous assaultiveness or destructiveness. The patients in this category who have been most frequently treated by neurosurgeons have been those whose senseless violence was a component of an illness that included temporal lobe epilepsy. Other groups of patients who may be abruptly destructive, even homicidal, are some paranoid schizophrenics, some who are mentally retarded, and a few who are classified more vaguely as psychopaths. Mark and his colleagues have studied such individuals who presented themselves either of their own will or after persuasion by friends, relatives, the clergy, or social workers.[38] Parallel with this, at Brandeis University there has been a study of group violence, as for example, in riots.[11] There appears to be essentially no overlap between the two groups of violent individuals. Those who have a personal problem with abrupt unreasoning rages apparently have little of the rioters' interest in solving group social problems by violence. Indeed, their recognition in their lucid phases of their difficulty provides the basis for their willingness to seek medical help. Others with this problem may, however, seek an outlet for their rages by joining either police or other standard law enforcement agencies on the one hand or groups attacking such agencies on the other hand.[12] Both types of group are well advised to screen their membership for such persons whose utterly irrational rages are likely to bring general discredit or failure to the group effort.

The pioneers in the neurosurgical treatment of these patients have been in Japan. Narabayashi and co-workers initiated the use of bilateral stereotaxic destruction of the amygdala, a procedure that has been done with success in at least 10 other countries in the world.[49] Mark and Ervin found that electrical stimulation of the medial amygdala worsened the patient's tendency to rage and "dyscontrol," whereas stimulation of the lateral amygdala had a calming effect.[37] Narabayashi and Shima have since sought to confine the target for destruction to the lateral part of the medial amygdala, with a substantial improvement in the results in respect to both assaultiveness and seizures when the latter were present.[48] The bilateral amygdalar lesions produce reduction in creative productivity and other modest psychological deficits as described in detail by Andersen.[1] Balasubramaniam and colleagues at the Institute of Neurology in Madras have the largest series of cases— 280 by 1975.[5,6]

In Japan, the mores require parents to take responsibility for their children. Thus when they beget an incorrigibly destructive and murderous child the only acceptable solution in the view of many Japanese parents is to kill all their children and then kill themselves. Sano noted such reports of mass family suicide for this reason in the Tokyo papers about once a year. He and his associates were led by these frightful tragedies to take the promethean step of making bilateral lesions in the posteromedial hypothalamus.[61,65] The rationale for the placement of these lesions was that ventromedial hypothalamic destruction in the cat usually produces an animal in continuous rage. If one then destroys the posteromedial hypothalamus, the animal is restored to a more placid state. Reasoning that the posteromedial hypothalamus was probably farther downstream in the effector pathways for rage than the amygdala, Sano made his lesions at that site. Even though stimulation there in the so-called ergotropic triangle evokes changes in blood pressure, pulse, respiration, and pupillary diameter, destruction there gave rise to only modest deficits of acceptable degree. There was "excellent or good" relief of the rage behavior in 95 per cent of 43 cases, a higher percentage than was achieved by bilateral amygdalotomy. Four other groups of workers have in general confirmed these results.[2,15,30,65] Cox and Brown have also treated patients with uncontrollably violent behavior by a multitarget operation bilaterally involving the cingulum, the subcaudate region, and the amygdala. There was modest to marked improvement in 16 of the 19 patients so treated, whereas modest improvement occurred in only 1 of 17 similar patients treated without operation.[18] The number of patients who have been studied critically needs to be increased, and all these operations for rage states probably are best classed as being still in the experimental phase.

A pure addiction to narcotics or alcohol has been treated by operation. This was tried after frontal leucotomies at various sites that were successful in relieving pain of organic cause also led typically to abrupt cessation of massive doses of narcotics without withdrawal symptoms. One of the earliest reports described 14 of 16 patients who were addicted to a narcotic prior to their electrocoagulative "cingulumotomy" in whom abrupt withdrawal after operation "resulted in only a minimal syndrome of withdrawal in five, and none was recognized in the remaining nine."[21] The most commonly performed operations with this objective are subcaudate tractotomy and cingulotomy. The latter procedure has been used by Balasubramaniam on 60 addicts.[5] He states that the psychopaths without much drive for cure are not much helped. The adventitious addicts, i.e., those who become addicted when given narcotics for pain or who are physicians, dentists, or nurses, do much better; 60 to 80 per cent of these narcotic addicts are relieved, as are a somewhat lower percentage of the alcoholics.

In an even more exploratory phase are hypothalamic operations in sexual offenders—either pedophilic homosexuals or those who repeatedly commit sexual crimes of violence. These operations have been reported from two groups in Germany and Czechoslovakia.[19,47,56,64]

The new knowledge of the monoaminergic and the peptidergic neurotransmitter mechanisms, and the increasing use of intracerebral electrical stimulation to improve such symptoms as pain, provide a basis on which to seek to benefit other forms of disordered behavior by nondestructive means.[66,71,72] Specific electrodes for the appropriate chemical neurotransmitter, its potentiator or inhibitor, and the proper electrical signal would be the neurosurgically manipulated devices to achieve these objectives. The vista of new fields to explore should not dim appreciation of the tremendous progress already achieved in the neurosurgical treatment of medically intractable affective mental disorders.

Acknowledgment. The author wishes to express his gratitude to the Neuro-Research Foundation for its financial support of the preparation of this manuscript.

REFERENCES

1. Andersen, R.: Differences in the course of learning as measured by various memory tasks after amygdalotomy in man. *In* Hitchcock, E., et al., eds.: Psychosurgery. Springfield, Ill., Charles C Thomas, 1972, pp. 177–183.
2. Arjona, V. E.: Stereotactic hypothalamotomy in erethic children. Acta Neurochir., *21*:185–191, 1974.
3. Arnot, R. E.: Clinical indications for pre-frontal lobotomy. J. Nerv. Ment. Dis., *109*:267–269, 1949.
4. Balasubramaniam, V.: Stereotactic surgery for behavior disorders. *In* Hitchcock, E., et al., eds.: Psychosurgery. Springfield, Ill., Charles C Thomas, 1972, pp. 156–163.
5. Balasubramaniam, V.: *In* Valenstein, E. S.: The Practice of Psychosurgery: A Survey of the Literature (1971–1976). Cited by Stevens, J. S., pp. I 150–158, Appendix Psychosurgery, U.S. Department of Health, Education and Welfare Publication No. (OS)77-0002, 1977, pp. 1–183.
6. Balasubramaniam, V., and Kanaka, T. S.: Amygdalotomy and hypothalamotomy—a comparative study. Confin. Neurol., *37*:195–201, 1975.
7. Ball, J., Klett, C. J., and Gresock, C. J.: The Veterans Administration study of prefrontal lobotomy. J. Clin. Exp. Psychopath., *20*:205–217, 1959.
8. Ballantine, H. T., Cassidy, W. L., Brodeur, J., and Giriunas, I.: Frontal cingulotomy for mood disturbance. *In* Hitchcock, E., et al., eds.: Psychosurgery. Springfield, Ill., Charles C Thomas, 1972, pp. 221–229.
9. Ballantine, H. T., Levy, B. S., Dagi, T. F., and Giriunas, I.: Cingulotomy for psychiatric illness: Report of 13 years' experience. *In* Sweet, W. H., et al., eds.: Neurosurgical Treatment in Psychiatry, Pain and Epilepsy. Baltimore, University Park Press, 1977, pp. 333–353.
10. Barraclough, B.: Evaluation of the surgical treatment of functional mental illness: Proposal for a prospective trial. *In* Sweet, W. H., et al., eds.: Neurosurgical Treatment in Psychiatry, Pain and Epilepsy. Baltimore, University Park Press, 1977, pp. 175–188.
11. Baskin, J. A., Lewis, A. G., Mannis, J. H., and McCullough, L. W., Jr.: The Long Hot Summer. An Analysis of Summer Disorders 1967–1971. Lemberg Center for the Study of Violence. Report No. 2. Brandeis University, Waltham, Mass., 1971.
12. Bazelon, Judge D. L.: Psychiatry's fear of analysis. The fear of psychiatrists: Leaving their protective shell. Washington Post, Sunday, June 24, 1973, pp. C1, C3.
13. Bingley, T., Leksell, L., Myerson, B. A., and Rylander, G.: Stereotactic anterior capsulotomy in anxiety and obsessive-compulsive states. Laitinen, L. V., and Livingston, K. E., eds.: Surgical Approaches in Psychiatry. Baltimore, University Park Press, 1973, pp. 159–164.
14. Bingley, T., Leksell, L., Myerson, B. A., and Rylander, G.: Long-term results of stereotactic anterior capsulotomy in chronic obsessive-compulsive neurosis. *In* Sweet, W. H., et al., eds.: Neurosurgical Treatment in Psychiatry, Pain and Epilepsy. Baltimore, University Park Press, 1977, pp. 287–299.
15. Black, P., Vemaesu, S., and Walker, A. E.: Stereotactic hypothalamotomy for control of aggressive behaviour. Confin. Neurol., *37*:187–188, 1975.
16. Bonis, A., Covello, L., Lempérière, T., et al.: Étude critique des indications d'interventions psychochirurgicales. Encéphale, *57*:439–473, 525–563, 1968.
17. Corkin, S., Twitchell, T. E., and Sullivan, E. V.: Safety and efficacy of cingulotomy in man for pain or psychiatric disorder. *In* Hitchcock, E. R., Ballantine, H. T., and Meyerson, B. A., eds.: Modern Concepts in Psychiatric Surgery. Am-

sterdam, Elsevier–North Holland Publishing Co., 1979, pp. 253–272.

17a. Neuropathological observations on yttrium implants and on undercutting in the orbitofrontal areas of the brain. *In* Laitinen, L. V., and Livingston, K. E., eds.: Surgical Approaches in Psychiatry. Baltimore, University Park Press, 1973.

18. Cox, A. W., and Brown, M. H.: Results of multitarget limbic surgery in the treatment of schizophrenic and aggressive states. *In* Sweet, W. H., et al., eds.: Neurosurgical Treatment in Psychiatry, Pain and Epilepsy. Baltimore, University Park Press, 1977, pp. 469–479.

19. Dieckmann, G., and Hassler, R.: Treatment of sexual violence by stereotactic hypothalamotomy. *In* Sweet, W. H., et al., eds.: Neurosurgical Treatment in Psychiatry, Pain and Epilepsy. Baltimore, University Park Press, 1977, pp. 451–462.

20. Evans, P.: Failed leucotomy with misplaced cuts: A clinicoanatomical study of two cases. Brit. J. Psychiat., *118*:165–170, 1971.

21. Foltz, E. L., and White, L. E., Jr.: Pain "relief" by frontal cingulumotomy. J. Neurosurg., *19*: 89–100, 1962.

22. Fulton, J. F.: Functional Localization in Relation to Frontal Lobotomy. London, Oxford University Press, 1949, pp. 81–93.

23. Fulton, J. F., and Jacobsen, C. F.: The functions of the frontal lobes, a comparative study in monkeys, chimpanzees and man. Abstr. 2nd Int. Neurol. Congr., 1935, pp. 70–71; see also Advances Mod. Biol. (Moscow), *4*:113–123, 1935.

24. Freeman, W., and Watts, J.: Psychosurgery. Springfield, Ill., Charles C Thomas, 1950.

25. Göktepe, E. O., Young, L. B., and Bridges, P. K.: A further review of the results of stereotactic subcaudate tractotomy. Brit. J. Psychiat., *126*:270–280, 1975.

25a. Hitchcock, E. R., Ballantine, H. T., Jr., and Meyerson, B. A., eds.: Modern Concepts in Psychiatric Surgery. Proceedings, Fifth World Congress of Psychiatric Surgery, August 21–25, 1978. Amsterdam, Elsevier–North Holland Publishing Co., 1979.

26. Hitchcock, E., Laitinen, L., and Vaernet, K., eds.: Psychosurgery. Proceedings of the Second International Congress of Psychosurgery, August 1970, Copenhagen, Denmark. Springfield, Ill., Charles C Thomas, 1972.

27. Hohne, H. H., and Walsh, K. W.: Surgical modification of the personality: Mental health research project. Victoria Mental Health Authority, Special Publication No. 2. Melbourne, Australia, 1970.

28. Knight, G. C.: Bi-frontal stereotactic tractotomy: An atraumatic operation of value in the treatment of intractable psychoneuroses. Brit. J. Psychiat., *115*:257–266, 1969.

29. Knight, G. C.: Further observations from an experience of 660 cases of stereotactic tractotomy. Postgrad. Med. J., *49*:845–854, 1973.

30. Kalyanaraman, S.: Some observations during stimulation of the human hypothalamus. Confin. Neurol., *37*:189–192, 1975.

31. Kullberg, G.: Differences in effect of capsulotomy and cingulotomy. *In* Sweet, W. H., et al., eds.: Neurosurgical Treatment in Psychiatry, Pain

and Epilepsy. Baltimore, University Park Press, 1977, pp. 301–308.

32. Laitinen, L. V., and Livingston, K. E., eds.: Surgical Approaches in Psychiatry. Proceedings of the Third International Congress of Psychosurgery, August 14–18, 1972, Cambridge, England. Baltimore, University Park Press, 1973.

33. Levin, H. S., O'Neal, J. T., Barratt, E. S., Adams, P. M., and Levin, E. M.: Outcome of stereotactic bilateral cingulotomy. *In* Sweet, W. H., et al., eds.: Neurosurgical Treatment in Psychiatry, Pain and Epilepsy. Baltimore, University Park Press, 1977, pp. 401–413.

34. Lhermitte, F., Derouesné, J., and Signoret, J. L.: Analyse neuropsychologique du syndrome frontal. Rev. Neurol. (Paris), *127*:415–440, 1972.

35. Lopez-Ibor, J. J., and Lopez-Ibor Alino, J. J.: Selection criteria for patients who should undergo psychiatric surgery. *In* Sweet, W. H., et al., eds.: Neurosurgical Treatment in Psychiatry, Pain and Epilepsy. Baltimore, University Park Press, 1977, pp. 151–162.

36. Luria, A. R.: The Working Brain. London, Penguin Books, Ltd., 1973.

37. Mark, V. H., and Ervin, F. R.: Violence and the Brain. New York, Harper & Row, 1970.

38. Mark, V. H., Sweet, W. H., and Ervin, F. R.: The effect of amygdalotomy on violent behavior in patients with temporal lobe epilepsy. *In* Hitchcock, E., et al., eds.: Psychosurgery. Springfield, Ill., Charles C Thomas, 1972, pp. 138–155.

39. Marks, I. M., Bingley, J. L. T., and Gelder, M. G.: Modified leucotomy in severe agoraphobia: A controlled serial inquiry. Brit. J. Psychiat., *112*:757–769, 1966.

40. Martin, W. L., McElhaney, M. L., and Meyer, G. A.: Stereotactic cingulotomy: Results of psychological testing and clinical evaluation preoperatively and postoperatively. *In* Sweet, W. H., et al., eds.: Neurosurgical Treatment in Psychiatry, Pain and Epilepsy. Baltimore, University Park Press, 1977, pp. 381–386.

41. McKenzie, K. G., and Kaczanowski, G.: Prefrontal leukotomy: A five-year controlled study. Canad. Med. Ass. J., *91*:1193–1196, 1964.

42. Meyer, A., Beck, E., and McLardy, T.: Prefrontal leucotomy: A neuro-anatomical report. Brain, *70*:18–49, 1947.

43. Milner, B.: Visually-guided maze learning in man: Effects of bilateral, hippocampal, bilateral frontal, and unilateral cerebral lesions. Neuropsychologia, *3*:317–338, 1965.

44. Mirsky, A. F., and Orzack, M. H.: Final report of psychosurgery pilot study. *In* Appendix Psychosurgery, U.S. Department of Health, Education and Welfare Publication No. (OS)77-0002, pp. II 1–160.

45. Mitchell-Heggs, N., Kelly, D., and Richardson, A. E.: Stereotactic limbic leucotomy: Clinical, psychological and physiological assessment at 16 months. *In* Sweet, W. H., et al., eds.: Neurosurgical Treatment in Psychiatry, Pain and Epilepsy. Baltimore, University Park Press, 1977, pp. 367–379.

46. Moniz, E.: Tentatives opératoires dans le traitement de certaines psychoses. Paris, Masson & Cie, 1936.

47. Nádvornik, P., Sřamka, M., and Patoprstá, G.:

Transventricular anterior hypothalamotomy in stereotactic treatment of hedonia. *In* Sweet, W. H., et al., eds.: Neurosurgical Treatment in Psychiatry, Pain and Epilepsy. Baltimore, University Park Press, 1977, pp. 445–449.

48. Narabayashi, H. M., and Shima, F.: Which is the better amygdala target, the medial or lateral nuclei? (For behavior problems and paroxysm in epileptics). *In* Sweet, W. H., et al., eds.: Neurosurgical Treatment in Psychiatry, Pain and Epilepsy. Baltimore, University Park Press, 1977, pp. 129–134.

49. Narabayashi, H. M., Nagao, T., Sato, Y., Yoshida, M., and Nagahata, M.: Stereotaxic amygdalotomy for behavior disorders. Arch. Neurol. (Chicago), 9:1–16, 1963.

50. National Commission for the Protection of Human Subjects of Biomedical and Behavioral Research: Report and Recommendations. Psychosurgery. U.S. Department of Health, Education, and Welfare Publication No. (OS)77-0001. Washington, D.C., U.S. Government Printing Office, 1977.

51. Nauta, W. J. H.: Some efferent connections of the prefrontal cortex in the monkey. *In* Warren, J. M., and Akert, K., eds.: Frontal Granular Cortex and Behavior. New York, McGraw-Hill Book Co., 1964, pp. 397–409.

52. Nauta, W. J. H.: The problem of the frontal lobe: A reinterpretation. J. Psychiat. Res., 8:167–187, 1971.

53. Poppen, J. L.: Technic of prefrontal lobotomy. J. Neurosurg., 5:514–420, 1948.

54. Post, F., Rees, W. L., and Schurr, P. H.: An evaluation of bimedial leucotomy. Brit. J. Psychiat., 114:1223–1246, 1968.

55. Robin, A. A.: A controlled study of the effects of leucotomy. J. Neurol. Neurosurg. Psychiat., 21:262–269, 1958.

56. Roeder, F., Orthner, H., and Muller, D.: The stereotactic treatment of pedophilic homosexuality and other sexual deviations. *In* Hitchcock, E., et al., eds.: Psychosurgery. Springfield, Ill., Charles C Thomas, 1972, pp. 87–111.

57. Rubio, E., Arjona, V., and Rodriguez-Burgos, F.: Stereotactic cryohypothalamotomy in aggressive behavior. *In* Sweet, W. H., et al., eds.: Neurosurgical Treatment in Psychiatry, Pain and Epilepsy. Baltimore, University Park Press, 1977, pp. 439–444.

58. Ryan, K. J.: *In* National Commission for the Protection of Human Subjects of Biomedical and Behavioral Research: Report and Recommendations. Psychosurgery. U.S. Department of Health, Education and Welfare Publication No. (OS)77-0001. Washington, D.C., U.S. Government Printing Office 725–852, 1977. pp. 7–11.

59. Rylander, G.: Personality analysis before and after frontal lobotomy. Proc. Ass. Res. Nerv. Ment. Dis., 27:691–705, 1948.

60. Rylander, G.: The renaissance of psychosurgery. *In* Hitchcock, E., et al., eds.: Psychosurgery. Springfield, Ill., Charles C Thomas, 1972.

61. Sano, K., Ogashiwa, M., and Ishijima, B.: Results of stimulation and destruction of the posterior hypothalamus in man. J. Neurosurg., 33:689–707, 1970.

62. Sano, K., Sekino, H., and Mayanagi, Y.: Results of stimulation and destruction of the posterior hypothalamus in cases with violent aggressive or restless behaviors. *In* Hitchcock, E., et al., eds.: Psychosurgery. Springfield, Ill., Charles C Thomas, 1972, pp. 57–75.

63. Schneider, G. E.: Growth of abnormal nerve connections following focal brain lesions: Constraining factors and functional effects. *In* Sweet, W. H., et al., eds.: Neurosurgical Treatment in Psychiatry, Pain and Epilepsy. Baltimore, University Park Press, 1977, pp. 5–26.

64. Schneider, H.: Psychic changes in sexual delinquency after hypothalamotomy. Ibid., pp. 463–468.

65. Schvarcz, J. R.: Results of stimulation and destruction of the posterior hypothalamus: A long-term evaluation. *In* Sweet, W. H., et al., eds.: Neurosurgical Treatment in Psychiatry, Pain and Epilepsy. Baltimore, University Park Press, 1977, pp. 429–439.

66. Smith, B. H., and Sweet, W. H.: Neuroscience for the neurosurgeon: Monoaminergic regulation of central nervous system function. I. Noradrenergic systems. Neurosurgery, 3:109–119, 1978.

67. Sourkes, T. L.: Nobel Prize Winners in Medicine and Physiology 1901–1965. 2nd Ed. London, Toronto, Abelard-Schuman, 1966.

68. Ström-Olsen, R., and Carlisle, S.: Bifrontal stereotactic tractotomy: A followup study of its effects on 210 patients. Brit. J. Psychiat., 118:141–154, 1971.

69. Ström-Olsen, R., and Northfield, D. W. C.: Undercutting of orbital cortex in chronic neurotic and psychotic tension states. Lancet, 1:986–991, 1955.

70. Sweet, W. H.: Treatment of medically intractable mental disease by limited frontal leucotomy—justifiable? New Eng. J. Med., 289:1117–1125, 1973.

71. Sweet, W. H.: Neuroscience for the neurosurgeon: The neuropeptides. Neurosurgery, 1:311–316, 1977.

72. Sweet, W. H., and Smith, B. H.: Neuroscience for the neurosurgeon: The neuropeptides and behavior. Neurosurgery, 2:62–69, 1978.

73. Sweet, W. H., Obrador, S., and Martin-Rodriguez, J., eds.: Neurosurgical Treatment in Psychiatry, Pain and Epilepsy. Proceedings of the Fourth World Congress of Psychiatric Surgery, September 7–10, 1975, Madrid, Spain. Baltimore, University Park Press, 1977.

74. Tan, E., Marks, I. M., and Marset, P.: Bimedial leucotomy in obsessive-compulsive neurosis: A controlled serial inquiry. Brit. J. Psychiat., 118:155–164, 1971.

75. Teuber, J. L., Corkin, S., and Twitchell, T. E.: A study of cingulotomy in man. *In* Appendix Psychosurgery. U.S. Department of Health, Education and Welfare Publication No. (OS)77-0002, 1977, pp. III 1–115.

76. Tucker, W. I.: Indications for modified leukotomy. Lahey Clin. Found. Bull., 15:131–139, 1966.

77. Valenstein, E. S.: The practice of psychosurgery. A survey of the literature (1971–1976). *In* Appendix Psychosurgery. U.S. Department of Health, Education and Welfare Publication No. (OS)77-0002, 1977, pp. I 1–183.

78. Van Hoesen, G. W., Pandya, D. N., and Butters, N.: Cortical afferents to the entorhinal cortex of

the rhesus monkey. Science, *175*:1471–1473, 1972.

79. Vilkki, J.: Late psychological and clinical effects of subrostral cingulotomy and anterior mesoloviotomy in psychiatric illness. *In* Sweet, W. H., et al., eds.: Neurosurgical Treatment in Psychiatry, Pain and Epilepsy. Baltimore, University Park Press, 1977, pp. 253–259.

80. Walsh, K. W.: Neuropsychological aspects of modified leucotomy. *In* Sweet, W. H., et al., eds.: Neurosurgical Treatment in Psychiatry, Pain and Epilepsy. Baltimore, University Park Press, 1977, pp. 163–174.

81. White, J. C., and Sweet, W. H.: Pain and the Neurosurgeon: A Forty Year Experience. Springfield, Ill., Charles C Thomas, 1969, pp. 703–704.

144

INDICATIONS FOR AND RESULTS OF HYPOPHYSECTOMY

HISTORICAL BACKGROUND

Hypophysectomy, defined as ablation of the normal pituitary gland, was first performed in 1934 to control malignant diabetes mellitus, and in 1935 to treat epilepsy.[20,29,30,107] Later, when corticotropin and cortisone became available to control the resulting hypoadrenalism, hypophysectomy was considered as a treatment for Cushing's syndrome, malignant hypertension, chronic glomerulonephritis with associated hypertension, disseminated malignant melanoma, metastatic carcinoma of the breast and prostate, and advancing diabetic retinopathy.[57-59,88,93,103]

Although pituitary ablation gave no therapeutic benefit to patients with epilepsy, hypertension, or malignant melanoma, it did ameliorate the effects of advancing diabetic retinopathy and metastatic carcinoma of the breast and prostate.[42,57-59] In this chapter, the current status of hypophysectomy as a treatment for these diseases is reviewed. Operative treatment of secreting and nonsecreting pituitary adenomas is discussed in Chapter 98.

HORMONE DEPENDENCY OF CERTAIN MALIGNANT TUMORS

The first reports on the possible benefits of oophorectomy as a treatment for cancer of the breast appeared in 1896. The endocrine approach to the treatment of cancer received little attention, however, until 1942, when orchiectomy was reported to cause regression of the skeletal metastases from mammary cancer in a man.[32] Hypophysectomy was first attempted for palliation of carcinoma of the prostate in 1948, and for carcinoma of the breast in 1951.[57,102] The beneficial effect of hypophysectomy in promoting objective remission of metastatic tumor deposits and relief of pain due to skeletal involvement in the patient who had undergone prior castration and adrenalectomy was thought to result from the elimination of growth hormone or prolactin secretion.

The metabolism and growth rate of breast and prostate carcinomas are influenced by endogenous hormones. Some cancer cells differ significantly from ancestral normal cells in their responses to modification of the hormonal environment. The growth, differentiation, and activity of normal mammary cells are predominantly regulated by estrogen and prolactin, but androgens, progesterone, corticoids, insulin, and growth hormone are also known to exert an influence on these functions.[65] Regardless of whether experimental mammary carcinomas are induced by radiation, by virus infection, or chemically with 7,12-dimethylbenzathracene (DMBA), or occur spontaneously, as they do in some strains of rats or mice, the frequency with which a neoplasm occurs is dependent upon endocrinological factors.[17] For example, ovariectomy prevents DMBA induction of mammary carcinoma in rats.[25] Established rat DMBA tumors will regress in 50 per cent of the animals after ovariectomy, but tumors will resume growth if estrogens are resupplied.

J. HARDY, P. R. WEINSTEIN, AND C. B. WILSON

Breast cancer has been produced in male mice by high-dosage estrogen treatment and in virgin female mice after repeated induction of pseudopregnancy.[54,73] In other studies, however, 52 per cent of mammary carcinomas in rats underwent regression following large doses of estradiol and progesterone.[44] The apparently contradictory results may be explained by postulating that estrogen interferes with prolactin stimulation of tumor growth, since the inhibitory effect of estrogen can be overcome by increasing the level of endogenous or exogenous prolactin.[69] Prolactin reactivates and increases the number and size of DMBA-induced tumors in adrenalectomized and ovariectomized rats, and antiprolactin antiserum induces regression of such tumors.[77,85,89] Prolactin binds to mouse and rabbit mammary gland cells and influences their metabolism.[68] Mammary gland cancer can be induced in mice subjected to implantation of multiple subcutaneous pituitary isografts, and the causative factor is thought to be prolactin secretion.

Pain due to skeletal metastases can be alleviated in breast cancer patients by administration of L-dopa, which reduces serum prolactin levels.[70] It is also of interest that administration of growth hormone in hypophysectomized patients reproduces metastatic skeletal pain that has been relieved by pituitary ablation.[21]

In addition to circulating androgens such as testosterone and dihydrotestosterone, hypophyseal secretions such as growth hormone and prolactin are required for development of prostatic carcinoma.[21] The dependence of prostatic cancer on androgens has been established clinically by the effects of orchiectomy and estrogen therapy. Similarly, plasma prolactin levels were higher in patients with tumors than in those with benign prostatic hypertrophy. Stilbestrol administration, which often inhibits growth of prostatic carcinoma, lowers plasma levels of testosterone, estradiol, follicle-stimulating hormone, and luteinizing hormone, but does not affect growth hormone and may increase prolactin levels.[40] Thus, the exact mechanism of action is unclear, but inhibition of androgen excretion is the most likely factor. Hypophysectomy or adrenalectomy results in a sustained decrease in the excretion of androgen metabolites, as measured by urinary 11-deoxy-17-ketosteroids, that correlates well with the postoperative clinical remission of prostatic carcinoma.[75]

PITUITARY INSUFFICIENCY AND DIABETIC RETINOPATHY

Evidence implicating the pituitary in the pathogenesis of diabetes mellitus dates back to 1930, when Houssay and Biasotti observed the ameliorating effect of pituitary ablation on the diabetes of pancreatectomized dogs.[43] In 1936, similar results were obtained in diabetic cats after adrenalectomy and hypophysectomy.[56] Although the first hypophysectomy for diabetes mellitus in man was performed by Puech in 1934, the specific role of the pituitary gland in diabetic retinopathy was not recognized until 1953, when it was reported that retinopathy disappeared in a diabetic woman after she developed postpartum pituitary insufficiency (Sheehan's syndrome).[20,90] This woman died from renal failure in 1960, and an autopsy revealed complete necrosis of the anterior lobe of the pituitary gland, sparing the neurohypophysis.[91]

Hypophysectomy to treat the retinopathy of diabetes was first explored in 1955, with encouraging results.[59] A number of reports on this subject followed, but enthusiasm faded quickly and the procedure was almost abandoned because its indiscriminate application produced disappointing results. Now, a critical reappraisal has clearly established the beneficial effect of hypophysectomy in diabetic patients who have been selected by strict ophthalmological criteria.[23,53]

Hypophysectomy appears to eliminate the presence of a pituitary factor that has diabetogenic activity, although the nature of this factor (or factors) is still not known. Although it is generally believed that pituitary growth hormone and adrenocorticotropic hormone possess diabetogenic activity, other pituitary factors may be equally important in the etiology of diabetic retinopathy. After experiments had shown that an adrenalectomized dog was less sensitive to insulin than one that had been subjected to both adrenalectomy and hypophysectomy, growth hormone was reported to be the major diabetogenic factor.[28] In other experiments, adrenocorticotropic hormone caused retinal changes in diabetic rabbits. The role of these hormones is questionable, however, because the frequency of diabetic retinopathy has not increased in humans in proportion to the widespread clinical use of ACTH and adrenal corticosteroids. Also, retinopathy rarely accompanies the diabetes of human acromegaly.[94] Posthypophysectomy improvement in retinopathy was reported to occur independently of growth hormone suppression in 31 insulin-treated diabetic patients.[92] Other studies, however, suggest that postoperative growth hormone suppression, as an indication of completeness of hypophysectomy, correlates well with clinical response.[2]

Increased platelet aggregation may be a factor in retinopathy; there is a lower incidence of retinal hemorrhage in diabetic patients with coincidental rheumatoid arthritis who are receiving large doses of aspirin, a known platelet agglutination inhibitor.[82] Of a group of diabetic patients with retinopathy, only those who had not been treated by hypophysectomy exhibited adenosine diphosphate (ADP)–induced platelet hyperaggregation; this phenomenon appeared to be related to a platelet plasma membrane factor rather than to a platelet factor in circulating plasma.[13]

OTHER CONSIDERATIONS CONCERNING HYPOPHYSECTOMY

It is well established that pituitary ablation does not palliate other diabetic complications such as neuropathy, peripheral vascular changes, and nephropathy.[1,47,48] A common endocrinological complication of hypophysectomy is diabetes insipidus. It is transient in 40 per cent of patients operated on by the micro-operative transsphenoidal technique and persists in 10 per cent. Urinary output can be adequately controlled by treatment with Pitressin hormone preparations.

Adult human pituitary cells lack significant regeneration capabilities. Since 10 per cent or more of the gland remaining in the sella is sufficient to support endocrine requirements under normal conditions, however, a functionally complete hypophysectomy requires the removal of more than 90 per cent of pituitary gland tissue.[55,112] Recurrence of diabetic retinopathy, after an initial favorable response to hypophysectomy, has been correlated with the presence of residual pituitary tissue; the benefits observed initially were attributed to the sudden, temporary depletion of pituitary hormones.[37] These observations support the view that more than 90 per cent of the gland must be removed or destroyed to achieve the long-lasting benefits of hypophysectomy.

As a treatment for cancers that respond to endocrine hormones, transsphenoidal hypophysectomy is superior to bilateral adrenalectomy because it is accompanied by significantly less discomfort and morbidity and a lower mortality rate. Each procedure has a similar initial effect on tumor growth if hypophysectomy is done by craniotomy, but better results can be expected with transsphenoidal techniques.[60] Many adrenalectomized patients experience additional palliation after hypophysectomy is performed in a second operation.

SELECTION OF PATIENTS

Now that acceptable techniques for total hypophysectomy are available, attention has focused on criteria for selecting patients most likely to benefit from pituitary ablation. Since the procedure itself carries little risk, a relatively low response rate is acceptable if the responsive patients experience regressions of good quality and long duration. A decision to perform pituitary ablation should be made only after other potentially effective but less drastic forms of therapy have been tried. In the past, candidates for hypophysectomy were selected from two groups of patients: those who had previously responded to endocrine manipulation, i.e., hormonal therapy, castration, or both; and any patient with advanced carcinoma, regardless of previous response to hormones and chemotherapy, for whom all other modalities of palliation had failed.[3,4,114] The response rate of cancer patients depends on four known variables: aggressiveness of the tumor (best expressed by the length of the disease-free interval between initial diagnosis and appearance of disseminated disease), age of the patient, location of metastases at the time of diagnosis (involvement of viscera predicts a poor response), and response to earlier endocrine ablative procedures (patients who have experienced remission after castration are more likely to respond to hypophysectomy than those in whom castration was ineffective).

EVALUATION OF RESPONSE

At the present time, there are no uniformly accepted objective criteria for evaluating postoperative tumor regression. The lowest regression rate after hypophysectomy for breast cancer was reported by Witt and co-workers, who used the rigid criteria of the Cooperative Breast Cancer Group.[36,116] Therapeutic effect was judged on the basis of quantitative shrinkage of visible tumor, radiographically demonstrated calcification and healing of osteolytic lesions, and absence of new lesions. Relief of pain without objective regression, commonly reported after hypophysectomy, was considered failure. By these criteria, hypophysectomy by transfrontal craniotomy achieved regression in 11 per cent of unselected postmenopausal patients. Obviously, if patients are selected on the basis of known previous responses and if the less traumatic transsphenoidal route is employed for ablation, the regression rate will be higher and morbidity and mortality rates will decrease. The inclusion of patients who were relieved of pain, with no tumor regression, would more than double the number of responders. Under less stringent criteria, a response rate of 87 per cent was reported among patients benefited by castration.[95] In another series of patients, unselected with respect to age and previous response, 40 per cent responded favorably to cryohypophysectomy.[115]

For precise and comprehensive reporting of the assessment of clinical response to endocrine therapy the following definitions have been recommended:

Regression—six months of subjective cessation of symptoms, with measurable decrease in size of metastatic lesions and without appearance of new lesions.

Arrest—six months of subjective cessation of symptoms without progression or appearance of new lesions.

Exacerbation—objective progression of disease in association with clinical deterioration.

Rebound—objective progression of disease after cessation of previously effective endocrine manipulation.[81]

CARCINOMA OF THE BREAST

Recurrent and metastatic breast cancer is a fatal disease, but often it can be controlled for extended periods of time. The median survival of untreated patients with primary lesions is 2.7 years, with 18 per cent surviving up to 5 years.[14] Only 20 per cent of treated women in whom four or more positive lymph nodes are found at operation will be alive and disease-free five years later. Endocrine therapy provides significant palliation in 20 to 40 per cent of unselected cases.[83]

Endocrine Sensitivity

In the past, unsuccessful attempts to predict responsiveness to endocrine manipulation in breast cancer patients have included measuring urinary excretion of estrogen and analyzing the histological characteristics or enzyme activity of excised tissue.[18,26,104] Although response to additive endocrine therapy is not correlated with response to other modalities, benefit from castration augurs significant palliation following hypophysectomy.[6] In more recent studies, hormone-responsive tumors exhibited greater uptake of radioisotope-labeled estradiol into the cell nuclei during in vitro incubation of tissue fragments.[66] These results led to further studies on hormonal regulation of cellular metabolism and growth.

Hormone Receptors

The cytoplasmic concentration of circulating estrogen in target organs, such as the uterus, results from the presence of a specific, high-affinity, estrogen-binding receptor protein (ERP) in the cytosol.[49] After binding to estrogen, the receptor enters the cell nucleus and may then initiate a specific sequence of RNA and protein synthesis.[65] Estrogen-binding receptor protein can be found in about 60 per cent of breast cancers but is not present in significant concentrations in the other 40 per cent.[67] Benign human breast tissue also lacks the protein receptors.

Currently, the most accurate indicator of responsiveness to hormone manipulation therapy is a positive assay for estrogen-binding receptor protein in primary or metastatic breast tumors. Results from a number of clinical studies indicate that there is a 60 to 70 per cent probability that patients with such tumors will respond to additive (estrogen or androgen) or ablative (oophorectomy, adrenalectomy, or hypophysectomy) endocrine manipulation, while those with tumors free of estrogen-binding receptor protein have a 5 to 8 per cent response rate.[67] There is an excellent correlation between a given patient's response and the presence of the receptor protein in primary or metastatic tumor tissue from that patient. There is no statistical correlation, however, between the presence of the receptor protein at either primary or metastatic sites and any of the following variables: menopausal status, stage of spread and node involvement, morphological tumor characteristics, site of recurrence, or length of disease-free interval. An estrogen-binding receptor protein assay is performed on at least 500 mg of tumor tissue that is quick-frozen in liquid nitrogen at the time of initial mastectomy or later biopsy of metastatic levels; levels of 2.5 femtomoles per milligram of protein, or higher, are considered positive.* Higher levels do not predict better response rates, however. It is valid to predict a positive response to hypophysectomy, performed after relapse following oophorectomy or additive endocrine therapy, if estrogen-binding receptor protein remains present in later biopsies.[17] Tumors that contain the protein are more likely to be curable.[67] Receptor proteins appear to be synthesized primarily by those neoplastic cells in which the growth-stimulating effects of hormones are reversible by hormone manipulation therapy.

Prolactin and progesterone receptors have been found in malignant animal tumors as well as in 30 and 60 per cent of human breast cancers respectively.[83] The clinical significance of these receptors is not known.[105] On the basis of all these observations, the presence of a complex endocrine regulatory system in normal mammary cells has been postulated.[21,65] When this system remains intact after malignant transformation as verified by measuring cytoplasmic estrogen-binding receptor protein content, it may be utilized to control unrestrained growth and replication of carcinoma cells. When the receptor protein disappears from the cancer cell, the tumor may have to be considered endocrinologically autonomous as the result of a biochemical lesion in the regulatory system.

Sequence and Results of Treatment

Hypophysectomy has a role in the sequential endocrine manipulation of recurrent or metastatic breast cancers. Although pituitary ablation as a prophylactic treatment has been considered in high-risk patients who have three or more positive axillary lymph nodes, its value cannot be estimated at present.[34] If estrogen-binding receptor protein determinations are not available, endocrine manipulation should be considered in all patients. High-risk patients or those with recurrent tumors that lack the receptor protein are usually treated initially with cytotoxic chemotherapy, since endocrine response is unlikely. Radiation therapy is useful for local control of solitary skeletal metastasis or invasion of the axilla or chest wall.

In premenopausal women the initial endocrine manipulation is oophorectomy. A 40 to 60 per cent favorable response rate can be expected in unselected cases.[83] The average duration of regression is 12 to 16 months.

Postmenopausal women and premenopausal patients who experience recurrence or fail to respond after oophorectomy may benefit from androgen therapy (additive); regression rates of 33 per cent with mean duration of 12 months are reported.[54,81] Estrogen therapy (additive) is successful in 34 per cent of cases, with a 16-month mean duration of regression. Exacerbation was observed in 36 per cent of estrogen-treated and 20 per cent of androgen-treated patients. The estrogen-binding receptor protein assay is a predictor of response to ovariectomy and androgen or estrogen therapy. Megestrol is a strong oral progestin and antiestrogen that has been effective in patients who fail to respond to androgen and estrogens; its effectiveness has not

---

* One femtomole equals 10^{-15} mole.

been correlated with the receptor protein levels.[17] Corticosteroids provide relatively weak and brief tumor regression rates, even at high dosage levels.[16] L-Dopa and certain ergot derivatives, such as bromocriptine, though known to suppress prolactin secretion, have been less effective in control of breast cancer dissemination than in relief of pain due to skeletal metastases.[17,70,71] L-Dopa response has been of some value in predicting endocrine sensitivity of metastatic breast cancer.[71]

Major ablative endocrine therapy should be considered only after these modalities have been explored. Hypophysectomy yields results that are as good as or better than can be achieved by adrenalectomy. In addition, when stereotaxic or microoperative transsphenoidal techniques are used rather than craniotomy, hypophysectomy can be performed more easily and safely.[5,41,104] Response rates vary from 10 to 50 per cent and may be raised to 70 per cent by selecting only those patients with positive estrogen-binding receptor protein assays.[17] The best results reported are those of Hardy, who documented relief of pain in 92 per cent of 160 breast cancer patients after total transsphenoidal hypophysectomy.[38] Sufficient data are not available to determine whether additional benefits will accrue from hypophysectomy performed in patients with progressive disease after adrenalectomy. Remissions average 14 months after pituitary ablation, and arrests lasting three to five years have been reported in 5 to 10 per cent of cases.[5] Patients who are postmenopausal but are under 65 years of age and have a longer disease-free interval, and those who have skeletal and soft-tissue, rather than visceral, metastasis are more likely to respond. Patients with pulmonary, hepatic, or visceral metastases without pain due to skeletal involvement have a response rate of less than 30 per cent.[14]

CARCINOMA OF THE PROSTATE

In 50 per cent of patients with prostatic carcinoma, the metastatic disease is present at the time of initial diagnosis.[40] There are 18,000 deaths per year from this disease in the United States.[75] Pelvic and vertebral metastases are the most common, and involvement at both sites is often associated with severe pain. The untreated patient with metastatic prostatic cancer survives an average of 19 months. Following antiandrogen therapy with orchiectomy and estrogens, the average survival is 65 months.[106] Relapse after successful estrogen therapy is followed by an average survival time of nine months.[78] Radiation therapy may offer useful local palliation.[98]

Endocrine Sensitivity

Lack of animal models for prostatic carcinoma has limited the endocrinological information available about this disease. Androgen receptors and a high concentration of dihydrotestosterone have been found in cytoplasm and nuclei of rat prostate cells, and this androgen metabolite appears to be responsible for inducing cell division in tissue culture.[9,64] Human receptor assays are not as yet available. Prostate glands in hypophysectomized rats are less responsive to testosterone, and the normal cell growth response to pituitary gonadotropins and growth hormone has been postulated but not demonstrated. Results of adrenalectomy are comparable to those of hypophysectomy, and sustained decrease in urinary excretion of 17-ketosteroids can be correlated with clinical response after either procedure.[46,101,106]

A more favorable response to pituitary ablation can be predicted by a history of previous response to endocrine manipulation. Thus, only a 14 per cent response rate can be expected in patients who have failed to respond to both previous orchiectomy and estrogen therapy, as compared with a 71 per cent response rate in those who benefited from orchiectomy and a 57 per cent rate in those with estrogen-induced remissions.[109]

Indications and Results

Patients with systemic metastases, an enlarging pelvic mass and urinary or intestinal obstruction, or diffuse intractable skeletal pain should be considered for pituitary ablation after failure of castration, estrogen therapy, and radiation.[101] Chemotherapy remains of limited value.[40]

In one series of 18 patients, 66 per cent experienced dramatic pain relief after cryohypophysectomy, while only 33 per cent exhibited objective tumor regression.[62] Other reports indicate that a 40 to 50 per cent objective remission rate can be expected after hypophysectomy by craniotomy.[76,93,96] Similar results have been reported following micro-operative transsphenoidal hypophysectomy, with relief of pain in up to 90 per cent of patients.[110] Duration of response ranged from two months to three years in one series. Prolonged painfree remission of six months to three years occurred in 20 per cent of these cases.[109] A mean duration of response of seven months was observed in another series.[62] Other effects of hypophysectomy may include relief of urinary obstruction and prolonged decrease in serum acid phosphatase levels.

Postoperative growth hormone assays performed after insulin-induced hypoglycemia to provide a measure of the extent of hypophysectomy indicated that a 73 per cent or greater decrease in growth hormone levels correlated well with significant clinical remission and prolongation of survival, while partial responses were observed when levels decreased from 22 to 73 per cent.[113] On the basis of this experience, it appears that anatomical or endocrinologically complete pituitary destruction is necessary to achieve a better remission rate in prostatic carcinoma also.

OTHER MALIGNANT TUMORS

To date, responsiveness to hormonal manipulation has been reported in carcinomas of the breast, prostate, thyroid, kidney, endometrium, and seminal vesicles, as well as in leukemias, lymphosarcomas, and certain melanomas.*

Hypophysectomies have been performed on patients with malignant melanomas, choriocarcinoma of the testes, multiple myeloma, hypernephroma, bronchial carcinoma, carcinoma of the ovary, leiomyosarcoma, and carcinoma of the thyroid.[31,103,111] The results in these cases have been discouraging. Therefore, at the present time, hypophysectomy cannot be advised for the control of malignant tumors other than disseminated carcinoma of the breast and prostate.

Pituitary ablation has, however, effectively relieved pain caused by metastases of a variety of endocrine-insensitive tumors.[72] Pain relief without objective tumor remission is also observed following hypophysectomy for breast and prostate carcinoma. This response remains unexplained but could be due to changes in hormonal balance or effects upon other pituitary-mediated factors such as prostaglandins or endorphins.

DIABETIC RETINOPATHY

Diabetes is now the most common cause of newly diagnosed blindness in patients 30 to 65 years of age.[52] It is accompanied by retinopathy in 40 to 95 per cent of long-term diabetics, depending on duration of illness, and 5 to 10 per cent of diabetics surviving 20 years after diagnosis will be blind.[52,82] The mean survival time after onset of retinopathy is five years, with death resulting from coincident nephropathy and cardiovascular disease. The pathogenesis of retinopathy has not been elucidated, but studies have been carried out on the roles of genetic factors, growth hormone, and microvascular changes in causing hypoxia.[52] It appears that adequate control of diabetes will lower the incidence of retinopathy or retard its progression.

Florid retinopathy is a rare occurrence that usually affects diabetic patients under the age of 40.[53] Its evolution can be documented by fundus photography and has been described as "rapid, bloody, and blinding."[11,52,80] Progression to blindness usually occurs in less than one year.[53] Grading systems are available for defining the natural history and results of treatment.[52]

Indications

Retinopathy may be conveniently classified as proliferative or nonproliferative. Currently, the diabetic patient with only nonproliferative retinopathy (i.e., microaneurysm, dot retinal hemorrhage, hard and soft exudates, and irregularities in retinal vessels) does not qualify for hypophysec-

---

* See references 7, 15, 32, 45, 50, 51, 87, 103.

tomy because such retinopathy poses little threat to vision.[33]

Quite different is the patient with proliferative disease, distinguished by characteristic new vessel formation (neovascularization) and associated vitreous and preretinal hemorrhage, changes that are followed by proliferation of fibrous tissue and retinal detachment. Loss of vision that is due to vascular edema and destruction of retinal tissue may not always correlate with findings on funduscopic examination. After neovascular changes appear, 30 to 40 per cent of younger patients and 40 to 60 per cent of older patients progress to legal blindness within five years, and approximately 75 per cent of these become blind during the first year.[35] In 90 per cent of cases, the diabetic patient who is already blind in one eye will eventually become blind in the remaining eye. Only 10 to 14 per cent of patients with proliferative retinopathy experience spontaneous arrest with preservation of useful vision.[12,19,28] Therefore, the onset of progressive visual loss due to florid proliferative retinopathy is an indication for operative treatment.

The ophthalmologist may first advise direct treatment. Photocoagulation, with the xenon arc or argon laser, can be utilized to coagulate bleeding vessels or to destroy proliferating vessels and scar tissue within the retina with minor risk of causing further retinal damage. Results of a recent controlled cooperative study, in which only the more severely affected eye of each patient was treated, indicate benefit in preventing loss of visual field and acuity over a two-year follow-up period.[28] Vitrectomy has been performed in patients with opacities following hemorrhage, with significant restoration of vision as long as retinal detachment had not occurred.[61]

Selection of Patients

Criteria for selecting patients for hypophysectomy have differed according to the method selected to achieve hypopituitarism, the more strict criteria applying to major operative procedures such as craniotomy, as compared with the nonoperative techniques such as heavy-particle irradiation. The five criteria generally used to select patients for hypophysectomy are:

1. The presence of proliferative retinopathy, the earliest indisputable evidence of which is neovascular change.

2. Progressive loss of vision that, untreated, can be expected to lead to blindness. Because the course of proliferative retinopathy is now so clearly documented, particularly in the patient with significantly impaired vision in one eye, the need to document progressive visual loss is open to question. Instead, the presence of neovascularization may be a sufficient indication for hypophysectomy.

3. At least one clinically healthy macula, with corrected vision not worse than 20/60 to 20/80.

4. Intellectual, social, and psychological characteristics that assure the patient's ability to cooperate and adhere to the medical management essential for survival in a state of hypopituitarism, with its fluctuations in insulin and steroid requirements.

5. Absence of serious cardiovascular and renal disease. This is of relative importance, depending on the risks of the method used to achieve the hypopituitaristic state.

Ray has suggested a sixth criterion:

6. An age limit of 40 years. The rationale for this limit is that older patients may be difficult to evaluate adequately, may tolerate an operation less well, and do not obtain the degree of benefit seen in younger patients.[97] While these statements are true, it also can be argued that the benefit an otherwise healthy older patient derives from hypophysectomy will usually override the added risk.

Results

According to recent reports, pituitary ablation arrests the progression of proliferative retinopathy in 60 to 80 per cent of diabetic patients.* Five years after hypophysectomy, 65 per cent of the patients retained a normal visual index.[39] Beneficial effects may also include some or all of the following: clearing of vitreous haze, which may begin within 48 hours after the ablation and become complete within a few weeks; cessation of hemorrhagic activity; loosening and resorption of fixed collections of blood

---

* See references 2, 22, 24, 37, 63, 95, 99, 100.

in preretinal spaces or vitreous fluid; decrease in the caliber of previously dilated retinal veins; self-occlusion of new vessels; reduction in size of macroaneurysms and disappearance of some microaneurysms; decrease in size and number of exudates, and migration of exudates outward from the macular region; flattening of and later spontaneous reattachment of the retina; regression of arteriolar tortuosity; and improvement of vision.

Patients who have total hypophysectomy seem to respond better than patients who have pituitary stalk section alone.[100] Although in most patients the insulin requirement declines following pituitary ablation, failure to observe a postoperative reduction in insulin dosage does not mean that vision will not benefit from hypophysectomy.[24]

Comparative studies suggest that pituitary ablation may be more effective than photocoagulation in preventing blindness.[8,53] In one group of 10 patients, 11 eyes with florid diabetic retinopathy were treated with photocoagulation; at one year six were blind and five had good vision.[53] Of 20 patients, with a total of 29 eyes with florid proliferative retinopathy, only 3 were blind at one year and 12 of 17 eyes had vision five years after hypophysectomy. Their visual acuity was significantly better one and two years after hypophysectomy than in the untreated group or those who had photocoagulation. Although hypophysectomy remains the treatment of choice for rapidly advancing, multifocal retinopathy, photocoagulation is recommended for early cases in which involvement is still restricted.[8] Since end-stage cases cannot be expected to benefit from pituitary ablation, however, the procedure should be performed before irreversible visual loss has occurred.

REFERENCES

1. Adams, D. A., Rand, R. W., Roth, N. H., et al.: Cryoablation of the pituitary in the treatment of progressive diabetic retinopathy. Diabetes, *17*:634–640, 1968.
2. Adams, D. A., Rand, R. W., Roth, N. H., et al.: Hypophysectomy in diabetic retinopathy. The relationship between the degree of pituitary ablation and ocular response. Diabetes, *23*:698–707, 1974.
3. Atkins, H., Bulbrook, R. D., Falconer, M. A., et al.: Ten years' experience of steroid assays in the management of breast cancer. A review. Lancet, *2*:1255–1260, 1968.
4. Atkins, H., Bulbrook, R. D., Falconer, M. A., et al.: Urinary steroids in the prediction of response to adrenalectomy or hypophysectomy. A second clinical trial. Lancet, *2*:1261–1263, 1968.
5. Atkins, H., Falconer, M. A., Hayward, J. L., et al.: Adrenalectomy and hypophysectomy for advanced cancer of the breast: A comparative study. Lancet, *1*:489–496, 1957.
6. Atkins, H., Falconer, M. A., Hayward, J. L., et al.: The timing of adrenalectomy and of hypophysectomy in the treatment of advanced breast cancer. Lancet, *1*:827–830, 1966.
7. Balme, H. W.: Metastatic carcinoma of the thyroid successfully treated with thyroxine. Lancet, *1*:812–813, 1954.
8. Balodimos, M. C.: Treatment of diabetic retinopathy. Pituitary ablation and retinal photocoagulation. Med. Clin. N. Amer., *55*:989–999, 1971.
9. Baulieu, E. E., Lasnitzki, I., and Robel, P.: Metabolism and testosterone and action of metabolites on prostate glands grown in organ culture. Nature, *219*:1155–1156, 1968.
10. Beatson, G. T.: On treatment of inoperable cases of carcinoma of mamma: Suggestions for new method of treatment, with illustrative cases. Lancet, *2*:104–107, 162–165, 1896.
11. Beaumont, P., and Hollows F. C.: Classification of diabetic retinopathy with therapeutic implications. Lancet, *1*:419–424, 1972.
12. Beetham, W. P.: Visual prognosis of proliferating diabetic retinopathy. Brit. J. Ophthal., *47*:611, 1963.
13. Bensoussan, D., Levy-Toledano, S., Passa, P., et al.: Platelet hyperaggregation and increased plasma level of Von Willebrand factor in diabetics with retinopathy. Diabetologia, *11*:307–312, 1975.
14. Bloom, H. J. G.: The natural history of untreated breast cancer. Ann. N.Y. Acad. Sci., *114*:747–754, 1964.
15. Bloom, H. J. G., Dukes, C. E., and Mitchley, B. C. V.: Hormone-dependent tumours of kidney: I. The oestrogen-induced renal tumour of Syrian hamster: Hormone treatment and possible relationship to carcinoma of kidney in man. Brit. J. Cancer, *17*:611–645, 1963.
16. Brennan, M. J.: Corticosteroids in the treatment of solid tumors. Med. Clin. N. Amer., *57*:1225–1239, 1973.
17. Brennan, M. J.: Endocrinology in cancer of the breast; status and prospects. Amer. J. Clin. Path., *64*:797–809, 1975.
18. Bulbrook, R. D., and Hayward, J. L.: The possibility of predicting the response of patients with early breast cancer to subsequent endocrine ablation. Cancer Res., *25*:1135–1139, 1965.
19. Caird, F. E., Burditt, A. F., and Draper, G. J.: Diabetic retinopathy. A further study of prognosis for vision. Diabetes, *17*:121, 1968.
20. Chabanier, H., Puech, P., Lobo-Onell, C., et al.: Hypophyse et diabète: A propos de l'ablation d'une hypophyse normale dans un cas de diabète grave. Presse Méd., *44*:986–989, 1936.

21. Chan, L., and O'Malley, B. W.: Mechanism of action of the sex steroid hormones. New Eng. J. Med., *294*:1322–1328, 1372–1381, 1430–1437, 1976.

22. Contreras, J. S., Field, R. A., Hall, W. A., et al.: Ophthalmological observations in hypophyseal stalk section. Report of 8 cases of advancing diabetic retinopathy. Arch. Ophthal., *67*:428–438, 1962.

23. Cullen, J. F., and Town, S. M.: Diabetic retinopathy. Review of 82 patients presenting with unilateral blindness. Trans. Ophthal. Soc. U.K., *95*:484–486, 1975.

24. Danowski, T. S., Sabeh, G., Alley, R. A., et al.: Pituitary ablation, insulin dosage, and course of diabetic retinopathy. Metabolism, *17*:953–965, 1968.

25. Dao, T. L. Y.: Endocrine environment and neoplasia. *In* Wissler, R. W., Dao, T. L. Y., and Woods, S., eds.: Endogenous Factors Influencing Host-Tumor Balance. Chicago, University of Chicago Press, 1967, pp. 75–97.

26. Dao, T. L. Y., and Libby, P. R.: Conjugation of steroid hormones by breast cancer tissue and selection of patients for adrenalectomy. Surgery, *66*:162–166, 1969.

27. DeBodo, R. C., and Sinkoff, M. W.: The role of growth hormone in carbohydrate metabolism. Ann. N.Y. Acad. Sci., *57*:23–60, 1953.

28. Diabetic Retinopathy Study Research Group: Preliminary report on effects of photocoagulation therapy. Amer. J. Ophthal., *81*:383–396, 1976.

29. Elden, C. A.: The pituitary-ovarian relationship in a human hypophysectomized female. Endocrinology, *20*:679–680, 1936.

30. Elden, C. A., and Kummer, A. J.: A clinical laboratory and pathological study of a partially hypophysectomized human female. J. Clin. Endocr., *3*:596–599, 1943.

31. Evans, J. P., Fenge, W., Kelly, W. A., et al.: Transcranial yttrium[90] hypophysectomy. Surg. Gynec. Obstet., *108*:393–405, 1959.

32. Farrow, J. H., and Adair, F. E.: Effect of orchidectomy on skeletal metastases from cancer of the male breast. Science, *95*:654, 1942.

33. Field, R. A., Schepends, C. L., Sweet, W. H., et al.: The effect of hypophyseal stalk section on advancing diabetic retinopathy. Report of thirteen cases. Diabetes, *11*:465–469, 1962.

34. Fisher, B.: Surgical adjuvant therapy for breast cancer. Cancer, *30*:1556–1564, 1972.

35. Goldberg, M. F., and Fine, S. L., eds.: Symposium on the treatment of diabetic retinopathy. Public Health Service Publication No. 1890, 1968.

36. Goldenberg, J. S. (Cooperative Breast Cancer Group): Testosterone propionate therapy in breast cancer. J.A.M.A., *188*:1069–1072, 1964.

37. Hardy, J., and Ciric, I.: Selective anterior hypophysectomy for treatment of diabetic retinopathy: A transsphenoidal microsurgical technique. J.A.M.A., *203*:73–78, 1968.

38. Hardy, J., Grisoli, F., Leclercq, T. A., and Somma, M.: Le traitement du cancer du sein métastatique par l'hypophysectomie transsphénoidale. Expérience de 160 cas. Un. Med. Canada, *104*:1557–1562, 1975.

39. Hardy, J., Panisset, A., Marchildon, A., and Lanthier, A.: Microsurgical selective anterior pituitary ablation for diabetic retinopathy. Canad. Med. Ass. J., *100*:785–792, 1969.

40. Harper, M. E., Peeling, W. B., Cowley, T., et al.: Plasma steroid and protein hormone concentrations in patients with prostatic carcinoma, before and during oestrogen therapy. Acta Endocr. (Kobenhavn), *81*:409–426, 1976.

41. Hayward, J. L., Atkins, H., Falconer, M. A., et al.: Clinical trials comparing transfrontal hypophysectomy with adrenalectomy and with transethmoidal hypophysectomy. *In* Joslin, C. A. F., and Gleave, E. N., eds.: Clinical Management of Advanced Breast Cancer. Second Tenovus Workshop. Cardiff 1970. Cardiff, Alpha Omega Alpha Publishing Co. 1971, pp. 50–53.

42. Hoge, A. F., Shaw, M. T., Bottomley, R. H., et al.: Therapeutic regimens in advanced breast cancer. J.A.M.A., *231*:1357–1360, 1975.

43. Houssay, B. A., and Biasotti, A.: La diabetes pancreatica de los perros hipofisoprivos. Rev. Soc. Argent. Biol., *6*:251–296, 1930.

44. Huggins, C. B.: Propositions in hormonal treatment of advanced cancer. J.A.M.A., *192*:1141–1145, 1965.

45. Huggins, C. B., and Hodges, C. V.: Studies on prostatic cancer: I. The effect of castration, of estrogen and of androgen injection on serum phosphatases in metastatic carcinoma of the prostate. Cancer Res., *1*:293–297, 1941.

46. Huggins, C. B., and Scott, W. W.: Bilateral adrenalectomy in prostatic cancer, clinical features and urinary excretion of 17-ketosteroids and estrogen. Ann. Surg., *122*:1031–1041, 1945.

47. Ireland, J. T., Patnaik, B. K., and Duncan, L. J. P.: Effect of pituitary ablation on the renal arteriolar and glomerular lesions in diabetes. Diabetes, *16*:636–642, 1967.

48. Isaacs, M., Pazianos, A. G., Greenberg, E., et al.: Renal function after pituitary ablation for diabetic retinopathy. J.A.M.A., *207*:2406–2410, 1969.

49. Jensen, E. V., Block, G. E., Smith, S., et al.: Estrogen receptors and breast cancer response to adrenalectomy. Nat. Cancer Inst. Monogr., *34*:55–70, 1971.

50. Kees, O. S. R.: Clinical improvement following estrogenic therapy in case of primary adenocarcinoma of the seminal vesicle. J. Urol., *91*:665–670, 1964.

51. Kelley, R. M., and Baker, W. H.: Progestational agents in treatment of carcinoma of the endometrium. New Eng. J. Med., *264*:216–222, 1961.

52. Kohner, E. M., and Oakley, N. W.: Diabetic retinopathy. Metabolism, *24*:1085–1102, 1975.

53. Kohner, E. M., Hamilton, A. M., Joplin, G. F., et al.: Florid diabetic retinopathy and its response to treatment by photocoagulation or pituitary ablation. Diabetes, *25*:104–110, 1976.

54. Lacassagne, A.: A comparative study of the carcinogenic action of certain oestrogenic hormones. Amer. J. Cancer, *28*:735–750, 1936.

55. Landolt, A. M.: Regeneration of the human pituitary. J. Neurosurg., *39*:35–41, 1973.

56. Long, C. N. H., and Lukens, F. D. W.: The effects of adrenalectomy and hypophysectomy upon experimental diabetes in the cat. J. Exp. Med., *63*:465–490, 1936.

57. Luft, R., and Olivecrona, H.: Experiences with hypophysectomy in man. J. Neurosurg., *10*:301–316, 1953.

58. Luft, R., Olivecrona, H., and Sjogren, B.: Hypofysektomi pa manniske [hypophysectomy in man]. Nord. Med., *47*:351–354, 1952.

59. Luft, R., Olivecrona, H., Ikkos, D., et al.: Hypophysectomy in man. Further experiences in severe diabetes mellitus. Brit. Med. J., *2*:752–756, 1955.

60. MacDonald, I.: Adrenalectomy and hypophysectomy in disseminated mammary carcinoma. A preliminary statement by the Joint Committee on endocrine ablative procedures in disseminated mammary carcinoma. J.A.M.A., *175*:787–790, 1961.

61. Machemer, R., and Norton, E. W. D.: A new concept for vitreous surgery. 3. Indications and results. Amer. J. Ophthal., *74*:134, 1972.

62. Maddy, J., Norrell, H., and Winternitz, W.: Cryohypophysectomy in the management of advanced prostatic cancer. Cancer, *28*:322–328, 1971.

63. Madsen, P. H.: Prognosis for vision and fundus changes in patients with proliferative diabetic retinopathy. Brit. J. Ophthal., *55*:372–382, 1971.

64. Mainwaring, W. I. P.: Androgen receptors, some aspects of the aetiology and biochemistry of prostatic cancer. *In* Proceedings of the Third Tenovus Workshop, Cardiff, 1970. Cardiff, Alpha Omega Alpha Publishing Co. 1971, pp. 109–114.

65. McGuire, W. L.: A new approach for selecting patients with metastatic breast cancer for hypophysectomy. Clin. Neurosurg., *21*:39–59, 1973.

66. McGuire, W. L., and Julian, J. A.: Comparison of macromolecular binding of estradiol in hormone dependent and hormone independent rat mammary carcinoma. Cancer Res., *31*:1440–1445, 1971.

67. McGuire, W. L., Carbone, P. P., and Vellmer, E. O., eds.: Estrogen Receptors in Human Breast Cancer. New York, Raven Press, 1975.

68. McGuire, W. L., Chamness, G. C., Costlow, M. E., and Shepherd, R. E.: Hormone dependence in breast cancer. Metabolism, *23*:75–100, 1974.

69. Meties, J., Cassell, E., and Clark, J.: Estrogen inhibition of mammary tumor growth in rats: Counteraction by prolactin. Proc. Soc. Exp. Biol. Med., *137*:1225–1227, 1971.

70. Minton, J. P.: Prolactin and human breast cancer. Amer. J. Surg., *128*:628–630, 1974.

71. Minton, J. P., and Dickey, R. P.: Levodopa test to predict response of carcinoma of the breast to surgical ablation of endocrine glands. Surg. Gynec. Obstet., *136*:971–974, 1973.

72. Moricca, G.: Chemical hypophysectomy for cancer pain. Advances Neurol., *4*:707–714, 1974.

73. Muhlbrock, O.: Studies on the hormone dependence of experimental breast tumors in mice. *In* Currie, A. K., ed.: Endocrine Aspects of Breast Cancer. Baltimore, Williams & Wilkins, 1958, pp. 291–296.

74. Muhlbrock, O., and Boot, L. M.: Induction of mammary cancer in mice without the mammary tumor agent by isografts of hypophyses. Cancer Res., *19*:402–412, 1959.

75. Murphy, G. P.: Prostate cancer. CA, *24*:282–288, 1974.

76. Murphy, G. P., Boctor, Z. N., Gailani, S., et al.: Hypophysectomy for disseminated prostatic carcinoma. J. Surg. Onc., *1*:81–95, 1969.

77. Nagaswa, H., and Yanai, R.: Effects of prolactin or growth hormone on growth of carcinogen-induced mammary tumors of adreno-ovariectomized rats. Int. J. Cancer, *6*:488–495, 1970.

78. Nesbit, R. M., and Baum, W. C.: Endocrine control of prostatic carcinoma. J.A.M.A., *143*:1317, 1950.

79. Norrell, H., Alves, A. M., Winternitz, W. W., et al.: A clinicopathologic analysis of cryohypophysectomy in patients with advanced cancer. Cancer, *25*:1050–1060, 1970.

80. Oakley, N., Hill, D. W., Joplin, G. F., et al.: Diabetic retinopathy. I. The assessment of severity and progress by comparison with a set of standard fundus photographs. Diabetologia, *3*:402–405, 1967.

81. Oberfield, R. A., Nesto, R., Cady, B., et al.: A multidisciplined approach for the treatment of metastatic carcinoma of the breast; A review of five years' experience. Med. Clin. N. Amer., *59*:425–430, 1975.

82. Palumbo, P. J., and Munoz, J. M.: Diabetic retinopathy. Amer. Fam. Physician, *14*:60–63, 1976.

83. Pearson, O. H.: Endocrine treatment of breast cancer. CA, *26*:165, 1976.

84. Pearson, O. H., Eliel, L. P., Rawson, R. W., et al.: ACTH and cortisone-induced regression of lymphoid tumors in man. A preliminary report. Cancer, *2*:943–945, 1969.

85. Pearson, O. H., Llerena, O., Llerena, L., et al.: Prolactin-dependent rat mammary cancer: A model for man? Trans. Ass. Amer. Physicians, *82*:225–237, 1969.

86. Pearson, O. H., Ray, B. S., Lipsett, M. B., Hood, H., and Greenberg, E.: Hypophysectomy in man. Arch. Surg. (Chicago), *77*:144–152, 1958.

87. Pearson, O. H., Ray, B. S., McLean, J. M., et al.: Hypophysectomy for the treatment of diabetic retinopathy. J.A.M.A., *188*:116–122, 1964.

88. Perrault, M., LeBeau, J., Klotz, B., et al.: L'hypophysectomie totale dans le traitement de cancer du sein: Premier cas français: Avenir de la méthode [Total hypophysectomy in the treatment of breast cancer: First French case: Future of the method]. Thérapie, *7*:290–300, 1952.

89. Pierpaoli, W., and Sorkin, E.: Inhibition of growth of methylcholanthrene-induced mammary carcinoma in rats by anti-adenohypophysis serum. Nature [New Biol.], *238*:58–59, 1972.

90. Poulsen, J. E.: The Houssay phenomenon in man. Recovery from retinopathy in a case of diabetes with Simmonds' disease. Diabetes, *2*:7–12, 1953.

91. Poulsen, J. E.: Diabetes and anterior pituitary insufficiency. Final course and postmortem study of a diabetic patient with Sheehan's syndrome. Diabetes, 15:73–77, 1966.

92. Powell, E. D. U., Frantz, A. G., Rabkin, M. T., et al.: Growth hormone in relation to diabetic retinopathy. New Eng. J. Med., 275:922–925, 1966.

93. Radley Smith, E. J., Gurling, K. L. J., and Baron, D. N.: The effect of hypophysectomy in advanced carcinoma of the prostate. Brit. J. Urol., 31:181–186, 1959.

94. Ranke, E. J.: Diabetic retinopathy and the pituitary. Arch. Ophthal., 62:859–863, 1959.

95. Ray, B. S.: The neurosurgeon's new interest—in the pituitary. J. Neurosurg., 17:1–21, 1960.

96. Ray, B. S.: Some inferences from hypophysectomy on four-hundred-fifty human patients. Arch. Neurol. (Chicago), 3:121–126, 1960.

97. Ray B. S., Pazianos, A. G., Greenberg, E., et al.: Pituitary ablation for diabetic retinopathy. I. Results of hypophysectomy. J.A.M.A., 203:79–84, 1968.

98. Ray, G. R., Cassady, J. R., and Bagshaw, M. A.: Definitive radiation therapy of carcinoma of the prostate. A report on 15 years of experience. Radiology, 106:407–418, 1973.

99. Saglam, S., Wilson, C. B., and Seymour, R. J.: Indications for hypophysectomy in diabetic retinopathy and cancer of the breast and prostate. Calif. Med., 113:1–6, 1970.

100. Schimek, R. A.: Pituitary ablation in progressive diabetic retinopathy. Arch. Otolaryng. (Chicago), 86:50–57, 1967.

101. Schoones, R., Bourke, R. S., Reynoso, G., et al.: Hypophysectomy for reactivated disseminated prostatic carcinoma. S. Afr. Med. J., 46:1278–1285, 1972.

102. Scott, W. W.: Role of pituitary in normal and abnormal prostatic growth. Trans. Amer. Ass. Genitourin. Surg., 46:33, 1954.

103. Shimkin, M. B., Boldrey, E. B., Kelly, K. H., et al.: Effects of surgical hypophysectomy in a man with malignant melanoma. J. Clin. Endocr., 12:439–453, 1952.

104. Shucksmith, H. S., Bonser, G. M., and Dossett, J. A.: A method of selection of patients with advanced breast cancer for hypophysectomy or adrenalectomy: A preliminary report. Proc. Roy. Soc. Med., 53:901–902, 1960.

105. Smithline, F., Sherman, L., and Kolodny, H. D.: Prolactin and breast carcinoma. New Eng. J. Med., 292:784–790, 1975.

106. Stanbitz, W. J., Oberkircher, O. J., and Lent, M. H.: Clinical results of the treatment of prostatic carcinoma over a ten year period. J. Urol., 72:939, 1954.

107. Stephens, D. J.: Chloride excretion in hypopituitarism with reference to adrenocortical function. Amer. J. Med. Sci., 199:67–75, 1940.

108. Tayler, S. G., III: Endocrine ablation in disseminated mammary carcinoma. Surg. Gynec. Obstet., 15:433–448, 1962.

109. Thompson, J. B., Greenberg, E., Pazianos, A., et al.: Hypophysectomy in metastatic prostate cancer. New York J. Med., 74:1006–1008, 1974.

110. Tindall, G. T., Christy, J. H., Nixon, D. W., et al.: Transsphenoidal hypophysectomy for disseminated carcinoma of the breast and prostate gland. In Allen, M., ed.: The Pituitary, A Current Review. New York, Academic Press, 1977.

111. Udvarhelyi, G. B., and Dickson, R. J.: Transsphenoidal radiation hypophysectomy with gold-198. Use of the Johns Hopkins image intensifier. J.A.M.A., 181:84–87, 1962.

112. Van Buren, J. M., and Bergenstal, D. M.: An evaluation of graded hypophysectomy in man. A quantitative functional and anatomical study. Cancer, 13:155–171, 1960.

113. West, C. R., and Murphy, G. P.: Pituitary ablation and disseminated prostatic carcinoma. J.A.M.A., 225:253–256, 1973.

114. Wilson, C. B., Winternitz, W. W., Bertan, V., et al.: Stereotaxic cryosurgery of the pituitary gland in carcinoma of the breast and other disorders. J.A.M.A., 198:587–590, 1966.

115. Wilson, C. B., Winternitz, W. W., Rush, B. F., et al.: Cryohypophysectomy—indications, technic, and results. Int. Surg., 48:28–40, 1967.

116. Witt, J. A., Gardner, B., Gordan, G. S., et al.: Secondary hormonal therapy of disseminated breast cancer. Comparison of hypophysectomy, replacement therapy, estrogens, and androgens. Arch. Intern. Med., 11:557–563, 1963.

145

TRANSSPHENOIDAL HYPOPHYSECTOMY

The transsphenoidal approach to the sella turcica is a relatively old operation that fell into disuse for several decades and has been revised and revived by modern technical advances. The binocular operating microscope allows increased precision and refinement of the manipulations required in the operation and enables the surgeon to avoid trauma to the surrounding structures. Televised radiofluoroscopic control allows rapid localization of instruments during the operative procedures in the cranial cavity and thus reduces the time consumed in obtaining repeated radiological verification of the instrument position, particularly in stereotaxic procedures.[5]

The author has performed more than 1000 transsphenoidal operations using these modern technical adjuvants for ablation of the normal pituitary, removal of pituitary fossa tumors, and treatment of various sellar and parasellar lesions. Continued experience and progressive improvements have resulted in a well-standardized procedure that offers several advantages. Among them are: (1) rapid access to the sella turcica through an extracranial route, (2) a relatively safe operation without manipulation of intracranial structures, and (3) a relatively benign and well-tolerated procedure without visible scarring due to the operation.

In this description of the transsphenoidal approach, particular emphasis is placed on the anatomy encountered during the operation and the technique for ablation of the normal pituitary gland. Discussion of the indications for hypophysectomy as a treatment for advanced metastatic carcinoma of the breast and prostate, and for the prevention of blindness in patients suffering from diabetic retinopathy, is given in Chapter 144.

OPERATIVE TECHNIQUE

Positioning

Proper positioning of the patient and the surgeon is important. The patient is placed in a semi-sitting position with the head firmly attached to the occipital head rest. The neck is slightly flexed to an angle of 20 degrees from the horizontal. The head should be tilted 40 degrees on the left shoulder and rotated to the right so that it remains vertical (Fig. 145–1A). This position allows the surgeon to face the patient straight on so that he can work in a strictly median sagittal plane and yet have the patient's body and the operating table out of his way.

A portable image intensifier should be placed at the side of the patient's head so that the horizontal beam is centered on the sella turcica. The television monitor should be behind and just above the patient's head. This set-up, which enables the surgeon to look at the television screen in line with the binocular eye pieces of the microscope, minimizes his head movement as he switches from the operative field to the screen (Fig. 145–1B).

The arrangement of the instrumentation and the location of members of the team are schematically represented in Figure 145–1C. Lead shielding and aprons should be

J. HARDY

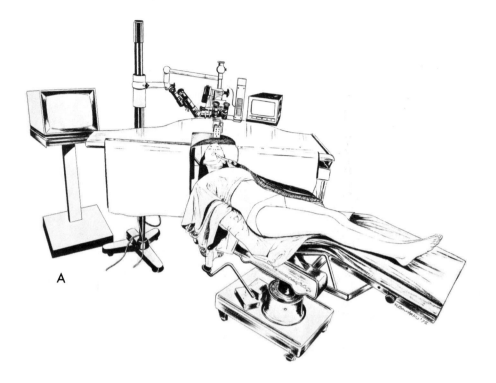

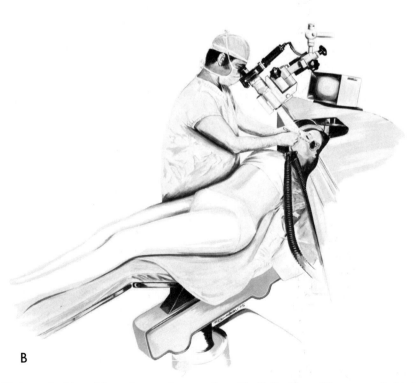

Figure 145–1   *A*. Position of the patient on the operating table. *B*. Position of the surgeon just in front of the patient's face.

Illustration continued on opposite page

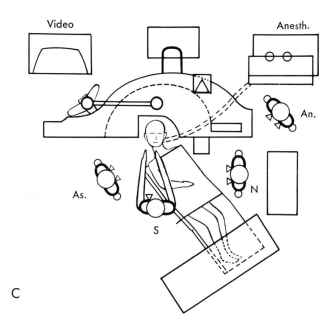

Video   Anesth.

An.

As.

N

S

C

Figure 145–1 (continued) C. Operative setup and position of the attending personnel: the surgeon, S, just in front of patient; the assistant, As., on the left; the scrub nurse, N, on other side of table; the anesthesiologist, An., behind the patient's head, controlling respiration through an extension tube. TV monitor and video-tape machine, Video, and anesthesiology equipment, Anesth., are behind the fluoroscopic apparatus. (Courtesy of Codman & Shurtleff, Inc.)

used to protect operating room personnel from secondary radiation. The radiofluoroscope is controlled by the left foot of the surgeon or by his assistant. It should be used sparingly during the operation. Proper placement of instruments decreases the time that the radiofluoroscope needs to be used at each stage of the procedure.

Preparation of the Patient

After the patient has been anesthetized with thiopental (Pentothal), an endotracheal tube is placed in the angle of the mouth to continue the administration of light general anesthesia. To prevent bronchial aspiration, the pharyngeal cavity should be packed with moist sponges. An aqueous aseptic solution is used to wash the face, mouth, and nasal cavities.

Infiltration of the nasal mucosa and upper gum with 0.5 per cent procaine containing epinephrine (1:200,000) facilitates the elevation of the mucosa and diminishes blood loss.

An adhesive plastic drape is used to cover the face, and additional draping of the entire operative field contributes to complete isolation and sterility. A hole is made in the drape at the level of the upper lip so that only the upper gingival margin is exposed.

Approach to the Sella

A horizontal incision extending to the canine fossa on either side is made just under the upper lip at the junction of the gum (Fig. 145–2A). The incision is made deep to the bone of the maxilla. The mucosa of the floor of the nose is first elevated on both sides with a small periosteal elevator to expose the nasal bony cavum (Fig. 145–2B). The sharp edge of the maxilla is then sheared off. If a wider operative field is needed, the lateral ascending branches of the maxilla can be sheared off to enlarge the opening. This can be accomplished with a down-biting punch rongeur (Fig. 145–2C). The mucosal elevator is introduced along the nasal septum to detach the mucosa from the cartilage (Fig. 145–2D). When the periosteal elevator has reached the bottom of the cavity, a check on the television screen will verify the proper direction toward the floor of the sphenoid sinus (Figs. 145–2E and 145–4).

The elevated mucosa is held in place by a long-handled blade retractor. This maneuver allows further mucosal elevation from the vomer in the deepest part of the operative field. The inferior third of the anterior cartilaginous septum is resected with a swivel knife (Fig. 145–2F). As the vomer comes into view it has the appearance of the keel of a boat. A self-retaining bivalve

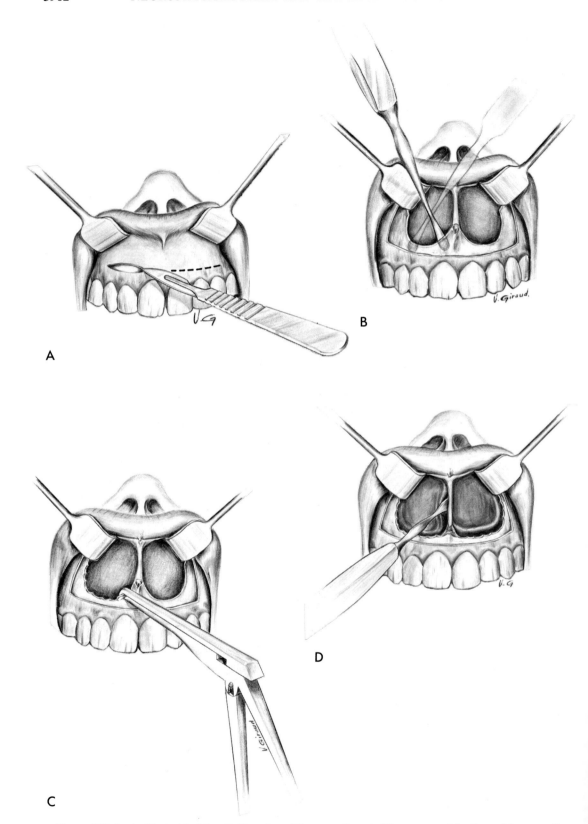

Figure 145–2   *A*. Gingival incision. *B*. Elevation of the upper lip and of the mucosa of the floor of the nose. *C*. Enlargement of the bony cavity. *D*. Elevation of the mucosa from the nasal septum (front view).

Illustration continued on opposite page

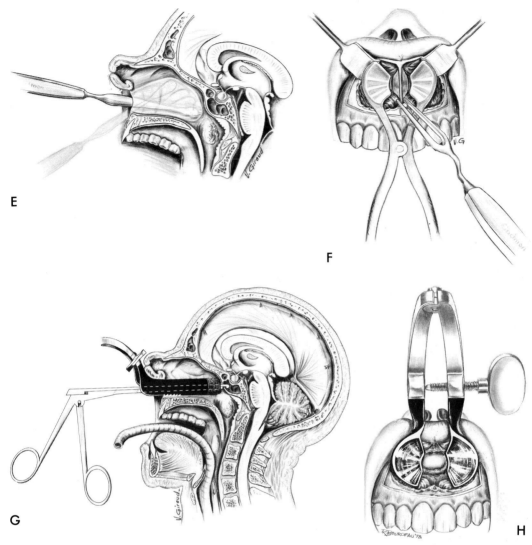

Figure 145–2 (*continued*) *E.* Elevation of the mucosa from the nasal septum (lateral view). *F.* Resection of the nasal cartilage with a swivel knife. *G.* Lateral view of bivalve speculum in place. Opening of the sphenoid sinus floor with punch rongeur. *H.* Enlargement of the opening in the sphenoid sinus floor with the new Codman bivalve speculum giving wide exposure into the sphenoid sinus. The sellar floor comes into view. (Courtesy of Codman & Shurtleff, Inc.)

nasal speculum is introduced and opened widely to hold the retracted mucosa out of the operative field. By this maneuver, a newly formed mucosal cavity is created and the entire floor of the sphenoid sinus is exposed (Fig. 145–2*G*).

Ordinarily, only minimal pressure is required to open the blade of the speculum. If the speculum cannot be opened wide enough, it is usually because of a narrow bony nasal orifice, which should be enlarged by further cutting of the ascending branches of the maxilla. Occasionally, hypertrophy of the turbinates, particularly in acromegalic patients, may require the use of a dilator, which presses the turbinate against the lateral wall of the maxilla. Next the vomer is detached with either the grasping forceps or a sphenoidal punch rongeur. Further resection of the sphenoidal floor gives a wide exposure to the entire sinus cavity (Fig. 145–2*H*).

Next the thin mucosa of the sinus is pierced and deflected. The bony septum is removed to expose the entire posterior aspect of the sinus and the floor of the sella turcica. The boundaries of the sella are carefully determined under direct vision

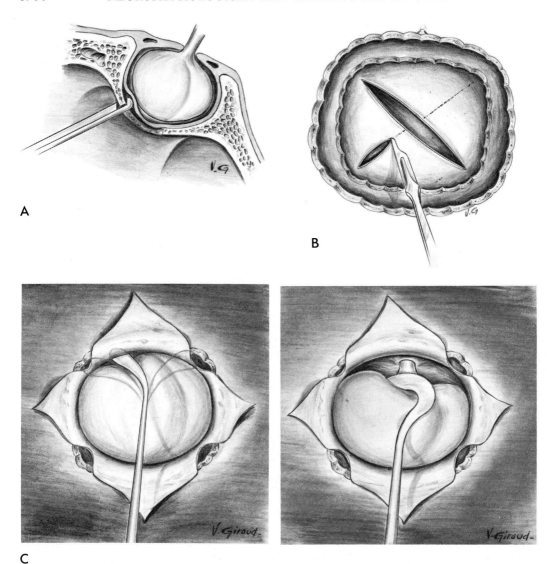

Figure 145–3 *A*. Opening of the sellar floor with sellar punches. *B*. Cruciate incision of the dura mater. *C*. Initiation of dissection at the superior surface of the gland, creating the extracapsular plane of cleavage. *D*. Identification of pituitary stalk.

Illustration continued on opposite page

with the microscope and appropriate fluoroscopic control. The upper recess beneath the tuberculum sellae defines the superior limit of the opening. Palpation with a blunt instrument will identify a groove formed by the bulging carotid artery on either side of the sella. At this stage, the binocular operating microscope should be moved into place.

Technique for Total Hypophysectomy

The floor of the sella is opened in the midline. Usually it is easily broken with a blunt-ended No. 4 dissector mounted on a bayonet handle. Small angulated punches are used to open a rectangular window about 1.5 cm wide and 1 cm high (Fig. 145–3*A*). This maneuver exposes the dural aponeurosis of the anterior aspect of the pituitary fossa.

A No. 11 knife blade is used to make an oblique cruciform incision in the dura mater (Fig. 145–3*B*). Care should be taken not to enter the pituitary capsule. The dural incision is enlarged to the edges of the sellar opening, and the dural flaps are further opened. This maneuver exposes the entire anterior aspect of the pituitary gland. The extracapsular plane of cleavage is identified

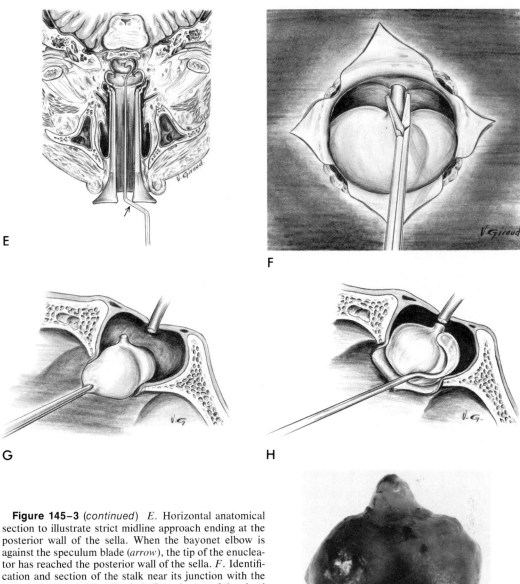

Figure 145–3 *(continued)* *E.* Horizontal anatomical section to illustrate strict midline approach ending at the posterior wall of the sella. When the bayonet elbow is against the speculum blade *(arrow)*, the tip of the enucleator has reached the posterior wall of the sella. *F.* Identification and section of the stalk near its junction with the superior surface of the gland. *G.* Detachment of the gland from posterior and lateral walls. *H.* Ablation of the gland in one piece, ensuring total hypophysectomy. *I.* Operative specimen of a pituitary gland totally removed in one piece. (Courtesy of Codman & Shurtleff, Inc.)

by gentle pressure on the superior surface of the pituitary (Fig. 145–3C).

A curved blade dissector is used to continue dissection until the stalk and diaphragmatic orifice are identified (Fig. 145–3D). It is important to have the instruments mounted on bayonet handles and to perform the operative maneuvers strictly in the median plane so that the instruments extend just to the posterior wall of the sella turcica. The length of the instrument should

be carefully calculated so that when the elbow of the bayonet handle touches the blade of the speculum, the tip of the dissector has reached the posterior wall; this precaution protects against penetration beyond the posterior limit of the sella turcica (Fig. 145–3E).

At this point a fluoroscopic check should be made to verify the proper position of the tip of the dissector (Fig. 145–4). This verification is particularly important when the di-

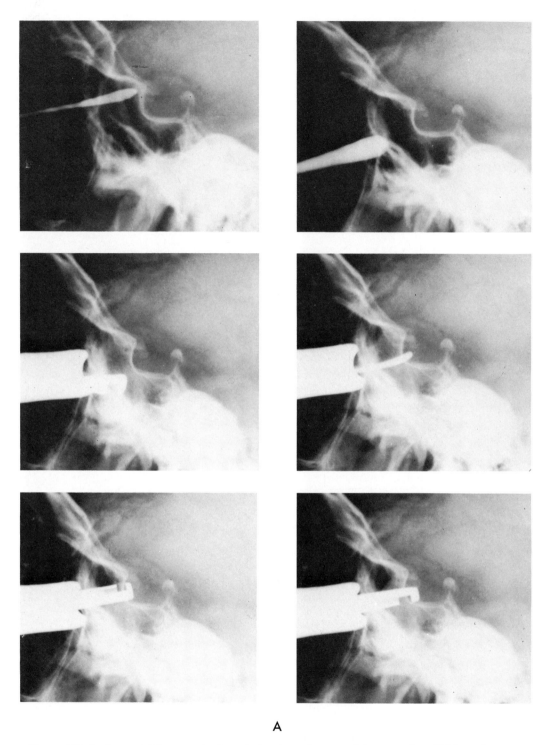

A

Figure 145–4   Sequential fluoroscopic views during the main steps of the transsphenoidal hypophysectomy. Only a few seconds of exposure are required each time. *A*. The approach.

Illustration continued on opposite page

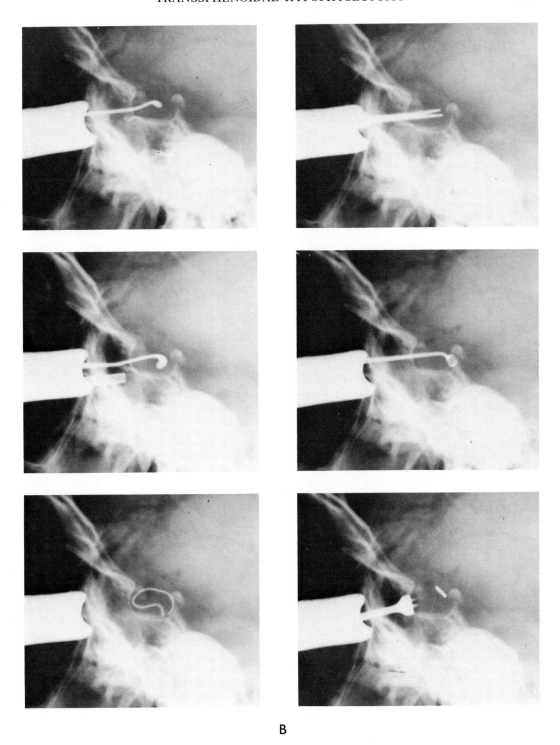

B

Figure 145–4 (*continued*) *B.* Control of the instrumental maneuvers. (Courtesy of Codman & Shurtleff, Inc.)

aphragmatic orifice is large. In this situation a diverticulum containing arachnoid may be present within the sellar cavity. When present, it is easily visualized and should be protected with a cotton pledget to prevent tearing that would permit leakage of the cerebrospinal fluid into the sella.

After the pituitary stalk has been identified, small blunt scissors are used to section the stalk near its junction with the superior surface of the gland (Fig. 145–3F). Occasionally a thin rim of yellow-orange tissue, the pars tuberalis, is seen like a collar around the inferior tip of the stalk. In this situation, the section is carried out just above the pars tuberalis. After being sectioned, the stalk retracts upward and hangs freely in the sella.

A blunt dissector is used to continue the dissection laterally, posteriorly, and then inferiorly on both sides to separate the entire pituitary surface from its dural attachments (Fig. 145–3G). Dissector blades have been designed with dimensions that correspond to the contour of the average-sized pituitary gland. There is one for detaching the gland on the right side, one for the left side, and a third for the inferior aspect. Small blade dissectors may be used but are not fitted to the contour of the pituitary gland. They have the disadvantage of frequently breaking its thin capsule, thus preventing the certainty of a complete ablation. With the curved instruments, the whole gland is enucleated with the capsule intact and falls into the sellar window,

allowing its removal in one piece (Fig. 145–3H and I). Should the capsule be broken and the gland have to be removed piecemeal, it is necessary to scrape the sellar cavity with angulated ring curets to insure total removal of the glandular tissue. Postage stamp–sized pieces of Gelfoam can be used to control the oozing of blood from the inferior pituitary vessels.

Closure

It is recommended that in all cases a watertight closure of the diaphragmatic orifice be used even though no leakage of cerebrospinal fluid is seen at the time of the operation. Closure is accomplished by using a small patch of fascia lata, which is applied beneath the diaphragma so that it extends from the lateral wall of both sides and from the tuberculum sellae to the posterior clinoid processes. A muscle patch of about the same volume as the pituitary gland is gently packed into the sella to support the fascia against the rim of the diaphragmatic orifice. The use of a too-large muscle patch should be avoided, since the fascia may herniate into the chiasmatic cistern (Fig. 145–5A). To save time, an assistant can obtain the fascia and muscle plug while the surgeon is positioning the patient's head and preparing the face for the operative procedure.

The cartilage of the nasal septum that was removed early in the operation is used

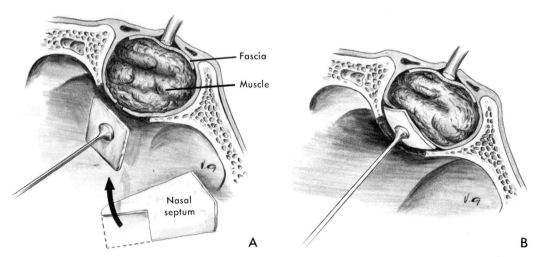

Figure 145–5 *A*. Watertight closure with fascia, muscle, and a piece of cartilage from the previously removed nasal septum. *B*. The cartilage graft is "snapped" into the sellar window in the extradural space, using the trident fork.

Illustration continued on opposite page

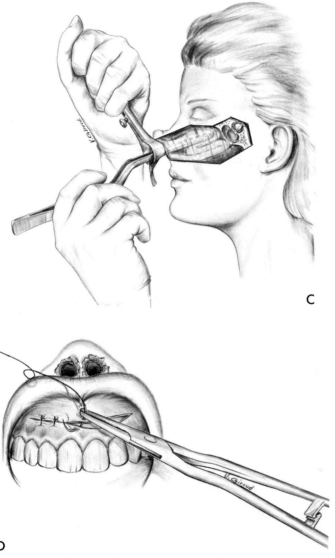

C

D

Figure 145-5 (*continued*) *C.* Nasal packing with petrolatum (Vaseline) gauze around the nasopharyngeal tubes. *D.* A few loose catgut sutures on the gingiva. (Courtesy of Codman & Shurtleff, Inc.)

as a graft to seal the floor of the sella to hold the muscle plug in place. The graft should be cut slightly larger than the sellar opening so that after it has been snapped into place, it remains firmly lodged against the inner rim of the sella in the extradural position (Fig. 145–5B). Placement of the graft is made with a trident fork that has been stuck into the cartilage. With the fork it is carried under pressure into the sellar window. It is unnecessary to pack the sphenoidal sinus, and indeed, it should be left empty in order to prevent unnecessary postoperative discomfort.

Antibiotic powder should be dusted into

the sphenoidal cavity. The nasal mucosa is reapproximated with endonasal packs (Fig. 145–5C). These packs are removed after 48 hours. Nasal pharyngeal tubes should be placed in each nostril to insure free nasal airways and thereby increase the comfort of the patient.

Loose catgut sutures are used to reapproximate the gingival mucosa (Fig. 145–5D). Because of a temporary numbness due to section of the small nerve endings on the gingival rim, this sublabial gingival approach is well tolerated and painless. Further, it produces no visible postoperative scar.

PITFALLS, DANGERS, AND COMPLICATIONS OF APPROACH TO THE SELLA TURCICA

A knowledge of the anatomical variations or incidental anomalies of the intrasellar contents and the surrounding neurovascular structures is important.[6] This knowledge reduces the risk of complications during the operative procedure. These rarely encountered variations do not obviate the advantages of the transsphenoidal approach as has been suggested by some authors.[2,11] Detailed operative reports of 266 consecutive cases undergoing transsphenoidal, open operative hypophysectomies have been reviewed.[7] A summary of the significant findings is as follows.

Anatomical Variations

Hamburger and colleagues have described three varieties of sphenoidal sinus cavities (Fig. 145–6).[4] These varieties can be identified preoperatively by tomographic studies of the sella turcica.

The *sellar* type was seen in 226 of the 266 cases (85 per cent). They have the ideal anatomical configuration for approach to the sella turcica, since the sella comes into direct view in the operative field. The obviously bulging floor enables the surgeon to recognize easily the area that should be penetrated first. After the initial opening, additional bone is removed in fragments with the sellar rongeur punch until an adequate-sized sellar window is achieved.

The *presellar* type has cancellous bone at the basisphenoid that extends upward underneath the sellar floor and does not allow easy recognition of the true position of the floor. This configuration was encountered in 32 of 266 cases (12 per cent). Fortu-

nately, accurate placement of the probe in the direction of the sellar cavity can be made by noting the lateral view of the sella turcica on the image intensifier, and the sella can be opened without further difficulty (cf. Fig. 145–4).

The *conchal* type is filled almost entirely by cancellous bone and has virtually no sphenoid sinus. It was encountered in 8 of 266 cases (3 per cent). This anatomical variation obliterates the view of the sella turcica and presents a troublesome bony barrier to entrance into the sella. The difficulty can be overcome by using a diamond air drill mounted on a 30-degree angle shaft. A tunnel is driven through the cancellous bone (Fig. 145–7). The drilling should be continuously monitored on the television screen to insure the proper trajectory to approach the sella. Since the bone is porous, there is continuous oozing of blood as the drilling is accomplished. The oozing is easily controlled by application of bone wax or cotton tamponade.

In cadaver studies, Reen and Rhoton have described the protrusion of the optic canal or the bulging of a carotid artery within the sphenoidal sinus.[11] The author has not encountered this abnormality in patients and does not believe that it would be a contraindication to the use of the procedure, since it is unnecessary to make a wide exposure of the sphenoidal sinus to accomplish the operation. Thus, the abnormalities described by Reen and Rhoton would be beyond the operative field.

In 24 cases (9 per cent), an anterior intercavernous sinus extending from one side to the other and just in front of the pituitary gland was encountered within the sella turcica. In nine cases the anterior intercavernous sinus was located high enough to allow enough room to begin the hypophysectomy through the incised dura mater

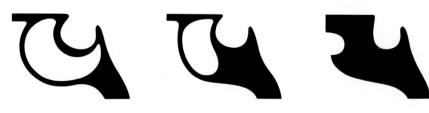

Sellar
226 (85%)

Presellar
32 (12%)

Conchal
8 (3%)

Figure 145–6 Varieties of sphenoid sinus. (From Hardy, J., and Maira, G.: Microsurgical anatomy in transsphenoidal hypophysectomy. J. Neurol. Sci., *21*:151–157, 1977. Reprinted by permission.)

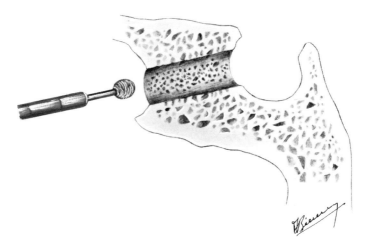

Figure 145-7 Method of approaching the sella turcica through a nonpneumatized "conchal" sphenoid bone by chiseling a tunnel with a diamond air drill. (Courtesy of Codman & Shurtleff, Inc.)

below. In 15 cases there was no alternative other than to incise the sinus, which resulted in continuous venous bleeding. In these situations, rapid dissection and removal of the gland was accomplished, and the hemorrhage was controlled by placing muscle inside the sella to produce pressure on the sinus. In only four cases was the bleeding so profuse that the gland had to be removed piecemeal instead of in the usual one piece.

A protrusion of a carotid artery within the sella was seen in 17 cases (6 per cent). In one case both carotids were inside the sella and distorted the gland into a dumbbell shape. In all these cases the bulging carotid artery was identified and trauma to it was avoided by dissection of the gland with a blunt enucleator. As a result the author does not regard this finding as a disadvantage to the approach to the sella from below.

A large diaphragmatic orifice (more than 5 mm) or absence of a diaphragma sellae was encountered in 76 cases (28.6 per cent). In 41 cases (15.4 per cent) there was an intrasellar herniation of the arachnoidal cistern. The arachnoidal sheath was torn in 26 cases. Tearing of the sheath permitted better identification of the pituitary stalk, but it also caused a leak of cerebrospinal fluid into the sella turcica. In all cases the standard method of duraplasty as previously described was used, fascia lata being placed beneath the diaphragm and followed by muscle packing and cartilaginous graft in the sellar window (see Fig. 145-5A and B). None of these patients had rhinorrhea postoperatively.

In the author's experience, neither the absence of the diaphragma nor a large diaphragmatic orifice has caused damage to neurovascular structures such as optic nerves, chiasma, or carotid or anterior cerebral arteries located above the sella. This infrequency of complication is attributed to the strict observance of technical maneuvers performed with the instruments under direct view through the microscope and the use of televised radiofluoroscopic control so that the instruments are never introduced higher than the interclinoid process line. It is apparent that the anomalies just described would be of consequence if the operation were performed as a blind procedure such as indirect destruction of the hypophysis after introduction of a probe for delivering heat, cold, ultrasound, or radioactive materials.* Fortunately, such damage is rarely reported. Rand and co-workers used stereotaxic cryohypophysectomy and never had permanent damage to the optic chiasm, optic nerves, extracranial nerves, or hypothalamus.[9] It is important to be aware of the presence of anomalies preoperatively, and both carotid and retrograde jugular injections for visualization of the cavernous sinus are justified.[8]

Pathological Findings

Of the 266 cases, 16 (6 per cent) had metastatic tissue from primary breast cancer in the sella turcica. The metastatic tissue was in the parenchyma of the tissue in some cases and localized to the sellar floor

---

* See references 1, 3, 9, 10, 12-14.

in others. When it involved the sellar floor, the opening of the sella was made easier, since the metastatic tissue made it softer than the normal bone of the sellar floor. Metastatic tissue within the sella makes it more difficult to find a plane of cleavage, however, and frequently the gland has to be removed piecemeal. Because of the increased vascular supply of the metastatic tissue, profuse bleeding may be encountered, and an infusion of blood may be necessary. Rapid dissection and removal of the gland will tend to prevent excessive bleeding and may obviate the need for transfusion.

If the floor of the sella has been destroyed by metastatic tissue, it may be impossible to reseal it in the standard manner with dura, muscle, and nasal cartilage. In these rare instances, the author has closed the area either with acrylic substance or with a stamp of lyophilized dura applied with a biological glue (Histoacryl Tissue Adhesive).*

Acknowledgment. The illustrations in this chapter have been reproduced from Signature Series 7, *Transsphenoidal Operations on the Pituitary,* with the permission of Codman & Shurtleff, Inc., Randolph, Massachusetts 02368. Credit is also given to V. Giraud and R. Bourdeau, medical artists, for their skillful professional assistance.

REFERENCES

1. Arslan, M.: Ultrasonic hypophysectomy. J. Laryngol., *80*:73–85, 1966.

2. Bergland, R. M., Ray, B. S., and Torack, R. M.: The surgical significances of the anatomic variations surrounding the pituitary. Presented at the Harvey Cushing Society Meeting, San Francisco, April, 1967.

3. Forrest, A. P. M., Blair, D. W., Brown, D. A., et al.: Radio-active implantation of the pituitary. Brit. J. Surg., *47*:61–70, 1959.

4. Hamburger, C. A., Hammer, G., Noorlen, G., and Sjogren, B.: Trans-sphenoidal hypophysectomy. Arch. Otolaryngol. *74*:2–8, 1961.

5. Hardy, J.: Televised radiofluoroscopic control in intracranial surgery. Un. Med. Canada, *92*:907, 1963.

6. Hardy, J.: Microneurosurgery of the hypophysis. Subnasal transsphenoidal approach, with television magnification and televised radiofluoroscopic control. *In* Rand, R. W., ed.: Microneurosurgery. St. Louis, C. V. Mosby Co., 1969, pp. 87–103.

7. Hardy, J., and Maira, G.: Microsurgical anatomy in transsphenoidal hypophysectomy. J. Neurol. Sci., *21*:151–157, 1977.

8. Rand, R. W., and Hanafee, W. N.: Cavernous sinus venography and stereotaxic cryohypophysectomy. J. Neurosurg., *26*:521–526, 1967.

9. Rand, R. W., Dashe, A. M., Paglia, D. E., et al.: Stereotactic cryohypophysectomy. J.A.M.A., *189*:255–259, 1964.

10. Rand, R. W., Dashe, A. M., Solomon, D. H., et al.: Stereotaxic yttrium-90 hypophysectomy for metastatic mammary carcinoma. Ann. Surg., *156*:986–993, 1962.

11. Reen, W. H., and Rhoton, A. L.: Microsurgical anatomy of the sellar region. J. Neurosurg., *43*:288–298. 1975.

12. Talairach, J., Szikla, G., Tournoux, P., et al.: La chirurgie stéréotaxique hypophysaire. Confin. Neurol., *22*:204–213. 1962.

13. Talairach, J., et al.: La chirurgie stéréotaxique de l'hypophyse non tumorale par les radioisotopes. Neurochirurgie, *12*:141–301, 1966.

14. Zervas, N. T.: Technique of radiofrequency hypophysectomy. Confin. Neurol., *26*:157–160, 1965.

* Trihawk International Co., P.O. Box 110-120, D-3508 Melsungen, West Germany.

146

STEREOTAXIC HYPOPHYSECTOMY

Three considerations favor stereotaxic hypophysectomy over open operation: patients with disseminated carcinoma and advanced diabetes often are in poor general condition, the cerebral vessels of diabetic patients may be more prone to injury because of arteriosclerosis, and total operative removal of the normal pituitary gland may be difficult if not impossible in some patients because of anatomical variations.

Stereotaxic operations were introduced in 1953 with the following objectives: (1) to accomplish a more complete if not total destruction of the pituitary gland; (2) to give the benefit of pituitary ablation to as many patients as possible, including those who were not acceptable risks for craniotomy or the transsphenoidal approach; (3) to reduce the morbidity associated with hypophysectomy; and (4) to reduce the risk of damaging important adjacent structures. Destructive stereotaxic techniques are applicable for ablation of the normal pituitary and also can be used to destroy functioning pituitary tumors confined to the sella turcica.

INTERSTITIAL RADIATION

Radioactive substances have been introduced into the sella turcica by stereotaxic approaches (transfrontal, transethmoidal, and transsphenoidal) and by craniotomy.[2,4,13] Radon was the first radioactive material to be implanted into the pituitary.[14] Because radon seeds emit poorly controlled gamma rays, radiation damage to parasellar structures was a frequent complication. Rasmussen and co-workers introduced the use of yttrium (^{90}Y) in 1955.[28] Subsequently, radioactive chromic phosphate, tritium, palladium, gold (^{198}Au), and strontium (^{90}Sr) have been used with varying success.[4,16,32] ^{90}Yttrium and ^{198}gold have definite advantages over the other radioactive substances.[13] Because ^{90}yttrium does not emit gamma radiation, it has the advantages of causing less parasellar damage than gold, but a larger amount of yttrium is required to achieve complete pituitary destruction.

Studies on the radiosensitivity of the normal hypophysis and parasellar structures have shown that the normal anterior pituitary is relatively resistant to the damaging effects of interstitial radiation, with 110,000 to 190,000 rep being required to produce necrosis.[19] The hypothalamus, optic chiasm or tract, and oculomotor nerves are less radioresistant. As little as 30,000 to 60,000 rep will produce oculomotor nerve palsy. Table 146–1 shows the energy characteristics of the two most commonly used radioactive materials.

Hypophysectomy by means of interstitial radiation is now performed only rarely because of three major disadvantages: (1) the difficulty of effecting clinically complete hypophysectomy at radiation levels free of complications; (2) damage to the optic nerve and to cranial nerves supplying extraocular muscles; and (3) early and late occurrence of cerebrospinal fluid rhinorrhea, with resulting meningitis or pituitary abscess.

EXTERNAL RADIATION

External radiation as a nonoperative alternative, with either conventional apparatus or the betatron, cannot achieve selec-

---

P. R. WEINSTEIN AND C. B. WILSON

TABLE 146–1 CHARACTERISTICS OF RADIOACTIVE GOLD AND YTTRIUM

ISOTOPE	RADIO-ACTIVE DECAY	HALF-LIFE (Hours)	BETA ENERGY (mev)	MAXIMUM RANGE IN WATER (mm)
[198]Gold	B.4	64	0.96	3.8
[90]Yttrium	B	61	2.18	11

tive destruction of the normal pituitary gland. This fact has been confirmed by clinical observations in humans and by experimental irradiation of the hypophysis in the rat and rabbit.[2,20,30] Patients undergoing irradiation to treat parasellar tumors show no evidence of hypopituitarism at the dosage commonly used for tumor destruction (i.e., 5000 to 6000 rads). Since hypothalamic neurons are more radiosensitive than cells in the normal pituitary gland, cases of postirradiation hypopituitarism are most probably due to hypothalamic nuclear degeneration.[29]

Because the 340-mev proton beam and 900-mev alpha particles have the advantage of greater penetration without scatter, the normal pituitary gland can be destroyed by heavy particles generated from the 184-inch cyclotron.[5] Heavy-particle irradiation, however, has three disadvantages: (1) full irradiation effect is delayed and pituitary function declines over a period of time; (2) although the incidence is low, adjacent structures can be damaged; and (3) the cyclotron is not widely available. Similar limitations apply to the use of a Leksell stereotaxic device for single high-dosage (20 krad) gamma radiation with [60]cobalt for hypophysectomy.[3]

RADIOFREQUENCY COAGULATION

Radiofrequency coagulation was recently introduced for pituitary ablation in patients considered poor candidates for other methods of hypophysectomy.[37] Under general endotracheal anesthesia and stereotaxic control, a 2.0-mm radiofrequency electrode is introduced into the sella turcica. Overlapping radial lesions are made by projecting lateral spring stylets at various angles around the main axis of the electrode. A Radionics Type 3 radiofrequency generator is used for this purpose. All le-

sions are made with generator outputs adjusted to reach the boiling point in two to four minutes. The end point is signified by an increase in tissue resistance as the boiling point is reached. Depending on the shape of the sella, 6 to 10 lesions usually are sufficient. The effectiveness and the complications of pituitary destruction by radiofrequency current cannot be compared with other methods because it has not received widespread application.

CRYODESTRUCTION

Stereotaxic transsphenoidal cryohypophysectomy was introduced in 1961 by Rand.[27] Clinical applications have been reviewed in later publications.[6,26,35] A metallic probe cooled at its tip by circulating liquid nitrogen was used by Tytus to destroy either benign or malignant tissue in the central nervous system, and the technique was applied by Cooper to stereotaxic thalamotomies.[8,9,10,31] Tissue destruction occurs during freeze-thaw cycles, even at temperatures above −50°C.[23] A steep tissue temperature gradient rising with distance from the probe tip has been measured with implanted thermocouples in the pituitary.[7] When the probe tip is cooled to −180°C, temperatures 7 mm away may be only −8 to −10°C, and pituitary tissue adjacent to the cavernous sinus and carotid arteries, which serve as a heat sink, probably cannot reach temperatures much below −20°C.[7,25] Cranial nerve palsies develop if advance of the adjacent ice ball results in exposure of the nerves to temperatures lower than +15°C during cryohypophysectomy. As the probe tip is warmed from −180° past −120°C these palsies usually disappear.[25]

Pathological studies of sellar contents and parasellar structures removed en bloc at autopsy of patients who had died of cancer after cryohypophysectomy have been reported. Norrell and co-workers found complete pituitary destruction in 3 of 18 cases studied. There was less than 1 per cent residual anterior lobe in one specimen and less than 10 per cent residual gland in 11 specimens. Of the remaining three cases, one patient had undergone reoperation and the other two had had clinical evidence of early postoperative pituitary insufficiency despite the finding at autopsy of 49 per cent and 28 per cent residual volume of the anterior lobe.[22] Conway found that complete pituitary destruction had been achieved in 12 of 16 cases. In the remaining four specimens 2 to 15 per cent of the most laterally situated portion of the adenohypophysis remained. Of interest was the finding of metastatic implants within the necrotic pituitary in seven cases.[7]

Histological evidence of partial or complete cryogenic damage to the hypophyseal stalk was found in all of Conway's cases, and the posterior gland was always completely destroyed.[7] Others, however, have found sparing of the neurohypophysis.[22,23] Norrell correlated postoperative endocrine function with findings at autopsy and found a rise in growth hormone levels in response to insulin-induced hypoglycemia to be the most reliable indicator of residual hypophyseal function, but it could be documented only in association with a finding of more than 10 per cent residual pituitary gland at autopsy. No evidence of cryonecrosis was found in the hypothalamus.[22] Histological alterations in the supraoptic and paraventricular nuclei were observed frequently, however, and were attributed to retrograde neuronal degeneration.[7] No evidence of cryogenic damage to the optic chiasm, oculomotor nerves, or other parasellar structures was observed.[7,22] Fibroblastic scar tissue had sealed perforation sites in the pituitary capsule and sellar floor, a finding that is consistent with results of earlier studies demonstrating that fibrocytes and collagen are relatively less susceptible to cryodestruction.[15]

The anatomical results of cryohypophysectomy compare favorably with findings reported in autopsy studies after open hypophysectomy by both craniotomy and the transsphenoidal approach. Residual pituitary tissue was found in 50 to 60 per cent of cases after open operation, although in most instances less than 10 per cent of the gland remained viable.[24] Anatomically complete destruction of the pituitary does not appear to be necessary to produce effective and prolonged remissions in metastatic carcinoma and diabetic retinopathy.* However, patients with total loss of pituitary function, as documented by failure of growth hormone response to insulin toler-

ance testing, are most likely to benefit.[1,22] Panhypopituitarism has been documented in 60 to 90 per cent of cryohypophysectomy patients.[1,22,26] No evidence of pituitary regeneration was found at autopsies performed from 4 to 30 months after cryohypophysectomy.[7,22]

The advantages of cryohypophysectomy over other methods of pituitary ablation are several. Cryohypophysectomy is performed under local anesthesia, and patients who would be poor candidates for craniotomy or a transsphenoidal micro-operative procedure usually tolerate the shorter and less stressful operation. The operative mortality rate is extremely low; only one death occurred among the authors' last 80 patients. The accuracy of the stereotaxic procedure allows complete pituitary ablation and avoids damage to adjacent vital structures.[36] The cavernous sinuses and subarachnoid cisterns around the sella serve as protective insulation for the surrounding neural tissues. As experience has increased, the occurrence of two complications, persistent diabetes insipidus and postoperative cerebrospinal fluid rhinorrhea, has been reduced to less than 10 per cent.

Although transient diabetes insipidus is common, only rarely is it permanent. It should not occur unless the neurohypophysis is damaged or destroyed, and should not persist unless irreversible damage to the upper pituitary stalk and hypothalamus has occurred.[12] With care, one can preserve the dural covering of the gland and reduce the frequency of rhinorrhea to less than 5 per cent. When rhinorrhea does occur, it is easily treated by stereotaxic placement of a muscle plug into the fistula.

Operative Technique

A stereotaxic hypophysectomy is performed in the operating room and requires two portable or wall-mounted x-ray tubes, or one x-ray tube and an image intensifier. The patient's head is aligned in the Todd-Wells stereotaxic frame and centered in the true anteroposterior plane as verified on Polaroid films taken at a tube-to-film distance of 40 inches. Four pointed screws assure fixation of the skull to the stereotaxic frame. The horizontal plane is collimated by using the image intensifier, with the

* See references 11, 17, 18, 21, 22, 24, 33.

image projected onto a television camera, amplified, and displayed on a 15-inch viewing screen. The headholder is adjusted to bring the midsellar perpendicular line onto the vertical axis of the stereotaxic arc. Figure 146–1 shows the equipment and the patient's head fixed in the stereotaxic apparatus. If an image intensifier is not available, a second x-ray tube is collimated in the horizontal plane at a tube-to-film distance of 10 feet, and the headholder is adjusted to bring the lower anterior quadrant of the sella turcica into the transverse axis of the stereotaxic arc. The focal point of the arc in any plane will then lie in the sagittal midline on a transverse axis through the midpoint of the anterior inferior quadrant of the pituitary fossa, as defined in the lateral view. The target can be moved in the transverse axis to either side of the midsagittal plane by appropriate adjustments on the tangent bar.

The nasal cavity is sprayed with lidocaine or cocaine and swabbed first with cocaine and then with bacitracin solution and phenylephrine on cotton pledgets. A long needle directed through the drill guide is used to anesthetize mucosa and periosteum at the point of entry into the sphenoid sinus and the sella turcica. For convenience, the procedure is performed through the right nasal cavity unless anatomical factors such as a deviated nasal septum interfere.

Through a cannula mounted on the tangent bar, the floor and roof of the sphenoid sinus are penetrated successively with a twist drill. Contact with the dura propria of the sella turcica causes severe but momentary pain in the forehead. If biopsy of the gland is not required, the dura propria is invaginated with the probe rather than opened, to reduce the risk of rhinorrhea. If biopsy is desired, the dura can be opened to admit a needle. Adequate specimens from

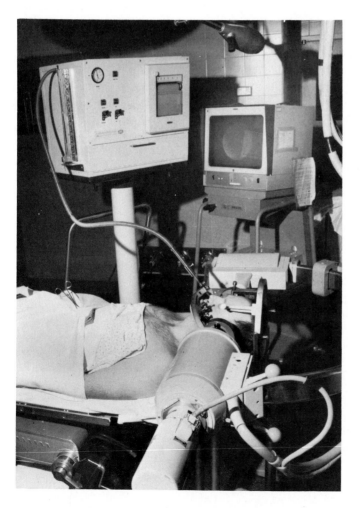

Figure 146–1 The cold probe is in position for freezing. Connection to the liquid nitrogen source is shown. The patient is fixed in the Todd-Wells stereotaxic instrument. A fluoroscopic tube with image intensifier allows continuous visualization of drill and probe in the lateral projection; an overhead tube for anteroposterior views is not shown. A television monitor for the image amplifier is seen on the patient's right.

pituitary tumors can be obtained in this manner.

After the position of the cannula has been confirmed radiographically, the drill is withdrawn and the 4.76-mm Linde cryoprobe is introduced. Because the cryoprobe is flexible and may be deflected slightly during introduction, its final position is confirmed by taking films in both planes before cooling the probe. Figure 146–2 shows x-ray control of the position of the cryoprobe in anteroposterior and lateral projections. The temperature of the probe is lowered to 0°C while the patient's vision and ocular movements are tested. In the absence of untoward effects, the temperature of the probe is lowered to −180°C for 15 minutes by the circulation of liquid nitrogen

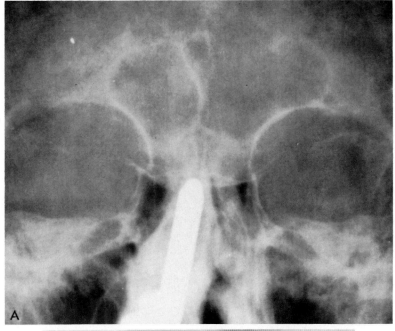

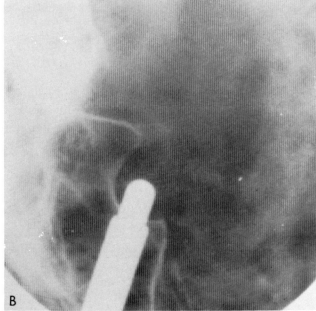

Figure 146–2   Anteroposterior, *A*, and lateral, *B*, views of the sella turcica show the 4-mm cryoprobe in position for freezing a normal pituitary gland in a patient with disseminated prostatic cancer.

from the Linde CE-2 cryogenic unit. The probe is allowed to warm to 0°C again before it is withdrawn. Visual fields and eye movements are checked every 30 seconds during freezing. The probe is warmed and repositioned if transient deficits are observed prior to completion of the lesion.

After the probe is removed, a dumbbell-shaped silicone rubber plug is forced through the cannula into the anterior wall of the sella at the point of probe penetration under fluoroscopic control; this is done to prevent a cerebrospinal fluid fistula. No nasal packing is required.

Postoperatively, the patient is cautioned not to blow his nose, but activities are otherwise unrestricted. Adrenal corticosteroid replacement therapy is continued by intramuscular injection for 24 hours, and then by oral administration in doses that are gradually decreased to a maintenance level of cortisone, 30 to 45 mg per day.

If cerebrospinal fluid rhinorrhea persists, it can be treated in the following manner. Under local anesthesia, the patient's head is repositioned in the stereotaxic guide, and the tip of the 4-mm diameter biopsy probe is directed into the sphenoid sinus through the original opening. A long strip of muscle obtained from the thigh and soaked in bacitracin solution is impacted in the sellar opening with a blunt obturator.

Position of Probe and Freezing Time

A single 15-minute lesion (−180°C) with the tip of the probe at the midline in the anterior inferior quadrant should produce a functionally complete hypophysectomy. Bilateral paramedian lesions, 8 to 10 minutes on each side, may produce more complete hypophysectomy regardless of the position of the probe in the lateral projection.[7,22]

In the authors' experience, the occurrence of diabetes insipidus did not correlate with high placement of the probe, perforation of the dura as indicated by rhinorrhea, or the duration of freezing. Nor can a correlation be established between cerebrospinal rhinorrhea and any of the following factors: position of the probe, period of freezing, number of openings into the pituitary fossa, osteoporosis or metastatic involvement of the sella turcica, or age of the patient.

Preoperative Preparation of the Patient

Preoperatively, all patients being treated for pituitary adenoma should receive a thorough endocrine evaluation in addition to routine laboratory studies. Baseline pituitary function studies before ablation of a normal gland are helpful for comparison with postoperative results. Pituitary-adrenal function is estimated by determining the plasma hydrocortisone level, urinary 17-ketogenic and 17-ketosteroid excretion, and the response to metyrapone or insulin-induced hypoglycemia. Thyroid stimulating hormone (TSH) levels are obtained, and thyroid function is assayed by means of triiodothyronine (T3) and levothyroxine (T4) levels. Pituitary gonadotropins are estimated by bioassay of urinary follicle stimulating hormone (FSH). Growth hormone is assayed in the fasting state and in response to insulin-induced hypoglycemia. Serum prolactin levels are measured, and suppression following L-dopa administration can be assayed.

Diabetes should be controlled with regular insulin before operation. Cortisone supplement therapy should be started preoperatively with 100 mg hydrocortisone administered intramuscularly just before operation.

Roentgenographic examination of the skull and sphenoid sinus serves two purposes: it forewarns the surgeon of anatomical abnormalities and excludes from consideration those patients with active sinusitis. During the three days before operation, the patient is given nose drops containing an equal mixture of bacitracin (500 units per milliliter) and phenylephrine (0.25 per cent) every four hours. The scalp is washed with hexachlorophene soap the day before operation.

Support During Operation

On the morning of the operation, preoperative medication includes meperidine, hydroxyzine (Vistaril), and atropine, the exact dosage of each being determined by the patient's age and condition. Normal saline containing soluble hydrocortisone, 100 mg per 1000 ml, is infused intravenously throughout the operation, and additional meperidine and hydroxyzine are administered intravenously as needed.

Postoperative Replacement Therapy

Following the operation, endocrine function studies are repeated at appropriate intervals. Hormone replacement therapy is continued, using 50 mg cortisone acetate or hydrocortisone intramuscularly every 6 hours for 24 to 48 hours, which is then adjusted to 30 to 45 mg per day orally.

Hypothyroidism, if it appears, is evident six to eight weeks after operation, and treatment is started at that time with either 120 to 180 mg desiccated thyroid or 100 to 200 mg of levothyroxine daily.

Postoperative insulin requirements in diabetics are unpredictable, but a major complication is hypoglycemia due to increase in insulin sensitivity. Regular insulin is given on a sliding scale with no attempt to maintain a sugar-free urine.

Diabetes insipidus is controlled with vasopressin (Pitressin). The aqueous preparation is used as needed to maintain a urinary volume of less than 150 ml per hour. After the first week, continuing polyuria is managed with Pitressin tannate in oil, 3 to 5 units intramuscularly every two to three days, or posterior pituitary powder by nasal insufflation three or four times a day.

Gonadal hormone replacement is rarely requested by older women but can be provided under supervision of the gynecologist for premenopausal women who wish to maintain a normal menstrual cycle. Men may be given testosterone propionate on request (50 mg per week intramuscularly).

SPECIAL PROBLEMS OF THE HYPOPHYSECTOMIZED PATIENT

Three major problems characterize hypophysectomized patients: (1) The insulin requirements of diabetic patients may be difficult to determine. The treatment of uncontrolled diabetes with the usual doses of insulin may easily cause hypoglycemic coma, since patients with hypopituitarism are particularly sensitive to insulin. (2) The dosage of steroids should be increased during any acutely stressful illness because of posthypophysectomy adrenocortical defi-

ciency. (3) Some patients who have difficulty conserving salt in the postoperative period may develop postural hypotension. Occasionally, liberal quantities of salt and small doses of 9-alpha-fluorohydrocortisone are needed. Glomerular filtration may be reduced by up to 20 per cent after hypophysectomy, and diabetic patients with advanced nephropathy may develop uremia.

REFERENCES

1. Adams, D. A., Rand, R. W., Roth, N. H., Dashe, A. M., Gipstein, R. M., and Heuser, G.: Hypophysectomy in diabetic retinopathy. The relationship between the degree of pituitary ablation and ocular response. Diabetes, 23:698–707, 1974.
2. Arnold, A.: Effects of x-irradiation on the hypothalamus: A possible explanation for the therapeutic benefits following x-irradiation of the hypophysial region for pituitary dysfunction. J. Clin. Endocr., 14:859–868, 1954.
3. Backlund, E. O., Rahn, T., Sarby, B., de Schryver, A., and Wennerstrand, J.: Closed stereotactic hypophysectomy by means of ⁶⁰Co gamma radiation. Acta Radiol. [Ther.] (Stockholm), 11:545–555, 1972.
4. Bauer, K. H., and Klar, E.: Zur Technik der percutanen Hypophysenausschaltung durch radioaktives gold. Chirurg, 29:145–159, 1958.
5. Cleveland, A., Braun-Cantilo, J., La Roche, G., Tobias, C., Constable, J., Sangalli, F., Carlson, R., and Lawrence, J. H.: Alpha-particle pituitary irradiation in metastatic carcinoma of the breast. Metabolic effects. Proceedings of the Conference on Research on the Radiotherapy of Cancer. Besthesda, Md., National Cancer Institute, 1961, pp. 190–198.
6. Conway, L. W., and Collins, W. F.: Results of transsphenoidal cryohypophysectomy for carcinoma of the breast. New Eng. J. Med., 281:1–7, 1969.
7. Conway, L. W., and Garcia, J. H.: Cryohypophysectomy: Postmortem findings in 16 cases. J. Neurosurg., 32:435–442, 1970.
8. Cooper, I. S.: Cryogenic surgery. A new method of destruction or extirpation of benign or malignant tissues. New Eng. J. Med., 268:743–749, 1963.
9. Cooper, I. S.: Involuntary movement disorders. Harper & Row, New York, 1969.
10. Cooper, I. S., and Hirose, T.: Application of cryogenic surgery to resection of parenchymal organs. New Eng. J. Med., 214:15–18, 1966.
11. Danowski, T. S., Sabeh, G., Alley, R. A., Robbins, T. J., Sarver, M. E., Parsons, J. A., Susen, A. F., and Narduzzi, J. V.: Pituitary ablation, insulin dosage, and course of diabetic retinopathy. Metabolism, 17:953–965, 1968.
12. Dingman, J. F., Jessiman, A. G., Despontes, R. H., Hammond, W. G., Matson, D. D., Emerson, K., Jr., and Moore, F. D.: Residual neurohypophyseal function in hypophysectomized man. New Eng. J. Med., 260:997–1001, 1959.

13. Evans, J. P., Fenge, W., Kelly, W. A., and Harper, P. V., Jr.: Transcranial yttrium[90] hypophysectomy. Surg. Gynec. Obstet., *108*:393–405, 1959.

14. Forrest, A. P., Brown, D. A. P., Morris, S. R., and Illingworth, C. F.: Pituitary radon implant for advanced cancer. Lancet, *1*:399–401, 1956.

15. Haas, G. M., and Taylor, C. B.: Quantitative hypothermic method for production of local injury in tissue. Arch. Path. (Chicago), *45*:563–580, 1948.

16. Harper, P. V., Strandjord, N., Paloyan, E., Moseley, R. D., Warner, N. E., and Lathrop, K. A.: Destruction of the hypophysis with a Sr[90] – Y[90] needle. Ann. Surg., *160*:743–751, 1964.

17. Harrold, B. P., Cates, J. E., and James, J. A.: Treatment of advanced cancer by transsphenoidal hypophysectomy. Brit. J. Cancer, *22*:19–31, 1968.

18. Hortling, H., af-Bjorkesten, G., and Hiisi-Brummer, L.: Experiences with hypophysectomy in mammary cancer patients. Acta Endocr. (Kobenhavn) (suppl.), *31*:289–293, 1957.

19. Kelly, W. A., Evans, J. P., Harper, P. V., and Humphreys, E. M.: The effect upon the hypophysis of radioactive yttrium. Surg. Gynec. Obstet. *106*:600–604, 1958.

20. Lawrence, J. H., Nelson, W. O., and Wilson, H.: Roentgen irradiation of the hypophysis. Radiology, *29*:446–454, 1937.

21. Luft, R., Olivecrona, H., Ikkos, D., Nilsson, L. B., and Ljunggren, H.: Hypophysectomy in the treatment of malignant tumors. Amer. J. Med., *21*:728–738, 1956.

22. Norrell, H., Alves, A. M., Winternitz, W. W., and Maddy, J.: A clinicopathologic analysis of cryohypophysectomy in patients with advanced cancer. Cancer, *25*:1050–1060, 1970.

23. Paglia, D. E.: Mechanisms of cryogenic injury in the pituitary: Observations on the pathologic changes associated with transsphenoidal cryohypophysectomy. *In* Rand, R. W., Rinfret, A. P., Von Leden, H., eds.: Cryosurgery. Springfield, Ill., Charles C Thomas, 1968, pp. 246–268.

24. Pearson, O. H., and Ray, B. S.: Hypophysectomy in the treatment of metastatic mammary cancer. Amer. J. Surg., *99*:544–552, 1960.

25. Rand, R. W.: Cryogenic technics in stereotaxic neurosurgery. Cryohypophysectomy and cryothalamectomy. Int. Surg., *49*:212–216, 1968.

26. Rand, R. W.: Hypophysectomy in endocrine disorders. Clin. Neurosurg., *17*:226–249, 1970.

27. Rand, R. W., Dashe, A. M., Paglia, D. E., Conway, L. W., and Solomon, D. H.: Stereotactic cryohypophysectomy. J.A.M.A., *189*:255–259, 1964.

28. Rasmussen, T. B., Harper, P. V., Yuhl, E., and Bergenstal, D. M.: The destruction of the pituitary gland in metastatic carcinoma with yttrium-90 pellets. Semiannual Report to the Atomic Energy Commission, Argonne Cancer Research Hospital, University of Chicago, *3*:1–17, 1955.

29. Tan, B. C., and Kunaratnam, N.: Hypopituitary dwarfism following radiotherapy for nasopharyngeal carcinoma. Clin. Radiol., *17*:302–304, 1966.

30. Tobias, C. A., Van Dyke, D. C., Simpson, M. E., Anger, H. E., Huff, R. L., and Koneff, A. A.: Irradiation of the pituitary of the rat with high energy deuterons. Amer. J. Roentgen., *72*:1–21, 1954.

31. Tytus, J. S., and Ries, L.: Further observations on rapid freezing and its possible application to neurosurgical techniques. Bull. Mason Clin., *15*:51–61, 1961.

32. Udvarhelyi, G. B., and Dickerson, R. J.: Transsphenoidal radiation hypophysectomy with gold-198. Use of the Johns Hopkins image intensifier. J.A.M.A., *181*:84–87, 1962.

33. Van Buren, J. M., and Bergenstal, D. M.: An evaluation of graded hypophysectomy in man. Cancer, *13*:155–171, 1960.

34. West, C. R., and Murphy, G. P.: Pituitary ablation and disseminated prostatic carcinoma. J.A.M.A., *225*:253–256, 1973.

35. Wilson, C. B., Winternitz, W. W., Rush, B. F., Walton, K. N., and Maddy, J. A.: Cryohypophysectomy. Int. Surg., *48*:28–40, 1967.

36. Winternitz, W. W., Maddy, J. A., Wilson, C. B., and Norrell, H.: Experience with the technique of pituitary freezing as a means of destruction of the gland. J. Kentucky Med. Ass., *66*:43–48, 1968.

37. Zervas, N. T.: Stereotaxic radiofrequency surgery of the normal and the abnormal pituitary gland. New Eng. J. Med., *280*:429–437, 1969.

147

HYPOPHYSECTOMY BY CRANIOTOMY

When adrenal corticosteroids to treat hypoadrenalism became available about 1950, total removal of the pituitary gland in man became feasible. Since that time hypophysectomy has been extensively employed in the management of breast and prostatic cancer, diabetic retinopathy, and certain pituitary tumors. A variety of techniques have been employed to ablate the pituitary gland, including the transnasal application of heat and cold, the implantation of radioactive isotopes, and operative excision. Of all these methods, removal of the gland under direct vision is preferable in most cases in order to assure that no functioning pituitary tissue is left behind.

Controversy about the best operative approach to the pituitary gland has existed for at least 75 years. The transcranial approach was favored by Luft and Olivecrona, and by Ray and co-workers, who reported the first substantial series of hypophysectomies in man.[12,16] The advent of the operating microscope renewed interest in the transnasal approach. Since patients generally tolerate the transnasal operation better than craniotomy, the former has currently gained favor.

There are circumstances, however, under which transfrontal hypophysectomy is preferable to the transnasal operation. The first is a developmental variation in which the sphenoid sinus fails to become aerated. Under these circumstances 1 or 2 cm of cancellous bone may separate the back of the nasal cavity from the sella turcica. How often this is observed is not entirely clear. Hammer and Radberg reported that the sphenoid sinus failed to become aerated in approximately 2.5 per cent of individuals.[6] These authors, however, made no statement about the age of their patients. The sphenoid sinus becomes aerated progressively, beginning at age 4 and usually finishing by age 13.[23] Possibly some of Hammer and Radberg's patients were children, in whom an unaerated sphenoid sinus may be anticipated but in whom the indications for operations on the pituitary gland are infrequent.

Other indications for transcranial hypophysectomy arise if hypophysectomy is to be employed in the management of a patient with pituitary tumor in whom an eccentric suprasellar extension exists. Patients with pituitary tumors in whom the sella is enlarged and the suprasellar extension is directly above the sella turcica can be operated on satisfactorily by the transnasal route. If the sella is of normal size, however, or if the tumor spills over into the anterior or middle cranial fossa, then complete tumor removal may be difficult or impossible from below and the transcranial approach assumes special advantages.

OPERATIVE PROCEDURE

The day prior to the hypophysectomy corticosteroids are administered in substantial doses such as 4 mg of dexamethasone every six hours, not only to replace the secretions of the adrenal gland but also to reduce postoperative cerebral swelling. An anticonvulsant drug, such as 32 mg of phenobarbital three times daily, is also given, in anticipation that it will be continued for the first postoperative week and then stopped.

The patient is positioned supine with one or two large-gauge spinal needles or a sub-

R. H. PATTERSON, JR.

arachnoid catheter in place in order to drain cerebrospinal fluid. A catheter should be present in the bladder in case diuresis occurs because of either the administration of diuretics or the onset of diabetes insipidus.

The incision is made in the hairline, extending from the right temple to perhaps 8 cm to the left of the midline. This will be a variable distance back from the eyebrows, depending on the position of the hairline. The head need not be completely shaved; only a strip of hair, perhaps 5 cm wide, need be removed. The opening in the skull should be about 5 cm square and must be flush with the roof of the orbit and reach the midline. The easily palpable ridge where the zygoma attaches to the frontal bone above the lateral margin of the orbit is a convenient landmark. The most important cut in the bone is from this point along the orbital ridge to the midline just above the glabella. A trephine opening can be placed near the midline at the glabella through the frontal sinuses. A second trephine opening about 2 cm posterior to the first and just to the right of the midline is also helpful. The important point is that the cut across the frontal bone must be as far forward and as low as possible. The surgeon must accept the fact that in most cases the frontal sinus will be opened. If the saw cut is too high, too much retraction of the frontal lobe will be necessary. Excessive retraction of the frontal lobe is the basis of most of the serious complications of the transfrontal operation.

In young people, in whom the brain is full, the administration of 50 to 100 gm of mannitol at the beginning of the procedure will reduce the necessity for retraction of the frontal lobe from the floor of the frontal fossa. In addition, all the spinal fluid can be removed by allowing the fluid to drain by gravity from the previously placed needles. The amount might total 100 to 175 ml. The fluid can be saved to be replaced at the end of the procedure, which the author prefers to do rather than substitute a mock cerebrospinal fluid.

Next in the operation, the olfactory nerve is divided, and a brain retractor is slipped over the tip of the frontal lobe down to the region of the sella. The retractor must be placed along the falx, because it is almost impossible to remove all the pituitary gland through an oblique approach.

The larger veins draining the tip of the frontal lobe into the sagittal sinus are saved, if possible. Should the brain be tight despite the administration of an osmotic diuretic and the withdrawal of cerebrospinal fluid, it is a better option to resect a small portion of the frontal lobe to obtain adequate exposure than to resort to heavy retraction. Any patient who appears drowsy the day following the operation can be assumed to have had too much retraction of the frontal lobe.

The arachnoid is stripped off the optic nerves, starting on the right side and continuing across in front of the chiasm to the left. This will allow exposure of the pituitary stalk, which is to be divided sharply at the level of the diaphragma sellae. If the optic nerves are short, it is necessary to resect the tuberculum sellae in front of them. The planum of the sphenoidal tuberculum is fractured with a chisel, and the bone between the optic nerves is removed with a delicate punch. It is possible to preserve the dura and avoid the bleeding that accompanies a tear in the circular sinus.

Next, the pituitary stalk is divided with a pair of fine scissors at the level of the diaphragm. The hole in the diaphragm for the pituitary stalk is enlarged with a blunt instrument to provide access to the gland. A variety of ring curets may then be used to remove the pituitary gland piecemeal. The most likely place to leave a fragment of gland unremoved is under the right optic nerve, so the surgeon should be particularly diligent in this area.

After all the gland appears to have been removed, any remaining glandular tissue can be destroyed by applying Zenker's solution. A rubber sponge placed in the sella is saturated by passing the solution through a small-gauge polyethylene catheter, one end of which is implanted in the sponge. A sucker is used to remove excess fluid that wells up from the sella.

Sudden bleeding from the sella sometimes occurs and may prove alarming. It is, however, almost always due to a small tear in the cavernous sinus. Packing the cavity with cottonoid patties for a few minutes usually will stop the bleeding and allow the surgeon to continue.

If the tuberculum has been removed, it is necessary to repair the hole in the sphenoidal sinus by packing muscle or fat into the cavity and sewing back the flap of dura to hold the packing in place. Then the spinal fluid is replaced, which flushes out any air or blood and allows the brain to come up against the floor of the frontal fossa. If possible, the dura is closed. Sometimes the dura is densely adherent to the inner surface of the skull, particularly in older people. In this case it is almost impossible to remove the bone plate without shredding the dura. Under these circumstances, it is acceptable to leave the dura open. Spinal fluid may temporarily collect under the scalp flap, but this soon disappears. It is important to close the frontal sinuses if they have been opened. Gelfoam, muscle, or fat is packed into the opening, and then a flap of pericranium is turned down from the coronal scalp flap and tacked to the dura along the brow. This closure will prevent a spinal fluid fistula. Gelfoam can be used to impact the bone plate against the brow and thereby keep the pericranium tight against the open sinus. Then the bone plate is replaced along with the trephine buttons. The author often uses silicone rubber cement of the kind that cardiac surgeons use on pacemaker wires to fill in the saw cuts and trephine openings and thereby prevent unsightly depressions under the scalp flap.

Besides steroids and anticonvulsants, the patient may require vasopressin postoperatively. This is given as Pitressin tannate in oil in a dose of 3 units if the urinary output exceeds 200 ml for two consecutive hours. After two or three days patients can be given vasopressin by nasal spray rather than by injection. Diabetes insipidus usually moderates rapidly postoperatively, and relatively few patients will need long-term management of the condition. Patients do require thyroid replacement, though the need for this is not apparent immediately but takes 10 to 20 days following hypophysectomy to become manifest. Patients generally receive 0.2 mg of thyroxine for maintenance.

Patients with diabetes mellitus are managed on a sliding scale of insulin depending on the extent of the glycosuria and ketoacidosis. The dose of insulin will need to be large at first when the dosage of corticosteroid is high, and will become progressively less as the dosage of corticosteroid is tapered in the postoperative interval.

Opinions vary about the usefulness of antibiotics as prophylaxis against postoperative infection. The case for using them after hypophysectomy is strong, since the para-nasal sinuses usually are entered and this development increases the opportunity for bacterial contamination of the wound. With their use, postoperative wound infection or meningitis is distinctly rare.

RESULTS

Completeness of Hypophysectomy

Pearson and Ray reported an autopsy study in which serial microscopic sections were made of the sella turcica in patients who had undergone transfrontal hypophysectomy.[15] In 60 per cent of 35 patients no residual pituitary cells were observed. In 29 per cent only a microscopic focus of pituicytes was found; in an equal number of patients the remaining gland was estimated at 1 to 2 per cent, and in 11 per cent of patients as much as 5 to 10 per cent of the gland remained.[11,15]

No similar morphological study has been made of patients undergoing the transsphenoidal operation, but Bates and co-workers did compare pituitary function in two groups of patients with disseminated breast cancer treated by transsphenoidal and transfrontal hypophysectomy. Perhaps unexpectedly, they found that ablation of the gland appeared most complete in the group of patients who had undergone hypophysectomy by craniotomy. Each group contained only 10 patients, however, and their results may not be representative.[2]

Operative Mortality Rates

An experienced surgeon operating on patients in good condition should be able to accomplish hypophysectomy with an operative mortality rate of 1 to 2 per cent, the deaths resulting from unexpected myocardial infarction, pulmonary embolism, and the like. The rate has been higher, however, in some reported series. Ray and Pearson reported a 30-day mortality rate of 6.6 per cent among their first 345 patients, and Kennedy and French had a mortality rate of 5.6 per cent in 71 cases.[7,15] The largest single contributing factor to the deaths is choosing to operate on patients with far-advanced disease who succumb to pulmonary or hepatic failure when subjected to the stress of operation. In a subsequent series of more carefully selected patients, Ray and Pearson reported performing 107 consecutive hypophysectomies with only one postoperative death, and Collins has reported comparable results.[4,17] Postoperative death as a consequence of operative manipulation usually results from undue traction on the frontal lobe with subsequent cerebral swelling; this can be avoided by techniques outlined elsewhere in this chapter.

Operative Morbidity

Serious loss of vision is rare following transfrontal hypophysectomy if certain precautions are taken, primarily those of approaching the chiasm along the falx and removing the tuberculum sellae if the optic nerves are short. A lateral approach to the sella forces the surgeon to operate over one optic nerve, which places the nerve in a vulnerable position. Trying to insert instruments into the sella when the nerves are short and the chiasm is close to the tuberculum likewise puts the visual apparatus at risk.

Rhinorrhea either from the opened frontal sinus or through the floor of the sella occurs in less than 1 per cent of cases. Meningitis has occurred in only 0.25 per cent of cases, perhaps because antibiotics have been used prophylactically when the paranasal sinuses are opened.

Anosmia due to dividing one olfactory nerve and stretching the other occurs in perhaps 10 to 40 per cent of cases. If spinal drainage and osmotic diuretics are employed, the left frontal lobe may fall back sufficiently to tear the left olfactory nerve, particularly in the elderly. If the exposure is achieved by resecting a wedge of frontal lobe without resorting to diuretics or spinal drainage, however, the left olfactory nerve is more likely to remain intact.

Convulsive seizures have occurred in less than 5 per cent of patients during the first 10 postoperative days. Late seizures are not a problem unless cerebral metastases are present.

Carcinoma of the Breast

The overall reported rate of remission following hypophysectomy has varied from 30 to 60 per cent and averages 45 per cent. The variation is partly accounted for by the selection of patients, because some patients are more likely to achieve remission than others. A second consideration is the criteria for what constitutes a remission. Tindall and associates report that as many as 83 per cent of patients may have relief of pain postoperatively, and they consider pain relief alone as ample indication for the operation.[22] Even though pain is relieved, in many patients the tumor will continue to grow, and life will not be prolonged. The Cooperative Breast Cancer Group required a remission to include, among other criteria, a decrease in size of the measurable lesions by more than 50 per cent. They discounted the healing of an ulcerated skin lesion or the clearing of a pleural effusion. By these criteria, approximately 32 per cent of 28 patients achieved a remission.[13] The average survival after hypophysectomy in patients who experience a remission is 24 months as compared with 5 months in those patients who do not. The average remission lasts about 18 months, though in some patients it may last many years.

Because the tumor will regress in less than half the patients following hypophysectomy, there is a substantial premium on identifying subgroups in which success or failure can be more reliably predicted. Of the various predictors, the best is the response to oophorectomy. Patients who have responded favorably for a time to castration stand a 90 per cent chance of a second remission from hypophysectomy. On the other hand, a premenopausal woman who fails to respond to oophorectomy has less than a 10 per cent chance of responding to subsequent pituitary ablation. Consequently, castration is a reasonable first therapeutic modality in a premenopausal woman with disseminated carcinoma of the breast. If she responds, hypophysectomy would be appropriate at a later date when the disease recurs.

A number of other bedside predictors of response are available. Robin and co-workers have shown that patients with a small amount of neoplastic tissue have a higher response rate than those who have a large amount of tumor tissue.[19] This speaks for resorting early to endocrine ablation rather than waiting until the patient has extensive disease. Patients in whom the disease is progressing slowly fare better than those in whom the growth is rapid; the response rate is only 33 per cent in those in whom the free interval between mastectomy and the diagnosis of a metastasis is less than one year, and it is 66 per cent if the free interval is longer than four years. The elderly appear to have a higher remission rate than those who are younger; it is 41 per cent among those who are 1 to 5 years postmenopausal and 56 per cent in those who are more than 10 years postmenopausal.

Whether or not mammary cancer responds to endocrine manipulation depends in part on whether the malignant cells have retained the population of hormonal receptor sites present in the normal cells. Cells that have lost these receptor sites appear to grow independently of their hormonal environment. Particular interest has centered on the presence or absence of estrogen receptors in the cell cytoplasm. Estrogen receptors are estimated by the uptake of tritium-labeled estradiol in the cytosol of biopsy specimens and reported in units of femtomoles per milligram of cytosol protein. If estrogen receptors are absent (taken as less than 3 femtomoles per milligram), the likelihood of a remission following any kind of endocrine manipulation is on the order of 5 per cent. If estrogen receptors are present, the reported remission rate from hypophysectomy ranges around 55 to 70 per cent. Therefore, the presence or absence of estrogen receptors more reliably predicts nonresponders than it does responders.[3,14]

Carcinoma of the Prostate

Relief of pain for varying lengths of time was achieved in 60 per cent of 47 patients subjected to hypophysectomy at the New York Hospital, but objective remission occurred in only 20 per cent of them.[21] Most of the patients are referred with far-advanced disease after other forms of therapy have failed, which probably accounts in part for the low incidence of remission when compared with that for patients with breast cancer.[8,20,22]

Diabetic Retinopathy

Diabetic retinopathy affects approximately 25 per cent of the several million di-

abetics in the United States and may be our leading cause of blindness. In juvenile diabetics it appears after the disease has been manifest for 10 to 15 years, but in patients who acquire diabetes late in life it may be present at the time the diabetes is diagnosed. The visual loss may be due to neovascularization that leads to preretinal vitreous hemorrhages and also to macular edema and the formation of exudates and microaneurysms; these are the changes that may be remedied by hypophysectomy. Patients with other causes of visual loss such as retinitis proliferans, retinal detachment, and cataracts are not benefited.[1]

Ray and associates reported that 67 per cent of 47 patients with the appropriate visual findings who were submitted to hypophysectomy showed improvement in the retinopathy, that the retinopathy was arrested in 13 per cent, and that no benefit was seen in 21 per cent.[18] Fager and coworkers reported similar results, with improvement occurring in 61 per cent of their 23 patients.[5]

Recent interest in the management of diabetic retinopathy has centered on photocoagulation of the new vessels, and the relative merits of the two forms of treatment remain unsettled.[1,10] Kohner and co-workers have presented recent evidence that pituitary ablation is superior to photocoagulation for the florid type of retinopathy with severe neovascularization but without advanced retinitis proliferans (Table 147–1).[9]

Unfortunately, most diabetics with se-

TABLE 147–1 PHOTOCOAGULATION COMPARED WITH PITUITARY ABLATION IN DIABETIC RETINOPATHY IN 34 PATIENTS (68 EYES)*

TREATMENT	NUMBER OF EYES WITH FLORID RETINOPATHY	BLIND AT 1 YEAR	MARKED IMPROVE-MENT
None	11	9	1
Photo-coagulation	11	6	0
Hypophy-sectomy	29	3	7

* Data from Kohner, E. M., Hamilton, A. M., Joplin, G. F., and Fraser, T. R.: Florid diabetic retinopathy and its response to treatment by photocoagulation or pituitary ablation. Diabetes, 25:104–110, 1976. The figures do not add up to 34 because some patients had one eye that was untreated and another eye that was treated with photocoagulation, and some patients who underwent hypophysectomy had one eye that was blind to begin with.

vere retinopathy also have advanced renal and cardiac disease. The hope that hypophysectomy would arrest vasculopathy in these critical organs and thereby prolong life has not been realized. This fact has detracted to a certain extent from the allure of this form of treatment. The presence of impaired renal and cardiac function also increases the risk of operation in these patients. Besides meeting the visual criteria already outlined, the patients should have a creatinine clearance rate greater than 50 ml per minute, a urea clearance of at least 50 per cent of normal, albuminuria of less than 5 gm per 24 hours, and no pyelonephritis. They should not have a history of angina pectoris, myocardial infarction, cardiac failure, severe hypertension, or advanced peripheral vascular disease. If these criteria are observed, hypophysectomy can be performed with a low mortality rate in diabetics.

REFERENCES

1. Balodimos, M. C.: Treatment of diabetic retinopathy. Pituitary ablation and retinal photocoagulation. Med. Clin. N. Amer., *55*:989–999, 1971.
2. Bates, T., Rubens, R. D., Bulbrook, R. D., et al.: Comparison of pituitary function and clinical response after transsphenoidal and transfrontal hypophysectomy for advanced breast cancer. Brit. J. Surg., *62*:654, 1975.
3. Brennan, M. J.: Endocrinology in cancer of the breast. Amer. J. Clin. Path., *64*:797, 1975.
4. Collins, W. F.: Hypophysectomy: Historical and personal perspective. Clin. Neurosurg., *21*:68–78, 1974.
5. Fager, C. A., Rees, S. B., and Bradley, R. F.: Surgical ablation of the pituitary in the treatment of diabetic retinopathy. J. Neurosurg., *24*:727–734, 1966.
6. Hammer, G., and Radberg, C.: The sphenoidal sinus. An anatomical and roentgenologic study with reference to transsphenoidal hypophysectomy. Acta Radiol. (Stockholm), *56*:401–422, 1961.
7. Kennedy, B. J., and French, L.: Hypophysectomy in advanced breast cancer. Amer. J. Surg., *110*:411–415, 1965.
8. Kennedy, B. J., and Kiang, D. T.: Hypophysectomy in the treatment of advanced cancer of the male breast. Cancer, *29*:1606–1612, 1972.
9. Kohner, E. M., Hamilton, A. M., Joplin, G. F., and Fraser, T. R.: Florid diabetic retinopathy and its response to treatment by photocoagulation or pituitary ablation. Diabetes, *25*:104–110, 1976.
10. Lancet: Photocoagulation for diabetic retinopathy. Lancet, *2*:77–78, 1976.
11. Linholm, J., Korsgaard, O., and Rasmussen, P.: Ectopic pituitary function. Acta Med. Scand., *198*:299, 1975.
12. Luft, R., and Olivecrona, H.: Experiences with hypophysectomy in man. J. Neurosurg., *10*:301, 1953.
13. McGuire, W. L.: Current status of estrogen receptors in human breast cancer. Cancer, *36*:638–644, 1975.
14. Pearson, O. H.: Endocrine treatment of breast cancer. Cancer, *26*:165, 1976.
15. Pearson, O. H., and Ray, B. S.: Hypophysectomy in the treatment of metastatic mammary cancer. Amer. J. Surg., *99*:544, 1960.
16. Pearson, O. H., Ray, B. S., Harold, C. D., et al.: Effects of hypophysectomy on neoplastic disease in man. J. Clin. Endocr., *14*:828, 1954.
17. Ray, B. S., and Pearson, O. H.: Hypophysectomy in the treatment of disseminated breast cancer. Surg. Clin. N. Amer., *42*:419–433, 1962.
18. Ray, B. S., Pazianos, A. G., Greenberg, E., et al.: Pituitary ablation for diabetic retinopathy. I. Results of hypophysectomy (A ten-year study). II. Results of yttrium 90 implantation in the pituitary gland. J.A.M.A., *203*:79–84, 85–87, 1968.
19. Robin, P. E., Powell, D. J., Waterhouse, J. A. H., et al.: Trans-sphenoidal hypophysectomy in disseminated carcinoma of the breast. Brit. J. Surg., *62*:85–91, 1975.
20. Silverberg, G. D.: Hypophysectomy in the treatment of disseminated prostate cancer. Cancer, *39*:1727–1731, 1977.
21. Thompson, J. B., Greenberg, E., Pazianos, A., and Pearson, O. H.: Hypophysectomy in metastatic prostate cancer. N.Y. State J. Med., *74*:1006–1008, 1974.
22. Tindall, G. T., Ambrose, S. S., Christy, J. H., and Patton, J. M.: Hypophysectomy in treatment of disseminated carcinoma of the breast and prostate. Southern Med. J., *69*:579, 1976.
23. Vidíc, B.: The postnatal development of the sphenoidal sinus and its spread into the dorsum sellae and posterior clinoid processes. Amer. J. Roentgen., *104*:177, 1968.

XIV

REHABILITATION

148

REHABILITATION FOLLOWING CENTRAL NERVOUS SYSTEM LESIONS

THE REHABILITATION TEAM

Comprehensive rehabilitation of the patient who has suffered a major paralysis, frequently one combined with loss of bowel and bladder control, requires a well-coordinated team approach. If at all possible, this treatment should be provided in a comprehensive rehabilitation center; however, many departments in general hospitals are able to provide outstanding rehabilitation services with small but enthusiastic teams of therapists, nurses, and physicians. A brief discussion of the structure of a typical rehabilitation team and the tasks of its members follows.

Rehabilitation Nursing

The nurse is the person who, of all the team members, has the most personal contact with the patient. She has to be very familiar with techniques for positioning and turning severely disabled patients. The nurse must be able not only to cope with the difficult task of helping the patient to understand and adjust to his disability but to help him cope with the problems of incontinence. Very close liaison must be maintained with the physical and occupational therapists in order to assure that ability to perform tasks learned in the therapy areas will be carried over.

Physical Therapy

The responsibility of the physical therapist is to maintain range of motion of all the joints, thus preventing contractures, as well as to record muscle strength after accurate manual muscle testing. Tests of muscle strength will be repeated and recorded at three- to four-week intervals during the patient's rehabilitation. Exercises for muscle strengthening include assistive exercise in which the therapist helps the patient to move the limb whose muscle grades are below the fair range. With stronger muscles the physical therapist can use certain mechanical devices or techniques for which only his supervision is required. Tilt board activities, mat exercises, and ambulation training as well as some activities of daily living are supervised by the physical therapist. In the later stages of rehabilitation, training for travel and ambulation in the community is also the responsibility of the physical therapist.

Occupational Therapy

The occupational therapist has a primary responsibility for patients with deficits in the upper extremities or perceptual problems. He provides exercises similar to those provided by the physical therapist; they are, however, directed primarily toward developing dexterity and immediate functional ability. Various upper extremity orthoses are used as indicated. Techniques for feeding, grooming, and self-care are introduced as soon as feasible. The use of the upper extremities for vocational activities is evaluated, and the occupational therapist gives instruction and supervises prevocational training. For many patients, home-making skills are of primary importance, and for these training should be started in specially equipped occupational therapy areas.

The rehabilitation nurse, the physical therapist, and the occupational therapist should combine and coordinate their efforts in teaching the patient such techniques as transfers, proper positioning and turning in bed, dressing, safe use of the bathroom, and other necessary tasks.

Speech Therapy

Patients with aphasia, dysarthria, and other speech disorders require the services of a speech pathologist. The speech deficit should be accurately assessed and the patient's progress monitored. Speech therapy is given individually or in groups as indicated.

Psychology

Every patient requiring intensive rehabilitative training as a result of a severe paralyzing disability should be evaluated in depth by a psychologist. After assessing the patient's ability to follow instructions, either verbal or demonstrated, the psychologist should communicate his findings to the rehabilitation team and make recommendations for the proper psychological approaches in the overall training program. The psychologist should also test patients with brain dysfunction for perceptual and cognitive problems, and cooperate with the occupational therapist in tailoring individual programs to meet specific needs. The psychologist is also responsible for providing supportive psychotherapy for the reactive depression so commonly seen in these patients.

Social Service

The social worker must be available for consultation with the patient and his family, and aid in securing financial sponsorship for his treatment if necessary. The social worker has a primary role in making discharge plans and in establishing liaison with appropriate community services.

Vocational Counseling

For young disabled patients, vocational counseling is of major importance. The vocational counselor helps the patient to make plans for continuing education and to find vocational placement, or advises him about vocational requirements and opportunities. The vocational counselor must be in touch with the patient's employer during the period of rehabilitation and must make contact with the Department of Vocational Rehabilitation for sponsorship of required training and equipment.

Driver Training

Most patients, even those with severe physical disabilities, are able to drive an automobile and should be trained before discharge from the rehabilitation program. Many rehabilitation centers have their own driver training programs; others use commercial driving schools. It is important also to assist these patients in obtaining their driver's licenses.

Home Planning

It is desirable to have a home planning consultant available who is familiar with the needs of a physically handicapped person. When necessary, this home planning consultant should visit the patient's home and recommend modifications if indicated, especially in the bathroom, kitchen, and entrance ways. Since many homes have stairs and other architectural barriers, the consultant may recommend major home modifications or may suggest a complete change to living quarters with a barrier-free environment.

Medical Supervision

All the activities discussed so far must be closely supervised by an experienced physician who is a specialist in the field of rehabilitation medicine. He should be the coordinator of rehabilitation services. This physician will maintain close contact with both the patient and the staff, and may of necessity consult with other specialists in order to treat concurrent medical problems. Such consultation will very often be with the urologist, since many patients with central nervous system dysfunction are incontinent. A close relationship with the referring neurologist or neurosurgeon is also required, and in addition, the rehabilitation specialist has to know when orthopedic surgery is indicated to improve function. Frequently an internist has to be consulted for medical problems such as respiratory or cardiac complications. A patient who is severely depressed or who had premorbid psychiatric problems requires supervision by a psychiatrist, although in the authors' experience not many patients undergoing rehabilitation for severe physical disabilities require psychiatric help. For the definitive management of homonymous hemianopia and diplopia or other ophthalmological complications, consultation with an ophthalmologist may on occasion be required. With so many consultants and members of the rehabilitation staff seeing the patient, the rehabilitation specialist, usually a physiatrist, has the responsibility of interpreting to the patient and his family both progress and problems.

REHABILITATION OF PATIENTS WITH INTRACRANIAL LESIONS

Hemiplegia

Immediate Rehabilitation Measures

Rehabilitation of the patient with hemiplegia should start as soon as possible after onset of the disability. Proper positioning in bed is of utmost importance in early care, particularly to prevent pressure sores and contractures. These complications can be avoided by turning the patient frequently, initially at least every two hours. When positioned on his side, the patient should have the shoulder on which he lies slightly protracted with the forearm in supination. Both knees should be flexed and they should be separated by a pillow. A relatively small pillow under the head is usually more comfortable than a large pillow that may force the neck into lateral flexion.

A footboard may be used to keep the blankets off the patient's feet to prevent

equinus deformity, but not necessarily to force the feet into 90 degrees of ankle dorsiflexion, which may cause pressure sores on the soles. In the supine position, hips and knee joints should be kept in extension. Prolonged hip and knee flexion in bed or the indiscriminate use of a water bed should be avoided, since they lead to contractures. When the patient's position is being changed, all peripheral joints should be passively moved through the complete range of motion by the nurse or the physical therapist. This routine not only will prevent contractures but also may prevent deep vein thrombosis. Patients who have hemianopia should be placed in beds where they can see the room and not only the wall. To prevent swelling of the paralyzed hand and eventual stiffness. the upper extremity should be elevated in bed by using pillows (Fig. 148–1).

Treatment of the Paralyzed Upper Extremity

In hemiplegia, paralysis of shoulder muscles may lead to painful subluxation of the glenohumeral joint. This may be prevented by using a tightly fitting arm sling. If the patient cannot tolerate an arm sling or spends most of his time in a wheelchair, a hemilapboard can be used. If the hand is edematous, the lapboard can be provided with a wedge to elevate the hand. Another alternative is to support the paralyzed upper extremity with an overhead sling that is attached to the wheelchair (Fig. 148–2).

Occasionally it is necessary to utilize upper extremity orthoses for the hemiplegic patient. For instance, in the presence of excessive wrist-drop that stretches the extensors and causes wrist pain, a relatively simple wrist extension orthosis is required. A flexion contracture of the hand and a tight thenar web space require an orthosis that places the wrist in a neutral position, the fingers in extension or slight flexion, and the thumb in maximal opposition. This orthotic device may be on either the volar or the dorsal aspect of the hand. If spasticity exists, a dorsal hand orthosis is recommended to avoid a spasticity-producing stimulus in the palm of the hand (Fig. 148–3).

If a painful shoulder-hand syndrome occurs, conservative treatment consisting of local heat to the painful joints, along with

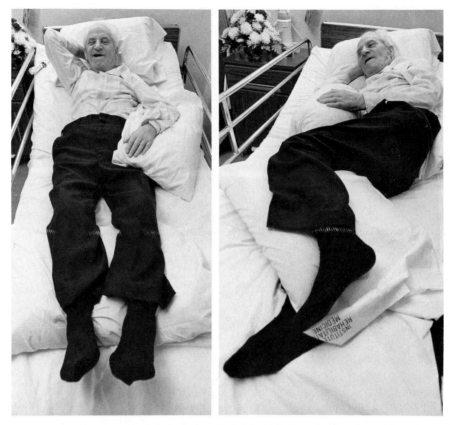

Figure 148–1 Correct bed positioning of patient with left hemiplegia. A footboard should not be used if daily range of motion exercises can be given.

aspirin, should be tried for a few days. Simultaneously, vigorous range of motion exercises of the entire upper extremity should be performed at least twice a day. If the condition does not improve or deteriorates, treatment with small doses of systemic steroids may be tried. When the upper extremity shows no return of motor function, it may be better to allow the shoulder to contract in a functional position, allowing 30 to 60 degrees of abduction and flexion.[7]

As neurological function returns in the upper extremity, the physical and occupational therapists may utilize several means of treatment. Daily range of motion exercise of all joints of the upper extremity should be continued and is an important part of the more conventional treatment technique. Muscle re-education may consist of assisted active movements of muscle groups that are too weak to overcome gravity. These movements may be performed with gravity eliminated, as on a powder board, in an overhead sling, or with the as-

sistance of a therapist. Return of muscle power will most likely, but not always, first occur in synergistic movements, especially in flexion synergy. The therapist in this case will encourage this flexion synergy by mechanically stimulating the skin over flexor muscles. In later stages of neurological recovery, the flexion synergistic movements may interfere with the function of the paretic upper extremity. In this case, not facilitory but inhibitory techniques are used for the flexor muscles while the antagonistic muscle groups are facilitated. The use of biofeedback is often helpful in these situations. The popular technique of squeezing a rubber ball should be discouraged, since it only overexercises the already relatively strong finger flexors.[1,11,15] Because the usefulness of many treatment techniques used by physical and occupational therapists is still being debated, especially when they are used exclusively, it is imperative to have the treatment supervised by an experienced and reliable therapist.

Concomitantly with the treatment of the

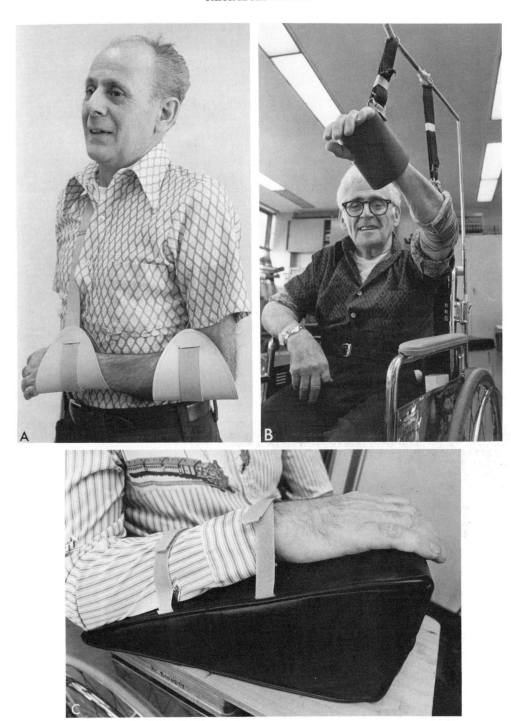

Figure 148–2 Support of the paralyzed upper extremity using, *A*, a regular arm sling, *B*, an overhead sling, and *C*, a hemi-lapboard with wedge.

paralyzed upper extremity, the nonparalyzed upper extremity should be strengthened, and new hand skills and dexterity developed, especially if it is the dominant limb that is paralyzed. As soon as possible the patient should be encouraged to use his unparalyzed hand for feeding, grooming, shaving, and the like. He should also help to dress himself, initially his upper body. When performing some of these activities, the patient may become aware of his homonymous hemianopia and should be en-

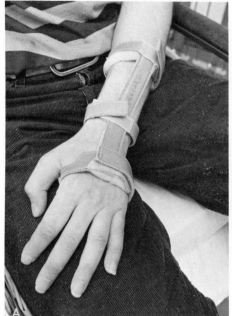
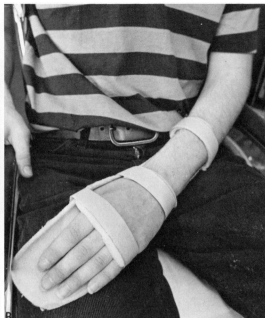

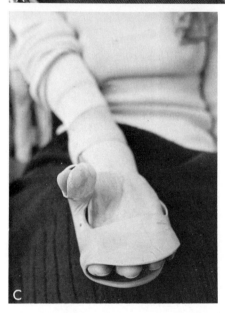

Figure 148–3 Orthoses to prevent contractures of hand and fingers in hemiplegia. *A*. Simple wrist extension orthosis. *B*. Volar hand extension splint. *C*. Dorsal laminated hand extension splint with opponens bar.

couraged to correct for it himself by learning to turn his head and use visual cues when scanning. If at all possible, he should wear his own clothes, rather than a hospital gown, when up in a wheelchair and receiving rehabilitation therapy. By becoming involved in personal hygiene and dressing himself, the patient will immediately see the functional goal of many of the exercises.

As soon as the vital signs are stable, the patient should be encouraged to be in the upright position. This is started in the sitting position, and exercises are given to increase trunk balance. Trunk balance, and later standing balance, can also be improved by using a tilt board. Even though the patient may not have any voluntary muscle contractions in the lower extremity, he may be able to use extension synergy of the knee and hip extensors that will enable him to support his body weight on the paralyzed limb. This can be tested by asking the supported patient to put his full weight on the paralyzed leg and palpating for muscle contractions of the knee and hip extensor.

Preambulatory training of more severely involved hemiplegic patients involves redevelopment of reciprocal movements of both lower extremities. In order to accomplish this, the restorator, and in later stages the Kinetron, can be utilized. On the restorator the paralyzed leg can be mobilized by the uninvolved leg by pedaling, as on a bicycle. When exercising on the Kinetron machine, the patient can be in either the sitting or the standing position, and he can monitor his own progress while essentially performing an isokinetic exercise (Fig. 148–4).

Patients with hemiplegia who undergo intensive rehabilitation training will quite frequently develop sufficient active hip and knee extension to obviate the need for long leg orthoses. Initially, however, a temporary long leg brace, such as a "Handee-Standee," can be utilized if knee extension is not sufficient for full weight-bearing ambulation. The patient has to be encouraged to use his weak lower extremity for full weight-bearing during the gait cycle.

Ambulation Training

Since most hemiplegic patients who receive a long leg brace will not utilize it for ambulation, every effort should be made to strengthen knee and hip extensors so that a below-knee orthosis will suffice. Conventionally, a double-bar short leg orthosis with 90-degree posterior ankle stops or a spring-loaded dorsiflexion assist is indicated. If considerable ankle and foot spasticity exists, a varus correction strap may have to be added to the orthosis (Fig. 148–5).

During the last few years, plastic orthoses have become increasingly popular and effective. The simplest plastic orthosis for the hemiplegic patient is the posterior leaf-spring orthosis. This unit requires active plantar flexion by the patient, which can be accomplished by having either adequate muscle power in the gastrocnemius-soleus group or a tight heel cord at approximately 90 degrees. If flaccid paralysis of the dorsiflexors and plantar flexors exists, a spiral below-knee orthosis is indicated. Patients with spasticity, especially of the in-

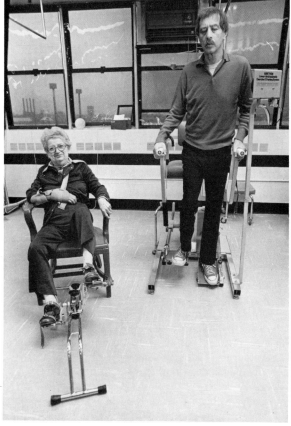

Figure 148–4 Restorator (*left*) and Kinetron (*right*) being used in rehabilitation training of hemiplegic patients not only to strengthen the lower extremities but to retrain reciprocal movements.

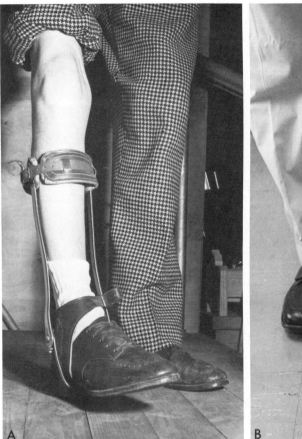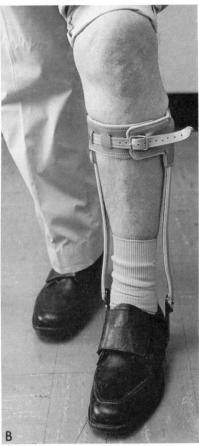

Figure 148–5 Conventional below-knee orthosis with varus correction strap, *A*, and with orthosis attached to shoe with Velcro closure for easier donning and doffing. *B*.

version type, who demonstrate a positive Strümpell sign with knee flexion require a hemispiral below-knee orthosis. This particular device will quite effectively counteract the frequently observed equinovarus deformity of the spastic hemiplegic patient. If spasticity is further increased, a solid-ankle below-knee orthosis may have to be considered. When ordering this plastic orthosis, it may also be necessary to prescribe a rocker-bottom shoe (Figs. 148–6 and 148–7).[16,22]

Gait training is usually started in the parallel bars. This method is especially helpful to the patient in orienting himself in the vertical position. Once he has achieved adequate standing balance, he should be provided with a wide-based quadripod cane. During further training he may use a narrower-based "quad cane" and later a regular J-line cane. As long as weakness or spasticity or both exist in the lower extremity, the use of a cane should be encouraged for both balance and safety.

Activities of Daily Living

All hemiplegic patients who can follow two- and three-step instructions should be able to learn most activities of daily living, including dressing. If the patient remains wheelchair-bound, he must of necessity learn how to transfer, either using a sliding board or performing a standing pivot transfer. He must learn first how to assist with his dressing and later how to dress himself independently. When an orthosis is prescribed, one should also remember that the patient should be able to don and doff his own orthotic device. Shoes may be laced in a special "hemi" fashion, or a Velcro closure may be used.

Speech Therapy

The speech disorder most frequently encountered in intracranial disorders is aphasia. Aphasia is generally classified as non-fluent or fluent, depending on its speech

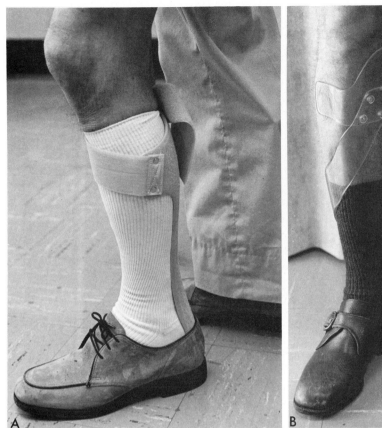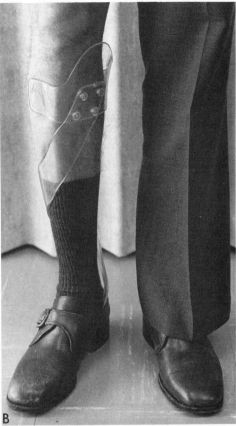

Figure 148-6 *A.* Plastic leaf-spring orthosis for hemiplegic patient with active plantar flexion or heel cord tightness. *B.* Institute of Rehabilitation Medicine spiral orthosis for patient with flaccid paralysis of dorsiflexors and plantar flexors.

characteristics. Most frequently there are such severe limitations in all modes of communication that the aphasia cannot be classified. It is then referred to as global aphasia. When a patient with a hemispheric lesion produces slow, labored speech with difficulty in articulation and many distorted sounds produced with marked inconsistency, the symptom is called verbal aphasia, more appropriately referred to as cortical dysarthria. Verbal apraxia is most often associated with aphasia and, in contrast to a typical brain stem dysarthria, is a cortical motor speech disorder.

One of the early tasks of the speech pathologist is to test the patient with a speech disorder accurately. While the physician in his examination will perform only relatively rough tests, asking the patient to identify common objects in the immediate surroundings or from the physician's pocket, the speech pathologist must test the patient initially and periodically during the rehabilitation course. Tests frequently adminis-

tered are the Schuell Test, also known as the Minnesota Test for the Differential Diagnosis of Aphasia, and the Functional Communication Profile developed by Martha Taylor Sarno, which is actually not a test but a rating scale.[18,22] The ratings are converted into percentages that represent the percentage of estimated premorbid communication ability retained by the patient. Other speech tests include the Language Modalities Test for Aphasia, the Boston Veterans Administration Diagnostic Aphasia Examination, the Token Test, the Neurosensory Center Comprehensive Examination for Aphasia, and the Porch Index of Communicative Ability.[20]

Speech therapy may be given individually or in groups. Daily half hour individual speech therapy sessions for patients with communication disorders are generally preferred. While the value of formal speech therapy in global aphasia is still being debated, there seems to be little doubt that speech therapy offers important psycholog-

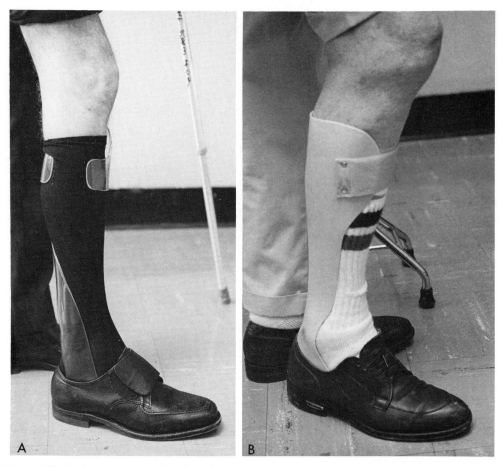

Figure 148–7 *A*. Plastic hemispiral orthosis for patients with moderate inversion spasticity. *B*. Solid-ankle below-knee orthosis for patients with considerable inversion and plantar flexion spasticity.

ical support for the patient with a severe communicative disorder.[21,23]

Often the speech pathologist will spend considerable time and effort helping the patient to understand and cope with his communication deficits and the psychological consequences of these impairments. Group therapy sometimes helps to provide a setting in which the patient can ventilate fears and frustrations and gain comfort from the support of fellow patients.

By interpreting the patient's communication problems to other members of the rehabilitation team, the speech pathologist helps to make it easier for other therapists and the nursing staff to help the patient. Members of the family and close friends also generally receive counseling by the speech pathologist concerning how best to deal with the patient's speech disorder, how to supplement speech therapy during visiting hours or at home, and how to spare the patient excessive frustration. For this, informative literature such as *Understanding Aphasia* can be extremely helpful.[19]

Perceptual Retraining

A considerable number of patients with hemiplegia have perceptual and cognitive problems. While damage to the dominant cerebral hemisphere is frequently accompanied by loss of language and ability to solve problems related to verbal skills, damage to the nondominant hemisphere is related to disturbances in visual spatial tasks. In addition to this, the patient may have a variety of behavioral problems—apathy, impulsivity, hostility, and unwillingness to acknowledge problems. Perceptual retraining can therefore be instituted only after initial orientation training in which the patient can become aware of his problems. Once the cognitive defects have been identified, a very individualized training program is given by a therapist who may be a specially trained psychologist or occupational therapist. Since cognitive problems appear very often in areas requiring great skill, these problems will be more apparent in individuals who previously were in intellectually demanding professions. With improvement in cognitive functioning, changes in emotional states have been noted as the patient learned to deal with life problems more easily. It may, therefore, be very important to continue perceptual retraining after the patient's discharge and especially when he returns to a vocation.[3,28]

Bladder and Bowel Training

An uninhibited neurogenic bladder and bowel can be very disturbing to the patient with hemiplegia and a very interfering factor in his rehabilitation. An intensive rehabilitation program will not allow the patient to return to his room or reach the next toilet in time for urination or a bowel movement. Many rehabilitation centers, therefore, utilize urinary collection devices, such as external drainage. On days when the patient is not taking part in an intensive rehabilitation program, as for instance on weekends, the external collecting device may be discontinued and voiding can be attempted on a prescribed schedule. The objective is to make the patient aware of bladder distention and to teach him that he should void every two to three hours. Frequently the problem of urination seems to be more evident in the hospital or rehabilitation center than at home where the patient feels more comfortable and is closer to a bathroom. Elderly patients with benign prostate hypertrophy frequently require transurethral resection of the prostate. The prolonged use of an indwelling catheter or a suprapubic cystostomy should be discouraged.

The patient with an uninhibited neurogenic bowel can usually be taught to adhere to a good bowel routine. It is important to teach him to empty his bowel regularly every day or every other day at precisely the same time, either in the evening or in the morning. It is desirable to use the gastrocolic reflex, and therefore the bowel movement should be scheduled after a meal. Stool softeners may be used, but the patient should be advised that stool softeners only work with an adequate fluid intake. Mild laxatives such as Senokot granules or tablets, or milk of magnesia, can be recommended. If necessary, suppositories can be used to initiate a mechanical stimulus for bowel emptying. Irritating suppositories should be avoided if they have to be used over a prolonged period.

Required Equipment for Use at Home

The ambulatory hemiplegic patient usually requires only minimal equipment after discharge. In addition to a cane and possibly an orthotic lower extremity device for ambulation, he may not need more than grab bars in the bathroom and possibly a tub shower chair for his bathtub. Patients who are not completely ambulatory will require a wheelchair with a footrest on the paralyzed side, an elevated toilet seat, or if necessary, a shower commode chair. A hand-shower attachment is quite useful for patients with hemiplegia. Since activities such as transferring, dressing in bed, and coming up to a sitting position can only be accomplished with ease in a bed with a relatively firm mattress, the patient should use a bed with fairly hard support and a firm 3- to 5-inch-thick foam rubber mattress. The bed should preferably be at the same height as the wheelchair. A hospital bed is usually not required and its use should be discouraged whenever possible as evidence of a further return to normality.

Ataxia, Extrapyramidal Symptoms, Brain Stem Dysfunction

In rehabilitation medicine, the patient with ataxia represents a difficult challenge. He requires a prolonged course of meticulous and repetitive training. The key to success lies in daily, repeated coordination exercises for upper as well as lower extremities, initially supine, later on in the sitting position, and eventually standing. Many patients require assistive devices that are weighted to assure additional stability. Despite all rehabilitation efforts, it is still very difficult for the ataxic patient to operate without visual or auditory cues. It is therefore quite obvious that these patients will not be able to function safely in the dark.

Patients with extrapyramidal symptoms may require instructions in safety for performing activities of daily living. Patients

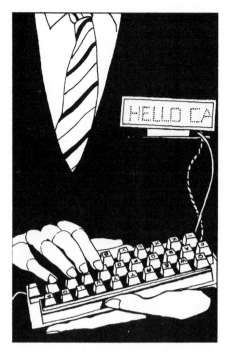

Figure 148–8   Talking Brooch to be used by anarthric or severely dysarthric patients who have residual upper extremity function. (Drawing by Deborah Rust originally appeared in Rehabilitation/WORLD. Reprinted by permission.)

with parkinsonism need instruction in daily range of motion exercises, in economical performance of their everyday energy-consuming tasks, and possibly in wheelchair activities.

Patients with brain stem dysfunction—for example, the "locked-in syndrome"—may require electronic devices for basic communication and the activities of daily living. The patient with severe dysarthria may need a simple spelling board or a Talking Brooch if he is able to use some fingers or one hand (Fig. 148–8).[2] Other electronic equipment available is described later.

REHABILITATION OF THE PATIENT WITH SPINAL CORD DYSFUNCTION

Early Management

Patients with traumatic spinal cord dysfunction, especially after fracture-dislocations of the spine, require early immobilization of the spine. During this period of immobilization it is of extreme importance to prevent skin breakdown by turning the

patient properly at least every two hours, either by log-rolling or by using a turning frame. At present the most commonly used technique is to immobilize and turn the patient on a Stryker frame. The once popular Circoelectric bed is now considered outdated for this purpose and useless if the patient needs cervical traction. Automatic beds that tilt or turn the patient have become quite popular but can never replace good nursing care, especially in the early phases of spinal cord dysfunction. When the patient is turned the skin should be inspected and cleaned carefully with soap and water, dried, and massaged lightly. A bland oil or neutral ointment may also be applied. If erythema of the skin appears that does not disappear after finger pressure, or if small decubitus ulcers have occurred, pressure on these areas should be eliminated until the skin returns to normal or healing has been accomplished. If the patient cannot be turned at all, bolsters have to be used and their location changed every two hours (Fig. 148–9). Every two hours, when the patient is being turned and repositioned, his lower extremities should be examined for circumferential differences to detect early signs of thrombophlebitis or ectopic bone formation.

Range of Motion

All joints of the affected extremities should be taken through their complete range of motion at least twice daily. Patients who have residual muscle power should be encouraged to move the joint actively as far as possible, and the therapist should complete the range of motion passively. Bed clothes should be kept loose over the foot of the bed in order to prevent shortened heel cords that might later interfere with proper foot positioning on the footrest of a wheelchair or with ambulation training.

Therapeutic Exercises

Muscle strengthening exercises should be started early with particular emphasis on conditioning the shoulder depressors, triceps, and latissimus dorsi. These are the muscles that most patients must use to perform push-ups in the wheelchair and, if in-

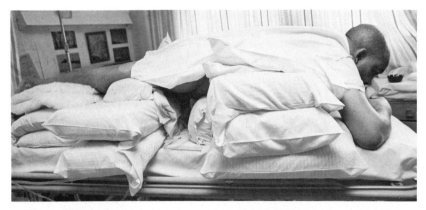

Figure 148-9   Quadriplegic patient positioned on bolsters in the prone position.

dicated, to ambulate with braces and crutches. Exercises for these muscles should be started early and increased in intensity as rapidly as possible (Figure 148–10). As soon as they can be tolerated, the patient will be started on mat activities to improve sitting balance and coordination. This may be done in a class and can make use of ball games (Fig. 148–11). The patient with quadriplegia will, in addition to this, require exercises taught by the occupational therapist that will help him to utilize existing musculature, and he will also learn to compensate for lost upper extremity function with or without adaptive devices.

Management of Spasticity

Spasticity that interferes with function should be treated. It is known that spasticity is aggravated by skin lesions, bladder problems (e.g., stones, infection), and muscle tightness. These aggravating factors should be eliminated if possible. All patients with spinal cord dysfunction and

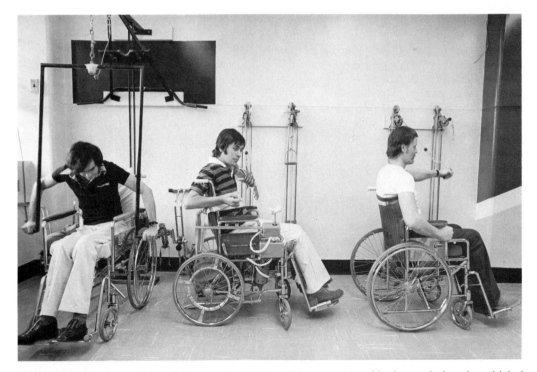

Figure 148-10   Progressive resistive exercises to strengthen upper extremities in paraplegic and quadriplegic patients. Latissimus bar on left, wall pulleys in middle and on right side. Note how elbow extension splint is used in order to exercise shoulder muscles of quadriplegic patient in middle.

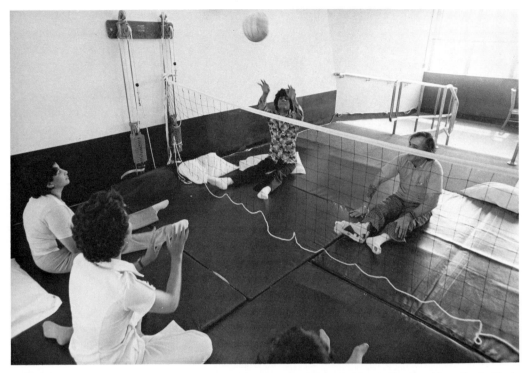

Figure 148–11   Mat class using ball game to promote sitting balance and coordination. (From Rusk, H. A.: Rehabilitation Medicine. 4th Ed. St. Louis, C. V. Mosby Co., 1977. Reprinted by permission.)

spastic paralysis experience muscle tightness on waking in the morning, but thorough stretching of the muscles seems to eliminate this effectively for the rest of the day and thus reduces spasticity and improves ability in activities of daily living. If spasticity still continues to interfere, medication with diazepam or dantrolene sodium should be considered. Dantrolene sodium is started with low dosages and increased gradually. Patients have to be carefully monitored for its possible hepatotoxic effects.

Destructive procedures such as subarachnoid phenol or alcohol blocks, as well as rhizotomies, should be considered only in rare cases, since they interfere with automatic bladder emptying and reflex erection in males.

Wheelchair Activities

Every paraplegic with strong upper extremities and adequate training should be completely independent in a wheelchair. This independence should not only include propelling the wheelchair and transferring independently from it to the bed and other furniture but should also include maintenance of the wheelchair and its use to jump curbs and small steps in either direction. This requires a good sense of balance and intensive training by an experienced physical therapist. Wheelchair training should include instructions in techniques for safely falling from the wheelchair and transferring into the chair from the floor (Fig. 148–12).

Erect Activities

It is important to stand the patient with spinal cord injury on a tilt board as soon as possible to help him overcome orthostatic hypotension as well as to improve trunk balance and coordination. Trunk exercises may be performed on tables with removable upper sections that support the hips and lower trunk only. Tilt table classes in which group ball games are played are excellent as balancing exercises (Fig. 148–13).

Braces are considered for many paraplegics. It should be recognized that functional ambulation can be achieved only with relatively low levels of paraplegia. The tenth

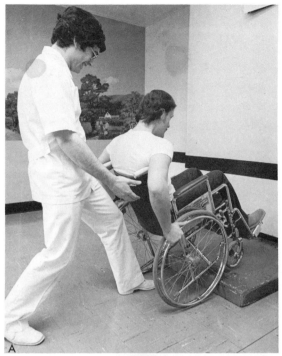

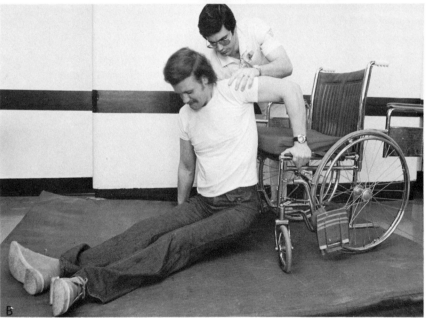

Figure 148–12 *A*. Patient with paraplegia performing "wheely" in order to climb small curb. *B*. Patient learning how to get into wheelchair from floor.

thoracic neurotome can be considered as a basic landmark. Conventional bracing consists of double-bar long leg orthoses with a pelvic band and a Knight spinal attachment for the back. These orthoses are usually fitted with sliding, box-type locks at the hip and knee joints. The ankle joints can have stirrup attachments with a 90-degree stop or may be the solid-ankle type for easier standing. Patients with preserved hip flexors and knee extensors (L3, L4 lesions) should become ambulatory with below-knee orthoses and two canes. The recently developed plastic orthoses are far more

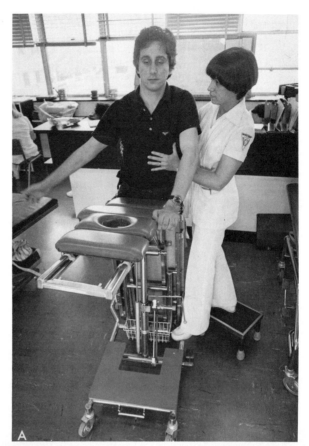

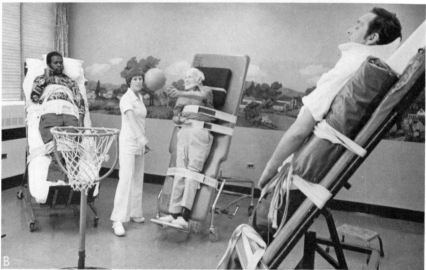

Figure 148–13   *A*. Swedish tilt table with removable sections can be used to strengthen trunk control in paraplegic patient. *B*. Tilt table class for patients with quadriplegia is being used to strengthen upper extremities and overcome orthostatic hypotension. (From Rusk, H. A.: Rehabilitation Medicine. 4th Ed. St. Louis, C. V. Mosby Co., 1977. Reprinted by permission.)

cosmetic than the usual metal orthoses.[10] Early ambulation with pneumatic orthoses allows the patient to try his ambulating ability before a more definitive orthosis is prescribed (Fig. 148–14).[13]

Driver Training

All paraplegics, as well as quadriplegics with intact C6 segments, should be able to learn how to drive an automobile. The automobile should be equipped with hand controls, and the quadriplegic may require some additional adaptive equipment. The paraplegic should learn to transfer into the automobile from the wheelchair to the driver's seat and be able to pull his wheelchair into the car afterward. The C6 quadriplegic may also be able to learn this procedure, but to eliminate the lengthy and difficult transfer procedure, he may alternatively use a van with an electric or hydraulic lift. In this case he can position the wheelchair behind the steering wheel and drive the van while seated in his own wheelchair (Fig. 148–15).

Functional Levels of Independence

In activities of daily living the patient is taught to take care of his own daily needs with transfers to the bed and the toilet, turning in bed, eating, and dressing and undressing as well as wheelchair activities, elevating, walking, climbing, and traveling. All paraplegic patients except those with severe spasticity should learn to become completely wheelchair independent in all activities of daily living. The chair should always be ordered carefully and with attention to individual problems. The patient with spinal cord dysfunction requires a bed with a foam rubber mattress on a firm support, which will allow him to sit up and roll in bed easily. The bed should be the same height as his wheelchair and should be positioned up against the wall. A grab bar should be attached to the wall for easier turning. The patient also requires a tub shower chair or a tub bench for showering in a bathtub or, preferably, a shower commode chair to be used as a toilet and for taking a shower in a roll-in cabinet-type shower. In addition to the foregoing, the patient needs urological equipment, frequently condom

drainage sets, leg bags, and drainage sets for bedside use for the male. A woman who requires intermittent catheterization can use a Walther sound. For skin protection many patients may require protective cushions in the wheelchair and occasionally also in bed. Alternating air mattresses are needed in only a very few cases, especially cases of high quadriplegia. For vocational and recreational pursuits, other adaptive equipment may be needed.

A C7 quadriplegic lacks intrinsic hand musculature as well as long finger flexors and extensors, and his wrist flexors are weak. He can, however, become completely independent in activities of daily living by using adaptive equipment, especially a short opponens orthosis to give him thumb opposition for tasks requiring dexterity. Some patients may benefit by reconstructive procedures in which fusion of thumb and finger joints may be combined with tendon transfers in order to provide a functional grasp and release mechanism. The time required for postoperative care and retraining by the occupational therapist is very long, however, and tends to delay the total rehabilitation process considerably.

The quadriplegic patient with an intact C6 neurotome will have basically intact shoulder musculature, elbow flexors, and wrist extensors. Approximately 50 per cent of such patients will achieve functional independence in a wheelchair if they are well motivated and able to start early on a rehabilitation program. These patients certainly need more adaptive equipment than has been mentioned. They are able to develop a tenodesis grasp, frequently aided by a wrist-driven prehension orthosis (Fig. 148–16). This group may require the most extensive and prolonged rehabilitation of all patients with spinal cord dysfunction. The patient with a C6 lesion should propel his own wheelchair manually if the wheelchair is adapted with vertical tips on the handrims. If, however, the patient needs to cover long distances either at college or at work, an electric wheelchair may be indicated.

Patients with a neurological lesion of the C5 segment and above require still more adaptive devices—for instance, a balanced forearm orthosis especially designed for feeding themselves, writing, and operating the electric wheelchair (Fig. 148–17). For those with even higher lesions, electronic

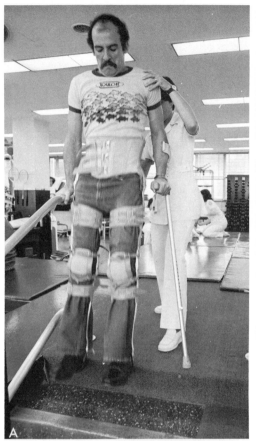

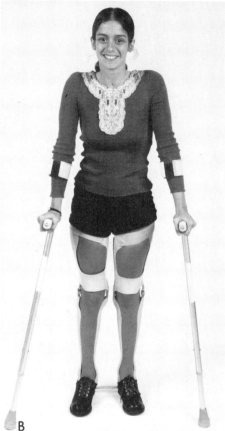

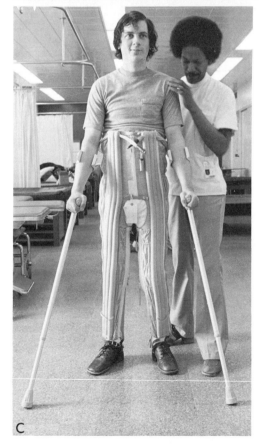

Figure 148–14 Lower extremity orthoses in paraplegia. *A*. Conventional double-bar long leg braces with Knight spinal attachment. *B*. Plastic laminated above-knee orthosis with solid ankle and rocker-bottom shoes. *C*. Pneumatic orthosis as a temporary device for early ambulation training. (*A* and *C* from Rusk, H. A.: Rehabilitation Medicine. 4th Ed. St. Louis, C. V. Mosby Co., 1977. Reprinted by permission.)

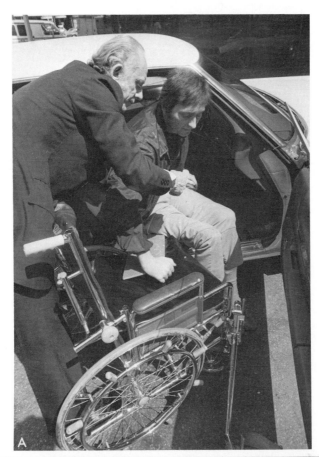

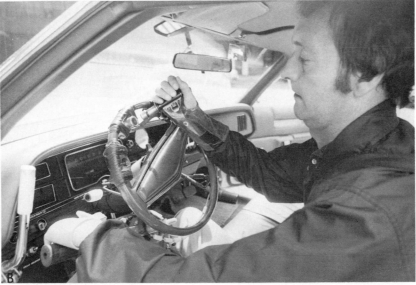

Figure 148–15   Driver training in quadriplegia. *A.* Transfer into two-door sedan from wheelchair by using sliding board. *B.* Use of adaptive devices and hand controls for driving. (From Rusk, H. A.: Rehabilitation Medicine. 4th Ed. St. Louis, C. V. Mosby Co., 1977. Reprinted by permission.)

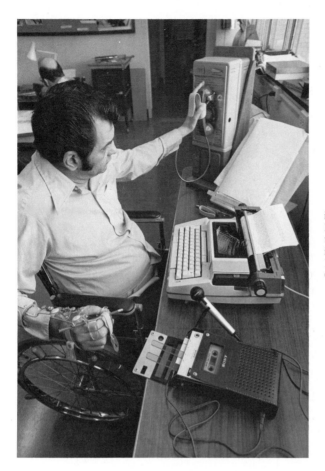

Figure 148–16 Quadriplegic patient with intact C6 neurotome using wrist-driven prehension orthosis on right hand and adaptations on tape recorder and telephone for easier use. (From Rusk, H. A.: Rehabilitation Medicine. 4th Ed. St. Louis, C. V. Mosby Co., 1977. Reprinted by permission.)

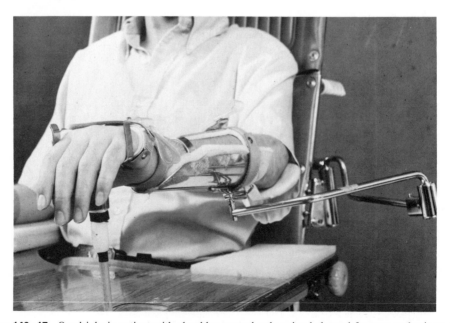

Figure 148–17 Quadriplegic patient with shoulder control only using balanced forearm orthosis to operate electric wheelchair.

devices are available that can be operated with pressure switches or microswitches or pneumatically. A wheelchair can be safely operated with these controls, and an environmental control unit allows the individual with high quadriplegia to perform some functions without help (Fig. 148–18). In the authors' experience, pneumatic "sip and puff" controls for wheelchairs and environmental units are favored by most patients with high quadriplegia. Environmental control units can be installed in home or office, and allow the quadriplegic patient to make telephone calls, operate radio and television sets, open and close curtains at windows, use a page turner and a tape recorder. Other systems allow the use of a typewriter, calculator, and computer terminals.

Management of Neurogenic Bladder and Bowel

At the time of injury or at the beginning of the spinal cord dysfunction, the bladder enters a stage of flaccid inactivity due to spinal shock. During this phase there is no reflex voiding; thus the bladder, unless catheterized, becomes greatly distended, emptying small amounts of urine by overflow incontinence.

It is known that during this stage of paralysis a degree of muscular activity persists through the action of autonomic nerve fibers within the bladder walls; hence the viscus is not truly atonic. This autonomic tonus plays a vital part in the functional evolution of some bladders and must be preserved. Overdistension quite promptly destroys this tonus and converts a partially functional detrusor into a hopelessly atonic sac. Prevention of overdistension is easily achieved by prompt catheterization.

Another factor of equal importance is the management of the catheter as a substitute for micturition. In the normal individual the bladder is an organ in continuous operation, specializing in filling and emptying itself while serving as a temporary reservoir for the excretory products of renal function. In the past, techniques such as tidal drainage or clamping of the catheter have been used to simulate bladder filling and emptying, but intermittent catheterization seems now to be the treatment of choice.[6] This is done every four to six hours, and a strict schedule for drinking fluids should be adhered to. When bladder automaticity occurs and the patient starts to void sponta-

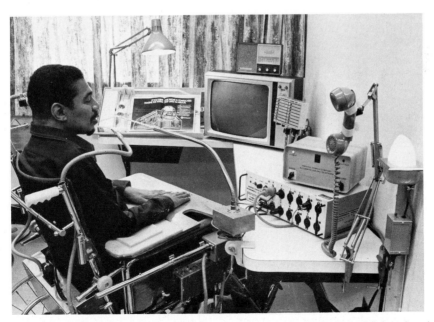

Figure 148–18 C4 quadriplegic using pneumatically controlled devices such as wheelchair and environmental control system. With the environmental control unit in this picture, the patient can operate (*left to right*) the light switch, a page turner, radio and television sets including channel change, opening and closing of curtain on window, telephone, and nurse call system. (From Rusk, H. A.: Rehabilitation Medicine. 4th Ed. St. Louis, C. V. Mosby Co., 1977. Reprinted by permission.)

neously, intermittent catheterization can be performed less frequently. Women with spinal cord injury may opt to continue with intermittent catheterization as a reliable means of controlling incontinence for the rest of their lives.

The man with a neurogenic bladder should learn to void without a catheter and to empty his bladder; an acceptable residual urine volume is 100 ml or less, depending upon bladder capacity. If residual urine volume remains high or if there is reflux, a transurethral bladder neck operation should be considered. External sphincterotomy seems to be the procedure of choice for patients who are unable to void or unable to achieve a low volume of residual urine.[14] It should be recognized, however, that this procedure will make the patient more incontinent and should preferably be performed only in male patients since they can use external collecting devices. This procedure should be combined with a transurethral resection of the prostate. A retrospective study covering a period of six years revealed that of 377 male patients with spinal cord injury, 24 per cent required transurethral operations to facilitate micturition.[9] Most of them underwent combined transurethral resection of the prostate and external sphincterotomy. The procedure is usually performed within six to twelve months of the onset of irreversible spinal cord dysfunction and is more frequently required by quadriplegic patients than by paraplegics.

In the urological rehabilitation of the patient with paraplegia, efforts are directed mainly toward complete or nearly complete emptying of the bladder. If this act can be accomplished at regular intervals, the patient should be considered as having satisfactory or balanced bladder function. The patient may aid emptying by straining and performing Credé maneuvers at reasonably regular times. The functionally adequate spastic reflex bladder is, however, a viscus of absolutely unpredictable action, dependent in some instances on peripheral spasms and in others on the stretch reflex within the detrusor muscle. The majority of these patients will require some sort of urinary apparatus for the involuntary and unpredictable evacuations characteristic of this type of erratic bladder function. External condom draining devices utilizing standard condoms attached via a drainage tube to a leg bag are the solution of choice for men. Most women will choose intermittent catheterization with a Walther metal sound. This sound is kept in a small tube with Zephiran solution. Intermittent catheterization can be performed either in bed or in a sitting position in a wheelchair.

In order to prevent complications of the urinary tract such as pyelonephritis, renal calculi, hydronephrosis with or without vesicoureteral reflux, and urethral diverticuli or fistulae, semiannual or annual urological re-evaluations are required. At this time an intravenous pyelogram should be performed together with a cystogram to outline both upper and lower urinary tracts. Cystoscopy is indicated, and any small bladder stones present should be removed at that time. The volume of residual urine after voiding should be determined, and cystometric studies should be performed. Cystometry can be combined with electromyographic examination of the rectal sphincter in order to ascertain the interaction of detrusor and sphincter. When the patient is catheterized for residual urine determination, urine for urinalysis and culture sensitivity studies should be obtained.

Most patients with a neurogenic bladder require agents to acidify the urine such as methenamine mandelate (Mandelamine) or methenamine hippurate (Hiprex) combined with vitamin C for a long time if not for lifetime. A diet low in calcium is recommended during the first few months of spinal cord dysfunction in order to avoid excessive calcium loading and to help prevent formation of urinary stones.

Management of the neurogenic bowel of the patient with spinal cord dysfunction is similar to treatment of the neurogenic bowel in the hemiplegic patient. Irritating laxatives or suppositories should be avoided whenever possible. Mild laxatives may be used 6 to 12 hours prior to bowel movement. Bowel movement may be initiated by a suppository, usually Vacuetts, Senokot, or glycerin suppositories. Later, digital stimulation may suffice to initiate evacuation of the lower bowel. It appears to be important that the patient empty his bowel in the sitting position either on the toilet or on a shower commode chair, preferably at the same time, either daily or every other day.

Management of Complications

Decubitus Ulcers

Decubitus ulcers should first be treated conservatively. The patient should not put any pressure on the ulcer. This means that in most instances he will be required to stay in bed until the ulcer has healed. If the decubitus ulcer is superficial, spontaneous healing may occur without operative intervention. The decubitus ulcer should be cleaned with soap and water or Betadine solution. If necessary, debridement of necrotic tissue may be performed either operatively or by using enzyme ointments. Occasionally hyperbaric oxygen can be used in cleaning and granulating a decubitus ulcer.[4] After the ulcer is clean and if spontaneous closure is unlikely within a reasonable time, plastic surgery should be considered. Preferably, a rotation flap should be constructed and should be advanced from as far away as possible in order to save tissue for further operative procedures. It is very important that the patient be taught to prevent further decubitus ulcers by frequent changes in position or by doing push-ups. When in bed, the patient with chronic spinal cord dysfunction may prefer to sleep in the prone position in order to avoid frequent changes from side to side during the night.[8]

Heterotopic Bone Formation

Extensive ectopic bone formation, sometimes referred to as paraosteoarthropathy or myositis ossificans, usually involving large segments of pelvic and thigh musculature, may be a troublesome complication of spinal cord dysfunction. Despite its impressive x-ray appearance, it usually does not produce grave symptoms. Excision may be considered if limiting joint contracture exists, but should, however, be considered only after the process has been stabilized as proved by bone scan and normal alkaline phosphatase values. Pharmacological treatment of ectopic bone formation and its prevention are still being investigated.[27]

Autonomic Hyperreflexia

A frequent complication is the occurrence of autonomic hyperreflexia. This condition is encountered in patients with spinal cord lesions above the level of the fifth thoracic neurotome and is the result of increased autonomic (mainly sympathetic) activity caused by a noxious stimulus below the level of the lesion. This stimulus is most frequently a distended bladder caused either by a spastic sphincter or by a blocked indwelling catheter. Other causes are urinary stones, severe bladder infections, bowel constipation, acute abdominal problems, or skin lesions such as inguinal rashes, ingrown toenails, and decubiti. With greatly elevated systolic and diastolic blood pressure, autonomic hyperreflexia presents with severe headache, profuse sweating, and bradykinesia, and can even lead to cerebral hemorrhage. Treatment should be geared to eliminating the noxious stimulus. Immediate bladder drainage will usually stop the autonomic crisis and make the patient more comfortable. The use of anticholinergic drugs should be allowed only if adequate bladder emptying can be assured. Recent biochemical studies have shown very high norepinephrine levels in the arterial blood during crises.[24,25]

Vocational Rehabilitation

Vocational rehabilitation of the patient with central nervous system lesions requires a highly individualized approach, involving negotiations with schools and employers. Only large rehabilitation centers are able to provide such counseling services to an optimal degree. Several studies conducted over the past decade reveal that more and more patients with severe disabling handicaps are returning to some form of gainful employment.

In a study conducted at the Institute of Rehabilitation Medicine, New York University Medical Center, 93 of 157 patients with brain injury were contacted after 15 years after injury, and 46 per cent were found to have returned to full employment.[17]

Vocational placement of quadriplegics seems to be even more promising. While a study conducted between 1948 and 1960 showed that only 39 per cent of rehabilitated quadriplegics were employed and 10 per cent were in college, a study conducted between 1962 and 1967 revealed that 34 per cent were in competitive employment, 2 per cent were homemakers, and 47 per cent were in school. Only 17 per cent were unemployed.[26] The authors' experience with quadriplegics who have successfully completed a college program indicates that this group has a highly successful employment record. It is quite obvious that vocational planning should start as early as possible in the rehabilitation process. It requires a dedicated effort not only by the rehabilitation team but also by the patient, his family, his employers, and his teachers.

Recreational Activities

A person with severe physical handicap is certainly limited in his choice of recreation. There are, however, many athletic activities that can be performed from a wheelchair. Every four years wheelchair athletes from around the world meet in the Para Olympic games and compete in various sports.[5] Many recreational activities can be modified, and the physically handicapped can participate in pursuits such as fishing, bowling, and riding. Paralyzed patients can join interest or consumer groups such as the National Paraplegic Foundation, the Paralyzed Veterans Association, or the Coalition for the Handicapped. These groups not only help the patient to maintain knowledge about development of new devices and ongoing research but also foster public awareness regarding architectural barriers, problems with public transportation systems, and various forms of discrimination.

Patient and Family Counseling

One of the most important tasks of the rehabilitation specialist is to guide the patient through the rehabilitation program. This can only be done with constant counseling of the patient and his family. The patient should not be considered a sick individual after his condition has stabilized following the acute stage. The physiatrist, as the leader of the rehabilitation team, should familiarize the patient with his condition as soon as possible—including the diagnosis and prognosis as well as sexual counseling —and help with his readjustment to social and family life.[12] The rehabilitation specialist should follow the disabled patient on a long-term basis and should act as a resource consultant for the neurosurgeon, the internist, or the general practitioner who follows the patient locally.

REFERENCES

1. Brudny, J., Korein, J., Grynbaum, B. B., Friedmann, L. W., Weinstein, S., Sachs-Frankel, G., and Belandres, P. V.: EMG feedback therapy; Review of treatment of 114 patients. Arch. Phys. Med., *57*:55–61, 1976.
2. Copeland, K., ed.: Aids for the Severely Handicapped. New York, Grune & Stratton, Inc., 1975.
3. Diller, L.: Perceptual and intellectual problems in hemiplegia: Implications for rehabilitation. Med. Clin. N. Amer., *53*:3:575–583, 1969.
4. Fischer, B. H.: Topical hyperbaric oxygen treatment of pressure sores and skin ulcers. Lancet, *2*:405, 1969.
5. Guttmann, L.: Textbook of Sport for the Disabled. Aylesbury, England. HM & M Publishers. Ltd. 1976.
6. Guttmann, L., and Frankel, H.: The value of intermittent catherization in the early management of traumatic paraplegia and tetraplegia. Paraplegia, *4*:63, 1966.
7. Hollander, J. L., and McCarty, D. J., Jr.: Arthritis and Allied Conditions. 8th Ed. Philadelphia, Lea & Febiger, 1972, pp. 1488–1499.
8. Kosiak, M.: Etiology and pathology of ischemic ulcers. Arch. Phys. Med., *40*:62–69, 1959.
9. Lee, I. Y., Ragnarsson, K. T., Sell, G. H., and Morales, P.: Transurethral bladder neck surgery in spinal cord injured patients. Arch. Phys. Med., *56*:549, 1975.
10. Lehneis, H. R.: New concepts in lower extremity orthotics. Med. Clin. N. Amer., *53*:3:585–592, 1969.
11. Licht, S.: Therapeutic Exercise. Baltimore, Waverly Press, Inc., 1965.
12. Mooney, O., Cole, T. M., and Chilgren, R. A.: Sexual Options for Paraplegics and Quadriplegics. Boston, Little, Brown & Co., 1975.
13. Ragnarsson, K. T., Sell, G. H., McGarrity, M., and Ofir, R.: Pneumatic orthosis for paraplegic patients: Functional evaluation and prescription considerations. Arch. Phys. Med., *56*:479–483, 1975.
14. Ross, J. C., Gibbon, N. O. K., and Damanski, M.: Division of external sphincter in the treatment of neurogenic bladder. A ten year review. Brit. J. Surg., *54*:627, 1967.
15. Rusk, H. A.: Rehabilitation Medicine. 4th Ed. St. Louis, C. V. Mosby Co., 1977, pp. 93–122.
16. Ibid., pp. 213–243.
17. Rusk, H. A., Block, J. M., and Lowman, E. W.: Rehabilitation of the brain injured patient. *In* Walker, A. E., Caveness, W. F., and Critchley, M., eds.: The Late Effects of Brain Injury. Springfield, Ill., Charles C Thomas, 1969.
18. Sarno, M. T.: The Functional Communication Profile Manual of Directions. Rehabilitation

Monograph 42. New York, Institute of Rehabilitation Medicine, New York University, 1969.

19. Sarno, M. T.: Understanding Aphasia. Patient Publication No. 2. New York, Institute of Rehabilitation Medicine, New York University Medical Center, 1973.

20. Sarno, M. T.: Disorders of communication in stroke. *In* Licht, S., ed.: Stroke and its Rehabilitation. Baltimore, Waverly Press, Inc., 1975, pp. 380–408.

21. Sarno, M. T., and Levita, E.: Natural course of recovery in severe aphasia. Arch. Phys. Med., *52*:175–179, 1971.

22. Schuell, H. M.: Minnesota Test for Differential Diagnosis of Aphasia. (Research Edition.) Minneapolis, University of Minnesota Press, 1955.

23. Schuell, H., Jenkins, J. J., and Jiminez-Pabon, E.: Aphasia in Adults. New York, Harper & Row, 1964.

24. Sell, G. H., Naftchi, N. E., Lowman, E. W., and Rusk, H. A.: Autonomic response in spinal man. Sixth International Congress of Physical Medicine, Barcelona, Spain, July 2–6, 1972. Madrid, Instituto Nacional de Previsión de Espana (Ministerio de Trabajo), 1974. Vol. I, pp. 723–727.

25. Sell, G. H., Naftchi, N. E., Lowman, E. W., and Rusk, H. A.: Autonomic hyperreflexia and catecholamine metabolites in spinal cord injury. Arch. Phys. Med., *53*:415–417, 1972.

26. Siegel, M. S.: The vocational potential of the quadriplegic. Med. Clin. N. Amer., *53*:3:713–718, 1969.

27. Stover, S. L., Hataway, C. H., and Zeiger, H. E.: Heterotopic ossification in spinal cord injured patients. Arch. Phys. Med., *56*:199–204, 1975.

28. Weinstein, E., ed.: Hemi-inattention in rehabilitation: The evolution of a rational remediation program. *In* Hemi-Inattention and Hemisphere Specialization. New York, Raven Press, 1977.

Index

In this index page numbers set in *italics* indicate illustrations. Page numbers followed by (t) refer to tabular material. Drugs are indexed under their generic names when dosage or action or special use is given. The abbreviation vs. is used to indicate differential diagnosis.

Abdomen, distention of, postoperative, 1106
  ganglioneuroma of, 3310
  in head injury in children, 2093
  in multiple trauma, 2520–2521
  in thoracic spinal injury, 2346
  pain in, in cancer, 3630, 3630(t)
    of unknown origin, 3631
Abdominal cutaneous nerve syndrome, 2463
Abducens nerve, anatomy of, orbital, 3027
  clinical examination of, 20
    in infants and children, 46, 56
  in percutaneous trigeminal rhizotomy, 3569, *3571*
  palsy of, 657, *657*
    in pseudotumor cerebri, 896
    increased intracranial pressure and, 878
Ablative procedures, 3769–3786
  in refractory pain, 3763–3765
ABLB test, 697, 2974
Abnormal movement disorders, 3821–3857. See also *Dyskinesias*.
Abscess. See also names of specific abscesses.
  actinomycotic, 3399
  brain, 3343–3355
    brain scanning in, 155(t), 159
    computed tomography in, 116, *118*, 3346, *3348*, 3355
    ultrasound in, 190
  epidural, 3333
    in head injury, 1915
  spinal, epidural, vs. viral encephalitis, 3360
    extradural, 3449–3451, *3450, 3451*
    subdural, 3451–3452, *3451*
  spinal cord, *3451*, 3452–3453, *3452*
  stitch, 1088
  subgaleal, 3328
Absence status, treatment of, 3878
Abulic trait, in normal-pressure hydrocephalus, 1424
Acceleration-deceleration injury, cervical, 2320, 2330–2332, 2338–2343, *2339*
Accident(s), care of spine in, cervical,
    thoracic, 2345
  cerebrovascular. See *Cerebrovascular accident* and *Stroke*.
Acetazolamide, cerebral blood flow and, 810(t)
  in pseudotumor cerebri, 3192
Acetylcholine, cerebral blood flow and, 808(t)
  metabolism of, 770
Achondroplasia, genetic aspects of, 1229, *1230, 1231*
  narrow spinal canal in, 2554
Acid-base balance, in multiple trauma, 2497–2500, *2498*, 2499(t)
Acid cholesteryl ester hydrolase deficiency, diagnosis of, 385(t)
Acidosis, metabolic, in multiple trauma, 2499
  respiratory, in head injury, in children, 2121
    in multiple trauma, 2500

Acoustic neuromas, 2967–3003
  angiography in, *317*, 2979–2985, *2982–2984*
  brain scanning in, 146, 150(t), 152, *153*
  computed tomography in, 122, *122*, 2976, *2977*
  diagnosis of, 2971–2992, *2974*
  operation(s) for, development of, 2968
    posterior fossa transmeatal, 2992–2997, *2992–2997*
    results of, *2998, 2999,* 2999–3000
  postoperative care in, 2997–2999
Acoustic reflex test, 700
Acrocephalopolysyndactyly, 1212–1213
Acrocephalosyndactyly, 1212–1213
Acrodysostosis, 1214
Acromegaloid appearance, vs. early acromegaly, 956
Acromegaly, 952–958
  diagnosis of, differential, 956
    potential pitfalls in, 955
  galactorrhea with, hormone secretion and, 964
  headache in, 3129
  histological study in, *3118*
  laboratory examination in, 953
  microadenoma in, 3124, *3125*
  pituitary tumor and, 952
  radiation therapy for, 3165, *3166*
  skull in, 3251
  study schedule for, 957
  treatment of, 956, 957(t)
    results of, 3146
  tumor herniation in, *3132*
Acrylic resin, cranioplasty with, 2236–2239, *2238–2240*
    advantages and complications of, 2241, *2241*
ACTH. See *Adrenocorticotropic hormone*.
Actinomycosis, 3398–3401
  meningitic, cerebrospinal fluid in, 462
Activities of daily living, in rehabilitation, 3996
Adamkiewicz, artery of, 553, *554, 556, 557, 561, 565*
Addison's disease, pseudotumor cerebri and, 3181(t)
Adenocarcinoma, ethmoid sinus, *3278,* 3279
  metastatic, tumor complexes of, *189*
  paranasal sinus, 3277
  scalp, 3319
Adenohypophysis, 935–970. See also *Anterior pituitary*.
  anatomy of, 3108
Adenoid cystic carcinoma, of paranasal sinuses, 3277
Adenoma, chromophobe, brain scanning in, *154*
  facial sebaceous, *1228*
  nonfunctioning chromophobe, radiation therapy of, 3164
  pituitary. See *Pituitary adenoma*.
Adenosine, cerebral blood flow and, 812(t)
Adenosine arabinoside, in herpes simplex encephalitis, 3363
Adenosine triphosphate, cerebral blood flow and, 812(t)

Adenosine triphosphate (*Continued*)
  depletion of, mechanisms retarding, 768, *769*
  production and utilization of, 767, *767*
Adenovirus, as carcinogen, 2675
Adie syndrome, genetic aspects of, 1223
  pupillary reactions in, 648, *649,* 649(t)
Adjustment reaction, "effected" pain and, 3498–3501
Adolescence, disc disease in, 2550
  epilepsy in, 3858–3909
Adrenal insufficiency, acute, preoperative, 1057
Adrenal steroids, urinary, in acromegaly, 955
Adrenalectomy, bilateral, vs. transsphenoidal hypophysectomy, 3949
  in Cushing's disease, 960
Adrenocortical dysfunction, pseudotumor cerebri and, 3185
Adrenocorticosteroids, in postoperative edema, 1091
Adrenocorticotropic hormone, cerebral blood flow and, 811(t)
  hypothalamic-pituitary relationship and, 943
  in afebrile seizures, 3876(t)
  insufficiency of, 945
  nature and function of, 939
  replacement of, in anterior pituitary failure, 949
Adrenoleukodystrophy, diagnosis of, 384(t)
Adult respiratory distress syndrome, in multiple trauma, 2487
Affective disorders, "effected" pain and, 3498–3501
  involving pain, 3727–3738
  primary, 3927–3943, *3930–3932,* 3934(t)–3936(t), *3938, 3939, 3941*
Age, as determinant of brain injury in children, 2088, *2089, 2090*
  brain abscess and, 3348
  brain tumor incidence and, *2682, 2683,* 2684, 2685(t), *2687*
  cerebral blood flow and, 799, 813, 826–827
  craniofacial operations and, 1470
  craniosynostosis operation and, 1464
  disc disease and, 2550–2551
  meningioma incidence and, 2936, 2937(t)
  post-traumatic epilepsy and, 2190
  prognosis after head injury and, 2141, 2142(t)
  supratentorial tumors and, in children, 2702, 2704(t)
Aggressiveness, pathological, epilepsy and, 3883
Agyria, during morphogenesis, 1211(t)
Air conduction audiometric testing, 695
Air embolism, Doppler ultrasound in, 738, *739, 740*
  during operative procedures, 1070
  following pneumoencephalography, 368
  sitting position and, 1132
Air encephalography. See *Pneumoencephalography.*
Air myelography, in spinal angioma, 578, *578*
  in stereotaxic cordotomy, 3676, *3676*
Airway, adequate, provision of, 1119
  in multiple trauma, 2476–2479
  obstruction of, acute respiratory failure and, 1014
Akathisia, in Parkinson's disease, 3838
Akinetic mutism, 63
Albers-Schönberg disease, of skull, 3255
Albumin, serum, intrathecal injection of, in cerebral death, 755(t)
Alcohol, absolute, administration of, 3658, *3658*
  as neurolytic agent, 3657
  in trigeminal neuralgia, 3559–3560
  results of, 3660
Alcoholism, cerebrospinal fluid in, 471
  chronic, cerebral blood flow in, 807
  operations for, 3942
Aldosterone, secretion of, post-traumatic, 992
Alexander disease, brain biopsy in, 386(t)
Aliquorrhea, cerebrospinal fluid in, 471
Alkaline phosphatase, serum, in acromegaly, 954
Alkalosis, metabolic, in head injury in children, 2121
  in multiple trauma, metabolic, 2499
  respiratory, 2500
Allergic reaction(s), intracranial hypertension in, 3180(t)
  postoperative, 1112
Alloplastic material, in cranioplasty, 2233–2241, *2234, 2235, 2238–2241,* 2245
  in maxillofacial injuries, 2296

n-Allylnormorphine, cerebral blood flow and, 811(t)
Alpers disease, brain biopsy in, 386(t)
Alpha adrenergic blocking agent, cerebral blood flow and, 809(t)
Alpha motoneuron, in dyskinesias, 3826
Alternate binaural loudness balance test, 697
  in acoustic neuroma, 2974
Aluminum, cranioplasty with, 2236
Alveolus, anatomy of, 1005
Alzheimer disease, brain biopsy in, 386(t)
  vs. normal-pressure hydrocephalus, 895
Amantadine, in Parkinson's disease, 3842
Amaurosis. See *Blindness.*
Amblyopia, suppression, definition of, 652
Ambulation, in hemiplegia, 3995, *3996–3998*
  in spina bifida aperta, 1273
Amebiasis, 3367–3370
Amenorrhea-galactorrhea syndrome, causes of, 3119
  invasive adenoma in, 3127, *3127*
American Association of Neurological Surgeons guidelines in cerebral death, 757
Amino acids, in cerebrospinal fluid, 451
  postischemic concentrations of, 778, *779*
Aminoglycosides, in bacterial infections, 3326
  inner ear changes and, 692
Aminophylline, cerebral blood flow and, 810(t)
  in cerebral vasospasm, 820
Amitriptyline, in anxiety and depression, 3500
  in chronic pain syndrome, 3758
  in compulsive personality, 3504
  in peripheral neuropathy, 3641
  in postherpetic neuralgia, 3642
  in spinal cord injury, 3624
Ammon's horn sclerosis, 3860
Ammonium chloride, cerebral blood flow and, 811(t)
Amnesia, following head injury, 2167
  in post-traumatic syndrome, 2181
  prognosis after head injury and, 2147
  transient global, in ischemic vascular disease, 1531–1532
Amobarbital-pentylenetetrazol, in children, 3896
Amphetamine sulfate, cerebral blood flow and, 808(t)
Amphotericin B, in blastomycosis, 3407
  in coccidioidomycosis, 3412
  in cryptococcosis, 3415
  in histoplasmosis, 3418
  in paracoccidioidomycosis, 3422
  in phycomycosis, 3426
Ampicillin, in bacterial infections, 3326
  in bacterial meningitis, 3339
Amputation, pain of, 3637, 3637(t)
Amygdalectomy, stereotaxic, for destructive behavior, 3942
  in temporal lobe epilepsy, 3925
Amygdalotomy, stereotaxic, in epilepsy, in children, 3897
Anal sphincter, electromyography of, 627
Analgesia, following mesencephalotomy, 3709
  following open cordotomy, 3696
Anaplastic astrocytoma, 2788
Anastomoses, arterial, extracranial to intracranial, 1584–1618
  cervical carotid to intracranial carotid bypass graft in, 1611
  to increase cerebral blood flow, 832
  posterior fossa revascularization by, 1611–1613
  superficial temporal artery to middle cerebral artery, 1585–1611, *1586–1593,* 1594(t)–1596(t), *1597–1599, 1601–1605, 1608–1610*
  micro-operative techniques in, 1169, 1585
Androgens, in anterior pituitary failure, 950
Anemia, cerebral blood flow in, 822
  hemolytic, familial, skull involvement in, 3261
  of infancy and childhood, skull in, 3261, *3263*
  pernicious, cerebrospinal fluid in, 468
  postoperative, 1099
  prognosis after head injury and, 2145, 2146(t)
  pseudotumor cerebri and, 3181(t), 3187
Anencephaly, 1219
  fetal, ultrasound scanning in, *721*
  incidence of, 1218(t)

Anencephaly (*Continued*)
  morpnogenetic timing of, 1211(t)
Anesthesia, 1119–1135
  conduction, diagnostic uses of, 3644, *3645–3647*
    in pain management, 3644–3663
    intrathecal neurolytic agents in, 3655, *3656*
  electroencephalography during, 227, *227, 228*
  epidural, 3648
    for relief of pain, 3652
  general, 1121
    in spinal operations, 1152
  in aneurysm procedures, anterior circulation, 1667
    posterior circulation, 1722
  in angiography, cerebral, 233
    of spine, 556
  in closed head injury, 2024
  in diagnostic procedures, 1124
  in electrocorticography, 1123
  in epilepsy in children, 3883
  in posterior fossa procedures, 1123
    for tumors in children, 2742–2743
  in stereotaxic procedures, 1123, 3673
  in temporal lobectomy, 3883
  increased intracranial pressure and, 901
  local, 1120
  monitoring in, 1130
  neuroleptanalgesia as. See *Neuroleptanalgesia.*
  position of patient for, 1131–1133
  premedication for, 1062, 1120
  principles of, 1119–1123
  special considerations in, 1123
  special techniques for, 1124–1131
Anesthesia dolorosa, following percutaneous rhizotomy, 3575
Anesthetics, cerebral blood flow and, 804–807
  postischemic survival and, 780
  reversible local, 3644–3655
    diagnostic uses of, 3644, *3645–3647, 3650, 3651*
    therapeutic uses of, 3652
  volatile, 1122
Aneurysms, 1663–1785
  angiography in, carotid, 289, *289, 290, 299, 300–304,*
    1665–1666
  anterior cerebral artery, 1682–1686, *1683,* 1684(t)
  anterior circulation, 1663–1714
    anatomy in, 1667
    carotid occlusion in, 1967–1711, *1702, 1705–1707,* 1710(t)
    clinical presentation of, 1664
    intracranial procedures in, 1663–1692
      adjuncts to, 1667
      micro-operative technique in, 1668, *1669, 1670–1673*
      results of, 1686, 1688(t)–1691(t)
      timing of, 1666
    radiological investigation of, 1665
  anterior communicating artery, 1682–1686, *1683,* 1684(t)
  anterior inferior cerebellar artery, 1741, *1743, 1744,* 1746(t)
  basilar artery, at anterior inferior cerebellar artery, 1741, *1743, 1744,* 1746(t)
    at bifurcation, 1729, 1739(t), *1743,* 1761(t)
    at superior cerebellar artery, 1740, 1742(t), *1743*
    at vertebral junction, 1745
  berry, genetic aspects of, 1224
  carotid artery, extracranial, as indication for operation, 1568–1569, *1569*
    internal, *1635,* 1677–1681, *1678–1680,* 1690(t), 1701
    intracavernous, 1678–1679, *1764,* 1766–1771
  cirsoid, of scalp, skull in, 3250
  clipping of, 1674–1675
  computed tomography in, 123, *124,* 138, *139,* 1666
    postoperative, 134
  extracranial to intracranial arterial anastomosis in, 1603, *1604*
  giant, anterior, carotid ligation in, 1701
    posterior, 1749, 1752(t), *1754, 1758*
    subarachnoid hemorrhage and, 1815–1816
  headache and, 1664, 3552

Aneurysms (*Continued*)
  ligation of, 1675
    middle cerebral artery, *1631, 1633,* 1681–1682, *1681, 1683,* 1684(t)
  multiple, anterior, 1665, 1676
    posterior, 1760
    subarachnoid hemorrhage and, 1814–1815
  mycotic, 1812–1814
  nonoperative treatment of, 1645–1653, 1646(t), 1649(t), 1650(t), *1650–1652,* 1652(t)
  posterior cerebral artery, 1738, 1740(t)
  posterior circulation, 1715–1761, *1716*
    anatomy in, 1717, 1717(t)
    clinical features of, 1719
    natural history of, 1718
    operative techniques in, 1721, *1727–1729, 1731, 1734, 1736*
    radiological diagnosis of, 1720
    results of, 1722(t), 1738, 1739(t), 1740, 1740(t), 1741, 1742(t), 1745, 1746(t), 1749, 1749(t)
    subtemporal approach to, 1724, 1726
  rupture of, 1676
    increased intracranial pressure and, 891
  sphenoid, parasellar involvement in, 3155
  subarachnoid hemorrhage and, 1630–1637, *1631–1633,* 1634(t), 1635, 1812–1816
  superior cerebellar artery, 1740, 1742(t), *1743*
  thrombosis of, induced, 1676
  traumatic, 1702
    of cavernous plexus, 1770–1771
    subarachnoid hemorrhage and, 1811–1812
  vertebral artery, 1746, 1746(t), *1747, 1748,* 1749(t)
    at basilar junction, 1745, 1746(t)
  wrapping (encasement) of, 1675
Aneurysmal bone cyst, embolization of, 1202
  of orbit, 3056
  spinal angiography in, 610–611
    in children, *3216*
Angiitis, noninfectious granulomatous, 1546
  cerebrospinal fluid in, 463
  in sarcoidosis, 3428
Angina pectoris, sympathectomy for, 3720, 3721
Angiofibroma, subungual, *1228*
Angiography, cerebral, 231–350
    abnormal angiogram in, 282–344, *285–295, 297–317, 319–327, 329–335, 337–344*
    approaches in, 232
    catheter preparation for, 242–244, *242, 243*
    catheterization techniques in, 246, 253
    contrast media in, 242
    equipment for, 232
    extracranial lesions and, 282, *283–295*
    interval between films in, 242
    normal angiogram in, 256–282, *256, 258–284*
    normal arterial anatomy in, 256, *256, 258–270, 272–279*
    normal venous anatomy in, 280, *280, 281*
    preparation and positioning of patient for, 233
    prognosis after head injury and, 2148, 2149(t)
    projections used in, 233–241, *234–241*
    technique of, 231–256
      percutaneous, 246, 253
      via carotid artery, 232, 244–256, *244, 246, 247.* See also *Carotid angiography.*
      premedication in, 1120
      via vertebral artery, 232, 252, *253, 254.* See also *Vertebral angiography.*
  in acoustic neuroma, 2980, *2982–2984, 2988*
  in aneurysms of anterior circulation, 1665–1666
    arterial buckling and, 289, *289, 290*
  in arachnoid cysts, 1439
  in arteriovenous fistulae, 291, *291, 292*
  in arteriovenous malformations, spinal, 562–604, 1854. See also *Angioma, spinal.*
  in astrocytomas, 2775
  in brain abscess, 3346, *3347, 3349*

INDEX

Angiography (*Continued*)
in carotid body tumors, 292, *294*
in cavernous plexus lesions, 3015, *3021*
in cerebral death, *751, 752*
in cerebral infarction, 1536
in congenital lesions, 292, *293*
in Dandy-Walker malformation, 1295–1296
in empty sella syndrome, 3173
in encephalocele, *1300,* 1302
in epilepsy, in children, 3873, *3874*
in glioblastoma, 2811, *2811*
in glomus jugulare tumor, 3288, *3288–3291*
in head injury, 1981–1987, *1982–1986,* 2023
in hemangioblastoma of brain, 2851, *2851*
in hydrocephalus, in children, 1396, *1396, 1397, 1403*
in intracerebral and intracerebellar hemorrhage, 1833
in intracranial aneurysms, 299, *300–304*
in intracranial lesions, 296–344, *297–317, 319–327, 329–335, 337–344*
in lymphoma of brain, 2841
in metastatic tumors, 2877
in meningioma, 2944
in orbital tumors, 3038
in pineal tumors, 2866
in pituitary adenoma, 3133, *3135*
in postoperative tissue edema, 1091
in pseudotumor cerebri, 3182, 3188
in spinal cord tumors, 3202, *3204*
in stroke, 1621, *1622*
in subarachnoid hemorrhage, 1630, 1630(t)
in subdural empyema, 3335, *3336*
in supratentorial brain tumors, in children, 2706, *2707*
in sylvian fissure cyst, 1439
in tuberculoma, 3443, *3443*
in vascular occlusive disease, 282, *285–288,* 296, *297–299,* 1573, 1597, *1597–1599*
of extracranial carotid artery, *1572,* 1573
in vertebromedullary tumors, 604–612, *604–608, 610, 611*
spinal cord, 551–616
abnormal angiograms in, 562–615, *563–588,* 589(t), *590–608, 610, 611, 613–615*
in ischemia from atheromatous or disc lesions, 612–615, *613–615*
normal anatomy in, 551–555, *551–556*
normal angiogram in, *558,* 559–562, *559–562*
technique of, 555–558, *556, 557*
Angioma(s). See also *Hemangioma* and *Lymphangioma*.
cavernous, 1637
spinal, 562–604
clinical classification of, 562, 563
clinical symptoms of, 563, *564–569*
distribution of, 588
draining veins of, 584, *587, 588*
embolization of, 589, *596–602,* 1199–1200, *1199*
general characteristics of, 579, *579*
intramedullary, classification of, 589(t), *590–595*
mass of, 582, *585–587*
mixed treatment of, 602, *603*
myelographic appearance of, *536*
nutrient vessels of, 579, *580–584*
radiological evaluation of, 569, *570–588,* 589(t)
angiography in, 579, *579–588*
gas myelography in, 578, *578*
plain and tomographic x-rays in, 569, *570–574*
positive contrast myelography in, 569, *575–577*
results of treatment of, 602
venous, 1638
Angiomatosis, hereditary, central nervous system in, 1224, 1225(t)
Angiostrongyliasis, 3395–3398
meningitic, cerebrospinal fluid in, 462
Angiotensin, vessel constriction and, 819
Angiotensin amide, cerebral blood flow and, 809(t)
Ankle, tibial nerve injury at, 2404

Ankylosing spondylitis, osteotomy in, 2641, *2644*
radiography of, 509, *509*
Anomalies, developmental and acquired, 1205–1508. See also *Malformations* and names of specific anomalies.
Anosmia, genetic aspects of, 1223
head injury and, 2165
hypophysectomy by craniotomy and, 3984
Anoxia, epileptogenic focus in, 3862
increased intracranial pressure in, 894
Anterior cerebral artery, aneurysms of, 1682–1686, *1683,* 1684(t), 1691(t)
occlusion of, 296
radiological anatomy of, 261, *262*
Anterior choroidal artery, radiological anatomy of, 261, *262*
Anterior communicating artery, aneurysm of, *301, 303,* 1682–1686, *1683,* 1684(t), 1691(t)
carotid ligation in, 1701–1702, *1702,* 1709
Anterior decompression, in craniovertebral anomalies, 1502
Anterior horn cell disease, electromyography in, 633, 634(t)
in neonates, 48
Anterior inferior cerebellar artery, aneurysms of, 1741–1744, *1743, 1744*
cranial nerve root compression by, 3778, *3778–3780*
in cisternal myelography, 527
radiological anatomy of, 275
Anterior interosseous nerve, entrapment of, 2449–2451, *2450*
Anterior pituitary, 935–970
failure of, 943
classification of causes of, 944(t)
detection of, schedule for, 951
laboratory studies in, 946, 946(t)
replacement therapy in, 948
hormones of, cells and, 935, 938(t)
nature and function of, 938
hyperfunction of, 951
hypothalamus and, 940
Anterior spinal artery, anatomy of, 554–555, *555*
angiography of, *558–561,* 559–561
Anterior spinal artery syndrome, *545*
Anthracene compounds, as carcinogens, 2673–2674
Antibiotics in bacterial infections, 3325–3327. See also names of specific drugs.
brain abscess and, 3349, 3350
in multiple trauma, 2529–2530
in postoperative wound infection, 1089
inner ear changes and, 692
intraoperative, 1063
preoperative, 1061
prophylactic, in pediatric hydrocephalus, 1409
Anticholinergics, in Parkinson's disease, 3842
Anticoagulation, in cerebral infarction, 1537, 1537(t)
of cerebrospinal fluid, 457
Anticonvulsants, in febrile seizures, 3875
in head injury, 2043, 2054
prophylactic, 2191–2193
in localized brain and skull injuries, 2054
in metastatic tumors, 2883
in supratentorial tumors in children, 2709
starting dosages of, 3877(t)
withdrawal of, to localize epileptogenic focus in children, 3870
Antidepressants, in chronic pain syndrome, 3758
tricyclic, in objective pain, 3489
Antidiuretic hormone, function of, 972
in neurohypophyseal diabetes insipidus, 975–977
inappropriate secretion of, 980–983, 980(t)
postoperative, 1100
subarachnoid hemorrhage and, 1658
synthesis of, 970
Antiemetics, as premedication, 1120
Antifibrinolytic agents, in subarachnoid hemorrhage, 1650–1652, 1650(t), *1650–1652,* 1652(t)
Antiganglionic agents, in detrusor hyperreflexia, 1041
Antihypertensive drugs, cerebral blood flow and, 809(t)
in intracerebral or intracerebellar hemorrhage, 1840–1841
in subarachnoid hemorrhage, 1649–1650

Antimicrobial agents, in bacterial infections, 3325–3327. See also *Antibiotics* and names of specific drugs.
Anuria, postoperative, 1105
Anxiety, ''effected'' pain and, 3481, 3498–3501
Aorta, coarctation of, subarachnoid hemorrhage and, 1807–1808
Apert syndrome, 1212
  characteristics of, 1471
Aphasia, as indication for carotid operation, 1565
  in intracranial disorders, 3996
  tests for, 3997
Aplasia cutis congenita, 1215
Apnea, episodic, Arnold-Chiari malformation and, 1286
  neonatal episodes of, 40
  posthyperventilation, in unconscious patient, 65
    prognosis after head injury and, 2153
  sleep, postcordotomy, 3698
Aponeurosis, scalp, anatomy of, 2299, *2299*
Apoplexy. See also *Stroke.*
  pituitary, 948, 3148
Aqueduct, in hydrocephalus, congenital stricture of, 1434
  stenosis of, 1430
  stenosis of, in childhood, 3364
Arachnoid, cysts of, 1436–1446
  cerebellopontine angle, cisternal myelography in, *528*
  clival, 1442
  computed tomography in, 136, *136*, 1439, *1441*, *1443*
  differential diagnosis of, 1436–1437, 1438
  distribution of, 1437, 1438(t), *1439*
  intracranial, 1439, *1440*, *1441*, *1443*
  parasellar, 3155
  pathogenesis of, 1437–1438, *1437*
  posterior fossa extra-axial, vs. Dandy-Walker malformation, 1293(t)
  post-traumatic, 2205–2208, *2206*, *2207*
  spinal, 1443, *1444*, *1445*
    of lumbar and sacral roots, 1445
  symptoms and signs of, 1438–1445
  thoracic spinal, ultrasound scanning of, *733*
  formation of, 1240
  villi of, cerebrospinal fluid absorption and, 428
Arachnoiditis, *3620*
  basal, 1492
  chronic adhesive, as complication of disc operation, 2549
    open cordotomy in, 3696
  in chronic low back pain, 3615, *3615*
Areflexia, detrusor, 1039–1040, *1039*, 1043–1045
Argyll Robertson pupil, 649
Arhinencephaly, morphogenetic timing of, 1211(t)
Arm, median nerve in, entrapment of, 2452
  paralyzed, rehabilitation of, 3991–3995, *3993*, *3994*
  radial nerve injury in, 2395–2396
Arnold-Chiari malformation, 1278–1288, 1489–1490, *1490*
  abnormal embryology of, 1280
  anatomical anomalies associated with, 1280(t)
  classification of, 1283, *1283*
  definition of, 1278
  management of, 1286, *1287*
  morphogenetic timing of, 1211(t)
  pathology of, 1278(t), 1281
  pneumoencephalography in, *360*
  spina bifida aperta with, 1253
  ultrasound scanning in, *722*
  vs. Dandy-Walker malformation, 1222, *1222*
Arnold's head, in cleidocranial dysplasia, 1213
Arsenic poisoning, intracranial hypertension in, 3180(t)
Arteriography. See also *Angiography.*
  carotid, brain scanning after, 161
    in brain tumors, results of, 168(t)
  in carotid artery occlusion, 1700
  in metastatic tumors, 2877
  in spinal angiography, 557
  postoperative, in superficial temporal to middle cerebral arterial anastomosis, 1608–1610, *1608–1610*
Arterioles, diameter of, cerebral blood flow and, 791

Arteriosclerosis, as contraindication to carotid ligation, 1703
  carotid-cavernous aneurysm and, 1768–1770
  cerebral, cerebrospinal fluid in, 466
  superficial temporal to middle cerebral arterial anastomosis in, 1600
  tic douloureux and, 3594
Arteriovenous fistulae, angiography in, 291, *291*, 292
  carotid-cavernous, 1764, 1771–1782, *1772*, 1773(t), *1776–1778*
  supplied by artery of Adamkiewicz, 575
Arteriovenous malformation(s), brain scanning in, 155(t), 159. *160*
  in children, 162
  cerebral blood flow in, 821, 828, *829*
  characteristics of, 1637
  computed tomography in, 123, *123*
    vs. radionuclide imaging, 167(t)
  dynamic vs. static imaging in, 163
  intracranial, embolization of, 1195, 1196, *1196–1198*
  of brain, 1786–1806
    diagnosis of, 1789
      neuropsychological, 711, 712
    etiology and pathophysiology of, 1787
    in newborn infant, 45
    pathology of, 1788
    treatment of, 1789, *1793–1803*
      nonoperative, 1653–1654, 1653(t)
  of spinal cord, 1850–1872
    anatomy in, 1850
    angiography of, 562–604. See also *Angioma, spinal.*
    cervical intramedullary, 1858, *1859*, 1869, *1871*
    classification of, 562–563, *563*, 1856, *1857*
    epidural, 1869, *1872*
    glomus, 1858, 1866, *1868*
    juvenile, 1858
    long dorsal, 1856, *1857*, 1863, *1863–1867*
    radiological investigation of, 1854, *1855*, *1856*
    syndromes and natural history, 1853
    treatment of, 1859, *1861–1868*, *1870–1872*
  orbital, 3055
  subarachnoid hemorrhage from, 1653–1654
Arteritis, cranial (temporal), 1550
  cephalic pain and, 3538–3539
Arteries. See also *Blood vessels* and names of specific arteries.
  aging of, cerebral blood flow and, 813, *814*
  anatomy of, normal radiological, 256, *256*, *258–270*, *272–279*
    orbital, 3026–3027, *3025*
  angiography of, 256. See also *Angiography.*
  buckling of, angiography in, 289
  extracranial, cerebral blood flow and, in hypertension, 828, *829*
  occlusions of, intracranial, operative management of, 1619–1626
    mechanisms of, 1515
  operation on, increased cerebral blood flow and, 831
  orbital, 3026
  radiculomedullary, *552*, *553*
  rupture of, cerebral blood flow and, 819
  spasm of, in subarachnoid hemorrhage, 819
  stenosis of, angiographic appearance of, *614*
    cerebral blood flow and, 814, *815*
Arthrosis, cervical spinal, etiology of, 2578–2591, *2579–2590*
Aseptic meningitis. See *Meningitis, aseptic.*
Aspartate, metabolism of, 771
Aspergillosis, 3402–3405
Asphyxia neonatorum, 2126
Aspiration, in acute respiratory failure, 1015
  of brain abscess, 3350, *3352*
  of cyst, in craniovertebral junction anomalies, 1500–1502, *1501*
  pneumonia from, in multiple trauma, 2483–2484
Assaultiveness, operations for, 3941
Astroblastoma, 2788
Astrocytoma, 2765–2779
  anaplastic, 2788

Astrocytoma (*Continued*)
  brain scanning in, 150, 150(t), *152, 2775*
    in children, 162(t)
  cerebellar, in children, 2746–2747, 2775
  cerebral hemisphere, in children, 2711–2712, *2711,* 2712(t)
  computed tomography in, 114, *114, 115,* 2775, *2775, 2776*
  cranial, malignant, chemotherapy of, 3065
    radiation therapy of, 3098, 3098(t), 3099(t)
  gemistocytic, 2769, *2769*
  grading of, 2769
  high-pressure hydrocephalus and, 1433
  hypothalamic, 139
  incidence of, 2765–2766
  investigation of, 2774–2776, *2774, 2776*
  location of, 395(t)
  pathogenesis of, 2766
  pathology of, 2766–2771, *2767–2769, 2771, 2772*
  pilocytic, 2779–2786, *2781, 2784–2786,* 3154
  radiation therapy of, 3098, 3098(t), 3099(t), 3212, 3224(t)
  spinal, 3197, 3197(t), 3206–3207
    in children, *3216*
    operative treatment of, 3210, *3210*
    ultrasound scanning of, *730, 731*
  static radionuclide image in, 149
  subependymal giant cell, 2786–2788
  suprasellar, in children, 2719
  supratentorial, in children, 2729–2730, 2729(t)
  tumor complexes of, *189*
Ataxia, acute cerebellar, in children, vs. cerebellar tumors, 3360
  hereditary, cerebrospinal fluid in, 468
  in posterior fossa tumors in children, 2736
  in supratentorial tumors in children, 2706
  rehabilitation of patient with, 3999
Atelectasis, multiple trauma and, 2487
  postoperative, 1094
  pulmonary contusion and, *1020*
Atherosclerosis, aortocranial, dementia in, 1529–1530
  cerebral, cerebral blood flow in, 816
  superficial temporal to middle cerebral arterial anastomosis in, 1600
  ultrasound scanning in, *735, 736*
Athetosis, clinical diagnosis of, in child, 39
Atlas, axis and, dislocation of, 1486, *1487*
  fusion of, in craniovertebral junction anomalies, 1502–1506, *1503–1505*
  development of, 1482, *1483*
  occipitalization of, 1484–1485, *1486, 1487*
Atony, sphincter, 1041, 1046
Atresia, congenital, of foramina of Magendie and Luschka, in Dandy-Walker malformation, 1288–1289
  venous sinus, in pseudotumor cerebri, 3181(t)
Atrophy, cerebral, computed tomography in, 132, *133*
  cranial defects and, 2230–2231, *2232*
  optic, in newborn, 46
Atropine, as premedication, 1120
  for therapeutic embolization, 1195
  as test, in cerebral death, 755, 755(t)
  in angiography, 233
Audiometric testing, 694–700, *696*
  in acoustic neuroma, 2972
Auditory canal, carcinoma of, 3281, *3282*
  internal, in cisternal myelography, *527*
Auditory meatus, internal, anatomy of, 680, *681, 682,* 2251
Autofluoroscope, invention of, 143
Autoimmune disease, ischemic vascular, 1543
Autonomic nervous system, spinal flow of, 3717, *3718*
Autopsy, brain, in cerebral death, 755(t), 756
Autoregulation, of cerebral blood flow, 792–794, *792*
  intracranial pressure and, 866–868
  metabolic, 793–794, 869
Avitaminoses, cerebrospinal fluid in, 471
Avulsion, nerve, in trigeminal neuralgia, 3561
  of scalp, 2302–2311, *2303–2309*

Axilla, median nerve injury at, 2389–2390
  radial nerve injury at, 2396
  ulnar nerve injury at, 2392–2393
Axis, development of, 1482, *1483*
  malformation of, 1486, *1487*
Axon, injury to, 2363–2365
  regeneration of, time and distance in, 2375
Axonotmesis, 2364
Ayala quotient, 431, 3188
Azamethonium, cerebral blood flow and, 808(t)

Bacitracin, in subdural empyema, 3337
  in subgaleal abscess, 3328
Back pain, chronic, 3613–3624. See also *Pain.*
  Hendler screening test for, 3488, 3490(t)
Bacterial infections, 3323–3357. See also names of specific infections.
  as clinical entities, 3327–3355
  basic considerations in, 3323–3327
  clinical features of, 3324
  diagnosis of, 3324
  focus, pathways, and results of, 3327, *3327*
  host factors in, 3323
  in spinal extradural space, 3449
  intracranial hypertension in, 3180(t)
Bacterial meningitis, 3337–3341
  coma in, 72
  intracranial hypertension in, 3180(t)
Bactericidal agents, 3325
Bacteriostatic agents, 3325
Balance, disturbances of, following thalamotomy, 3837
Ballism, physiological basis of, 3827
Balloon, intracranial, 873, 874
Barbiturates, cerebral blood flow and, 804
  in angiography, 233
  in chronic pain, 3526, 3527, 3758
  in hypoxia, 774
  in increased intracranial pressure, 915
  postischemic survival and, 780
Basal angle, of Boogaard and McRae, *1486*
Basal cell carcinoma, of ear, 3281
  of scalp, 3317, *3319*
Basal ganglia, tumors of, in children, 2721–2722, 2721(t)
Basilar artery, aneurysms of, angiography of, *304*
  at bifurcation, *1716,* 1729–1738, *1731, 1734–1736,* 1739(t)
  at superior cerebellar artery, *1636,* 1740–1745, 1742(t), *1743, 1744*
  at vertebral junction, 1745–1746, 1746(t)
  morbid anatomy in, 1717–1718, 1717(t)
  in cisternal myelography, *527*
  radiological anatomy of, *268,* 271, *274*
Basilar impression, 1483–1485, *1483–1485*
  cerebrospinal fluid in, 467
  radiography in, 491, *492*
Basilar vein, *280,* 282
Batten disease, diagnosis of, 384(t)
Battered child, 2127–2129
BCNU, tumor chemotherapy, 3083–3084, 3083(t), 3088
Bed rest, in subarachnoid hemorrhage, 1848–1849, 1849(t)
Beery Developmental Form Sequence test, 706
Behavior, destructive, operations for, 3941
  disorders of, following head injury, 2168
  epilepsy and, in children, 3880–3883, 3895
Behçet's disease, cerebrospinal fluid in, 463
Békésy audiometry, in acoustic neuroma, 2972
Bell's palsy, 3771, 3778–3782, *3778–3780*
Bell's phenomenon, in cerebral death, 750
Bender Motor Gestalt test, 706
Benton Visual Retention Test, 706
Benzhexol, in Parkinson's disease, 3842
Benzodiazepine(s), in objective pain, 3489
Benzothiazide compounds, in neurohypophyseal diabetes insipidus, 977

Berry aneurysms, genetic aspects of, 1224
Bertrand leukotome, 3806
Bertrand stereotaxic instrument, 3804
Beta-lipotropin, bovine, *937*
Beta-melanocyte–stimulating hormone, synthesis of, *937*
Bethanechol chloride, in detrusor areflexia, 1043
  in postoperative genitourinary tract complications, 1104
Bielschowsky head tilt test, 654
Bilirubin, in cerebrospinal fluid, 437
Binder, head, angiographic, 233
Binocular microscope, *1164, 1167, 1169*
Biopsy, 382–422
  brain, alternatives to, 384(t)–386(t)
    complications of, 390, 390(t)
    diseases diagnosed by, 384(t)
    indications for, 383, 383(t)
    operative techniques in, 389, *389*, 390(t)
    site in, 389, *389*, 390(t)
    tissue handling in, 393, 393(t)
      tissues suitable for, 383(t)
  peripheral nerve, 405–410, 406(t), *407*, 407(t), 409(t)
  skeletal muscle, 410–415, 412(t), 413(t)
  tumor, 395–405
    intraoperative diagnosis in, 399
    tissue techniques in, 400, 400(t), 402(t)
Bipolar coagulator, 1179–1181, *1180*
Birth defect(s). See also *Midline fusion defects.*
  definition of, 1207
  incidence of, 1210(t)
Birth history, in examination of infant, 40
Bithionol, in paragonimiasis, 3390
Bladder, urinary. See *Urinary bladder.*
Blastomycosis, 3405–3407
  meningitic, cerebrospinal fluid in, 462
Bleeding. See also *Hemorrhage* and *Subarachnoid hemorrhage.*
  disorders of, in multiple trauma, 2522–2524, 2523(t)
    intraoperative, 1069
    postoperative, 1093
Bleomycin, [57]cobalt-labeled, in brain scanning, 145
Blepharospasm, encephalitis and, 641
Blindness, following ventriculography, 379
  pupil in, 650–651, *650, 651*
Block anesthesia. See also names of specific blocks.
  alcohol, in trigeminal neuralgia, 3559–3560
  diagnostic, in pain, 3752, 3644–3655, *3645–3647*
  facet, 3618
  increased cerebral blood flow and, 831
  peripheral, in chronic low back pain, 3617
  trigger point, in refractory pain, 3763
Blocking agents, neuromuscular, in semicoma, 915
Blood, bedside administration of, 1108
  cerebral flow of, 786–832. See also *Blood flow, cerebral.*
  disorders of, pseudotumor cerebri and, 3187
  evaluation of, in neurosurgical patient, 1057
  loss of, intraoperative, 1069
    low perfusion and, 1068
  metastasis via, in spinal cord tumors, 3220, 3220(t)
  tests of, in transient ischemic attack, 1523
  viscosity of, cerebral blood flow and, 830
Blood ammonia, in cerebrospinal fluid, 451
Blood flow, cerebral, 786–832. See also *Cerebral blood flow.*
  aging and, 826
  amount of, 786–788, 787(t), 788(t)
  anesthesia and, 1133
  anesthetics and, 804
  autoregulation of, 792–794, *792*, 866–868
    carbon dioxide tension and, 805
    metabolic, 793–794, 869
  blood pressure and, 792
  carbon dioxide and, 800, *800*, 801(t)
  carotid ligation and, 1700
  collateral system and, 794–800
  control of, 791–794, *792*
  drugs and, 800–813
  epileptogenic focus and, 3862

Blood flow (*Continued*)
  cerebral, factors affecting, 788–791, *789–791*
    following subarachnoid hemorrhage, 893
    hypotension and, 1126
    impaired, in diffuse cerebral ischemia, 1540–1541, *1541*
    in anemia and polycythemia, 822
    in carotid artery occlusion, 1700
    in cerebral death, 751–752, *751*, 755(t)
    in cerebral trauma, 825
    in cerebrovascular disease, 813, *814, 815*
    in dementia, 827
    in disease and abnormal conditions, 813–829
    in head injury 883, 885(t), *886–888*
    in headache, 822
    in hypoglycemia, 771
    in hypoxia, 774
    in ischemia, 774
    in miscellaneous diseases, 828
    increased cerebral activity and, 826
    intracranial mass lesions and, 873
    intracranial pressure and, 823, 866–875, *870*
      in head injury, 825, 1925–1927, *1926*
    measurement of, 853
    methods of increasing, 829–832
    monitoring of, Doppler ultrasound in, 740, *741, 742*
    oxygen and, 803, 804(t)
      jugular bulb levels as index of, 1131
    position of head and, 827
    postischemic, irreversible brain cell damage and, 780
    prognosis after head injury and, 2154–2156
    regional, 787
    respiratory gases and, 800–813
    retinal, in ischemic vascular disease, 1520
    sleep and, 804
    systemic drugs and, 807, 808(t)
Blood gases, in acute respiratory failure, 1024, 1025
  prognosis after head injury and, 2153
Blood groups, in etiology of brain tumors, 2669
Blood plasma, constituents of, cerebrospinal fluid and, 432
Blood pressure, arterial, in acute respiratory failure, 1023
  carotid ligation and, 1698–1700, 1710
  cerebral blood flow and, 792, 799, 801(t)
  control of, in operative procedures, 1067
  elevation of, for increased cerebral blood flow, 832
  evaluation of, neurosurgical, 1054
  in acute respiratory failure, 1025
  in ischemic vascular disease, 1518
  increased intracranial pressure and, 861
  venous, spinal cord malformations and, 1853
Blood vessels, cerebral, in trauma, 1898, 1907
  intrinsic disease of, embolism and, 1516
  cerebral blood flow and, 789, *789, 790*, 814, *815*
    operations on, 831–832
  deliberate sacrifice of, superficial temporal to middle cerebral
    arterial anastomosis in, 1601–1604, *1603–1605*
  impressions of, in skull, 3250
  in aneurysm procedures, 1670–1671
  in craniopagus twins, 1211
  injury to, as complication of disc operation, 2549
  intracavernous, 1764–1782
  lesions of, sympathectomy in, 3721
  malformations of, genetic aspects of, 1224–1227
    headache and, 3552
    in subarachnoid hemorrhage, 1637–1641
  of scalp, 2299, *2300*
  peripheral, in multiple trauma, 2490–2491
    preoperative evaluation of, 1059
  small, diffuse ischemic disease of, 1543–1548
  spasm of. See *Vasospasm.*
Blood-brain barrier, cerebrospinal fluid barrier and, 431
  in bacterial infections, 3325
  in brain scanning, 146
  in trauma, 1898
Blood–cerebrospinal fluid barrier, in bacterial infections, 3325

Body fluids, agents affecting, cerebral blood flow and, 811(t)
  normal, 2494
Body temperature, cerebral metabolism and, 769, *769*
  control of, during operative procedures, 1067
  intracranial pressure and, 913, *914*
Bohr effect, 1125
Bone. See also names of specific bones.
  autogenous, cranioplasty with, 2242–2247, *2243–2247*
    grafting with, in facial fractures, 2286–2296, *2290–2296*
  heterotopic, spinal cord dysfunction and, 4011
  injury to, in cervical spine injury, 2323–2330
  necrosis of in operative procedures, prevention of, 1076
  pain in, malignant disease and, 3628
Bone conduction audiometric testing, 695
Bone flap(s), in craniotomy, 1141, *1141*, 1147, *1147, 1148*
  in meningioma, 2945, *2946, 2947*
  in operative procedures, 1075
Botulism, cerebrospinal fluid in, 471
Bounet-Dechoume-Blanc syndrome, 1803
Bowel, in spinal cord dysfunction, rehabilitation of, 4009–4010
  training of, in hemiplegia, 3999
Braces, in paraplegia, 4002
Brachial artery, carotid angiography via, 250, *250*
Brachial plexus, entrapment of, 2457–2462, *2458, 2461*
  injury to, 2396–2401, *2397, 2400–2402*
    in newborn infants, 48, 49
  lesions of, electromyography in, 632, 635(t)
  malignant disease and, pain in, 3627–3628
  schwannoma of, benign, 3301
    malignant, 3304
Brachycephaly, trigeminal nerve in, 3593
Bradykinesia, gamma system and, 3826
  in Parkinson's disease, 3838
Brain, arteriovenous malformations of, 1786–1806
  autopsy of, in cerebral death, 755(t)
  biopsy of, 383–395. See also *Biopsy, brain.*
  blood flow in, 786–832. See also *Blood flow, cerebral.*
  cells of, characteristics of, 765
    damage in, mechanisms of, 780, 781(t)
    selective vulnerability of, 766
  circulatory system of, collateral, 794
  cold lesions of, intracranial pressure and, 874
  contusion of. See *Contusion(s), cerebral.*
  death of. See *Cerebral death.*
  edema of, 846
    in head injury, 1914–1915, *1914*
    infarction and, operative treatment of, 1623–1625
    intracranial hypertension and, 874
    intraoperative, acute, 1071, 2034
    vs. vascular brain swelling, 2048
  energy production within, 766–767, *766*, 766(t)
  energy utilization within, 767–768, *767*
  formation of, 1241–1242
  growth of, from conception, *2087*
  hemorrhage in, spontaneous, 1821–1844
  herniation of, in head injury, 1916, 1917(t), 1918–1921, *1920, 1921*
    intracranial pressure in, 858, 1924
  in craniotomy, exposure and resection of, 1139, *1140–1146*
    intraoperative complications of, 1078–1079
    irrigation of, 1145
  infarction of. See *Infarction, cerebral.*
  inflammatory disease of, computed tomography in, 132, *134, 135*
    in children, brain scanning in, 162
  injury to, in head injury, 1897–1904
    electrical activity of, 1993–2010
    evoked potentials of, 1998–2000, *1999–2005*, 2002(t), 2004(t), 2006(t), *2007*, 2008
    in children, 2115–2123, *2118, 2120*
    in post-traumatic epilepsy, 2188
    ischemia in, 1927–1928
    major determinants of, 2086–2091, *2087, 2089, 2090*
    primary damage in, 1897, *1900–1902, 1904*
    secondary damage in, 1909–1927

Brain (*Continued*)
  injury to, in head injury, secondary displacement of, 1916
    localized, 2048
    prior, in prognosis after head injury, 2142
    psychological testing after, 2195–2203
    vs. malingering, 713
  ischemia and anoxia of intracranial pressure and, 894–895
  laceration of, 1903, 2053
  lesion of, increased intracranial pressure and, 881, 881(t)
  lymphomas of, 2836–2844
  metabolism in, 765–785. See also *Metabolism, cerebral.*
  midline echo of, in cerebral death, 752
  missile injuries of, 1903, 2055–2068, *2055, 2058, 2060, 2062–2067*
  parenchymal vessels of, collateral blood supply and, 798
  penetrating injuries of, 1903
  perforating wounds of, 2054
  protection of, as indication for cranioplasty, 2229
  "respirator," 756
  stimulation of, in chronic pain, 3623
  surface retraction of, 1078
  temperature of, in cerebral death, 755(t)
  tumors of. See *Brain tumors* and names of specific tumors.
  weeping, in pseudotumor cerebri, 3189
Brain abscess, 3343–3355, *3343*
  amebiasis and, 3368
  angiography in, 324
  candidiasis and, 3408
  causative organisms of, 3348, *3349*
  clinical presentation of, 3344
  craniofacial operation for cancer and, 3274
  diagnosis of, 3345, *3346–3348*
    vs. viral encephalitis, 3359
  management of, 3350, *3352–3354*
Brain compression-decompression syndromes, 1084
Brain fungus, following operative procedures, 1087
Brain mantle index, in sonoventriculography, 183, *184*
Brain retractors, in micro-operative procedures, 1181, *1182*
Brain scan. See also *Radionuclide imaging.*
  appearance of diseases in, 149, *150–154*, 154(t), 155(t), *156–160*
  in astrocytoma, 2775
  in brain abscess, 3345, *3346*
  in cerebral infarction, 1535
  in Dandy-Walker malformation, 1294
  in dural fistulae, 2218, *2218, 2219*
  in glioblastoma, 2810, *2810*
  in ischemic vascular disease, 1535
  in lymphoma of brain, 2841
  in orbital tumors, 3039
  in posterior fossa tumors in children, 2737, *2738*
  in subdural empyema, 3335, *3335*
  in supratentorial tumors in children, 2707, *2707*
  in transient ischemic attack, 1523
  indications for, 144, 144(t)
  normal, 147–149, *149*
  post-treatment, 154
  radiopharmaceuticals for, 148(t)
  vs. computed tomography, 165, 167(t), 168(t)
Brain stem, abnormalities of, electroencephalography in, 215, 221
  astrocytoma of, 2770, 2774
  disease of, opticokinetic nystagmus in, 661
  dysfunction of, prognosis after head injury and, 2147
    rehabilitation in, 4000
  evoked response from, audiometry by, 698–700, *699*
    in acoustic neuroma, 2972
    in head injury, 2008–2010, *2009*
  glioma of, in children, 2751–2752
  in ascending pain pathway, 3466–3467
  in Dandy-Walker malformation, 1290
  in head injury, 880, 1899
    contusion of, in children, 2117
    evoked potentials in, 2008–2010, *2009*
    injury to, 1899
      irreversible coma and, 879

Brain stem (*Continued*)
  investigation of, 2776
  lesions of, coma in, 68
  responses of, in cerebral death, 755
  reticular formation of, 3466
  treatment of, 2779
  tumors of, radiation therapy of, 3102
Brain stem evoked response audiometry, 698–700, *699*
Brain tumors. See also names of specific tumors.
  biochemistry of, 2691
  biology of, 2666–2693, *2676, 2682, 2683,* 2685(t)–2687(t), *2687, 2688*
  cerebral blood flow in, 828, *829*
  chemotherapy of, 3065–3095
  classification of, 2659–2666, *2661,* 2664(t), 2759–2761, 2761(t)
  diagnostic tests for, 168(t)
  dyskinesia and, 3821
  electroencephalography in, 221, 2707
  etiological agents in, 2666–2676
  glial, 2759–2801
  grading of, 2661–2663
  growth mechanisms of, 2676–2682
  immunobiology of, 2688–2690
  incidence of, 2682–2688, *2682, 2683,* 2685(t), 2761–2762
  intracranial pressure in, increased, 889
  investigation of, 2763–2764. See also names of specific tumors.
  lymphomas as, 2836–2842
  meningeal, 2936–2966
  metastatic, 2872–2895
  neuronal, 2801–2835
  of disordered embryogenesis, 2899–2935
  operative treatment of, 2764–2765. See also names of specific tumors.
  posterior cranial fossa, in children, 2733–2758
  radiation therapy of, 3096–3106
  sarcomas as, 2845, 2855–2858
  sellar and parasellar, 3107–3155
  subarachnoid hemorrhage and, 1816
  supratentorial, in children, 2702–2732
  vascular, 2845–2855
  vs. viral encephalitis, 3360
Breast, carcinoma. See under *Carcinoma.*
Breathing. See *Respiration.*
Briquet's syndrome, "effected" pain and, 3507–3511, 3509(t), 3510(t)
Bromide psychosis, cerebral blood flow in, 829
Bromocriptine, in acromegaly, 957
  in hyperprolactinemia, 968
5-Bromo-2'-deoxyuridine, intra-arterial administration of, 3073
Bronchoscopy, fiberoptic, in atelectasis, 1019, *1019*
Bronchospasm, as postoperative complication, 1095
Brown's multitarget operation, in psychiatric disorders, 3938, *3939*
Brucellosis, cerebrospinal fluid in, 462
  intracranial hypertension in, 3180(t)
Bruising. See *Contusion.*
Bruit, carotid, asymptomatic, as indication for operation, 1567
  intracranial, in infants and children, 41, 45
BUdR, intra-arterial administration of, 3073
Burr holes, exploratory, in head injury, 1992
Burst fracture, cervical, 2319, *2320*
Butorphanol, in inappropriate secretion of antidiuretic hormone, 982

CAA 40, cerebral blood flow and, 809(t)
Caesarean section, in prevention of epilepsy, 3865
Caffeine, cerebral blood flow and, 810(t)
Calcification(s), in skull radiography, as pseudolesions, 77–80, *79,* 88, *89*
  pathological, 100, 100(t), *101–103*
  in spinal angioma, *574*

Calcification(s) (*Continued*)
  intracranial, genetic aspects of, 1227
Calcium, abnormalities of, in multiple trauma, 2501
  in cerebrospinal fluid, 450
  serum, in acromegaly, 954
Caloric test, in cerebral death, 755(t)
  of vestibular function, 683, *684*
Calvarium, defects of, 1215
Campotomy, 3829
Canavan disease, brain biopsy in, 386(t)
Cancer. See also names of specific types of cancer.
  craniofacial operation for, 3274
  endocrine treatment of, 3947
  visceral, pain in, 3627–3630
Candidiasis, 3407–3410
  meningitic, cerebrospinal fluid in, 461
Candidiosis, 3407
Candidosis, 3407
Capillary hemangioblastoma, posterior fossa, in children, 2754, *2755*
Capillary hemangioma. See *Hemangioma.*
Capsulotomy, bilateral anterior, in psychiatric disorders, 3835, 3936(t)
  vs. cingulotomy, 3936(t)
Caput succedaneum, transillumination in, 41
Carbamazepine, in afebrile seizures, 3876, 3876(t)
  in neurohypophyseal diabetes insipidus, 977
  in trigeminal neuralgia, 3558
  starting dosages of, 3877(t)
Carbenicillin, in bacterial infections, 3326
Carbon dioxide, cerebral blood flow and, 800, *800,* 801(t), 818, 830
  in acute respiratory failure, 1024
  in general anesthesia, 1123
  response to, prognosis after head injury and, 2153
Carbon monoxide poisoning, vascular ischemia in, 1542–1543, 1543(t)
Carcinoma, breast, hypophysectomy in, 3950–3952, 3984–3985
    posthypophysectomy (by craniotomy), 3984
  bronchial, hypophysectomy in, 3953
  bronchogenic, of conus, myelographic appearance of, *534*
  extracranial primary, brain scanning in, 152
  head and neck, mesencephalotomy for, 3707
  pain in, 3536–3538, *3536, 3537*
  metastatic, to skull, 3239, *3240, 3241,* 3244
  of ear, 3281, *3282, 3283*
  of scalp, 3316, *3319*
  orbital, 3059
  pancreatic, reversible nerve block in, 3655
  paranasal sinus, 3277, *3278–3281*
  prostate, hypophysectomy in, 3952–3953, 3985
Carcinogens, biological, 2675–2676, *2676*
  chemical, 2673–2675
Carcinomatosis, meningeal, cerebrospinal fluid in, 463
  chemotherapy for, 3090(t)
Cardiac arrest, in diffuse cerebral ischemia, 1540–1541
  in multiple trauma, 2492–2494
  intraoperative, 1073
  postoperative, 1097
Cardiac dysrhythmias, as postoperative complication, 1097
  in ischemic vascular disease, 1215
  intraoperative, 1072
Cardiac output, in acute respiratory failure, 1023
Cardiogenic shock, pathophysiology of, 2505
Cardiopulmonary physiology, clinical application of, formulas for, 1008(t)
  symbols in, 1007(t)
Cardiorespiratory disorders, intracranial hypertension in, 3180(t)
Cardiovascular disease, cerebrospinal fluid in, 469
Cardiovascular system, evaluation of, 1054
  in head injury in children, 2093
  in multiple trauma, 2490–2491
Carisoprodol, in histrionic personality, 3507
  in objective pain, 3489
  in psychogenic tissue tension pain, 3497

Carotid angiography, 244–256
  approaches in, 232
  brain scanning after, 161
  catheterization techniques for, 246–252, *247, 248, 250, 251*
    direct puncture, 244–246, *244, 246, 247*
  premedication in, 1120
Carotid artery (arteries), anastomoses between, 796
  aneurysms of, angiography in, 289, *290*
  anomalies of, 292
  arteriovenous fistulae of, 291
  berry aneurysms of, headache in, 3552
  buckling of, *288, 289*
  cerebral angiography via, 244–256. See also *Carotid angiography.*
  clamping of, tolerance to, 831, 1698, 1703
  endarterectomy of, 1569–1581, *1572, 1575–1577,* 1580(t)
  external, stenosis of, operation in, 1567
  extracranial, directional Doppler scanning of, 741, *742*
    occlusive disease of, 1559–1583, *1560–1562*
  in collateral circulatory system, 795
  in percutaneous rhizotomy, 3569
  internal, aneurysms of, 1677–1681, *1677, 1678, 1680*
    ligation in, 1701–1703, 1708
    exposure of, in glomus jugulare tumor, *3296, 3297*
    kinking of, cerebral blood flow and, 815
    sitting position and, 1132
  intracavernous, vascular lesions of, 1764–1785
    classification of, 1768
    ligation of, 1701–1710
  occlusion of, in aneurysms of anterior circulation, 1697–1714
  radiological anatomy of, 257–261, *258–261*
  radiography in, 283, *286–288*
  transient ischemic attacks and, 1520–1530, *1521,* 1522(t), 1524(t), 1525(t)
  trauma to, 2314–2317, *2315, 2316*
  ultrasound scanning of, 734, *735–737,* 1524
  vertebral-basilar anastomoses in, 278, *279*
Carotid body, tumors of, angiography of, 292, *294*
  catecholamines in, 3287
Carotid-cavernous fistula, 1771–1782, *1772,* 1773(t), *1776–1778*
Carotid endarterectomy, 1569–1579, 1580(t)
  electroencephalography during, 226, *227, 228*
Carotid sinus, massage of, in ischemic vascular disease, 1518–1519
Carotid siphon, 257
Carpal tunnel syndrome, electromyographic studies in, 630
  in acromegaly, 955
  median nerve in, 2447–2449
Carpenter syndrome, 1212
Catecholamines, cerebral blood flow and, 807
  synthesis of, 770
Catheter(s), cup, in measurement of intracranial pressure, 852
  for angiography, preparation of, 242, *242, 243*
  urethral, in neurosurgical patient, 1058
  ventricular, obstruction of, in hydrocephalus, 1415–1416, *1416*
Catheterization, for carotid angiography, 244
    nonselective (aortic arch studies), 252
    segmental selective, 250, *250, 251*
    Seldinger, 248, *248*
    vertebral, 255, *255*
  in total parenteral nutrition, 1001
  of bladder, in multiple trauma, 2528
    in spinal cord dysfunction, 4010
    intermittent, in detrusor areflexia, 1043
    postoperative, complications of, 1104
    preoperative, 1058
Cauda equina, tumors of, pathophysiology of, 3199
Caudal regression syndrome, 1356–1358
Causalgia, in peripheral nerve injury, 2421–2423, 3628
  neuromodulation in, 3638
  reversible local anesthesia in, 3653–3654
  sympathectomy for, 3628, 3628(t), 3720
Causalgic syndromes, anesthetic diagnosis of, 3649
  pain in, 3628
Cavernous hemangioma. See *Hemangioma.*

Cavernous plexus, 3004–3023
  anatomy of, 1764–1768, *1765–1767, 1769,* 3005, *3006–3013,* 3111, 3112
  aneurysms of, 1768–1771
  fistulae of, 1771–1782, *1772,* 1773(t), *1776–1778,* 1780
  lesions of, 3004, 3014–3021
Cavum veli interpositi, *352*
CCNU, tumor chemotherapy, 3085, 3088, 3089(t)
Celiac ganglia, neurolytic injections of, 3661
Celiac plexus block, 3651–3652
Cell(s), brain, in head injury, 1897, *1900, 1901*
    mechanisms of injury to, 780–781, 781(t)
  in cerebrospinal fluid, 438–440
    counts of, 457–458
  pituitary, hormones and, 935–938, 938(t)
  tumor, biopsy identification of, 396–397, 397(t)
    kinetics of, chemotherapy and, 3070–3071
    proliferation of, as growth mechanism, 2677
Cellulitis, orbital, in phycomycosis, 3424
Central nervous system, anomalies of, epidemiology of, 1210
  cerebrospinal fluid and, 432
  diseases of, photophobia in, 641(t)
    urological problems associated with, 1031–1050
    vertigo and, 687
  embryology of, 1236–1242
  lesions of, electrolyte and metabolic regulation in, 989
    rehabilitation following, 3989–4013
  leukemia of, radiation therapy in, 3104
  malformations of, 1236–1380
  metastatic disease in, radiation therapy of, 3104
  parasitic and fungal infections of, 3366–3440
  radiation tolerance of, 3097–3098
  stimulating drugs for, cerebral blood flow and, 810(t)
Cephalea, 3564
Cephalgia, of psychological origin, 3545–3546
  post-traumatic, 3541–3542, *3542, 3543*
Cephalhematoma, 3245
  echoencephalography in, 181
  in head injury in children, 2096
  of newborn, 45, 2096, 3245, *3248*
Cephalhematoma deformans, 3245
  anatomy and physiology of, 3531–3532
  atypical facial neuralgia as, 3543–3545, *3544, 3545*
  dental disorders and, 3532–3534, *3534*
  migraine as, 3546–3550
  occipital neuralgia as, 3540–3541
  of psychological origin, 3545–3546
  postherpetic neuralgia as, 3542–3543
  post-traumatic cephalgia as, 3541–3542, *3542, 3543*
  referral patterns in, 3532
  temporal arteritis as, 3538
  temporomandibular joint in, 3539–3540
  tumor-related headaches as, 3550–3552, *3551*
  vascular headaches as, 3546–3550
Cephalic reflexes, in cerebral death, 758
Cephalometry, in midface retrusion, 1471, *1472*
Cephalosporins, in bacterial infections, 3326
  in bacterial meningitis, 3339
Cephalothin, in temporal lobectomy, 3883
Ceramidase deficiency, diagnosis of, 385(t)
Cerebellar vein, precentral, 282
Cerebellar vermis, stimulation of, in cerebral palsy, 3850
Cerebellopontine angle, anatomy of, acoustic neuroma and, 2975
  arachnoid cysts of, 1442
  examination of, with Pantopaque, 372–373, *373*
  meningioma of, 2942, 2959–2960
Cerebellum, arteries of. See names of specific arteries.
  connections of, in neonate, 49
  disease of, ocular signs of, 656
  hemorrhage in, spontaneous, 1821, *1824, 1830, 1837*
  in Arnold-Chiari malformation, 1283, *1283,* 1284
  in Dandy-Walker malformation, 1290
  normal embryology of, 1279
  parenchymous degeneration of, cerebrospinal fluid in, 468
  stimulation of, in epilepsy in children, 3898

Cerebellum (*Continued*)
  tonsillar herniation of, in head injury, 1921, *1921*
  tumors of. See Brain *tumors* and names of specific tumors.
Cerebral abscess, brain scanning in, 155(t)
Cerebral aneurysms, 1630–1637
  polycystic kidney and, 1808–1809
Cerebral angiography, 231–350. See also *Angiography, cerebral.*
Cerebral blood flow, 786–845. See also *Blood flow, cerebral.*
Cerebral death, 746–761
  characteristics of, 750–756, *752*
  discussion with survivors in, 759–760
  formal criteria of, 756–759
  legal aspects of, 748, 749(t)
  moral aspects of, 748–749
  world acceptance of, 749–750, 749(t)
Cerebral dematiomycosis, cerebrospinal fluid in, 462
Cerebral depression, bilateral, coma in, 68
Cerebral hemispheres, astrocytoma of, 2776–2778, 2777(t)
  destruction of, death and, 747
  lesions of, opticokinetic nystagmus in, 661
  tumors of, 2709
    in children, 2709–2714
Cerebral infarction, anticoagulants for, 1537, 1537(t)
  brain scanning in, 155(t)
  computed tomography in, 118, *119, 120*
    vs. radionuclide imaging in, 167(t)
  of carotid territory, 1525
Cerebral palsy, 3849
  incidence of, 1210(t)
  porencephaly and, 2127, *2128*
Cerebral vasodilatation, stimuli to, 868
Cerebral vasomotor paralysis, 874
Cerebral veins, deep, radiological anatomy of, 282, *283, 284*
  internal, *280*
  superficial middle, *280*
Cerebral venous pressure, relationship of, to intracranial
  cerebrospinal fluid pressure, 871
Cerebral vessels, intrinsic disease of, and arterial occlusion, 1516
  sympathetic innervation of, 867
Cerebritis, 3343, 3346
  brain scanning in, 159
  treatment of, 3354
Cerebrospinal fluid, 423–486
  absorption of, 428, 1381
    as test, in normal-pressure hydrocephalus, 1428
  acid-base balance of, 448
  biology of, 426–435, 434(t)
  blood-brain barrier and, 431
  cellular analysis of, 438
  chlorides in, 448
  circulation of, hydrocephalus and, 1381
  coagulation of, 436
  composition of, 432, 434(t)
  drainage of, in cranial operations, 1137
    in craniotomy, 1143
  flow of, obstruction to, 430
  formation of, 427
  function of, 433
  glucose and intermediates in, 447
  hemorrhagic, 436
  in acromegaly, 955
  in acute transverse myelitis, 466
  in bacterial meningitis, 3338
  in benign intracranial hypertension, 471
  in brain tumors, 2692
  in cardiovascular diseases, 469
  in degenerative disease, 470
  in demyelinating disease, 469
  in developmental defects, 467
  in hepatic disease, 469
  in hypoliquorrhea, 471
  in immunological disease, 469
  in infancy and prematurity, 451
  in infections, 460
  in inherited diseases, 468

Cerebrospinal fluid (*Continued*)
  in lymphoma of brain, 2840
  in meningism, 465
  in metabolic systemic diseases, 468
  in neoplastic disease, 467
  in normal-pressure hydrocephalus, 471
    pressure of, 1423
  in osteomyelitis of spine, 465
  in paroxysmal disorders, 471
  in polyneuropathy, 471
  in pseudotumor cerebri, 3189
  in renal disease, 469
  in rhinorrhea and otorrhea, 472
  in spinal angioma, 565
  in spinal epidural abscess, 465
  in trauma, 467
  in vascular lesions, 466
  in viral encephalitis, 3361
  leakage of, following craniotomy, 1151
    in aneurysms, 1691
    from ear, 2254
    in basilar skull fractures, 2254
    in head injury in children, 2100, *2101*
    in operative procedures, 1075, 1086
    in pseudomeningoceles, 1086
    nonoperative management of, 2223(t)
  lipids in, 449, 2692
  metastasis via, in spinal cord tumors, 3220(t), 3221
  microbes in, 440
  nature of, 435–452
  neurotransmitters in, 449
  postmortem findings in, 452
  pressure of, 429
    fluctuations in, intracranial lesions and, 875
    intracranial pressure and, 858
      cerebral venous pressure and, 871
      passive hyperventilation and, 1125
    prior lumbar puncture and, 472
    prognosis after head injury and, 2154
  protein in, 441
  radionuclide studies of, 163–165, *165*
  serology of, 446
  solid in, 450
  standardized laboratory tests of, 457–459
  turbidity of, 435
  xanthochromia in, 437
Cerebrospinal fluid space, anatomy of, 426
  puncture of, 452–457
Cerebrotendinous xanthomatosis, diagnosis of, 385(t)
Cerebrovascular accident. See also *Stroke.*
  brain scanning in, 155, *155(t) 156, 156(t), 157*
    in children, 162
  dynamic vs. static imaging in, 163
  electromyographic studies in, 633
  vs. tumor, 155
Cerebrovascular disease, brain scanning in, 155
  cerebral blood flow in, 813, *814, 815*
  superficial temporal to middle cerebral arterial anastomosis in,
    1597, *1597–1599*
  sympathectomy for, 3720
Cerebrovascular insufficiency, cerebrospinal fluid in, 466
Cerebrovascular lesions, static radionuclide image in, 150
Cerebrum, abscess of, brain scanning in, 155(t)
  arteries of. See *Artery(ies)* and names of specific arteries.
  atrophy of, computed tomography in, 132, *133*
    cranial defects and, 2230–2231, *2232*
  bilateral destruction of, death and, 747
  blood flow in, 786–832. See also *Blood flow, cerebral.*
  contusions of, brain scanning in, 161
    computed tomography in, 126, *126*
      vs. radionuclide imaging in, *167(t)*
  echinococcosis of, 3377
  edema of, following craniotomy, 1152
  electrical potentials of, 203–215
  function of, hyperventilation and, 1125

Cerebrum (*Continued*)
hemorrhage in, spontaneous, 1821–1844, *1822, 1823, 1826, 1827*
diagnosis of, 1830, *1831, 1832, 1834–1838*
management of, 1837
in craniopagus twins, 1212
in inflammatory disease of, in children, brain scanning in, 162
injury to, acute respiratory failure and, 1016
ischemia in. See *Ischemia, cerebral.*
lesions of, focal, electroencephalography in, 220–222
hypernatremia and, 989
metabolism in, 765–785. See also *Metabolism, cerebral.*
metastases to, 2872–2888
diagnosis of, 2874
differential, 2879
treatment of, 2880, 2881(t)
oxygen consumption in, cerebral death and, 755(t)
paragonimiasis of, 3388
phycomycosis of, 3424
schistosomiasis of, 3384
swelling in, craniotomy and bone flap replacement in, 1148
tuberculoma of, 3441–3445, *3442–3445*
Ceroid-lipofuscinosis, diagnosis of, 384(t)
Ceruminoma, 3281
Cervical artery, 553, *554*
Cervical pain syndromes, 2598–2609
Cervical paravertebral somatic block, 3648
Cervical rib, 1216
syndrome of, brachial plexus in, 2457–2460
Cervical spine. See *Spine, cervical.*
Chamberlain's line, in normal skull, *1484*
Charcot's spine, 506
Charcot-Marie-Tooth disease, 1209
Chemicals, in etiology of brain tumors, 2673–2675
in stereotaxic lesion making, 3800
Chemodectoma, 3312
vs. paraganglioma, 3285
Chemosis, in orbital tumors, 3030
Chemotherapy, 3065–3095. See also names of specific tumors and specific drugs.
agents used in, abbreviations for, 3066(t)
new, clinical evaluation of, 3077, 3077(t), 3079(t)–3081(t)
anatomical considerations in, 3066–3068
animal models in, 3065–3066, 3066(t), 3067(t)
clinical trials in, initial and recurrent tumors and, 3077–3082, 3077(t), 3079(t)–3081(t)
combination, 3087–3088, 3089(t)
immunotherapy in, 3090
in acromegaly, 957
in cerebral metastases, 2887
in Cushing's disease, 959
in hyperprolactinemia, 968
in leptomeningeal metastases, 2892, 2893(t)
pharmacology and pharmacokinetics in, 3070–3071
radiosensitizers in, 3089
routes of administration in, 3071–3076
selection of drugs in, 3090, 3090(t)
specific drugs in, 3082–3087
steroids in, 3089–3090
tumor cell population kinetics in, 3068–3070, 3068(t)
Chest, flail, 2479–2480
injuries to, in multiple trauma, 2479, 2482
wall of, in malignant disease, pain in, 3627
wounds of, multiple trauma and, 2482
Cheyne-Stokes respiration, 66
increased intracranial pressure and, 863
Chiari malformation, 1489, *1490.* See also *Arnold-Chiari malformation.*
Chiari-Frommel syndrome, 965
Chiasm, optic. See *Optic chiasm.*
Child(ren), acromegaly in, differential diagnosis of, 956
acute cerebellar ataxia in, vs. cerebellar tumors, 3360
anemia in, skull in, 3261, *3263*
anterior pituitary failure in, adrenal corticosteroid replacement in, 949

Child(ren) (*Continued*)
bacterial meningitis in, 3339
battered, 2127–2129
brain scanning in, 161–162, 162(t)
brain tumors in, posterior fossa, 2733–2758
supratentorial, 2702–2732, 2703(t), 2704(t), *2705, 2707,* 2709–2711(t), *2709, 2710, 2712–2720,* 2718(t), 2721(t), *2721–2727,* 2723(t), 2726(t), 2728(t), 2729(t)
cerebrospinal fluid pressure in, 429
clinical examination in, 39–62
concussion in, 2115
contusion in, 2116
development of, Gesell's major fields of, 40
normal, 42(t)
disc disease in, 2550
epilepsy in, 3858–3909
eyes in, examination of, 643
facial fractures in, 2286
focal cerebral lesions in, electroencephalography in, 220
general anesthesia in, 1122
gonadal insufficiency in, 944
gross motor capacities of, 40
head injury in, 2084–2136
pathophysiology of, 883
hydrocephalus in, 1381–1422
ultrasound in, *727*
infections in, spinal, 505
intracranial hematomas in, brain scanning in, 157
intradiploic cyst in, 3245
intraoperative blood loss in, 1068
lymphoblastic leukemia in, radiation therapy of, 3104
mental status of, evaluation of, 61
middle cerebral artery in, radiological anatomy of, 264
motor nerve conduction values in, 625(t)
multiple trauma in, 2524–2525
neuroblastoma in, 3307
neurological examination in, 41–44
neuropsychological assessment in, 706
ocular deviations in, 652
pneumoencephalography in, premedication for, 354, 354(t)
porencephaly in, 2127
pseudo-subluxation of C2 and C3 in, 505, *505*
retropharyngeal abscess in, *505*
rhabdomyosarcoma in, 644
scoliosis in, angiography in, *573*
sensory examination in, 61
skeletal traction in, 1081
sonoventriculography in, 183, *185,* 186
spinal cord tumors in, 3215–3221
subdural empyema in, 3334
ventricular shunt in, in hydrocephalus, 1404–1409, *1405–1408*
postoperative care of, 1409–1418
ventriculography in, 378
viral encephalitis in, 3359
visual acuity in, 642
wide spinal canal in, radiography of, 569, *571*
Chloramphenicol, in bacterial infections, 3327
in bacterial meningitis, 3339
in brain abscess, 3350
Chlordiazepoxide, in objective pain, 3489
Chlorides, in cerebrospinal fluid, 448
^{203}Chlormerodrin, 143
in brain scanning, 144
Chloroform, cerebral blood flow and, 805
Chlorothiazide, in neurohypophyseal diabetes insipidus, 977
Chlorphenesin carbamate, in trigeminal neuralgia, 3558
Chlorpromazine, cerebral blood flow and, 812(t)
in acromegaly, 957
in cerebral vasospasm, 820
in objective pain, 3489
in postoperative hiccough, 1105
in psychogenic tissue tension pain, 3497
vs. extensive lobotomy, 3928
Chlorpropamide, in neurohypophyseal diabetes insipidus, 977
Chlorthalidone, in pseudotumor cerebri, 3192

Cholesteatoma, vertigo and, 686
  vs. trigeminal neuralgia, 3557
Cholinergics, cerebral blood flow and, 808(t)
Chondroma, angiographic appearance of, 612
  of skull, 3229
Chondrosarcoma, of skull, 3229(t), 3234, *3234*
  transdural sonography in, 188, *189*
Chordoma, location of, 395(t)
  of sacrum, *514*
  of skull, 3236
    vs. chondroma, 3229
  posterior fossa, in children, 2754
  spinal, 3209
Chorea, Huntington's, 3851
    vs. Parkinson's disease, 3841
  Sydenham's, cerebrospinal fluid in, 470
Choreoathetosis, 3849–3851
  as dyskinesia, 3821
  physiological basis of, 3827
Choriocarcinoma, of testes, hypophysectomy in, 3953
Chorioretinitis, in newborn, 46
Choristoma, 3154
Choroid plexus, absorptive capacity of, 428
  anatomy of, 427
  in Dandy-Walker malformation, 1290
  papilloma of, 2798–2801, *2799, 2800*
    in posterior fossa, in children, 2754
Choroidal artery, anterior, 261, *262*
  posterior, *275, 276, 278*
Chromatolysis, in brain injury, 1897
Chromomycosis, cerebrospinal fluid in, 462
Chromophobe adenoma, nonfunctioning, radiation therapy of, 3164
Chronic low back cripple, 3613–3624
Chronic pain syndrome, 3758
Cigarette smoking, cerebral blood flow and, 809(t)
Ciliary ganglion, in orbit, 3028
Ciliospinal reflex, 67
Cingulotomy, anterior, 3941, *3941*
  in alcoholism, 3943
  in psychiatric disorders, *3930,* 3933, 3934(t)
    vs. capsulotomy, 3936(t)
  mesencephalotomy with, 3709
  rostral, in affective disorders, 3733–3737, *3733–3736*
Circle of Willis, anatomy of, 3113, *3115*
  collateral circulation and, 796
Circulation, of blood. See *Blood flow.*
Cirsoid aneurysm, of scalp, skull in, 3250
Cisterna magna, *352*
  arachnoid cyst of, 1443, *1443*
Cisternography, controlled overpressure in, 164
  in acoustic neuroma, 2978, *2978–2981*
  isotope, in dural fistulae, 2218, *2218, 2219*
    in normal-pressure hydrocephalus, 1428
  of spine, 527, *527, 528*
  radiopharmaceuticals for, 148(t)
Cisterns, subarachnoid, *352*
Cladosporiosis, 3410–3411
Clavicle, fracture of, in newborn, 49
Cleft palate, incidence of, 1210(t)
  morphogenetic timing of, 1211(t)
Cleidocranial dysplasia, 1213, *1213*
Clivus, arachnoid cysts of, 1442
Clofibrate, in neurohypophyseal diabetes insipidus, 977
Clonazepam, in afebrile seizures, 3876(t), 3877
  starting dosages of, 3877(t)
Clonidine, in migraine. 3549
Clorazepate, in objective pain, 3489
Cloxacillin, 3326
Club foot, incidence of, 1210(t)
Coagulation, disturbances of, following hypothermia, 1129
  radiofrequency, hypophysectomy by, 3974
Coarctation of aorta, subarachnoid hemorrhage and, 1807–1808
Cobb's syndrome, spinal angioma and, *564, 565*

Cocaine test, in oculosympathetic paralysis, 647, *648*
Cocarboxylase, cerebral blood flow and, 811(t)
Coccidioidomycosis, 3411–3413
  meningitic, cerebrospinal fluid in, 461
Coccydynia, 3616
Cochlea, anatomy of, 676–678, *677–679*
  hearing and, 693–700
Cogan's syndrome, endolymphatic hydrops in, 689
Cold, in stereotaxic lesion making, 3800, 3810–3811
Collapsing cord sign, 529, *541*
Collateral circulation, of brain, 794–800
Collier's sign, 643
Colloid cyst, 2923–2928
  computed tomography in, 135, *136, 2926, 2926*
  pneumoencephalography in, *367*
Coloboma, acquired, 46
Coma, 63–72
  airway in, 1119
  clinical examination in, 64, 64(t), 65(t)
  dehydration in, 994
  drug-induced, electroencephalography in, 223, *223*
    vs. postanoxic, 217
  electroencephalography in, 222–226, *223, 225*
  encephalitis and, 224, *225*
  hyperosmolal extracellular fluid in, 994
  hypoglycemic, cerebral metabolism in, 771
  in cerebral infarction, 1534
  in newborn, 44
  in post-traumatic syndrome, 2181
  increased intracranial pressure and, 878
    hyperbaric oxygen in, 830
    management of, 898
  irreversible, brain stem injury and, 879
    definition of, 747
  metabolic disorders causing, 65(t), 72
  motor function in, 69
  of unknown origin, diagnosis in, 63(t)
  parenteral fluids in, 994
  physical signs in, 64(t)
  prognosis after head injury and, 2147
  pupillary abnormalities in, 66
  reflex eye movements in, 67
  subtentorial lesions causing, 71–72
  supratentorial lesions causing, 69–71, 70(t)
  traumatic, management of, 899
Comitancy, definition of, 652
Commissural myelotomy, 3693, 3695
Commissurectomy, anterior, 3923
Commissurotomy, in epilepsy in children, 3898
Communicating arteries, anterior, aneurysms of, *301, 303,* 1682–1686
  posterior, radiological anatomy of, 268, 278, *279*
Compression, foramen magnum syndrome of, in Arnold-Chiari malformation, 1287–1288, *1287*
  from spinal cord tumor, in children, 3220(t), 3221
  in occult spinal dysraphism, 1319
  ischemia and, in peripheral nerve injury, 2367, *2367, 2368*
  spinal cord and nerve root, from benign lesions, cervical, 2574–2609
    lumbar, 2535–2555
    thoracic, 2562–2572
    vertebral artery, anterior approach in, 2619
  wound hematoma and, 1085
Compression fracture, local anesthesia in, 3653
  of lumbar spine, 2356–2358, *2357–2359*
Compulsive personality, "effected" pain and, 3503–3504
Computed tomography, 111–142
  anesthesia in, 1124
  clinical applications of, 113–139
  general considerations in, 112–113
  in acoustic neuroma, 2977, *2977*
  in aneurysms of anterior circulation, 1666
  in anterior sacral meningocele, 1352
  in astrocytomas, 2775, *2775, 2776*
  in brain abscess, 116, *118,* 3346, *3348,* 3355

Computed tomography (*Continued*)
  in brain masses, extra-axial, 121, *121–125*
    in malignant intraparenchymal, 113, *114, 115*
  in cerebral contusion, 126, *126*, 2118, *2118*
  in cerebral death, 752, 755(t)
  in cerebral infarction, 118, *119, 120*, 1535
  in cerebral tuberculoma, 3444, *3444*
  in choroid plexus papilloma, 2800, *2800*
  in craniopharyngioma, 138, *138*, 2906, *2906, 2908*
  in cysts, 135, *136*
    colloid, 2926, *2926*
    epidermoid, 2921, *2921*
    neonatal intracranial, *725*
    of sylvian fissure, 1439, *1441*
  in Dandy-Walker malformation, 1294, *1294*
  in dural fistulae, 2220, *2220*
  in echinococcosis, 3379
  in empty sella syndrome, 3173, *3175*
  in encephalocele, *1300, 1302*
  in epilepsy, 3873, *3873*
  in glioblastoma, 2811, *2811*
  in glomus jugulare tumor, *3291*
  in head injury, 125, *126*, 1915, *1915*, 1951–1981, *1953–1982, 1987, 1988*, 2020–2023, *2020–2022*
  in hemangioblastoma of brain, 2850, *2851*
  in hematomas, epidural and subdural, 127, *127–131*
    evolving, in head injury, 1961, *1962*
  in high-pressure hydrocephalus, 1434
    in children, 1393–1396, *1394, 1395*
    neonatal, *723, 727, 728*
    normal-pressure, 1425, *1425–1427*
    pediatric chronic subdural, 2109, *2110, 2111*
  in inflammatory brain disease, 132, *134*
  in intracerebral and intracerebellar hemorrhage, 1831–1833, *1831, 1832, 1834, 1835*
  in ischemic vascular disease, 1535
  in lumbosacral lipoma, *1335*, 1337
  in lumbosacral myelomeningocele, *1260*
  in lymphoma of brain, 2841, *2841*
  in meningioma, 2944, *2944*
  in metastatic disease, 116, *116, 117*
    cerebral, 2875, *2876, 2877*
    leptomeningeal, 2891, *2892*
  in myelomeningocele, *1260*
  in orbital tumors, 3033, 3037, *3035–3037, 3036–3038*
  in pineal tumors, 2866, *2866*
  in pituitary adenoma, 3136, *3136, 3137*
  in posterior fossa tumors in children, 2739–2740, *2739, 2740*
  in pseudotumor cerebri, *3186*, 3188
  in sellar and juxtasellar lesions, 136, *136–139*
  in spinal cord tumors, 3202
  in spinal eosinophilic granuloma, *515*
  in subarachnoid hemorrhage, 893
  in subdural empyema, 3335
  in supratentorial brain tumors, in children, *2705*, 2708, 2711, 2713, 2714.
  in ventricular enlargement, 129, *131, 133*
  in viral encephalitis, 3361, *3362*
  partial volume effect in, 1958–1961, *1959, 1960*
  post-therapeutic, 133, *134, 135*
  prognosis after head injury and, 2148, *2149*, 2149(t), 2150(t)
  radionuclide imaging and, 165–168, 167(t), 168(t)
  spinal, 139–141, *140*
Concussion, at nerve level, 1877, *1878*
  cerebral, clinicopathologic correlation of, 1881, *1884–1893*
    in children, 2115
    mechanisms of, 1877, 1879–1895, *1880, 1881*
  spinal cord, in arteriovenous malformations, 1852–1853
Conduction anesthesia, intrathecal neurolytic agents in, 3655, *3656*
Conduction velocity, as diagnostic study, 624–627, 625(t), 626(t), 628
  in nerve entrapment, 2442–2445, *2443*
Condyle, third occipital, 1483
Confrontation test, visual field and, 663, *663*

Confusion, postoperative, 1112
  prolonged, after head injury, 2167
Congenital disorders, as cause of cranial defect, 2229
  heart disease as, cyanotic, brain abscess and, 3343, 3344, 3345
    treatment of, 3353, *3354*
  malformations as, 1210–1222, 1210(t), 1211(t)
    cerebral angiography in, *267*, 292, *293*
  midline fusion defects as, 1236–1360
  spinal cord tumors as, 3220, 3220(t)
Congestive heart failure, intracranial hypertension in, 3180(t)
  postoperative, 1098
Connective tissue, disease of, cerebrospinal fluid in, 469
  genetic aspects of, 1229–1232
  of scalp, 2298, *2299*
Consciousness, state of, differential diagnosis of, 63–73
  in head injury, 1943
    in children, 2091, *2092*
  in post-traumatic syndrome, 2181
  in transtentorial herniation syndrome, 70(t)
  physiology and pathology of, 64–65
Consensual reflex, pupillary, 647
Constipation, intrathecal neurolytic agents and, 3659
Continuous pressure monitoring, in diagnosis of normal-pressure hydrocephalus, 1426
Contrast media, angiographic, 242, 569
  enhancement by, in computed tomography, 113, *114–124, 130, 131, 134, 135, 137–140*
    in intracerebral and intracerebellar hemorrhage, 1833, *1834, 1835*
  radiographic, cerebral blood flow and, 813
  ventriculography with, in hydrocephalus, 1398, *1399*
    in stereotaxic localization, 3787
Contusion(s), cerebral, brain scanning in, 161
  computed tomography in, 126, *126*, 2118, *2118*
    vs. radionuclide imaging, 167(t)
  in children, 2116–2123, *2118, 2120*
  management of, 2033, 2053
  mechanisms of, 1877–1895
  peripheral nerve, 2365–2366
  scalp, 2301
  echoencephalography in, 181
Conus medullaris, tumors of, pathophysiology of, 3199
Conversion, aggravated pain and, 3515–3519, 3756
Convulsions, intracranial hypertension in, 430
Cooley's anemia, skull in, 3261, *3263*
Cooper stereotaxic instrument, 3802, *3803*
Coordination, in child, 60
Copper, in cerebrospinal fluid, 450
Cor pulmonale, intracranial hypertension in, 3180(t)
Cordotomy, in chronic pain syndrome, 3764
  in malignant visceral disease, 3627–3630
  open, 3686–3699
    anterior cervical, 3691, *3692*
    complications of, 3697–3698
    indications for, 3689
    posterior high cervical, 3691
    posterior thoracic, 3689, *3690*
    results of, 3694–3697
    technique for, 3689–3694, *3690, 3692*
  percutaneous, 3672–3684. See also *Stereotaxic procedures, cordotomy as.*
  in nonmalignant visceral pain, 3630
  stereotaxic, 3672–3684. See also *Stereotaxic procedures, cordotomy as.*
  transcutaneous electrical, 3712
Corneal reflex, in cerebral death, 750
  in newborn, 46
Corneal ulceration, sympathectomy for, 3720
Coronal suture, synostosis of, 1450, *1451, 1452–1457*, 1460, *1465*
  widened, in skull radiographs, 80, *81*
Corpus callosum, agenesis of, genetic aspects of, 1222
  in Dandy-Walker malformation, 1291
  morphogenetic timing of, 1211(t)
  cistern of, *352*

Corpus callosum (*Continued*)
  lipoma of, in children, 2713, *2714*
  section of, in generalized convulsions, 3923
Corpus cerebelli, dysraphism of, in Dandy-Walker malformation, 1289
Cortex, destruction of, death and, 747
  epileptogenic focus in, 3859
  function of, in newborn, 44
  in Arnold-Chiari malformation, 1285
  in ascending pain pathway, 3468
  resection of, in epilepsy, 3879–3891
  superficial veins of, radiological anatomy of, 280, *280*
  venous infarction of, 1539
Corti, organ of, 677, *679*
Corticosteroids, in afebrile seizures, 3876(t)
  in brain scanning, 154
  in metastatic tumors, 2880–2883
  in neurosurgical patient, 983–985
  in posterior fossa tumors in children, 2742
  in pseudotumor cerebri, 3192
    withdrawal of, 3181(t)
Corticotropic adenoma, 3123
  gross pathology of, 3124
Cortisone acetate, in cranial operations, 1136
  in neurosurgical patient, 983
Cosmetic indications, for cranioplasty, 2229
  violation of, complications of, 1075
Costochondral epiphyses, in acromegaly, 955
Costoclavicular syndrome, 2461–2462
Costotransversectomy, in spinal osteomyelitis, 3454, *3455*
Costovertebral dysplasia, characteristics of, 1214
Cough headache, 3550, *3551*
Counseling, family, in posterior fossa tumors in children, 2742
  genetic, 1209–1210
  in rehabilitation program, 4012
    vocational, 3990, 4011
Cover test, in ocular examination, 654
Cramps, muscle, in Parkinson's disease, 3838
Cranial arteritis, 1550–1552
Cranial fossa, posterior. See *Posterior fossa.*
Cranial nerves. See also names of specific nerves.
  congenital defects of, 1223–1224
  examination of, 20
    in infants and children, 45, 52, 55
  in cavernous plexus, 3007
  in cerebral death, 750
  in head injury in children, 2099
  in orbit, *3025*, 3027
  in posterior fossa tumors in children, 2736
    in medulloblastoma, 2746
  palsies of, isolated, 657, *657*, 658(t), *659*, 659(t)
  regeneration of, ocular motility and, 660–661, *660*, 661(t)
  root compression syndromes of, 3771–3784
    hyperactive dysfunction in, *3773*, 3774(t), *3775*, 3777(t), *3776*
    hypoactive dysfunction in, 3778–3782, *3778–3780*
    vascular decompression in, 3772
Craniectomy, bilateral, in increased intracranial pressure, 916
  in craniosynostosis, 1455, *1455–1457*, 1459–1462, *1459*, *1460*
  in penetrating craniocerebral wounds, 2061
  retromastoid, in micro-operative decompression in trigeminal neuralgia, 3597, *3597*
    for vascular decompression, 3772
  suboccipital, in glomus jugulare tumor, 3295, *3295*
    in glossopharyngeal neuralgia, 3605, *3606*
Craniocerebral injury. See *Head injury.*
Craniocerebral topography, 1137, *1137*
Craniodiaphyseal dysplasia, characteristics of, 1214
Craniofacial region, developmental anatomy of, 1468–1470, *1468, 1469*
  dysostosis of, 1471–1472, *1472*
  malformations of, 1212, 1467–1481
    evaluation of, 1470–1474, *1470, 1472, 1473*
    historical background of, 1467–1468
    morphogenetic timing of, 1211(t)

Craniofacial region (*Continued*)
  malformations of, operative techniques in, 1474–1480, *1475–1479*
    postoperative management of, 1480
  neoplasia of, 3269–3284
  penetrating wounds of, 2066, *2066, 2067*
  team approach to, 1468
Craniolacuna(e), definition of, 1219
  myelomeningocele and, 1254, 1259
Craniopagus twins, 1211
Craniopathy, metabolic, 3256
Craniopharyngioma, 2899–2914
  brain scanning in, 150(t), 162(t), 2906
  computed tomography in, 138, *138*, 2906, *2906, 2908*
  in adults, 3153
  in children, 2718–2719, 2718(t)
  incidence of, 2900
  investigation of, 2905, *2906–2908*
  pathology of, 2901, *2901, 2903*
  pneumoencephalography in, *366*
  radiation therapy in, 2912, 3167–3168
  signs and symptoms of, 2902
  transgressing posterior fossa, in children, 2755
  treatment of, 2908, 3153
Cranioplasty, in cranial defects, 2229–2231
  in craniotomy infection, 1148
  in skull fractures, 2053
  methods of, 2233–2247, *2234, 2235, 2238–2241, 2243–2247*
  preoperative management of, 2231–2233
  timing of, 2231
Craniospinal space, anatomy and physiology of, 846
Craniosynostosis, 1447–1466, *1448*
  deformities of, 1447–1455, *1449–1454*
  development of suture in, *1454*, 1455, *1455*
  etiology of, 1447, *1448*
  genetic aspects of, 1212
  mortality and morbidity in, 1462–1463
  operation in, indications for, 1457–1458
    recent modifications in, 1464, *1465*
    results of, 1463, *1463*
    techniques for, 1459–1462, *1459, 1460*
  postshunt, 1416
  recommendations in, 1465–1466
  reoperation in, indications for, 1463–1464, *1463*
  surgical principles in, 1458–1459, *1458*
  total, 1464–1465, *1465*
Craniotomy, approach to lesion in, 1145
  basic incisions in, 1138, *1138*
  brain abscess and, 3344
  brain scanning following, 154
  closure of operative defect in, 1147, *1147–1149*
  defects from, vs. recurrent cerebral neoplasms, 161
  exposure and resection of brain in, 1139, *1140–1146*
  hypophysectomy by, 3981–3986
  in aneurysms of anterior circulation, 1671
  in chronic subdural hematoma, 2073
  in glomus jugulare tumor, 3295, *3295*
  in penetrating craniocerebral wounds, 2061
  infections following, 1089
  large trauma, technique of, 2026, *2027–2029*
  local anesthesia in, 1120
  meningitis following, 3341
  osteomyelitis following, 3330, *3330, 3332, 3333*
  position of patient for, 1131
  postoperative considerations in, 1151
  postoperative water retention and, 992
  specific operative approaches in, 1149
  standard, technique for, *1138*, 1139, *1140–1149*
  suturing in, 1148, *1148, 1149*
  temporal, in trigeminal neuralgia, 3580–3585, *3581–3583*
Craniovertebral junction, anomalies of, 1215, 1482–1508
  absence of odontoid process as, 1489
  anterior decompression in, 1502
  asymptomatic, 1482–1483
  atlantoaxial fusion in, 1502, *1503–1505*

Craniovertebral junction (*Continued*)
  anomalies of, axis malformation as, 1486, *1487*
    basal arachnoiditis as, 1492
    basilar impression as, 1483, *1483–1485*
    Chiari malformation as, 1489, *1490*
    cyst aspiration and drainage in, 1500, *1501*
    Dandy-Walker malformation as, 1490, *1491, 1492*
    diagnosis of, 1495–1496, *1495–1498*
    dural closure in, 1500, *1500*
    embryology of, 1482, *1483*
    occipitalization of atlas as, 1484, *1486, 1487*
    platybasia as, 1484, *1486*
    posterior decompression in, 1496, *1499*
    separate odontoid process as, 1487, *1487–1489*
    symptomatic, 1483–1494
    symptoms and signs of, 1494–1495
    syringomyelia as, 1492, *1493*
    treatment of, 1496–1506
    ventricular drainage in, 1502
Cranium. See *Skull.*
Cranium bifidum occultum, 1219
Creatinine, clearance of, in acromegaly, 955
  in cerebrospinal fluid, 451
Creutzfeldt-Jakob disease, brain biopsy in, 386(t)
  cerebrospinal fluid in, 465
Crista ampullaris, 679, *680*
Crouzon's disease, characteristics of, 1471
Crush injury, in multiple trauma, 2518–2520
Cryofibrinogenemia, pseudotumor cerebri and, 3181(t), 3184
Cryohypophysectomy, 3974–3979, *3976, 3977*
  transsphenoidal, in acromegaly, 3165
Cryptococcosis, 3413–3416
  meningitic, cerebrospinal fluid in, 461
Cultures, cerebrospinal fluid, 458
Cushing reflex, 823, 864
Cushing's disease, 958–961
  laboratory diagnosis of, 958
  microadenoma in, 3125
  postoperative assessment in, 960
  treatment of, 959
    radiation therapy in, 3166–3167
    results of, 3147
    special considerations in, 960
Cushing's syndrome, 958
  cerebrospinal fluid in, 468
  differentiation of, 959(t)
  investigation of, schedule for, 961
  laboratory diagnosis of, 958
Cutaneous nerves, abdominal, syndromes of, 2463
  lateral femoral, entrapment of, 2463–2464, *2464*
Cyanosis, neonatal, 40
Cyclandelate, cerebral blood flow and, 807, 809(t)
Cyclopia, 1469
Cyclopropane, cerebral blood flow and, 805
Cyproheptadine, in Cushing's disease, 959
  in migraine, 3549
  in Nelson's syndrome, 963
Cyst(s). See also names of specific cysts.
  aneurysmal, of bone. See *Aneurysmal bone cyst.*
  arachnoid, 1436–1446. See also *Arachnoid cysts.*
    post-traumatic, 2205–2208
  aspiration and drainage of, in craniovertebral anomalies,
    1500–1502, *1501*
  computed tomography in, 135, *136,* 1439, *1441, 1443,* 2926,
    2926
  Dandy-Walker, 1289
  intradiploic, in children, 3245
  leptomeningeal, in children, 3245, *3249*
  perineurial, 1355
  porencephalic, pneumoencephalography in, *364*
  posterior fossa, in children, 2753–2754
  spinal extradural, 1355
    incidence of, 1219
Cystic fibrosis, pseudotumor cerebri and, 3181(t)

Cysticercosis, 3373–3376
  cerebrospinal fluid in, 462
Cystometry, gas, 1035, *1035*
Cystourethrogram, voiding, in urinary bladder malfunction, 1038
Cytomegalic inclusion disease, in newborn, 46
Cytosine arabinoside, in viral encephalitis, 3363

Dandy-Walker malformation, 1288–1298, 1293(t), *1294, 1295,*
    1297(t), 1490, *1491, 1492*
  clinical evaluation of, 1292
  definition of, 1288
  embryology of, abnormal, 1288
  genetic aspects of, 1221, *1222*
  morphogenetic timing of, 1211(t)
  pathology of, 1290
  prognosis in, 1297, 1297(t)
  treatment of, 1296
    results of, 1297, 1297(t)
  vs. arachnoid cyst, 1293(t)
Dantrolene, in objective pain, 3489
  in spastic urinary sphincter, 1045
DDAVP, in diabetes insipidus, 976
Deafness, head injury and, 2165–2166
  evoked potentials in, 2006
  post-percutaneous rhizotomy for trigeminal neuralgia, 3576
Death, cerebral, 746–761. See also *Cerebral death.*
Decompression, anterior, in craniovertebral junction anomalies,
    1502
  external, as cause of cranial defect, 2229
  in increased intracranial pressure, 916
  of trigeminal nerve, in temporal craniotomy, 3584–3585
    micro-operative, in trigeminal neuralgiaa 3589–3603
  posterior, in craniovertebral junction anomalies, *1490,*
    1496–1500, *1499, 1501*
Decubitus ulcers, 4011
  postoperative, 1113
Degenerative disease, cerebral blood flow in, 828, *829*
  cerebrospinal fluid in, 470
Dehydration, in coma, 994
  postoperative, 1099
Del Castillo syndrome, 965
Delirium tremens, cerebral blood flow in, 807
Dematiomycosis, cerebrospinal fluid in, 462
Demeclocycline, in inappropriate secretion of antidiuretic
  hormone, 982
Dementia, cerebral blood flow in, 827
  hydrocephalic, 1423
Demyelinating disease, cerebrospinal fluid in, 469
Denervation, suprasensitivity test, in urinary bladder malfunction,
  1038
Dental disorders, cephalic pain and, 3532–3534, *3534*
  vs. trigeminal neuralgia, 3558
Deoxyribonucleic acid, in cerebrospinal fluid, 451
Dependent personality, "effected" pain and, 3501–3503
Depression, "effected" pain and, 3498–3501
  of visual field, definition of, 666
  pain as symptom of, 3755
Dermal sinus, congenital, cranial, 1312–1317
  spinal, 1325–1330
Dermatomes, spinal, 3666, *3667*
  somatic pain and, 3645
Dermoid cyst, 2914
  cerebrospinal fluid in, 463
  locations of, 395(t)
  posterior fossa, in children, 2753–2754, *2753*
  sellar, 3154
  spinal, 3208, *3209*
    in children, *3216*
Dermoid tumor, of cranium, 3232
  of orbit, 3058
Desmosterol, in brain tumor diagnosis, 2692
Detrusor areflexia, 1039, *1039,* 1043

Detrusor hyperreflexia, 1039
  cystometrogram in, *1035*
Detrusor muscle, urinary bladder evacuation and, 1045
Detrusor reflex, dysfunction of, 1039, *1039,* 1041, *1042, 1043*
  micturition center for, 1032, *1032*
Detrusor-sphincter dyssynergia, urinary flow rate in, 1038, *1038*
  with detrusor hyperreflexia, 1040, *1040*
Development, arrest of, theory of, in Arnold-Chiari malformation, 1281
  in encephalocele, 1298
  in spina bifida aperta, 1246
  infant and child, 40
Devic's disease, cerebrospinal fluid in, 470
Dexamethasone, adrenal corticosteroid therapy and, 949
  cranial operations and, 1136
  embolization and, 1195
  head injury and, 899
  in supratentorial tumors in children, 2709
  intracranial pressure and, increased, 910
  lobectomy and, temporal, 3883
  meningismus and, postoperative, 1111
  spinal tumors and, 3211
  status epilepticus and, 3878
  thalamotomy and, 3834
  tissue edema and, postoperative, 1091
  trigeminal neuralgia and, 3596
Dextran, and cerebral blood flow, 813
Diabetes insipidus, 973
  causes of, 975(t)
  cryohypophysectomy and, 3975, 3979
  diagnosis of, 973
  hypophysectomy and, 3983
  in pineal tumors, 2864
  management of, 978
  neurohypophyseal, 973
  postoperative, 978, *979,* 1101–1103
  thirst sensation loss and, 996
  treatment of, 975
Diabetes mellitus, acromegaly and, 954
  cerebral blood flow in, 829
  cerebrospinal fluid in, 468, 471
  electromyographic studies in, 633
  evaluation of, 1056
  hypophysectomy and, 3983
  retinopathy in, hypophysectomy in, 3953–3954, 3985, 3985(t)
    photocoagulation vs. pituitary ablation in, 3985(t)
    pituitary insufficiency and, 3948–3949
Dianhydrogalactitol, in tumor chemotherapy, 3087
Diaphragma sellae, *936*
  anatomy of, 3112, *3113*
  defects of, 3171
Diastematomyelia, 496, *496,* 1339–1346, *1342, 1344*
  radiography in, 496, *496*
  spina bifida aperta and, 1250
Diastrophic dwarfism, genetic aspects of, 1229
Diatrizoate sodium, in ventriculography, 3788
Diazepam, dosages of, 3877(t)
  in absence status, 3878
  in afebrile seizures, 3876(t), 3877
  in chronic pain, 3526, 3527, 3758
  in febrile seizure, 3875
  in neonatal seizures, 3874
  in objective pain, 3489
  in pain relief, 3481
  in status epilepticus, 3878
  local anesthesia and, 1120
  prior to embolization, 1195
Dicloxacillin, 3326
Diethyl ether, cerebral blood flow and, 805
Diethylstilbestrol, in anterior pituitary failure, 950
  in acromegaly, 957
Digital nerves, injury to, 2410
Dihydroergotamine, cerebral blood flow and, 809(t)
Dihydroergotoxine, cerebral blood flow and, 809(t)

Dihydrostreptomycin, inner ear damage and, 691, 691(t)
Dimer-X, in ventriculography, 3788
Dimethylamino ethanol, cerebral blood flow and, 812(t)
Diphenylhydantoin, dosages of, 3877(t)
  in absence status, 3878
  in afebrile seizures, 3876, 3876(t)
  in febrile seizures, 3875
  in inappropriate secretion of antidiuretic hormone, 982
  in status epilepticus, 3878
  in trigeminal neuralgia, 3558
  temporal lobectomy and, 3889
Diphtheria, cerebrospinal fluid in, 471
Diplopia, history in, 639
  mesencephalotomy and, 3709
  rhizotomy for trigeminal neuralgia and, 3576
Disc, cervical, osteoarthritis and, 509
  disease of, angiography in, 612, *613*
    cervical, 2574–2609
      anterior approach in, 2620–2621
        evaluation for, 2623–2627
    discography in, 2544
    electromyography in, 628–630, 2544
    lumbar, 2540–2552
    myelography in, 2543–2544
    prevention of, 2545
    radiography in, 2543
    thoracic, 2562–2572, *2565, 2567–2571,* 2572(t)
    treatment of, 2545–2552, *2566–2571,* 2572(t)
  embryonic, formation of, 1237
  herniated. See *Herniation, disc.*
  intervertebral, 2535–2552
    anatomy and function of, 2536
    biochemistry of, 2539
    disease of, 628, 2540, 2546
    infections of, 3457
    rupture of, 2578–2591, *2579–2590*
  thoracic, *548*
Disc space, infection of, 3457, *3457*
Discography, 2544
Disease. See names and types of specific diseases.
Dislocation, atlantoaxial, 500, *510*
  C2–C3, 2326, *2327, 2330*
  thoracic spine, 2348, *2349*
Disuse, pain of, 2424
  physical inactivity in, 3525–3526
Diuretics, in craniotomy, 1143
  in posterative tissue edema, 1091
  preoperative, 1063
Diverticulum(a), arachnoid, 1445
  porencephalic, 378
  sacral, *546*
  subarachnoid, *538*
Dizziness, in basilar skull fracture, 2257
  in post-traumatic syndrome, 2176, 2179, 2184, 2185
DNA, in cerebrospinal fluid, 451
Dolichocephaly, trigeminal nerve in, 3593
Doll's head maneuver in cerebral death, 750
L-Dopa, cerebral blood flow and, 812(t)
  in dyskinesias, 3826
Dopamine, cerebral blood flow and, 812(t)
  synthesis of, 770
Doppler ultrasound, 738–743, *739–743*
  in cerebral infarction, 1536
  in transient ischemic attack, 1524
  pulsed, 743, *743*
Dorsal rhizotomy, in pain, 3664–3670, 3665(t), *3665–3667, 3669*
Doxepin, in chronic pain syndrome, 3758
  in compulsive personality, 3504
  in objective pain, 3489
Draping, patient, for cranial operations, 1136
  for spinal operation, 1152
Driver training, in rehabilitation, 3990
  in spinal cord dysfunction, 4005, *4007*
Droperidol, in dyskinesias, 3828

Droperidol (*Continued*)
  in increased intracranial pressure, 901
Droperidol-fentanyl, with local anesthesia, 1120
Drugs. See also *Chemotherapy* and names of specific drugs.
  addiction to, operations for, 3942
  in chronic pain, 3526–3527, 3526(t)
  in trigeminal neuralgia, 1558
  increased cerebral blood flow and, 831
  injection of, in peripheral nerve injury, 2369, *2370*
  instillation via Ommaya reservoir of, 2893(t)
  intraoperative, in supratentorial tumors in children, 2709
  poisoning by, eye movement in, 69
  reaction to, in pseudotumor cerebri, 3187
  sympathectomy by, 3724
  systemic, cerebral blood flow and, 807, 808(t)–812(t)
Duane syndrome, genetic aspects of, 1223
Dura mater, arteriovenous malformation of, 1802–1803, *1803*
    embolization of, 1200, *1200*
    headache and, 3552
  closure of, in craniovertebral junction anomalies, 1500, *1500*
    in missile injuries, 2063, *2063*
    in spina bifida aperta, 1267–1268, *1269*
  fistula(e) of, 2209–2224
    etiology of, 2210, *2210*, 2211(t)
    nontraumatic, 2214, *2215*
    prognosis in, 2224
    symptoms and diagnosis of, 2214, *2216–2220*, 2218(t)
    traumatic, 2211, *2212, 2213*
    treatment of, 2220, *2222, 2223*, 2223(t)
  formation of, 1240
  in Arnold-Chiari malformation, 1285
  in Dandy-Walker malformation, 1291
  in diastematomyelia, 1342
  in encephalocele, 1299
  incision of, 1144, *1144*
  repair of, for myelopathy, 2604, *2605*
    in skull fractures, 2053
  trauma to, in head injury, 1907–1908
  tumors of, in children, 2728–2729
  venous sinuses of. See *Venous sinus(es)*.
Dwarfism, diastrophic, genetic aspects of, 1229
  in growth hormone insufficiency, 944
Dwyer instrumentation, in spinal deformities, 2639, *2640, 2642*
Dysarthria, head injury and, 2166
  management of, 4000, *4000*
Dysautonomia, in newborn, 48
Dysesthesias, cordotomy and, 3682
  lancinating pain vs., 3673
  mesencephalic, postoperative, 3710
Dysgerminoma, suprasellar, computed tomography in, 116
Dysgraphesthesia, 61
Dyskinesias, 3821–3857
  operations in, indications for and results of, 3837–3853
    physiological basis of, 3823–3828
    thalamic, 3834
    techniques in, 3828–3837, *3829–3831*
Dysmenorrhea, management of, 3632
  presacral neurectomy for, 3722
Dysostosis, definition of, 1212
Dysphasia, following head injury, 2163
  thalamotomy and, 3835
Dysplasia, definition of, 1212
  fibromuscular, superficial temporal to middle cerebral arterial
    anastomosis in, 1600
  of skull, 1213–1215
    fibrous, *3264, 3265, 3265*
Dysraphism, cerebellar, in Dandy-Walker malformation, 1289
  cranial, 1237(t)
  definition of, 1236
  epidemiology and etiology of, 1217, 1218(t)
  genetic counseling in, 1218
  spinal, 1237(t)
    hydrodynamic theory of, 1247
    occult, 1318–1325, *1320*, 1320(t), *1322*
  spinal deformity and, 2648–2649

Dysraphism (*Continued*)
  syndromes of, 1219–1220
Dystonia musculorum deformans, 3845–3846
  as dyskinesia, 3821
  physiological basis of, 3827
Dystrophy, myotonic, in newborn, 45
  reflex sympathetic, pain in, 3639–3640, *3639*

Ear(s), anatomy of, 676–680, *677–682*
    cochlear system in, 693–700
    vestibular system in, 680–692
      tests for, 683
  bleeding from, head injury and, 2254
  carcinoma of, 3281, *3282, 3283*
  cerebrospinal fluid leakage from, 2254
  examination of, in vertigo, 686
  injury to, 2270, *2273*
  inner, anatomy of, 676–680, *677–682*
    toxic injury to, 691, 691(t)
  physiology of, 680
Early's foraminotomy, 2606–2607
Echinococcosis, 3376–3383. See also *Hydatid disease*.
Echocardiography, in transient ischemic attack, 1523
Echoencephalography, 176–194. See also *Ultrasound*.
  definition of, 176
  diagnostic technique in, 178–180, *179, 180*
  findings in, 180–183, *181–183*
    in cerebral death, 755(t)
    in cerebral infarction, 1535
    in craniopharyngioma, 2906
    in hydrocephalus, 1393
    in intracerebral and intracerebellar hemorrhage, 1830–1831
    in ischemic vascular disease, 1535
    in supratentorial brain tumors, in children, 2707
  principles of, 177–178, *178*
  properties of, 178, 178(t)
  sonoventriculography in, 183–186, *184, 185*
  transdural sonography in, 186–192, *187–189, 191–193*
  value of, 193
Ectopalin, in stereotaxic surgery, 3808
Edema, head injury and, computed tomography in, 1964
  postoperative, in posterior fossa tumors in children, 2745
  pulmonary. See *Pulmonary edema*.
  reactive, postoperative radiotherapy and, 3081
  tissue, postoperative, 1090
Edinger-Westphal nucleus, 66
Edrophonium chloride test, in myasthenia gravis, 658
"Effected" pain, 3493–3511, 3509(t), 3510(t)
Effusion, subdural, of infancy, 1912
Ehlers-Danlos syndrome, 1549
  genetic aspects of, 1229
  intracranial bleeding in, 1809
Elbow, median nerve at, entrapment of, 2449–2452, *2450*
    injury to, 2388–2389, *2389*
  radial nerve at, injury to, 2394–2395
  ulnar nerve at, entrapment of, 2452–2454
    injury to, 2391–2392
Electrical activity, brain, head injury and, 1993
Electrical cordotomy, transcutaneous, 3712
Electrical impedance, in stereotaxic surgery, 3799
Electrical stimulation, for epilepsy, 3886
  in chronic pain syndrome, 3620, *3621*, 3760
  in hemicorticectomy, 3892
  in stereotaxic surgery, 3796
  intracerebral, for chronic pain, 3739–3748
  of midbrain, in stereotaxic mesencephalotomy, 3706–3707,
    3707(t), *3707, 3708*
  transcutaneous, 3628, 3634
Electricity, in peripheral nerve injury, 2369, *2370*
Electrocardiography, in cerebral death, 752
  in serum potassium abnormalities, 991
  in transient ischemic attack, 1523
Electrocerebral silence, definition of, 753

Electrocoagulation, in trigeminal neuralgia, 3574, 3574(t)
Electroconvulsive therapy, in psychiatric disorders, 3940
Electrocorticography, in adult epilepsy, 3912, *3913–3917,*
3919–3922
in hemicorticectomy, 3892
in temporal lobectomy, 3885, *3885,* 3888
neuroleptanalgesia in, 1121
nitrous oxide in, 1122
Electrode(s), implantation of, in epileptogenic focus localization,
3871, *3871*
in thalamic stimulation for chronic pain, 3740–3745, 3741(t),
3742(t)
Electrodiagnosis, neuromuscular, 617–635. See also
Electromyography.
clinical applications of, 628–636
nerve conduction studies in, 624–627, 625(t), 626(t)
Electroencephalography, 195–230, 3911
benefits of, 229
cerebral potentials in, 203–217
abnormal, 206, *207–214*
normal, 203, *204, 206*
concepts and definitions of, 195–196
extracerebral potentials in, 201–203, *202*
in astrocytomas, 2774
in brain tumors, 168(t)
in carotid artery occlusion, 1700
in cerebral death, 753, *754,* 755(t)
in cerebral infarction, 1535
in cerebral lesions, 220–222
in coma, 222–226, *223, 225*
in craniopharyngioma, 2906
in encephalopathies, 222–226, *223, 225*
in epilepsy, 207, *209–211,* 216, 217–220, 2191
in children, 3868, *3868,* 3870
in head injury, 1994–1998, *1995, 1996*
evoked potentials and, 2000
in herpes simplex encephalitis, *213, 214,* 222
in hydrocephalus, 1393, 1428
in hypoglycemia, 771, 772(t)
in ischemic vascular disease, 1535
in Jakob-Creutzfeldt disease, 207, *213,* 222
in lymphoma of brain, 2841
in metastatic tumors, 2877
in panencephalitis, 207, *212,* 222
in paragonimiasis, 3390
in Sturge-Weber syndrome, 207, *207,* 221
in supratentorial brain tumors, in children, 2708
in viral encephalitis, 3361
interpretations in, 214
intraoperative, 226–229, *227, 228*
nasopharyngeal, 3870
normal tracings in, 196–201, *197, 199*
procedures and stimuli in, 215, *216*
prognosis after head injury and, 2156–2159, *2157, 2158*
sphenoidal, 3870
Electroimmunodiffusion, of cerebrospinal fluid, 459
Electrolysis, in stereotaxic surgery, 3805
Electrolyte(s), administration of, in head injury, 2044
derangement of, in neurosurgical patient, 993–999, 993(t)
evaluation of, preoperative, 1053
management of, in multiple trauma, 2494–2501
postoperative disturbances of, 989, 1098–1104
Electromyography, 619–624, 620(t), *621*
anal sphincter, 627
in disc disease, 2544
dorsal, 2566
lumbar, 2544
in nerve entrapment, 2435, 2438–2442, *2439, 2440*
in peripheral nerve injury, 2377
in spinal cord tumors, 3202
in urinary bladder malfunction, 1036, *1036, 1037*
sphincter, methods of, 1035
technique for, 619, *621, 624*
Electroneurography, in peripheral nerve injury, *2374,* 2378–2379
Electronystagmography, in cerebral death, 755(t)

Electronystagmography (*Continued*)
in vestibular function, 684, *685*
Electroretinogram, 201, *202*
Elimination, maintenance of, in intracerebral or intracerebellar
hemorrhage, 1840
Embolectomy, intracranial, 1619–1623, *1622, 1623*
Embolism, air. See *Air embolism.*
arterial occlusion by, 1515–1516, 1515(t)
superficial temporal to middle cerebral arterial anastomosis
in, 1601, 1603
cardiac, in carotid infarction, 1526
cerebral, cerebrospinal fluid in, 466
intracranial hypertension in, 3180(t)
fat, 1548–1549
in multiple trauma, 2521–2522
paradoxical, in carotid infarction, 1526
pulmonary, in multiple trauma, 2483–2487
postoperative, 1096
reversible nerve block in, 3654
retinal, in ischemic vascular disease, 1519, 1519(t)
vs. thrombosis, 299
Embolization, in glomus jugulare tumor, 1200–1201, *1201*
selective, 3292
in interventional neuroradiology, 1194
applications of, 1195–1202, *1196–1201*
of spinal cord arteriovenous malformations, 589, *596–602,*
1859
Embryoma, 2914
Embryonic disc, formation of, 1237
Emergency care, in head injury, 2014–2018, 2016(t), *2017, 2018*
in cerebral infarction, 1534
medical system review in, 1051
Empty sella syndrome, 3170–3178, *3171, 3173–3175*
computed tomography in, 136, *136,* 3173, *3175*
operative treatment for, *3151*
primary vs. secondary, 3149–3151, *3150, 3151*
vs. pseudotumor cerebri, 3190
Empyema, subdural, 3333–3337, *3334–3336*
in head injury, 1915
vs. viral encephalitis, 3359
Encephalitis, acute, 3358
blepharospasm and, 641
coma and, 224, *225*
computed tomography in, 132, *134*
epidemic, cerebrospinal fluid in, 464
herpes simplex, electroencephalography in, *213, 214,* 222
necrotizing, acute, 3362
Parkinson's disease and, 3840
sporadic, cerebrospinal fluid in, 465
viral, 3358–3365, *3362*
diagnosis of, 385(t), 3359
Encephalocele, 1298–1312, *1300*
basal, 1306, 1309, 1311
classification of, 1298(t)
definition of, 1298
embryology of, abnormal, 1298
frontoethmoidal, 1306, *1307,* 1311
frontosphenoidal, 1310
in sinus system, 3536
occipital, 1219, 1299, *1300*
of cranial vault, 1304
orbital, 3053–3054
spheno-ethmoidal, 1309
spheno-orbital, 1310
transethmoidal, 1309
transsphenoidal, 1309
parasellar involvement and, 3155
Encephalography, 351–374
air, anesthesia in, 1124
in astrocytomas, 2776
in craniopharyngioma, 2907
in intracerebral hemorrhage, 1836
in supratentorial brain tumors, in children, 2706
Encephalomeningocele, 1308
Encephalomyelitis, 3358

Encephalomyelitis (*Continued*)
  cerebrospinal fluid in, 470
Encephalopathy, alcoholic, cerebral blood flow in, 828, *829*
  electroencephalography in, 222–226, *223, 225*
  hepatic, glutamine levels in, 451
  hypertensive, 1547–1548
    pathophysiology of, 3180(t)
  metabolic, coma in, 72
    pupillary abnormalities in, 67
  post-traumatic, cerebral blood flow in, 828, *829*
  spongiform, brain biopsy in, 386(t)
  transient, postoperative radiotherapy and, 3081
Endarterectomy, carotid, contraindications to, 1569–1571
Endocrine function, 931–988
  evaluation of, 1056
  hypothermia and, 1129
  in empty sella syndrome, 3175
  in pineal tumors, 2864
  in supratentorial tumors, in children, 2706
  multiple, adenomatosis and, 947
  pseudotumor cerebri and, 3185, *3186*
Energy, impaired substrate for, in diffuse cerebral ischemia,
    1541–1543, 1543(t)
  production and use of in brain, 766–770, *766*, 766(t), *767,
    769, 770*
Enflurane, as general anesthetic, 1122
  in increased intracranial pressure, 901
Engelmann's disease, osteopetrosis vs., 3255
Enterostomy, feeding, in multiple trauma, 2526–2528
Environment, genetics and, in neural tube malformations,
    1242–1243
Enzymes, lysosomal, in brain tumors, 2691
  in ischemia, 781
Eosinophilic granuloma, of spine, *515*
  ultrasound scanning in, *730*
Eosinophilic meningitis, 3395
  ventricular, anatomy of, 428
Eosinophils, in cerebrospinal fluid, 440
Ependymal cyst, arachnoid cyst vs., 1436
Ependymal veins, 282, *283*
Ependymitis, pneumoencephalography in, *368*
Ependymoblastoma, cerebral hemisphere, in children, 2712, *2713*
Ependymoma, adult, 2792–2797, *2793–2796*
  brain scanning in, 150(t), 152, 162(t)
  cauda equina, angiography in, *608, 609*
  cerebral hemisphere, in children, 2712
  computed tomography in, 116, 2795, *2795, 2796*
  conus, myelography in, *533*
  exophytic, headache and, 3551, *3551*
  high-pressure hydrocephalus and, 1433
  intracranial, radiation therapy of, 3101, 3101(t)–3102(t)
  locations of, 395(t)
  lumbar vertebrae scalloping in, *3201*
  posterior fossa, in children, 2750–2751
  recurrent, chemotherapy for, 3090(t)
  spinal, *3197*, 3197(t), 3205–3206, *3206*
    chemotherapy for, 3213
    fusiform defect in, *3204*
    in children, *3216*
    operative treatment of, 3211
    radiation therapy for, 3212, 3223(t)
Ephedrine, cerebral blood flow and, 808(t)
  in atonic urinary sphincter, 1046
Epidermoid cyst(s), 2914
  cerebrospinal fluid in, 463
  incidence of, 2915
  locations of, 395(t)
  parasellar, 3154
  posterior fossa, in children, 2753–2754
  spinal, 3208
    myelography in, *535*
Epidermoid tumor, of cranium, 3232, *3233*
Epidural abscess, 3333
  in head injury, 1915
  spinal, cerebrospinal fluid in, 465

Epidural anesthesia, 3648, 3650
  diagnostic, in somatic pain, 3645
  in stereotaxic cordotomy, 3676, *3676*
  therapeutic, for pain, 3652
Epidural fibrosis, pain in, 3614, *3614*
Epidural hematoma. See *Hematoma, epidural.*
Epilepsia partialis continua, 3878
Epilepsy, 3858–3925
  alcoholic, cerebral blood flow in, 828, *829*
  behavioral aspects of, 3880–3883, 3895
  brain abscess and, 3355
  causes of, 3865–3867, 3865(t)
  deterioration from, 3881
  early, 3866
  electroencephalography in, *209*, 210, 215, 217–220,
    3868–3871, *3868*, 3911
  in posterior fossa tumors in children, 2736
  Lafora familial myoclonic, 384(t)
  late, 3866
    preventive treatment of, 3875
  localization of focus in, 3867. See also *Epileptogenic focus.*
  myoclonus with, 3852
  pediatric, causes of, 3865, 3865(t)
    clinical diagnosis of, 3867
    cortical resections in, 3879–3897
    medical treatment of, 3874–3879, 3876(t), 3877(t)
      complications of, 3878
    operative treatment of, 3879-3898
      cortical resections in, 3896
      hemicorticectomy in, 3892, *3892, 3894*
      temporal lobectomy in, 3883, *3885, 3888*
    prognosis in, 3878
  post-traumatic, 2166, 2167(t), 2188–2194
  pupils in, 651
  secondary brain damage from, in head injury, 1928
  seizures in, cerebral blood flow in, 828, *829*
    cerebral metabolism during, 770
    classification of, 3864, 3865, 3865(t)
  spina bifida aperta and, 1274
  sympathectomy for, 3720
  temporal lobe, cortical excision in, 3891
    depth electrode localization in, 3917
    stereotaxic management of, 3924
  vertiginous, 687
Epileptic neurons, 3861
Epileptic psychosis, 3882
Epileptogenic focus, chemistry of, 3863, *3864*
  excision of, 3912–3923
  localization of, in adults, electrocorticography in, 3912–3923
    in children, 3867–3871
  morphology of, 3859
  physiology of, 3861
  viral encephalitis and, 3363
Epinephrine, anesthesia and, general, 1123
    local, 1120
  cerebral blood flow and, 808(t)
  in temporal lobectomy, 3884
Epiphyses, costochondral, in acromegaly, 955
Epipodophyllotoxin, in tumor chemotherapy, 3087
Episodic syndromes, altered consciousness in, 72
  clinical diagnosis of, 38
Epsilon-aminocaproic acid, in intraoperative bleeding, 1070
Erb's palsy, in newborn infant, 49
Ergot alkaloids, cerebral blood flow and, 809(t)
Erythrocytes, in cerebrospinal fluid, 436
Esthesioneuroblastoma, 3275, *3276*
Estrogens, in anterior pituitary failure, 950
Ethacrynic acid, inner ear damage and, 691, 691(t)
Ethanolism, electromyographic studies in, 633
Ethinyl estradiol, in anterior pituitary failure, 950
Ethmoid block, *3271*
Ethmoid sinus, anatomy of, 3269, *3270, 3271*
  carcinoma of, 3279, *3279*
Ethmoidectomy, in esthesioneuroblastoma, 3276
Ethosuximide, dosages of, 3877(t)

Ethosuximide (*Continued*)
in absence status, 3878
in afebrile seizures, 3876(t), 3877
Ethyl alcohol, cerebral blood flow and, 807, 810(t)
Ethyl ether, as anesthetic, disadvantages of, 1122
Ethylnitrosourea, as carcinogen, 2654
Evoked response, brain, in head injury, 1998–2010, *1999–2005,*
2002(t), 2004(t), 2006(t), *2007, 2008*
in prognosis after head injury, 2159–2163, *2160–2162,*
2162(t)
brain stem, audiometry by, 689–700, *699*
in cerebral death, 755
in electroencephalography, 201, *202,* 216–217, *216*
in stereotaxic surgery, 3798–3800
Ewing's tumor, of spinal cord, in children, *3217*
skull metastasis and, 3242
Examination, clinical, 3–38
in infancy and childhood, 39–62
history in, 39–41
regional localization of lesions in, 9
syndromes of specific functions in, 6
in extracranial carotid occlusive disease, 1571
neurological, 41–44
in head injury, 1944–1951, 1945(t)
in spina bifida aperta, 1255–1260, 1256(t), 1259(t)
tests and, in cervical pain, 2596
neurovascular, in ischemic disease, 1517–1521, *1517,* 1519(t)
Exophthalmos, causes of, 644, *645*
in tumors of orbit, 3029(t), 3030
Extracellular fluid, hypertonicity of, 993, 993(t)
hypotonicity of, 997
Extradural space, abscess of, 3449–3451, *3450, 3451*
cyst of, spinal, in children, *3216*
measuring intracranial pressure from, 851
Extrapyramidal symptoms, rehabilitation in, 3999
Extremities, lower, muscles of, in spina bifida aperta, 1253,
1256(t), 1259(t)
pain in, in occult spinal dysraphism, 1323
post-traumatic, sympathectomy in, 3720
paralyzed, rehabilitation of, 3991–4004
schwannoma of, benign, 3301
malignant, 3304, 3305
sympathetic innervation of, 3718–3719
Eye(s), care of, percutaneous trigeminal rhizotomy and, 3576
examination of, 639, *640,* 641(t), 642–645, 644(t), *645*
in head injury, 1945, 1946
in pineal tumors, 2864, *2865*
ocular motility in, 651–663
ophthalmoscopy in, 671–675
pupil in, 645–651, *648–651,* 649(t), 650(t)
visual acuity determination in, 641–642
visual fields in, 663–671
exposure keratinitis of, 47
in posterior fossa tumors in children, 2735
movements of, in head injury, 1946–1949
reflex, in coma, 67
newborn, clinical examination of, 46
nystagmoid movements of, 662
red, causes of, 645
Eyelids, examination of, 643
injury to, 2270, *2272*

Face, congenital anomalies of, 1212–1215, 1467–1480. See also
names of specific abnormalities.
deformity of, in encephalocele, 1312
developmental anatomy of, 1468, *1468, 1469*
fractures of, 2275–2296, *2275–2296*
lower, triangular oris muscle and, 46
paralysis of, in basilar skull fracture, 2254–2257, *2255–2257*
penetrating wounds of, 2066, *2066, 2067*
schwannoma of, 3300
soft-tissue injuries of, 2263–2274, *2264–2274*
turning of, in ocular examination, 652

Face (*Continued*)
weakness of, following head injury, 2165
Facet block, in chronic low back pain, 3618
Facet denervation, in chronic low back pain, 3617, 3618(t)
Facet syndrome, 3617
Facial bone, fractures of, 2274–2286
Facial nerve, clinical examination of, 20
in infants and children, 46, 58
in Bell's palsy, 21, 3782
injury to, 2409
in basilar skull fractures, 2251–2260, *2256*
in soft-tissue wounds of face, 2266
misdirection of, 661
pain in. See *Facial neuralgia.*
palsy of, eye disorders and, 643
Facial neuralgia, atypical, 3543–3545, *3544, 3545*
vascular compression in, 3771, 3776
vs. trigeminal neuralgia, 3557
Falx cerebri, *936*
in Arnold-Chiari malformation, 1285
meningioma of, 2941, 2945–2949, *2948, 2949*
Family, counseling of, in posterior fossa tumors in children, 2742
interaction with, in post-traumatic syndrome, 2183
preoperative discussion with, 1060
Farber lipogranulomatosis, diagnosis of, 385(t)
Fasciculations, muscular, 622
Fat embolism, 1548
in multiple trauma, 2521–2522
Fecal impaction, postoperative, 1107
Feeding, difficulties with, in neonatal period, 40
enterostomy for, in multiple trauma, 2526–2528
Femoral nerve, entrapment of, 2463–2464
injury to, 2407–2408
palsy of, 2464
traction test of, 2542
Femtomole, 3951
Fentanyl, in dyskinesias, 3828
in increased intracranial pressure, 901
Fetal hydantoin syndrome, 1223
Fetus, activity pattern of, 40
head injury in, 2123
myelomeningocele in, detection of, 1274
risks to, 40
ultrasound scanning of, *720, 721, 723–732, 724, 725*
Fever, in intracranial hemorrhage, 1840
in multiple trauma, 2528–2529
postoperative, 1110, 1112
Fibrillation potentials, of muscle fiber, 621
Fibrinogen, in cerebrospinal fluid, test for, 459
Fibrolipoma, with spina bifida aperta, 1250
Fibroma, orbital, 3056
skull, 3231
Fibromuscular dysplasia, superficial temporal to middle cerebral
arterial anastomosis in, 1600
Fibromuscular hyperplasia, 1550
as indication for extracranial carotid operation, 1568, *1568*
Fibromyxoma, spinal cord, in children, *3216*
Fibrosarcoma, skull, 3235, *3235*
spinal cord, in children, *3216*
Fibrosing osteitis, of skull, 3250
Fibrosis, epidural, pain in, 3614, *3614*
Fibrous dysplasia, of orbit, 3055
of skull, *3264,* 3265, *3265*
Film changer, angiographic, 232
Fincher's syndrome, 3205
Fingers, tremors of, 48
Fischgold's line, in normal skull, 1484, *1485*
Fistula(e), arteriovenous. See *Arteriovenous fistula(e).*
dural. See *Dura mater, fistulae of.*
labyrinthine, test for, 686
subarachnoid mediastinal, 505
wound, postoperative, 2068
Flail chest, 2479–2480
Flame nevus, in infants and children, 41
Flavectomy, for cervical myelopathy, 2602–2604

Fludrocortisone acetate, 984
  in anterior pituitary failure, 951
Fluids, administration of, in head injury, 2044
    in intracerebral or intracerebellar hemorrhage, 1839
    intraoperative, 1066–1067
  body, derangements of, 993–999
      extracellular, hypertonicity of, 993, 993(t)
        hypotonicity of, 997
      in multiple trauma, 2494–2501
      normal, 2494
      postoperative complications and, 1098
      preoperative evaluation of, 1054–1054
    cerebrospinal, 423–472. See also *Cerebrospinal fluid.*
    corrosive and sclerosing, in stereotaxic lesion making, 3807
    subdural, in infants and children, 41
Fluorine intoxication, skull and, 3253
5-Fluorocytosine, in cryptococcosis, 3415
5-Fluorouracil, in tumor chemotherapy, 3086
Fluoxymesterone, in anterior pituitary failure, 950
Fluphenazine, in peripheral neuropathy, 3641
  in postherpetic neuralgia, 3642
  in spinal cord injury, 3624
Flurazepam, in objective pain, 3489
Folate concentration, of cerebrospinal fluid, 451
Follicle-stimulating hormone, hypothalamic-pituitary relationship
    and, 943
  insufficiency of, 944
  nature and function of, 940
Fontanel, anterior, encephalocele at, 1305
    vs. pseudotumor cerebri, 3190, 3191(t)
    clinical examination of, 41
  posterior, encephalocele at, 1304
Foramen (foramina), of Magendie and Luschka, in Dandy-Walker
    malformation, 1288–1289, 1290
  ovale and spinosum, in skull radiography, 80, 81, 109
    shallow, 2581
  vertebral, depth of, in radiculopathy, 2581–2586, 2582–2587
Foramen magnum, compression syndrome of, in Arnold-Chiari
    malformation, 1287–1288, 1287
  meningioma of, 2942–2943, 2960, 2960
Foraminotomy, for cervical myelopathy, 2605–2607, 2606
Forbes-Albright syndrome, 965
Forceps, micro-operative 1184, 1184, 1187, 1188, 1190, 1191
Foreign body (bodies), cerebral, in children, 2123
  in penetrating wounds, 2066, 2066, 2067
  intraventricular, 2067
  postoperative rejection of, 1087
Foster Kennedy syndrome, 673, 673
  clinical examination in, 17
Fovea ethmoidalis, 3270
Fracture(s). See also names of specific bones.
  compression, local anesthesia in, 3653
  hangman's, 2326, 2326
  in multiple trauma, 2521–2522
  Jefferson, 500, 2324
  malignant disease and, 3628
  rib, local anesthesia in, 3653
  skull, computed tomography in, 125, 126
    in head injury, 1905–1907, 1906(t), 1907(t)
    leptomeningeal cyst and, in children, 3245, 3249
  radiography of, 86, 95, 96–100
  spinal, cervical, 500, 498–503
    computed tomography in, 140
    lumbar, 2356–2359, 2357–2358
    radiography in, 496, 498–503
    thoracic, 2348
  temporal bone, 2251–2259, 2252, 2253, 2255–2257
  thoracic-lumbar, 500, 502
Fracture-dislocation, cervical, 2326, 2327
  mechanism of, 2319, 2320, 2321
  radiography in, 501, 502
  lumbar, 2358
  rehabilitation in, 4000
  thoracic, 2348, 2349

Freezing, in stereotaxic lesion making, 3810
  in hypophysectomy, 3974–3979, 3975, 3976
Friedreich's ataxia, cerebrospinal fluid in, 468
Froin's syndrome, 441
Frontal lobe, lesions of, clinical examination in, 13–14, 13
  evoked potentials in, 2007
Frontal sinus, anatomy of, 3270, 3271, 3272
Frontalis nerve, in orbit, 3028
Frostbite, sympathectomy for, 3720
Full Range Picture Vocabulary test, 706
Function, altered, in posterior fossa tumors in children,
    2735–2736
  brain, disturbed, in systemic trauma, 1909
  bulbar and cranial nerve, in posterior fossa tumors in children,
    2736
  deficits of, in astrocytoma, 2773
    in brain tumors, 2763
  intellectual, psychological testing of, 703–705, 704
  pulmonary, in scoliosis, 2633
  sexual, in spina bifida aperta, 1273
  social, disorders of, after head injury, 2168
    in spina bifida aperta, 1273
  useful, after peripheral nerve injury, 2418–2420, 2418, 2420
  ventilatory, in multiple trauma, 2479–2483
  weakness of, electromyography in, 633
Fungal infections, 3366–3440. See also names of specific
    infections.
  aneurysms from, subarachnoid hemorrhage and, 1812–1814
  cerebrospinal fluid in, 441–443
  spinal, 3456
Funicular pain, in spinal cord tumors, 3199
Furosemide, in inappropriate antidiuretic hormone secretion, 982
  in postoperative tissue edema, 1091
Fusion(s), spinal, in deformities, 2637–2638
    osteotomy of, 2639, 2643

Gait, characteristic disorders of, 60(t)
  in normal-pressure hydrocephalus, 1424
  in Parkinson's disease, 3838
  stereotaxic lesions and, 3843
Gait training, in hemiplegia, 3996
Galactokinase deficiency, pseudotumor cerebri and, 3181(t), 3188
Galactorrhea, in acromegaly, 954
  hormone secretion and, 964
Galactosemia, pseudotumor cerebri and, 3181(t), 3188
Galea aponeurotica, anatomy of, 2299, 2299
Galen, vein of, malformation of, 1796–1802, 1802
Gallbladder, pain in, 3631
Gallium citrate, in brain scanning, 146
Galvanic skin reflex, 3649, 3650
Gamma camera, in cerebral death, 755(t)
Gamma globulin, in cerebrospinal fluid, 442–445
  determination of, 459
Gamma system, in dyskinesias, 3825
Gamma-amino butyric acid, cerebral blood flow and, 812(t)
  metabolism of, 771
Gangliocytoma, as neuronal tumor, 2801
Ganglioglioma, as neuronal tumor, 2801
  cerebral hemisphere, in children, 2713
  posterior fossa, in children, 2754
Ganglion (ganglia), basal, tumors of, in children, 2721–2722,
    2721(t)
  celiac, neurolytic injection in, 3661–3662
  ciliary, in orbit, 3028
  dorsal, of spinal cord, 3657, 3657
    in ascending pain pathway, 3463–3464
  excision of, sympathetic innervation following, 3719
  Scarpa's, 679
  sympathetic, neurolytic injections in, 3661
Ganglioneuroblastoma, 2801, 3310
  sympathoblast and, 3307
Ganglioneuroma, 2801, 3310
  biochemical assay in, 2692

Ganglioneuroma (*Continued*)
  spinal cord, in children, *3216*
  sympathoblast and, 3307
Ganglionic blocking agents, cerebral blood flow and, 807, 808(t)
Ganglionic stimulating drugs, cerebral blood flow and, 809(t)
Gangliosidosis, diagnosis of, 385(t)
Gangrene, paradoxical, following sympathectomy, 3724
Gas(es), blood, in respiratory failure, 1024, 1025
  normal transport of, 1011
  cystometry with, 1035, *1035*
  myelography with, in Arnold-Chiari malformation, 1287, *1287*
    in separate odontoid process, *1488*
    in spinal angioma, 578, *578*
Gastrointestinal system, postoperative complications in, 1105–1108
  preoperative evaluation of, 1055–1056
Gaucher disease, diagnosis of, 385(t)
Gemistocytic astrocytoma, 2769
Genetic disorders, neurosurgical aspects of, 1207–1235. See also names of specific disorders.
  counseling in, 1209–1210
  in dysraphias, 1218, 1218(t)
Genetics, as predisposing factor in brain tumors, 2666–2671
  environment and, in neural tube malformations, 1242–1243
Geniculate neuralgia, 3605–3607, *3607*
Genitourinary systems, postoperative complications of, 1104–1105
  preoperative evaluation of, 1058–1059
Gentamicin, 3327
  in bacterial meningitis, 3339
  inner ear damage and, 691, 691(t)
Geographic skull, 3258
Geography, brain tumor incidence and, 2685–2688, 2686–2687(t)
Germinoma, 2716
  location of, 395(t)
  suprasellar, 3153
    in children, 2719, *2719*
  supratentorial, in children, 2716
Gerstmann's syndrome, clinical examination in, 16
Gesell's stages of infant and child development, 42(t)
Giant cell tumor, angiographic appearance of, 612
  astrocytoma as, subependymal, 2786–2788
  benign, of skull, 3231
Gigantism, 953. See also *Acromegaly.*
  cerebral, vs. acromegaly, 956
  intrasellar adenoma in, 3131, *3131*
Glasgow coma scale, in head injury, *1943*, 1944, *1945*
  in prognosis after head injury, 2138, 2139(t), 2141(t)
    neurological signs and, 2146, 2146(t), 2147(t)
Glaucoma, low-tension, 674
  sympathectomy for, 3720
Glioblastoma, brain scanning in, 2810, *2810*
  in children, 162(t)
  cell death in, 3068
  computed tomography in, 114, *114*, 2811, *2811*
  in adult, 2802–2817
  necrosis of, 3067
Glioblastoma multiforme, brain scanning in, *152*
Glioma(s), 2759–2823. See also names of specific glial tumors.
  anaplasia in, 2770
  anaplastic, brain scanning following, 154
  brain scanning in, 150(t)
  brain stem, in children, 2751–2752
  computed tomography vs. radionuclide imaging in, 167(t)
  cranial, cerebral blood flow in, 825
  intracerebral, skull defects and, 3251
  intracranial, intracranial pressure monitoring in, 890
  radiation therapy of, 3099, 3099(t)
    treatment of, dexamethasone in, 910
  malignant, infiltration by, 3066
    kinetic parameters of, 3068, 3068(t)
    recurrent or untreated, chemotherapy for, 3090(t)
  mixed, in adult, 2771
  of spinal cord, angiography in, *608*, 609

Glioma (*Continued*)
  of spinal cord, myelographic appearance of, *533*
    radiation therapy of, 3212, 3224(t)
  optic, 644, 3042–3046, *3043–3047*
    computed tomography in, 139, 2724, *2725*, *2726*
    in children, 2722–2727, *2722–2726*, 2724(t), 2726(t)
      brain scanning in, 162(t)
    temporal lobe, and headache, 3552
    widening of spinal canal and, 512
Gliomatosis cerebri, 2823
Globoid cell leukodystrophy, diagnosis of, 385(t)
Glomus jugulare tumor, 3285–3298
  arterial supply to, 3292, *3293*
  classification of, 3285–3287
  clinical experience in, 3289–3290
  death and morbidity in, 3290
  diagnosis of, 3287–3289, *3287–3291*
  extracranial, embolization of, 1201, *1202*
  treatment of, 3290–3297, *3291*, *3293–3296*
"Glomus" malformation, of spinal cord, 1858, 1866–1869, *1868*
Glossopharyngeal nerve, clinical examination of, 20
  in infants and children, 47, 59
  pain in, 3604–3605, *3606*, 3775, *3776*
    percutaneous rhizotomy in, 3609–3612, *3610*, *3611*
    vascular decompression in, 3771, 3775–3776, *3776*
    with trigeminal neuralgia, posterior approach for, 3587
Glucocorticocoids, in tumor chemotherapy, 3089–3090
Glucose, cerebrospinal fluid, 447
  determination of, 459
  oxidative metabolism and, 765
  plasma, in anterior pituitary failure, 947
  serum, in acromegaly, 954
Glutamate, metabolism of, 771
Glutamine, in cerebrospinal fluid, 451
Glycerol, in craniotomy, 1143
  in increased intracranial pressure, 909
  in pseudotumor cerebri, 3192
Glycogenoses, diagnosis of, 385(t)
Glycolysis, energy yield of, 766, *766*
Goiter, exophthalmic, sympathectomy for, 3720
Gold, radioactive, characteristics of, 3974(t)
Gonadotropin, insufficiency of, 944–945
  replacement of, in anterior pituitary failure, 949–950
  secretion of, by pituitary tumors, 964
Gradenigo's syndrome, 3329
Grafts, nerve, in peripheral nerve injury, 2146–2147, *2147*
Graham-Kendall Memory for Designs Test, 706
Grand mal. See *Epilepsy.*
Granulocytic sarcoma, orbital, 3058
Granuloma, eosinophilic, spinal, *515*
  orbital, 3061–3062
  parasellar, 3155
Granulomatous angiitis, cerebrospinal fluid in, 463
  in sarcoidosis, 3428
  noninfectious, 1546
Graphesthesia, 61
Grass cortical electrode assembly, 3885, *3885*
Graves' disease, proptosis and, 3059
Great occipital nerve, entrapment of, 2462–2463
Great vein of Galen, *280*, 282
Grief, pain as symptom of, 3756
Growth hormone, hypothalamic-pituitary relationship and, 941
  in pituitary tumors, 952–958, 957(t)
  insufficiency of, 944
  nature and function of, 938(t), 939
  replacement of, in anterior pituitary failure, 948
  serum, measurement of, in acromegaly, 953
Guillain-Barré syndrome, cerebrospinal fluid in, 436, 471
  vs. acute transverse myelitis, 3359
Guiot stereotaxic instrument, 3804
Gumma, cerebral, 3445–3446
Gyrus (gyri), cerebral, absence of, 1211(t)
  hippocampal, in craniotomy, 1147
  in Arnold-Chiari malformation, 1285

Hallervorden-Spatz syndrome, brain biopsy in, 386(t)
Halo traction, in cervical injuries, 2329
  in spinal deformities, 2642–2646, *2646*
Haloperidol, in organic brain syndrome, 3496
Halothane, as general anesthetic, 1122
    electroencephalographic monitoring of, 227
  cerebral blood flow and, 805
Hand, paralyzed, rehabilitation of, 3991–3995, *3993, 3994*
Hand-Schüller-Christian disease, skull in, 3258
Handee-Standee, 3995
Hangman's fracture, 2326, *2326*
Harelip, incidence of, 1210(t)
Harrington instrumentation, in lumbar spinal fracture, 2357
  in spinal deformities, 2638–2639, *2638, 2640, 2641*
  in thoracic spinal injury, 2348, *2349*
Harvard criteria for brain death, 756–757
Head, carcinoma of, mesencephalotomy for, 3707
  circumference of, in hydrocephalus, 1387, *1387–1391*
  examination of, in infants and children, 41
  fixation of, in aneurysm procedures, 1671
    in angiography, 233
    in micro-operative procedures, 1181, *1183*
  injury to, 1896–2174. See also *Head injury.*
  pain-sensitive structures in, anatomy and physiology of, 3531–3532
  position of, cerebral blood flow and, 827, 830
    in ocular examination, 652
  schwannoma of, benign, 3300
    malignant, 3304
  size of, deviation in, 1220
    in posterior fossa tumors in children, 2735
  transillumination of, 41
Head binder, angiographic, 233
Head injury, 1896–2174
  airway in, 1119
  angiography in, 326, *326, 327*
  carotid-cavernous fistula and, 1772–1781, *1776–1778, 1780*
  cavernous plexus aneurysms and, 1770–1771
  closed, management of, 2010–2018, 2011(t), 2012(t), *2013,* 2016(t), *2017*
    operative treatment of, 2018
    psychiatric complications with, 2199
  coma and, 64(t)
  computed tomography in, 125–127, *126,* 1951–1981, *1953–1982,* 2020–2023, *2020–2022*
  diagnostic evaluation of, 1941–2010, *1943–1945,* 1945(t)
    in children, 2091–2096, *2092, 2094*
  electronencephalography in, 1994–1998, *1995, 1996*
  epidemiology of, 1939–1940, 2084–2086, *2085*
  hydrocephalus and, 1429
  in adults, 1938–2083
  in children, 2084–2136
    specific entities in, 2096–2123
  increased intracranial pressure in, 880–889, 881(t), 882(t), 885(t), *886–888*
    causes of, 1922
  management of, in adults, 883, 889, 2010–2070
    in children, 2091–2096
    intensive medical, 2036–2048, *2038–2042*
    operative, 2018–2037, *2020–2022, 2027–2029, 2031–2033, 2035, 2036*
    steroids in, 911
  mechanisms of, 1877–1894
    in children, 2090
  metabolic response to, 989
  missile injuries as, 2055–2068, *2055, 2058, 2060, 2063–2067*
    orbital-facial-cranial wounds as, 2066
  pathophysiology of, 1896–1937
    damage to related structures in, 1904, 1906(t), 1907(t)
    ischemic brain damage in, 1927
    preinjury status in, 1896, 1897(t)
    primary brain damage in, 1897, *1900–1902, 1904*
    secondary brain damage in, 1909, *1910, 1914,* 1917(t), 1918(t)
  post-traumatic cephalic pain and, 3541–3542, *3542, 3543*

Head injury (*Continued*)
  prenatal and perinatal, 2123–2127
  prevention of, 1940–1941
  prognosis after, 2137–2174
    clinical factors in, 2141, 2142(t), 2143(t), 2146(t), 2147(t)
    data required for, 2138, 2139(t), 2141(t)
    diagnostic studies and, 2148, *2149,* 2149(t), 2150(t), *2151, 2152, 2157, 2158, 2160–2162*
    in children, 2129–2130
    quality of survival in, 2163–2170
  pseudotumor cerebri and, 3181(t)
  psychological testing after, 2195–2204
  superficial temporal to middle cerebral arterial anastomosis in, 1601
  tangential, management of, 2064
  vascular complications of, 2070
Headache, aneurysm-related, 3552
  cerebral blood flow in, 822, 828, *829*
  eye disorders and, 641
  in astrocytomas, 2772
  in brain tumors, 2762
  in pituitary adenoma, 3129
  in posterior fossa tumors in children, 2734
  in post-traumatic syndrome, 2176, 2177, 2184, 2185
  in sylvian fissure cyst, 1439
  increased intracranial pressure and, 877
  pneumoencephalography and, 368
  severe focal, neuropsychological assessment in, 710
  tension, 3546
  tumor-related, 2762, 2772, 3550–3552, *3551*
  vascular, 3547–3550
    arteriovenous anomalies and, 3552
Hearing, in newborn, 47
  loss of, head injury and, 2165–2166
    in basilar skull fractures, 2257–2258
  physiology of, 693
  tests of, 693–700, *696, 698, 699*
    in acoustic neuroma, 2972–2974, *2974*
    in head injury, 2006
Heart. See also entries beginning *Cardiac* and *Cardio-.*
  auscultation of, in ischemic vascular disease, 1517–1518, *1517*
  congenital cyanotic disease of, skull in, 3261
  congestive failure of, postoperative, 1098
  disease of, pain in, 3631
  injury to, in multiple trauma, 2491–2492
  lesions of, cerebral embolization incidence and, 1515(t)
  malformation of, incidence of, 1210(t)
  open procedures on, neurological abnormalities after, 1549
Heart rate, increased intracranial pressure and, 863
Heat, in stereotaxic lesion making, 3800, 3808–3810, *3809*
Hemangioblastoma, 2846–2853, 2846(t), *2849, 2851*
  brain scanning in, 153
  capillary, in posterior fossa, in children, 2754, *2755*
  location of, 395(t)
  spinal, 3208, *3209*
    angiography in, 604–609, *604–607*
    operative treatment of, 3211, *3211*
  subarachnoid hemorrhage and, 1642, *1642*
  tumor complexes of, 190, *193*
Hemangioendothelioma, benign, orbital, 3054
  spinal cord, in children, *3216*
Hemangioma, capillary, orbital, 3054
  cavernous, cerebral hemisphere, in children, 2713
    orbital, 3054
  skull, 3231, *3232*
  spinal, embolization of, 1202
    hourglass defect of, 3201, *3203*
    radiographic appearance of, *514*
Hemangiopericytoma, of brain, 2853–2855, *2854*
  orbital, 3055
Hematocrit, neonatal, 40
Hematoma, acute, early epilepsy and, 3866
  chronic, 2070–2073
  computed tomography vs. radionuclide imaging in, 167(t)
  echoencephalography in, 181, *181,* 182, *183,* 190, 192

Hematoma (*Continued*)
  epidural, angiography in, *331,* 332–341, *334, 335*
    brain scanning in, 155(t)
    cerebrospinal fluid in, 466
    computed tomography in, 127, *127,* 1975, *1978, 1979*
    in head injury, 1909, 1975, *1978, 1979,* 2030
    prognosis after head injury and, 2144
    traumatic, in children, 2103–2107, *2105, 2106*
  intra-axial, computed tomography in, 129, *129, 130*
  intracerebral, adjacent to aneurysm, intracranial pressure in, 893
    as contraindication to carotid ligation, 1703
    brain scanning in, 155(t), 159
    cerebral blood flow and, 886, *886*
    in head injury, 1913–1914, 2033
      computed tomography in, 1961, *1962,* 1965, *1968, 1969, 1978, 1979*
      operative management of, 2030
    traumatic, in children, 2113–2114, *2114*
    vs. intracerebral contusions, 161
  intracranial, brain scanning in, 156, *159*
    postoperative, in aneurysms, 1960
  intraspinal, 1085
  posterior fossa, computed tomography in, 129
    in neonate, 2125
  spinal cord, myelographic appearance of, *533*
  subdural, angiography in, 328–332, *329, 330, 332, 333*
    cerebrospinal fluid in, 466
    chronic, 2070–2073, 2108
    chronic relapsing juvenile, 1439
    computed tomography in, 127, *127–129,* 1969–1975, *1969–1977,* 2109, *2110, 2111*
    following pneumoencephalography, 368
    in head injury, 1911–1939, 1969–1975, *1969–1977,* 2030, *2031*
      in children, 2107–2113, *2109–2111*
    post-shunt, 1416, *1417*
    prognosis after head injury and, 2144
    sylvian fissure cyst with, 1439
  tumor complexes of, *189*
  wound, postoperative, 1083–1085
Hemianopia, bitemporal, 668, *668*
  definition of, 665, *666*
  rehabilitation of patient with, 3991
  transient homonymous, migraine and, 640
Hemiballism, 3851
  thalamotomy and, 3837
Hemichorea, 3851
Hemicorticectomy, in epilepsy, in children, 3892–3896, *3892, 3894*
Hemifacial spasm, vascular decompression in, 3773–3775, *3773,* 3774(t), 3775(t)
Hemimyelomeningocele, 1245
Hemiparesis, as indication for carotid operation, 1565
  in head injury, evoked potentials in, 2006
  in newborn, signs of, 48, 49
Hemiplegia, as indication for carotid operation, 1565
  in head injury, 2166
    evoked potentials in, 2006
  infantile, electroencephalography in, 221
    epilepsy and, 3919–3923
  manipulation, temporal lobectomy and, 3890
  rehabilitation in, 3991–3999, *3992–3998*
Hemisphere(s), cerebral, dysfunction of, electroencephalography in, 224–226, *225*
  in head injury, evoked potentials from, 2006, 2008–2010
Hemispherectomy, in epilepsy, results of, 3892
  in infantile hemiplegia, 3920
Hemivertebra(e), 491, *494*
  angiography of, 562, *562*
  excision of, 2641–2642, *2645*
Hemoglobin, in acute respiratory failure, 1023
Hemolytic uremic syndrome, 1547
Hemophilia, operative procedures in, bleeding control in, 1070
Hemophilus influenzae brain abscess, 3348

Hemorrhage, acute cerebral, cerebrospinal fluid in, 466
  coma in, 71
  apoplectic, 3148
  cerebral, brain scanning in, 155
    cerebrospinal fluid and, 436–437
  gastrointestinal, postoperative, 1106
  hypertensive, 1822–1830
  in basal skull fractures, 2254
  in dural sinus exposure, 1076
  in thalamotomy, 3835
  intracerebral and intracerebellar, spontaneous, 1821–1849, *1822–1824*
    diagnosis of, 1830, *1831, 1832, 1834–1838*
    management of, 1837
  intracranial, in supratentorial tumors, in children, 2704
    neonatal, 48, 2125
    vs. viral encephalitis, 3360
  intraventricular, computed tomography in, 1975, *1980*
  meningeal, traumatic, in children, 2103
  neonatal, 40
    retinal, 46
  postcraniotomy, 1152
  postoperative, causes of, 1093
    in posterior fossa tumors in children, 2745
  postventriculography, 379
  reduction of, carotid ligation in, 1708–1710
  spinal meningeal, in angiomas, 563
  subarachnoid. See *Subarachnoid hemorrhage.*
Hemosiderosis, central nervous system, cerebrospinal fluid in, 462
Hemothorax, in multiple trauma, 2480–2482
Hendler screening test, in chronic back pain, 3488, 3490(t)
Hensen's node, formation of, 1237
Heparin, in postoperative venous thrombosis, 1109
  prophylactic use of, 1059
Hepatic disease, cerebrospinal fluid in, 469
Hepatitis, postoperative, 1107
Hepatolenticular degeneration, intention tremor in, 3852
Herniation, brain, computed tomography in, 126
  head injury and, 1917
  intracranial pressure in, 858, 1924
  lumbar puncture and, 456
    in brain abscess, 3346
  secondary, in encephalocele, 1299
  disc, air myelography in, *529*
    blocked vertebrae and, myelographic appearance of, *547*
    cerebrospinal fluid in, 467
    metrizamide myelography in, 525, *525*
    myelographic appearance of, 530
    recurrent, in chronic low back pain, 3613
    sacral and iliac destruction in, *513*
  incisural, uncal, in craniotomy, 1147
  of invasive adenoma, 3132, *3132*
  tentorial, 1917(t), 1918–1921, *1920*
    angiography in, *316,* 324, 325, *325*
    cerebral edema and, 878
    clinical diagnosis of, 879
    in newborn, 46
    syndromes of, 70(t)
  tonsillar, 1921, *1921*
    angiography in, *316,* 325
    pneumoencephalography and, 363
Herpes simplex, Bell's palsy and, 3782
  encephalitis in, 3362
    cerebrospinal fluid in, 465
    electroencephalography in, *213,* 214, 222
  tic douloureux and, 3594
    percutaneous trigeminal rhizotomy and, 3577
    temporal craniotomy for trigeminal neuralgia and, 3583
Herpes zoster, acute, reversible nerve block in, 3655
  cerebrospinal fluid in, 465
  neuralgia following, 3542–3543, 3641–3642, *3642*
Herpesvirus hominis infection, brain biopsy in, 388
Hertwig-Magendie position, 656
Hexamethonium, cerebral blood flow and, 808(t)

Hexamethonium (*Continued*)
in deliberate hypotension, 1127
Hiccough, postoperative, 1105
Hindbrain, in Arnold-Chiari malformation, 1283, *1283, 1284*
Hippocampal gyrus, craniotomy and, 1147
Hirschsprung's disease, sympathectomy in, 3720
Histamine, cerebral blood flow and, 809(t)
Histiocytoma, fibrous, of orbit, 3057
Histiocytosis X, anterior pituitary failure and, 948
infiltration of, in parasellar region, 3154
skull in, 3258, *3260*
Histoplasmosis, 3416–3419
cerebrospinal fluid in, 461
History taking, 1, 4–6
in children, 39–41
in head injury, 1943, *1943, 1944*
ophthalmological, 639–641
preoperative review of, 1060
Histrionic personality, "effected" pain and, 3505–3507
Hodgkin's disease, skeletal involvement in, *514,* 3244
Home, in rehabilitation, 3990
rehabilitation equipment in, 3999
Homeostasis, general care and, 762–1117
neurophysiological, suffering and, 3729–3733, *3730, 3731*
Homosexuality, pedophilic, neurosurgery for, 3943
Hormones. See also names of specific hormones.
anterior pituitary, 935–943, 937(t), 938(t)
in cerebrospinal fluid, 435, 451
malignant tumor dependency on, 3947–3948
post-traumatic secretion of, 992–993
production of, embryology and, 3108
replacement of, gonadal, following cryohypophysectomy, 3979
Horner's syndrome, in ganglioneuroma, 3310
pupillary reactions in, 647, *648*
symptoms of, in newborn, 46
Host, susceptibility of, in bacterial infection, 3323
Hot stroke phenomenon, 156, *158*
Humerus, fracture of, in newborn, 49
injury to, radial nerve in, 2395
Hunterian ligation, in giant aneurysms of posterior circulation, 1750
Huntington's chorea, 3851
vs. Parkinson's disease, 3841
Hyaline bodies, of optic nerve, 672, *672*
Hydatid disease, 3376–3383
cerebral, 3377
cerebrospinal fluid in, 462
cranial, 3380
vertebral, 3381
Hydranencephaly, genetic aspects of, 1221
transillumination in, 41
1-Hydrazinophthalazine, cerebral blood flow and, 809(t)
Hydrocephalus, 1381–1435
arrested, diagnostic criteria for, *1418,* 1419–1420, *1419*
clinical features of, 1383–1385, *1384*
computed tomography in, 129–132, *131,* 1393–1396, *1394–1395,* 1404, *1405, 1406*
postoperative, 133, *134, 135*
congenital, cerebrospinal fluid in, 467
definition of, 1381
diagnosis of, 1385–1400, *1386–1400,* 1386(t)
etiology of, 1383
fetal, ultrasound scanning in, *720*
genetic aspects of, 1221, *1221*
head circumference in, 1387, *1387–1391*
high-pressure, 1433–1434
idiopathic, selection of patients for operation in, 1428
in adults, 1423–1435
in Arnold-Chiari malformation, 1282, *1283,* 1286
in children, 1381–1422
treatment of, 1400–1409
in Dandy-Walker malformation, 1291
in encephalocele, 1301
in head injury, computed tomography in, 1980, *1981*

Hydrocephalus (*Continued*)
in infant, echoencephalography in, 186
ultrasound scanning in, *722, 728*
in neonate, *44*
in posterior fossa tumors in children, 2746
in sarcoidosis, 3427
in spina bifida aperta, 1259, 1270, 1272
control of, 1263
postoperative, 1270
incidence of, 1210(t)
lumbar cerebrospinal fluid pressure in, *850*
myelomeningocele and, 1259
noncommunicating, cerebrospinal fluid in, 430
normal pressure, 164, *166,* 1423–1433
cerebrospinal fluid in, 471
clinical presentation of, 1424
diagnostic tests for, 1425
etiology and pathology of, 1423
increased intracranial pressure in, 895, 1426
operative treatment of, 1430, *1430–1432*
selection of patients for, 1428
postoperative evaluation of, 1433
vs. Alzheimer's disease, 895
vs. cerebral atrophy dementia, 827
obstructive, cerebrospinal fluid in, 430
postoperative, intracranial pressure monitoring in, 891
subarachnoid hemorrhage and, 1658
otitic, pseudotumor cerebri and, 3182
pathogenesis of, 1382, *1382,* 1382(t)
pathophysiology of, 3180(t)
pneumoencephalography in, *368*
postoperative, in aneurysms, 1691
subarachnoid hemorrhage and, 1816–1817
transillumination of skull in, 41, 1387
vs. pseudotumor cerebri, 3189
x-ray landmarks in, 3795
Hydrocortisone, as prophylaxis for steroid deficiency, in neurosurgical patient, 1057
in anterior pituitary failure, 949
in postoperative steroid insufficiency, 1103
Hydrodynamics, theory of, in Arnold-Chiari malformation, 1280
in Dandy-Walker malformation, 1289–1290
in encephalocele, 1299
in spina bifida aperta, 1247–1248
Hydroflumethiazide, in treatment of pseudotumor cerebri, 3192
Hydromyelia, computed tomography in, 139
Hydrops, endolymphatic, secondary, 689
vertigo in, 688, *689*
Hydrostatic expulsion, in echinococcosis, 3380
Hydroxyproline, urinary, in acromegaly, 955
5-Hydroxytryptamine, cerebral blood flow and, 809(t)
Hydroxyurea, in tumor chemotherapy, 3087
Hydroxyzine, in histrionic personality, 3506
in objective pain, 3489
in pain relief, 3481
in stereotaxic cordotomy, 3673
Hygroma, subdural, in head injury, 1913
post-traumatic, in children, 2112
Hyperabduction syndrome, 2460–2461, *2461*
Hyperactive dysfunction syndromes, 3772–3778
Hyperbaric oxygen, cerebral blood flow and, 818, 830
in increased intracranial pressure, 903–905
Hyperbilirubinemia, in crush injury, 2519–2520
Hypercalciuria, in acromegaly, 954
Hypercapnia, cerebrovascular responsivity to, 888
Hypercarbia, intracranial pressure in, 868
Hyperchloremia, cerebral lesions and, 989
Hyperchloruria, 997
Hyperemia, in head injury, 885, 885(t)
Hyperextension-hyperflexion injury, of cervical spine, 2320, 2330–2332, 2338–2343, *2339*
of lumbar spine, 2358
Hyperglycemia, in acromegaly, 954
Hyperhidrosis, sympathectomy for, 3720

Hyperkalemia, electrocardiography in, 991
Hyperkinesias, following thalamotomy, 3837
Hypernatremia, cerebral lesions and, 989
　in coma, 994
　postoperative, 1103
Hypernatruria, 997
Hypernephroma, hypophysectomy in, 3953
　metastatic, chemotherapy for, 3090(t)
Hyperosmotic agent, in craniotomy, 1143
Hyperostosis, infantile cortical, skull in, 3256
　skull radiography in, 92–94, 100–110, 107
Hyperostosis corticalis generalisata, 3255
Hyperostosis frontalis interna, 3256, 3257
Hyperparathyroidism, primary, acromegaly and, 957
　skull in, 3251, 3252
Hyperperfusion phenomenon, 156, 158
Hyperplasia, fibromuscular, 1550
　as indication for extracranial carotid operation, 1568, 1568
Hyperprolactinemia, 965–969
　conditions associated with, 966(t)
　radiation therapy in, 3167
Hyperpyrexia, brain damage from, in head injury, 1929
　postoperative, 1112
Hyperreflexia, autonomic, spinal cord dysfunction and, 4011
Hypertelorism, 1470–1471, 1470
　development of, 1469
　operative techniques in, 1474–1476, 1475–1477
Hypertension, cerebral infarction and, 817
　encephalopathy in, 1547–1548
　　pathophysiology of, 3180(t)
　hemorrhage in, 1822–1830, 1822–1825
　in coma, 64(t)
　intracranial, 846–930. See also Intracranial pressure,
　　increased.
　sympathectomy for, 3720
　thoracolumbar resection for, 3723
Hyperthermia, in coma, 64(t)
　postoperative, 1112
Hypertonic solutions, cerebrovascular and metabolic responses to,
　909
　in increased intracranial pressure, 905–910
　saline, in inappropriate antidiuretic hormone secretion, 981
Hypertonicity, of extracellular fluid, 993, 993(t)
Hyperventilation, apnea following, in unconsciousness, 65
　　prognosis after head injury and, 2153
　as anesthetic, 1124–1126
　cerebral blood flow and, 802, 806
　in electroencephalography, 215
　in increased intracranial pressure, 901–903
　therapeutic, and cerebral blood flow, 825, 830
Hyperviscosity, neonatal, 40
Hypervitaminosis A, pseudotumor cerebri and, 3181(t), 3187
　skull in, 3253
Hypervitaminosis D, skull in, 3253
Hypoactive dysfunction syndromes, 3778–3782
Hypocalcemia, in newborn, 48, 49
Hypocapnia, cerebrovascular responsivity to, 888
Hypochloremia, 997
Hypochondria, cephalic pain and, 3546
Hypoglossal nerve, clinical examination of, 20
　in infants and children, 47
　disease of, 3782
　injury to, 2410
Hypoglycemia, anterior pituitary failure and, 945
　brain damage from, in head injury, 1928
　in ischemic vascular disease, 1543
　cerebral metabolism in, 771–772
　in acromegaly, 954
　in neonate, 40
Hypoliquorrhea, cerebrospinal fluid in, 471
Hyponatremia, 997–998
　following open cordotomy, 3697
　postoperative, 1103
Hypoparathyroidism, pseudotumor cerebri and, 3181(t), 3186

Hypophosphatasis, pseudotumor cerebri and, 3181(t), 3188
Hypophyseal cachexia, 943
Hypophysectomy, by craniotomy, 3981–3986, 3985(t)
　diabetes insipidus and, 3949
　evaluation of response following, 3950
　in breast carcinoma, 3950–3952, 3984–3985
　in diabetic retinopathy, 3948–3949, 3953–3955, 3985–3986,
　　3985(t)
　　vs. photocoagulation, 3955, 3985(t)
　in metastatic bone pain, 3628
　in prostate carcinoma, 3952–3953
　indications for, 3947–3958
　malignant tumor hormone dependency and, 3947–3948
　results of, 3947–3958
　selection of patients for, 3949–3950
　special problems following, 3979
　stereotaxic, 3973–3980
　transsphenoidal, 3959–3972
　　technique for, 3959–3969, 3960–3969
　　vs. bilateral adrenalectomy, 3949
Hypophysis, microscopic anatomy of, 3116, 3116
　pharyngeal, embryology of, 3107
Hypopituitarism, 943
　unitropic, 945
Hyposexuality, temporal lobe epilepsy and, 3881
Hypotension, deliberate, as anesthetic technique, 1126–1128
　in aneurysm procedures, 1668
　monitoring during, 1130
　following cordotomy, 3698
　in coma, 64(t)
　postoperative, 1098
　postural, following hypophysectomy, 3979
　profound, in diffuse cerebral ischemia, 1541, 1541
　prognosis after head injury and, 2145, 2146(t)
Hypothalamico-neurohypophyseal system, 970–983, 971
Hypothalamus, anterior pituitary and, 940–943
　blood supply of, 934
　posteromedial, lesions in, in primary affective disorders,
　　3942
Hypothermia. See also Cryo- entries.
　deliberate, as anesthetic technique, 1128–1130
　　for stereotaxic lesion making, 3810
　　hypotension with, 1127
　　in aneurysm procedures, 1668
　　monitoring during, 1130
　in coma, 64(t)
　in increased intracranial pressure, 912–915
　postischemic survival and, 780
Hypothyroidism, following cryohypophysectomy, 3979
Hypotonia, in newborn, 45, 47
Hypoventilation, cerebral blood flow and, 806
　generalized, acute respiratory failure and, 1015
　postoperative, 1094
　pulmonary, intracranial hypertension in, 3180(t)
Hypovitaminosis A, pseudotumor cerebri and, 3181(t), 3187
Hypovolemia, postoperative, 1098
　shock in, pathophysiology of, 2502–2504
　therapy in, 2506–2509
Hypoxemia, increased intracranial pressure and, 866
　prognosis after head injury and, 2145
　secondary brain damage from, in head injury, 1928
Hypoxia, cerebral metabolism in, 772–774, 773
　hypoxemic, in diffuse cerebral ischemia, 1541–1542
　hypoxic, function effects of, 772, 773
　in newborn, 45, 48, 49
　intracranial pressure in, 868

Iatrogenic problems, in chronic pain, 3527
Image intensifier, angiographic, 232
Imipramine, in atonic urinary sphincter treatment, 1046

Immune status, brain abscess and, 3349
 cerebrospinal fluid and, 469
Immunoglobulins, in cerebrospinal fluid, 442–445
 determination of, 459
Immunotherapy, in brain tumors, 3090
 in cerebral metastases, 2887
 in glioblastoma, 2817
 sympathectomy by, 3724
Impact, physical, in concussion, 1880, *1881*
 in post-traumatic syndrome, 2181
Impedance studies, auditory, 2972
 in stereotaxic surgery, 3799–3800
Incisions, craniotomy, 1138, *1138*
 for meningioma operations, 2945, *2946, 2947*
 intraoperative complications and, 1074
 postoperative pain from, reversible nerve block in, 3653
Incisural sclerosis, 3860
Inclusion tumors, 2914–2923
Incontinence, in normal-pressure hydrocephalus, 1424
 rectal, intrathecal neurolytic agents and, 3659
Indium DTPA, in brain scanning, 145, 148(t)
Indomethacin, pseudotumor cerebri and, 3181(t), 3187
Infant, anemia in, skull in, 3261, *3263*
 cerebrospinal fluid in, 451
 cervical spine in, *493*
 cortical hyperostosis in, 3256
 countercurrent aortography in, 251
 examination of, clinical, 39–62
 neurological, 41–44, 1255–1260
 full anterior fontanel in, vs. pseudotumor cerebri, 3190, 3191(t)
 hemiplegia in, epilepsy associated with, 3919
 hydrocephalus in, echoencephalography in, 186
 hypervitaminosis A in, 3253
 neuroaxonal dystrophy in, diagnosis of, 384(t)
 normal development of, 40, 42–43(t)
 prophylactic administration of vitamin K₁ to, 1058
 spina bifida aperta in, 1243
 subdural empyema in, 3334
 sylvian fissure cyst in, 1441
Infarction, cerebral, cerebral blood flow in, 816–818, 828, *829*
 computed tomography in, 118–120, *119, 120,* 1535
 in head injury, 1981
 hemodynamic, and arterial occlusion, 1516
 management of, 1534–1538, 1537(t)
 of carotid territory, 1525–1529, 1525(t)
 of vertebrobasilar territory, 1533–1534
 venous, 1538–1540
 intracranial hypertension in, 3180(t)
 myocardial, postoperative, 1098
Infection(s). See also names of specific infections.
 as cause of cranial defect, 2228
 bacterial intracranial, 3323–3357
 biopsy in, 388
 blocked vertebrae and, *495*
 cerebrospinal fluid in, 460–465
 clinical examination in, 37
 dural fistula following, 2213–2214
 during craniotomy, 1148
 following ventriculography, 378
 fungal, 3366–3440. See also names of specific diseases.
 in acute respiratory failure, 1028
 in head injury, 1915–1916
 in penetrating craniocerebral wounds, 2057
 intracranial hypertension in, 3180(t)
 of spine and spinal cord, 3449–3458
 radiography in, 505–506, *506*
 parasitic, 3366–3440. See also names of specific diseases.
 pericranial, and brain abscess, 3345
 postoperative, disseminated, 1110
 in aneurysms, 1691
 in craniofacial operation for cancer, 3274
 in disc operation, 2549
 in ventricular shunt operation, 1411, *1411,* 1412(t)
 preoperative evaluation of, 1076

Infection(s) (*Continued*)
 pulmonary, multiple trauma and, 2487
 spinal abnormalities and, 505
 wound, postoperative, 1088
 in carotid ligation, 1708
Inferior sagittal sinus, *280*
Inflammation, brain, computed tomography in, 132, *134, 135*
 chronic, angiographic appearance of, 611
 focal, electroencephalography in, 220, 221
 in occult spinal dysraphism, 1319
 in vasculitis, intracranial hypertension in, 3180(t)
 intracerebral, brain scanning in, 159
 in children, 162
 muscular, biopsy in, 410
 orbital, 3059–3061
 vascular, collagen diseases with, 1543–1546, 1544(t), 1545(t)
 postoperative, 1108–1110
Infraorbital nerve, avulsion of, in trigeminal neuralgia, 3561
Infratemporal fossa, anatomy of, 3272, *3273*
Infundibulum, embryology of, 3107
Infusion(s), as cerebrospinal fluid absorption test, 455
 cerebral blood flow and, 813
Iniencephaly, characteristics of, 1219
Injections, in angiography, 233, 245, 255
 in stereotaxic lesion making, 3807–3808
Injector, automatic, angiographic, 233
Injury. See *Trauma* and specific types of injury, e.g., *Head injury.*
Instruments, micro-operative, 1178–1192, *1180, 1182–1184,* 1183(t), *1186–1190, 1192*
Intellectual status, following head injury, 2167
 in myelomeningocele, 1272, 1272(t)
Intelligence quotient, following thalamotomy, *3836*
 neuropsychological evaluation and, 702
Intention tremor, 3852
Intercanthal distance, in craniofacial malformations, 1472
Intercostal nerve block, 3646, *3646, 3647*
Interorbital distance, in craniofacial malformations, 1473
Interosseous nerve(s), entrapment of, anterior, 2449–2451, *2450*
 posterior, 2456–2457
Interpupillary distance, in craniofacial malformations, 1472
Intervertebral disc, 2535–2552. See also *Disc, intervertebral.*
Intoxication. See also *Poisoning.*
 drug, inner ear injury from, 691, 691(t)
 fluorine, skull in, 3253
 water, postoperative, 1100–1101
"Intracerebral steal" phenomenon, cerebral blood flow and, 821–822
 hyperventilation and, 902
 in ischemic vascular disease, 1532–1533
Intracranial aneurysms, nonoperative treatment of, 1645–1653
Intracranial hemorrhage. See *Hemorrhage, intracranial.*
Intracranial hypertension, 846–930. See also *Intracranial pressure, increased.*
Intracranial pressure, body temperature and, 913, *914*
 cerebral blood flow and, 823–824, 829, 866, 1925
 control of, in intracranial hemorrhage, 1648, 1841
 hyperventilation and, 1124
 halothane and, 1122
 increased, 846–930
 A waves in, 430
 anatomy and physiology in, 846–860
 anesthesia in, 901
 barbiturate therapy in, 915
 benign, 3179
 cerebral blood flow in, 824
 cerebrospinal fluid in, 471
 brain abscess and, 3345
 brain swelling from, 874
 causes of, 897
 cerebral circulation and, 823, 846–930
 cerebral death and, angiography in, *751*
 cerebral ischemia and, 876

Intracranial pressure (*Continued*)
  increased, clinical diagnosis of, 17, 876–880
    definition of, 900
    disturbed brain function and, 860, *860*
    hyperbaric oxygen in, 903
    hypertonic solutions in, 905
    hyperventilation in, 901
    hypothermia in, 912
    incidence and significance of, 880–897
    in brain ischemia and anoxia, 894
    in brain tumors, 889
      of posterior fossa, in children, 2734–2735
      supratentorial, in children, 2704
    in comatose patient, 898
    in head injury, 880, 881(t), 882(t), 885(t), *886–888*,
      1922–1927, *1922–1924*, 2045–2048
      in children, 2119, *2120*
    in normal-pressure hydrocephalus, 895, 1426
    in pseudotumor cerebri, 896
    in Reye's syndrome, 895
    in subarachnoid hemorrhage, 891, *892*
    lumbar puncture in, 850
    nitrous oxide and, 1121
    operative decompression in, 916
    pathology of, 860–876
    pressure waves of, 875
    prognosis after head injury and, 2150–2152, *2151, 2152*
    pulmonary edema with, 864
    respiratory failure and, 1016
    signs and symptoms of, 876
    sinus occlusion and, in cerebral infarction, 1539, 1540
    steroids in, 910
    tentorial pressure cone in, 878
    treatment of, 897–916
    vital signs and, 861
  intracranial volume and, 853, *854–856*
  measurement of, in head injury, 1989–1992
    methods of, 850
  monitoring of, postoperative, in closed head injury,
    2037–2042, *2038–2042*
  neuroleptanalgesia and, 1121
  normal, 847, *848–850*
  pressure/volume index of, 855
  tests for, in cerebral death, 755(t)
  transmission of, 857
Intracranial space, pain-sensitive structures in, 877
  volume/pressure response for elastance of, 854
Intracranial tap, percutaneous, in pediatric hydrocephalus, 1400,
  1400
Intracranial tumors, enlarged ventricles and, 1429
  increased intracranial pressure in, 889
  vs. trigeminal neuralgia, 3557
Intracranial vascular disease, postoperative vasospasm and, 1092
Intracranial vessels, manipulation of, in operative procedures,
  1080
Intracranial volume, reduction of, for operation, 1667
Intradiploic cyst, 3245
Intravenous pyelogram, in urinary bladder malfunction, 1038
Intravenous thiopental test, 3492
Intraventricular foramen, *353*
Intraventricular space, measurement of intracranial pressure from,
  852
Intubation, in multiple trauma, endotracheal, 2476–2477
  nasogastric, 2526–2528
Iophendylate, in ventriculography, 3788
IQ. See *Intelligence quotient.*
Iron, in cerebrospinal fluid, 450
Iron deficiency anemia, and pseudotumor cerebri, 3181(t), 3187
  skull involvement in, 3261
Irradiation necrosis, delayed, ultrasound in, 190
Irrigation, in cerebral resections, 1146
Ischemia. See also *Ischemic vascular disease.*
  brain damage in, in head injury, 1927–1928
  cerebral, definition of, 774

Ischemia (*Continued*)
  cerebral, diffuse, 1540–1549, *1541,* 1543–1545(t)
    increased intracranial pressure and, 876, 894–895
    metabolism in, 774–781
    pathophysiology of, 1513–1516, 1515(t)
    transient, carotid, 1520–1530
      cerebral blood flow in, 828, *829*
      vertebrobasilar, 1530–1531
    complete, 777, *778, 779*
    coronary, pain in, dorsal rhizotomy in, 3668
    in peripheral nerve entrapment, 2433–2435, *2433–2437*
    in peripheral nerve injury, 2367, *2367, 2368*
    incomplete, 775, *776*
    postoperative, in carotid ligation, 1708
    recovery following, factors affecting, 780
Ischemic stroke, acute, operative management of, 1619–1626
Ischemic vascular disease, cerebral, 1511–1553
  clinical evaluation of, 1516–1520, *1517,* 1519(t)
  definitions and classification of, 1511–1513
  epidemiology of, 1513
  focal, 1514, 1520–1534
  kinking of carotid artery and, 816
  management of, 1534–1538
  mechanisms of, 1512, 1512(t), 1513(t), 1515–1516
  pain management in, 3632
  pathophysiology of, 1513, 1515(t)
  time course of, 1512
  unusual arterial disorders in, 1549–1553
  venous infarction in, 1538–1540
Isoproterenol, cerebral blood flow and, 808(t)
Isotope scan. See *Brain scan* and *Radionuclide imaging.*
Isoxsuprine hydrochloride, cerebral blood flow and, 808(t)

Jakob-Creutzfeldt disease, brain biopsy in, 386(t)
  cerebrospinal fluid in, 465
  electroencephalography in, 207, *213,* 222
Jaundice, neonatal, 40
  postoperative, 1107
Jefferson's fracture, 500, 2324
Joints, range of motion of, in rehabilitation, 4000
Juvenile malformations, of spinal cord, 1858, *1859,* 1869

Kanamycin, in bacterial infections, 3327
  in cerebral vasospasm, 821
  inner ear damage and, 691, 691(t)
Katzman cerebrospinal fluid absorption test, 455
Keratinitis, in lower facial weakness, 47
Keratitis, exposure, tarsorrhaphy in, 643, *643*
  post–craniotomy for trigeminal neuralgia, 3583
Kernig test, 2542
Kernohan notch, supratentorial mass lesion and, 879
Ketamine, as general anesthetic, 1122
  cerebral blood flow and, 805
  in increased intracranial pressure, 901
Ketoacidosis, diabetic, intracranial hypertension in, 3180(t)
Ketone bodies, in cerebral metabolism, 767
Kidney(s), hypothermia and, 1129
  pain in, 3632
  polycystic, cerebral aneurysm and, 1808–1809, 1808(t)
  spinal metastasis from, 512
Kiloh-Nevin syndrome, 659, *660*
Kindling, 3862
Kinetron machine, 3995
Kinking, vascular, angiography in, *288,* 289, *289*
  cerebral blood flow and, 815–816
Klippel-Feil syndrome, 491, *494,* 1215
Klippel-Trenaunay syndrome, 565, *568, 569*
Klumpke's palsy, in neonate, 49
Klüver-Bucy syndrome, clinical examination in, 15
Knee, peroneal nerve injury at, 2402–2404

Knee (*Continued*)
  tibial nerve injury at, 2404–2405
Krabbe disease, 385(t)
Krause's corpuscles, 3461
Kuru, cerebrospinal fluid in, 465
Kyphoscoliosis, spinal osteomyelitis and, 3454
Kyphosis, 2629–2655
  congenital, 1258
  etiology of, 2631, 2632(t)
  natural history of, 2633–2635, *2634, 2635*
  neurosurgical problems in, 2648
  nonoperative treatment of, 2635, *2636*
  operative treatment of, 2637, *2638–2646*
  orthopedic problems in, 2648
  thoracolumbar myelomeningocele, and, 1252, *1252, 1253*

Laboratory tests, in anterior pituitary hyperfunction, 953–955
  in anterior pituitary failure, 946–947, 946(t)
  in cerebral death, 751
  in metastatic tumors, of brain, 2875
    of leptomeninges, 2891
  of cerebrospinal fluid, 457–459
Labyrinth, acoustic, sound transmission in, 693
  vestibular, anatomy of, *677, 678–680, 680–682*
    toxic injury to, 691, 691(t)
Labyrinthine fistula test, in vertigo, 686
Labyrinthitis, 690
Laceration, brain, in head injury, 2033
  peripheral nerve, 2365
  scalp, 2301, *2301–2303*
Lacrimal gland tumors, 3058–3059
Lacrimal nerve, in orbit, 3027
Lactate, tissue concentrations of, in ischemia, 777, *778*
Lactotropic microadenoma, 3125
Lacunar infarcts, carotid, 1529
Lacunar skull, of newborn, 1219
Lamaze technique, 3481
Lambdoid suture, synostosis of, 1447, *1450, 1453*, 1461
Lamina terminalis, cistern of, *352*
Laminagraphy, in acoustic neuroma, 2975, *2977, 2989–2991*
Laminectomy, for cervical myelopathy, 2602–2604
  in thoracic spinal cord injuries, 2350
  infections in, 1089
Language, ventrolateral thalamus and, 3835
Larsen syndrome, characteristics of, 1214
Lateral femoral cutaneous nerve, entrapment of, 2463–2464, *2464*
Lead poisoning, intracranial hypertension in, 3180(t)
Leber, optic atrophy of, 667
LeFort fractures, 2279, *2282, 2283*
Leg. See *Extremities, lower.*
Leiomyosarcoma, hypophysectomy in, 3953
Leksell anterior capsulotomy, 3931, *3931, 3932*
Leksell stereotaxic instrument, 3805, *3806*
Leptomeninges, arteries of, in collateral circulatory system, 797
  cyst of, in children, 3245, *3249*
  development of, *1437*
  metastases to, 2888–2894, *2892, 2893*, 2893(t)
Leptomeningitis, brain abscess and, 3344
  diagnosis of, 3324
Leptospiral meningitis, cerebrospinal fluid in, 462
Lethargy, 63, 3834
Letterer-Siwe disease, skull in, 3258
Leucoencephalopathy, progressive multifocal, cerebrospinal fluid in, 465
Leucotomy, bimedial, 3928
  prefrontal, 3927
Leukemia, calvarial lesions in, 3244
  cerebrospinal fluid in, 467
  orbital, 3058
  radiation therapy in, 3104
  spinal cord tumors and, in children, *3216*
Leukodystrophy, metachromatic, cerebrospinal fluid in, 468

Leukodystrophy (*Continued*)
  metachromatic, diagnosis of, 385(t)
    sudanophilic, brain biopsy in, 386(t)
Leukoencephalitis, hemorrhagic, 3358, 3361, 3363
Leukotome, 3806
Levodopa, in Parkinson's disease, 3841
Levothyroxine sodium, in anterior pituitary failure, 949
Lévy-Roussy syndrome, cerebrospinal fluid in, 468
Lidocaine, in cerebral vasospasm, 820
Ligament of Struthers, electromyography of, 631
Lighting, for operating microscope, *1165*, 1171, *1171*
Limb, deformities of, spina bifida aperta and, 1257–1259, 1259(t)
Limbic system, 3730, *3731*, 3929
  lesions of, clinical examination in, 14–15, *15*
Lindstrom's ultrasonic radiation procedure, in psychiatric disorders, 3938, *3939*
Linear pressure regression, of cerebrospinal fluid, technique for, 455
Link's IgG index, 444
Lipid(s), in brain tumors, 2692
  in cerebrospinal fluid, 449
Lipidosis, electroencephalography in, 216, *216*, 222
Lipogranulomatosis, Farber, 385(t)
Lipoma, corpus callosum, 2713–2714, *2714*
  intracranial, 2928, *2928*
  lumbosacral, 1333–1339, *1334, 1335, 1337*
  spinal, 3208, *3208, 3216*
    computed tomography in, 139
    myelographic appearance of, *535*
Lithium carbonate, in inappropriate antidiuretic hormone secretion, 982, 1101
Litigation, chronic pain and, 3528–3529
Liver. See also *Hepatic.*
  disease of, glutamine levels in, 451
  hypothermia and, 1129
  necrosis of, postoperative, 1107
Lobectomy, temporal, in adult epilepsy, 3917, *3919–3922*
  in children and adolescents, 3883, *3885, 3888*
Lobotomy, frontal, for pain, 3732
Locked-in syndrome, 63
  rehabilitation in, 4000
Lombroso-Erba Pentothal activation test, 3896
Long thoracic nerve, entrapment of, 2462
Lordosis, 2629–2655
  development of, 1258
  etiology of, 2631, 2631(t), 2632(t)
  natural history of, 2633–2635, *2634, 2635*
  neurosurgical problems in, 2648
  nonoperative treatment of, 2635, *2636*
  operative treatment of, 2637, *2638–2646*
  orthopedic problems in, 2648
Lower motor neuron, paralysis of, clinical diagnosis of, 7–8
Lückenschädel skull deformity, in myelomeningocele, 1259
Lumbar canal, narrow, *508, 509*
Lumbar disc, failed, dorsal rhizotomy in, 3668
Lumbar drainage, in craniotomy, 1143
Lumbar paravertebral nerve block, 3646, *3647*
Lumbar puncture, 452–457
  alternatives to, 457
  cerebrospinal fluid response to, 472
  complications of, 456
  contraindications for, 452
  in brain abscess, 3346
  in cerebral infarction, 1535
  in hydrocephalus, 1426
  in intracranial hypertension, 850
  in post-traumatic meningitis, 3341
  in pseudotumor cerebri, 3188, 3191
  in spinal cord tumors, 3200
  in subdural empyema, 3335
  indications for, 452
  technique of, 453
Lumbar subarachnoid pressure, intracranial pressure and, 858
Lumbosacral lipoma, 1333–1339, *1334, 1335, 1337*
Lumbosacral plexus, pelvic metastasis to, 3629, 3629(t)

Lung(s), anatomy of, 1005
  care of, in intracerebral and intracerebellar hemorrhage, 1840
  edema of, production of, 1016
  innervation of, 1006
  shock, in multiple trauma, 2487–2490
  skull metastases from, *3240,*
  vascular supply to, 1006
Lupus erythematosus, disseminated, 1543–1545, 1544(t), 1545(t)
  cerebrospinal fluid in, 469
Luschka, foramen of, atresia of, 1288
Luteinizing hormone, hypothalamic-pituitary relationship and, 943
  insufficiency of, 944
  nature and function of, 938, 940
Luxury perfusion phenomenon, 156
  definition of, 874
  hyperventilation and, 902
Lymph, scalp drainage of, 2300
Lymphangioma, orbital, 3054
Lymphoma, brain, 2836–2844, *2839–2844*
  cerebrospinal fluid in, 462, 2840
  computed tomography in, 116, *117,* 2841, *2841*
  orbital, 3057–3058
  scalp, 3316, *3317*
  skeleton in, 3244
  spinal, chemotherapy for, 3213
Lysine-8-vasopressin, in neurohypophyseal diabetes insipidus, 976
Lysosomal enzymes, in ischemia, 781
Lytic cocktail, 1129

Macrocephaly, characteristics of, 1220
  in achondroplasia, 1232
Macrodex, cerebral blood flow and, 811(t)
Macroelectrode recording, in stereotaxic procedures, 3798
Macular sparing, definition of, 666
Magendie, foramen of, *353*
  atresia of, 1288
Magnesium, in cerebrospinal fluid, 450
Magnesium sulfate, in neonatal seizures, 3874
Magnification, operative, 1161
  microscope in, 1163, *1164–1166,* 1168(t), *1169–1171*
Malformation, craniofacial, congenital, 1467–1480
  neural, in spina bifida aperta, 1248–1251, 1251(t), *1249, 1250*
  vascular. See also *Arteriovenous malformation.*
    in subarachnoid hemorrhage, 1637–1640, *1638–1640,*
    1640(t)
    of brain, 1786–1805
    of spinal cord, 1850–1873
Malignancy, determination of, in biopsy in, 397, 397(t)
  grading of, in astrocytomas, 2769
  in tumors, 2760
Malignant disease, visceral pain from, 3627–3630, 3629(t),
  3630(t)
Malingering, affected pain in, 3512–3515
  vs. brain damage, psychological testing in, 713
Mammary cancer, hormone dependency of, 3947
Mandible, fractures of, 2285–2286, *2286–2289*
Manganese, in cerebrospinal fluid, 451
Manipulation, complications of, 1080
  hemiplegia from, temporal lobectomy and, 3890
Manipulative patient, pain and, 3756–3757
Mannitol, cerebral blood flow and, 811(t)
  in craniotomy, 1143
  in head injury, 900
  in hypophysectomy by craniotomy, 3982
  in increased intracranial pressure, 907–909
  in micro-operative decompression in trigeminal neuralgia, 3596
  in status epilepticus, 3878
  in supratentorial tumors in children, 2709
Marcus Gunn phenomenon, 650, *650, 651,* 661
  genetic aspects of, 1224
Marie syndrome, cerebrospinal fluid in, 468

Marie-Strumpell disease, 509, *509*
Mass lesions, intracranial, angiography in, 341–344
  computed tomography in, 113–115, *114, 115,* 121–125,
    121–125
  in head injury, 1909–1916, *1914*
    brain herniation and, 1916–1921, 1917(t), 1918(t), *1920,*
      1921
    early operation for, 2019, 2024–2036, *2027–2029, 2031,*
      2033, 2035, 2036
  in congenital dermal sinus, cranial, 1315
    spinal, 1328
  in prognosis after head injury, 2143, 2143(t)
  intracranial pressure and, 873–874
Massa intermedia, in Arnold-Chiari malformation, 1285
Masserman cerebrospinal fluid formation test, 455
Masseter muscle, in neonate, 46
Mastoiditis, pseudotumor cerebri and, 3181(t), 3182, *3183*
Matas test, in carotid ligation, 1704–1705
Maxilla, fractures of, 2276–2279, *2282*
  hypoplasia of, 1477–1480, *1478, 1479*
Maxillary sinus, anatomy of, 3269, *3270*
  carcinoma of, 3277–3279, *3278–3281*
Maxillofacial injuries, 2261–2297
  fractures in, 2274, *2275–2296*
  soft-tissue, 2263–2274
  triage in, 2261–2263
McGregor's line, 491, *1484*
Mecamylamine hydrochloride, in detrusor hyperreflexia, 1041
Meckel's cave, 3591
Median nerve, entrapment of, 2446–2452, *2446, 2450*
  electromyography in, 630
  injury to, 2386–2390, *2387, 2389*
  ulnar nerve and, 2393–2394
Mediastinum, schwannoma of, benign, 3301
  malignant, 3304
Medroxyprogesterone, in acromegaly, 957
  in anterior pituitary failure, 950
Medulloblastoma, 2817–2823, *2819, 2820*
  brain scanning in, 150, *150(t), 162(t)*
  cerebellar, in children, 2748–2750, 2755
  computed tomography in, 116, *117,* 2821, *2821*
  radiation therapy of, 3100, 3100(t)
  recurrent, chemotherapy for, 3090(t)
  spinal, chemotherapy for, 3213
Medulloepithelioma, 2823
Megalencephaly, idiopathic, 1220
Meglumine iothalamate, cerebral blood flow and, 812(t)
  in ventriculography, 3788
Melanoma, malignant, hypophysectomy in, 3953
  scalp, 3320, *3320*
  spinal cord, in children, *3217*
Melzack-Wall pain theory, 3761
Memory deficits, verbal, post-thalamotomy, 3836
Menadione sodium bisulfate, in biliary disease, 1058
Menarche, pseudotumor cerebri and, 3181(t)
Mendelian traits, basic, 1207–1209
Ménière's disease, differential diagnosis of, 689
  vascular decompression in, 3771
  vertigo in, 688, *689*
  vs. vascular accident, 688
Meninges, formation of, 1240
  hemorrhage from, in head injury in children, 2103–2114
  in spina bifida aperta, 1251
  metastases to, 2888–2894, *2892, 2893,* 2893(t)
  tumors of, 2936–2966. See also *Meningioma.*
Meningioma, 2936–2965, 3236, *3237, 3238*
  angiography in, cerebral, *307, 309, 312,* 318–321, *319–322*
    spinal, 609
  blood-brain barrier in, 146
  brain scanning in, 149, 150, 150(t), *151*
  clinical presentation of, 2939–2943
  computed tomography in, 121, *121, 122,* 138, *138*
    vs. radionuclide imaging, 167(t)
  convexity, 2949, *2950*
  cerebellar, 2942

INDEX

Meningioma (*Continued*)
  convexity, cerebral, 2941
  cranial, cerebral blood flow in, 825
    radiation therapy of, 3103, 3103(t)
  diagnosis of, 2943, *2943, 2944*
  fibrous, tumor complexes of, *189*
  foramen magnum, air myelography in, *529*
  in children, 2728
  incidence of, 2936, 2937(t)
  locations of, 395(t), 2937, 2937(t)
  orbital, 3046–3049, *3047–3049*
    transcranial approach to, 2960, *2961*
  parasagittal, neuropsychological assessment in, 713
  parasellar, operation for, 3151
  pathology of, 2937, *2938–2940*
  pterion, embolization of, 1202
  recurrence of, 2960–2962
  skull, benign secondary, 3226, *3227, 3228*
    vs. chondroma, 3229
  spinal, 512, *3197*, 3197(t), 3204–3205, *3204*
    myelography in, *532, 3202*
    operation for, 3212
      ultrasound scanning in, *734*
    survival in, 2962, *2962–2965*
  tentorial, myelographic appearance of, *537*
  vertebromedullary, angiography in, 609
  vs. trigeminal neuralgia, 3557
Meningism, cerebrospinal fluid in, 465
  in posterior fossa tumors in children, 2736–2737
  postoperative, 1110–1112
Meningitis, aseptic, cerebrospinal fluid in, 464
  in medulloblastoma in children, 2746
  pneumoencephalography and, 368
  radionuclide cerebrospinal fluid studies and, 163
  bacterial, 3337–3341
    coma in, 72
    intracranial hypertension in, 3180(t)
  basal, in sarcoidosis, 3427
  brain damage from, in head injury, 1929
  brain scanning in, 159
  cerebrospinal fluid in, 461–463
  coccidioidal, 3412
  computed tomography in, 133
  eosinophilic, 3395
  in congenital dermal sinus, cranial, 1315
    spinal, 1328
  postcraniotomy, 3341
  post–hypophysectomy by craniotomy, 3984
  postoperative, in spina bifida aperta, 1270
  post-traumatic, 3340, *3340*
  serous, 3179
  subarachnoid space obliteration following, 1429
  tuberculous, cerebrospinal fluid in, 461
Meningocele, orbital, 3053–3054
  spinal, 1274–1278, *1276*
    distribution of, 1248(t)
    incidence of, 1210(t)
    intrasacral, 1219
      occult, 1353–1355
    intrathoracic, 1219
    nondysraphic, 1355–1356
    sacral, anterior, 1350–1353
    spina bifida and, 496, *497*
Meningoencephalitis, aseptic, chronic, cerebrospinal fluid in, 462
  bacterial, acute, cerebrospinal fluid in, 460
  cryptococcosis and, 3414
  infectious, chronic, cerebrospinal fluid in, 461
  Toxoplasma, cerebrospinal fluid in, 462
  viral, cerebrospinal fluid in, 464
    coma in, 72
Meningomyelocele. See *Myelomeningocele.*
Mental disorders, organic, "effected pain" and, 3494–3496
Mental status, changes in, in astrocytoma, 2773
  evaluation of, in child, 61
    normal-pressure hydrocephalus, 1424

Mephenesin carbamate, in trigeminal neuralgia, 3558
Mephentermine, cerebral blood flow and, 808(t)
Mephenytoin, in afebrile seizures, 3876(t), 3877
Mephobarbital, in afebrile seizures, 3876(t)
Meprobamate, in chronic pain, 3527
Mercury chlormerodrin, in brain scanning, 148(t)
Mesencephalon. See *Midbrain.*
Mesencephalotomy, in chronic pain syndrome, 3765
  stereotaxic, 3702–3710, 3704(t), *3705, 3706*
Mesial temporal sclerosis, 3860
Metabolism, cerebral, 765–785
  characteristics of, 765–766
  energy production in, 766–767, *766*
  energy utilization in, 767–770, *767, 770*
  in anesthesia, 1133
  in hypoglycemia, 771–772
  in hypoxia, 772–774, *773*
  in ischemia, 774–781
  of transmitter compounds, 770–771
  oxygen, rate of, temperature dependence of, 769, *769*
  disorders of, biopsy in, 410
    clinical examination in, 37–38
    coma and, 65(t), 72
    intracranial hypertension in, 3180(t)
    skull in, 3251
  in autoregulation of cerebral blood flow, 793–794, 869
  in head injury, in children, 2121
  inborn errors of, biopsy in, 387–388
  oxidative, in brain tumors, 2691
  rate of, basal, in acromegaly, 955
  response of, to hypertonic agents, 909–910
  vitamin, in pseudotumor cerebri, 3187
Metal(s), cranioplasty with, 2234–2239, *2234, 2235, 2240*
  poisoning by, cerebrospinal fluid in, 471
Metaraminol, cerebral blood flow and, 808(t)
Metastasis (metastases), brain, 2872–2895
  angiography in, 321, *323*
  diagnosis of, 2874, 2874(t), 2875(t), *2876–2878*
  incidence of, 2872, 2873(t)
  radiation therapy of, 3104
  treatment of, 2880, 2880(t)–2885(t), *2886,* 2887(t)
  brain scanning in, *150(t),* 152, *153*
  computed tomography in, 116, *116, 117*
    vs. radionuclide imaging, 167(t)
  leptomeningeal, 2888–2894, *2892, 2893,* 2893(t)
  of pituitary adenoma, 3127
  spinal cord, *3197,* 3197(t), 3207–3208, *3207*
    in children, 3220–3221, 3220(t)
    radiotherapy of, 3224–3225
  spinal tumors and, 512
Metergoline, in hyperprolactinemia, 968
Methacholine test, in pupillary disorders, 649, 650(t)
Methadone, cerebral blood flow and, 811(t)
  in chronic pain syndrome, 3758
Methantheline bromide, in detrusor hyperreflexia, 1041
Methemoglobin, in cerebrospinal fluid, 438
Methicillin, 3326
Methiodal sodium, in ventriculography, 3788
Methohexital, in epileptogenic focus localization, 3871
  in temporal lobectomy, 3884
Methotrexate, in brain tumors, 3086
  in leptomeningeal metastasis, 2892, 2893(t)
  in spinal cord tumors, 3213
  intra-arterial administration of, 3073
Methoxyflurane, cerebral blood flow and, 805
  disadvantages of, 1122
Methsuximide, in afebrile seizures, 3876(t)
Methyl alcohol, cerebral blood flow and, 810(t), 813
Methylglucamine diatrizoate, cerebral blood flow and, 812(t)
  for angiography, 242
Methylnitrosourea, as carcinogen, 2674
Methyphenidate hydrochloride, cerebral blood flow and, 810(t)
Methylprednisolone, in arachnoiditis, 3616
  in chronic pain syndrome, 3763
  in cranial operations, 1136

Methylprednisolone (*Continued*)
  in trichinosis, 3395
Methysergide maleate, in migraine, 3548
Metopic suture, synostosis of, *1452*, 1454, 1459, *1459, 1460*
Metrizamide, in cerebrospinal fluid, 425
  in empty sella syndrome, 3175
  in myelography, 518–527, *524–526*
    advantages of, 525
    in anterior sacral meningocele, 1352
    in diastematomyelia, 1344
    in lumbosacral lipoma, *1327*
    side effects of, 1526
  in ventriculography, 370
Meynert's commissure, in Arnold-Chiari malformation, 1285
Miconazole, in cryptococcosis, 316
Microadenoma, pathology of, 3124, *3125, 3126*
  pituitary, 969, *970*, 984
  subclinical, 3129
Microbes, in cerebrospinal fluid, 440–441
Microcephaly, characteristics of, 1220
Microelectrode recording, in stereotaxic procedures, 3798
Microembolism, retinal, identifying features of, 1519, 1519(t)
  syndromes of, 1548–1549
Microglioma, locations of, 395(t)
  tumor complexes of, *189*
Microgyria, in Arnold-Chiari malformation, 1285
  morphogenetic timing of, 1211(t)
Microscope, operative, 1163–1178, *1164–1166, 1169–1177*
    accessories for, 1175, *1175–1177*
    care of, 1174
    eyepieces and focus for, 1167
    for aneurysms, 1671
    light system for, 1171, *1171*
    magnifications with, 1168(t)
    magnification changer for, 1170
    mount for, 1172, *1173*
    objective fields with, 1168(t)
    objective lens for, 1169
    sterilization of, 1171
    zoom, 1170, *1170*
Micro-operative technique, 1160–1193
  advantages and disadvantages of, 1160
  definition of, 1160
  in aneurysm procedures, 1668–1674, *1669, 1670, 1672, 1673*
  instruments in, 1178–1192, 1671
    bayonet forceps, 1184, *1184*
    bipolar coagulator, 1179, *1180*, 1671
    brain retractors, 1181, *1182*
    cup forceps, 1191
    curets, 1191
    cutters, 1185, *1188*
    dissectors, 1191, *1192*
    drills, 1190, 1671
    head-fixation devices, 1181, *1183*, 1671
    irrigation equipment, 1185, *1186*
    needles, 1181, 1183(t), *1184*
    needle holders, 1181, 1183(t), *1184*
    suction equipment, 1185, *1186*
    suture holders, 1181, 1183(t), *1184*
  microscope in, 1163–1178, *1164–1166, 1169–1177*
  nursing in, 1162–1163
  training in, 1161–1162
Microsuture technique, training in, 1162
Micturition, anatomy and physiology of, 1031–1035
  central pathways in, 1031, *1032, 1033*
  normal, 1034
Midbrain, anatomy of, 3703
  disease of, Collier's sign in, 643
  electrical stimulation in, in stereotaxic mesencephalotomy, 3706–3707, 3707(t), *3707, 3708*
  in Arnold-Chiari malformation, 1285
  infarction of, coma in, 71
  injury to, hyperpnea in, 994
    metabolic response to, 989
  pain pathways of, 3703

Middle cerebral artery, anastomosis of, to superficial temporal artery, 1585–1611, *1586–1593*, 1594(t), 1595(t), *1596–1599, 1601–1605, 1608–1610*
  aneurysms of, *301*, 302, *1631, 1633*, 1681–1682, *1681*, 1691(t)
    carotid ligation in, 1702, 1709
    headache and, 3552
    operative treatment of, 1681–1682
  angiography of, *258*, 262–264, *263–265*, 342
  bifurcation of, embolectomy at, 1620, *1623*
Midline fusion defects, 1236–1380
Migraine, 3546–3550
  cerebral blood flow in, 822
  sympathectomy for, 3720
  transient homonymous hemianopia in, 640
Milwaukee brace, in spinal deformity, 2636, *2636*
Mineralocorticoids, in anterior pituitary failure, 950
Miosis, pupillary reactions in, 649–650
Missile injuries, of brain and skull, 2055–2068, *2055, 2058, 2060, 2062–2067*
Mithramycin, in brain tumors, 3087
MLB test, 697
Möbius syndrome, in neonate, 47
Mollaret's meningitis, cerebrospinal fluid in, 463
Monaural loudness balance test, 697
Mongolism, in neonate, 45
  incidence of, 1210(t)
Moniliasis, 3407
Monitoring, in anesthesia, 1130–1131
  of blood flow, ultrasound in, 740–742, *741, 742*
Monoiodomethane sulfanate, in ventriculography, 3788
Monro-Kellie doctrine, 429, 791
Moro reflex, in neonate, 49
Morphine, cerebral blood flow and, 811(t)
Motion, range of, in rehabilitation, 4000
Motoneuron, alpha, in dyskinesias, 3826
Motor function, cerebral death and, 751
  contralateral weakness of, postmesencephalotomy, 3709
  in children, 53–55, *54*, 59–60, 60(t), 61(t)
  in coma, 69
  in head injury, 1949
  in neonate, 47–51, *48, 50, 51*
  in nerve entrapment, 2442, *2443*
  in spina bifida aperta, 1255–1256, 1256(t)
  in transtentorial herniation syndrome, 70(t)
  psychological testing and, 705
  subcortical hemispheric paratonic rigidity and, 69
Motor nerve conduction, studies in, 624, 625(t)
Moyamoya disease, 1550
  cerebrovascular, extracranial to intracranial arterial anastomosis in, 1600–1601, *1601*
Mucocele(s), paranasal sinus, exophthalmos and, 3058
  sphenoid sinus, skull in, 3261, *3262*
    with parasellar involvement 3155
Mucolipidosis, diagnosis of, 385(t)
Mucopolysaccharidoses, diagnosis of, 385(t)
Mucor, brain abscess and, 3349
Mucormycosis, cerebral, 3423
Multiceps multiceps meningitis, cerebrospinal fluid in, 462
Multiple myeloma, hypophysectomy in, 3953
  of skull, *3243*, 3244
  of spine, 512, *516*
Multiple sclerosis, cerebrospinal fluid in, 469
  diagnosis of, 385(t)
  intention tremor in, 3852
  intracranial hypertension in, 3180(t)
  trigeminal neuralgia and, 3556
  vertigo in, 688
  visual field loss in, 667
Muscle(s), cramps of, in Parkinson's disease, 3838
  extraocular, anatomy of, 3025
    electromyographic studies of, 627
    paretic, identification of, 654, 654(t)
  facial, weakness of, in head injury, 2165
  lower extremity, in spina bifida aperta, 1253

Muscle(s) (*Continued*)
  lower extremity, innervation of, 1256, 1256(t)
    nerve and root supply to, 620(t)
  mass of, in child, 60
  ocular, action of, 652
    tests of, 653–654, *653, 654*(t)
  paresis of, rhizotomy for trigeminal neuralgia and, 3576
  power of, in children, 60
  skeletal, biopsy of, 410–415, *412*(t), *413*(t)
    lesions of, clinical examination in, 35
  smooth, epinephrine sensitivity in, 3719
  strength of, grading of, 60(t)
  tone of, in cerebral death, 758
    in children, 60
  upper extremity, nerve and root supply to, 620(t)
Mutism, akinetic, 63
Myasthenia gravis, electromyographic studies in, 634, 635(t)
  neonatal, 45
  ocular signs of, 658
Mydriasis, traumatic, pupillary reactions in, 650
Myelin, abnormalities of, in cranial nerve syndromes, 3777
Myelitis, acute transverse, 3359
  cerebrospinal fluid in, 466
  viral, 3359
Myelodysplasia, 1243
  in occult spinal dysraphism, 1319
Myelography, 512–530, *515–517, 519–548*
  air, 529, *529, 541, 545*
    in spinal angiomas, 578, *578*
    in stereotaxic cordotomy, 3676, *3676*
  cisternography, in 527, *527, 528*
  in arteriovenous malformations, 1854, *1855, 1856*
  in craniovertebral junction anomalies, 1495, *1496, 1497*
  in diastematomyelia, 1344, *1344*
  in disc disease, lumbar, 2543–2544
    thoracic, 2564–2566, *2565*
  in leptomeningeal metastases, 2891
  in lumbosacral lipoma, 1337, *1337*
  in spinal arachnoid cysts, 1444, *1445*
  in spinal cord tumors, 3201, *3202–3204*
  in viral encephalitis, 3362
  lesions in, 529, *530–548*
  metrizamide in, 518, *524–526*
    advantages of, 525
    side effects of, 526
  positive contrast, in spinal angiomas, 569, *575–577*
  radionuclide tracers in, 163
  technique of, 517, *519–523, 540*
Myeloma, multiple. See *Multiple myeloma*.
Myelomeningocele, *1244*, 1245
  antenatal detection of, 1274
  assessment of, 1254
  distribution of, 1248(t)
  hydrocephalus with, 1259
  intellectual development with, 1272, 1272(t)
  management of, 1263, *1263–1267*
  morphogenetic timing of, 1211(t)
  neurological complications of, delayed, 1274, *1275*
  neurological examination in, 1255, 1256(t), 1259(t)
  operative treatment of, 1264, *1264–1267*
  radiography in, 496, *497*, 1259
Myelopathy, spondylotic, 2597–2598
Myeloschisis, 1243–1244, *1244*
  developmental arrest in, 1246
Myelotomy, commissural, 3693, 3695
  in spinal angioma, *603*
  midline, for perineal pain, 3629
Myocardial infarction, postoperative, 1098
Myoclonus, 3851–3852
  oculopalatopharyngeal, 663
Myofascial pain syndromes, anesthetic diagnosis of, 3652
  pain relief in, 3752
  reversible nerve block in, 3654
Myogenic theory, of cerebral blood flow autoregulation, 792

Myoglobinuria, in crush injury, 2518–2519
Myoneural junction, diseases affecting, 658, *660*
Myopathies, biopsy in, 410
  electromyographic studies in, 634, 635(t)
  nerve conduction in, 636
Myositis ossificans, spinal cord dysfunction and, 4011
Myotonia, 622
  percussion, in neonate, 48
Myotonic dystrophy, in neonate, 45

Nafcillin, 3326
Nalidixic acid, 3181(t), 3187
Naloxone, in chronic pain, 3746
Narcotic antagonists, in inappropriate antidiuretic hormone
    secretion, 982
Narcotics, in chronic pain, 3527, 3758
Nasociliary nerve, in orbit, 3028
Nasogastric tube, in multiple trauma, 2526–2528
Nasopharynx, anatomy of, 3272, *3273*
  carcinoma of, skull in, 3244, *3246*
  tumors of, vs. trigeminal neuralgia, 3557
Nausea, increased intracranial pressure and, 877
Neck, aneurysms in, 289
  arteriovenous fistulae in, 291
  carcinoma of, mesencephalotomy for, 3707
  pain syndromes in, 2598–2609, *2605, 2606*
  schwannoma of, benign, 3300
    malignant, 3304
  venous obstruction in, in pseudotumor cerebri, 3184
  vessels of, false occlusive patterns of, 295, *295*
Necrosis, aseptic, vs. osteomyelitis of bone flap, 3332
  bone, prevention of, 1076
  liver, postoperative, 1107
  radiation, computed tomography in, 135, *135*
    of skull, 3250
  tissue, postoperative, 1088
Needle biopsy, 398, 412
Nelson's syndrome, 963
  adenoma in, 3123, *3126*
  treatment of, 3148
Nelson-Salassa syndrome, 963
Neocortex, somatosensory areas of, in nociception, 3468
Neocortical death, 747
Neomycin, in bacterial infections, 3326
  in subdural empyema, 3337
  in subgaleal abscess, 3328
  inner ear damage and, 691, 691(t)
Neonate, bacterial meningitis in, 3339
  cephalhematoma of, 3245, *3248*
  cerebrospinal fluid pressure in, 429
  clinical history of, 40
  hemorrhage in, intraventricular, 1641
  hydrocephalus in, 1383, *1384*
    ultrasound scanning in, *722, 728*
  neoblastoma in, 3307
  seizures in, 3865
    treatment of, 3874
  skull of, lacunar, 1219
    ultrasonic scanning of, 720–732, *722, 723, 728, 729*
Neoplasm(s). See also *Tumors* and names of specific tumors.
  as cause of cranial defect, 2228
  benign, of skull, 3228, 3228(t)
  blood vessel, 2845–2862
  central nervous system, locations of, 395(t)
  cerebral, brain scanning in, 153, *154*(t)
    recurrent, vs. craniotomy defects, 161
  cerebrospinal fluid in, 467
  clinical examination in, 36
  craniofacial, 3269–3284
  extracranial to intracranial arterial anastomosis in, 1601
  metastatic, locations of, 395(t)
  radionuclide imaging in, 150, 150(t), *151–154*

Neoplasm(s) (*Continued*)
  spinal, computed tomography in, 140
  subarachnoid hemorrhage and, 1642
  vascular, embolization of, 1200–1202
Neostigmine, in detrusor areflexia, 1043
Nerve(s), avulsion of, in trigeminal neuralgia, 3561
  conduction velocity studies in, 624–628, 625(t), 626(t)
  cranial. See *Cranial nerves* and names of specific nerves.
  entrapment of, 2430–2470. See also *Nerve entrapment.*
  grafting of, 2416
  lesions of, repair of, 2410–2418
  mobilization of, 2412
  of scalp, 2299, *2300*
  of Wrisberg, *3607*
  peripheral, injury of, 2362–2470. See also *Peripheral nerves, acute injury of* and names of specific nerves.
  resection and suture of, 2413
  stimulators for, implantable, for chronic back pain, 3621, *3622, 3623*
Nerve block(s), alcohol, in trigeminal neuralgia, 3559–3560
  in deliberate hypotension, 1127
  increased cerebral blood flow and, 831
  sacral, in detrusor hyperreflexia, 1041, *1042*
  in spastic urinary sphincter, 1046
Nerve entrapment, 2430–2470
  electrophysiological investigation in, 2435, *2438–2440, 2443*
  etiology of, 2432
  incidence of, 2445
  pressure and ischemia in, 2433, *2433–2437*
  structure and function in, 2430, *2431, 2432*
  syndromes of, 2446–2470. See also names of specific nerves and syndromes.
Nerve root(s), arachnoid cysts of, 1445
  compression of, from benign lesions, cervical, 2574–2612
    dorsal, 2562–2573
    lumbar, 2535–2561
    vascular, cranial, 3771–3782
  disease of, cervical, 2593–2597, *2594, 2595, 2597*
    foraminotomy for, 2605–2607, *2606*
  in ascending pain pathway, 3463–3464
  in disc disease, cervical, 2589–2591
  injury to, in chronic low back pain, 3614
  lesions of, electromyographic studies in, 634(t)
  manipulation of, in operations, 1079
  sympathetic innervation and, 3719
  trigeminal, in tic douloureux, micro-operative decompression of, 3589–3601, 3772
    percutaneous rhizotomy of, 3564–3578
    section of, in posterior fossa, 3586–3588
      temporal extradural, 3580–3584
      temporal intradural, 3584–3585
Nerve root sleeve, amputation of, myelographic appearance of, *546*
Nerve sheath, tumors of, 3300–3306
  malignant, 3303
  myelography in, *3202*
  operative treatment of, 3211, *3212*
Neural arch, intact, 2553
Neural crest, development of, 1240, 1468, *1468*
Neural ectoderm, diastematomyelia and, 1339
Neural plaque, myeloschisis and, 1248–1251, *1249, 1250*
Neural tube, defects of, 1217–1220, 1218(t)
  formation of, 1237, *1238–1240*
  malformations of, 1242–1243
Neuralgia, atypical facial, 3543–3545, *3544, 3545*
  vs. trigeminal neuralgia, 3557
  geniculate, 3605–3607, *3607*
  glossopharyngeal, 3587, 3604–3605, *3606*
    posterior approach in, 3587
  nervus intermedius, 3606
  occipital, 3540–3541
  postherpetic, 3542–3543
    pain in, 3641, *3642*
  vs. trigeminal neuralgia, 3557

Neuralgia (*Continued*)
  postsympathetic, 3724
  trigeminal. See *Trigeminal neuralgia.*
  vasomotor, vs. trigeminal neuralgia, 3557
Neurapraxia, 2363
Neurectomy, in chronic pain syndrome, 3764
  presacral, 3724
Neurenteric canal, defects of, 1220
  formation of, 1237
  in diastematomyelia, 1340
Neurenteric cyst, 1346–1350
  of spinal cord, in children, *3216*
Neurilemoma. See also *Tumors, spinal cord.*
  in children, *3216*
  of orbital peripheral nerves, 3050
  operative treatment of, 3211, *3212*
Neuritis, optic, causes of, 674(t)
    visual field loss and, 667
  postirradiation, percutaneous cordotomy in, 3629
  retrobulbar, cerebrospinal fluid in, 470
  spinal, *3197,* 3197(t), 3202–3204, *3205*
Neuroblastoma, 3307
  skull metastasis from, 3241, *3242*
  spinal cord, in children, *3216*
  sympathoblast and, 3307
Neuroectodermal dysplasias, skull involvement in, 3261
Neuroectodermal tumors, in children, 2713
Neuroendocrinology, 931–988. See also *Endocrine function.*
  adenohypophysis in, 935–970
  adrenal corticosteroids in, 983–985
  hypothalamico-neurohypophyseal system in, 970–983
  pituitary gland in, 931–935, *932, 934*
Neurofibroma, 3301–3303
  locations of, 395(t)
  of orbital peripheral nerves, 3049, 3050, *3050, 3051*
  plexiform, 3303
  solitary, 3302
  spinal, 512, *516,* 3202–3204
    computed tomography in, 139, *140*
    in children, *3216*
  vs. benign schwannoma, 3300
Neurofibromatosis, von Recklinghausen's, 3302–3303
  computed tomography in, *123*
  dural ectasia in, 512
  genetic aspects of, 1227–1228, 1227(t)
  of spine, *516*
  skull in, 3261
Neurofibrosarcoma, of orbital peripheral nerves, 3051
  of spinal cord, in children, *3216*
Neurogenic shock, in multiple trauma, 2504, 2509–2510
Neurogenic theory of cerebral blood flow autoregulation. 793
Neurohypophysis, 970
  tumors of, 3128, 3154
Neuroleptanalgesia, 1121
  in dyskinesias, 3828
  in electrocorticography, 1123
  in supratentorial tumors in children, 2709
Neurolysis, 2411
Neurolytic agents, in pelvic metastasis, 3629
  intrathecal, in pain, 3655–3662
Neuroma(s), acoustic, 2967–3003. See also *Acoustic neuroma.*
  crush injury and, objective pain in, 3491
  in continuity, 2372–2375, *2372, 2373*
    peripheral nerve pain and, 3636, *3636*
  pain in, 2423
  peripheral nerve pain and, 3636, *3636*
  vertebromedullary, angiography in, 609, *610*
  vs. trigeminal neuralgia, 3557
Neuromodulation, brain stimulation in, 3623
  in abdominal pain, 3630, 3630(t)
  in chronic low back pain, 3620, *3621–3623*
  in pelvic pain, 3630
  in peripheral nerve injury, *3621, 3622,* 3634–3636, 3635(t), *3635, 3636*

Neuromodulation (*Continued*)
  spinal cord stimulation in, 3621, *3622, 3623*
  transcutaneous, 3620, *3621*
Neuromuscular junction, disorders at, electromyographic studies
  in, 634
Neuromusculoskeletal syndrome, in occult spinal dysraphism,
  1321
Neuromyelitis optica, cerebrospinal fluid in, 470
  visual field loss in, 667
Neuromyotonia, 622
Neuron(s), epileptic, 3861
  mechanisms of, *3864*
  injury to, 2362, *2363*
  periventricular heterotopias of, morphogenetic timing of,
    1211(t)
  tumors of, 2801–2835
  of brain, 2759, 2835
Neuronitis, vestibular, 3782
  vertigo in, 690
Neuropathy, entrapment, electromyographic studies in, 630,
  635(t)
  ischemic optic, loss of visual field in, 667
  peripheral, pain in, 3641
  vs. papilledema, 673, *673*
Neurophthalmology, 639–675. See also *Eye(s), examination of*
  and *Vision*.
Neurophysins, secretion of, 971
Neuropsychological assessment, after head injury, 2195–2203
  in epilepsy in children, 3872–3873
  indications for, 703
  procedures in, 706–709
  techniques in, 703–706, *704*
  testing in, 709–714
Neuropsychology. See also *Psychological evaluation.*
  evolution of, 701–703
Neuroradiology, interventional, 1194–1204
  complications of, 1202
  embolization in, 1195–1202, *1196–1201*
  materials in, 1194–1195
  technical considerations in, 1194–1195
Neurosarcoidosis, 3426
Neuroschisis, theory of, in Arnold-Chiari malformation, 1281
  in Dandy-Walker malformation, 1289
  in encephalocele, 1299
  in spina bifida aperta, 1248
Neurosis (neuroses), anxiety and depressive, "effected pain" and,
  3498
  obsessive-compulsive, stereotaxic anterior capsulotomy in,
    3936(t)
  pain, 3530, 3530(t)
  traumatic, in post-traumatic syndrome, 2181
Neurosyphilis, cerebrospinal fluid in, 463
Neurotmesis, 2364
Neurotology, 676–700. See also *Ear(s), examination of* and
  Hearing.
Neurotransmitters, in cerebrospinal fluid, 449
  metabolism of, 770
Nicotinamide, cerebral blood flow and, 811(t)
Nicotine hydrochloride, cerebral blood flow and, 809(t)
Nicotinic acid, cerebral blood flow and, 807, 809(t), 811(t)
Niemann-Pick disease, cerebrospinal fluid in, 468
  diagnosis of, 385(t)
Nikethamide, cerebral blood flow and, 811(t)
Nitrazepam, in afebrile seizures, 3876(t)
Nitrogen, in metabolic response to trauma, 991–992
Nitrogen mustard, inner ear damage and, 691, 691(t)
  intra-arterial, 3073
Nitroprusside, in cerebral vasospasm, 820
N-nitroso compounds, as carcinogens, 2674
Nitrosureas, in tumor chemotherapy, 3082
Nitrous oxide, as general anesthetic, 1121
  in air encephalography, 1124
Nocardiosis, 3419–3421
  brain abscess in, 3349
  cerebrospinal fluid in, 462

Nociceptor, 3461
  in physiology of pain, 3461
Nonapeptide, 970
Noradrenalin, cerebral blood flow and, 808(t)
  synthesis of, 770
Norepinephrine, cerebral blood flow and, 808(t)
Nose, fractures of, 2276, *2280–2282*
  in phycomycosis, 3424
  injury to, 2270, *2274*
Notocord, split, in diastematomyelia, 1340
Nuclei ventralis posterior, stimulation of, in chronic pain, 3740,
    3741(t), 3742(t)
  in stereotaxic surgery, 3798
Nucleus caudalis, of trigeminal complex, 3464
Nursing, microneurosurgical, 1162–1163
  rehabilitation, 3989
Nutrition, 989–1002
  in intracerebral or intracerebellar hemorrhage, 1839
  parenteral, 999–1002
  preoperative, in posterior fossa tumors in children, 2741
  status of, evaluation of, 1052
Nylidrin, cerebral blood flow and, 807, 808(t)
Nystagmus, classification of, 683
  in neonate, 46
  in posterior fossa tumors in children, 2736
  in supratentorial tumors in children, 2706
  in vestibular disorders, 683
  opticokinetic, evaluation of, 661
    vestibular function and, 685
  positional testing for, 685, *685*
  vs. oscillopsia, 639

Obesity, pseudotumor cerebri and, 3181(t)
Obtundation, definition of, 63
Obturator nerve, entrapment of, 2465–2466, *2465*
Occipital lobe, lesions of, evoked potentials in, 2008
  visual field loss in, 669, *670*
Occipital neuralgia, 3540–3541
Occipital tunnel syndrome, 2462–2463
Occipital vertebra, 1482
Occipitalization, of atlas, 491, *492,* 1484, *1486, 1487*
Occiput, development of, 1482, *1483*
  encephalocele of, 1219
Occlusive disease, angiography in, 296–299, *297–299*
  false patterns of, 295
  cerebral blood flow in, 816
  extracranial, of carotid artery, 1559–1583
  intracranial, operative management of, 1619–1626
  vascular, pain of, 3640
Occupational therapy, 3989
Octapeptides, 970
Ocular bobbing, 69
Ocular defects, mesencephalotomy and, 3709
Ocular motility, disorders of, 651–663
  abnormal vertical responses in, 661
Ocular motor apraxia, 655, 655(t)
Ocular muscles, action of, 652
  weakness of, tests for, 653, *653,* 654(t)
Oculocephalic reflex(es), 68
  in cerebral death, 750
  in transtentorial herniation syndrome, 70(t)
Oculomotor nerve, clinical examination of, 20
  in infants and children, 46, 56
  in percutaneous trigeminal rhizotomy, 3569, *3571*
  misdirection of, ocular signs of, 660, *660,* 661(t)
  orbital, *3025, 3027*
  palsy of, 657, 658(t)
    in supratentorial tumors in children, 2706
    transtentorial herniation and, 878
Oculopalatopharyngeal myoclonus, 663
Oculosympathetic paresis, pupil in, 644(t), 647–648, *648*
Oculovestibular reflex, 68
  in neonate, 47

Oden's syndrome, 3661
Odontoid process, absence of, 1489
  fracture of, *498*, 2324, *2324*
  radiography of, 491, *493, 498*
  separate, 1487–1488, *1487–1489*
Olfactory groove, meningioma of, 2941, 2952–2955, *2955*
Olfactory nerve, congenital defects in, 1223
  in children, 55
Oligodendroglioma, 2789–2792, *2790*
  brain scanning in, 150(t), 152, *2791*
  cerebral hemisphere, in children, 2713
  radiation therapy in, 3102
Oligodendroma, common locations of, 395(t)
  cranial, radiation therapy of, 3102
Oliguria, postoperative, 1105
Olivopontocerebellar atrophy, cerebrospinal fluid in, 468
Ommaya reservoir, in leptomeningeal metastasis, 2892, *2893*
Oncocytoma, 3124
Oncornavirus, as carcinogen, 2675
Operative procedure(s), 1062–1082. See also names of specific
    procedures.
  air embolism during, 1070
  bleeding diatheses during, 1069
  blood pressure control during, 1067
  body temperature control during, 1067
  bone exposure, removal, and replacement in, 1075
  brain swelling during, 1071
  cardiac arrest during, 1073
  complications of, 1068
    intraoperative, 1081
    postoperative, 1082–1113
      alimentary, 1105
      blood and transfusion-related, 1108
      cardiac, 1097
      electrolyte, 1098
      genitourinary, 1104
      hormonal, 1098
      respiratory, 1093
      skin margin, 1082
      wound, 1082, 1090
    wound-related, 1074
  exposures in, extradural, 1077
    intradural, 1078
  incision in, 1074
  infection following, 1110
  instrument use in, 1066
  low perfusion states during, 1068
  open heart, neurological abnormalities after, 1549
  parenteral fluid administration in, 1066
  positioning for, 1064
  preparation of patient for, 1060
  prophylactic measures during, 1062
  prostheses in, 1080
  stereotaxic, neurological complications of, 1080
  sterile inflammatory responses following, 1110
  sterile site for, 1066
  transfusion reaction during, 1070
  venous thromboses and inflammation following, 1108
  wound dehiscence and disruption in, 1082
  wound dressing and support in, 1082
  wound hematoma in, 1083
Operative technique, 1117–1204
  cranial, 1136–1152
    approaches in, 1149
  general, 1136–1159
  spinal, 1152–1157
    approaches in, 1154
Ophthalmic artery, blood flow of, monitoring of, 740, 741
  in collateral circulatory system, 796
  radiological anatomy of, 257, *260*
Ophthalmic nerve, in orbit, 3027
Ophthalmofacial-hypothalamic malformations, 1803, *1804, 1805*
Ophthalmoplegia, internuclear, 655
  ocular signs of, 659, *660*
  transdural sonography in, 188, *189*

Ophthalmoscopy, 671–675, *672, 673,* 674(t)
  in tumors of orbit, 3031
  modification by, 3469–3471
Opiate(s), as pain modifiers, 3469
  receptors for, 3732
Opsoclonus, 662
Optic canal, radiography of, 84–86, *84–86*
Optic chiasm, anatomy of, 3112, *3114, 3115*
  diseases affecting, visual field loss in, 668, *668*
Optic disc, atrophy of, 674, 674(t)
  genetic aspects of, 1223
  in neonate, 46
  of Leber, 667
  primary, 673, *673*
  congenital anomalies of, 667
  myelinated nerve fibers in, 672, *672*
Optic nerve, *936*
  anatomy of, 3025
  arachnoid cysts of, 1442
  congenital defects of, 1223
  glioma of, 3042–3046. See also *Glioma, optic.*
  hyaline bodies of, 672, *672*
  in infants and children, 45, 56
  visual field disturbance and, 666–668, *667*
Optic tract, visual field loss and, 668, *669*
Opticokinetic nystagmus, ocular motility and, 661–663
  vestibular function and, 685–686
Oral contraceptives, pseudotumor cerebri and, 3181(t), 3185
Orbit, anatomy of, 3024–3029, *3025, 3026*
  cellulitis of, in phycomycosis, 3424
  congenital malformations of, 1474–1477, *1475–1477*
    measurements in, 1472, *1473*
  dystopia of, 1476
  encephalocele of, 1310, 3053–3054
  fractures of, 2282–2285, *2284, 2285*
  penetrating wounds of, 2066, *2066, 2067*
  tumors of, 3024–3064. See also names of specific tumors.
    angiography in, 324
    diagnosis of, 3030–3040, *3032–3039*
    incidence of, 3029–3030
    treatment of, 3039–3042, *3041*
    types of, 3042–3062
Orbital undercutting procedure, Scoville's, for psychiatric
    disorders, 3938, *3938*
Orotic acid, cerebral blood flow and, 811(t)
Orthoses, in hemiplegia, 3991, *3994, 3996–3998*
  in paraplegia, 4002, *4006, 4008*
  in quadriplegia, *4008*
Oscillopsia, nystagmus vs., 639
Osmoregulatory defects, 996
Osteitis, alveolar, occult, 3533
  fibrosing, of skull, 3250
  tuberculous, of skull, 3330
Osteitis deformans. See *Paget's disease.*
Osteitis fibrosa disseminata, skull in, 3266
Osteoarthritis, spinal abnormalities and, 506, *507–509*
Osteoblastic metastases, to skull, 3239, *3241*
Osteoclastic metastases, to skull, 3239, *3240*
Osteogenesis imperfecta, characteristics of, 1214
Osteogenic sarcoma, of orbit, 3056
  of skull, 3234
    vs. fungal infection, 3456
Osteoma, of orbit, *3026,* 3055
  of skull, 3230, *3230, 3231*
Osteomyelitis, cranial, 3253, *3254, 3255,* 3329, *3329, 3330,*
    3332, 3333
  brain abscess and, 3344
  spinal, 3453–3454, *3453–3455*
    cerebrospinal fluid in, 465
Osteopetrosis, of skull, 3255, *3256*
Osteophytes, cervical, anterior approach to, 2619
Osteoporosis, of skull, hyperparathyroidism and, 3251, *3252*
Osteoporosis circumscripta, 3258
Osteosarcoma, of skull, 3234
Otitis media, suppurative, vertigo and, 686

Otolith organ, 679
Otorrhea, in head injury in children, 2100, *2101*
  postoperative, in penetrating wounds, 2068
  radionuclide study of, 164, *165*
  secretions of, cerebrospinal fluid vs., 472
Otosclerosis, endolymphatic hydrops in, 689
Ototoxicity, 691
Outpatient care, brain scan in, 144
Ovary, carcinoma of, hypophysectomy in, 3953
Overgrowth, theory of, in Arnold-Chiari malformation, 1281
  in diastematomyelia, 1339
  in spina bifida aperta, 1246
Oxacillin, in bacterial infections, 3326
Oxazepam, in objective pain, 3489
Oxilorphan, in inappropriate antidiuretic hormone secretion, 982
Oxychlorosene therapy, reversible nerve block in, 3655
Oxygen, cerebral blood flow and, 803, 804(t)
  hyperbaric, cerebral blood flow and, 818, 830
    in increased intracranial pressure, 903–905
  poisoning by, postoperative, 1095
  values for, in acute respiratory failure, 1024
Oxyhemoglobin, in cerebrospinal fluid, 437
Oxytocin, function of, 972

Pachydermoperiostosis, acromegaly vs., 956
Pachygyria, morphogenetic timing of, 1211(t)
Paget's disease, basilar impression in, *1483*
  basilar invagination in, *492*
  cerebrospinal fluid in, 468
  pseudotumor cerebri and, 3181(t), 3188
  skull involvement in, 3258, *3259*
  spinal abnormalities and, 509, *509, 511*
  vs. acromegaly, 956
Pain, 3459–3768
  acute, definition of, 3523–3524, 3749–3750
  affected, psychiatric aspects of, 3512–3519
  affective disorders involving, 3727–3738
  anatomy and physiology of, 3461–3471
    pain-sensitive structures in head and, 3531–3532
  as indication for cranioplasty, 2230
  as symptom of depression, 3755
  ascending pathways of, 3461–3468
  back, in occult spinal dysraphism, 1323
    intractable, evaluation of, 3752
  central, mesencephalotomy for, 3709
    vs. peripheral, 3644, *3645*
  cephalic, 3531–3553
  cervical, syndromes of, treatment of, 2598–2609, *2605, 2606*
  chronic, behavior phases in, 3524, 3524(t)
    definition of, 3749–3750
    drug misuse and abuse in, 3626(t)
    effects of, 3525–3529
    iatrogenic, 3527
    legal system and, 3528
    low back, 3613–3624
    management of, 3523–3530, 3524(t), 3526(t), 3757–3765
    manipulative patient with, 3756–3757
    pain neurosis in, 3530, 3530(t)
    psychological factors in, 3752
    psychological intervention in, 3758
    refractory, management of, 3749, 3757–3765
    social aspects of, 3529
    treatment of, 3529, 3757–3765
    vs. psychogenic pain, 3755
  classification of, 3523–3525
  clinical course of, 3483–3488
  conduction anesthesia in, 3644–3662
    intrathecal neurolytic agents in, 3655, *3657–3659*, 3661(t)
    reversible local agents in, 3644, *3645–3647*
  conversion symptom of, 3756
  cordotomy in, open operative, 3686–3699, *3687, 3690, 3692*
    stereotaxic, 3672–3684, *3674–3678*, 3680(t), 3681(t)
  definition of, 3749–3750

Pain (*Continued*)
  delusional, 3755
  dental, vs. trigeminal neuralgia, 3558
  dorsal rhizotomy in, 3664–3670, 3665(t), *3665–3667, 3669*
  exaggerated (effected), psychiatric aspects of, 3493–3513, 3509(t), 3510(t)
  funicular, in spinal cord tumors, 3199
  glossopharyngeal and vagal, rhizotomy for, 3609–3612, *3610, 3611*
  in intracerebral or intracerebellar hemorrhage, 1840
  in occult spinal dysraphism, 1323
  in scoliosis in adult, 2633
  incisional, postoperative, 3653
  indifference to, congenital, 1224
  intracerebral stimulation in, 3739–3747
  lancinating vs. dysesthesias, 3673
  mesencephalotomy in stereotaxic, 3702–3710, 3704(t), *3705, 3706*, 3707(t), 3708(t)
  modification of, 3468–3471
    neuromodulation in, peripheral nerve, 3634–3636
      spinal, 3620–3624, *3621–3623*
  nerve injury, 2421
  neurolytic agents in, 3655–3662
  objective, psychiatric aspects of, *3484–3487*, 3490–3491(t)
  of disuse, 2424
    physical inactivity in, 3525–3526
  of undetermined origin, 3625
    thiopental test in, 3492–3493
  peripheral nerves in, 3461–3463
    injury to, 2421–2424, 3634–3643
    vs. central, diagnosis of, 3644, 3645
  peripheral neural events and, 3462
  personality in, 3501, 3503, 3505
  phantom limb, 2423–2424
  post-laminectomy, 3764
  psychiatric aspects of, 3480–3519
  psychopathophysiology of, 3727–3729
  psychosomatic, 3497–3498, 3545–3546
  referral patterns of, 3532
  spinal, 3613–3625, *3614, 3615*, 3618(t), *3619–3623*
    paraplegia and, 3624
    postincisional, 3624
  sympathectomy in, 3717–3724, *3718*
  tabetic, 3673
  temporary relief of, therapeutic uses of, 3652
  traumatic, local anesthesia in, 3653
  trigeminal, 3554–3603. See also *Trigeminal neuralgia.*
  trigeminal tractotomy in, 3710–3714, *3711–3714*
  vascular disease in, 3640
  visceral, 3627–3633, 3629(t), 3630(t)
    neurolytic injections in, 3661
    vs. somatic, anesthetic diagnosis of, 3651
Pain neurosis, 3530, 3530(t)
Palate, myoclonus of, 3852
Palladium-109, in stereotaxic surgery, 3813
Palsy (palsies), abducens, 657, *657*
  Erb's, in neonate, 49
  Klumpke's, in neonate, 49
  oculomotor, 657–658, 658(t)
  "Saturday night," 2457
  sensory and motor, in ulnar nerve entrapment, 2455–2456
  supranuclear gaze, 654–657, 655(t)
  trochlear, 658, *659*, 659(t)
Pancreas, carcinoma of, reversible nerve block in, 3655
Pancreatitis, acute, reversible nerve block in, 3655
  pain of, management of, 3631
Panencephalitis, subacute sclerosing, 3358
  cerebrospinal fluid in, 465
  diagnosis of, 385(t)
  electroencephalography in, 207, *212*, 222
Pangamic acid, cerebral blood flow and, 811(t)
Pansinusitis, chronic, 3535
  subdural empyema and, *3334–3336*
Pantopaque, in cerebellopontine angle examination, 372–373, *373*
  in myelography, 512, 569, *575–577*

Pantothenic acid, cerebral blood flow and, 811(t)
Papaverine, cerebral blood flow and, 807, 809(t)
Papilledema, in pituitary adenoma, 3130
  in pseudotumor cerebri, 3180, 3188
  increased intracranial pressure and, 878
  ophthalmoscopy in, 671, 672
  visual field loss in, 667
Papillitis, ophthalmoscopy in, 671, 674(t)
Papilloma, choroid plexus, 2798–2801, 2799, 2800
  in posterior fossa, in children, 2754
Papovavirus, as carcinogen, 2675
Paracoccidioidomycosis, 3421–3423
  cerebrospinal fluid in, 462
Paraganglioma, 3311–3313
  vs. chemodectoma, 3285
Paragonimiasis, 3387–3393
  cerebral, 3388
  diagnosis of, 3389(t)
  spinal, 3391
Paraldehyde, in status epilepticus, 3878
Paralysis, cerebral vasomotor, 874
  facial, in temporal bone fractures, 2254
  lower neuron, clinical examination in, 7–8
  oculosympathetic, clinical signs of, 644(t)
    differential diagnosis in, 648
    pupillary reactions in, 647, 648
  spinal curvature and, 2633–2635, 2635
    coexistent unrelated, 2650–2652
  upper motor neuron, clinical examination in, 6–7
  vasomotor, computed tomography in, 125
Paramethadione, in afebrile seizures, 3876(t)
Paranasal sinuses, carcinoma of, 3277, 3278–3281
  skull in, 3244
  treatment of, 3279, 3280, 3281
  mucocele of, 3058
  skull in, 3261
Paranoia, "effected" pain and, 3496–3497
Paraosteoarthropathy, spinal cord dysfunction and, 4011
Paraplegia, braces in, 4002
  pain of, 3624–3625
  rehabilitation in, 4000, 4001–4004, 4006–4009
  spastic, sympathectomy for, 3720
  spinal angiomas of, embolization of, 597, 598
  tilt table in, 4002, 4004
  tuberculosis and, 3456
  urological rehabilitation in, 4010
  with spinal curvature, 2649–2650, 2650, 2651
Parasitic infections, 3366–3440. See also names of specific
  infections.
  intracranial hypertension in, 3180(t)
Parathormone, serum, in acromegaly, 954
Parathyroid disease, cerebrospinal fluid in, 468
Paratonic rigidity, 69
Paravertebral nerve block, cervical, 3648
  lumbar, 3647
  lumbar sympathetic, 3649, 3651
Parenteral therapy, 989–1003
  in coma, 994
  intra-operative, 1066–1067
  nutrition by, 999–1002
Paresis, abductor vocal cord, in Arnold-Chiari malformation, 1286
  lower facial, post-thalamotomy, 3834
  oculosympathetic, 647–648, 648
  postoperative, in open cordotomy, 3697
    in percutaneous trigeminal rhizotomy, 3576
    in stereotaxic cordotomy, 3681
    postictal, 1112
Paresthesia, postcordotomy, 3698
  post–temporal craniotomy for trigeminal neuralgia, 3583
Parietal lobe, lesions of, evoked potentials in, 2007, 2007
  visual field loss in, 669, 670
  syndromes of, clinical examination in, 15–16
Parkinson's disease, 3837–3845

Parkinson's disease (Continued)
  as dyskinesia, 3821
  cerebrospinal fluid in, 470
  diagnosis of, 3839
    differential, 3841
  etiology of, 3840
  management of, medical, 3841
    operative, 3842, 3843
  neuropsychological assessment in, 706
  progression of, 3841
  rehabilitation in, 4000
  symptoms of, 3837
Parotid gland, injury to, 2268, 2269–2271
Parotiditis, postoperative, 1107
Paroxysmal disorders, cerebrospinal fluid in, 471
  electroencephalography in, 217–220
Pars distalis, of adenohypophysis, cells of, 935
Pars tuberalis, embryology of, 3107
Patient, total care of, in multiple trauma, 2526
Peabody test, 706
Pelizaeus-Merzbacher disease, brain biopsy in, 389
Pelvic girdle, benign schwannoma of, 3301
Pelvic nerve, in neurolytic procedures, 3659
Pelvic plexus, injury to, 2408–2409
Pelvis, ganglioneuroma of, 3310
  malignant disease of, pain in, 3628–3630, 3629(t)
  viscera of, in anterior sacral meningocele, 1351
Penetrating injury, of brain, 1903, 2055–2068, 2055, 2058, 2060,
    2062–2067
  electroencephalography in, 1998
  vs. blunt, in prognosis after head injury, 2145
  of lumbar spine, 2359
  of thoracic spine, 2352–2353
  perforating, of skull, 1907, 2054, 2054
Penicillin(s), in actinomycosis, 3400
  in bacterial infections, 3326
  pseudotumor cerebri and, 3181(t), 3187
Penicillin G, in bacterial meningitis, 3339
  in brain abscess, 3350
Pentazocine, in chronic pain, 3526
Pentobarbital, in angiography, 233
  in head injury, 900
Pentolinium, in deliberate hypotension, 1127
Pentylenetetrazol, cerebral blood flow and, 807, 810(t)
  in electroencephalography, 216
  in epileptogenic focus localization, 3871
Perceptual training, in hemiplegia, 3998
Percussion myotonia, in neonate, 48
Percutaneous rhizotomy, in glossopharyngeal and vagal neuralgia,
    3609–3612, 3610–3611
  in trigeminal neuralgia, 3564–3578
Percutaneous stimulation, in peripheral nerve injury, 3634
Perfusion, low, intraoperative, 1068–1069
  pulmonary, 1009
    physiological dead space and, 1021
    ventilation and, 1009–1011, 1010
Perhexiline maleate, pseudotumor cerebri and, 3181(t), 3187
Pericranium, anatomy of, 2299
Periorbita, anatomy of, 3025
Peripheral nerve(s). See also names of specific nerves.
  biopsy of, 405–410, 406(t), 407(t), 409(t)
  congenital defects of, 1223–1224
  in neonate, 48
  injury of, acute, 2362–2425
    axon in, 2363, 2366
    electromyography in, 630–633, 634–635(t)
    management of, 2383, 2410–2418, 2413–2415, 2417
    mechanisms of, 2365, 2367, 2368, 2370, 2371
    neuroma in continuity, 2372, 2372–2374
    neuron in, 2362, 2363
    regeneration in, 2374, 2375, 2376–2382
    rehabilitation in, 2418, 2419, 2420
    specific injuries in, 2386, 2387, 2389–2391, 2397,
      2400–2402, 2406, 2407
  entrapment, 2430–2474

Peripheral nerve(s) (*Continued*)
  injury of, entrapment, ischemia and pressure and, 2433–2435
    nerve conduction in, 618, 630
    in basilar skull fracture, 2251–2260
    pain of, 3534–3643
      causes of, 3636
      neuromodulation in, 3634
    rehabilitation in, 2418–2425
  lesions of, clinical examination in, 31–35, *32, 33,* 34(t)
  orbital, tumors of, 3049–3053
  receptors and, in pain, 3461–3462
  stimulators for, implantable, 3635, *3636*
  tumors of, 3299–3315
    neuronal, 3306–3311
    of Schwann cell origin, 3303–3306
  urinary bladder and sphincter, 1033–1034
Peripheral neuropathy, 3641
Peripheral paroxysmal vertigo, benign, 690
Peripheral vascular system, injuries to, in multiple trauma, 2490
  preoperative evaluation of, 1059
Peroneal nerve, electromyography of, 632
  entrapment of, 2467–2469, *2468*
  injury to, 2401–2404
    tibial nerve and, 2405–2407, *2406, 2407*
Perorbital projection, angiographic, 238, *239*
Perphenazine, in compulsive personality, 3504
  in histrionic personality, 3506, 3507
  in objective pain, 3489
  in psychogenic tissue tension pain, 3497, 3498
Personality, changes in, in supratentorial tumors in children, 2705
  compulsive, effected pain and, 3503
  constriction of, in post-traumatic syndromes, 2182
  dependent, effected pain and, 3501
  histrionic, effected pain and, 3505
Petechiae, in coma, 64(t)
Petit mal. See *Epilepsy.*
Petriellidiosis, 3401–3402
Phakomatoses, in supratentorial tumors, in children, 2704, *2705*
  nervous system neoplasia in, 1227, 1227(t)
Phantom limb pain, 2423–2424, 3637, 3637(t)
  mesencephalotomy in, 3709
  neuromodulation techniques in, 3637
Phantom target stereotaxic instrument, 3802, *3804*
Pharyngeal reflex, in cerebral death, 750
Phenacemide, in afebrile seizures, 3876(t)
Phenobarbital, in absence status, 3878
  in afebrile seizures, 3876, 3876(t)
  in febrile seizures, 3875
  in neonatal seizures, 3874
  in status epilepticus, 3878
  post–temporal lobectomy, 3889
  starting dosages of, 3877(t)
Phenol, in chronic pain syndrome, 3763
  in glycerol, administration of, 3658, *3659, 3661*
    as neurolytic agent, 3656
    results of, 3660, 3661(t)
Phenoxybenzamine, cerebral blood flow and, 809(t)
  in spastic urinary sphincter, 1045
Phenylalanine mustard, intra-arterial, 3073
Phenylephrine, cerebral blood flow and, 808(t)
  in atonic urinary sphincter, 1046
Pheochromocytoma, 3311
  glomus jugulare tumor with, 3287
Phlebitis, postoperative, 1108
Phoria, definition of, 652
Phosphatase, serum alkaline, in acromegaly, 954
Phosphate, inorganic, serum, in acromegaly, 954
Phosphocreatine, ischemia and, 777, *778*
Phosphorus, in cerebrospinal fluid, 450
Photocoagulation, in diabetic retinopathy, vs. hypophysectomy, 3955
    vs. pituitary ablation, 3985(t)
Photophobia, in acromegaly, 3129
  in central nervous system diseases, 641(t)
Phrenic nerve, electromyography of, 632

Phycomycosis, 3423–3426
Physical therapy, 3989
Pia, formation of, 1240
Pick disease, brain biopsy in, 386(t)
Picrotoxin, cerebral blood flow and, 807, 810(t)
Pilocytic astrocytoma, 2779–2786, 3154
Pilonidal sinus, 1330
Pineal gland, in head injury, 1989
Pineal region, tumors of, 2863–2871
  angiography in, 324
  in children, 2714–2717, *2715–2717*
    in posterior fossa, 2755
  radiation therapy of, 3103, 3103(t)
Pinealoma, brain scanning in, 153
  pediatric, 162(t)
  computed tomography in, 116
Pineoblastoma, in children, 2716
Pipradol, cerebral blood flow and, 812(t)
Pitressin tannate, postcryohypophysectomy, 3979
  post–hypophysectomy by craniotomy, 3983
Pituitary abscess, 3154
Pituitary adenoma, 3107–3151
  anterior pituitary failure and, 948
  brain scanning in, 150(t), 152, *154*
  classification of, architectural, 3117, *3118, 3119*
    functional, 3121, 3122(t)
  computed tomography in, 137, *137, 138*
  corticotropic, 3123
  cryohypophysectomy in, 3978
  endocrine-active, 3122
  endocrine-inactive, 3124
  etiology of, 3128
  extrasellar expansion and invasion of, 3125
  in children, 2727–2728, *2727*
  metastasis of, 3127
  microscopic, 3124
    incidental, 969, *970*
    treatment of, 984
  pathology of, 3117, *3118–3121,* 3124, *3125, 3126*
  polysecretory, 964
  secretory properties of, 3119, *3120, 3121*
  staining properties of, 3117
  symptoms and findings in, 3129
  thyrotropic, 3123
  treatment of, 3137, 3137(t)
    complications of, 3148, 3148(t)
    medical, 3137(t), 3142
    methods of, 3143, 3144(t), *3145*
    operative, 3137(t), 3138
    radiotherapy in, 3137(t), 3142
    results of, 3144, 3147(t), 3148(t)
  ultrasound in, 190
Pituitary apoplexy, 948, 3148
Pituitary extract, posterior, cerebral blood flow and, 811(t)
Pituitary gland, 931–935
  ablation of. See *Hypophysectomy.*
  abscess of, 3154
  adenoma of, 3107–3151. See also *Pituitary adenoma.*
  anatomy of, 3107, *3109–3116*
    microscopic, 3116, *3116*
  anterior, 935–970. See also *Anterior pituitary.*
  blood supply of, 933, *934,* 3113
  embryology of, 931, *932,* 3107
  hormones of, 935–943
    deficiency of, diabetic retinopathy and, 3948–3949
    radiation therapy and, 3164
  structures adjacent to, 935, *936*
  structures of, 3107
  transsphenoidal approaches to, 3140
  tumors of. See also *Pituitary adenoma.*
    etiology of, 3128
    gonadotropin-secreting, 964
    hormone secretion and, 952
    management of, 957(t)
      early diagnosis and, 969

Pituitary gland (*Continued*)
 tumors of, prolactin-screening, 965
  radiation therapy of, 3163–3169
  thyrotropin-secreting, 963
  vs. empty sella turcica, 3172
Plaque, neural, in spina bifida aperta, 1248–1251, *1249, 1250*
Plasma, blood, cerebrospinal fluid and, 432
 cells of, in cerebrospinal fluid, 440
Plateau waves, in increased intracranial pressure, 889
Platybasia, 1484, *1486*
Pleuritis, pain in, 3631
Pneumocranium, post-traumatic meningitis and, 3340, *3340*
Pneumoencephalography, 351–369
 brain tumor, results of, 168(t)
 cerebrospinal fluid in, 472
 in acoustic neuroma, 2985, *2985*
 in craniopharyngioma, 2907, *2907*
 in empty sella syndrome, 3150, *3150,* 3172, *3173*
 in epidermoid cysts, 2921, 2922
 in hydrocephalus, normal-pressure, 1426
  in children, 1399, *1399*
 in intracerebral and intracerebellar hemorrhage, 1836–1897, *1838*
 in orbital tumor, 3037, *3038*
 in pituitary adenoma, 3132, *3133, 3134, 3135*
 in stereotaxic localization, 3786, *3787*
 in supratentorial tumors, in children, 2706
 premedication in, 1120
 preparation for, 351, 354(t)
 technique of, 354, *355–362, 364–368*
Pneumonia, as postoperative complication, 1095
 aspiration, multiple trauma and, 2483–2484
Pneumothorax, 1019, *1020*
 in multiple trauma, 2480–2482
 intercostal nerve block and, 3646, *3647*
 postoperative complication of, 1096
Pneumoventriculography, vs. ultrasound, *184,* 186
Poiseuille's law, 790, 871
Poisoning, arsenic, intracranial hypertension in, 3180(t)
 carbon monoxide, vascular ischemia in, 1542–1543, 1543(t)
 drug, eye movement in, 69
 heavy metal, cerebrospinal fluid in, 471
Poliodystrophy, progressive, brain biopsy in, 386(t)
Poliomyelitis, cerebrospinal fluid in, 465
Polyarteritis nodosa, 1545–1546
 cerebrospinal fluid in, 469
Polycystic kidney, cerebral aneurysm and, 1808–1809, 1808(t)
Polycythemia, cerebral blood flow in, 822, 829
 pseudotumor cerebri and, 3181(t)
Polydipsia, primary, vs. postoperative diabetes insipidus, 1102
Polyethylene, cranioplasty with, 2239–2241
 film, in craniectomy for synostosis, 1458, *1458*
Polymorphonuclear cells, in cerebrospinal fluid, 440
Polymyositis, electromyographic studies in, 634
 fibrillation potentials in, 621
Polymyxins, 3327
 in subdural empyema, 3337
 in subgaleal abscess, 3328
Polyneuropathies, cerebrospinal fluid in, 471
 diffuse, electromyography in, 633
Polyradiculopathy, vs. acute transverse myelitis, 3359
Polyuria, causes of, 973(t)
Pompe's disease, in neonate, 47
Pons, hemorrhage in, 1829–1830
 infarction of, coma in, 71
 perforating arteries to, radiological anatomy of, 275
Pontomesencephalic vein, anterior, 282
Porencephaly, in children, 2127, *2128*
 needle, ventricular tap and, *1398*
 pneumoencephalography in, *364*
 ventriculography in, *371*
 vs. arachnoid cyst, 1436
Porphyria, acute, cerebrospinal fluid in, 469
Positional tests, of vestibular function, 685, *685*

Positioning, for angiography, 223
 for cranial operation, 1136
 for operative procedures, 1064–1066
  anesthesia and, 1131–1133
  for cervical pain, 2601–2602
  for posterior fossa tumors in children, *2743*
  spinal, 1152–1157
 of head, cerebral blood flow and, 827–828, 830
Postconcussional syndrome, 2167
Posterior cerebral artery, aneurysms of, 1738, 1740(t)
 occlusion of, angiography in, 296
 radiological anatomy of, *274,* 275–276, *275–277*
Posterior choroidal arteries, radiological anatomy of, *275,* 276–278, *278*
Posterior communicating arteries, radiological anatomy of, *268,* 278, *278, 279*
Posterior decompression, in craniovertebral junction anomalies, 1496, *1499, 1501*
Posterior fossa, exploration of, anesthesia in, 1123
  monitoring during, 1130
  patient position in, 1132
 hematoma of, postoperative, 1085
  subdural, in children, 2112, 2125
 in Dandy-Walker malformation, 1290
 lesions of, clinical examination in, 20–22
 revascularization of, extracranial to intracranial arterial anastomosis in, 1611–1613
 transmeatal approach to, 2992
 tumors of. See *Brain tumors* and names of specific tumors.
 veins of, 282
Posterior inferior cerebellar artery, cranial nerve root compression by, 3773, *3773*
 radiological anatomy of, 271, *272, 273, 275*
Posterior intermedius nerve, entrapment of, 2456–2459
Posterior pituitary powder, in neurohypophyseal diabetes insipidus, 975
Posterior tibial nerve, entrapment of, 2466–2467, *2466*
 injury to, 2404–2405
  nerve conduction in, 631
 peroneal nerve and, 2405–2407, *2406, 2407*
Postherpetic neuralgia, 3542–3543
 pain in, 3641, *3642*
 trigeminal neuralgia vs., 3557
Post–lumbar puncture syndrome, 456
 cerebrospinal fluid in, 472
Post-thoracotomy syndrome, pain in, 3624
Post-traumatic epilepsy, 2188–2194
Post-traumatic syndrome, 2175–2187
 description of, 2176–2177
 diagnosis of, 2184–2185
 pathogenesis of, 2177–2184
 treatment of, 2185–2186
Potassium, abnormalities of, in multiple trauma, 2500
 in cerebrospinal fluid, 450
 post-traumatic imbalance of, 991
Potassium perchlorate, in brain scanning, 147
Pott's disease, 3455
Pott's puffy tumor, 3253, *3254*
Prednisolone phosphate, 984
 in Cushing's disease, 960
Pregnancy, cerebrospinal fluid in, 471
 pseudotumor cerebri and, 3181(t)
 risks to fetus in, 40
 subarachnoid hemorrhage in, 1809–1811
Pregnancy-cell adenoma, 3117
Prematurity, cerebrospinal fluid in, 451
Premedication, for operative procedure, 1062
 for pneumoencephalography, 1120
Prenatal history, in clinical examination, 39
Preoperative evaluation, 1051–1116
Pressure, blood. See *Blood pressure.*
 cerebrospinal fluid, 429–431
  linear regression in, 455
 in peripheral nerve entrapment, 2433–2435, *2433–2437*
 in stereotaxic lesion making, 3800

Pressure, (*Continued*)
  intracranial. See *Intracranial pressure*.
Pressure cone, tentorial, 878–880
Pressure-fits, 430
Primary affective disorders. See *Psychiatric disorders*.
Primidone, in afebrile seizures, 3876, 3876(t)
Procaine, cerebral blood flow and, 810(t)
  in stereotaxic operations, 3808
  starting dosages of, 3877(t)
Procarbazine, in tumor chemotherapy, 3085–3086, 3088, 3089(t)
Progesterone, in anterior pituitary failure, 950
Progressive diaphyseal dysplasia, vs. osteopetrosis, 3255
Projector light test, in visual field evaluation, 664, *664, 665*
Prolactin, hypothalamic-pituitary relationship and, 942
  measurement of, in acromegaly, 954
  nature and function of, 939
Prolactinoma, 3123
  angiography in, *3135*
  etiology of, 3128
  histology of, *3121, 3122*
  tomography in, 3130, *3130, 3134*
  treatment of, 3147, 3147(t)
Promethazine hydrochloride, in dyskinesias, 3828
Pronator teres syndrome, 2451
  electromyography in, 631
Propantheline bromide, in detrusor hyperreflexia, 1041
Propoxyphene, in chronic pain, 3526
Propranolol, in migraine, 3549
Prostaglandins, cerebral blood flow and, 812(t)
  in cerebrospinal fluid, 449
Prostate, carcinoma of, hormone dependency of, 3947
    hypophysectomy in, 3952–3953
    metastases to skull from, *3241*
    metastases to spine from, 512
    post–hypophysectomy by craniotomy, 3985
Prostheses, intraoperative complications with, 1080
  urinary sphincter, 1046–1047, *1047*
Protein, in cerebrospinal fluid, 424, 441–446
Pseudocyst, postoperative radiotherapy and, 3082
Pseudohypoparathyroidism, skull in, 3251
Pseudomeningoceles, postoperative, 1086
Pseudomonas aeruginosa, in brain abscess, 3348
Pseudopapilledema, ophthalmoscopy in, 671
Pseudotumor, idiopathic inflammatory, of orbit, 3060
Pseudotumor cerebri, 3179–3195, *3180(t)*
  cerebral blood flow in, 824
  diagnosis of, 3188–3190
    differential, 3190–3191, 3191(t)
  etiology of, 3181(t), 3182–3188, *3183, 3186*
  follow-up in, 3192–3193
  increased intracranial pressure in, 877, 896
  signs and symptoms of, 3179–3182, 3180(t), 3181(t)
  treatment of, 3191–3192, 3191(t)
Pseudoxanthochromia, 438
Psychiatric disorders, cephalic pain and, 3545
  epilepsy and, 3881
  following head injury, 2168
  operations for, 3927, 3937, 3941. See also *Psychiatric*
    disorders, treatment of.
  sites of lesions in, 3929, *3930, 3940*
  pain and, 3480–3519, 3525
    patient evaluation in, 3753
  treatment of, bimedial leucotomy in, 3928
    capsulotomy vs. cingulotomy in, 3936(t)
    lobotomy in, 3928
    stereotaxic operations in, 3929
    techniques for, 3931
Psychogenic disorders, in post-traumatic syndrome, 2176, 2179,
  2185, 2186
  pain as, 3755–3756
  tissue tension pain as, 3494, 3497
Psychological deficits, following head injury, 2167
Psychological evaluation, in chronic pain, 3755
  in epilepsy in children, 3872
  in rehabilitation, 3990

Psycho-organic syndrome, following aneurysm operations, 1692
Psychosis, bromide, cerebral blood flow in, 829
  epileptic, 3881, 3882
Psychosomatic pain, 3497–3498, 3545–3546
Psychosurgery, 3927
Pterygoid canal, nerve of, 3269
Pterygoid muscle, in neonate, 46
Pterygopalatine fossa, *3270*
Ptosis, causes of, 643
  unilateral, ganglionectomy for, 3720
Pudendal nerves, section of, in spastic urinary sphincter, 1046
Pulmonary artery, pressure in, respiratory failure and, 1023
Pulmonary edema, as postoperative complication, 1096
  increased intracranial pressure and, 864–866
  production of, 1016
  vascular congestion and, 1019, *1021*
Pulmonary embolism, in multiple trauma, 2484–2487
  postoperative, 1096
  reversible nerve block in, 3654
Pulmonary function, 1004–1028
  circulatory failure and, 1015
  complications of, 1004
  disorders of, as contraindication to cordotomy, 3673
  in malignant visceral disease, 3627
  in multiple trauma, 2487
  in scoliosis, 2633
  normal, 1005–1012
  perfusion in, 1009
  ventilation in, 1009
    failure of, 1014
    regulation of, 1011
Pulpitis, occult, 3533, *3534*
Pulse(s), in ischemic vascular disease, 1517
  rate of, in acute respiratory failure, 1023
Pulsed Doppler examination, 742–743, *743*
Pupil(s), amaurotic, 650, *650, 651*
  Argyll Robertson, 649
  examination of, 645–651, *648–651*, 649(t), 650(t)
    in head injury, 1945
  fiber pathways in, 646
  in cerebral death, 758
    light reflex of, 750
  in coma, 66–67
  in epilepsy, 651
  in transtentorial herniation syndrome, 70(t)
  in unconscious patient, 66
  miotic, 649
  tonic, 648, *649*, 649(t)
Pure-tone audiometry, 694–695
Purpura, in coma, 64(t)
  thrombotic thrombocytopenic, 1546–1547
Putamen, hemorrhage in, 1828–1829
Pyelogram, intravenous, in urinary bladder malfunction, 1038
Pyocele, 3261
Pyocephalus, 3342
Pyogenic infections, cerebrospinal fluid in, 441
  of vertebrae, 505, *506*
Pyramiditis, petrous, 3329
Pyridoxine, in neonatal seizures, 3874

Quadrigeminal plate region, arachnoid cysts of, 1442
Quadriplegia, rehabilitation in, 4000–4012, *4001–4004,*
  4006–4009
  tilt table in, *4004*
  vocational placement of patient with, 4011
Queckenstedt test, in pseudotumor cerebri, 3188
  spinal cord tumors, 3201
  technique of, 453, 454–455

Rabies, cerebrospinal fluid in, 465
Race, brain tumor incidence and, 2685–2688, *2687*

Rachischisis, of arch of atlas, 1482
Radial nerve, entrapment of, 2456–2457
  electromyography in, 631
  injury to, 2394
  palsy of, in newborn, 49
Radiation, central nervous system tolerance of, 3097–3098
  hypophysectomy by, 3973, 3974(t)
  in etiology of brain tumors, 2673–2674
  in stereotaxic lesion making, 3812–3814
  necrosis from, computed tomography in, 135, 135
  of skull, 3250
  postoperative radiotherapy and, 3082
Radiculopathy, cervical, 2575, 2591–2597
  dynamic factors in, 2586–2591, 2588–2590
  foraminotomy for, 2605–2607, 2606
Radiofrequency coagulation, hypophysectomy by, 3974
  in psychiatric disorders, 3931
  in stereotaxic lesion making, 3800, 3808–3810, 3809
  in stereotaxic trigeminal tractotomy, 3711, 3711
  neurotomy by, in chronic low back pain, 3618, 3618(t)
Radiography. See also specific radiological procedures, e.g.,
    Angiography.
  contrast agents for, cerebral blood flow for, 813
  in acoustic neuroma, 2975, 2976
  in acute respiratory failure, 1019, 1019–1021, 1025
  in anterior sacral meningocele, 1352
  in arachnoid cysts, 1439, 1440, 1444
  in astrocytomas, 2774
  in basilar skull fractures, 2258
  in brain abscess, 3345
  in brain tumors, results of, 168(t)
  in carotid cavernous fistula, 1774–1775, 1781–1782
  in cavernous plexus aneurysms, 1771
  in cavernous plexus lesions, 2015, 3017
  in craniopharyngioma, 2905
  in craniosynostosis, 1450–1453
  in disc disease, lumbar, 2543
    thoracic, 2564
  in dural fistulae, 2217, 2217, 2221
  in epilepsy, in adults, 3911
    in children, 3873–3874, 3873, 3874
  in glomus jugulare tumor, 3287, 3287
  in head injury, 1987–1989, 1988
  in hydrocephalus, high-pressure, 1434
    in children, 1392, 1392, 1393, 1404, 1405–1408
  in meningioma, 2943, 2943
  in metastatic tumors, 2877, 2878
  in myelomeningocele, 496, 497, 1259
  in orbital tumors, 3032
  in pineal tumors, 2865
  in pituitary adenoma, 3130
  in posterior fossa tumors in children, 2737
  in pseudotumor cerebri, 3188
  in stereotaxic localization, 3785–3796
  in sylvian fissure cyst, 1439, 1440
  in transient ischemic attack, 1524
  skull, 77–110
    calcifications in, 77, 79
    extracalvarial structures simulating lesions in, 77, 78
    in skull tumors, 3227, 3229(t)
    in supratentorial brain tumors, in children, 2706
    prognosis after head injury and, 2148, 2149(t)
    pseudolesions in, 77
  spinal, 487–550
    in angiomas, 569, 570–574
    in arteriovenous malformations of cord, 1854–1856
    in cord tumors, in adults, 3200, 3200, 3201
    in diastematomyelia, 1344
    in lumbosacral lipoma, 1337, 1337
Radionuclide imaging, 143–175. See also Brain scan.
  after carotid arteriography, 161
  appearance of disease in, 149–161, 150(t), 151–154,
    154(t)–156(t), 156–160
  cerebrospinal fluid studies in, 163–165, 165
  cisternography in, 164

Radionuclide imaging (Continued)
  computed tomography and, 165–168, 167(t), 168(t)
  dynamic, 162–163
  in arteriovenous malformation, 159, 160
  in brain tumors, results of, 168(t)
  in cerebrovascular accidents, 155, 155(t), 156, 156(t), 157
  in children, 161–162, 162(t)
  in Dandy-Walker malformation, 1294
  in intracerebral hemorrhage, 1831
  in intracerebral inflammatory disease, 159
  in intracranial hematoma, 156, 159
  in neoplastic lesions, 150, 150(t) 151–154
  in nonneoplastic disease, 154, 155(t)
  in pediatric hydrocephalus, 1393, 1393
  in skull lesions, 161
  in spinal cord tumors, 3202
  in trauma, 161
  indications for, 144, 144(t)
  instrumentation in, 146–147
  normal appearance in, 147–149, 149
  post-treatment, 154
  radiopharmaceuticals in, 144–146, 148(t)
  static and dynamic images in, 149
  technique in, 147
  value of, 168, 168(t)
  ventriculography in, 164
Radiosensitizers, in treatment of brain tumors, 3089
Radiotherapy, in acromegaly, 956
  in brain tumors, 3096–3106
    BCNU and, 3084
  in cerebral metastasis, 2882(t), 2883(t), 2887, 2887(t)
  in glioblastoma, 2815–2816
  in glomus jugulare tumor, 3290
  in hyperprolactinemia, 968
  in pituitary tumor, 2912, 3163–3169
  in spinal cord tumor, 3222–3226
    in adults, 3212–3213
  postcraniotomy, in intracranial tumor, 1152
  postoperative, diagnostic confusion of, 3081
Railroad nystagmus, 685
Rathke's pouch, embryology of, 3107
Rauwolfia alkaloid, cerebral blood flow and, 809(t)
Raynaud's phenomenon, pain in, 3640–3641
  sympathectomy for, 3721
Reading, dominant hemisphere, cerebral blood flow and, 826
Recreational activities, in paraplegia and quadriplegia, 4012
Recruitment tests of hearing, 697
Rectal incontinence, intrathecal neurolytic agents and, 3659
Rectus abdominis syndrome, 2463
Red eye, causes of, 645
Red-glass test, for ocular muscle weakness, 653, 653
Reflex(es), acoustic, test of, 700
  in child, 60, 61(t)
  in newborn, 49
  nerve conduction studies of, 628
  pupillary, 647–651, 648–651
  spinal, in cerebral death, 757
Reflex sympathetic dystrophy, 3639, 3639
Refsum's syndrome, vs. chronic progressive external
    ophthalmoplegia, 660
Regeneration, axonal, 2374, 2375–2383, 2376–2382
  cranial nerve, misdirection in, 660–661, 660, 661(t)
Rehabilitation, 3987–4013
  after brain injury, 3991–4000
    psychological testing in, 2202
  bimedial leucotomy and, 3929
  in peripheral nerve injury, 2418–2425, 2419, 2420
  nursing in, 3989
  planning of, neuropsychological assessment in, 709
  team approach to, 3989–3991
  vocational, 4012–4013
Reissner's membrane, 677, 678
Reitan-Indiana Screening Test, 706
Renal disease, cerebrospinal fluid in, 469
Renal failure, acute, in multiple trauma, 2511–2518

Renal failure (*Continued*)
  acute, postoperative, 1105
Renal rickets, skull in, 3253
Rendu-Osler angiomatosis, spinal angioma and, 565, *565, 566*
Reserpine, cerebral blood flow and, 809(t)
  in cerebral vasospasm, 821
Resistance, host, in bacterial infections, 3323
Respiration, arrest of, in multiple trauma, 2482–2483
  energy yield of, 766, *766*
  failure of. See *Respiratory failure.*
  gas transport in, 1011
  in coma, 65–66
  in head injury, management of, 2043
    in children, 2093
  in multiple trauma, 2476–2490
  in transtentorial herniation syndrome, 70(t)
  in unconscious patient, 65
  increased intracranial pressure and, 863
  intracranial hypertension and, 876
  normal, 1005–1012
  physiology of, 1006
  postoperative complications of, 1093–1097
    following cordotomy, 3698
    following stereotaxic cordotomy, 3682
  preoperative evaluation of, 1054
  prognosis after head injury and, 2145, 2152–2154
  ventilation-perfusion relationships in, 1009, *1010*
Respirator brain, 756
Respiratory distress, 40
Respiratory failure, acute, 1004, 1012–1028
  clinical course of, 1017
  complications of, 1028
  diagnostic studies in, 1018, *1019–1023*
  etiology of, 1014
  management of, 1025
  pathophysiology of, 1012, *1012, 1013*
  predisposing factors in, 1018
  prevention of, 1024
  treatment of, 1024
    equipment in, 1021, *1021*
Restlessness, in intracerebral or intracerebellar hemorrhage, 1840
Reticulum cell sarcoma, vertebral body, *514*
  vs. Ewing's tumor, 3243
Retina, evoked potentials from, 201–203, *202*
  in diabetes mellitus, hypophysectomy and, 3953–3955,
    3985–3986, 3985(t)
  in newborn, 46
  lesions of, visual field disturbance in, 666–668
  vascular status of, in ischemic disease, 1519–1520, 1519(t)
Retinal artery, pressure in, carotid ligation and, 1699–1700,
    1706, *1707*
Retinitis pigmentosa, sympathectomy in, 3720
Retractors, brain, micro-operative, 1181, *1182*
Retrobulbar neuritis, cerebrospinal fluid in, 470
Retropharyngeal abscess, in children, *505*
Rewarming shock syndrome, 1129
Reye's syndrome, increased intracranial pressure in, 895
Rhabdomyosarcoma, in children, 644
  of orbit, 3057
Rheomacrodex, cerebral blood flow and, 811(t)
  in cerebral vasospasm, 820
Rheumatoid arthritis, of spine, 509, *510*
Rhinorrhea, post-hypophysectomy by craniotomy, 3984
  postoperative, in penetrating wounds, 2068
  radionuclide study of, 164, *165*
  secretions of, vs. cerebrospinal fluid, 472
Rhinotomy, in esthesioneuroblastoma, 3276, *3276*
Rhizotomy, dorsal, 3664–3671, 3665(t), *3665–3667, 3669*
  in chronic pain syndrome, 3764
  in spasmodic torticollis, 3847
  percutaneous, in trigeminal neuralgia, 3564–3579
    vagoglossopharyngeal pain, 3609–3612, *3610, 3611*
  posterior, in malignant visceral disease, 3627
  sacral, in detrusor hyperreflexia, 1042, *1043*
Rhomboencephalography, 373–374

Rib, cervical, 1216
  formation of, 1241
  fracture of, local anesthesia in, 3653
Richmond screw, 899
Rickets, renal, skull in, 3253
Rieckert stereotaxic instrument, 3803, *3804*
Rigidity, in Parkinson's disease, 3838
  paratonic, 69
Rinne test, 693
Robin Hood syndrome, 322
Rolando, fissure of, 1138
Roseola infantum, pseudotumor cerebri and, 3181(t), 3188
Rostral cingulotomy, in affective disorders, 3733–3737,
    3733–3736
Rotation injury, of lumbar spine, 2358
Ruffini's endings, 3461

Sacral dimple, in infants and children, in clinical examination, 41
Sacral meningocele, anterior, 1350–1353
Sacral nerve block, in detrusor-sphincter dyssynergia, *1038,* 1046
Sacrococcygeal region, in congenital spinal dermal sinus, 1325,
    1327, *1327*
  teratoma of, 1358–1360, *1359*
Sacrum, fractures of, 2360
  in anterior sacral meningocele, 1351
Sagittal sinus, *936*
  lesions near, clinical examination in, *15,* 17–19, *18*
  occlusion of, in cerebral infarction, 1539–1540
Sagittal suture, meningioma near, 2941, 2945–2949, *2948, 2949*
  synostosis of, 1447, *1448–1450, 1453, 1454,* 1461
Salbutamol, in cerebral vasospasm, 820
Saline solution, cerebral blood flow and, 811(t)
Sanger-Brown syndrome, cerebrospinal fluid in, 468
Saphenous nerve, entrapment of, 2465
Sarcoidosis, 3426–3430
  anterior pituitary failure and, 948
  cerebrospinal fluid in, 463
  pseudotumor cerebri and, 3181(t), 3188
  skull in, 3258
  vertebral, 3429
Sarcoma, brain, 2845, 2855–2858, *2858*
  brain scanning in, 153
  botryoid, of spinal cord, in children, *3217*
  dural, in children, 2728
  granulocytic, of orbit, 3058
  of scalp, 3319
  osteogenic, of orbit, 3056
  of skull, 3234
Saturday night palsy, 2457
Scala media, 677, *678*
Scalp, anatomy of, 2298–2300, *2298, 2300*
  avulsion of, 2302, *2304–2310*
  blood supply to, 2299, *2300*
  congenital defects of, 1215
  contusion of, echoencephalography in, 181
  incisions in, craniotomy, 1138, *1138,* 1139
  injuries of, 2298–2313
    evaluation of, 2300–2301
    management of, 2301, *2301–2312*
    primary, in head injury, 1904
    thermal and irradiation, 2311
  intravenous fluid infiltration of, transillumination in, 41
  nerve supply to, 2299, *2300*
  tumors of, 3316–3320, *3317–3320*
Scanners, for brain scan, 146–147
Scarpa's ganglion, 679
Schilder disease, brain biopsy in, 389
  cerebrospinal fluid in, 470
  intracranial hypertension in, 3180(t)
  visual loss in, 667
Schistosomiasis, 3383–3386
Schizophrenia, paranoid, "effected" pain and, 3496–3497
Schwabach test, for hearing, 694

Schwannoma, benign, 3300–3301
  dural, in children, 2728
  location of, 395(t)
  malignant, 3303–3306
  of orbital peripheral nerves, 3050, *3051, 3052*
  spinal, 512
Schwartz-Jampel syndrome, neuromyotonia in, 622
Sciatic nerve, entrapment of, 2466
    electromyographic studies in, 632
  injury to, 2405–2407, *2406, 2407*
Scintillation camera, invention of, 143
Schizophrenia, paranoid, effected pain and, 3496
SCL-90 test, for pain, 3483, *3484–3487*
Sclerosis, Ammon's horn, 3860
  amyotrophic lateral, cerebrospinal fluid in, 470
    electromyographic studies in, 633
    myelographic appearance of, *542*
  mesial, asphyxia and, 3918
  multiple. See *Multiple sclerosis.*
  tuberous, genetic aspects of, 1228, *1228*
Scoliosis, 2629–2655
  coexistent paralysis in, 2650
  congenital, anomalies in, 1217
  development of, 1258
  etiology of, 2631, 2631(t)
  in children, angiography in, *573*
  in occult spinal dysraphism, 1323
  natural history of, 2633–2635, *2634, 2635*
  neurosurgical problems in, 2648
  nonoperative treatment of, 2635, *2636*
  operative treatment of, 2637, *2638–2646*
  orthopedic problems in, 2648
Scotoma, definition of, 665
Scoville's orbital undercutting procedure, 3938, *3938*
Secobarbital, in temporal lobectomy, 3883
Sedation, excessive, in neonate, symptoms of, 45
Sedative drug poisoning, eye movement in, 69
Seizure(s). See also *Epilepsy.*
  afebrile, medical treatment of, 3875, 3876(t)
  as indication for cranioplasty, 2230
  classification of, 3864, 3865(t)
  clinical examination in, 10
  electroencephalography in, 207, *209–211,* 2191, 3868–3871, *3868*
  febrile, in infants, 3866
    medical treatment of, 3875
  genetic aspects of, 1222–1223
  in astrocytoma, 2772–2773
  in brain tumors, 2673
  in children, etiology of, 3865, 3865(t)
    pathological causes of, 3871, *3873, 3874*
    prognosis in, 3878–3879
  in pituitary adenoma, 3130
  in sarcoidosis, 3427
  in supratentorial tumors, in children, 2702
  in ventriculography, 378
  neonatal, in clinical examination, 40, 46, 49
    medical treatment of, 3874
  neurobiology of, 3859–3864
  post-hypophysectomy by craniotomy, 3984
  postoperative, 1112
  post-traumatic, 2189
  procedures to limit spread of, 3923–3925
  prognosis after head injury and, 2145
  prolonged, in children, 3877
  psychical, 3882
  serial, treatment of, 3877
  tumor regrowth and, 3082
Seldinger catheterization, 248, *248*
Sella turcica, anatomy of, 3110, *3110, 3111*
  approach to, complications of, 3970–3972, *3970, 3971*
    in transsphenoidal hypophysectomy, 3961–3964, *3962, 3963*
  arachnoid cysts of, 1441–1442
  ballooned, microadenoma and, 3125
  congenital tumors of, 3154

Sella turcia (*Continued*)
  embryology of, 3017
  empty. See *Empty sella syndrome.*
  enlarged, 3170
    causes of, 3171(t)
  evaluation of, computed tomography in, 136, *136*
  radiography of, 90–95, *91–94,* 95(t)
    pseudolesions in, 77, *79,* 80–84, *82, 83*
  tumor of, and anterior pituitary failure, 947
    in adults, 3107–3162. See also names of specific tumors.
    in children, 2717
      radiation therapy of, 3103, 3103(t)
Sensitivity reactions, allergic, postoperative, 1112
Sensory function, clinical evaluation of, in infants and children, 51, 53, 61
  disturbance of, in percutaneous rhizotomy for trigeminal neuralgia, 3575–3576, 3575(t)
  in nerve entrapment, *2443,* 2444
  in peripheral nerve injury, aberrant, 2423
    recovery of, 2380–2381, *2380–2382*
  in sensation of pain, 3462–3463
  in spina bifida aperta, 1256
  nerve conduction studies of, 625, 626(t)
  perceptual function and, psychological testing of, 705
  post–dorsal rhizotomy, *3665, 3666*
  responses in cerebral death, 751
Sensory root, in trigeminal neuralgia, decompression and compression of, 3584
Septal vein, *280*
Septic shock, in multiple trauma, 2504–2505, 2510–2511
Septum, in diastematomyelia, 1341, *1342*
Septum pellucidum, *353*
Serotonin, cerebral blood flow and, 812(t)
  synthesis of, 771
  vessel constriction and, 819
Serous labyrinthitis, 690
Serratus anterior palsy, 2462
Serum sickness, intracranial hypertension in, 3180(t)
Sexual crimes, violent, ablative procedures and, 3943
Sexual function, in spina bifida aperta, 1273
Sheehan's syndrome, 943, 3948
Shingles. See *Herpes zoster.*
Shivering, in hypothermia, 1129
Shock, in multiple trauma, 2501–2511
    classification of, 2502(t)
  in post-traumatic syndrome, 2181
  prognosis after head injury and, 2145
Shock lung, in multiple trauma, 2487–2490
Short increment sensitivity index, 697, 2974
Shoulder-hand syndrome, neuromodulation techniques in, 3640
  pain management in, 3632, 3640
  rehabilitation in, 3991
Shunt(ing), arteriovenous, collateral blood supply and, 799
  cerebrospinal fluid, in posterior fossa tumors in children, 2741
  ventricular, in Dandy-Walker malformation, 1297
    in hydrocephalus, 1430, *1430–1432*
      in children, 1404–1409, *1405–1408*
Sialorrhea, in Parkinson's disease, 3839
Sickle cell disease, skull in, 3261
  spine in, *516*
Sigmoid sinus, obstruction of, pseudotumor cerebri and, 3181(t)
Silastic spheres, embolization with, 1195
Silicone, liquid, in glomus jugulare tumor embolization, 3292
Silver-slipper syndrome, 3505
Simmonds' disease, 943
Sinus. See also names of specific sinuses.
    cavernous. See *Cavernous plexus.*
    congenital cranial dermal, 1312–1317, *1313, 1315*
    dural venous. See *Venous sinus(es).*
    maxillary, anatomy of, 3269, *3270*
    paranasal. See *Paranasal sinuses.*
    pilonidal, 1330
    sagittal. See *Sagittal sinus.*
    sphenoid. See *Sphenoid sinus.*
Sinus pericranii, 3251

Sinusitis, cephalic pain and, 3534–3536, *3535*
  in phycomycosis, 3424
SISI test, 697, 2974
Sitting position, problems with, 1065–1066
Skeletal muscle, biopsy of, 410–415, 412(t), 413(t)
  disorders of, clinical examination in, 35
Skew deviation, in cerebellar disease, 656
Skin, care of, in intracerebral or intracerebellar hemorrhage, 1840
  in occult spinal dysraphism, 1320, *1321*
  in spina bifida aperta, 1251
    closure of, 1268–1270, *1269*
  of scalp, 2298
  postoperative complications of, 1082
Skull, anomalies of, structural, 1212–1215, *1213*
  bacterial infections of, 3323–3357
  decompression of, in increased intracranial pressure, 916
  defects of, as indications for cranioplasty, 2229–2231
    etiology of, 2228–2229
    in operative procedures, 1075
    in scalp injuries, 2311, *2311, 2312*
    reconstruction of, 2311, *2311, 2312*
    repair of, 2231–2248, *2232, 2234, 2235, 2238–2241,
      2243–2247*
  delayed ossification in, 1213, *1213*
  dermal sinus of, congenital, 1312–1317, *1313, 1315*
  fetal and neonatal, ultrasound scanning of, 723
  formation of, 1242
  fracture of, basilar, linear, 1906, 2099
    nerve injuries in, 2099–2100, 2251–2260
    computed tomography in, 125, *126, 2049*
    depressed, 1906, 2049–2054, *2049, 2052,* 2102–2103
    in head injuries in children, 2096–2103, *2097, 2098, 2100,
      2101*
  geographic, 3258
  in Arnold-Chiari malformation, 1286
  in encephalocele, 1299, 1304, 1312
  lacunar, of newborn, 1219
  lesions of, brain scanning in, 161
  metabolic diseases affecting, 3251
  missile injuries of, 2055
  newborn, normal sutures in, *1448*
  operations on, 1136–1152. See also *Craniectomy* and
    Craniotomy.
  Paget's disease of, basilar impression in, *1483*
  penetrating wounds of, 2066, *2066, 2067*
  perforating wounds of, 1907
    management of, 2054
  radiographic lines in, 491, *1484*
  radiology of, 77–110. See also *Radiography, skull.*
  transillumination of, 40, 1387
  trauma to, 1905–1907, 1906(t), 1907(t)
    in children, 2096
    localized, 2048
  tumors of, 3227–3268, 3228(t)
    benign, 3228, 3236
    diagnostic techniques in, 3227–3228
    malignant, 3234, 3239
    nonneoplastic lesions simulating, 3245–3266
    primary, 3228–3236
    radiographic classification of, 3229(t)
    secondary, 3236–3245
  vascular impressions in, 3250
Skull unit, angiographic, 232
Sleep, apnea during, following cordotomy, 3698
  cerebral blood flow and, 804
  electroencephalography and, 205–206, *206*
  in epileptogenic focus localization, 3870
  intracranial pressure during, 877, 889
Sleeves, in peripheral nerve injury, 2417–2418
Smoking, cigarette, cerebral blood flow and, 809(t)
Social function, chronic pain and, 3529
  disorders of, after head injury, 2168
Social service, in rehabilitation, 3990
Sodium, body, excessive loss of, 997
  in cerebrospinal fluid, 450

Sodium (*Continued*)
  post-traumatic, retention of, 990
Sodium acetrizoate, cerebral blood flow and, 812(t)
Sodium bicarbonate, cerebral blood flow and, 811(t)
Sodium diatrizoate, cerebral blood flow and, 812(t)
  in angiography, 242
Sodium dipropylacetate, in afebrile seizures, 3876
Sodium fluorescein, in brain scanning, 143
Sodium hydrocortisone hemisuccinate, in neurological operations,
  984
Sodium nitroprusside, cerebral blood flow and, 805
  in deliberate hypotension, 1127
  in increased intracranial pressure, 901
Sodium perchlorate, in brain scanning, 147
Sodium phenobarbital, in status epilepticus, 3878
Sodium thiopental. See *Thiopental.*
Soft tissue, injuries of, scalp, 2302, *2302–2304*
Somatomedin, in acromegaly, 955
Somatostatin, in acromegaly, 957
Somatotropic adenoma, 3122
  pathology of, 3125
Sonography, intraoperative, 177, 186
  transcalvarial, 177
  transdural, 186–192, *187–189, 191–193*
Sonoventriculography, 183–186, *184, 185*
Sotos disease, 1220
Spasm, arterial, as contraindication to carotid ligation, 1703
  in aneurysm procedures, 1676
  in subarachnoid hemorrhage, cerebral blood flow and, 819
  as complication of disc operation, 2549
  bronchial, postoperative, 1095
  hemifacial, vascular decompression in, 3773–3775, *3773,*
    3774(t), 3775(t)
  vs. vascular occlusive disease, radiological differentiation of,
    295
Spasticity, 3849–3851
  post-mesencephalotomy, 3709
  rehabilitation in, 4001–4002
  sphincter, treatment of, 1045
Speech, disorders of, rehabilitation in, 3990, 3996–3998
  dominant hemisphere in, cerebral blood flow and, 826
  ventrolateral thalamotomy and, 3835
Speech audiometry, 697
Sphenoid bone, anatomy of, 3108, *3109–3111*
  radiography of, 80, *81,* 86, *86*
  tumors of, parasellar involvement in, 3154
  wing of, meningioma of, 2940, *2940,* 2950–2952, *2951–2953*
Sphenoid sinus, anatomical types of, 3108, *3109,* 3970, *3970*
  carcinoma of, 3279
  mucocele of, skull in, 3261, *3262*
Sphenoparietal sinus, *936*
Spherocytosis, hereditary, skull in, 3261
Sphincter(s), electromyography of, 1035
  in occult spinal dysraphism, 1322
  in spina bifida aperta, 1257, 1273
  urinary, atonic, 1041
    treatment of, 1046
    dysfunction of, treatment of, 1045–1047
      prosthetic, 1046, *1047*
    innervation of, 1033–1034
    spastic, 1040, *1040*
Sphingolipidosis, cerebrospinal fluid in, 468
Spiegel-Wycis stereotaxic instrument, 3802
Spina bifida. See also *Spina bifida aperta* and *Spina bifida
  occulta.*
  anterior, anterior sacral meningocele in, 1350
  combined anterior and posterior, 1350
  incidence of, 1210(t)
  meningocele with, 496, *497*
  meningomyelocele with, 496, *497*
  of arch of atlas, 1482
Spina bifida aperta, 1243–1274
  abnormal embryology in, 1246
  clinical evaluation in, 1254
  congenital anomalies associated with, 1254

INDEX

Spina bifida aperta (*Continued*)
  definition of, 1243
  initial management of, 1254
  intraspinal abnormalities with, 1250
  neurological examination in, 1255, 1256(t), 1259(t)
  pathology of, 1248
  prognosis in, 1271, 1271(t)
  survival in, 1271, 1271(t)
  treatment of, 1263, *1263–1267, 1269*
    complicating spinal deformity in, 1268
    historical perspective of, 1260
    results of, 1271
Spina bifida occulta, 1317–1318
  incidence of, 1219
  radiography in, *494*
Spinal accessory nerve, clinical examination of, 21
  in infants and children, 47, 59
  injury to, 2410
Spinal anesthesia, diagnostic, in central vs. peripheral pain, 3644, *3645*
Spinal arteries, anterior, anatomy of, 554
  in normal angiogram, *558, 559, 559–561*
  occlusion of, vs. viral encephalitis, 3360
  posterior, in normal angiogram, 561, *562*
Spinal artery syndrome, *545*
Spinal canal, developmental shallowness of, 2581–2586, *2582–2587*
  lesions of, clinical examination in, 22–31, *23–25*
  narrow, 2553–2555
  widening of, in children, radiography of, 569, *571*
Spinal cord, abscess in, *3451,* 3452–3453, *3452*
  anatomy of, 22–31, *23–25,* 3197
  angiography of, 551–616. See also *Angiography, spinal cord.*
  arteriovenous malformations of, 1850–1874
    embolization of, 1199, *1199*
  atrophy of, myelographic appearance of, *541*
  cervical, injuries to, 2318–2337
      compound, 2334, *2334*
      incomplete, 2332, *2333*
      mechanisms of, 3319–3320, *3320, 3321*
  clinical examination of 22–31, *23–25*
  compression of, from benign lesions, cervical, 2574–2612
    dorsal, 2562–2573
    lumbar, 2535–2561
    in cervical spine injury, 2320
    stages of, 3198
  disease of, cervical, 2575
    dynamic factors in, 2586–2589, *2588–2590*
    intraoperative complications and, 1079
    spondylotic, 2597–2598
    treatment of, 2598–2609, *2605, 2606*
  dorsal ganglia of, *3657, 3657*
  dorsal horn of, 3464
  dysfunction of, complications of, 4011
    functional levels of independence in, 4005–4008, *4009*
    rehabilitation in, 4000–4012, *4001–4004, 4006–4009*
  embryology of, vertebral column development and, 1239, *1239*
  enlarged, myelographic appearance of, *541*
  entry of dorsal roots into, 3464
  ependymomas of, radiation therapy of, 3223(t)
  in anterior sacral meningocele, 1351
  in Arnold-Chiari malformation, 1283, *1283, 1284*
  in diastematomyelia, 1339, 1340
  in occult spinal dysraphism, 1319
  in spina bifida aperta, 1248–1251, 1248(t), *1249, 1250,* 1265, *1265–1267*
  incomplete lesions of, 2332, 2353
  infections of, 3449–3458
  injuries to, cervical, 2318–2337
    electromyographic studies in, 633
    in neonate, symptoms of, 48, 49
    lumbar, injuries to, 2356–2361, *2357–2359*
    pain in, 3624–3625
    pulmonary edema in, 865

Spinal cord (*Continued*)
  ischemia of, from atheromatous or disc lesions, angiography in, 612–615, *613–615*
  neoplasms of, cerebrospinal fluid in, 467
  pain pathways in, 3464–3466, 3687, *3687*
  paragonimiasis of, 3391
  schistosomiasis of, 3385
  stimulation of, for urinary bladder evacuation, 1045
    in chronic low back pain, 3621–3623, *3622, 3623*
  tethered, syndrome of, 1331–1333
  thoracic, injuries to, 2344–2353, *2347*
    penetrating wounds of, management of, 2352
    transthoracic approaches to, 2351
  transection of, clinical examination in, 29
    complete thoracic, 2352
    neurolytic agents following, 3662
  tumors of, chemotherapy of, 3213
    diagnostic tests for, 3199–3202, *3200–3204,* 3218, *3219*
    glial, angiography in, *608, 609*
    in adults, 3196–3214
    in children, 3215–3221
    incidence of, 3196–3197, 3197(t), *3197,* 3215, *3216,* 3216(t)
    metastatic, 3207, 3207(t)
      operative treatment of, 3212
    operative treatment of, 3210–3212, *3210–3212,* 3219, 3219(t), 3220(t)
      anterior approach for, 2618–2619
    pathophysiology of, 3198–3199
    radiation therapy of, 3212–3213, 3222–3226
    radiography of, 512, *513–516*
    surgical anatomy of, 3197–3198
    vs. viral encephalitis, 336, 3360
  vascular disease of, vs. viral encephalitis, 3360
  vasculature of, anatomy of, 551–555, *551–555,* 1850–1852
  widening of, myelographic appearance of, *548*
Spinal dermatomes, 3666, *3667*
  somatic pain and, 3645
Spinal muscular atrophy, progressive, electromyography in, 633
Spinal nerve block, differential diagnostic, 3649
Spinal reflexes, in cerebral death, 751, 758
Spinal root deficit, syndromes of, in angiomas, 563
Spinal tap. See *Lumbar puncture.*
Spine, abnormalities of, radiographic appearance of, 491–512
  arachnoid cysts of, 1443–1445
  benign lesions of, 2533–2656
  cervical, anomalies of, 1215
    in Arnold-Chiari malformation, 1286
    anterior operative approach to, 2613–2628, *2614, 2615, 2623–2626*
    evaluation of, 491
    fractures of, 500
    infant, *493*
    injuries to, 2318–2337
      hyperextension, 2330
      hyperflexion and, 2338–2343
      vertigo from, 692
    normal, *488, 491*
    stability of, assessment of, 750
  clinical examination of, in infants and children, 41
  computed tomography of, 139–141, *140*
  congenital dermal sinus of, 1325–1330, *1327*
  congenital strictures of, 2554
  defects of, 1215
  deformity of, in diastematomyelia, 1342
    in infants and children, 41
    in spina bifida aperta, complicating treatment, 1268
    kyphosis and lordosis and scoliosis as, 2629–2654, 2630(t)–2632(t)
      development of, 1258
    neurological level and, 1257
    postlaminectomy, 2652–2654, *2652, 2653*
  extradural cyst of, 1355
    congenital, 1219
  fractures of, 496, *498–503*
    cerebrospinal fluid in, 467

INDEX

Spine (*Continued*)
   fractures of, cervical, 500, 2323–2330
      lumbar, 2356–2359, *2357–2359*
      sacral, 2360
   fusions of, in chronic low back pain, 3616
      in deformities, 2637–2638
   infections of, 3449–3458
   intramedullary lesions of, 512, *534*
   lumbar, injuries to, 2356–2361, *2357–2359*
      normal, *490*
   operations on, 1152–1157. See also names of specific
      techniques.
      specific approaches in, 1154
   osteomyelitis of, cerebrospinal fluid in, 465
   radiology of, 487–550
   rheumatoid arthritis of, 509, *510*
   segmental anomalies of, 1216
   stenosis of, as complication of disc operation, 2549
      computed tomography in, 140, *140*
   thoracic, injuries to, 2344–2353, *2345–2347, 2349*
      normal, *489*
   ultrasound scanning of, 730, *730–734*
Spinocollicular tract, pain and, 3703
Spinotectal tract, pain and, 3703
Spinothalamic tract, anatomy of, 3688
   pain and, 3703
Splanchnicectomy, in gallbladder and stomach pain, 3631
Splenius capitis syndrome, reversible nerve block in, 3654
Spondylitis, ankylosing, osteotomy in, 2641, *2644*
   radiography of, 509, *509*
Spondylolisthesis, *504, 505*, 2552–2553
   myelographic appearance of, *540*
Spondylolysis, 2552–2553
   myelographic appearance of, 530, *542–544*
Spondylosis, small spinal canal and, 2554–2555
Spongioblastoma, primitive polar, 2823
Sprains, of lumbar spine, 2359–2360
Sprengel's deformity, radiography in, 491, *494*
Squamous cell carcinoma, cephalic pain and, *3537*
   of ear, 3281, *3282*
   of maxillary sinus, 3278, *3279*
   of paranasal sinuses, 3277
   of scalp, 3316, *3317, 3318*
   vs. trigeminal neuralgia, 3557
Stanford-Binet test, in children, 40
Staphylococcus aureus, brain abscess and, 3348
Status epilepticus, in neonate, medical treatment of, 3874
   intracranial hypertension in, 3180(t)
   treatment of, 3877
Steal phenomena, in arteriovenous malformations of spinal cord,
   1852
   in ischemic vascular disease, 1532–1533
   intracerebral, cerebral blood flow and, 821–822
      hyperventilation and, 902
Steel, stainless, cranioplasty with, 2235, 2237, *2240*
Stellate ganglion block, 3650
Stenosis, aqueductal, in childhood, 3364
   in hydrocephalus, 1430
   arterial, cerebral blood flow and, 814, *815*
   carotid, extracranial, as indication for operation, *1562*, 1567,
      1569, 1570, 1572
   spinal, as complication of disc operation, 2549
      computed tomography in, 140, *140*
   venous sinus, pseudotumor cerebri and, 3181(t)
Stereotaxic procedure(s), 3785–3820
   anesthesia for, 1123
   computer aids in, 3796
   cordotomy as, 3672–3685
      equipment for, 3674–3675, *3674*
      results of, 3679, 3680(t), 3681(t)
      technique for, 3675–3679, *3675–3678*
   hypophysectomy as, 3973–3979, *3976, 3977*
   in cerebral palsy, 3849
   in dyskinesias, 3828
   in epilepsy, in adults, 3924

Stereotaxic procedure(s) (*Continued*)
   in epilepsy, in children, 3897
   in intention tremor, 3852
   in Parkinson's disease, 3843
   in spasmodic torticollis, 3848
   instruments for, 3801–3805, *3803–3804*
   lesion production in, 3805–3814, *3806, 3807, 3809*
   mesencephalotomy as, 3702–3710, 3704(t), *3705, 3706*
   neurological complications of, 1080
   principles of, 3785–3820
   x-ray localization in, 3785–3791, *3787–3790*
      landmarks for, 3785, 3791–3796, *3792–3795*
      physiological adjuncts to, 3796–3801
Sternocleidomastoid muscle, evaluation of, in newborn infants, 47
Sternocleidomastoid syndrome, reversible nerve block in, 3654
Steroids. See also *Corticosteroids.*
   adrenal, urinary, in acromegaly, 955
   in cranial operations, 1136
   in head injury, 911, 2043
   in increased ultracranial pressure, 910–912
   in tumor chemotherapy, 3089–3090
   neuronal and glial function and, 912
   posthypophysectomy, 3979
   postoperative insufficiency of, 1103
   preoperative administration of, 1063
      prophylactic, 1057
   prior therapy with, evaluation of, 1056
Sterrognosis, 61
Stewart-Morel-Morgagni syndrome, 3256
Stimulation, chronic, cerebellar, in epilepsy, in adults, 3925
   in children, 3898
   in atonic urinary sphincter, 1046
   in detrusor areflexia, 1045
   intracerebral, in chronic pain, 3739–3747, 3741(t), 3742(t)
   intraoperative, in epilepsy in children, 3886, 3892–3893
   in stereotaxic surgery, 3796–3797
   midbrain, in stereotaxic trigeminal tractotomy, 3706–3707,
      3707(t), *3707, 3708*
   nerve, in peripheral nerve injury, 2377, *2377, 2378*
   transcutaneous, in chronic pain, 3761–3763
Stimulator, brachial plexus, 3628
Stitch abscess, 1088
Stomach, pain in, 3631
Strabismus, incidence of, 1210(t)
Straight sinus, *280*
Strength, evaluation of, in neonate, 48
Streptococcus viridans, brain abscess and, 3348
Streptomycin, in bacterial infections, 3326
   inner ear damage and, 691, 691t
Stress ulcers, in multiple trauma, 2525–2526
Stretch, as mechanism of nerve injury, 2366–2367
Stroke, acute, computed tomography in, 118, *119*
   anticoagulants in, 1537
   dexamethasone in, 911
   extracranial to intracranial arterial anastomosis in, 1593,
      1594(t)–1596(t)
   ischemic, acute, operative management of, 1619–1626, *1622,
      1623*
   occlusive arterial disease in, 285
Strychnine, cerebral blood flow and, 807, 811(t)
Stump, amputation, painful, 3637
Stupor, definition of, 63
   in post-traumatic syndrome, 2181
   metabolic causes of, 72
Sturge-Weber syndrome, electroencephalography in, 207, *207,
   221*
   epilepsy in, 3897
   genetic aspects of, 1225, 1225(t), *1226*
Subarachnoid bolt, in measurement of intracranial pressure, 852
Subarachnoid cisterns, *352*
Subarachnoid hemorrhage, aneurysms in, 1630–1637, *1631–1633,*
   1634(t), *1635, 1636*, 1645–1652, 1646(t), 1649(t), 1650(t),
   1650–1652, 1652(t), 1811–1816
   arteriospasm in, 819
   brain tumors and, 1816

Subarachnoid hemorrhage (*Continued*)
  cerebral blood flow in, 818–821, 893
  cerebrospinal fluid in, 436
    lumbar pressure of, *850*
  coarctation of aorta and, 1807–1808
  coma in, 72
  complications of, 1655–1659, *1656*
  computed tomography in, 124–125, *125*
  Ehlers-Danlos syndrome and, 1809
  headache prior to, 3552
  hydrocephalus and, 1429, 1816–1817
  in head injury, computed tomography in, 1980
  in neonate, vs. cerebellar injury, 49
  increased intracranial pressure in, 891–894, *892*
  intraventricular hemorrhage and, 1641, *1641*
  neurological grading of, 1646(t)
  nonoperative treatment of, 1645–1662, 1946(t), 1949(t),
    1950(t), *1950–1952,* 1952(t), 1953(t), *1956*
  of unknown origin, 1630, 1654–1655
  pathophysiology and clinical evaluation of, 1627–1644
  polycystic kidney and, 1808–1809, 1809(t)
  pregnancy and, 1809–1811
  special problems associated with, 1807–1820
  spontaneous, computed tomography in, 124, *125*
  vascular malformations in, 1637–1641, *1638–1640,* 1640(t),
    1653–1655, 1653(t)
  ventricular enlargement in, operative treatment of, 1429
  xanthochromia in, 437
Subarachnoid pressure, lumbar, intracranial pressure and, 858
Subarachnoid space, anesthetic injection into, cerebrospinal fluid
    following, 472
  development of, *1437*
  disruption of, traumatic, 505, *538*
  hemorrhage in. See *Subarachnoid hemorrhage.*
  in aneurysm procedures, 1669–1670, *1669, 1670*
  radiological examination of, 425
Subcaudate tractotomy, in psychiatric disorders, 3935
Subclavian artery, occlusive disease of, 286
Subclavian steal syndrome, 288, 822
Subdural effusion, of infancy, 1912
Subdural empyema, 3333–3337, *3334–3336*
  in head injury, 1915
  in viral encephalitis, 3359
Subdural hematoma. See *Hematoma, subdural.*
Subdural hygroma, in head injury, 1913
  in children, 2112
Subdural space, spinal, abscess of, 3451–3452, *3451*
Subdural tap, in hydrocephalus, in children, 1400, *1400*
Subependymoma, 2797–2798, *2798*
Subgaleal abscess, 3328
Subluxation, of vertebral bodies, 496
Submentovertical projection, angiographic, 238, *240*
Suction equipment, micro-operative, 1185
Suffering, pain and, 3729–3733, *3730, 3731,* 3756
Sulfamethoxazole, pseudotumor cerebri and, 3181(t), 3187
Sulfonamides, in bacterial infections, 3327
Superficial temporal artery, anastomosis of to middle cerebral
    artery, 1585–1611, *1586–1593,* 1594(t)–1596(t), *1597–1599,*
    1601–1605, 1608–1610
Superior cerebellar artery, aneurysms of, 1740–1741, 1742(t)
  cranial nerve root compression by, 3773, *3773*
  radiological anatomy of, 275
Superior sagittal sinus, *280*
Suppression amblyopia, 652
Supraclavicular nerve, entrapment of, 2460
Supraorbital nerve, avulsion of, in trigeminal neuralgia, 3561
Suprascapular nerve, entrapment of, 2460
Suprasellar tumors, in children, 2717
  radiation therapy of, 3103, 3103(t)
Supratentorial tumors, in children, 2702–2732
Sural nerve, biopsy of, 407–410, *407,* 409(t)
  entrapment of, 2467
Survival, in myelomeningocele, 1271, 1271(t)
  posterior fossa tumors in children and, 2756
  quality of, after head injury, 2163–2170, *2164,* 2167(t)

Susceptibility, host, in bacterial infections, 3323
Suture, cranial, development of, *1454–1457,* 1455–1457
  normal, in infant skull, *1448*
  resection and, in peripheral nerve injury, 2413–2416,
    2413–2415
    delayed, 2385–2386
  synostosis of, 1447–1466. See also *Craniosynostosis.*
Swallowing, difficulty in, in Parkinson's disease, 3839
  in neonate, 48
Sweating, in peripheral nerve injury, 2379–2380
  sympathetic innervation and, 3719
Sydenham's chorea, cerebrospinal fluid in, 470
  pseudotumor cerebri and, 3181(t), 3188
Sylvius, aqueduct of, *353*
  congenital stricture of, and hydrocephalus, 1433
  fissure of, 1137
    arachnoid cysts of, 1439, *1440, 1441*
    malformations of, 1795, *1799*
Sympathectomy, 3717–3726
  in peripheral neuralgias, 3638, 3638(t)
  in vasospastic conditions, 3654
Sympathetic nervous system, anatomy and physiology of,
    3717–3720, *3718*
  diagnostic nerve block in, 3649–3651, *3650, 3651*
  ganglia of, neurolytic injections of, 3661–3662
  influence of, on pupil, 646
  syndromes of, anesthetic diagnosis of, 3649, *3650, 3651*
    local anesthesia in, 3653
  tumors of, 3299–3315
Sympathomimetic agents, cerebral blood flow and, 808(t)
Symptom Check List of Ninety Questions, for pain, 3483,
    3484–3487
Synchrony, secondary bilateral, 3870
Syncope, orthostatic, vs. epilepsy, 687
Syndrome. See names of specific syndromes.
Synostosis, primary, 1447
  total, 1464–1465, *1465*
  types of, *1449–1454*
Syphilis, cerebral gumma in, 3445–3446
  cerebrospinal fluid in, 463–464
  congenital, endolymphatic hydrops in, 689
  of spinal cord, 3457
  osteomyelitis of skull and, 3253, *3255*
  test for, in transient ischemic attack, 1253
Syringes, angiographic, 233
Syringobulbia, hydrodynamic theory of, *1493*
Syringohydromyelia, in Arnold-Chiari malformation, 1287–1288,
    1287
  in spina bifida aperta, 1250
Syringomyelia, 1492–1494, *1493*
  cerebrospinal fluid in, 468
  computed tomography in, 139
Syringomyelomeningocele, 1245, *1245*
Systemic lupus erythematosus, cerebrospinal fluid in, 469
Systems, review of, in clinical examination of children, 40

Tabes dorsalis, sympathectomy for, 3720
Takayasu's disease, 1552–1553
Talking Brooch, 4000, *4000*
Tangential missile wounds, 2064, *2065*
Tangential projection, angiographic, 238, *241*
Tantalum, cranioplasty with, 2234–2235, *2234, 2235*
Tarlov cyst, 1355
Tarsorrhaphy, for exposure keratitis, 643, *643*
Tay-Sachs disease, cerebrospinal fluid in, 468
  diagnosis of, 385(t)
  foam cells in, 440
^{99m}Technetium compounds, in brain scanning, 145–147, 148(t),
    149
Tectorial membrane, 678
Teeth, cephalic pain and, 3532–3533, *3534*
  vs. trigeminal neuralgia, 3558
Telangiectasia, 1637

INDEX

Telangiectasia (*Continued*)
  familial hemorrhagic, brain abscess and, *3349*
Telencephalon, of promammalian brain, 3730, *3730*
Temperature, body. See *Body temperature.*
Temporal arteritis, 1550–1552
  cephalic pain and, 3538–3539
Temporal artery, superficial, anastomosis of to middle cerebral
    artery, 1585–1611, *1586–1593*, 1594(t)–1596(t),
    1597–1599, 1601–1605, 1608–1610
  carotid catheterization via, 250
Temporal bone, anatomy of, 2251, 2252, *3272, 3274, 3275*
  fractures of, diagnosis of, 2254, *2255–2257*
    treatment of, 2259
    types of, 2251, *2253*
  resection of, in ear carcinoma, 3282, *3283*
Temporal lobe, contused, cerebral blood flow and, 888, *888*
  in children, 2116
  epilepsy and, 3917–3919, *3919–3922*
  excision of, in epilepsy in children, 3883–3892, *3885, 3888,*
    3891(t)
  lesions of, clinical examination in, 14
    evoked potentials in, 2007, *2008*
    visual field loss in, 668, *669*
Temporomandibular joint pain, 3539–3540
Tendon(s), herniation through, in head injury, 1917(t),
    1918–1921, *1920*
  reflexes of, in cerebral death, 751
    in infants and children, 60, 61(t)
  transfer of, after peripheral nerve injury, 2420
Tensilon test, in myasthenia gravis, 658
Tension headache, 3546
Tentorial pressure cone, in increased intracranial pressure,
    878–880
Tentorium cerebelli, herniation of. See *Herniation, tentorial.*
  in Arnold-Chiari malformation, 1285
  meningioma of, 2957–2959, *2958*
    myelographic appearance of, *537*
Teratoma, incidence of, 2915
  juxtasellar, computed tomography in, 139
  parapituitary, 3154
  pineal, 2863
  sacrococcygeal, 1358–1360, *1359*
  spinal, 3208
    in children, *3216*
  suprasellar, in children, 2719
  supratentorial, in children, 2716
Ter-Pogossian camera, 143
Terson's syndrome, subarachnoid hemorrhage and, 1658
Test(s). See names of specific tests.
Testosterone, in acromegaly, 957
  in anterior pituitary failure, 949
Tethered cord syndrome, 1331–1333
Tetracaine, in central vs. peripheral pain, 3644
Tetracyclines, in actinomycosis, 3400
  in bacterial infections, 3327
  pseudotumor cerebri and, 3181(t), 3187
Thalamic syndrome, mesencephalotomy in, 3709
Thalamostriate vein, *280, 282*
Thalamotomy, avoidance of complications in, 3834
  in chronic pain, 3747
  in dyskinesias, 3828
  in intention tremor, 3853
  in myoclonus, 3852
  in Parkinson's disease, 3842
  neuroleptanalgesia in, 1121
  ventrolateral, in cerebral palsy, 3849
    in hemiballism, 3851
    in Parkinson's disease, 3842
Thalamus, astrocytoma of, 2770, 2773
  investigation of, 2776
  treatment of, 2779
  coronal section of, *3829*
  hemorrhage in, 1829
  in ascending pain pathway, 3467–3468
  limbic cortex and, 3732

Thalamus (*Continued*)
  operations on, in dyskinesias, 3828–3837, *3829–3831*
  stimulation of, in chronic pain, 3739–3747, 3741(t), 3742(t)
  tumors of, in children, 2721–2722, 2721(t)
  ventrolateral, language processes and, 3835
    stimulation of, 3832
Thalassemia, skull involvement in, 3261, *3263*
Theophylline, cerebral blood flow and, 810(t)
Thermography, in chronic pain, 3492
Thiabendazole, in trichinosis, 3395
Thiamine, cerebral blood flow and, 811(t)
Thigh, lateral femoral cutaneous nerve of, entrapment of,
    2463–2464, *2464*
  peroneal nerve injury at, 2403–2404
Thioctic acid, cerebral blood flow and, 811(t)
Thiopental, cerebral blood flow and, 805
  in physical vs. psychological pain, 3492
Thirst sensation, loss of in coma, 996
Thoracic artery, superior, 553, *554*
Thoracic cavity, ganglioneuroma of, 3310
Thoracic outlet syndrome, electromyographic studies in, 631
Thoracolumbar resection, 3723
Thorax, anatomy of, 1005
  venous obstruction in, in pseudotumor cerebri, 3184
Thorazine, in paranoid schizophrenia, 3497
Threshold tone decay test, in acoustic neuroma, 2973
Thromboangiitis obliterans, 1549
Thrombocytopenia, pseudotumor cerebri and, 3181(t)
Thrombocytopenic purpura, thrombotic, 1546
Thrombophlebitis, in multiple trauma, 2484–2487
Thrombosis, cerebral, anterograde extension of, embolism and,
    1516
  cerebrospinal fluid in, 466
  in arteriovenous malformations, of spinal cord, 1852
  induced, in aneurysms, 1676
  venous, cortical, 1539
    postoperative, 1108–1110
  venous sinus, in head injury in children, 2103, *2104*
    in pseudotumor cerebri, 3184
  vs. embolism, radiological differentiation of, 299
Thyroid, carcinoma of, hypophysectomy in, 3953
    spinal metastasis in, 512
  disease of, cerebrospinal fluid in, 468
    ocular, 659
      exophthalmos in, 644, *645*
  function of, in transient ischemic attack, 1524
  insufficiency of, 945
  replacement of, in anterior pituitary failure, 949
Thyroid-stimulating hormone, hypothalamic-pituitary relationship
    and, 942
  nature and function of, 940
Thyroid suppression test, Werner, 645
Thyrotropic adenoma, 3123
Thyrotropin, failure of, 945
  secretion of, by pituitary tumors, 963
Thyroxine, post–hypophysectomy by craniotomy, 3983
TIA. See *Transient ischemic attack.*
Tibial nerve, posterior. See *Posterior tibial nerve.*
Tic douloureux. See *Trigeminal neuralgia.*
Tidal volume, in acute respiratory failure, 1021, 1025
Tietze syndrome, objective pain in, 3492
Tilt table, in paraplegia, 4002, *4004*
Timing, of operation, in subarachnoid hemorrhage, 1647–1648
Tinel's sign, in peripheral nerve injury, 2379
Tinnitus, in basilar skull fracture, 2257–2258
  in ototoxicity, 692
  vascular decompression and, 3776
Titanium, cranioplasty with, 2235
Todd-Wells stereotaxic frame, 3711, *3711, 3713, 3976*
Toes, "tremor"-type movements of, in neonate, 48
Tolazoline hydrochloride, cerebral blood flow and, 809(t)
Tomography, computed, 111–142. See also *Computed*
    tomography.
  in glomus jugulare tumor, 3287, *3287*
  in orbital tumors, 3033, *3034*

Tomography (*Continued*)
    in pituitary adenoma, 3130, *3130, 3131*
    in spinal arachnoid cysts, *1444*
Tone, in neonate, 48
Tone decay test, 698
Tongue, atrophy of, in neonate, 47
    carcinoma of, mesencephalotomy for, 3708
Tonsil(s), cerebellar, herniation of, in head injury, 1921, *1921*
Torcular Herophili, *280*
Torticollis, spasmodic, 3821, 3846–3849
    physiological basis of, 3827
Towne's view, angiographic, 234, *236*
Toxoplasmosis, 3370–3373
    in neonate, 46
Tracers, radiopharmaceutical, 144–146, 148(t)
    accumulation and retention of, 146
Tracheostomy, in multiple trauma, 2477–2479
    postoperative complications requiring, 1094
Traction, in occult spinal dysraphism, 1318
    skeletal, in operative procedures, 1081
    theory of, in Arnold-Chiari malformation, 1280
Tractotomy, subcaudate, in alcoholism, 3943
    in psychiatric disorders, 3934, 3934(t)
    trigeminal, 3710–3714, *3711–3714*
Tranexamic acid, in subarachnoid hemorrhage, 1651
Tranquilizers, cerebral blood flow and, 812(t)
Transducers, in increased intracranial pressure, 851
Transfusion, intraoperative, reactions to, 1070
    postoperative complications and, 1108
Transient ischemic attack, as indication for carotid operation, 1563–1565
    brain scanning in, 156, 156(t)
    carotid territory in, 1520–1530, *1521*, 1522(t), 1524(t), 1525(t)
    superficial temporal to middle cerebral arterial anastomosis in, 1593, 1594(t)–1596(t)
    vertebrobasilar territory in, 1530–1531, 1530(t)
Transillumination, of skull, 41, 45
    in pediatric hydrocephalus, 1387
Transmitter compounds, in cerebral metabolism, 770–771
Trans-sacral injection, 3648
Transtentorial herniation, cerebral edema and, 878
    clinical diagnosis of, 879
    in neonate, 46
    syndrome of, 70(t), 71
Transverse myelitis, clinical examination in, 29
Traube-Herring-Mayer waves, in increased intracranial pressure, 875
Trauma, 1875–2532
    abdominal, 2520–2521
        head injury and, in children, 2093
    acute respiratory failure in, 1025
    arachnoid cysts after, 2205–2208
    as cause of cranial defect, 2228
    aspiration in, prevention of, 1025
    brain scanning in, 161
    carotid artery, 2314–2317, *2316, 2317*
        cavernous plexus aneurysm and, 1770–1771
    cerebral, cerebral blood flow in, 825
    cerebrospinal fluid in, 467
    coma in, management of, 899
    craniocerebral, epidemiology of, 1939–1940
        metabolic response to, 990–993
    epilepsy following, 2188–2193
    focal cerebral lesions in, electroencephalography in, 220, 221
    head, 1896–2174. See also *Head injury.*
    in etiology of brain tumors, 2671–2672
    intracranial hypertension in, 3180(t)
    maxillofacial, 2261–2296
    multiple, 2475–2530
        abdomen in, 2520
        acute renal failure in, 2511–2518
        bleeding disorders in, 2522–2524
        cardiovascular injuries in, 2490
        crush injuries in, 2518
        fat embolism in, 2521

Trauma (*Continued*)
    multiple, fluid and electrolyte management in, 2494, *2498*
        fractures in, 2521
        in child, 2524
        respiratory function in, 2476–2490
        shock in, 2501
        stress ulcers in, 2525
        total patient care in, 2526
    neural, as complication of disc operation, 2548
    pain of, reversible nerve block in, 3652–3655
    post-traumatic syndrome after, 2175–2186
    pupils in, 650
    skull, nonneoplastic tumors from, 3245
    spinal, radiography in, 496–505, *498–504, 540*
    spinal abnormalities and, 496
    systemic, brain dysfunction and, 1909
    vascular, as complication of disc operation, 2549
Tremor, in Parkinson's disease, 3837
    intention, 3852
Trendelenburg position, cerebral blood flow in, 828
Trephined, syndrome of, as indication for cranioplasty, 2230
Triangle of Reil, *258, 259*
Triangularis oris muscle, absence of, vs. lower facial weakness in neonate, 46
Trichinosis, 3393–3395
Trichloroethylene, cerebral blood flow and, 805
    in anesthesia, disadvantages of, 1122
Triethylenethiophosphoramide, intra-arterial administration of, 3073
Trigeminal artery, persistent, collateral blood supply and, 795
Trigeminal dysesthesia, mesencephalotomy in, 3709
Trigeminal nerve, anatomy of, in posterior fossa, 3591–3596
        orbital, *3025, 3027*
    in infants and children, 46, 56
    pain in. See *Trigeminal neuralgia.*
    pain-sensitive structures of head and, 3531
    stimulation of, ventricular arrhythmias and, 1130
    visualization of, in cisternal myelography, *527*
Trigeminal neuralgia, 3554–3603
    alcohol block in, 3559–3560
    atypical, sympathectomy for, 3720
    characteristics of, 3556–3557
    clinical findings in, 3589–3591
    comparative techniques in, 3577, 3578(t)
    differential diagnosis of, 3557–3558
    etiology of, 3555–3556
    medical treatment of, 3554, 3558
    micro-operative decompression in, 3589–3603
        complications of, 3600(t)
        findings in, clinical, 3589
            operative, 3594, 3595(t)
        indications for, 3596
        nerve avulsion in, 3561
        postoperative course in, 3599, 3600(t)
        technique of, 3596, *3597–3599*
    percutaneous rhizotomy in, 3564–3579, *3565*
        recurrence following, 3577
        results of, 3574, 3574(t)
        side effects of, 3574–3577, 3575(t)
        technique of, 3566–3574, *3567, 3568, 3570–3573*
        vs. other operative procedures, 3577–3578, 3578(t)
    postganglionic section in, 3560–3561
    sensory root section in posterior fossa in, 3586–3588
    temporal craniotomy in, 3580–3585, *3581–3583*
    vascular decompression in, 3772, *3773*
Trigeminal neuropathy, 3782
Trigeminal tractotomy, 3710–3714, *3711–3714*
Trigeminothalamic pathway, and pain, 3703
Trigger point block, in chronic pain syndrome, 3763
Trimethadione, in absence status, 3878
    in afebrile seizures, 3876(t), 3877
    starting dosages of, 3877(t)
Trimethaphan, as drip, in thalamotomy, 3835
    cerebral blood flow and, 808(t)
    in deliberate hypotension, 1127

Trismus, in rhizotomy for trigeminal neuralgia, 3576
Trochlear nerve, in infants and children, 46, 56
 in percutaneous trigeminal rhizotomy, 3569, *3571*
 orbital, 3027
 palsy of, 658, *659*, 659(t)
Tropia, definition of, 652
Trunk, schwannoma of, benign, 3301
 malignant, 3304
Trypanosomiasis, 3373
L-Tryptophan, cerebral blood flow and, 812(t)
Tuberculoma, cerebral, 3441–3445, *3442–3445*
 spinal, intradural, 3456
Tuberculosis, angiographic appearance of, 611
 cerebral, 3441
 meningitic, cerebrospinal fluid in, 461
 skull, osteitis in, 3330
 osteomyelitis in, 3253
 spinal, 3454–3456
 radiography of, 506, *506*
 vs. fungal infection, 3456
Tuberculum sellae, meningioma of, 2942, 2955, *2956*
Tuberous sclerosis, genetic aspects of, 1227(t), 1228, *1228*
Tullio phenomenon, 686
Tumors, 2657–3320. See also names of specific tumors.
 biopsy of, 395–405
 pathology report in, 396, 396(t)
 procedure for, 398
 brain. See also *Brain tumors* and names of specific tumors.
 biology of, 2666–2693, *2676, 2682, 2683,* 2685(t)–2687(t), *2687, 2688*
 classification of, 2659–2665, *2661,* 2664(t)
 carotid body, angiography for, 292, 294
 chemotherapy of, 3065–3095
 genetic aspects of, 1227–1229, 1227(t), 2666–2671
 inclusion, 2914–2923
 intracranial, cerebrospinal fluid in, 467
 headache and, 3550, *3551*
 hydrocephalus and, 1429
 vs. trigeminal neuralgia, 3557
 malignant, hormone dependency of, 3947–3948
 nerve sheath, 3300–3306
 orbital, 3024–3064
 vascular, 3054–3055
 peripheral and sympathetic nerve, 3299–3315
 pineal region, 2863–2871
 in children, 2714–2717, *2715–2717*
 puffy, Pott's, 3253, *3254*
 scalp, 3316–3320, *3317–3320*
 secondary, of peripheral nerve sheaths, 3306
 sellar and parasellar, 3107–3162
 computed tomography vs. radionuclide imaging in, 167(t)
 nonneoplastic, 3154–3155
 nonpituitary, 3151–3154
 pituitary, 3107–3151. See also *Pituitary adenoma*.
 skull, 3227–3268
 spinal, computed tomography in, 139–140
 spinal cord. See also *Spinal cord, tumors of*.
 in adults, 3196–3214
 in children, 3215–3221
 subarachnoid hemorrhage and, 1642
 suprasellar, in children, 2717–2719, *2718,* 2719(t)
 radiation therapy of, 3103, 3103(t)
 supratentorial, in children, 2702–2732
 vertebral, cervical, anterior approach to, 2619
 vertebroepidural, angiography in, 610, *611*
 vertebromedullary, angiography in, 604–612, *604–608, 610, 611*
 vs. cerebrovascular accident, brain scanning in, 155
Tumor-echo complex, 186, *188*
Tuning fork tests, 693
Turbidity, of cerebrospinal fluid, 435
Twinning, in diastematomyelia, 1339
Twins, craniopagus, 1211
Tympanometry, 698
Tympanum, transformer mechanism of, 693

Ulcers, decubitus, management of, 4011
 postoperative, 1113
 gastrointestinal, postoperative, 1106
 stress, in multiple trauma, 2525–2526
Ulnar nerve, entrapment of, 2452–2456, *2452*
 electromyographic studies in, 631
 injury to, 2390–2393, *2390, 2391*
 median nerve and, 2393–2394
Ultrasonic lesion, in stereotaxic surgery, 3811
Ultrasonic radiation procedure, Lindstrom's, in psychiatric disorders, 3938, *3939*
Ultrasound, 176–194. See also *Echoencephalography*.
 B-scan, 723–738
 of carotid artery, 734, *735–737*
 of fetal and neonatal cranium, *720–725,* 723, *727–730*
 of spine, *730, 732, 733, 734*
 Doppler, 738–743, *739–743*
 in anterior sacral meningocele, 1352
 in cerebral infarction, 1536
 in intracerebral hemorrhage, 1830–1831
 in orbital tumors, 3039
 in stereotaxic lesion making, 3801, 3811–3812
 in transient ischemic attack, 1523, 1524
 neurosurgical applications of, 717–745
 physical principles of, 717–723, *719*
Umbradil, cerebral blood flow and, 812(t)
Unconsciousness. See also *Coma* and *Consciousness*.
 clinical examination in, 64–69, 64(t), 65(t)
 episodic, 72
Upper motor neuron, lesions of, electromyography in, 633, 634(t)
 paralysis of, clinical examination in, 6–7
Urea, in cerebrospinal fluid, 451
 in increased intracranial pressure, 905–907
 oral, in pseudotumor cerebri, 3192
Uremia, chronic, intracranial hypertension in, 3180(t)
Urethral pressure profilometry, 1037, *1037*
Uric acid, in cerebrospinal fluid, 451
Urinary bladder, denervation of, in detrusor hyperreflexia, 1042
 disease of, neurological, findings in, 1039–1041, *1039, 1040*
 treatment of, 1041–1047
 efferent pathways to, 1033, *1033*
 function of, in occult spinal dysraphism, 1321
 in spina bifida aperta, 1257
 in spinal cord dysfunction, 4009
 malfunction of, central nervous system disease and, 1031–1047
 diagnostic methods in, 1035–1039, *1035–1038*
 consultation in, 1038
 pain in, 3632
 peripheral innervation of, 1033
 training of, in hemiplegia, 3999
Urinary diversion, in neurogenic bladder disease, 1043
Urinary flow rates, 1037, *1038*
Urinary sphincter, dysfunction of, 1040, *1040*
 treatment of, 1045
 prosthetic, 1046, *1047*
Urination, difficulty with, post–open cordotomy, 3697
Uroflowmetry, 1037, *1038*

Vacuum sinus, 3535
Vagus nerve, clinical examination of, 21
 in infants and children, 47, 59
 pain of, percutaneous rhizotomy in, 3609–3612, *3610, 3611*
 vascular compression of, 3776
Van Buchem's disease, 3255
Van Buren stereotaxic instrument, 3805, *3807*
Vancomycin, inner ear damage and, 691, 691(t)
Varices, 1637
Vascular accident, vertigo in, 688
Vascular disorders, 1509–1874. See also *Blood vessels* and names of specific disorders.
 cerebrospinal fluid in, 466
 clinical examination in, 36
 computed tomography in, 123, *123–125*

Vascular disorders (*Continued*)
electroencephalography in, 220, 221
intracranial hypertension in, 3180(t)
ischemic, 1511–1558. See also *Ischemic vascular disease.*
occlusive, angiography in, 282, *285–288, 296, 297–299*
brain scanning in, 163
pain of, 3640
vs. spasm, radiological differentiation of, 295
of extremities, sympathectomy for, 3721
seizures in children and, 3866
Vascular headache, 3546–3550
cerebral blood flow in, 822
sympathectomy in, 3720
transient homonymous hemianopia in, 640
Vascular system, peripheral, preoperative evaluation of, 1059
Vasculitis, inflammatory, intracranial hypertension in, 3180(t)
Vasoactive drugs, cerebral blood flow and, 808(t)
Vasodilatation, cerebral, stimuli to, 868
in sympathetic nerve block, 3649
Vasogenic shock, in multiple trauma, 2504–2505
Vasomotor paralysis, computed tomography in, 125
Vasopressin, cerebral blood flow and, 811(t)
in neurohypophyseal diabetes insipidus, 976
in postoperative diabetes insipidus, 1102
secretion of, 972
Vasospasm, cerebral, as contraindication to carotid ligation, 1703
cerebral blood flow in, 818–821
postoperative, 1092
prevention and management of, 820
subarachnoid hemorrhage and, 1655–1657
sympathetic nerve block in, 3654
Vein(s), anatomy of, intracavernous, *1765, 1766, 1768*
cerebral, deep, radiological anatomy of, 282
epidural, angiography of, in disc disease, 2544
in collateral circulation, 789
orbital, 3027
spinal, angiography of, 588
radiological anatomy of, 280, *280, 281*
thrombosis of, postoperative, 1108–1110
Vein of Galen, malformations of, 1796–1802, *1802*
Vein of Labbé, 282
Vein of Rosenthal, 282
Vein of Trolard, 282
Velum interpositum, *352*
Venous sinus(es), in Dandy-Walker malformation, 1291
in encephalocele, 1299
in head injury, 2068–2069, *2069*
in children, 2103, *2104*
in pseudotumor cerebri, 3182–3188, *3183*
injury to, management of, 2068
normal embryology of, 1279
radiological anatomy of, 280, *280*
syndromes of, clinical examination in, 18–21
Ventilation, assisted, in cerebral infarction, 1537
controlled, definition of, 1124
failure of, in acute respiratory failure, 1014–1015
in multiple trauma, 2479–2483
in normal respiration, 1009–1012
Ventricle(s), cerebral, *273*
collapse of, hematoma following, 1085
dilatation of, pathophysiology of, 3180(t)
drainage of, in craniovertebral junction anomalies, 1502
enlarged, computed tomography in, 129, *131, 133*
foreign bodies in, 2067
hemorrhage in, subarachnoid hemorrhage and, 1642
lateral, meningioma of, 2955–2957, *2956, 2957*
meningioma within, 2941
puncture of, in hydrocephalus, in children, 1400, *1400*
in increased intracranial pressure, 851
shunts in. See *Ventricular shunt.*
third, obstruction of, causes of, 1433
tumors of, in children, 2719–2720
Ventricular arrhythmias, trigeminal nerve stimulation and, 1130
Ventricular shunt, in Dandy-Walker malformation, 1297
in hydrocephalus, 1430, *1430–1432*

Ventricular shunt (*Continued*)
in hydrocephalus, in children, 1404–1409, *1405–1408*
complications of, 1411
function of, 1413
malfunction of, 1413, *1413–1416*
postoperative care in, 1409–1418
Ventriculitis, bacterial, 3341–3343
diagnosis of, 3324
postoperative, in spina bifida aperta, 1270
Ventriculography, 369–371, *371*
complications of, 378–380
in brain tumors, of pineal region, *2865, 2866*
of posterior fossa, in children, 2737–2739, *2738*
results of, 168(t)
supratentorial, in children, 2706
in colloid cyst, 2925
in craniopharyngioma, 2907
in Dandy-Walker malformation, 1295, *1295,* 1491, *1491*
in head injury, 1989, 1992, *1990–1992,* 2023
in hydrocephalus, in children, *1391,* 1396–1398, *1398, 1399*
in stereotaxic localization, 3787–3790, *3789, 3790*
in tuberculoma, 3444, *3444*
indications for and contraindications to, 375–376
prognosis after head injury and, 2148, 2149(t)
radionuclide, 164
surgical considerations of, 375–381
techniques for, 376–378, *377*
Ventriculomegaly, in myelomeningocele, 1282
Ventriculoperitoneal shunt, 1432, *1432*
Ventriculostomy, fourth, direct, in Dandy-Walker malformation, 1296
Ventriculovenous shunt, placement of, in adult, 1430, *1430–1432*
Veratrum viride, cerebral blood flow and, 809(t)
Vertebra(e), anomalies of, types of, 1216, *1216*
blocked, 491, *494*
acquired, *495*
anomalies of, types of, 1216, *1216*
cervical, anomaly of, *493*
anterior operative approach to, 2619
formation of, 1241
fractures of, 496, *499–501,* 2326, *2326, 2327*
lumbar, 2356–2359
thoracic, 2348, *2349*
hydatidosis of, 3381
in spina bifida aperta, 1251–1253, *1252–1254*
occipital, 1482
pyogenic infection of, 505, *506*
sarcoidosis of, 3429
tumors of, *514*
Vertebral angiography, 252–256
approaches in, 232
in acoustic neuroma, 2979, *2982–2984*
techniques for, catheterization, 255, *255*
direct puncture, 253, *253*
Vertebral artery (arteries), anastomoses of, with carotid tree, 278, *278, 279*
aneurysms of, *1636, 1716,* 1745–1749, 1746(t), *1747, 1748,* 1749(t)
angiography via, 252–256. See also *Vertebral angiography.*
anomalies of, 292, *293*
arteriovenous fistulae of, 291
caliber of, 270, *270*
compression of, anterior approach in, 2619
cranial nerve root compression by, 3773, *3773, 3775*
in cisternal myelography, 527
in collateral circulatory system, 795
occlusion of, 285
radiological anatomy of, 264–270, *265–270*
Vertebral block, spondylosis and, myelographic appearance of, *544*
Vertebral body, Hodgkin's disease of, *514*
Vertebrobasilar arterial tree, aneurysms of, *1716*
morbid anatomy in, 1717–1718
insufficiency of, vertigo in, 688
transient ischemic attacks and, 1530–1531, 1530(t)

Vertigo, cervical, 692
definition of, 683
differential diagnosis of, 686
endemic, 690
in basilar skull fracture, 2257
in posterior fossa tumors in children, 2736
of central origin, 687
of peripheral origin, 688
positional, 690
vascular decompression and, 3776
Vestibulocochlear nerve, anatomy of, 676, 2251
dysfunction of, auditory tests of, 2972, 3775, *3775*
vascular decompression in, 3775, *3775*
in infants and children, 47, 59
injury to, in basilar skull fractures, 2251–2260
Vestibular system, 680–692
anatomy of, 678, *680–682*
function of, tests of, 683
labyrinth of, *679,* 678–680, *680–682*
physiology of, 680
supranuclear connections of, 680, *681*
Vidian nerve, 3269
Vinblastine sulfate, in tumor chemotherapy, 3086
intra-arterial administration of, 3073
Vinca alkaloids, in tumor chemotherapy, 3086
Vincristine, in tumor chemotherapy, 3086
intra-arterial administration of, 3073
Viomycin, inner ear damage and, 691, 691(t)
Virchow-Robin perivascular spaces, 435
Virus(es), as carcinogens, 2675, *2676*
infection by, cerebrospinal fluid in, 441, 464–465
encephalitis as, 3358–3365, *3362*
diagnosis of, 385(t), 3359
intracranial hypertension in, 3180(t)
primary myelitis as, 3359
Viscus (viscera), disease of, malignant, pain in, 3627–3630
nonmalignant, pain in, 3630–3632
injury to, in disc operation, 2549
Vision, acuity of, 641–642
fields of, evaluation of, 663–671
in supratentorial tumors in children, 2705
following head injury, 2165
in pituitary adenoma, loss of, 3129
post-treatment improvement in, 3146
in pseudotumor cerebri, 3180
in supratentorial tumors in children, 2705
retrobulbar dysfunction of, evoked potentials in, 2005
transient loss of, 640
ventriculography and, 379
Vital capacity, in respiratory failure, 1021, 1025
Vital signs, increased intracranial pressure and, 861–864
Vitamin(s), metabolism of, in pseudotumor cerebri, 3187
skull and, 3253
Vitamin B₁, cerebral blood flow and, 811(t)
Vitamin C, in cerebrospinal fluid, 451
Vitamin D deficiency, rickets from, pseudotumor cerebri and, 3181(t), 3187
skull in, 3253
Vitamin K₁, prophylactic, 1058
Vocal cord, paresis of, in Arnold-Chiari malformation, 1286
Vocational counseling, in rehabilitation, 3990
Vocational rehabilitation, 4011
Vogt-Koyanagi-Harada syndrome, cerebrospinal fluid in, 463
Volume/pressure relationships, in intracranial pressure, 853–857, *854–856*
Vomiting, in astrocytoma, 2772
in posterior fossa tumors in children, 2734
postoperative, 1105
von Hippel-Lindau disease, genetic aspects of, 1224–1225, 1225(t)
von Recklinghausen's neurofibromatosis, 3302
genetic aspects of, 1227–1228, 1227(t)

von Recklinghausen's neurofibromatosis (*Continued*)
vs. orbital tumor, 3031
with spinal angioma, 565, *567*

Walker stereotaxic instrument, 3802, *3803*
Water, contrast media soluble in. See *Metrizamide.*
embedding media soluble in, for biopsy, 403–404
intoxication by, postoperative, 1100–1101
loss of, postoperative, 992, 1100, 1100(t)
retention of, excessive, 998
post-traumatic, 992
Weakness, functional, electromyography in, 633, 634(t)
Weber test, for hearing, 694
Wechsler-Bellevue test, in normal-pressure hydrocephalus, 1424
Wechsler Intelligence Scale, 703, *704*
for children, 40
subtests, of, 706
Weight, evaluation of, 1052
Werdnig-Hoffman disease, 40
heterogeneity in, 1209
in neonate, 47
symptoms of, 45
Werner thyroid suppression test, 645
Wheelchair activities, in spinal cord dysfunction, 4002, *4003*
Willis, circle of, anatomy of, 3113, *3115*
in collateral circulatory system, 796
Wilson's disease, intention tremor in, 3852
Wiskott-Aldrich syndrome, pseudotumor cerebri and, 3181(t), 3187
Wolman disease, diagnosis of, 385(t)
World Health Organization classification of tumors, 2760, 2761(t)
Wound(s), chest, in multiple trauma, 2482
compound, of cervical spine, 2334
delayed healing of, in spina bifida aperta, 1270
fistula of, postoperative, 2068
intraoperative complications of, 1074–1082
penetrating, of lumbar spine, 2359
of thoracic spine, 2352–2353
postoperative complications of, 1081–1093, *1090*
in carotid endarterectomy, 1578
in carotid ligation, 1708
soft-tissue, maxillofacial, 2263, *2264–2274*
Wrapping, in peripheral nerve injury, 2417–2418
of aneurysm, 1675–1676
Wrisberg, nerve of, *3607*
Wrist, median nerve at, entrapment of, 2446–2449
injury to, 2386–2388, *2387*
ulnar nerve at, entrapment of, 2454–2456
injury to, 2390–2391, *2390, 2391*
Wrist-drop, in hemiplegia, rehabilitation of, 3991

Xanthines, cerebral blood flow and, 807
Xanthochromia, of cerebrospinal fluid, 437–438
Xanthomatosis, cerebrotendinous, diagnosis of, 385(t)
X-rays, diagnostic. See *Radiography.*
in stereotaxic localization, 3785
therapeutic. See *Radiotherapy.*

¹⁶⁹Ytterbium DTPA, characteristics of, 3974(t)
in brain scanning, 145, 148(t)
⁹⁰Yttrium, in stereotaxic procedures, 3813

Zeiss binocular diploscope, 1176, *1176*
Zinc, in cerebrospinal fluid, 450
Zoom microscope, 1170
Zygoma, fractures of, 2279–2282, *2284, 2285*